The Molecular and Genetic Basis of Neurologic and Psychiatric Disease

The Molecular and Genetic Basis of Neurologic and Psychiatric Disease

Third Edition

Edited by

Roger N. Rosenberg, M.D.

Abe(Brunky), Morris, and William Zale Distinguished Chair in Neurology
and Professor of Neurology
Director, Alzheimer's Disease Center
Attending Neurologist, Zale-Lipshy University Hospital
and Parkland Memorial Hospital
The University of Texas Southwestern Medical Center
Dallas, Texas

Stanley B. Prusiner, M.D.

Director, Institute for Neurodegenerative Diseases
Professor of Neurology and Biochemistry
University of California, San Francisco, School of Medicine
San Francisco, California

Salvatore DiMauro, M.D.

Lucy G. Moses Professor of Neurology
Columbia University College of Physicians and Surgeons
New York, New York

Robert L. Barchi, M.D., Ph.D.

Provost and Professor of Neurology and Neuroscience
University of Pennsylvania
Philadelphia, Pennsylvania

Eric J. Nestler, M.D., Ph.D.

Lou and Ellen McGinley Distinguished Professor and Chairman
Department of Psychiatry
The University of Texas Southwestern Medical Center
Dallas, Texas

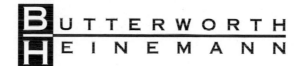

An Imprint of Elsevier Science

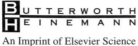

An Imprint of Elsevier Science

625 Walnut Street
Philadelphia, PA 19106

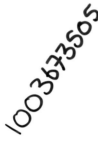

Notice

Neurology is an ever-changing field. Standard safety precautions must be followed but as new research and clinical experience broaden our knowledge, changes in treatment and drug therapy may become necessary or appropriate. Readers are advised to check the most current product information provided by the manufacturer of each drug to be administered to verify the recommended dose, the method and duration of administration, and contraindications. It is the responsibility of the treating physician, relying on experience and knowledge of the patient, to determine dosages and the best treatment for each individual patient. Neither the Publisher nor the author assumes any liability for any injury and/or damage to persons or property arising from this publication.

The Publisher

First Edition 1993. Second Edition 1997.

Library of Congress Cataloging in Publication Data
The molecular and genetic basis of neurologic and psychiatric disease / edited by Roger N. Rosenberg ... [et al.].– 3rd ed.
     p. ; cm.
   Rev. ed. of: The molecular and genetic basis of neurological disease. 2nd ed. 1997.
   Includes bibliographical references and index.
   ISBN 0-7506-7360-5
     1. Nervous system–Diseases–Molecular aspects. 2. Nervous system–Diseases–Genetic aspects.
   3. Molecular neurobiology. 4. Neurogenetics. I. Rosenberg, Roger N. II. Molecular and genetic basis of neurological disease.
     [DNLM: 1. Nervous System Diseases–genetics. 2. Mental Disorders–genetics. 3. Molecular Biology. WL 140 M718 2003]
   RC347.M59 2003
   616.8'0442–dc21   2003040308

Acquisitions Editor: Susan Pioli
Developmental Editor: Kimberley Cox
Senior Project Manager: Peter Faber

Printed in the United States of America.
Last digit is the print number: 9 8 7 6 5 4 3 2 1

We dedicate this text to our colleagues, who, by perseverance and dedication, have provided essential new scientific knowledge about the molecular and genetic basis of neurologic and psychiatric disorders and, in so doing, have conceptualized important insights into disease causation and therapies for the future.

Contents

Contents ix

Contributing Authors

Rita Alam, PhD
Senior Research Assistant
Department of Molecular Genetics
MD Anderson Cancer Center
Houston, Texas

Valerie Askanas, MD, PhD
Professor of Neurology and Pathology
University of Southern California,
Keck School of Medicine
Co-Director, USC Neuromuscular Center
Good Samaritan Hospital
Los Angeles, California

Robert L. Barchi, MD, PhD
Professor of Neurology and Neuroscience
University of Pennsylvania School of Medicine
Philadelphia, Pennsylvania

Rita Barresi, PhD
Postdoctoral Fellow
Department of Physiology and Biophysics
University of Iowa
Iowa City, Iowa

M. Flint Beal, MD
Anne Parrish Titzel Professor and Chairman
Neurology and Neuroscience
Weill Medical College of Cornell University
New York, New York

Merrill D. Benson, MD
Professor of Medicine, Pathology, and Laboratory
   Medicine
Indiana University School of Medicine
Indianapolis, Indiana

Vladimir M. Berginer, MD, PhD
Professor Emeritus
Faculty of Health Sciences
Ben Gurion University of the Negev
Consulting Neurologist
Soroka Medical Center
Beer-Sheva, Israel

Thomas D. Bird, MD
Professor, Neurology and Medicine
University of Washington
Research Neurologist
Geriatrics Research Education and Clinical Center
VA Puget Sound Health Care System
Seattle, Washington

D. Montgomery Bissell, MD
Professor of Medicine
University of California, San Francisco
Attending Physician
University of California Hospitals and Clinics
San Francisco, California

Eduardo Bonilla, MD
Professor of Clinical Neurology
Columbia University
College of Physicians and Surgeons
New York, New York

David R. Borchelt, MD
Associate Professor of Pathology and Neuroscience
Johns Hopkins School of Medicine
Baltimore, Maryland

Roscoe O. Brady, MD
Chief, Developmental and Metabolic Neurology
   Branch
Clinical Center
National Institute of Neurological Disorders and
   Stroke
National Institutes of Health
Bethesda, Maryland

Vicky L. Brandt, MD
Department of Pediatrics
Baylor College of Medicine
Houston, Texas

Edward S. Brodkin, MD
Assistant Professor of Psychiatry
Center for Neurology and Behavior
University of Pennsylvania School of Medicine
Attending Psychiatrist
Hospital of the University of Pennsylvania
Philadelphia, Pennsylvania

Maja Bucan, PhD
Associate Professor of Genetics
University of Pennsylvania School of Medicine
Philadelphia, Pennsylvania

Jeffrey R. Buchhalter, MD, PhD
Associate Professor of Neurology
Mayo Medical School
Rochester, Minnesota

Huaibin Cai, PhD
Research Associate
Department of Pathology
Johns Hopkins University School of Medicine
Baltimore, Maryland

Kevin P. Campbell, PhD
Professor
Department of Physiology and Biophysics
University of Iowa, Howard Hughes Medical Institute
Iowa City, Iowa

Arthur L. Caplan, PhD
Chair, Department of Medical Ethics
University of Pennsylvania
Philadelphia, Pennsylvania

George A. Carlson, PhD
Director, McLaughlin Research Institute
Great Falls, Montana

Phillip F. Chance, MD
Chief, Division of Genetics and Development
Professor of Pediatrics and Neurology
University of Washington School of Medicine
Seattle, Washington

David T. Chuang, PhD
Professor of Biochemistry
University of Texas Southwestern Medical Center
Dallas, Texas

Jacinta L. Chuang, MS
Senior Research Scientist, Biochemistry
UT Southwestern Medical Center
Dallas, Texas

Rody P. Cox, MD
Professor of Internal Medicine
University of Texas Southwestern Medical Center
Associate Director of Internal Medicine Residency
St. Paul University Hospital
Dallas, Texas

John C. Crabbe, Jr., PhD
Professor, Behavioral Neuroscience
Oregon Health Science University
Director, Portland Alcohol Research Center
VA Medical Center
Portland, Oregon

M. L. Cuccaro, MD
Associate Professor of Psychiatry
Assistant Professor of Medicine
Center for Human Genetics
Duke University Medical Center
Durham, North Carolina

Stephen J. DeArmond, MD, PhD
Professor of Pathology and Neuropathology
Institute for Neurodegenerative Diseases and
   Department of Pathology
University of California, San Francisco
San Francisco, California

Antonio V. Delgado-Escueta, MD
Professor of Neurology
Geffen School of Medicine
University of California, Los Angeles
Senior Neurologist
Greater Los Angeles Veterans Administration Medical
   Center
Los Angeles, California

Robert J. Desnick, MD, PhD
Professor and Chairman
Department of Human Genetics
Mount Sinai School of Medicine
Attending Physician
Mount Sinai Hospital
New York, New York

Darryl C. DeVivo, MD
Sidney Carter Professor of Neurology
Neurology and Pediatrics
Columbia University College of Physicians and
    Surgeons
Director Emeritus, Pediatric Neurology
Columbia Presbyterian Medical Center
New York, New York

Marc A. Dichter MD, PhD
Professor of Neurology
University of Pennsylvania
Philadelphia, Pennsylvania

Stefano DiDonato, MD
Scientific Director
Istituto Nazionale Neurologico C. Besta
Milan, Italy

Salvatore DiMauro, MD
Lucy G. Moses Professor of Neurology
Columbia University College of Physicians and
    Surgeons
New York, New York

Louis J. Elsas II, MD
Professor and Director
The Dr. John T. Macdonald Foundation Center for
    Medical Genetics
University of Miami
Attending Physician
Jackson Memorial Hospital
Miami, Florida

W. King Engel, MD
Professor of Neurology and Pathology
University of Southern California
Keck School of Medicine
Co-Director, USC Neuromuscular Center
Good Samaritan Hospital
Los Angeles, California

Charles J. Epstein, MD
Professor of Pediatrics
Chief, Division of Medical Genetics
University of California, San Francisco
San Francisco, California

Stanley Fahn, MD
H. Houston Merritt Professor of Neurology
Columbia University College of Physicians and
    Surgeons
Director, Movement Disorders Group
Attending Physician
New York Presbyterian Hospital
New York, New York

Martha J. Farah, MD
Professor of Psychology
Director, Center for Cognitive Neuroscience
University of Pennsylvania
Philadelphia, Pennsylvania

Nelson B. Freimer, MD
Professor of Psychiatry and Human Genetics
University of California, Los Angeles
Los Angeles, California

Theodore Friedmann, MD, MA
Professor, Pediatrics/Molecular Genetics
University of California, San Diego
San Diego, California

Robert C. Griggs, MD
Professor and Chair, Neurology
University of Rochester School of Medicine
Neurologist in Chief
Strong Memorial Hospital
Rochester, New York

Christina A. Gurnett, MD, PhD
Pediatric Neurology Fellow
Department of Neurology
Washington University School of Medicine
Department of Neurology, St. Louis Children's
    Hospital
St. Louis, Missouri

David H. Gutmann, MD, PhD
Donald O. Schnuck Family Chair in Neurology
Director, Neurofibromatosis Program
Washington University School of Medicine
St. Louis, Missouri

Richard Harold Haas, M.B., B.Chir., M.R.C.P.
Professor of Neurosciences and Pediatrics
University of California, San Diego
Attending Physician
UCSD Medical Center and
Children's Hospital and Health Center
San Diego, California

Anita Harding, MD, FRCP*
Professor of Clinical Neurology, Institute of Neurology
The National Hospital for Neurology and
    Neurosurgery
Middlesex University College of Physicians and
    Surgeons
London, England

Juliette M. Harris, PhD, MS
Staff Associate, Department of Neurology
Division of Movement Disorders
Columbia University College of Physicians and
    Surgeons
New York, New York

Stephen L. Hauser, MD
Professor and Chairman, Department of Neurology
University of California, San Francisco
San Francisco, California

Michio Hirano, MD
Associate Professor, Neurology
Columbia University College of Physicians and
    Surgeons
Associate Attending Physician, Neurology
New York Presbyterian Hospital and
Columbia Presbyterian Medical Center
New York, New York

Eric P. Hoffman, PhD
Director, Center for Genetic Medicine
A. James Clark Professor of Pediatrics
Children's National Medical Center
Washington, DC

Yadong Huang, MD, PhD
Staff Research Investigator
Gladstone Institute of Cardiovascular Disease
Staff Research Investigator
Gladstone Institute of Neurological Disease
Assistant Professor, Department of Pathology
University of California, San Francisco
San Francisco, California

Susan T. Iannaccone, MD
Professor of Neurology
The University of Texas Southwestern Medical Center
Director, Division of Neuromuscular Disease and
    Rehabilitation
Medical Director of Cellular Pathology
Texas Scottish Rite Hospital for Children
Dallas, Texas

Ken Inoue, MD, PhD
Assistant Professor, Molecular and Human Genetics
Baylor College of Medicine
Houston, Texas

William G. Johnson, MD
Professor of Neurology
Director, Division of Neurogenetics
UMDNJ, Robert Wood Johnson Medical School
Attending Neurologist
Robert Wood Johnson University Hospital
New Brunswick, New Jersey

Heinz Jungbluth, MD
Clinical Research Fellow, Paediatrics
Imperial College
London, England

Vassilis E. Kaliatsos, MD
Associate Professor
Pathology, Neurology, Neuroscience, and Psychiatry
    and Behavioral Sciences
Johns Hopkins University School of Medicine
Baltimore, Maryland

John P. Kane, MD, PhD
Professor of Medicine
Professor of Biochemistry and Biophysics
Associate Director, Cardiovascular Research Institute
Director, Lipid Clinic
University of California, San Francisco
San Francisco, California

Kleopas A. Kleopa, MD
Clinical Instructor, Neurology
University of Pennsylvania School of Medicine
Philadelphia, Pennsylvania

Edwin H. Kolodny, MD
Bernard A. and Charlotte Mardey Professor and
    Chairman, Department of Neurology
New York University School of Medicine
Chairman, Department of Neurology
Tisch Hospital
New York, New York

Agne Larsson, MD, PhD
Professor and Chairman, Department of Pediatrics
Karolinska Institutet
Huddinge University Hospital
Stockholm, Sweden

Michael K. Lee, MD
Assistant Professor, Department of Pathology
John Hopkins University School of Medicine
Baltimore, Maryland

*Deceased

Virginia M.-Y. Lee, PhD
Co-Director, Center for Neurodegenerative Disease
  Research
Pathology and Laboratory Medicine
University of Pennsylvania School of Medicine
Philadelphia, Pennsylvania

David A. Lewis, MD
Professor, Psychiatry and Neuroscience
University of Pittsburgh
Pittsburgh, Pennsylvania

K. H. Lewis, MA
Assistant Editor
Center for Human Genetics
Duke University Medical Center
Durham, North Carolina

Paul J. Lombroso, MD
Associate Professor
Child Study Center
Yale University School of Medicine
New Haven, Connecticut

James R. Lupski, MD
Cullen Professor of Molecular and Human Genetics
Professor of Pediatrics
Baylor College of Medicine
Houston, Texas

Mia MacCollin, MD
Assistant Professor, Neurology
Harvard Medical School
Director, Neurofibromatosis Clinic
Massachusetts General Hospital
Boston, Massachusetts

Robert W. Mahley, MD, PhD
Professor of Pathology and Medicine
Director, Gladstone Institute of Cardiovascular Disease
University of California, San Francisco
San Francisco, California

Mary J. Malloy, MD
Clinical Professor of Medicine and Pediatrics
Director, Pediatric Lipid Clinic
University of California, San Francisco
San Francisco, California

Giovanni Manfredi, MD, PhD
Assistant Professor, Neurology and Neuroscience
Weill Medical College of Cornell University
New York, New York

Ami K. Mankodi, MD
Department Fellow, Neurology
University of Rochester Medical Center
Strong Memorial Hospital
Rochester, New York

Kimberlee Michals Matalon, RD, PhD
Associate Professor, Human Development
University of Houston
Houston, Texas
Associate Professor of Pediatrics
University of Texas Medical Branch
Galveston, Texas

Reuben Matalon, MD, PhD
Professor of Pediatrics
University of Texas Medical Branch
Galveston, Texas

Carol A. Mathews, MD
Assistant Professor in Residence, Psychiatry
University of California, San Diego
La Jolla, California

Richard Mayeux, MD, MSc
Gertrude H. Sergievsky Professor of Neurology,
  Psychiatry, and Epidemiology
Director, Sergievsky Center
Co-Director, Taub Institute
Columbia University College of Physicians and
  Surgeons
Attending Physician, Neurology
New York Presbyterian Hospital
New York, New York

John H. Menkes, MD
Professor Emeritus, Neurology and Pediatrics
University of California, Los Angeles
Director Emeritus, Cedars-Sinai Medical Center
Los Angeles, California

Giovanni Meola, MD
Professor and Chair of Neurology
University of Milan
Chairman of Neurology
Istituto Policlinico San Donato
San Donato Milanese, Milan, Italy

Marcos T. Mercadante, MD, PhD
Associate Professor of Pervasive Development Disorder
    Program
Mackenzie Presbyterian University
Sao Paulo, Brazil
Affiliate Researcher, Child Study Center
Yale University Medical School
New Haven, Connecticut
Affiliate Researcher, Psychiatry Department
Sao Paulo University Medical School
Sao Paulo, Brazil

Hugo W. Moser, MD
University Professor of Neurology and Pediatrics
Johns Hopkins University
Director, Neurogenetics Research Center
Kennedy Krieger Institute
Balitmore, Maryland

Richard T. Moxley III, MD
Helen Aresty-Fine and Irving Fine Professor of
    Neurology
Associate Chair, Department of Neurology
University of Rochester School of Medicine and
    Dentistry
Director, Neuromuscular Disease Center
University of Rochester Medical Center
Rochester, New York

Francesco Muntoni, MD
Professor of Paediatric Neurology
Paediatrics and Neonatal Medicine
Imperial College
Consultant in Paediatric Neurology
Hammersmith Hospital
London, England

Charles B. Nemeroff, MD, PhD
Reunette W. Harris Professor and Chairman
Psychiatry and Behavioral Sciences
Emory University School of Medicine
Atlanta, Georgia

Orit Neudorfer
NORD/Roscoe Brady Lysosomal Storage Diseases
    Fellow
New York University School of Medicine
New York, New York

Ichizo Nishino, MD, PhD
Director, Department of Neuromuscular Research
National Institute of Neuroscience
National Center of Neurology and Psychiatry
Tokyo, Japan

Robert L. Nussbaum, MD
Chief, Genetics Disease Research Branch
National Human Genome Research Institute
Bethesda, Maryland

William L. Nyhan, MD, PhD
Professor of Pediatrics
University of California, San Diego
UCSD Medical Center and Children's Hospital and
    Health Center
San Diego, California

Jorge R. Oksenberg
Associate Professor of Neurology
University of California, San Francisco
San Francisco, California

Massimo Pandolfo, MD
Professor of Neurology
Faculty of Medicine
Université Libre de Bruxelles
Department Head, Neurology
Hôpital Erasme
Brussels, Belgium

Juan Pascual, MD, PhD
Assistant Professor
Neurology and Pediatrics
Columbia University College of Physicians and
    Surgeons
Assistant Attending Physician
Neurology (Pediatric Neurology)
Children's Hospital of New York
New York, New York

Shailendra Patel, BM, BCh, PhD
Associate Professor, Department of Medicine
Medical University of South Carolina
Charleston, South Carolina

Marc C. Patterson, MD
Professor of Clinical Neurology and Pediatrics
The Neurological Institute of New York
Columbia University College of Physicians and
    Surgeons
Director of Pediatric Neurology
Children's Hospital of New York
New York, New York

Henry L. Paulson, MD, PhD
Associate Professor, Department of Neurology
Roy J. and Lucilla A. Carver College of Medicine
University of Iowa Hospitals and Clinics
Iowa City, Iowa

Margaret A. Pericak-Vance, PhD
James B. Duke Professor of Medicine
Director, Center for Human Genetics
Duke University Medical Center
Durham, North Carolina

Donald L. Price, MD
Professor of Pathology, Neurology, and Neuroscience
Department of Pathology, Division of Neuropathology
Johns Hopkins University School of Medicine
Baltimore, Maryland

Stanley B. Prusiner, MD
Professor of Neurology
Professor of Biochemistry
Director, Institute for Neurodegenerative Diseases
University of California, San Francisco
San Francisco, California

Kerry J. Ressler, MD, PhD
Assistant Professor, Psychiatry and Behavioral Sciences
Emory University School of Medicine
Atlanta, Georgia

Victor I. Reus, MD
Professor of Psychiatry
University of California, San Francisco School of
    Medicine
Attending Physician, Langley Porter Hospital/
    Moffitt-Long Hospital
San Francisco, California

Ellinor Ristoff, MD
Medical Doctor, Department of Pediatrics
Karolinska Institute
Children's Hospital, Huddinge University Hospital
Stockholm, Sweden

Roger N. Rosenberg, MD
Abe(Brunky), Morris, and William Zale Distinguished
    Chair in Neurology
Professor of Neurology
The University of Texas Southwestern Medical Center
    at Dallas
Attending Neurologist
Zale-Lipshy University Hospital
Parkland Memorial Hospital
Dallas, Texas

David S. Rosenblatt, MD
Chairman and Professor, Human Genetics
McGill University
Director, Division of Medical Genetics
McGill University Health Center
Montreal, Quebec, Canada

Gerald Salen, MD
Professor of Medicine
Chief of Gastroenterology
UMD-New Jersey Medical School
Newark, New Jersey

Lawrence Scahill, MSN, PhD
Associate Professor of Nursing and Child Psychiatry
Child Study Center and School of Nursing
Yale University
New Haven, Connecticut

Gerard D. Schellenberg, PhD
Research Professor of Medicine and Neurology
Research Affiliate, Center on Human Development
    and Disability
University of Washington
Seattle, Washington

Stephen S. Scherer, MD, PhD
William N. Kelley Professor of Neurology
University of Pennsylvania, School of Medicine
Philadelphia, Pennsylvania

Raphael Schiffmann, MD
Chief, Clinical Investigations Section
Developmental and Metabolic Neurology Branch
National Institute of Neurological Disorder and Stroke
Bethesda, Maryland

Detlev Schindler, MD
Associate Professor
Department of Human Genetics
University of Wurzburg
Wurzburg, Germany

Eric A. Schon, PhD
Professor of Genetics and Development
Department of Neurology
Columbia University College of Physicians and
    Surgeons
New York, New York

Dennis Selkoe, MD
Vincent and Stella Coates Professor of Neurologic
    Diseases
Department of Neurology
Harvard Medical School
Director, Center for Neurologic Diseases
Brigham and Women's Hospital
Boston, Massachusetts

Serenella Servidei, MD
Associate Professor of Neurology
Catholic University
Rome, Italy

Caroline A. Sewry, PhD, MRC Path
Reader, Paediatrics
Imperial College
Honorary Consultant, Paediatrics
Hammersmith Hospital
London, England

Michael Shevell, MD, CM, FRCP
Associate Professor, Neurology/Neurosurgery and
    Pediatrics
McGill University
Montreal Children's Hospital, McGill University
    Health Center
Montreal, Quebec, Canada

Kunihiko Suzuki, MD
Director Emeritus, Neuroscience Center
Professor of Neurology and Psychiatry
Neuroscience Center
University of North Carolina School of Medicine
Chapel Hill, North Carolina

Franco Taroni, MD
Director, Laboratory of Cellular Pathology
Division of Biochemistry and Genetics
Department of Experimental Research and Diagnostics
Istituto Nazionale Neurologico C. Besta
Milan, Italy

Rabi Tawil, MD
Associate Professor of Neurology
University of Rochester Medical Center
Rochester, New York

John Q. Trojanowski, MD, PhD
Professor of Pathology and Laboratory Medicine
University of Pennsylvania, School of Medicine
Co-Director, Center for Neurodegenerative Disease
    Research
University of Pennsylvania Medical Center
Philadelphia, Pennsylvania

Seiichi Tsujino, MD
Section Chief, Department of Inherited Metabolic
    Disease
National Institute of Neuroscience, National Center of
    Neurology and Psychiatry
Tokyo, Japan

David W. Volk, PhD
Student Researcher, Neuroscience
University of Pittsburgh
Pittsburgh, Pennsylvania

Lewis J. Waber, MD, PhD
Associate Professor
The University of Texas Southwestern Medical Center
Director, Metabolism Service
Children's Medical Center of Dallas
Dallas, Texas

Ching H. Wang, MD, PhD
Associate Professor
Neurology and Neurological Sciences
Stanford University
Attending Physician in Pediatric Neurology
Neurology and Pediatrics
Stanford Hospital and Lucile Packard Children's
    Hospital
Stanford, California

Dong Wang, MD
Research Scientist, Neurology
Columbia University
New York, New York

David A. Wenger, PhD
Professor of Neurology
Jefferson Medical College
Philadelphia, Pennsylvania

Kristine M. Wiren, PhD
Associate Professor, Behavioral Neuroscience
Oregon Health Science University
Research Biologist
VA Medical Center
Portland, Oregon

Barry Wolf, MD, PhD
Director of Research, Associate Chair, and Professor of
    Pediatrics
University of Connecticut School of Medicine
Farmington, Connecticut
Director of Research, Pediatrics
Connecticut Children's Medical Center
Hartford, Connecticut

Philip C. Wong, PhD
Associate Professor, Pathology
Johns Hopkins University School of Medicine
Baltimore, Maryland

Frank M. Yatsu, MD
Professor and Chairman Emeritus, Neurology
University of Texas, Houston Medical School
Houston, Texas

Huda Y. Zoghbi, MD
Professor, Departments of Pediatrics, Neurology,
    Neuroscience, and Molecular and Human Genetics
Baylor College of Medicine
Houston, Texas

Introduction

In the introductions to the first and second editions of *The Molecular and Genetic Basis of Neurologic Disease*, published in 1993 and 1997, respectively, we said, "The remarkable achievements made in the fields of molecular and cellular neurobiology and molecular neurogenetics have been applied to genetic neurologic disease with equally dramatic results. The study of molecular pathogenesis of neurologic disease is a recent development, and it is fair to say that most of the scientific material presented here was not available even five years ago. This surge of molecular data on neurologic disease is a strong testimony to the vitality of investigators in the field." These statements are still true and the 3rd edition of our book contains molecular and genetic information about diseases of the nervous system elucidated only recently.

Again, we wish to emphasize that the determination of the molecular pathogenesis of genetic neurologic disease is indispensable to the development of pharmacologic or gene therapy for these disorders. Our ultimate goal is therapy for patients with the disorders described herein, and we see progress in this area as just beginning. Experimental new therapies are being tested in several areas such as glycogen storage disease, lipoprotein disorders, lysosomal disorders, Duchenne muscular dystrophy, genetic forms of epilepsy, membrane excitability disorders, prion disorders, mitochondrial diseases, Alzheimer's disease, Friedreich ataxia, and the major psychiatric diseases.

The third edition includes a new section on Inherited Psychiatric Diseases edited by Eric Nestler. Clearly, genetic diseases of the nervous system expressing major psychiatric symptoms and signs should now be included in an overall textbook dedicated to genetic diseases of the nervous system. It is an arbitrary distinction to cite separately neurologic or psychiatric disease, and it is our view that an integrated and comprehensive text for all molecular and genetic diseases of the nervous system is now essential. The new section on Psychiatric Diseases includes the chapters "Psychiatric Diseases: Challenges in Psychiatric Genetics" by Maja Bucan and Edward S. Brodkin; "Depression" by Kerry J. Ressler and Charles B. Nemeroff; "Bipolar Disorder" by Carol A. Mathews, Victor I Reus, and Nelson B. Freimer; "Schizophrenia" by David W. Volk and David A. Lewis; "Obsessive-Compulsive Disorder and Tourette's Syndrome" by Paul J. Lombroso, Marcos T. Mercadante, and Larry Scahill; "Molecular and Genetic Bases of Addictions" by John C. Crabbe, Jr., and Kristine M. Wiren and "Autism" by M.L. Cuccaro, K.H. Lewis, and M.A. Pericak-Vance.

The second edition of our book published in 1997 coincided with the awarding of the 1997 Nobel Prize in Medicine to our co-editor Stanley B. Prusiner for his research defining the molecular and genetic basis of the spongiform encephalopathies and the expression of the prion gene under both physiologic and pathologic conditions. Thus, it is appropriate that our third edition includes two new chapters authored by Dr. Prusiner, "Degenerative Diseases and Protein Processing" and "Prion Diseases."

In 2001, the initial analysis and sequence of the human genome was published by two groups, the International Human Genome Consortium directed by Francis Collins, and Celera Genomics headed by Craig Venter. The information contained in the initial sequence of the human genome has provided the means to find new genes and new genetic susceptibility factors for human diseases of the nervous system. The initial analysis of this genetic information will provide insights for our understanding of gene structure and the evolution of the human genome. Information from the database of both groups has demonstrated that genes expressed in the fruit fly and nematode nervous systems providing fitness and survival have been maintained by natural selection through evolution and are expressed in the human nervous system. Thus, these ancient and conserved genes such as the presenilin I and II genes and the amyloid precursor protein gene causal of dominantly inherited Alzheimer's disease in human's have their origins in the genome of invertebrates and early vertebrates that evolved 500 million years ago. These data and insights have been incorporated in three new chapters in this edition, "The Human Genome Project" by Robert Nussbaum; "Gene Therapy for Central Nervous System Disorders" by Theodore Friedmann; and "Emerging Ethical Issues in Neurology, Psychiatry, and the Neurosciences" by Arthur Caplan and Martha J. Farah.

The advances in clinical and molecular genetics have made it necessary to include entirely new chapters on the following subjects: "Triplet Repeat Disease: General Concepts and Mechanisms of Disease" by Vicky L. Brandt and Huda Y. Zoghbi; "Selected Genetically Engineered Models Relevant to Human Neurodegenerative Disease" by Donald L. Price, David R. Borchelt, Michael K. Lee, and Philip C, Wong; "Gene Mapping to Gene Targeting: Application of Mouse Genetics to Human Disease" by George Carlson; "Triplet Repeats: Genetics, Clinical Features, and Pathogenesis" by Vicki L. Brandt and Huda Y. Zoghbi; "Genotype-Phenotype Correlations" by Thomas D. Bird and Gerard D. Schellenberg; "Mitochondrial Disorders Due to Mutations in the Nuclear Genome" by Michio Hirano; "Mitochondria in Neurodegenerative Disorders" by Giovanni Manfredi and M. Flint Beal; "Lysosomal Membrane Disorders—LAMP-2 Deficiency" by Ichizo Nishino; "Alzheimer's Disease" by Dennis Selkoe; "Genetics of Movement Disorders" by Juliette M. Harris and Stanley Fahn; "The Molecular Genetic Basis of Spinal Muscular Atrophies" by Ching H. Wang; "Limb Girdle Muscular Dystrophies" by Rita Barresi and Kevin Campbell; "The Congenital Myopathies" by Heinz Jungbluth, Caroline A. Sewry, and Francesco Muntoni; "Hereditary Inclusion Body Myopathies" by Valerie S. Askanas and W. King Engel; "Facioscapulohumeral Dystrophy" by Rabi Tawil; "The Phakomatoses" by Mia MacCollin; "Disorders of Galactose Metabolism" by Louis J. Elsas, II,; "Disorders of Glucose Transport" by Darryl C. DeVivo, Dong Wang; and Juan M. Pascual; "Metabolic Disorders—Congenital Disorders of Glycosylation" by Marc C. Patterson; "Disorders of Glutathione Metabolism" by Ellinor Ristoff and Agne Larsson; "Friedreich's Ataxia and Iron Metabolism" by Massimo Pandolfo, and "The Influence of α-Tocopherol, Caloric Restriction, and Genes on Life Span" by Richard Mayeux. Importantly, the number of new genetic loci for dominant, recessive, and X-linked neurologic disease have increased significantly since our second edition as described in "A Neurologic Gene Map."

The editors are most grateful to all the contributing authors for their participation in this large undertaking. Each author is an authority and scholar in the field and, as such, has greatly enhanced the quality of this work.

The first edition of our book appeared at the beginning of the "Decade of the Brain," a resolution of the United States Congress signed by President George H.W. Bush in 1989, and the second edition of our book appeared in the latter years of this decade. Now, the third edition is published in 2003, at the start of the new millennium. By virtue of the publication of the initial sequence and analyses of the human genome, it is now possible to embark upon a new beginning. This new beginning, genomic neurology and psychiatry, represents a paradigm shift in the conceptualization of and our thinking on neurogenetics. Our previous orientation to clinical and molecular neurogenetics has been to ascribe function to a single gene and its immediate biochemical pathway causal of a neurologic or psychiatric disease. Now the emphasis has shifted to consider the consequences of the expression of every gene in the nervous system, normal or mutant, to the genome in its totality. Complex neurologic diseases involving multiple genes interacting with environmental stimuli can be analyzed for quantitative and coordinate levels of gene expression involving thousands of genes. We now have the information and technical ability to make these measurements. We must consider the genomic consequence of the ability of a single gene's mutation to cause a neurologic and psychiatric disease and the effect it has on many or all genes expressed in the nervous system. How each gene influences the pattern of expression of many other genes, simultaneously and coordinately, will be determined. Thousands of newly discovered and defined genes specific to the functioning of the nervous system will be identified in the next few years by virtue of the success of the human genome project, revolutionizing our understanding of gene action in both neurological function and disease.

The successes of the sequencing and analysis of the human genome will provide the means for identification of the genes responsible for inherited neurologic and psychiatric diseases and, even more important, the genes that underlie human behaviors, including the many-faceted components that compose human intelligence. We believe it is a magnificent time in science for the genetic exploration of the human nervous system and for defining the genotypes of all inherited neurologic and psychiatric diseases. We will soon be in a position to develop pharmacological and even pharmacogenomic drugs based on specific nucleotide polymorphisms in a patient's genome, as well as gene and stem cell therapies to treat neurologic and psychiatric disease and possibly to enhance specific human behaviors. Major ethical issues are involved in implementing these approaches and we need to be cautious in how we proceed.

The third edition of our book incorporates the most recent advances in the molecular and genetic understanding of diseases of the nervous system. The third edition incorporates major chapter revisions and new chapters to accommodate the dramatic increase in knowledge that has occurred in the past six years. Neurogenetics has become a mature and defined molecular field in neuroscience and in clinical medicine. Neurogenomics is just beginning and will serve as a catalyst to rapidly identify new genes, new gene functions and expressions, and new insights into disease causation and potential therapies. We believe the Golden Age of Neurology and Psychiatry has arrived as evidenced by the exponential increase in knowledge and insights into the molecular and genetic basis of human disease of the nervous system and the potential of the published sequence of the human genome.

The material in the third edition will be of value to clinicians caring for patients with hereditary neurologic, and psychiatric disorders and to investigators concerned with the scientific issues that these disorders pose. In addition, we hope that the body of information described here will serve to stimulate the next generation of neurologists, psychiatrists, and neuroscientists to enter this field and to move forward aggressively toward a clearer understanding of the molecular and genetic basis of neurologic and psychiatric disease well into the 21st century.

Finally, we wish to express our gratitude to Susan Pioli, Executive Publisher, Global Medicine, Elsevier Science, and to Kimberley Cox, Senior Developmental Editor, Elsevier Science, for their creative and constant support of the arduous efforts made by all of the authors and Editors to achieve a thoroughly updated and comprehensive review of *The Molecular and Genetic Basis of Neurologic and Psychiatric Disease.*

Roger N. Rosenberg, M.D.
Stanley B. Prusiner, M.D.
Salvatore Di Mauro, M.D.
Robert L. Barchi, M.D., Ph.D.
Eric Nestler, M.D., Ph.D.

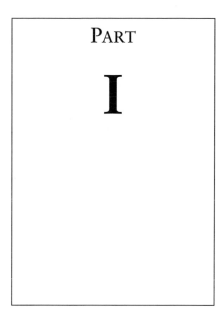

PART

I

GENERAL CONCEPTS OF MECHANISMS OF DISEASE

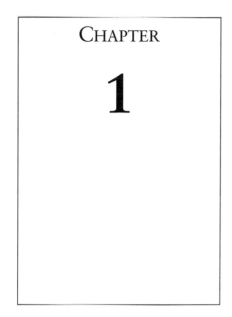

CHAPTER

1

Triplet Repeat Disease: General Concepts and Mechanisms of Disease

Vicky L. Brandt and Huda Y. Zoghbi

DYNAMIC REPEATS

A reliable assumption of mendelian genetics is that mutations are stably transmitted from parent to offspring. So solidly established was this assumption that evidence to the contrary was largely dismissed as ascertainment bias until 1991, when the gene responsible for fragile X was found to contain a trinucleotide repeat sequence that was anything but stable. Rather than being passed on from parent to offspring in its original form, this mutation could expand from a few dozen triplets to a thousand in one generation. This new kind of "dynamic" mutation turned out to be a not uncommon exception to the mendelian rule.

Dynamic mutations can involve anything from a series of trinucleotides to a complex sequence of pentanucleotides or dodecamer repeats (Table 1–1). In this chapter we will concentrate on diseases of triplet repeat expansions (Tables 1–2 and 1–3). We will cover several

general concepts important for understanding dynamic mutation diseases, then examine specific mechanisms that underlie the pathogenesis of different disorders. For these purposes, it is convenient to classify the diseases into two broad categories: untranslated repeats (see Table 1–2), which can interfere with DNA structure, transcription, or RNA-protein interactions, and translated polyglutamine (CAG) repeats (see Table 1–3), which alter the conformation of a given protein and impair its clearance.

GENERAL CONCEPTS

Repeat Instability. The most fundamental question, how and why repeat sequences expand, remains unanswered despite a decade of study and speculation. There are a few diseases that involve mild repeat sequence expansions that are *not* unstable; oculopharyngeal muscular dystrophy is one example. In most cases, however, the repeat sequences

TABLE 1–1. Diseases Caused by Dynamic Mutations Other Than Triplet Repeats

Disorder	Inheritance	Gene	Chromosome	Repeat	Normal repeat #	Mutant	Location	Effect*	Parental bias
Myotonic dystrophy type 2/proximal myotonic myopathy (PROMM)	AD	ZNF9	3q21	CCTG*	<26 without interruptions	75–11,000	intron 1	GOF (RNA)	—
Progressive myoclonus epilepsy 1	AR	CSTB	21q22.3	C_4GC_4GCG	2–3	35–80	5′ flanking	LOF*	paternal
SCA10	AD	SCA10	22q13	ATTCT	10–22	800–4500	intron 9	?	paternal

*The wild-type sequence is a complex, interrupted repeat motif: (TG)n(TCTG)n(CCTG)n;
GOF = gain of function; LOF = loss of function

TABLE 1–2. Diseases Caused by Noncoding Triplet Repeat Expansions

Disorder	Inheritance	Gene	Chromosome	Repeat	Normal repeat	Mutation range	Location	Effect	Parental bias
Fragile X syndrome	XL	FMR1	Xq27.3	CGG	6–52	premutation: 60–200 full mutation: 230–1000+	5'UTR	LOF	maternal
Fragile XE mental retardation	XL	FMR2	Xq28	GCC	7–35	premutation: 130–150 full mutation: 230–750+	5'UTR	LOF	?
Friedreich ataxia	AR	FRDA1	9q13–21.1	GAA	6–34	80 premutation, 112–1700+ full mutation	intron 1	LOF	maternal
Myotonic dystrophy	AD	DMPK	19q13	CTG	5–37	50–3000+	3'UTR	GOF (RNA); other	<100, paternal; maternal for large repeats
SCA8	AD	SCA8	13q21	CTA/CTG	15–37	typically 80–250, but 71–800 possible*	3'UTR (antisense)	GOF (RNA)	maternal
SCA12	AD	PPP2R2B	5q31-q33	CAG	7–28	66–78	5'UTR	?	?
Huntington disease–like 2	AD	JPH3	16q24.3	CAG/CTG	6–28	49–57	3'UTR	?	?

*Pathogenic range varies between families.
GOF = gain of function; LOF = loss of function

TABLE 1–3. Diseases Caused by Coding Triplet Repeat Expansions

Disorder	Inheritance	Gene	Chromosome	Repeat	Normal repeat #	Mutation range	Effect	Parental bias
Spinobulbar muscular atrophy	XL	*AR*	Xq13-21	CAG	11–33	38–66	GOF, LOF	—
Dentatorubropallidoluysian atrophy (DRPLA)	AD	*DRPLA*	12p13.31	CAG	6–35	49–88	GOF	paternal
Huntington disease	AD	*HD*	4p16.3	CAG	6–39*	36–121	GOF	paternal
Spinocerebellar ataxia type 1 (SCA1)	AD	*SCA1*	6p23	CAG	6–44*	36–81	GOF	paternal
SCA2	AD	*SCA2*	12q24.1	CAG	14–31	35–64	GOF	paternal
SCA3	AD	*SCA3*	14q32.1	CAG	12–41*	40–84	GOF	paternal
SCA6	AD	*CACNA1A*	19p13	CAG	7–18	21–33	GOF	?
SCA7	AD	*SCA7*	3p12-13	CAG	4–35	37–460	GOF	paternal
SCA17	AD	*TBP*	6q27	CAG	29–42	47–63	GOF	paternal

*Alleles with 21 or more repeats are interrupted by 1–3 (CAT) units; disease alleles contain pure CAG tracts.
GOF = gain of function; LOF = loss of function

are not only unstable but they have a bias for expansion: although they can lose nucleotides, the tracts are much more likely to add repeats. Interestingly, the bias toward expansion even shows up in comparisons between species: tandem repeats in humans, for example, tend to be longer than their homologues in chimpanzees.[1]

It is noteworthy that expansions can be quite unstable during mitosis, but they are remarkably unstable during meiosis. The degree of repeat instability varies among diseases; a quick glance at the tables reveals how extensive this variability is. This is partly because the instability of a repeat expansion increases with the size of the tract (the larger the expansion, the more likely it is to undergo further expansion). *Cis* elements (sequences flanking the repeat) also contribute to instability, however. Flanking sequences likely explain the varying degrees of stability of similar-length CAG tracts at different disease loci.

Several models have been proposed to explain how expansions might occur: slippage during DNA replication, misalignment and subsequent excision repair, and unequal crossing-over. Accumulating evidence suggests that the long repeats form secondary structures on Okazaki fragments, which then block or stall progression of the replication fork, increasing the likelihood of further expansion.[2] Cleary and coworkers[3] propose that a long repeat tract at the end of an Okazaki fragment might facilitate the formation of hairpins or slipped strand structures, whose metabolism might result in error-prone processing by replication, repair, or recombination proteins. This model neatly explains the existence of a small overlap in size between normal and disease-causing alleles in some triplet repeat disorders. Normal alleles have a sequence of one triplet interrupted occasionally by another (e.g., a normal string of CAG repeats is interrupted by a few CAT sequences), but disease-causing alleles lose those intervening triplets (becoming, for example, a pure string of CAG repeats). It has been established that these intervening triplets stabilize the tract; it is reasonable to think that they do so by preventing the formation of secondary structures on the Okazaki fragments.

Anticipation. The progressively earlier onset of symptoms and greater severity of disease in successive generations of a family was first documented in 1918 by Fleischer, a German physician who had been studying families afflicted with myotonic dystrophy (DM, for dystrophia myotonica).[4] The implications of Fleischer's genealogical work, that something was causing the same disease to take on a more virulent form as it was transmitted from one generation to the next, was generally accepted for about thirty years until Penrose compared a variety of different genetic disorders and was able to show varying degrees of anticipation in most.[5] Penrose proposed that a combination of phenotypic variability and ascertainment bias could account for the phenomenon, most of whose appearances were just that—appearance. (This conclusion was no doubt correct in a majority of cases.) Unfortunately, these arguments were compelling enough to quell a search for biological explanations of anticipation. It took another forty years or so for documentation of the severe congenital form of DM and parallels with fragile X syndrome to be made in order for "ascertainment bias" to be proven inadequate as an explanation. The discovery of unstable repeat tracts settled matters unequivocally.

Phenotype-Genotype Correlations. If continued repeat expansions over generations are responsible for anticipation, how close is the link between genotype and phenotype? The correlation between repeat size and either symptom severity or age of onset is definite but loose. In the case of DM, for example, there is a large gap between the repeat tract lengths that produce the minimal form of the disease (100 to 250 base pairs, which might cause only cataracts very late in life) and those that cause congenital disease (>2500 base pairs). Nonetheless, typical adult onset cases show a tremendous variability in expansion size that overlaps with each of these categories of disease, and clinically discordant twins with the same repeat number have been reported in studies of certain disorders. Conversely, genetically confirmed monozygotic twins have been found to have dramatically different expanded alleles.[6] In the polyglutamine diseases, it is not uncommon to see symptoms appear ten years later in one patient than in another bearing the same length CAG tract. The triplet repeat expansion is, therefore, not the only factor that determines onset and course, although no specific modifying factors have yet been identified. The clinically important conclusion to draw from this information is that repeat size cannot be used for individual prognosis in the majority of cases. Patients with expansions at the lowest or highest end of the range for their particular disease are, of course, likely to reliably follow either the mildest or most dismal course of progression.

Physicians should note that precise phenotype-genotype correlations are particularly elusive in the case of the coding repeat diseases, which are typified by enormous expansions. In these cases (1) there is tremendous somatic instability of the repeat tracts, so that different tissues bear quite different expansions; (2) somatic expansions also occur over time, that is, the same tissue may develop larger repeats as an individual ages; and (3) lymphocytes bear no direct relationship to the tissues manifesting clinical abnormalities, so the repeat expansions measured by blood tests may be quite different from those in disease tissue. Notwithstanding this imprecision, the unavoidable fact of anticipation makes genetic counseling as crucial as it is delicate: prospective parents must understand the risk of having children with much worse disease than they themselves experience.

Parent of Origin Effects. In general, large expansions seem to be more common in male meioses, whereas alleles transmitted by females usually undergo only modest increases in repeat tract length. This paternal bias, which holds for the CAG repeat diseases (see Table 1–3), is not surprising, because sperm undergo at least six times as many cell divisions to zygote than do ova. Yet most discussions of noncoding repeats disorders claim a maternal, not a paternal, bias, because the dramatic expansions leading to the most severe phenotypes are usually passed through the mother. Myotonic dystrophy provides an excellent means of examining this apparent contradiction.

Consider these three facts: (1) the severe, congenital form of DM is almost always transmitted by the mother; (2) there is a preponderance of asymptomatic or minimally affected males in the earliest generations of DM

families; (3) studies covering the entire range of repeat lengths show no clear sex difference in intergenerational expansion. This rather confusing state of affairs becomes understandable when the repeat length-dependence of expansion instability is taken into account. With smaller repeats (<100), the tendency for the DM disease allele to expand is greater in male transmissions. Note that this repeat range is responsible for both the mild form of DM (and other noncoding repeat diseases) and the severe, juvenile-onset forms of polyglutamine disease, which also show a paternal bias. Thus, the pattern for all triplet repeats in this expansion range seems to be for instability to be greater in male transmissions. The predominantly maternal transmission of extremely large expansions in DM results from a selective disadvantage for sperm carrying thousands of repeats (and decreased male fertility in this expansion range). What makes DM and other noncoding repeat disorders seem to be exceptions to the paternal bias rule is that individuals with extremely large expansions of hundreds or thousands of repeats are viable, and females with these large expansions are fertile.[7] In the polyglutamine diseases, CAG tract expansions of only 80 repeats or so cause early death.

We will now examine the pathogenetic mechanisms underlying specific repeat diseases to see how these principles are embodied in different disorders.

NONCODING REPEAT DISORDERS

Loss of Function through Hypermethylation: Fragile X Syndrome and Fragile XE Mental Retardation

Fragile X syndrome (FRAXA) is an X-linked disorder that is probably the single most common cause of mental retardation, with an incidence estimated at about 1:4000. As its name implies, it was originally associated with a folate-sensitive fragile site at Xq27.3 in affected patients. Sequence analysis of cosmids and cDNAs coincident with this fragile site revealed a polymorphic $(CGG)_n$ repeat in the 5′–untranslated region of the fragile X mental retardation gene (FMR1). There are four classes of alleles, referred to as normal, intermediate, premutation, and full mutation. Normal alleles typically contain about 30 CGG repeats punctuated by one or more AGG triplets, and this tract length is generally stable. Loss of the interspersed AGGs seems to destabilize the tract, rendering it susceptible to expansions, usually into the premutation range of 50 to 200 repeats. Premutation carriers usually do not manifest overt signs of disease—although it is becoming clear that there is a subtle premutation phenotype in both males and females —but they are at high risk for having fully affected children. Hyperexpansion is associated exclusively with maternal transmission, and the risk of expansion to more than 230 repeats is dependent on the size of the premutation in female carriers. Females with premutations of less than 60 repeats (the intermediate range) may transmit an allele that is expanded by only a few repeats, but females carrying premutations of more than 90 repeats have a high risk of transmitting a disease causing expansion to their children.

Expansion of the CGG repeat beyond 230 usually leads to hypermethylation of the CGG repeat as well as a CpG island within the FMR1 promoter region, which, in turn, recruits the transcriptional silencing machinery to the *FMR1* gene, preventing its expression. The FMR1 gene product, FMRP, is a selective RNA binding protein that shuttles between the nucleus and the cytoplasm. In the cytoplasm, FMRP forms messenger ribonucleoprotein (mRNP) complexes and associates with polyribosomes or endoplasmic reticulum-associated ribosomes. FMRP's association with the translational machinery in dendritic spines suggests it may play a role in modulating the localization or translation (or both) of its target mRNAs. Regulation of localized protein synthesis is important in cell growth, polarity, and the synaptic plasticity that underlies processes related to learning and memory. Some work used the discovery that FMRP has an affinity for intramolecular G quartets to identify mRNAs encoding proteins involved in synaptic function or dendritic growth that harbor FMRP binding elements.[8,9] Most of these mRNAs that harbor FMRP binding elements show altered polysome association in fragile X patient cells. This work is a tremendous advance toward characterization of the physiologic targets of FMRP and their role in mediating the mental retardation phenotype.[10] The other phenotypic features associated with fragile X syndrome could result from pleiotropic effects of abnormal RNA metabolism. This model has been supported by studies in mice lacking the *Fmr1* gene, which exhibit cognitive and behavioral deficits, macroorchidism, and hyperactivity, all of which are features of the human disease.

Fragile XE mental retardation (FRAXE) is milder than fragile X syndrome, and does not cause the morphologic features of the fragile X phenotype. FRAXE is caused by an expansion of a polymorphic CGG repeat in a folate-sensitive fragile site immediately adjacent to a CpG island, 600 kb distal to the FRAXA locus. The repeat size varies from 6 to 35 copies on normal alleles that are relatively stable on transmission, whereas repeat sizes in the premutation range (61 to 200) may expand to the full mutation (>200). Parent-of-origin effects are similar to those described earlier with FRAXA, but reductions in repeat number are frequently observed in FRAXE on germline transmission, and males with the full mutation can have affected daughters with full mutations.

The FRAXE CGG repeat resides in the promoter region of a gene termed *FMR2*. As in fragile X, the expanded repeats are abnormally methylated. The cognitive and behavioral deficits in FRAXE result from *FMR2* transcriptional silencing and subsequent loss of FMR2 protein function.[11] Although FMR2's precise function(s) are unknown, its putative role as a transcriptional activator and its high level of expression in areas of the brain involved in learning, memory, and emotion suggest that the pathogenic mechanism underlying FRAXE entails alterations in the regulation of neuronal genes.

Loss of Function through Transcriptional Interference: Friedreich Ataxia

Friedreich ataxia (FRDA), the most prevalent inherited ataxia, is autosomal recessive and usually manifests by late adolescence. The disease is caused by a large intronic GAA repeat expansion—the most common identified thus far, with a carrier frequency of 1 in 85—located in the center of an Alu repeat in FRDA1 (also known as *frataxin*). FRDA is unique among the triplet repeat disorders in that the repeat is located in an intron, and the repeat sequence is AT-rich rather than GC-rich. Normal alleles usually contain 5 to 34 repeats, but alleles containing 33 to 55 trinucleotides interrupted by a (GAGGAA)n sequence that stabilizes the tract are also normal. Intermediate or premutation alleles containing 34 to 65 pure (uninterrupted) GAA repeats are compatible with normal frataxin expression and function but can expand to 300 to 650 repeats in a single generation. The unstable GAA repeat can expand or contract on maternal transmission but usually contracts when passed through the father (although this depends on the size of the paternal allele). As with most other triplet repeat disorders, the disease-causing range of repeats may change as more patients are studied, and determination of test results in borderline cases is complicated by the fact that the GAA expansion in leukocytes is not necessarily the same as that contained in relevant tissues. Nonetheless, larger GAA expansions (particularly the size of the smaller of each pair of alleles) correlate with earlier age of onset and shorter times to loss of ambulation, as well as the appearance of certain features (e.g., cardiomyopathy). In general, alleles with fewer than 500 repeats are associated with disease onset after 25 years of age.

The correlation between disease severity, onset, and expansion size is directly reflected in FRDA molecular pathogenesis. The GAA trinucleotide repeat expansion interferes with transcription and causes a severe deficiency of normally spliced FRDA mRNA, and thus of the frataxin protein. The longer the GAA repeat on the shorter of the two alleles, the more severe the frataxin deficiency. In support of the notion that FRDA results from partial loss of frataxin function, patients who carry only one expanded allele and one truncating point mutation on the second allele have all the clinical features of typical FRDA. Interestingly, sequences with more than 59 repeats form a higher order triplex structure that directly interferes with transcription. In other words, it is the expanded GAA tract itself that hinders transcription, not a secondary event such as the hypermethylation that occurs in fragile X. There is no in vivo evidence for mis-splicing or altered RNA processing; RNase protection assays and in vitro transcription experiments show all portions of frataxin mRNA are reduced. Moreover, heterozygous carriers express mRNA at a level intermediate between wild-type and affected individuals with similar repeat lengths.

Frataxin localizes to the mitochondrial membrane and has well-conserved homologues in many lower organisms. Yeast deficient for the frataxin homologue (Yfh1) lose mitochondrial DNA and develop abnormal accumulation of mitochondrial iron and respiratory deficiency. These early studies led investigators to suspect that mitochondrial iron accumulation was likely to be the primary defect, followed by a secondary deficiency of iron sulfur cluster enzymes mediated by oxidative damage. But more recent research in mice presents a different picture. Inactivation of the mouse homologue causes early embryonic lethality without iron accumulation; more importantly, a conditional, tissue-specific knockout mouse develops respiratory deficiency and tissue pathology before intramitochondrial iron deposition.[12] The most convincing evidence to date that mitochondrial iron overload is a secondary development, however, comes from Chantrel-Groussard and coworkers,[13] who found that fibroblasts from individuals with FRDA or the conditional frataxin knockout mouse have difficulty inducing superoxide dismutase or the iron-import machinery in response to oxidative stress. It is thus most likely that a defect in mitochondrial oxidative phosphorylation underlies FRDA.

Haploinsufficiency, Gene Dysregulation, and Toxic RNA: Myotonic Dystrophy

Myotonic dystrophy type 1 (DM, for the Latin *dystrophia myotonica*) is the most common and most variable of the muscular dystrophies. It is a dominantly inherited multisystem disorder that can cause not only muscle hyperexcitability, weakness, and wasting, but also cataracts, kidney failure, hyperinsulin secretion, cardiac conduction abnormalities, and, in males, premature baldness and testicular atrophy.

DM1 is caused by an expanded CTG repeat that lies in both the 3′ untranslated region of the dystrophia myotonica protein kinase (*DMPK*) gene and the promoter region of the adjacent homeodomain gene *SIX5*. Three mechanisms have been suggested to explain how this CTG expansion causes the complex phenotype of DM; in fact, it has seemed most reasonable to believe that all three mechanisms act in concert to produce the diverse features of the syndrome. The three mechanisms are readily remembered as operating at the protein, DNA, and RNA levels.

The first hypothesis, that DM results from a protein kinase deficiency, was prompted by the observation that

DM patients exhibit reduced phosphorylation of membrane proteins in muscle tissue and red blood cells. DMPK haploinsufficiency is proposed to result when the expansion is transcribed from a CTG sequence to a CUG sequence in RNA (replacing the thymine with a uracil) and the mutant RNA fails to enter the cytoplasm, thereby preventing mRNA from being translated into protein. The evidence supporting this mechanism is mixed: a *DMPK* knockout mouse manifests DM1-like cardiac abnormalities[14] but none of the multisystem defects that are characteristic of the disease. Other mechanisms must be involved.

The second proposed mechanism, operating at the DNA level, neatly addresses the unusual diversity of features. In this model, the CTG expansion alters regional chromatin in the nucleus and suppresses expression of *SIX5* and other nearby genes. Indeed, two groups independently showed that mice deficient in *SIX5* develop cataracts,[15,16] and another study suggests that methylation-induced disruption of DM1 insulator function causes dysregulation of gene expression.[17] Unfortunately, the type of cataracts formed in the *SIX5* mice differs from that seen in patients, so the explanatory power of this mechanism, too, is limited.

The third proposed mechanism entails toxic RNA: the mutant RNA binds to other proteins, disrupting nuclear activities. Specifically, accumulation of the expanded RNA into nuclear foci is thought to alter the regulation of CUG-binding proteins. In support of this model, transgenic mice expressing mRNA (unrelated to the DMPK protein) with a CUG tract of about 250 repeats develop myotonia and myopathy.[18] Furthermore, there is evidence that CUG repeat-induced changes in CUG-binding protein (CUG-BP) disrupts RNA splicing of *insulin receptor* (*IR*)[19] and *cardiac troponin T* (*cTNT*)[20]; perturbations in the functions of these genes could certainly contribute to the insulin insensitivity and cardiac abnormalities seen in DM. In short, the DM expansion can be thought of as a toxic gain-of-function mutation in RNA.

Although it is conceivable that all three mechanisms are at work, the balance has been tipped toward the toxic RNA model. Liquori and coworkers[6] discovered that a tetramer repeat expansion underlies DM2, a multisystem disease quite similar to DM1 but milder in its manifestations. DM2 was not even recognized as a distinct entity until the genetic defect in DM1 failed to appear in a subset of DM patients. The clinical parallels between DM1 and DM2 point strongly to a common pathogenetic mechanism, yet the DM2 protein bears no apparent relation to DMPK. The DM2 expansion is located in a transcribed but untranslated portion of the *zinc finger protein 9* (*ZNF9*) gene, whose product is a nucleic acid binding protein. Not only is ZNF9 completely unrelated to DMPK, but genes in the DM2 region have no discernible relationship to genes at the DM1 locus. Both DM1 and DM2 do, however, bear evidence of RNA toxicity. The

RNA foci in both syndromes cause colocalization of the CUG-binding protein muscleblind.[21] Furthermore, the insulin-resistant spliced form of *IR* is thought to underlie the hyperinsulinemia seen in both DM1 and DM2. RNA toxicity thus seems almost certain to play an important role in the multisystemic character of DM; it may also be at work in other noncoding repeat disorders, such as SCA8 and possibly SCA10.

Altered RNA Regulation: Spinocerebellar Ataxia Type 8

Like DM1, SCA8 is caused by an untranslated CTG expansion. In this case, the repeat lies near the 3′ end of a processed, noncoding mRNA.[22] The 5′ end of the SCA8 gene overlaps the 5′ end of *Kelch-like 1* or *KLHL1*,[23] which encodes an actin-binding protein that is transcribed in the opposite direction. The location of the CTG repeat in the antisense KLHL1 transcript suggests that the SCA8 transcript may be an endogenous antisense RNA that regulates KLHL1 expression. Although the normal function of KLHL1 in the brain is not understood, its POZ/BTB protein-protein domains, actin-binding domain, and similarities to a brain-specific gene, *NRP/B*, believed to be involved in neuronal process formation could account for the CNS-specific phenotype of SCA8.

The SCA8 expansion violates several principles of dynamic mutations outlined earlier. Disease-causing repeats tend to be passed on by the mother, and paternal transmissions have a strong tendency to contract dramatically (in one case, from 800 to 100!). Very large expansions between 250 and 800 repeats can leave an individual entirely unaffected, just like the 20 to 30 repeats present in the normal population: it seems to be a range of repeats between 100 and 250 that is pathogenic. Although this phenomenon is not yet fully understood, it is possible that very large repeats interfere with SCA8 expression or alter RNA processing or stability so that there is no toxic gain of function when the CUG tract is more than 250 repeats.

Mechanisms Unknown: Sca12 and Huntington Disease–Like 2

SCA12 is a rare disease affecting only a few families to date. It is caused by a noncoding CAG trinucleotide repeat expansion in the 5′UTR of the *PPP2R2B* gene,[24] which encodes a brain-specific regulatory subunit of protein phosphatase 2A (PP2A-PR55). This protein has numerous cellular functions, but the precise role of the PP2A-PR55 subunit is unknown. Although the repeat is flanked by transcriptional start sites and conserved promoter elements, it is not clear whether the expanded CAG tract interferes with or increases transcription of *PPP2R2B*.

Huntington disease–like 2, recognized as a distinct clinical entity after patients with Huntington disease–like

symptoms tested negative for the HD mutation, is caused by a CAG/CTG repeat expansion in the gene encoding junctophilin-3. The repeat is thought to lie in an alternatively spliced exon and to encode polyalanine or polyleucine.

Translated Repeats Confer Toxic Gains of Function: The Polyglutamine Diseases

As might be expected for autosomal dominant disorders, the polyglutamine neurodegenerative diseases (see Table 1–3) result from a toxic gain of protein function. The expansion of unstable CAG trinucleotide repeats coding for polyglutamine tracts in the respective proteins is thought to alter the conformation of the native protein, inducing neuronal dysfunction in any of several ways. An aberrant conformation might augment the protein's normal function in the cell, as in the case of mutant CACNA1A in SCA6, in which the channel has enhanced calcium current activity; the mutant protein might also interact more intensely with normal protein partners, perhaps diverting these partners from their normal functions or sequestering them in inappropriate subcellular compartments. The misfolded protein could also tie up the cell's degradation machinery, causing added cellular stress and modifying levels of key cellular proteins, which would further compromise cell function.

The CAG repeat tracts are polymorphic and vary in their instability: the *SCA7* gene, for example, may expand by hundreds of repeats in one intergenerational transmission, whereas the *SCA6* gene is relatively stable, and the difference in length between the wild-type and mutant CAG tract is only three repeats. But in all these diseases, CAG repeats exceeding the normal range for a given protein cause progressive neuronal dysfunction and death within 10 to 20 years in adult onset cases, with longer repeat tracts causing earlier age of onset and more severe disease (and death within only a few years for juvenile-onset patients). The normal functions of these proteins are unknown in most cases, the exceptions being the androgen receptor (spinobulbar muscular atrophy), the α_{1A}-voltage-dependent calcium channel (SCA6), and the TATA-binding protein (SCA17). Given this diversity of functions, the similarities in the phenotypes resulting from CAG expansions in these proteins are surprising.

Curiously, despite the widespread expression of polyglutamine-containing proteins throughout the brain and other tissues, only a certain subset of neurons is vulnerable to dysfunction in each of these diseases; also rather curiously, the cerebellum is usually one of the tissues vulnerable to degeneration. The variability in cell-specific degeneration despite overlapping expression patterns is lost when very large expansions lead to severe, juvenile-onset disease. In these cases neurodegeneration is widespread, and the few distinctions that can be made clinically between the various ataxias practically disappear. This loss of cell specificity with large expansions is intriguing, and hints that toxicity is probably much more widespread through neuronal and non-neuronal cells that have been thought to be spared when the repeat sizes are moderately expanded. It also suggests that repeat expansions are smaller in the coding repeat disorders because of selective pressure against the very large expansions, which are likely to be lethal during embryogenesis.

In most of the polyglutamine diseases, the mutant protein accumulates into visible aggregates in the nucleus. Because these aggregates also cause colocalization of portions of the cell's protein refolding and degradation machinery—chaperones, ubiquitin, and proteasomal subunits—it has been suspected that impaired protein clearance underlies the pathogenesis of SCA1 and related diseases. The polyglutamine expansion is thought to alter the conformation of the native protein, rendering it more resistant to degradation. At least two lines of evidence support this hypothesis. First, studies in both flies and mice have demonstrated that overexpression of chaperone proteins, which help refold proteins or target them for degradation, mitigates neurodegeneration.[25,26] Second, neuronal degeneration is considerably worse when ubiquitination is impaired in SCA1 transgenic mice, even though aggregation is diminished.[26] This suggests, in fact, that aggregates have a protective effect by sequestering the toxic protein. In this regard, it should be noted that in both patient tissue and a knock-in model of SCA1,[27] the cells that are the least vulnerable to disease develop aggregates very early on, whereas the most vulnerable neurons are unable to form aggregates until quite late in the disease. Variations in levels of chaperones or other proteins involved in protein folding or degradation could thus explain the selective neuronal vulnerability that typifies the polyglutamine diseases. In other words, although these proteins are ubiquitously expressed, different neuronal groups have greater or lesser abilities to curtail the mutant proteins' toxic effects by forming aggregates. Variations in the levels of the mutant proteins themselves could also play a role, of course.

It is striking that the polyglutamine diseases are not the only disorders resulting from impaired protein clearance: Alzheimer, amyotrophic lateral sclerosis (ALS), and Parkinson disease all involve the gradual accumulation of mutant proteins. Improving proper folding and degradation of the relevant proteins might be beneficial in all these cases. Molecular chaperones have already proved to be an effective means of moderating the aggregation and toxicity of mutant SOD-1 (the protein mutated in familial ALS) in cells; fly studies have similarly shown the beneficial effects of chaperones on mutant alpha-synuclein (the protein causing Parkinson disease). It appears that the potential applications for chaperones in neurodegeneration might be very broad.

There are two other main pathogenetic pathways that seem to provide likely therapeutic targets, at least for the polyglutaminopathies. There is evidence that the earliest step in polyglutamine pathogenesis is alteration of gene expression, and many polyglutamine proteins redistribute transcriptional regulators to the sites of aggregation. Because several of the polyglutamine-containing proteins interact with CBP, which has histone acetylase activity, histone deacetylase inhibitors (HDACs) were studied in cell lines and *Drosophila* expressing an expanded polyglutamine tract and were found to suppress cell death and improve viability. Caspase inhibitors have likewise been found to extend the life span of mice expressing an expanded Huntington peptide. The availability of several pathways for attempting therapeutic intervention certainly provides grounds for hope that these diseases can be treated or even cured in the not-too-distant future.

CONCLUSION

What began as a couple of puzzling exceptions to mendelian inheritance has become a class of diseases that defy easy generalizations. Although dominantly inherited diseases are usually caused by mutations that confer a gain of function on the altered protein, DM and SCA8 involve a toxic gain of RNA function instead. The intronic pentanucleotide repeat in SCA10 could also involve toxic RNA, or it could have effects like the FRDA repeat or even act on neighboring genes through chromatin alterations. The CAG expansion disorders, which do involve a gain of protein function, are dominantly inherited, except for SBMA, which is X-linked (and involves, paradoxically, at least a partial loss of androgen receptor function). In general, noncoding repeats expand to many hundreds of triplets, but SCA12 so far been has reported to occur with only 66 to 78 repeats. The noncoding repeat diseases are typically multisystem disorders whose pathogenic mechanisms vary according to the location of the repeat sequence within a given gene; nevertheless, the SCA8 phenotype is limited to the central nervous system. The polyglutamine diseases involve proteins that are ubiquitously expressed, and thus might well be expected to cause widespread pathology, but the expanded CAG repeats target specific groups of neurons in each disease. If the expansions are particularly large by polyglutamine standards, the neuropathology is broader but still confined to the CNS except in the case of SCA7 (in which infantile cases suffer patent ductus arteriosus). Despite this pattern of exceptions, however, there is one theme emerging among the coding and noncoding repeat diseases whose mechanisms are at least partially understood: the repeat expansion seems to interfere with transcription.

The discovery of dynamic mutations has clearly had a profound effect on the practice of neurology. It is now possible to provide an accurate diagnosis for all of these diseases with a simple DNA test; family members can receive informed genetic counseling. Most importantly, studying these mutations in animal models has yielded insight into the pathogenesis of these disorders and is beginning to provide opportunities for interventional trials.

REFERENCES

1. Rubinsztein DC, Amos W, Leggo J, et al: Microsatellite evolution-evidence for directionality and variation in rate between species. Nat Genet 1995; 10(3):337–343.

2. Pearson CE, Sinden RR: Trinucleotide repeat DNA structures: Dynamic mutations from dynamic DNA. Curr Opin Struct Biol 1998;8:321–330.

3. Cleary JD, Nichol K, Wang YH, Pearson CE: Evidence of cis-acting factors in replication-mediated trinucleotide repeat instability in primate cells. Nat Genet 2002;31(1):37–46.

4. Fleischer B: Über myotonische Dystrophie mit Katarakt. Albercht von Graefes. Arch Klin Ophthalmol 1918;96:91–133.

5. Penrose LS: The problem of anticipation in pedigrees of dystrophia myotonica. Ann Eugenics 1948; 14:125–132.

6. Liquori CL, Ricker K, Moseley ML, et al: Myotonic dystrophy type 2 caused by a CCTG expansion in intron 1 of ZNF9. Science 2001;293(5531):864–867.

7. Sullivan AK, Crawford DC, Scott EII, et al: Paternally transmitted FMR1 alleles are less stable than maternally transmitted alleles in the common and intermediate size range. Am J Hum Genet 2002; 70(6): 1532–1544.

8. Darnell JC, Jensen KB, Jin P, et al: Fragile X mental retardation protein targets G quartet mRNAs important for neuronal function. Cell 2001;107(4): 489–499.

9. Brown V, Jin P, Ceman S, et al: Microarray identification of FMRP-associated brain mRNAs and altered mRNA translational profiles in fragile X syndrome. Cell 2001;107(4):477–487.

10. Huber KM, Gallagher SM, Warren ST, Bear MF: Altered synaptic plasticity in a mouse model of fragile X mental retardation. Proc Natl Acad Sci U S A 2002;99(11):7746–7750.

11. Gu Y, McIlwain KL, Weeber EJ, et al: Impaired conditioned fear and enhanced long-term potentiation in Fmr2 knock-out mice. J Neurosci 2002;22(7): 2753–2763.

12. Puccio H, Simon D, Cossee M, et al: Mouse models for Friedreich ataxia exhibit cardiomyopathy, sensory nerve defect and Fe-S enzyme deficiency followed by intramitochondrial iron deposits. Nat Genet 2001; 27:181–186.

13. Chantrel-Groussard K, Geromel V, Puccio II, et al: Disabled early recruitment of antioxidant defenses in Friedreich's ataxia. Hum Mol Genet 2001;10: 2061–2067.

14. Reddy S, Smith DB, Rich MM, et al: Mice lacking the myotonic dystrophy protein kinase develop a late onset progressive myopathy. Nat Genet 1996;13:325–335.

15. Klesert TR, Cho DH, Clark JI, et al: Mice deficient in Six5 develop cataracts: Implications for myotonic dystrophy. Nat Genet 2000;25:105–109.

16. Sarkar PS, Appukuttan B, Han J, et al: Heterozygous loss of Six5 in mice is sufficient to cause ocular cataracts. Nat Genet 2000;25:110–114.

17. Galina N, Filippova GN, Cortlandt P, et al: CTCF-binding sites flank CTG/CAG repeats and form a methylation-sensitive insulator at the DM1 locus. Nat Genet 2001;28:335–343.

18. Mankodi A, Logigian E, Callahan L, et al: Myotonic dystrophy in transgenic mice expressing an expanded CUG repeat. Science 2000;289:1769–1773.

19. Savkur RS, Philips AV, Cooper TA: Aberrant regulation of insulin receptor alternative splicing is associated with insulin resistance in myotonic dystrophy. Nat Genet 2001;29(1):40–47.

20. Philips AV, Timchenko LT, Cooper TA: Disruption of splicing regulated by a CUG-binding protein in myotonic dystrophy. Science 1998;280:737–741.

21. Mankodi A, Urbinati CR, Yuan QP, et al: Muscleblind localizes to nuclear foci of aberrant RNA in myotonic dystrophy types 1 and 2. Hum Mol Genet 2001;10(19):2165–2170.

22. Koob MD, Moseley ML, Schut LJ, et al: An untranslated CTG expansion causes a novel form of spinocerebellar ataxia (SCA8). Nat Genet 1999;21(4): 379–384.

23. Nemes JP, Benzow KA, Moseley ML, et al: The SCA8 transcript is an antisense RNA to a brain-specific transcript encoding a novel actin-binding protein (KLHL1). Hum Mol Genet 2000;9(10):1543–1551.

24. Holmes SE, O'Hearn EE, McInnis MG, et al: Expansion of a novel CAG trinucleotide repeat in the 5′ region of PPP2R2B is associated with SCA12. Nat Genet 1999;23(4):391–392.

25. Warrick JM, Chan HY, Gray-Board GL, et al: Suppression of polyglutamine-mediated neurodegeneration in Drosophila by the molecular chaperone HSP70. Nat Genet 1999;23(4):425–428.

26. Cummings CJ, Sun Y, Opal P, et al: Over-expression of inducible HSP70 chaperone suppresses neuropathology and improves motor function in SCA1 mice. Hum Mol Genet 2001;10(14):1511–1518.

27. Watase K, Weeber EJ, Xu B, et al: A long CAG tract in the mouse Sca1 locus replicates human SCA1 and reveals the impact of mutant protein solubility on selective neuronal vulnerability. Neuron 2002;34: 905–919.

CHAPTER

2

Prions

Stanley B. Prusiner

The prion concept developed in the aftermath of many unsuccessful attempts to decipher the nature of the scrapie agent. In some respects, the early development of the prion concept mirrors the story of deoxyribonucleic acid (DNA).[1-3] Before the acceptance of DNA as the genetic material,[4,5] many scientists asserted that DNA preparations must be contaminated with protein, which is the true genetic material.[6] For more than half a century, many biologists thought that genes were made of protein and that proteins were reproduced as replicas of themselves.[7,8] The prejudices of these scientists were similar in some ways to those of investigators who have disputed the prion concept. But scientists who attacked the hypothesis that genes are composed of DNA had no likely alternative; they had only a set of feelings derived from poorly substantiated data sets that genes are made of protein. In contrast, those who attacked the hypothesis that the prion is composed only of protein had more than 30 years of cumulative evidence showing that genetic information in all organisms on our planet is encoded in DNA. Studies of viruses, and eventually viroids, extended this concept to these small infectious pathogens[9] and showed that genes could also be composed of ribonucleic acid (RNA).[10,11]

It is with this background that investigators working on scrapie began to unravel the curious and often puzzling properties of this infectious pathogen. The resistance of the scrapie agent to inactivation by formalin and heat treatments,[12] which were commonly used to produce vaccines against viral illnesses, was an important clue that the scrapie agent might be different from viruses, but it came before the structure of viruses was understood. Later, this resistance was dismissed as an interesting observation but of little importance, since some

viruses could be shown to survive such treatments; indeed, this was not an unreasonable viewpoint. Two decades were to pass before reports of the extreme radioresistance of the scrapie agent to inactivation again trumpeted the puzzling nature of this infectious pathogen.[13,14]

What Might Have Been: An Alternative Path of Discovery

By 1930, the high incidence of familial (f) Creutzfeldt-Jakob disease (CJD) in some families began to be recorded,[15,16] but almost 60 years passed before the significance of this finding could be appreciated.[17-20] CJD remained a curious, rare neurodegenerative disease of unknown etiology throughout this period.[21] Only with transmission of disease to apes by the inoculation of brain extracts prepared from patients who died of CJD did the story begin to unravel.[22]

Once CJD was shown to be a transmissible disease, relatively little attention was paid to the familial form of the disease because most cases were not found in families.[17] It is interesting to speculate how the course of scientific investigation might have proceeded if transmission studies had not been performed until after the molecular genetic lesion was identified. If the prion protein (PrP) gene had been identified in families with prion disease by positional cloning or through the purification and sequencing of PrP in amyloid plaques before brain extracts were shown to be transmissible, the prion concept, which readily explains how a single disease can have a genetic or infectious etiology, might have been greeted with much less skepticism.[23]

Within the scenario of finding mutations in the PrP gene before learning that prion diseases are transmissible, it seems likely that investigators would have focused their efforts on explaining how a mutant gene product might stimulate modification of the wild-type (wt) protein after inoculation into a susceptible host.[24] The modified wt protein would in turn stimulate production of more of its modified self. Less likely would have been the postulate that a mutant protein unrelated to immune defenses would render the host more susceptible to an infectious pathogen with a foreign genome, such as a virus, bacterium, or fungus.

Prions

Prions are infectious proteins. In mammals, prions reproduce by recruiting the normal, cellular isoform of the prion protein (PrP^C) and stimulating its conversion into the disease-causing isoform (PrP^{Sc}).

A major feature that distinguishes prions from viruses is the finding that both PrP isoforms are encoded by a chromosomal gene.[25] In humans, the PrP gene is designated *PRNP* and is located on the short arm of chromosome 20. Limited proteolysis of PrP^{Sc} produces a smaller, protease-resistant molecule of approximately 142 amino acids, designated PrP 27–30; under the same conditions, PrP^C is completely hydrolyzed (Fig. 2–1). In the presence of detergent, PrP 27–30 polymerizes into amyloid.[26] PrP amyloid formed by limited proteolysis and detergent extraction (Fig. 2–2) is indistinguishable from the filaments that aggregate to form PrP amyloid plaques in the central nervous system (CNS). Both the rods and the PrP amyloid filaments found in brain tissue exhibit similar ultrastructural morphology and green-gold birefringence after staining with Congo red dye.

PrP^C is rich in α-helix and has little β-sheet content whereas PrP^{Sc} is less rich in α-helix and has high β-sheet content. Comparisons of the secondary structures of PrP^C and PrP^{Sc} were performed on the proteins purified from Syrian hamster (SHa) brains.[27] Based on these data, structural models for PrP^C and PrP^{Sc} were proposed.[28] Subsequently, nuclear magnetic resonance (NMR) solution structures of recombinant SHa and mouse PrPs produced in bacteria showed that it is likely that PrP^C has three α-helices and not four as predicted by molecular modeling.[29,30] The computational model of PrP^{Sc} is supported by studies with recombinant antibody fragments (recFabs), which have been used to map the surfaces of PrP^C and PrP^{Sc}.[31] This α-to-β transition in PrP structure is the fundamental event underlying prion diseases, which are disorders of protein conformation. Much has been learned about the basic biology of prions using yeast, in which two different proteins unrelated to PrP form prions.[32,33]

Transmission of Scrapie to Mice

The transmission of the scrapie agent to mice[34] made a series of radiobiological studies possible.[13,14] With reports of the extreme resistance of the scrapie agent to inactivation by ultraviolet (UV) and ionizing radiation came a flurry of hypotheses to explain these curious observations. In some cases, these postulates ignored the lessons learned from the studies of DNA while others tried to accommodate them in rather obtuse but sometimes clever ways.

As the number of hypotheses about the molecular nature of the scrapie agent began to exceed the number of laboratories working on the problem (Table 2–1), the need for new experimental approaches became evident.

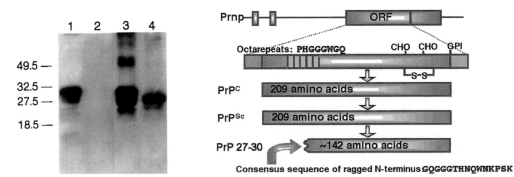

FIGURE 2–1. Prion protein isoforms. *A,* Western immunoblot of brain homogenates from uninfected (lanes 1 and 2) and prion-infected (lanes 3 and 4) Syrian hamsters (SHa). Samples in lanes 2 and 4 were digested with 50 µg/ml of proteinase K for 30 min at 37°C. PrP^C in lanes 2 and 4 was completely hydrolyzed under these conditions whereas approximately 67 amino acids were digested from the N-terminus of PrP^{Sc} to generate PrP 27–30. After polyacrylamide gel electrophoresis (PAGE) and electrotransfer, the blot was developed with anti-SHaPrP RO73 polyclonal rabbit antiserum.[158] Molecular-size markers are in kilodaltons (kDa). *B,* Bar diagram of SHaPrP gene, which encodes a protein of 254 amino acids. After processing of the N- and C-termini, both PrP^C and PrP^{Sc} consist of 209 residues. After limited proteolysis, the N-terminus of PrP^{Sc} is truncated to form PrP 27–30 (composed of approximately 142 amino acids), the N-terminal sequence of which was determined by Edman degradation.

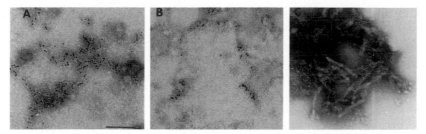

FIGURE 2–2. Electron micrographs of negatively stained and immunogold-labeled PrP^C (*A*) and PrP^{Sc} (*B*). Neither PrP^C nor PrP^{Sc} forms are recognizable, ordered polymers. *C*, Prion rods composed of PrP 27–30 were negatively stained. The prion rods are indistinguishable from many purified amyloids. Bar = 100 nm. (Copyright 1993 National Academy of Sciences, USA.)

Much of the available data on the properties of the scrapie agent had been gathered using brain homogenates prepared from mice with clinical signs of scrapie. These mice had been inoculated 4 to 5 months earlier with the scrapie agent, which had originated in sheep but had been passaged multiple times in mice.[35,36] Once an experiment was completed on these homogenates, an additional 12 months was required using end-point titration in mice. Typically, 60 mice were required to determine the titer of a single sample. These slow, tedious, and expensive experiments discouraged systematic investigation.

Sedimentation Studies

Although many studies had been performed on the physicochemical nature of the scrapie agent using the mouse end-point titration system,[37] few systematic investigations had been performed on the fundamental characteristics of the infectious scrapie particle. In fact, 12 years after the introduction of the mouse bioassay, there were no extensive data on the sedimentation behavior of the scrapie particle. Because differential centrifugation is frequently a very useful initial step in the purification of many macromolecules, some knowledge of the sedimentation properties of the scrapie agent under defined conditions seemed mandatory.[38] To perform such studies, Swiss mice were inoculated intracerebrally with the Chandler isolate of scrapie prions and the mice sacrificed approximately 30 and 150 days later when the titers in their spleens and brains, respectively, were at maximum levels.[39,40] The two tissues were homogenized, extracted with detergent, and centrifuged for increasing durations and at increasing speeds. The disappearance of scrapie infectivity was measured in supernatant fractions by end-point titration, which required 1 year to score as described earlier. Thus, a single set of experiments required 18 months from the beginning to obtaining results. This long time frame severely retarded progress.

Probing the Molecular Structure of Prions

The incubation time assay transformed investigations on the development of effective purification schemes for enriching fractions for scrapie infectivity.[41,42] It provided a quantitative means to assess those fractions that were enriched for infectivity and those that were not. Such studies rather rapidly led to the development of a protocol for separating scrapie infectivity from most proteins and nucleic acids. With an approximately

TABLE 2–1. Hypothetical Structures Proposed for the Scrapie Agent

1. Sarcosporidia-like parasite
2. "Filterable" virus
3. Small DNA virus
4. Replicating protein
5. Replicating abnormal polysaccharide with membrane
6. DNA subvirus controlled by a transmissible linkage substance
7. Provirus consisting of recessive genes generating RNA particles
8. Naked nucleic acid similar to plant viroids
9. Unconventional virus
10. Aggregated conventional virus with unusual properties
11. Replicating polysaccharide
12. Nucleoprotein complex
13. Nucleic acid surrounded by a polysaccharide coat
14. Spiroplasma-like organism
15. Multicomponent system with one component quite small
16. Membrane-bound DNA
17. Virino (viroid-like DNA complexed with host proteins)
18. Filamentous animal virus (SAF)
19. Aluminum-silicate amyloid complex
20. Computer virus
21. Amyloid-inducing virus
22. Complex of apo- and co-prions (unified theory)
23. Nemavirus (SAF surrounded by DNA)
24. Retrovirus

100-fold purification of infectivity relative to protein, greater than 98% of the proteins and polynucleotides were eliminated, which permitted more reliable probing of the constituents of these enriched fractions than was previously possible using crude preparations. As reproducible data began to accumulate, indicating that scrapie infectivity could be reduced by procedures that hydrolyze or modify proteins but was resistant to procedures that alter nucleic acids, a family of hypotheses about the molecular architecture of the scrapie agent began to emerge.[43] These data established for the first time that a particular macromolecule was required for infectivity and that this macromolecule was a protein. These experimental findings also extended the earlier observations on the resistance of scrapie infectivity to UV irradiation at 250 nm in two respects: (1) four procedures were used to probe for a nucleic acid based on physical principles that were independent of UV radiation damage, and (2) demonstration of a protein requirement provided a reference macromolecule. No longer could the scrapie agent be considered phlogiston or linoleum!

Once the requirement for a protein was established, it was possible to revisit the long list of hypothetical structures that had been proposed for the scrapie agent (see Table 2–1) and to eliminate carbohydrates, lipids, and nucleic acids as the infective elements within a scrapie agent devoid of protein.[43] No longer could structures such as a viroid-like nucleic acid, a replicating polysaccharide, or a small polynucleotide surrounded by a carbohydrate be entertained as reasonable candidates to explain the seemingly enigmatic properties of the scrapie agent.[43] But the family of hypotheses that remained was still large and required continued consideration of all possibilities in which a protein was a critical element. Thus, the prion concept evolved from a family of hypotheses in which an infectious protein was only one of several possibilities. With the accumulation of experimental data on the molecular properties of the prion, it became possible to discard an increasing number of hypothetical structures. In prion research as well as many other areas of scientific investigation, a single hypothesis is too often championed at the expense of a reasoned approach that involves continuing to entertain a series of complex arguments until one or more can be discarded on the basis of experimental data.[44]

Radiobiology of Scrapie

The experimental transmission of scrapie from sheep to mice[34] gave investigators a more convenient laboratory model, which yielded considerable information on the nature of the unusual infectious pathogen that causes scrapie.[13,14,45–48] Yet progress was slow because quantification of infectivity in a single sample required holding 60 mice for 1 year before accurate scoring could be accomplished, as noted earlier.[34]

Resistance to UV Radiation

The extreme resistance of the scrapie agent to both ionizing and UV irradiation suggested this infectious pathogen was quite different from all known viruses. The D_{37} value for irradiation at 254 nm was 42,000 J/m^2, which argued that the target was unlikely to be a nucleic acid. Irradiation at different wavelengths of UV light showed that scrapie infectivity was equally resistant at 250 and 280 nm.[14] Because proteins in general and aldolase in particular[49] are more sensitive to UV irradiation at 280 nm than at 250 nm, Alper and her colleagues concluded that the scrapie agent was unlikely to contain protein.[14] The sensitivity of proteins to inactivation at 280 nm is usually attributed to the destruction of amino acids with aromatic side chains. Later, the scrapie agent was found to be 6 times more sensitive to inactivation at 237 nm than at either 250 nm or 280 nm.[50] This finding reinforced the arguments that the scrapie agent contains neither a protein nor a nucleic acid. While the data were not sufficiently precise to eliminate protein as a candidate, a polysaccharide or polynucleotide composed of numerous modified nucleosides seemed more likely. Ironically, the inactivation spectrum of trypsin, which was published in the same paper with the data on aldolase,[49] was not recognized to be similar to that of the scrapie agent. The increased sensitivity of trypsin to inactivation by UV irradiation at 237 nm relative to 250 nm and 280 nm is due to the modification of cysteine (Cys) residues.[49]

Target Size

Inactivation by ionizing radiation gave a target size of approximately 150,000 Da,[13] which was later revised to 55,000 Da.[51] These data argued that the scrapie agent was as small as the viroids and prompted speculation that a viroid might be the cause of scrapie.[52] Later, when purified preparations of prions became available, their properties were compared with those of viroids. The properties of prions and viroids were found to be antithetical—consistent with the notion that viroids are composed of polynucleotides and prions are proteins (Table 2–2).[53] Because inactivation by ionizing radiation of viruses had given spurious results due to repair of double-stranded genomes, the size of the putative scrapie virus was thought to be substantially larger than 150,000 Da.[54,55] Once a protein was thought to be the most likely target of ionizing radiation, such arguments faded.[51]

Hypotheses about the Nature of the Scrapie Agent

As noted earlier, a fascinating array of structural hypotheses (see Table 2–1) was offered to explain the unusual features, first of the disease and later of the infectious agent; speculation was enhanced by the extreme resistance of the scrapie agent to both ionizing and UV

Table 2–2. Stabilities of Prions and Viroids after Chemical and Enzymatic Treatment

Chemical treatment	Concentration	PSTV*	Scrapie agent
Et$_2$PC	10–20 mM	(−)	+
NH$_4$OH	0.1–0.5 M	+	−
Psoralen (AMT)	10–500 mg/ml	+	−
Phenol	Saturated	−	+
SDS	1–10%	−	+
Zn^{2+}	2 mM	+	−
Urea	3–8 mM	−	+
Alkali	pH 10	(−)	+
KSCN	1 M	−	+
RNase A	0.1–100 mg/ml	+	−
DNase	100 mg/ml	−	−
Proteinase K	100 mg/ml	−	+
Trypsin	100 mg/ml	−	+

*Potato spindle tuber viroid.
"+" indicates sensitivity.

irradiation. Among the earliest hypotheses was the notion that scrapie was a disease of muscle caused by the parasite *Sarcosporidia*.[56,57] With the successful transmission of scrapie to animals, the hypothesis that scrapie is caused by a "filterable" virus became popular.[58,59] With the radiobiological findings of Alper and her colleagues described earlier, a myriad of hypotheses on the chemical nature of the scrapie agent emerged. Among the hypothetical structures proposed were a small DNA virus,[60] a replicating protein,[48,61–63] a replicating abnormal polysaccharide with membranes,[46,64] a DNA subvirus controlled by a transmissible linkage substance,[65,66] a provirus consisting of recessive genes generating RNA particles,[67,68] and a naked nucleic acid similar to plant viroids.[52] As already noted, subsequent investigations showed the viroid suggestion to be incorrect[53] whereas many other studies argued that the scrapie agent is composed only of a protein that adopts an abnormal conformation[27,69,70] as previously proposed.[61]

Unconventional Viruses and More

The term *unconventional virus* was proposed, but no structural details were ever given with respect to how these unconventional virions differ from the conventional viral particles.[71] Some investigators suggested that the term obscured the ignorance that continued to shroud the molecular nature of infectious pathogens causing scrapie and CJD.[72] Other suggestions included an aggregated conventional virus with unusual properties,[73] a replicating polysaccharide,[74] a nucleoprotein complex,[50] a nucleic acid surrounded by a polysaccharide coat,[75–77] a spiroplasma-like organism,[78,79] a multicomponent system with one quite small component,[80,81] membrane-bound DNA,[82]

and a virino (viroid-like DNA complexed with host proteins).[83] Small spherical particles approximately 10 nm in diameter were found in fractions said to be enriched for infectivity; these particles were thought to represent the smallest possible virus but were later shown to be ferritin.

PRION PROTEIN STRUCTURE

Once complementary DNA (cDNA) probes for PrP became available, the PrP gene was found to be constitutively expressed in adult, uninfected brain.[84,85] This finding eliminated the possibility that PrP^{Sc} stimulated production of more of itself by initiating transcription of the PrP gene as proposed nearly two decades earlier.[61] Determination of the structure of the PrP gene eliminated a second possible mechanism that might explain the appearance of PrP^{Sc} in brains already synthesizing PrP^C. Since the entire protein-coding region was contained within a single exon, there was no possibility that the two PrP isoforms were the products of alternatively spliced messenger RNAs (mRNAs).[86] Next, a posttranslational chemical modification that distinguishes PrP^{Sc} from PrP^C was considered but was not found in an exhaustive study,[69] and I considered it likely that PrP^C and PrP^{Sc} differed only in their conformations, a hypothesis also proposed earlier.[61]

When the secondary structures of the PrP isoforms were compared by optical spectroscopy, they were found to be markedly different.[27] Fourier transform infrared (FTIR) and circular dichroism (CD) spectroscopy studies showed that PrP^C contains approximately 40% α-helix and little β-sheet while PrP^{Sc} is composed of approximately 30% α-helix and 45% β-sheet.[27] That the two PrP isoforms have the same amino acid sequence runs counter to the widely accepted view that the amino acid sequence specifies only one biologically active conformation of a protein.[87]

Before comparative studies on the structures of PrP[C] and PrP[Sc], metabolic labeling studies showed that the acquisition of protease resistance by PrP[Sc] is a post-translational process.[88] In a search for chemical differences that would distinguish PrP[Sc] from PrP[C], we identified ethanolamine in hydrolysates of PrP 27–30, which signaled the possibility that PrP might contain a glycosylphosphatidyl inositol (GPI) anchor.[89] Both PrP isoforms were found to carry GPI anchors, and PrP[C] was found on the surface of cells where it could be released by cleavage of the anchor. Subsequent studies showed that PrP[Sc] formation occurs after PrP[C] reaches the cell surface[90] and is localized to caveolae-like domains.[91,92]

Nuclear Magnetic Resonance Structures of Recombinant PrPs

Modeling studies and subsequent NMR investigations of a synthetic PrP peptide containing residues 90 to 145 suggested that PrP[C] might contain an α-helix within this region.[93] This peptide contains residues 113 to 128, which are most highly conserved among all species studied and correspond to a transmembrane region of PrP that was delineated in cell-free translation studies. A transmembrane form of PrP was found in the brains of patients with Gerstmann-Sträussler-Scheinker syndrome (GSS) caused by the A117V mutation and in transgenic (Tg) mice overexpressing either mutant or wt PrP.[94] That no evidence for an α-helix in this region has been found in NMR studies of recombinant PrP in an aqueous environment[29,95,96] suggests that these recombinant PrPs correspond to the secreted form of PrP that was also identified in the cell-free translation studies. This contention is supported by studies with recFabs showing that GPI-anchored PrP[C] on the surface of cells exhibits an immunoreactivity profile similar to that of recombinant PrP prepared with an α-helical conformation.[31,97]

The NMR structure of recombinant SHaPrP (90–231) was determined after the protein was purified and refolded (Fig. 2–3A). Residues 90 to 112 are not shown because marked conformational heterogeneity was found in this region whereas residues 113 to 126 constitute the conserved hydrophobic region that also displays some structural plasticity.[95] Although some features of the structure of SHaPrP(90–231) are similar to those reported earlier for the smaller recombinant mouse (Mo) PrP(121–231) fragment,[29] substantial differences were found. For example, the loop at the N-terminus of helix B is defined in SHaPrP(90–231) but is disordered in MoPrP(121–231); in addition, helix C is composed of residues 200 to 227 in SHaPrP(90–231) but extends only from 200 to 217 in MoPrP(121–231). The loop and the C-terminal portion of helix C are particularly important, as described later. Whether the differences between the two recombinant PrP fragments are due to (1) their dif-

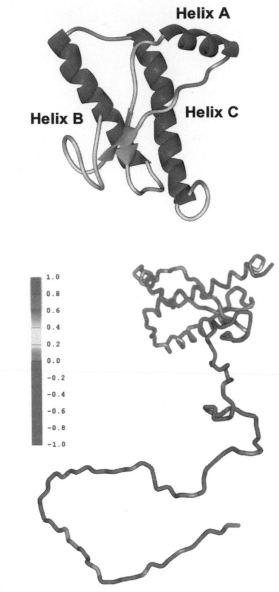

FIGURE 2–3. (See Color Plate I) Structures of the cellular isoform of the prion protein. A, NMR structure of recombinant Syrian hamster (SHa) PrP(90–231). Presumably, the structure of the α-helical form of SHaPrP(90–231) resembles that of PrP[C]. SHaPrP (90–231) is viewed from the interface where PrP[Sc] is thought to bind to PrP[C]. α-Helices A (residues 144 to 157), B (172 to 193), and C (200 to 227), strand S1 (residues 129 to 134), and strand S2 (residues 159 to 165) are shown. The arrows span residues 129 to 131 and 161 to 163, as these show a closer resemblance to β-sheet.[95] B, Schematic diagram showing the flexibility of the polypeptide chain for PrP(29–231).[96] The structure of the portion of the protein representing residues 90 to 231 was taken from the coordinates of PrP(90–231).[95] The remainder of the sequence was hand-built for illustration purposes only. The color scale corresponds to the heteronuclear {[1]H}-^{15}N NOE data: from red for the lowest (most negative) values, where the polypeptide is most flexible, to blue for the highest (most positive) values in the most structured and rigid regions of the protein. (Reprinted with permission from Proc Natl Acad Sci U S A 1997;94:13452–13457. Copyright 1997 National Academy of Sciences.)

ferent lengths, (2) species-specific differences in sequences, or (3) the conditions used for solving the structures remains to be determined.

NMR studies of MoPrP(23–231) and SHaPrP (29–231) showed, like the shorter fragments described earlier, that full-length PrP is also a three-helix-bundle protein with two short anti-parallel β-strands. The three helices form a globular C-terminal domain while the N-terminal domain is highly flexible and lacks identifiable secondary structure under the experimental conditions employed (Fig. 2–3*B*).[96] Studies of SHaPrP (29–231) indicate transient interactions between the C-terminal end of helix B and the highly flexible, N-terminal random-coil containing the octarepeats (residues 29–125).[96]

The NMR structures of more than 10 PrPs from different species have been determined (Table 2–3). The structures of all these PrP molecules are quite similar. Even the structure of mouse doppel (Dpl) is similar to that of mouse PrP even though the two proteins are only 25% homologous (Fig. 2–4).

Electron Crystallography of PrP^Sc

Because the insolubility of the PrP^Sc has frustrated structural studies by x-ray crystallography and NMR spectroscopy, we used electron crystallography to characterize the structure of two infectious variants of PrP. Isomorphous, two-dimensional (2D) crystals of the N-terminally truncated PrP^Sc (PrP 27–30) and a miniprion (PrP^Sc106) were identified by negative-stain electron microscopy. Image processing allowed the extraction of limited structural information to 7 Å resolution. By comparing projection maps of PrP 27–30 and PrP^Sc106, we visualized the 36-residue internal deletion of the miniprion and localized the N-linked sugars (Fig. 2–5). The dimensions of the monomer and the locations of the deleted segment and sugars were used as constraints in the construction of models for PrP^Sc. Only models featuring parallel β-helices as the key element could satisfy the constraints.

Previous endeavors to model the structure of PrP^Sc attempted to fit sequence-specific conformational preferences with spectroscopic, antibody-binding, and other biological data. Originally, we postulated an anti-parallel β-sheet formed from residues 90 to 170 packed against the two C-terminal α-helices.[28] The results obtained from the 2D crystals, the existence of PrP^Sc106 (implying the spatial colocalization of residues 140 and 177), and increasing data pointing to parallel β-sheet structure in amyloid-forming proteins[98,99] caused us to revisit this model.[28]

A single anti-parallel β-sheet was not consistent with the observed densities in the projection maps obtained from the 2D crystals. Specifically, the sheets were far too wide to fit into the observed hexameric arrangement. Efforts to adjust the sheet morphology to fit the density required the use of shorter strands. The amount of β-structure in these altered β-sheets was no longer compatible with the amounts of β-sheet observed by FTIR spectroscopy.[100,101] Furthermore, anti-parallel β-sheets typically have a twist of approximately 20

TABLE 2–3. Structures for PrP and Dpl

Species	Protein	How	PDB accession codes	Publication
Mouse	recPrP(121–231)	NMR	1AG2	29
Mouse	recPrP(23–231)	NMR	data not released	160
Syrian hamster	recPrP(90–231)	NMR	1B10, updated 1999	95
Syrian hamster	recPrP(29–231)	NMR	data not released	96
Syrian hamster	synthetic PrP(104–113) in complex with 3F4	NMR	1CU4 in complex with 3F4	161
Syrian hamster	recPrP(90–231)	NMR	used to update 1B10	30
Human	recPrP(23–230)	NMR	1QLX and 1QLZ	162
Human	recPrP(90–230)	NMR	1QM0 and 1QM1	162
Human	recPrP(121–230)	NMR	1QM2 and 1QM3	162
Cattle	recPrP(121–230)	NMR	1DWY and 1DWZ	163
Cattle	recPrP(23–230)	NMR	1DX0 and 1DX1	163
Human	recPrP(121–230,M166V)	NMR	1E1G and 1E1J	163
Human	recPrP(121–230,S170N)	NMR	1E1P and 1E1S	163
Human	recPrP(121–230,R220K)	NMR	1E1U and 1E1W	163
Human	recPrP(90–231,E200K)	NMR	1QM0, 1FKC, and 1FO7	164
Human	recPrP(90–231)	X-ray	1I4M	165
Mouse	recDpl(26–157)	NMR	1I17	166

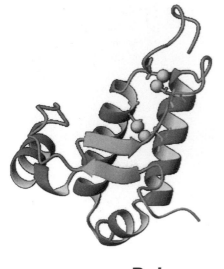

**mouse Dpl
(Mo et al., 2001)**

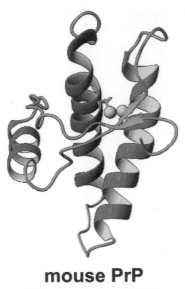

**mouse PrP
(Riek et al., 1996)**

FIGURE 2–4. (See Color Plate I) NMR structures of Dpl and PrP from mice. (Figure prepared by Jane Dyson and Peter Wright.)

degrees per strand. A six- to eight-stranded β-sheet would be difficult to accommodate in the electron density. Parallel β-sheets are commonly observed in protein structures as part of planar α/β folds, α/β barrels, and parallel β-helices. Planar α/β folds encounter the same problems as twisted anti-parallel β-sheets. α/β Barrels have alternating α-helices and β-strands with the fraction of α-helical residues exceeding that of the β-stranded residues. This would be in conflict with the FTIR results for both PrP 27–30 and PrP^{Sc}106. While we cannot exclude a novel protein fold for the structure of PrP^{Sc}, the parallel β-helix is the only known fold that provides the necessary β-sheet content, parallel β-architecture, and room to accommodate the α-helices that are expected at the C-terminus of the molecule.

PrP^{Sc} was modeled as a parallel β-helical fold (Fig. 2–6), placing the structurally conserved C-terminal α-helices and the glycosylation sites (N181 and N197) on the periphery of the oligomer and with the highly flexible N-linked sugars pointing above and below the plane of the oligomer (see Fig. 2–6). In this conformation, PrP^{Sc} is compact and fits readily into the density observed by electron microscopy (see Fig. 2–5). Because there is very little twist or bend to parallel β-helices, the modeled oligomers have relatively planar faces that permit stacking along the fibril axis. The β-helices also provide flat sheets for lateral assembly into disc-like oligomers and filamentous assemblies.[102,103] The deletion of 36 residues in PrP106 correlates favorably with exactly two turns of an average left-handed β-helix. Therefore, the orientation of the α- and β-helices, the sugars, as well as the fold of the oligomeric face, could be retained in this deletion mutant. This would allow full-length PrP^{Sc} as well as PrP^{Sc}106 to template the replication of PrP^{Sc}106. Furthermore, the shape and location of the β-helical deletions in our mod-

els are consistent with the different densities observed between the 2D crystals of PrP 27–30 and PrP^{Sc}106. Finally, the PrP sequence can be threaded onto the β-helical folds in a register that is consistent with secondary structure predictions, mutational information, and the negative electrostatic potential at the center of the oligomers.

PRION REPLICATION

In an uninfected cell, PrP^{C} with the wt sequence exists in equilibrium in its monomeric α-helical, protease-sensitive state or is bound to an auxiliary factor, provisionally designated protein X (Fig. 2–7). We denote the conformation of PrP^{C} that is bound to protein X as PrP*[104]; this conformation is likely to be different from that determined under aqueous conditions for monomeric recombinant PrP. The PrP*/protein X complex will bind PrP^{Sc}, thereby creating a replication-competent assembly. Order-of-addition experiments demonstrate that for PrP^{C}, protein X binding precedes productive PrP^{Sc} interactions.[105] A conformational change takes place wherein PrP*, in a shape competent for binding to protein X and PrP^{Sc}, represents the initial phase in the formation of infectious PrP^{Sc}.

Several lines of evidence argue that the smallest infectious prion particle is an oligomer of PrP^{Sc}, perhaps as small as a dimer.[51] On purification, PrP^{Sc} tends to aggregate into insoluble multimers that can be dispersed into liposomes.[106] Insolubility does not seem to be a prerequisite for PrP^{Sc} formation or prion infectivity, as suggested by some investigators[107,108]; a protease-resistant PrP^{Sc} that is soluble in 1% Sarkosyl was generated in scrapie-infected neuroblastoma (ScN2a) cells by expression of a PrP deletion mutant consisting of 106 residues.[109]

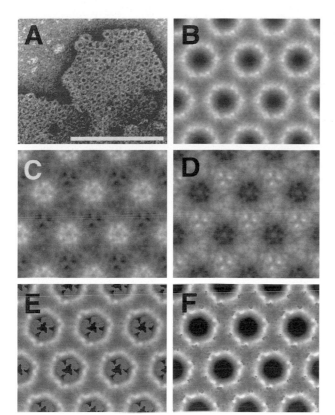

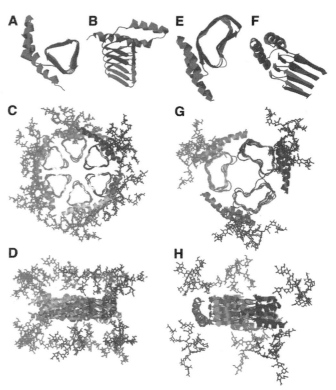

FIGURE 2–5. (See Color Plate II) Two-dimensional crystals of PrP^Sc. *A,* A 2D crystal of PrP^Sc106 stained with uranyl acetate. Bar = 100 nm. *B,* Image processing result after correlation-mapping and averaging followed by crystallographic averaging. *C and D,* Subtraction maps between the averages of PrP 27–30 and PrP^Sc106 *(panel B)*. *C,* PrP^Sc106 minus PrP 27–30 and *D,* PrP 27–30 minus PrP^Sc106, showing major differences in lighter shades. *E and F,* The statistically significant differences between PrP 27–30 and PrP^Sc106 calculated from panels *C* and *D* in red and blue, respectively, and overlaid onto the crystallographic average of PrP 27–30. (Copyright 2002 National Academy of Sciences, USA.)

FIGURE 2–6. (See Color Plate II) β-helical models of PrP 27–30. *A and B,* Top and side views, respectively, of PrP 27–30 modeled with a left-handed β-helix. The β-helical portion of the model is based on the *Methanosarcina thermophila* γ-carbonic anhydrase structure. *C and D,* Top and side views, respectively, of the trimer-of-dimer model of PrP 27–30 with left-handed β-helices. *E and F,* Top and side views, respectively, of PrP 27–30 modeled with a right-handed β-helix. The β-helical portion of the model is based on the most regular helical turns of *Bordetella pertussis* P.69 pertactin. *G and H,* Top and side views, respectively, of the trimer model of PrP 27–30 with right-handed β-helices. The structure of the α-helices was derived from the solution structure of recombinant SHaPrP. In the single molecule images (*A, B, E,* and *F*), residues 141 to 176 that are deleted in PrP106 are colored blue. (Copyright 2002 National Academy of Sciences, USA.)

In attempts to form PrP^Sc *in vitro*, PrP^C exposed to 3 M GdnHCl and then diluted 10-fold binds to PrP^Sc.[110,111] Based on these results, we presume that exposure of PrP^C to GdnHCl converts it into a PrP*-like molecule. Whether this PrP*-like protein is converted into PrP^Sc is unclear. Although the PrP*-like protein bound to PrP^Sc is protease-resistant and insoluble, it has not been re-isolated in order to assess whether or not it was converted into PrP^Sc. It is noteworthy that recombinant PrP can be refolded into either α-helical or β-sheet forms but none has been found to possess prion infectivity as judged by bioassay.

Cell Biology of PrP^Sc Formation

In prion-infected cells, PrP^C molecules destined to become PrP^Sc exit to the cell surface before conversion into PrP^Sc.[88–90] Like other GPI-anchored proteins, PrP^C

appears to re-enter the cell through a subcellular compartment bounded by cholesterol-rich, detergent-insoluble membranes, which might be caveolae or early endosomes.[91,92,112–114] Within this cholesterol-rich, non-acidic compartment, GPI-anchored PrP^C can be either converted into PrP^Sc or partially degraded.[92] Subsequently, PrP^Sc is trimmed at the N-terminus in an acidic compartment in scrapie-infected cultured cells to form PrP 27–30.[115] In contrast, N-terminal trimming of PrP^Sc is minimal in the brain, where little PrP 27–30 is found.[26]

Mechanism of Prion Propagation

From the foregoing formalism, I consider the rate-limiting step in prion formation. First, the impact of the

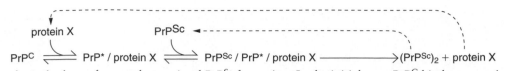

FIGURE 2–7. Hypothetical scheme for template-assisted PrP^{Sc} formation. In the initial step, PrP^{C} binds to protein X to form the PrP*/protein X complex. Next, PrP^{Sc} binds to PrP*, which has formed a complex with protein X. When PrP* is transformed into a nascent molecule of PrP^{Sc}, protein X is released and a dimer of PrP^{Sc} remains. The inactivation target size of an infectious prion suggests that it is composed of a dimer of PrP^{Sc}.[51] In the scheme depicted here, a fraction of infectious PrP^{Sc} dimers dissociates into uninfectious monomers as the replication cycle proceeds while most of the dimers accumulate in accordance with the increase in prion titer that occurs during the incubation period. Another fraction of PrP^{Sc} is cleared, presumably by cellular proteases. The precise stoichiometry of the replication process remains uncertain. (Copyright 1998 Cell Press.)

concentration of PrP^{Sc} in the inoculum, which is inversely proportional to the length of the incubation time, must be considered. Second, the sequence of PrP^{Sc} that forms an interface with PrP^{C} might play a role. When the sequences of the two isoforms are identical, the shortest incubation times are observed. Third, we must consider the strain-specific conformation of PrP^{Sc}. Some prion strains exhibit longer incubation times than others; the mechanism underlying this phenomenon is not understood. From these considerations, there exists a set of conditions under which initial PrP^{Sc} concentrations can be rate-limiting. These effects presumably relate to the stability of the PrP^{Sc}, its targeting to the correct cells and subcellular compartments, and its ability to be cleared. Once infection in a cell is initiated and endogenous PrP^{Sc} production is operative, then the following discussion of PrP^{Sc} formation seems most applicable. If the assembly of PrP^{Sc} into a specific dimeric or multimeric arrangement was difficult, then a nucleation-polymerization (NP) formalism would be relevant. In NP processes, nucleation is the rate-limiting step and elongation or polymerization is facile. These conditions are frequently observed in peptide models of aggregation phenomena[108]; however, studies with Tg mice expressing foreign PrP genes suggest that a different process is occurring.

Template-Assisted Prion Formation

From investigations with mice expressing both the SHaPrP transgene and the endogenous MoPrP gene, it is clear that PrP^{Sc} provides a template for directing prion replication, in which a template is defined as a catalyst that leaves its imprint on the product of the reaction.[116] Inoculation of these mice with SHaPrP^{Sc} leads to the production of nascent SHaPrP^{Sc} and not MoPrP^{Sc}. Conversely, inoculation of the Tg(SHaPrP) mice with MoPrP^{Sc} results in MoPrP^{Sc} formation and not SHaPrP^{Sc}. Even stronger evidence for templating has emerged from studies of prion strains passaged in Tg(MHu2M)$Prnp^{0/0}$ mice expressing a chimeric mouse-human PrP gene as described in more detail later.[117,118] Even though the conformational templates were initially generated with PrP^{Sc} molecules having different sequences in patients with inherited prion diseases, these templates are sufficient to

direct replication of distinct PrP^{Sc} molecules when the amino acid sequences of the substrate PrPs are identical. If the formation of this template were rate-limiting, then an NP model could apply. However, studies of PrP^{Sc} formation in ScN2a cells point to a distinct rate-limiting step.

Another line of evidence for template-assisted prion replication comes from studies of fatal insomnia (FI). In the inherited form of FI (FFI), the protease-resistant fragment of PrP^{Sc} after deglycosylation has an M_r of 19 kDa when measured by immunoblotting of brain extracts either from patients with FFI or from Tg(MHuM)$Prnp^{0/0}$ mice that were inoculated with FFI brain homogenate. In both humans and inoculated Tg(MHuM)$Prnp^{0/0}$ mice on both first and second passage, PrP^{Sc} is confined largely to the thalamus.[117] These findings argue that the conformation of PrP^{Sc} that yields a 19 kDa polypeptide after deglycosylation is propagated both in humans and in mice expressing an artificial chimeric transgene; in addition, the prion propagation process is confined to the thalamus. Additional evidence supporting these assertions comes from a patient who died after developing a clinical disease similar to FFI. Because both PrP alleles encoded wt human PrP sequence and a Met at position 129, we labeled this case sporadic fatal insomnia (sFI). At autopsy, the spongiform degeneration, reactive astrogliosis, and PrP^{Sc} deposition were confined to the thalamus.[119–122] These findings argue that the clinico-pathologic phenotype is determined by the conformation of PrP^{Sc} and not the amino acid sequence. Additionally, the FI strain of prions can be replicated with mutant human PrP(D178N), wt human PrP, or chimeric human-mouse PrP as the substrate. With all these different PrPs as substrates, the conformation of PrP^{Sc} must be faithfully copied. Template-assisted prion replication provides a mechanism for such a process.

Evidence for Protein X

Protein X was postulated to explain the results of the transmission of human prions to Tg mice (Table 2–4).[123,124] Mice expressing both Mo and HuPrP were resistant to human prions whereas those expressing only HuPrP were susceptible. These results argue that MoPrP^{C} inhibited transmission of human prions (i.e., the formation of nas-

TABLE 2–4. Evidence for Protein X from Transmission Studies of Human Prions[*]

Inoculum	Host	MoPrP gene	Incubation time [days ± SEM] (n/n_0)[†]
sCJD	Tg(HuPrP)	$Prnp^{+/+}$	721 (1/10)
sCJD	Tg(HuPrP)	$Prnp^{0/0}$	263 ± 2 (6/6)
sCJD	Tg(MHu2M)	$Prnp^{+/+}$	238 ± 3 (8/8)
sCJD	Tg(MHu2M)	$Prnp^{0/0}$	191 ± 3 (10/10)

[*]*Data with inoculum RG from reference 124.*
[†]*n, number of ill mice; n_0, number of inoculated mice.*

cent HuPrP^{Sc}). In contrast to the foregoing studies, mice expressing both MoPrP and chimeric MHu2MPrP were susceptible to human prions and mice expressing MHu2MPrP alone were only slightly more susceptible. These findings contend that MoPrP^C has only a minimal effect on the formation of chimeric MHu2MPrP^{Sc}.

When the data on human prion transmission to Tg mice were considered together, they suggested that MoPrP^C prevented the conversion of HuPrP^C into PrP^{Sc} by binding to another protein but had little effect on the conversion of MHu2M PrP into PrP^{Sc}. Based on these results, it was proposed that MoPrP^C binds to this protein with a higher affinity than does HuPrP^C. MoPrP^C was also postulated to have little effect on the formation of PrP^{Sc} from MHu2M (see Table 2–4) because MoPrP and MHu2M share the same amino acid sequence at the C-terminus. This also suggested that MoPrP^C only weakly inhibited transmission of SHa prions to Tg(SHaPrP) mice because SHaPrP is more closely related to MoPrP than is HuPrP.

To extend the foregoing findings in Tg mice, an expression vector with an insert encoding chimeric mouse-hamster PrP (MHM2) was transfected into ScN2a cells. MHM2 carries two SHa residues, which create an epitope recognized by the anti-SHaPrP 3F4 mAb that does not react with mouse PrP.[125] Substitution of a human residue at position 214 or 218 in MHM2 prevented formation of MHM2PrP^{Sc} in ScN2a cells.[105] The side chains of these residues protrude from the same surface of the C-terminal α-helix, forming a discontinuous epitope with residues 167 and 171 in an adjacent loop. Like MHM2(Q218K), substitution of a basic residue at position 167 or 171 prevented PrP^{Sc} formation. When MHM2PrP and MHM2PrP(Q218K) were co-expressed, the conversion of MHM2 PrP^C into PrP^{Sc} was inhibited, arguing that MHM2PrP(Q218K) is acting as a dominant negative. Similar results were obtained when studies were performed with MHM2PrP(Q167R).

Dominant-Negative Inhibition

One interpretation of dominant-negative inhibition of prion propagation is that mutant PrP^C binds more avidly

to another factor that participates in prion replication than does wt PrP. In this scenario, mutant PrP^C binds to protein X, which results in wt PrP^C being unable to bind. This explanation is also consistent with the protective effects of basic polymorphic residues in PrP of humans and sheep. The E219K substitution seems to render humans resistant to sCJD[126] and Q171R renders sheep resistant to scrapie.[127,128] The E219K and Q171K mutations correspond to Q218K and Q167R mutations, respectively, in MHM2.

To determine whether dominant-negative inhibition of prion formation occurs *in vivo*, Tg mice expressing PrP with either the Q167R or Q218K substitutions alone or in combination with wt PrP were produced.[129] Tg(MoPrP, Q167R)$Prnp^{0/0}$ mice expressing mutant PrP at levels equal to non-Tg FVB mice remained healthy for more than 550 days, indicating that inoculation with prions did not initiate a process sufficient to cause disease. Immunoblots of brain homogenates and histologic analysis did not reveal abnormalities. Tg(MoPrP, Q167R)$Prnp^{+/+}$ mice expressing both mutant and wt PrP did not exhibit neurologic dysfunction, but their brains revealed low levels of PrP^{Sc} and sections showed numerous vacuoles and severe astrocytic gliosis at 300 days after inoculation. Both Tg(MoPrP,Q218K)$Prnp^{0/0}$ and Tg(MoPrP,Q218K)$Prnp^{+/+}$ mice expressing high levels of the transgene product remained healthy for more than 300 days after inoculation. Neither PrP^{Sc} nor neuropathologic changes were found. These studies demonstrate that although dominant negative inhibition of wt PrP^{Sc} formation occurs, expression of the dominant-negative PrP at the same level as wt PrP does not completely prevent prion formation. However, expression of dominant-negative PrP alone had no deleterious effects on the mice and did not support prion propagation.

Is Protein X a Molecular Chaperone?

Cell biologic and transgenetic investigations argue for the existence of the chaperone-like molecule protein X that is required for PrP^{Sc} formation.[124] As described later, mutagenesis experiments have created dominant-negative forms of PrP^C that inhibit the formation of wt PrP^{Sc} by binding protein X.[105] This implies that the rate-limiting step in prion replication *in vivo* under conditions in which PrP^{Sc} is sufficient must be the conversion of PrP^C to PrP* because a dominant negative derived from a single point mutation could gate only a kinetically critical step in a cellular process. In the template-directed model, the conversion of PrP^C to PrP* is a first-order process. By contrast, NP processes follow higher-order kinetics ([monomer]^m in which m is the number of monomers in the nucleus). The experimental implications of these rate relationships are apparent in transgenetic studies; if first-order kinetics operate, halving the gene dose (hemizygotes) should double the incubation time while doubling the dose of a transgene array should halve the time to disease. This quantitative behavior has been observed in several studies in mice with altered levels of PrP expression.[116,130–132] The existence of prion strains that are conformational isoforms of PrP^{Sc} with distinct structures, incubation times, and neurohistopathology must also be considered in an analysis of the kinetics of PrP^{Sc} accumulation. Because the rate-limiting step in PrP^{Sc} formation cannot involve the unique template provided by a strain, differential rates of intercellular spread, cellular uptake, and clearance seem most likely to account for the variation in incubation times. This is consistent with the different patterns of protease sensitivity and glycosylation for distinct prion strains.[117,133–136]

However, I hasten to add that NP models can provide a useful description of other biologic phenomena. Under conditions in which the monomer is relatively rare and/or the conformational change is facile (e.g., short peptides), the NP model will dominate. However, when the monomer is sufficiently abundant or the conformational conversion is difficult to accomplish, the template assistance formalism provides a more likely description of the process.

STRAINS OF PRIONS

The existence of prion strains raised the question of how heritable biological information can be enciphered in any molecule other than nucleic acid.[137] Strains or varieties of prions were defined by incubation times and the distribution of neuronal vacuolation.[137,138] Subsequently, the patterns of PrP^{Sc} deposition were found to correlate with vacuolation profiles and these patterns were also used to characterize strains of prions.[135,139,140]

The typing of prion strains in C57Bl, VM, and F1 (C57Bl × VM) inbred mice began with isolates from sheep with scrapie. The prototypic strains called Me7 and 22A gave incubation times of approximately 150 days and approximately 400 days, respectively, in C57Bl mice.[137] The PrPs of C57Bl and I/Ln (and later VM) mice differ at two residues and control incubation times.[132,141]

For many years, support for the hypothesis that the tertiary structure of PrP^{Sc} enciphers strain-specific information[142] was minimal except for the DY strain isolated

from mink with transmissible encephalopathy.[133] PrP^{Sc} in DY prions showed diminished resistance to proteinase K (PK) digestion as well as an anomalous site of cleavage. The DY strain presented a puzzling anomaly since other prion strains exhibiting similar incubation times did not show this altered susceptibility to PK digestion of PrP^{Sc}.[143] Also notable was the generation of new strains during passage of prions through animals with different PrP genes.[143,144]

PrPSc Conformation Enciphers Variation in Prions

Persuasive evidence that strain-specific information is enciphered in the tertiary structure of PrP^{Sc} comes from transmission of two different inherited human prion diseases to mice expressing a chimeric MHu2MPrP transgene.[117] In FFI, the protease-resistant fragment of PrP^{Sc} after deglycosylation has an M_r of 19 kDa; in fCJD(E200K) and most sporadic prion diseases, this fragment is 21 kDa.[145] This difference in molecular size was shown to be due to different sites of proteolytic cleavage at the N-termini of the two human PrP^{Sc} molecules, reflecting different tertiary structures.[145] These distinct conformations were not unexpected since the amino acid sequences of the PrPs differ.

Extracts from the brains of FFI patients transmitted disease into mice expressing a chimeric MHu2MPrP gene about 200 days after inoculation and induced formation of the 19 kDa PrP^{Sc}, whereas fCJD(E200K) and sCJD produced the 21 kDa PrP^{Sc} in mice expressing the same transgene.[117] On second passage, Tg(MHu2M) mice inoculated with FFI prions showed an incubation time of ~130 days and a 19 kDa PrP^{Sc} while those inoculated with fCJD(E200K) prions exhibited an incubation time of ~170 days and a 21 kDa PrP^{Sc} (Table 2–5).[118] The experimental data demonstrate that MHu2MPrP^{Sc} can exist in two different conformations based on the sizes of the protease-resistant fragments, yet the amino acid sequence of MHu2MPrP^{Sc} is invariant.

Not only are patients with sFI instructive with respect to the mechanism of prion replication but they

TABLE 2–5. Distinct Prion Strains Generated in Humans with Inherited Prion Diseases and Transmitted to Transgenic Mice*

Inoculum	Host species	Host PrP genotype	Incubation time [days ± SEM] (n/n_0)†	PrP^{Sc} (kDa)
None	Human	FFI(D178N,M129)		19
FFI	Mouse	Tg(MHu2M)	206 ± 7 (7/7)	19
FFI (Tg(MHu2M))	Mouse	Tg(MHu2M)	136 ± 1 (6/6)	19
None	Human	fCJD(E200K)		21
fCJD	Mouse	Tg(MHu2M)	170 ± 2 (10/10)	21
fCJD(Tg(MHu2M))	Mouse	Tg(MHu2M)	167 ± 3 (15/15)	21

*Data from references 25, 117.

†n, number of ill mice; n0, number of inoculated mice.

also provide important information about prion strains. As described earlier, the brain extract of a patient who died of sFI contained a deglycosylated, protease-resistant PrP^{Sc} fragment of 19 kDa. Moreover, spongiform degeneration, reactive astrogliosis, and PrP^{Sc} deposition were confined to the thalamus; both PrP alleles encoded the wt sequence and Met at codon 129.[119–122] These findings provide yet another line of evidence arguing that the clinicopathologic phenotype is determined by the conformation of PrP^{Sc} and not by the amino acid sequence of PrP.

The results of these studies argue that PrP^{Sc} acts as a template for the conversion of PrP^C into nascent PrP^{Sc}. Imparting the size of the protease-resistant fragment of PrP^{Sc} through conformational templating provides a mechanism for both the generation and propagation of prion strains.

Interplay between the Species and Strains of Prions

Studies on the role of the primary and tertiary structures of PrP in the transmission of disease have given new insights into the pathogenesis of prion diseases. The amino acid sequence of PrP encodes the species of the prion (Table 2–6),[124,146] and the prion derives its PrP^{Sc} sequence from the last mammal in which it was passaged.[143] Whereas the primary structure of PrP is likely to be the most important or even sole determinant of the tertiary structure of PrP^C, existing PrP^{Sc} seems to function as a template in determining the tertiary structure of nascent PrP^{Sc} molecules as they are formed from PrP^C.[104,142] In turn, prion diversity appears to be enciphered in the conformation of PrP^{Sc} and prion strains may represent different conformers of PrP^{Sc}.[117,133,143]

Evidence for Different Conformations of PrPSc in Eight Prion Strains

Using a highly sensitive conformation-dependent immunoassay for the measurement of PrP^{Sc} in tissue homogenates, eight different prion strains passaged in Syrian hamsters were examined.[147] Brains from Syrian hamsters were collected when the animals displayed signs of neurologic dysfunction; the incubation times for the prion strains varied from 70 to 320 days. Most of the PrP

in the brains of Syrian hamsters with signs of neurologic disease was PrP^{Sc}, as defined by the β-sheet conformation. The level of PrP^{Sc} in the brains of these clinically ill animals exceeded that of PrP^C by 3- to 10-fold (Fig. 2–8A). The highest levels of PrP^{Sc} were found in the brains of Syrian hamsters infected with the Me7-H strain; in contrast, the lowest levels were found in the brains of Syrian hamsters inoculated with the SHa(Me7) strain (see Fig. 2–8A). Interestingly, the Me7-H and SHa(Me7) strains, which were both derived from Me7 passaged in mice,[143,144] possessed similar denatured/native PrP ratios, but they accumulated PrP^{Sc} to quite different levels (see Fig. 2–8). The highest denatured/native PrP ratio of all tested strains was from SHa(RML).

The apparent independence of the ratio of denatured/native PrP from the concentration of PrP^{Sc} became apparent after plotting both parameters in a single graph (see Fig. 2–8B). Each strain occupied a unique position, indicating differences in the conformations of accumulated PrP^{Sc}. Because the PrP^C concentration in each strain was less than or equal to 5 μg/ml and the PrP ratio for PrP^C was less than or equal to 1.8, the expected impact of the presence of PrP^C on the final PrP ratio was less than or equal to 15%.

Because only the most tightly folded conformers of PrP^{Sc} are likely to be protease-resistant, brain homogenates were digested with PK before measuring the ratio of denatured/native PrP (Fig. 2–8C). As shown, the positions of many strains changed when the protease-sensitive conformers of PrP^{Sc} were enzymatically hydrolyzed (see Fig. 2–8C). Most notable was the DY strain, which was readily detectable before limited proteolysis by immunoassay (see Fig. 2–8B) but became almost undetectable after digestion (see Fig. 2–8C), in accordance with earlier Western blot studies.[133,148] Equally important, strains such as Sc237 and HY were marginally separated before PK digestion (see Fig. 2–8B) but became quite distinct afterward (see Fig. 2–8C). These findings argue that Sc237 and HY are distinct strains even though they exhibit similar incubation times of ~70 d when passaged in Syrian hamsters.[143] It is noteworthy that limited proteolysis of PrP^{Sc} from Sc237- and HY-infected brains produced PrP 27–30 proteins that were indistinguishable by migration in sodium dodecyl sulfate polyacrylamide gel electrophoresis (SDS-PAGE).[143]

TABLE 2–6. Influence of Prion Species and Strain on Transmission from Syrian Hamsters to Hamsters and Mice*

Inoculum	Recipient	Sc237 prions Incubation time [days ± SEM] (n/n$_0$)†	139H prions
SHa→SHa	SHa	77 ± 1 (48/48)	167 ± 1 (94/94)
SHa→SHa	Non-Tg mice	>700 (0/9)	499 ± 15 (11/11)
SHa→SHa	Tg(SHaPrP)81 mice	75 ± 2 (22/22)	110 ± 2 (19/19)

*The species of prion is encoded by the primary structure of PrP^{Sc} and the strain of prion is enciphered by the tertiary structure of PrP^{Sc}. We recognize that the primary structure as well as the post-translational chemical modifications determine the tertiary structure of PrP^C, but we argue that the conformation of PrP^C is modified by PrP^{Sc} as it is refolded into a nascent molecule of PrP^{Sc}.117
†n, number of ill animals; n$_0$, number of inoculated animals.

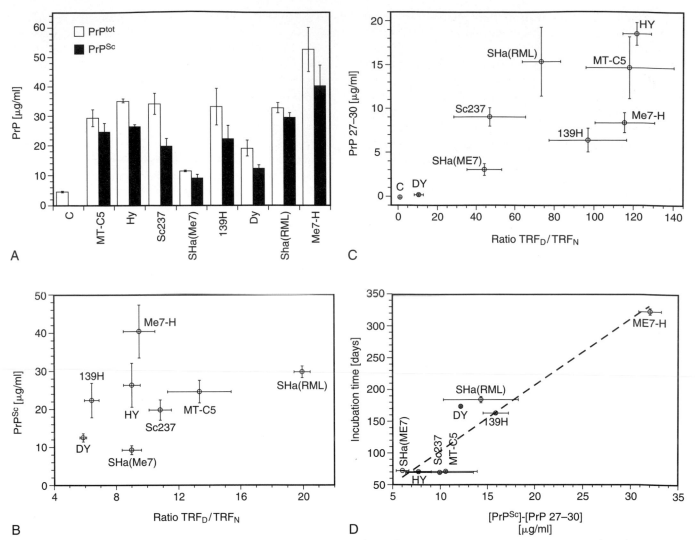

FIGURE 2–8. Eight prion strains distinguished by the conformation-dependent immunoassay. *A,* Concentration of total PrP and PrP^{Sc}. The columns and bars represent the average ± SEM obtained from three different brains of LVG/LAK Syrian hamsters infected with different prion strains and measured in three independent experiments. *B,* Ratio of antibody binding to denatured/native PrP and a function of concentration of PrP^{Sc} in the brains of Syrian hamsters infected with different prion strains. *C,* Brain homogenates of Syrian hamsters inoculated with different prion strains and uninoculated controls, denoted C, were digested with 50 µg/ml of proteinase K for 2 h at 37°C before detection by the conformation-dependent immunoassay. *D,* Incubation time plotted as a function of the concentration of the proteinase K-sensitive fraction of PrP^{Sc} ([PrP^{Sc}]–[PrP 27–30]). (Copyright 1998 Nature Publishing Group.)

When the incubation times of these eight strains were plotted as a function of either the concentration of PrP^{Sc} or PrP 27–30, no relationship could be discerned. Incubation times were also plotted as a function of the ratio of denatured/native PrP and, again, no correlation was found.

To assess the fraction of PrP^{Sc} that is sensitive to proteolysis during limited PK digestion, the protease-resistant PrP 27–30 fraction (see Fig. 2–8C) was subtracted from total PrP^{Sc} (see Fig. 2–8B) for each of the eight prion strains. It was asked whether the PK-sensitive fraction of PrP^{Sc} ([PrP^{Sc}] - [PrP 27–30]) might reflect those PrP^{Sc} molecules that are most readily cleared by cellular proteases. The clearance of PrP^{Sc} is of considerable inter-

est with respect to control of the length of the incubation time and other phenotypic features of prion strains.[149] When the PK-sensitive PrP^{Sc} fraction was plotted as a function of incubation time, a linear relationship was found with an excellent correlation coefficient ($R = 0.94$) (Fig. 2–8D).

These results demonstrate that eight different strains possess at least eight different conformations (see Fig. 2–8B, C). Additional data argue that each strain is composed of a spectrum of conformations as revealed by limited protease digestion and GdnHCl denaturation studies.[147] These findings contrast with the former notion that the primary structure of a protein determines a single tertiary structure.[87]

As noted by the studies described earlier, PrP^Sc must act as a template in the replication of nascent PrP^Sc molecules, and it seems likely that the binding of either PrP^C or the metastable intermediate PrP* to protein X is the initial step in PrP^Sc formation, which serves as the rate-limiting step in prion replication.[105,149,150] PrP^Sc interacts with PrP^C but not protein X in the PrP^C/protein X complex. When PrP^C or PrP* is converted into a nascent PrP^Sc molecule, protein X is released.

FUNGAL PRIONS

Although prions were originally defined in the context of an infectious mammalian pathogen,[43] it is becoming widely accepted that prions are elements that impart and propagate variability through multiple conformers of a normal cellular protein. Such a mechanism must surely not be restricted to a single class of transmissible pathogens. Indeed, it is likely that the original definition needs to be extended to encompass other situations in which a similar mechanism of information transfer occurs.

Two prion-like determinants, [URE3] and [PSI], have been described in yeast and a third, denoted [Het-s*], was reported in fungus.[32,151,152] Studies of prion proteins in yeast may prove to be particularly helpful in dissecting some of the events that feature in PrP^Sc formation. Interestingly, different strains of yeast prions have been identified.[153] Conversion to the prion-like [PSI] state in yeast requires the molecular chaperone Hsp104; however, no homologue of Hsp104 has been found in mammals.[151] The N-terminal prion domains of Ure2p and Sup35 that are responsible for the [URE3] and [PSI] phenotypes in yeast, respectively, have been identified. In contrast to PrP, which is a GPI-anchored membrane protein, both Ure2p and Sup35 are cytosolic proteins.[154] When the prion domains of these yeast proteins were expressed in *Escherichia coli*, the proteins were found to polymerize into fibrils with properties similar to those of proteolytically trimmed PrP and other amyloids.[155]

Whether prions explain some other examples of acquired inheritance in lower organisms is unclear.[156] For example, studies on the inheritance of positional order and cellular handedness on the surface of small organisms have demonstrated the epigenetic nature of these phenomena but the mechanism remains unclear.[157]

CONCLUDING REMARKS

Four new concepts have emerged from studies of prions. First, prions are the only known examples of infectious pathogens that are devoid of nucleic acid. All other infectious agents possess genomes composed of either RNA or DNA that direct the synthesis of their progeny. Second, prion diseases may manifest as infectious, genetic, or sporadic disorders. No other group of illnesses with a single etiology presents with such a wide

spectrum of clinical manifestations. Third, prion diseases result from the accumulation of PrP^Sc, the conformation of which differs substantially from that of its precursor PrP^C. Fourth, PrP^Sc can exist in a variety of different conformations, each of which seems to specify a disease phenotype. The mechanism by which a specific conformation of a PrP^Sc molecule is imparted to PrP^C during prion replication to produce nascent PrP^Sc with the same conformation is unknown. Additionally, it is unclear which factors determine where in the CNS a particular PrP^Sc molecule will be deposited and thus result in neurologic dysfunction.

Acknowledgments

I am especially grateful to Holger Wille for helping assemble some critical pieces of this chapter. I also want to acknowledge the help of Drs. Fred Cohen, Stephen DeArmond, Jane Dyson, and Peter Wright. This work was supported by grants from the National Institutes of Health.

REFERENCES

1. Avery OT, MacLeod CM, McCarty M: Studies on the chemical nature of the substance inducing transformation of pneumococcal types. Induction of transformation by a deoxyribonucleic acid fraction isolated from pneumococcus type III. J Exp Med 1944;79:137–157.

2. Stanley WM: The "undiscovered" discovery. Arch Environ Health 1970;21:256–262.

3. McCarty M: The Transforming Principle: Discovering that Genes Are Made of DNA. New York, WW Norton, 1985.

4. Hershey AD, Chase M: Independent functions of viral protein and nucleic acid in growth of bacteriophage. J Gen Physiol 1952;36:39–56.

5. Watson JD, Crick FHC: Genetical implication of the structure of deoxyribose nucleic acid. Nature 1953;171:964–967.

6. Mirsky AE, Pollister AW: Chromosin, a deoxyribose nucleoprotein complex of the cell nucleus. J Gen Physiol 1946;30:134–135.

7. Stanley WM: Isolation of a crystalline protein possessing the properties of tobacco mosaic virus. Science 1935;81:644–645.

8. Haurowitz F: Protein Synthesis. Chemistry and Biology of Proteins. New York, Academic Press, 1950.

9. Diener TO: Viroids and Viroid Diseases. New York, John Wiley, 1979.

10. Fraenkel-Conrat H, Williams RC: Reconstitution of active tobacco virus from the inactive protein and nucleic acid components. Proc Natl Acad Sci U S A 1955;41:690–698.

11. Gierer A, Schramm G: Infectivity of ribonucleic acid from tobacco mosaic virus. Nature 1956;177:702–703.

12. Gordon WS: Advances in veterinary research. Vet Res 1946;58:516–520.

13. Alper T, Haig DA, Clarke MC: The exceptionally small size of the scrapie agent. Biochem Biophys Res Commun 1966;22:278–284.

14. Alper T, Cramp WA, Haig DA, Clarke MC: Does the agent of scrapie replicate without nucleic acid? Nature 1967;214:764–766.

15. Meggendorfer F: Klinische und genealogische Beobachtungen bei einem Fall von spastischer Pseudosklerose Jakobs. Z Gesamte Neurol Psychiatr 1930;128:337–341.

16. Stender A: Weitere Beiträge zum Kapitel "Spastische Pseudosklerose Jakobs." Z Gesamte Neurol Psychiatr 1930;128:528–543.

17. Roos R, Gajdusek DC, Gibbs CJ Jr: The clinical characteristics of transmissible Creutzfeldt-Jakob disease. Brain 1973;96:1–20.

18. Masters CL, Gajdusek DC, Gibbs CJ Jr: Creutzfeldt-Jakob disease virus isolations from the Gerstmann-Sträussler syndrome. Brain 1981;104:559–588.

19. Hsiao K, Baker HF, Crow TJ, et al: Linkage of a prion protein missense variant to Gerstmann-Sträussler syndrome. Nature 1989;338:342–345.

20. Prusiner SB: Scrapie prions. Annu Rev Microbiol 1989;43:345–374.

21. Kirschbaum WR: Jakob-Creutzfeldt Disease. Amsterdam, Elsevier, 1968.

22. Gibbs CJ Jr, Gajdusek DC, Asher DM, et al: Creutzfeldt-Jakob disease (spongiform encephalopathy): Transmission to the chimpanzee. Science 1968;161:388–389.

23. Prusiner SB: The prion diseases. Sci Am 1995;272:48–51,54–57.

24. Prusiner SB: Prions (Les Prix Nobel Lecture). In Frängsmyr T (ed): Les Prix Nobel. Stockholm, Almqvist & Wiksell International, 1998.

25. Prusiner SB: Prions. Proc Natl Acad Sci U S A 1998;95:13363–13383.

26. McKinley MP, Meyer RK, Kenaga L, et al: Scrapie prion rod formation in vitro requires both detergent extraction and limited proteolysis. J Virol 1991;65:1340–1351.

27. Pan K-M, Baldwin M, Nguyen J, et al: Conversion of α-helices into β-sheets features in the formation of the scrapie prion proteins. Proc Natl Acad Sci U S A 1993;90:10962–10966.

28. Huang Z, Prusiner SB, Cohen FE: Scrapie prions: A three-dimensional model of an infectious fragment. Fold Des 1995;1:13–19.

29. Riek R, Hornemann S, Wider G, et al: NMR structure of the mouse prion protein domain PrP (121–231). Nature 1996;382:180–182.

30. Liu H, Farr-Jones S, Ulyanov NB, et al: Solution structure of Syrian hamster prion protein rPrP (90–231). Biochemistry 1999;38:5362–5377.

31. Peretz D, Williamson RA, Matsunaga Y, et al: A conformational transition at the N terminus of the prion protein features in formation of the scrapie isoform. J Mol Biol 1997;273:614–622.

32. Wickner RB: [URE3] as an altered URE2 protein: Evidence for a prion analog in Saccharomyces cerevisiae. Science 1994;264:566–569.

33. Sparrer HE, Santoso A, Szoka FC Jr, Weissman JS: Evidence for the prion hypothesis: Induction of the yeast [PSI+] factor by in vitro-converted Sup35 protein. Science 2000;289:595–599.

34. Chandler RL: Encephalopathy in mice produced by inoculation with scrapie brain material. Lancet 1961;1:1378–1379.

35. Chandler RL: Experimental scrapie in the mouse. Res Vet Sci 1963;4:276–285.

36. Eklund CM, Hadlow WJ, Kennedy RC: Some properties of the scrapie agent and its behavior in mice. Proc Soc Exp Biol Med 1963;112:974–979.

37. Hunter GD: Scrapie: A prototype slow infection. J Infect Dis 1972;125:427–440.

38. Prusiner SB: An approach to the isolation of biological particles using sedimentation analysis. J Biol Chem 1978;253:916–921.

39. Prusiner SB, Hadlow WJ, Eklund CM, Race RE: Sedimentation properties of the scrapie agent. Proc Natl Acad Sci U S A 1977;74:4656–4660.

40. Prusiner SB, Hadlow WJ, Eklund CM, et al: Sedimentation characteristics of the scrapie agent from murine spleen and brain. Biochemistry 1978;17:4987–4992.

41. Prusiner SB, Groth DF, Cochran SP, et al: Molecular properties, partial purification, and assay by incubation period measurements of the hamster scrapie agent. Biochemistry 1980;21:4883–4891.

42. Prusiner SB, Cochran SP, Groth DF, et al: Measurement of the scrapie agent using an incubation time interval assay. Ann Neurol 1982;11:353–358.

43. Prusiner SB: Novel proteinaceous infectious particles cause scrapie. Science 1982;216:136–144.

44. Chamberlin TC: The method of multiple working hypotheses. Science [Old Series] 1890;15:92–97.

45. Alper T, Haig DA, Clarke MC: The scrapie agent: Evidence against its dependence for replication on intrinsic nucleic acid. J Gen Virol 1978;41:503–516.

46. Gibbons RA, Hunter GD: Nature of the scrapie agent. Nature 1967;215:1041–1043.

47. Millson G, Hunter GD, Kimberlin RH: An experimental examination of the scrapie agent in cell membrane mixtures. II. The association of scrapie infectivity with membrane fractions. J Comp Pathol 1971;81:255–265.

48. Pattison IH, Jones KM: The possible nature of the transmissible agent of scrapie. Vet Rec 1967;80:1–8.

49. Setlow R, Doyle B: The action of monochromatic ultraviolet light on proteins. Biochim Biophys Acta 1957;24:27–41.

50. Latarjet R, Muel B, Haig DA, et al: Inactivation of the scrapie agent by near monochromatic ultraviolet light. Nature 1970;227:1341–1343.

51. Bellinger-Kawahara CG, Kempner E, Groth DF, et al: Scrapie prion liposomes and rods exhibit target sizes of 55,000 Da. Virology 1988;164:537–541.

52. Diener TO: Is the scrapie agent a viroid? Nature 1972;235:218–219.

53. Diener TO, McKinley MP, Prusiner SB: Viroids and prions. Proc Natl Acad Sci U S A 1982;79:5220–5224.

54. Rohwer RG: Scrapie infectious agent is virus-like in size and susceptibility to inactivation. Nature 1984;308:658–662.

55. Rohwer RG: Estimation of scrapie nucleic acid molecular weight from standard curves for virus sensitivity to ionizing radiation. Nature 1986;320:381.

56. M'Gowan JP: Investigation into the Disease of Sheep Called "Scrapie." Edinburgh, William Blackwood and Sons, 1914.

57. M'Fadyean J: Scrapie. J Comp Pathol 1918;31:102–131.

58. Cuillé J, Chelle PL: Experimental transmission of trembling to the goat. C R Seances Acad Sci 1939;208:1058–1060.

59. Wilson DR, Anderson RD, Smith W: Studies in scrapie. J Comp Pathol 1950;60:267–282.

60. Kimberlin RH, Hunter GD: DNA synthesis in scrapie-affected mouse brain. J Gen Virol 1967;1:115–124.

61. Griffith JS: Self-replication and scrapie. Nature 1967;215:1043–1044.

62. Lewin P: Scrapie: An infective peptide? Lancet 1972;1:748.

63. Lewin P: Infectious peptides in slow virus infections: A hypothesis. Can Med Assoc J 1981;124:1436–1437.

64. Hunter GD, Kimberlin RH, Gibbons RA: Scrapie: A modified membrane hypothesis. J Theor Biol 1968;20:355–357.

65. Adams DH, Field EJ: The infective process in scrapie. Lancet 1968;2:714–716.

66. Adams DH: The nature of the scrapie agent: A review of recent progress. Pathol Biol 1970;18:559–577.

67. Parry HB: Scrapie: A transmissible and hereditary disease of sheep. Heredity 1962;17:75–105.

68. Parry HB: Scrapie—Natural and experimental. In Whitty CWM, Hughes JT, MacCallum FO (eds): Virus Diseases and the Nervous System. Oxford, Blackwell Publishing, 1969.

69. Stahl N, Baldwin MA, Teplow DB, et al: Structural analysis of the scrapie prion protein using mass spectrometry and amino acid sequencing. Biochemistry 1993;32:1991–2002.

70. Telling GC, Haga T, Torchia M, et al: Interactions between wild-type and mutant prion proteins modulate neurodegeneration in transgenic mice. Genes Dev 1996;10:1736–1750.

71. Gajdusek DC: Unconventional viruses and the origin and disappearance of kuru. Science 1977;197:943–960.

72. Pattison IH: Fifty years with scrapie: A personal reminiscence. Vet Rec 1988;123:661–666.

73. Rohwer RG, Gajdusek DC: Scrapie—Virus or viroid: The case for a virus. In Boese A (ed): Search for the Cause of Multiple Sclerosis and Other Chronic Diseases of the Central Nervous System. Weinheim, Germany, Verlag Chemie, 1980.

74. Field EJ: The significance of astroglial hypertrophy in scrapie, kuru, multiple sclerosis, and old age together with a note on the possible nature of the scrapie agent. Dtsch Z Nervenheilk. 1967;192:265–274.

75. Adams DH, Caspary EA: Nature of the scrapie virus. BMJ 1967;3:173.

76. Narang HK: Ruthenium red and lanthanum nitrate a possible tracer and negative stain for scrapie "particles"? Acta Neuropathol (Berl) 1974;29:37–43.

77. Siakotos AN, Raveed D, Longa G: The discovery of a particle unique to brain and spleen subcellular fractions from scrapie-infected mice. J Gen Virol 1979;43:417–422.

78. Bastian FO: Spiroplasma-like inclusions in Creutzfeldt-Jakob disease. Arch Pathol Lab Med 1979;103:665–669.

79. Humphery-Smith I, Chastel C, Le Goff F: Spirosplasmas and spongiform encephalopathies. Med J Aust 1992;156:142.

80. Hunter GD, Kimberlin RH, Collis S, Millson GC: Viral and non-viral properties of the scrapie agent. Ann Clin Res 1973;5:262–267.

81. Somerville RA, Millson GC, Hunter GD: Changes in a protein-nucleic acid complex from synaptic plasma membrane of scrapie-infected mouse brain. Biochem Soc Trans 1976;4:1112–1114.

82. Marsh RF, Malone TG, Semancik JS, et al: Evidence for an essential DNA component in the scrapie agent. Nature 1978;275:146–147.

83. Dickinson AG, Outram GW: The scrapie replication-site hypothesis and its implications for pathogenesis. In Prusiner SB, Hadlow WJ (eds): Slow Transmissible Diseases of the Nervous System, vol 2. New York, Academic Press, 1979.

84. Chesebro B, Race R, Wehrly K, et al: Identification of scrapie prion protein-specific mRNA in scrapie-infected and uninfected brain. Nature 1985;315:331–333.

85. Oesch B, Westaway D, Wälchli M, et al: A cellular gene encodes scrapie PrP 27–30 protein. Cell 1985;40:735–746.

86. Basler K, Oesch B, Scott M, et al: Scrapie and cellular PrP isoforms are encoded by the same chromosomal gene. Cell 1986;46:417–428.

87. Anfinsen CB: Principles that govern the folding of protein chains. Science 1973;181:223–230.

88. Borchelt DR, Scott M, Taraboulos A, et al: Scrapie and cellular prion proteins differ in their kinetics

of synthesis and topology in cultured cells. J Cell Biol 1990;110:743–752.

89. Stahl N, Borchelt DR, Hsiao K, Prusiner SB: Scrapie prion protein contains a phosphatidylinositol glycolipid. Cell 1987;51:229–240.

90. Caughey B, Raymond GJ: The scrapie-associated form of PrP is made from a cell surface precursor that is both protease- and phospholipase-sensitive. J Biol Chem 1991;266:18217–18223.

91. Gorodinsky A, Harris DA: Glycolipid-anchored proteins in neuroblastoma cells form detergent-resistant complexes without caveolin. J Cell Biol 1995;129:619–627.

92. Taraboulos A, Scott M, Semenov A, et al: Cholesterol depletion and modification of COOH-terminal targeting sequence of the prion protein inhibits formation of the scrapie isoform. J Cell Biol 1995;129:121–132.

93. Huang Z, Gabriel J-M, Baldwin MA, et al: Proposed three-dimensional structure for the cellular prion protein. Proc Natl Acad Sci U S A 1994;91:7139–7143.

94. Hegde RS, Tremblay P, Groth D, et al: Transmissible and genetic prion diseases share a common pathway of neurodegeneration. Nature 1999;402:822–826.

95. James TL, Liu H, Ulyanov NB, et al: Solution structure of a 142-residue recombinant prion protein corresponding to the infectious fragment of the scrapie isoform. Proc Natl Acad Sci U S A 1997;94:10086–10091.

96. Donne DG, Viles JH, Groth D, et al: Structure of the recombinant full-length hamster prion protein PrP(29–231): The N terminus is highly flexible. Proc Natl Acad Sci U S A 1997;94:13452–13457.

97. Williamson RA, Peretz D, Smorodinsky N, et al: Circumventing tolerance to generate autologous monoclonal antibodies to the prion protein. Proc Natl Acad Sci U S A 1996;93:7279–7282.

98. Benzinger TLS, Gregory DM, Burkoth TS, et al: Propagating structure of Alzheimer's β-amyloid$_{(10-35)}$ is parallel β-sheet with residues in exact register. Proc Natl Acad Sci U S A 1998;95:13407–13412.

99. Antzutkin ON, Balbach JJ, Leapman RD, et al: Multiple quantum solid-state NMR indicates a parallel, not antiparallel, organization of β-sheets in Alzheimer's β-amyloid fibrils. Proc Natl Acad Sci U S A 2000;97:13045–13050.

100. Wille H, Zhang G-F, Baldwin MA, et al: Separation of scrapie prion infectivity from PrP amyloid polymers. J Mol Biol 1996;259:608–621.

101. Supattapone S, Bosque P, Muramoto T, et al: Prion protein of 106 residues creates an artificial transmission barrier for prion replication in transgenic mice. Cell 1999;96:869–878.

102. Seckler R: Folding and function of repetitive structure in the homotrimeric phage P22 tailspike protein. J Struct Biol 1998;122:216–222.

103. Schuler B, Rachel R, Seckler R: Formation of fibrous aggregates from a non-native intermediate: The isolated P22 tailspike beta-helix domain. J Biol Chem 1999;274:18589–18596.

104. Cohen FE, Pan K-M, Huang Z, et al: Structural clues to prion replication. Science 1994;264:530–531.

105. Kaneko K, Zulianello L, Scott M, et al: Evidence for protein X binding to a discontinuous epitope on the cellular prion protein during scrapie prion propagation. Proc Natl Acad Sci U S A 1997;94:10069–10074.

106. Gabizon R, McKinley MP, Groth D, Prusiner SB: Immunoaffinity purification and neutralization of scrapie prion infectivity. Proc Natl Acad Sci U S A 1988;85:6617–6621.

107. Gajdusek DC: Transmissible and non-transmissible amyloidoses: Autocatalytic post-translational conversion of host precursor proteins to β-pleated sheet configurations. J Neuroimmunol 1988;20:95–110.

108. Caughey B, Kocisko DA, Raymond GJ, Lansbury PT Jr: Aggregates of scrapie-associated prion protein induce the cell-free conversion of protease-sensitive prion protein to the protease-resistant state. Chem Biol 1995;2:807–817.

109. Muramoto T, Scott M, Cohen FE, Prusiner SB: Recombinant scrapie-like prion protein of 106 amino acids is soluble. Proc Natl Acad Sci U S A 1996;93:15457–15462.

110. Kocisko DA, Come JH, Priola SA, et al: Cell-free formation of protease-resistant prion protein. Nature 1994;370:471–474.

111. Kaneko K, Wille H, Mehlhorn I, et al: Molecular properties of complexes formed between the prion protein and synthetic peptides. J Mol Biol 1997;270:574–586.

112. Vey M, Pilkuhn S, Wille H, et al: Subcellular colocalization of the cellular and scrapie prion proteins in caveolae-like membranous domains. Proc Natl Acad Sci U S A 1996;93:14945–14949.

113. Kaneko K, Vey M, Scott M, et al: COOH-terminal sequence of the cellular prion protein directs subcellular trafficking and controls conversion into the scrapie isoform. Proc Natl Acad Sci U S A 1997;94:2333–2338.

114. Naslavsky N, Stein R, Yanai A, et al: Characterization of detergent-insoluble complexes containing the cellular prion protein and its scrapie isoform. J Biol Chem 1997;272:6324–6331.

115. Caughey B, Raymond GJ, Ernst D, Race RE: N-terminal truncation of the scrapie-associated form of PrP by lysosomal protease(s): Implications regarding the site of conversion of PrP to the protease-resistant state. J Virol 1991;65:6597–6603.

116. Prusiner SB, Scott M, Foster D, et al: Transgenetic studies implicate interactions between homologous PrP isoforms in scrapie prion replication. Cell 1990;63:673–686.

117. Telling GC, Parchi P, DeArmond SJ, et al: Evidence for the conformation of the pathologic isoform

of the prion protein enciphering and propagating prion diversity. Science 1996;274:2079–2082.

118. Prusiner SB: Prion diseases and the BSE crisis. Science 1997;278:245–251.

119. Mastrianni J, Nixon F, Layzer R, et al: Fatal sporadic insomnia: Fatal familial insomnia phenotype without a mutation of the prion protein gene. Neurology 1997;48 [Suppl]:A296.

120. Mastrianni JA, Nixon R, Layzer R, et al: Prion protein conformation in a patient with sporadic fatal insomnia. N Engl J Med 1999;340:1630–1638.

121. Parchi P, Capellari S, Chin S, et al: A subtype of sporadic prion disease mimicking fatal familial insomnia. Neurology 1999;52:1757–1763.

122. Gambetti P, Parchi P: Insomnia in prion diseases: Sporadic and familial. N Engl J Med 1999;340:1675–1677.

123. Telling GC, Scott M, Hsiao KK, et al: Transmission of Creutzfeldt-Jakob disease from humans to transgenic mice expressing chimeric human-mouse prion protein. Proc Natl Acad Sci U S A 1994;91:9936–9940.

124. Telling GC, Scott M, Mastrianni J, et al: Prion propagation in mice expressing human and chimeric PrP transgenes implicates the interaction of cellular PrP with another protein. Cell 1995;83:79–90.

125. Scott MR, Köhler R, Foster D, Prusiner SB: Chimeric prion protein expression in cultured cells and transgenic mice. Protein Sci 1992;1:986–997.

126. Shibuya S, Higuchi J, Shin R-W, et al: Protective prion protein polymorphisms against sporadic Creutzfeldt-Jakob disease. Lancet 1998;351:419.

127. Hunter N, Goldmann W, Benson G, et al: Swaledale sheep affected by natural scrapie differ significantly in PrP genotype frequencies from healthy sheep and those selected for reduced incidence of scrapie. J Gen Virol 1993;74:1025–1031.

128. Westaway D, Zuliani V, Cooper CM, et al: Homozygosity for prion protein alleles encoding glutamine-171 renders sheep susceptible to natural scrapie. Genes Dev 1994;8:959–969.

129. Perrier V, Kaneko K, Safar J, et al: Dominant negative inhibition of prion replication in transgenic mice. Proc Natl Acad Sci U S A (in press).

130. Prusiner SB, Groth D, Serban A, et al: Ablation of the prion protein (PrP) gene in mice prevents scrapie and facilitates production of anti-PrP antibodies. Proc Natl Acad Sci U S A 1993;90:10608–10612.

131. Büeler H, Raeber A, Sailer A, et al: High prion and PrPSc levels but delayed onset of disease in scrapie-inoculated mice heterozygous for a disrupted PrP gene. Mol Med 1994;1:19–30.

132. Carlson GA, Ebeling C, Yang S-L, et al: Prion isolate specified allotypic interactions between the cellular and scrapie prion proteins in congenic and transgenic mice. Proc Natl Acad Sci U S A 1994;91:5690–5694.

133. Bessen RA, Marsh RF: Distinct PrP properties suggest the molecular basis of strain variation in transmissible mink encephalopathy. J Virol 1994;68:7859–7868.

134. Collinge J, Sidle KCL, Meads J, et al: Molecular analysis of prion strain variation and the aetiology of "new variant" CJD. Nature 1996;383:685–690.

135. DeArmond SJ, Sánchez H, Yehiely F, et al: Selective neuronal targeting in prion disease. Neuron 1997;19:1337–1348.

136. Somerville RA, Chong A, Mulqueen OU, et al: Biochemical typing of scrapie strains. Nature 1997;386:564.

137. Dickinson AG, Meikle VMH, Fraser H: Identification of a gene which controls the incubation period of some strains of scrapie agent in mice. J Comp Pathol 1968;78:293–299.

138. Fraser H, Dickinson AG: The sequential development of the brain lesions of scrapie in three strains of mice. J Comp Pathol 1968;78:301–311.

139. DeArmond SJ, Mobley WC, DeMott DL, et al: Changes in the localization of brain prion proteins during scrapie infection. Neurology 1987;37:1271–1280.

140. Bruce ME, McBride PA, Farquhar CF: Precise targeting of the pathology of the sialoglycoprotein, PrP, and vacuolar degeneration in mouse scrapie. Neurosci Lett 1989;102:1–6.

141. Moore RC, Hope J, McBride PA, et al: Mice with gene targeted prion protein alterations show that *Prn-p, Sinc,* and *Prni* are congruent. Nat Genet 1998;18:118–125.

142. Prusiner SB: Molecular biology of prion diseases. Science 1991;252:1515–1522.

143. Scott MR, Groth D, Tatzelt J, et al: Propagation of prion strains through specific conformers of the prion protein. J Virol 1997;71:9032–9044.

144. Kimberlin RH, Walker CA, Fraser H: The genomic identity of different strains of mouse scrapie is expressed in hamsters and preserved on reisolation in mice. J Gen Virol 1989;70:2017–2025.

145. Monari L, Chen SG, Brown P, et al: Fatal familial insomnia and familial Creutzfeldt-Jakob disease: Different prion proteins determined by a DNA polymorphism. Proc Natl Acad Sci U S A 1994;91:2839–2842.

146. Scott M, Foster D, Mirenda C, et al: Transgenic mice expressing hamster prion protein produce species-specific scrapie infectivity and amyloid plaques. Cell 1989;59:847–857.

147. Safar J, Wille H, Itri V, et al: Eight prion strains have PrPSc molecules with different conformations. Nat Med 1998;4:1157–1165.

148. Bessen RA, Marsh RF: Biochemical and physical properties of the prion protein from two strains of the transmissible mink encephalopathy agent. J Virol 1992;66:2096–2101.

149. Prusiner SB, Scott MR, DeArmond SJ, Cohen FE: Prion protein biology. Cell 1998;93:337–348.

150. Cohen FE, Prusiner SB: Pathologic conformations of prion proteins. Annu Rev Biochem 1998;67: 793–819.

151. Chernoff YO, Lindquist SL, Ono B, et al: Role of the chaperone protein Hsp104 in propagation of the yeast prion-like factor [psi+]. Science 1995;268:880–884.

152. Coustou V, Deleu C, Saupe S, Begueret J: The protein product of the het-s heterokaryon incompatibility gene of the fungus Podospora anserina behaves as a prion analog. Proc Natl Acad Sci U S A 1997;94: 9773–9778.

153. Derkatch IL, Chernoff YO, Kushnirov VV, et al: Genesis and variability of [PSI] prion factors in Saccharomyces cerevisiae. Genetics 1996;144: 1375–1386.

154. Wickner RB: A new prion controls fungal cell fusion incompatibility [Commentary]. Proc Natl Acad Sci U S A 1997;94:10012–10014.

155. Paushkin SV, Kushnirov VV, Smirnov VN, Ter-Avanesyan MD: In vitro propagation of the prion-like state of yeast Sup35 protein. Science 1997;277:381–383.

156. Landman OE: The inheritance of acquired characteristics. Annu Rev Genet 1991;25:1–20.

157. Frankel J: Positional order and cellular handedness. J Cell Sci 1990;97:205–211.

158. Serban D, Taraboulos A, DeArmond SJ, Prusiner SB: Rapid detection of Creutzfeldt-Jakob disease and scrapie prion proteins. Neurology 1990;40: 110–117.

159. Wille H, Michelitsch MD, Guénebaut V, et al: Structural studies of the scrapie prion protein by electron crystallography. Proc Natl Acad Sci U S A 2002;99: 3563–3568.

160. Riek R, Hornemann S, Wider G, et al: NMR characterization of the full-length recombinant murine prion protein, mPrP(23–231). FEBS Lett 1997;413: 282–288.

161. Kanyo Z, Pan K-M, Williamson A, et al: Antibody binding defines a structure for an epitope that participates in the PrP^C Æ Prp^{Sc} conformational change. J Mol Biol 1999;293:855–863.

162. Zahn R, Liu A, Lührs T, et al: NMR solution structure of the human prion protein. Proc Natl Acad Sci U S A 2000;97:145–150.

163. García FL, Zahn R, Riek R, Wüthrich K: NMR structure of the bovine prion protein. Proc Natl Acad Sci U S A 2000;97:8334–8339.

164. Zhang Y, Swietnicki W, Zagorski MG, et al: Solution structure of the E200K variant of human prion protein. Implications for the mechanism of pathogenesis in familial prion diseases. J Biol Chem 2000;275: 33650–33654.

165. Knaus KJ, Morillas M, Swietnicki W, et al: Crystal structure of the human prion protein reveals a mechanism for oligomerization. Nat Struct Biol 2001;8: 770–774.

166. Mo H, Moore RC, Cohen FE, et al: Two different neurodegenerative diseases caused by proteins with similar structures. Proc Natl Acad Sci U S A 2001;98: 2352–2357.

CHAPTER

3

Mendelian, Nonmendelian, Multigenic Inheritance, and Complex Traits

Ken Inoue

James R. Lupski

It has been a widely accepted idea that genetics plays a major role in the pathophysiology of most human diseases, if not all. Such genetic influence can be the only sufficient factor required to manifest a disease phenotype, or it can be one relatively minor component of many different disease-associated factors. Perhaps the best example of the former is monogenic mendelian disorders with complete penetrance wherein a mutation in a single disease-causing gene always results in a relatively uniform disease phenotype. The latter pattern can be observed in many common diseases in which genetic factors contribute a portion of the risk and may play a role in either increasing or decreasing disease susceptibility. Between these extremes of genetic pathophysiology, however, there is a continuum of genetic influence on disease pathophysiology.

Mendelian traits represent the most basic and simple pattern of inheritance. Mutations in a gene encoded on an autosome or sex chromosome result in specific inheritance patterns. Nonmendelian traits reveal some complexity in their mode of inheritance, in which the classic pattern of inheritance may not always apply and epigenetic factors are often associated with disease mechanisms. Furthermore, in some diseases one gene is not sufficient to cause the clinical phenotype, but when two or more genes are involved, a particular disease becomes apparent. This latter mechanism is usually referred to as multigenic inheritance. Finally, complex traits involve multiple genes as susceptibility or protective factors, but also require internal factors including other health conditions as well as external factors such as environment, habit, diet, accident, infection, and drug exposure.

Regardless of the mode of inheritance, defining specific genetic factors that are associated with certain diseases and their functional role in phenotypic manifestations are very important for patient management and genetic counseling as well as for molecular understanding enabling insights into disease mechanisms and ultimately developing new therapeutic approaches. Molecular diagnostics by itself contributes to patient management by establishing a secure diagnosis, enabling the availability of presymptomatic or prenatal diagnosis, providing prognostic information, and further refining more general diagnostic labels. It is estimated that approximately one third of all human genes are expressed in the nervous systems, and thus neurogenetic phenotypes are common.[1] In this chapter, we review the modes of inheritance that can be observed in various human neurologic and psychiatric diseases.

MENDELIAN TRAITS

Mendel's Laws

Mendelian or monogenic traits refer to those that result from alterations at a single locus. The basic rules of inheritance were discovered by Gregor Mendel in his observation of the segregation of traits in the common garden pea, *Pisum sativum*.[2] Mendel's first law, the principle of independent segregation, referred to the ability of genes, which he called factors, to segregate independently during the formation of gametes or sex cells. Mendel's second law, the principle of independent assortment, was derived from his observations using peas that differed by more than one characteristic or trait. Mendel postulated that only one factor from each pair was independently transmitted to the gamete during sex-cell formation, and any one gamete contains only one type of inherited factor from each pair. There is no tendency for genes arising from one parent to stay together. Of course, we now know that this latter principle is true only for unlinked genes. Genes or loci that are linked, or physically located in close proximity on the same chromosome, do not assort independently. The closer these loci are, the more frequently they will cosegregate. Linkage analysis is a quantitative measurement of this cosegregation (expressed as a LOD score or $\log_{10}$ of the odds ratio for cosegregation versus independent assortment)[3] and has been utilized as a powerful tool in human genetics to map genes for disease traits to particular regions in the human genome.

Chromosomes

The chromosomal theory of heredity expounded by Sutton emphasized that the diploid chromosome group consists of a morphologically similar set, a homologous pair, for each chromosome and that during meiosis every gamete receives only one chromosome of each homologous pair. This observation was used to explain Mendel's results by assuming that genes, or factors, were part of the chromosome. Genes are arranged in a linear order on the chromosome, each having a specific position or locus. There are two copies for each gene at a given locus, one on each chromosome homologue. These two copies, or alleles, may be identical or homozygous at the specific autosomal locus. Alternatively, the two gene copies at a particular locus may be different and represent heterozygous alleles. When only one copy is physically present, either because of deletion or the special circumstances of the X chromosome in XY males, this condition is referred to as a hemizygous allele. The genes are passed to the next generation through parental gametes, which contain only one of the two alternative gene copies. A particular gamete may contain alleles from different chromosome homologues because of chromosome crossover and recombination of alleles that occur during meiosis.

Mendelian Inheritance

There are three major patterns of mendelian inheritance: autosomal dominant, autosomal recessive, and X-linked (Fig. 3–1). They represent the segregation patterns observed within a family for a specific trait. Mendelian inheritance patterns refer to observable traits and not to genes. Some alleles at a specific locus may encode a trait that segregates in a dominant manner, whereas another allele may encode a similar or the same trait, but segregate as a recessive. The identical or similar trait may actually be caused by mutations in different genes at different loci; this is known as *genetic heterogeneity*. The molecular basis of genetic heterogeneity is diverse but may be explained by abnormalities in different genes that function in the same biologic process. This may involve genes that encode various enzymes in the same metabolic pathway (e.g., GM2 gangliosidoses), abnormalities in genes that code for discrete subunits of a functional protein complex (e.g., leukodystrophy with vanishing white matter—MIM #603896), or a macromolecular structure such as myelin (Charcot-Marie-Tooth disease type 1). Different types of mutations in a single gene may result in the same clinical disease phenotypes. This phenomenon is referred to as *allelic heterogeneity*. It has been recognized more recently that different mutations in the same gene may give distinct clinical phenotypes—*allelic affinity* (e.g., Duchenne and Becker muscular dystrophies). Generally, disorders within a single family represent neither genetic nor allelic heterogeneity.

Autosomal dominant alleles exert their effect despite the presence of a corresponding normal allele on the homologous chromosome. The pattern observed in the pedigree is a vertical transmission pattern, with the trait manifested in approximately one half of the individuals in each generation (see Fig. 3–1A). An affected individual will have a 50% chance of transmitting the disease to each independent offspring, which is a reflection of whether the mutant or normal allele is segregated in the gamete used for fertilization. Usually, unaffected members of the family do not carry the mutant allele; thus they cannot transmit a disease allele to the next generation. If an affected male transmits the disease to his son, this is considered proof of autosomal dominant inheritance. Male-to-male transmission is inconsistent with X-linked inheritance because a father normally contributes the Y-chromosome or no X-chromosome to all his sons.

In autosomal recessive inheritance, both alleles must be abnormal for the disease trait to be expressed. The unaffected parents of an affected child are obligate heterozygote carriers for the recessive mutant allele. Affected children may be homozygous for a specific recessive mutant allele, as is more commonly observed with consanguineous matings, or they may be compound heterozygotes for two different mutations. Couples who are heterozygous carriers of a recessive mutant allele have a 25% risk of having an affected child with each pregnancy. The pattern of transmission observed in the pedigree is horizontal with multiple members of one generation affected (see Fig. 3–1B). The unaffected siblings have a 66% chance of being a carrier for the mutant allele.

X-linked inheritance patterns reflect special circumstances regarding sex chromosomes. Females have two X-chromosomes, while males have one X-chromosome and one Y-chromosome. In X-linked recessive inheritance, a mutation in a gene located on the X-chromosome may not express itself in females because of the normal copy on the other X-chromosome. However, all males who inherit the mutant allele will be affected. An important feature of X-linked inheritance is that male-to-male transmission never occurs, but all female offspring of affected males inherit the abnormal gene. Therefore, affected fathers will have genetically normal sons and obligate carrier daughters (see Fig. 3–1C).

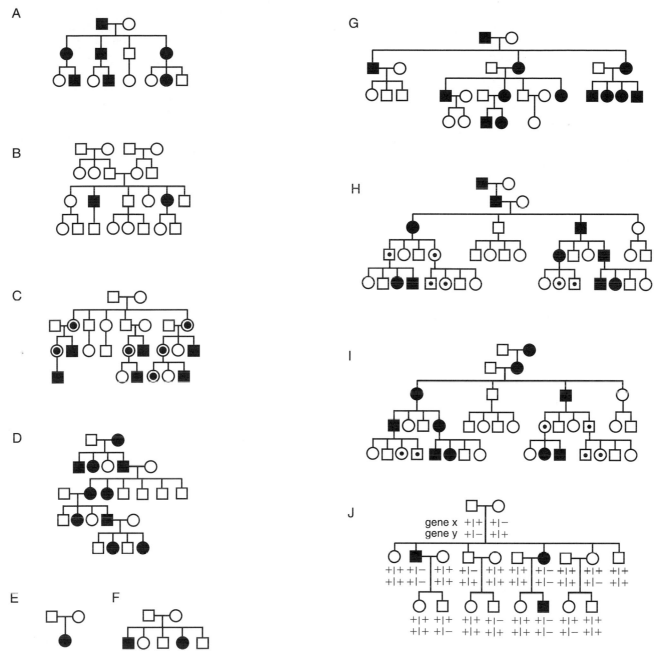

FIGURE 3–1. Pedigrees representing different patterns of inheritance that can be observed for disease traits in families. Unaffected males *(open squares)* and females *(open circles)* are shown. Completely filled symbols represent individuals manifesting the trait. Inheritance patterns include *A,* autosomal dominant; *B,* autosomal recessive; *C,* X-linked recessive showing individuals who carry the mutant gene but do not manifest the disease trait *(filled-in symbols with large dot in center); D,* X-linked dominant; *E,* sporadic or new mutation or autosomal recessive; *F,* new mutation with gonadal mosaicism or autosomal recessive; *G,* maternal or mitochondrial inheritance; *H,* dominant maternally imprinted showing individuals who carry the mutant imprinted gene on the nonexpressing allele and do not manifest the disease trait *(filled-in symbols with small dot in center); I,* dominant paternally imprinted; and *J,* digenic inheritance showing wild-type and mutant alleles at disease loci X *(plus signs)* and Y *(minus signs).*

X-linked recessive disorders may sometimes be observed in females because of a skewing in the process of *Lyonization* or *X-inactivation.*[4] Usually the expression of one of the two X-chromosomes in females is suppressed randomly in each cell early in embryonic development. If nonrandom or skewed X-inactivation occurs, such that the X-chromosome carrying a mutant allele for an X-linked recessive trait is predominantly the active X-chromosome, then a phenotype will be manifested in a carrier female. In normal females, a "bell-shaped" or Gaussian distribution represents X-inactivation patterns with a 50:50 average ratio. Therefore, a skewed inactivation pattern is not rare in normal females. A ratio of 80:20 or greater can be observed in 5% to 10% of normal females. This skewing may not result in a phenotype unless one has a deleterious mutation in a gene that is subject to X-inactivation. Alternatively, rare conditions such as mutations in *XIST* (a master regulatory gene of X-inactivation) or X-autosome translocation (which separates translocated genes from the regulation by *XIST)* result in skewed X-inactivation. In addition, X-linked recessive traits may be expressed in females with a 45,X karyotype and Turner syndrome phenotype.

In X-linked dominant inheritance, females who carry a mutation in a gene on the X-chromosome will express the disease phenotype but usually will have a milder clinical course than males with the mutation. Approximately twice as many females as males will be affected in a multigenerational pedigree. There will be no instance of male-to-male transmission (see Fig. 3–1D). Whether a trait is considered X-linked recessive or X-linked dominant may sometimes be a matter of how the phenotype is scored. For instance, the X-linked form of Charcot-Marie-Tooth disease may have subtle or no clinical features on neurologic examination of a female patient, but electrophysiologic studies may reveal reduced motor nerve conduction velocities. Some X-linked dominant disorders may be lethal in males and therefore may be observed only in females. Examples of X-linked dominant neurologic disorders that are usually lethal in males include incontinentia pigmenti (MIM #308300), Aicardi syndrome (MIM #304050), bilateral periventricular nodular heterotopia (MIM #300049) and Rett syndrome (MIM #312750).

Mechanisms of Mutations

Specific mutations in each gene may behave differently in disease pathogenesis and associated phenotypic expression.[5] Mutations may result in an inactive gene product and are thus referred to as *loss-of-function* mutations. Null alleles result from complete absence or loss-of-function of the protein product, whereas mutations resulting in some retention of protein function are considered *hypomorphic alleles*. Loss-of-function mutations explain most recessive traits in which phenotypes become evident only when both alleles are mutated. Heterozygous carriers may have no disease-associated phenotypes but may present with subtle biochemical defects or reduced levels of protein expression that may result in dominant susceptibility to a milder trait (e.g., homozygous or compound heterozygous *ABCA4* mutations are identified in all recessive Stargardt macular dystrophy (MIM #248200) patients, whereas heterozygous *ABCA4* mutations are identified in a fraction of patients with age-related macular degeneration [MIM #153800]). Some genes may require two wild-type alleles for normal function. In such case, heterozygotes for loss-of-function mutations may reveal phenotypes that can transmit as

dominant traits because of the insufficient amount of gene products (*haploinsufficiency*).

Two other mutational mechanisms can explain a dominant inheritance pattern. When a translated mutant protein interferes with the function of a normal (wild-type) protein that is produced from the normal allele, the condition is referred to as resulting from a *dominant-negative* effect (or *antimorphic mutations*). Dominant-negative alleles occur when the encoded proteins compose a subunit structure (homodimer, heterodimer, or other multimeric complex formation) or when they interact with other proteins (ligand-receptor) or DNA (transcription factors). In contrast, *gain-of-function* is the mechanism in which mutant proteins abnormally enhance the normal function, or acquire novel functions that are toxic to cells without interfering with the wild-type allele function (also referred to as *neomorphic alleles*). Many neurodegenerative disorders with dominant inheritance are likely associated with gain-of-function mutations (e.g., polyglutamine diseases, prion disorders) that may prevent proteins from proper cellular processing, such as folding, transport, or degradation. A unique example of gain-of-function mutation is the inappropriate gene activation that results from deletion of a variable number of tandem repeats (VNTR) at the subtelomeric region of chromosome 4q35 (*D4Z4*) and causes facioscapulohumeral muscular dystrophy (MIM #158900).[6]

Factors That Modify Classic Mendelian Inheritance Patterns

New Mutations, Mosaicism, and Somatic Mutation

In certain dominant alleles, new mutations or de novo mutations may have tremendous clinical significance (e.g., tuberous sclerosis [MIM #191100], neurofibromatosis type 1 [MIM #162200], Alexander disease [MIM #203450]). Such cases may present as sporadic occurrences in families (see Fig. 3–1E) and may not be recognized to involve hereditary factors if the phenotypes resemble nongenetic diseases. New mutations that are point mutations result from DNA replication/repair errors and frequently occur in germ cells of males with advanced age (e.g., paternal age effect observed in achondroplasia).

Mosaicism refers to the mixture of two or more different cell populations carrying either heterozygous mutant or homozygous normal alleles in the somatic cells generated by de novo mutations during mitosis. It is clinically significant when somatic mutations occur early in organogenesis and the organs comprise a reasonable ratio of mutant cells. Somatic mosaicism may not result in a phenotype, but its presence in germ line cells (gonadal mosaicism) may cause recurrence of affected offspring despite the parents' having no detectable mutation in DNA isolated from blood (see Fig. 3–1F). In the case of

Duchenne muscular dystrophy (MIM #310200), somatic mosaicism can account for a recurrence rate up to approximately 15%. A single somatic mutation may result in a tumor-associated phenotype when it arises in the context of an existing cellular recessive mutation on the other allele ("two-hit" model).[7] *NF1* and *RB1* mutations in neurofibromatosis type 1 (MIM #162200) and retinoblastoma (MIM #180200), respectively, are representative examples of cellular recessive mutations in dominantly inherited disorders that require somatic mutation events to manifest the phenotype.

Penetrance and Expressivity

We often observe differences in the severity of clinical manifestation within a pedigree (intrafamilial variablity) or between different pedigrees (interfamilial variability). *Penetrance* is a term that describes the proportion of individuals with the disease allele that present with any manifestations of the disorder. If one observes individuals who have genotypes that usually result in disease but are present with no sign of disorder over a lifetime, the condition is referred to as nonpenetrant. A family with nonpenetrant individuals may represent reduced penetrance.

The use of these terms is sometimes confusing. *Expressivity* illustrates the range of phenotypic expression in individuals who carry an identical mutation. Variation in age of onset may be included in the expressivity, but it may also be considered as age-dependent penetrance.[1] In the strictest sense, penetrance is qualitative (step function) while expressivity is quantitative and reflects variability in degree (continuous function).

NONMENDELIAN INHERITANCE

Mitochondrial Inheritance

In addition to the nuclear genome, mitochondria contain DNA that transmits genetic information to subsequent generations. Because of the cytoplasmic localization and high copy number of mitochondria, mitochondrial DNA (mtDNA) or the mitochondrial genome has a unique inheritance pattern (see Chapter 14). MtDNA is a circular genome of approximately 16.6 kilobase pairs (kb) located within the mitochondrial matrix in the cytoplasm of the cell. It encodes 13 polypeptides of subunits of the mitochondrial respiratory chain and oxidative phosphorylation system, 2 rRNAs, and 22 tRNAs. Each human cell contains hundreds of mitochondria, and each mitochondrion contains 5 to 10 mitochondrial genomes.

Traits that result from mtDNA mutations show a specific segregation pattern in a pedigree referred to as *maternal inheritance* (see Fig. 3–1 G). This is due to the fact that the ovum supplies the total complement of mtDNA, while there are effectively no mitochondria that can be transmitted from sperm. However, rare examples of paternal inheritance of mitochondrial mutations have been reported. Thus, paternal inheritance should be considered when no mutations were found in the maternal mtDNA.[8] Disorders resulting from mtDNA mutations can have tremendous variability in clinical expression because such mutations may present as a mixed intracellular population of mutant and normal molecules. This is referred to as *heteroplasmy,* wherein different tissues may have a different percentage of a mutant mitochondrial genome. In contrast, the condition wherein all mtDNA in a cell or organ represent either wild-type or mutant mtDNA is referred to as *homoplasmy.* Furthermore, during mitotic growth, the large number of mtDNA can result in asymmetric distribution of mutant versus normal copies (replicative segregation). Thus, the heteroplasmy ratio may change over time and the percentage of a mutant mtDNA in different cell lineages can be directed toward homoplasmy of either mutant or wild-type mtDNA. Moreover, different tissues have different requirements for the energy generated by oxidative phosphorylation, which contributes further to the tremendous clinical heterogeneity of mitochondrial disorders. Each of these variant features presents a significant challenge for genetic counseling in such families.

Imprinting

Genetics of Imprinting

Genomic imprinting refers to parent-of-origin effects on gene expression and may result from parental-origin–dependent methylation of CpG sites in DNA that result in a gene being transcribed from only one parental allele (monoallelic expression).[9] There have been approximately 50 imprinted genes identified in humans, and such genes continue to be described. These genes tend to cluster in particular chromosomal regions called "imprinted domains" and are likely to be involved in growth, behavior, and placental development. Imprinting can be uniform in all cells in the body or it can be tissue-specific. The effects of genomic imprinting become evident as clinical phenotypes when a lack of expression of one of these genes occurs (due to deletion, mutation, or other genetic defect) or one of these genes is overexpressed (due to duplication, relaxation of imprinting, or loss of imprinting control).[10] In families with such diseases, phenotypic expression depends on which parent transmitted the gene or allele responsible for the trait.

An inheritance pattern in which expression of a disease depends on which parent transmitted the mutant allele is referred to as a *parent-of-origin effect.* Pedigrees in Figure 3–1 *H, I* show families with defects in a maternally or paternally imprinted gene, respectively. In the former family, the gene is only expressed when inherited from the father and a mutant allele transmitted from mother is inactive. Therefore, the disease phenotype is only apparent when the mutant allele is inherited from the father. Similarly, in the latter family, the gene is expressed only when inherited from the mother. Thus, a mutant allele transmitted from the father is inactive. Of note, a female who inherited a paternally imprinted allele will switch this allele to a maternal imprint when she transmits it to her offspring. Likewise, a male who inherited a maternally imprinted allele will switch to the paternal imprint when he transmits it to his offspring. This reflects the fact that although imprinting is strictly maintained through numerous somatic cell divisions required to generate a human body, it is reversed during gametogenesis. Thus, an imprint from the previous generation is erased and a new imprint that is appropriate to the gender is established in either spermatogenesis or oogenesis.

Mechanisms for Imprinting

Imprinting is an epigenetic marking placed on certain genes or genomic regions as a result of passage through male or female gametogenesis for which the biochemical processes remain largely unknown. To date, allele-specific DNA methylation at the cytosine residue in CpG dinucleotides has been identified in the genomic regions adjacent to the majority of imprinted genes and has been proposed as the most likely candidate for a primary role in the regulation of imprinting. It is apparent from observations and analyses of mice lacking DNA methyltransferase that DNA methylation is necessary for maintaining the allelic difference of imprinted genes in somatic cells.[11] In addition, DNA methylation possibly plays a role as an initial mark to establish an imprint in gametes.

Several events must occur in the normal course of imprinting.[9,10] First, the imprint from the previous generation (one maternally and one paternally imprinted chromosome) that has been strictly maintained is erased in the germline cells. Second, a new imprint that is suitable for the sex of the gamete is established (i.e., only maternally imprinted chromosomes in oogenesis and only paternally imprinted chromosomes in spermatogenesis). Third, the complete genome with an appropriate imprint is transmitted to the zygote. Fourth, alleles with maternal and paternal imprints are stably inherited through somatic cell division in embryogenesis. Fifth, imprinting is properly inherited and maintained in the somatic cells that require monoallelic expression in a parent-of-origin specific manner. Failure in any of these requirements for the process of imprinting may in turn result in a human disorder or developmental error.[9,10]

Imprinting and Neuropsychiatric Disorders

Prader-Willi syndrome (PWS; MIM #176270) and Angelman syndrome (AS; MIM #105830) are phenotypically distinct neurobehavior syndromes that result from mutations in chromosome 15q11.2–q13, a region in which a number of imprinted genes are localized. PWS is

characterized by hypotonia and failure to thrive in infancy, small hands and feet, hypogonadism, mild mental retardation, and obesity. AS is characterized by developmental delay including absence of speech, severe mental retardation, ataxia with jerky arm movements, hyperactivity, seizures, aggressive behavior, and excessive inappropriate laughter. PWS results from loss of the paternal contribution of genes in the 15q11.2–q13 region, whereas AS is caused by failure of a maternal contribution of the same region. In both disorders, a large chromosomal deletion that spans 4.0 to 4.5 megabases (Mb) in 15q11.2–q13 has been identified in 60% to 70% of patients. A deletion in the paternally derived chromosome 15 results in PWS, and the same deletion in the maternally derived chromosome 15 causes AS.

An alternative mechanism resulting in absence of one parental contribution at a specific locus is to inherit both copies of a homologous pair from one parent. This is referred to as *uniparental disomy* (UPD). UPD accounts for 20% to 30% of PWS patients and approximately 5% of AS patients. UPD of maternal chromosome 15 results in a lack of a paternal contribution, causing PWS. Conversely, UPD of paternal chromosome 15 results in a lack of a maternal contribution, causing AS. Rare balanced chromosomal translocations involving paternally derived chromosome 15 also cause PWS. In approximately 10% of patients with AS, the disease results from maternally derived intragenic mutations in the *UBE3A* gene, which encodes ubiquitin ligase. No such single gene mutation has been found in PWS to date. These findings suggest that AS is a single-gene disorder owing to loss of maternal expression of *UBE3A*, whereas PWS likely results from lack of two or more contiguous paternally expressed genes. These genetic abnormalities for PWS and AS can be categorized as defects in the transmission of the imprinted genome to the embryo. In addition, in approximately 5% of PWS and AS patients, the disease results from imprinting defects in which uniparental DNA methylation and gene expression occur despite biparental chromosome inheritance. Some patients with imprinting defects have submicroscopic deletions of a genetic element termed the *imprinting center*. It is hypothesized that a defective imprinting center results in a failure of erasure and re-establishment of imprinting. However, studies reveal that the molecular mechanisms underlying imprinting center mutation are more complex than initially thought and require further exploration.[12]

Uniparental Disomy as a Mechanism for Disease

According to Mendel's first law, only one of two "factors" in a parent is transmitted to the next generation. UPD is an exception to this segregation rule. As mentioned in the previous section, UPD describes chromosomal inheritance of both copies of homologous chromosomes from only one parent.[13,14] Because UPD maintains numerical and structural features of diploid chromosomes, it may not always be associated with a phenotype unless additional genetic components (such as imprinting or a recessive allele) occur on the same chromosome. Thus, UPD may be more frequent than we observe because it may not produce a recognizable clinical phenotype.

Recessive Diseases in Isodisomy

When UPD results from two copies of a single chromosome homologue that was present in one biologic parent, this condition is referred to as *uniparental isodisomy*. In contrast, *heterodisomy* is the inheritance of the two different chromosomes for one homologous pair derived from one parent. Consequently, in the isodisomic condition, a homozygous allele for a recessive mutation can be transmitted from a heterozygous carrier parent, resulting in a nonmendelian inheritance pattern for a recessive mutation. At least 22 such diseases have been reported in which UPD results in reduction to homozygosity for a recessive mutation. These include UPD 5 and UPD X isodisomy causing spinal muscular atrophy (MIM #253300) and Duchenne muscular dystrophy, respectively.[15] UPD has been observed for almost all chromosomes, and for some chromosomes a specific phenotype is manifested.[15] However, this UPD phenomenon can theoretically occur for each chromosome and be responsible for any recessive disease condition.

UPD and Imprinted Genes

Parental-origin–specific monoallelic expression or imprinting occurs for several human chromosomal regions. UPD of these chromosomal regions leads to alteration of the normal imprinting pattern and can result in chromosome-specific and parental-origin–specific syndromes. As described in the previous section, maternal UPD of chromosome 15 (mUPD15) results in PWS, whereas paternal UPD of chromosome 15 (pUPD15) causes AS. UPD of imprinted loci also results in other genetic disorders including transient neonatal diabetes (pUPD6), Russell-Silver syndrome (MIM #180860, mUPD7), and Beckwith-Wiedemann syndrome (MIM #130650, pUPD11). UPD14 presents with a different phenotype depending on the parental origin: paternal UPD14 yields short stature and precocious puberty, while maternal UPD14 results in dwarfism, skeletal dysplasia, and thoracic narrowing.[15]

Chromosomal Mechanisms for UPD

Four distinct mechanisms were originally proposed to potentially result in UPD, and each has been later recognized.[14] Understanding of these mechanisms is important as each results in a different form of UPD: isodisomy/heterodisomy and uniform/mosaic.

Trisomy Rescue. Meiotic nondisjunction often results in a disomic gamete. Fusion of a disomic gamete with a normal gamete results in a trisomic zygote that is often spontaneously aborted unless the supernumerary chromosome is removed early during development. Of the zygotes that survive by trisomy rescue, statistically one third will have UPD (Fig. 3–2B). As most nondisjunction occurs in meiosis I, heterodisomic UPD is more common in this mechanism. Because trisomic cells can often persist in somatic tissue, mosaicism may be variable. This mechanism, such as that seen in nondisjunction trisomy 21 causing Down syndrome, is often associated with advanced maternal age. Familial or de novo Robertsonian translocations may also result in UPD via trisomy rescue.

Monosomy Rescue. Fertilization of a nullisomic germ cell with a normal gamete results in a monosomic zygote, which is usually lethal unless complemented by postzygotic duplication of a monosomic chromosome. UPD by this mechanism results in isodisomy. Mosaicism is unlikely, due to the lethality of monosomic somatic cells (see Fig. 3–2C).

Gamete Complementation. UPD can result from fusion of chromosomally complementary gametes (e.g., an egg with a duplication of a chromosome and a sperm missing the same chromosome) In this mechanism, the resulting zygote inherits two heterozygous chromosomes from one parent and is heterodisomic (see Fig. 3–2D).

Postfertilization Errors. UPD may derive from a normal biparental disomic zygote. Loss of one chromosome resulting from mitotic nondisjunction can be repaired by mitotic duplication of a chromosome (endoduplication), which leads to isodisomic UPD.

In addition, fertilization and early postfertilization errors resulting in UPD of entire chromosomes or segmental UPD can occur in somatic cells. Somatic interchromosomal recombination events (reciprocal homologous recombination or gene conversion) result in segmental UPD (see Fig. 3–2E). This somatic UPD is often present in a mosaic state. Such mechanisms can contribute to somatic loss-of-heterozygosity or loss-of-imprinting associated with some cancers, in addition to inherited diseases showing mosaicism.

CHROMOSOMAL INHERITANCE AND CHROMOSOMAL DISORDERS

In contrast to mendelian diseases in which alteration or mutation at a single locus, and usually within a single gene, is responsible for the disease phenotype, chromosomal disorders may involve loss or gain of an entire chromosome or a portion of a chromosome that usually contains multiple genes. There are 23 pairs of different chromosomes. Abnormalities in segregation of each member of the pair in

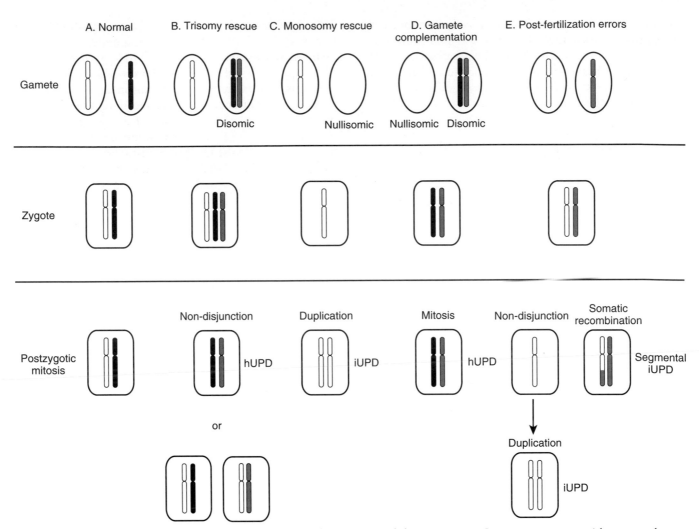

FIGURE 3–2. Schematic models of molecular mechanisms for uniparental disomy (UPD). Gametes may carry either normal (monosomic) or abnormal (nullisomic or disomic) chromosomes. Each chromosome originated in gametes is shown in a different shade *(white, shaded, and black)*. Isodisomy (iUPD; *chromosomes with same color)* and heterodisomy (hUPD; *chromosomes with different shades)* are shown. A, Normal zygote; B, Trisomy rescue (one third of rescued zygotes may result in UPD); C, Monosomy rescue; D, Gamete complementation; E, Postzygotic errors (monosomy resulting from mitotic nondisjunction may be rescued by duplication, while mitotic recombination may lead to formation of segmental isodisomy).

either meiosis or mitosis may result in genetic disorders that display distinct modes of inheritance.

A metaphase spread is used to identify specific chromosomes. In metaphase, the chromosomes are completely compacted in mitosis and can be visualized when stained with specific dyes. Giemsa or G-banding is commonly used in clinical cytogenetics laboratories. The average number of G bands that can be resolved in metaphase chromosomes is 400 to 500 bands per haploid set. In a high-resolution prometaphase chromosome banding analysis, up to 1000 bands can be resolved.

Fluorescent in situ hybridization (FISH) is a powerful cytogenetic technique used to investigate specific genomic regions of chromosomes in greater detail by hybridizing a fluorescent-labeled DNA probe of interest. FISH is continuously gaining widespread clinical applicability. Telomere FISH can simultaneously examine the

presence of subtelomeric deletions using a set of probes specific to the telomere for each chromosome arm. Using telomere FISH, reports identify abnormalities in greater than 5% of samples from patients with mental retardation whose previous G-banding karyotypes were normal. Detection of a balanced translocation carrier in such a family enables accurate recurrent risk and prenatal diagnosis.

Other technologies that will likely be applied clinically in the near future strive to gain better resolution of the human genome in specific patients. These include *comparative genome hybridization* to compare a patient sample with a normal control to evaluate for loss or gain of genetic information, and *genome microarrays* to interrogate multiple genomic regions simultaneously.

Chromosomal disorders can be classified into four major groups: aneuploidy; translocations; rearrangements including deletion, duplication, and inversion; and isochromosome formation. Constitutional chromosome rearrangements are usually observed in 100% of the cells when they are inherited from parents or occur in gametes. Alternatively, mosaicism of two or more different karyotypes may be observed in an individual when the chromosomes were rearranged in somatic cells during mitosis.

Aneuploidy

Chromosome aneuploidy is defined as a complement with an abnormal number of chromosomes. Trisomy refers to three copies of a single chromosome or the one extra chromosome. The most common trisomy in live births is for chromosome 21, which is associated with a Down syndrome phenotype (MIM #190685—karyotype 47,XX+21 in females or 47,XY+21 in males). This occurs in approximately 1:660 live births, making this a much more frequently observed mutational mechanism than alteration at a single locus. There is an increased frequency of trisomy with advanced maternal age. Monosomy refers to the absence of one chromosome from the pair. Monosomy is most frequently observed for the sex chromosomes, most notably the 45,X karyotype associated with Turner syndrome. Sex chromosome aneuploids, such as 47,XXY and 47,XXX, are relatively common occurring at a frequency of approximately 1:1000 live births. However, because at least 90% of 45,X conceptuses are spontaneously aborted, the incidence of this aneuploidy is only 1:5000. Marker chromosomes are small additional structurally abnormal chromosomes often derived from chromosomes X, 15, and 22.

Translocations

Translocation is an exchange of chromosomal segments or whole arms between two (or more, in rare cases) different chromosomes. The most frequent type is robertsonian translocations. These are whole-arm exchanges between the acrocentric chromosomes (chromosomes 13, 14, 15, 21, and 22), which are found in 1:1000 individuals. In contrast, reciprocal translocations, a segmental exchange between two chromosomes, are mostly unique and appear to occur randomly at any location and on all chromosomes. Translocation carriers who have the proper amount of genetic information (balanced translocation) have no abnormal clinical phenotype unless the translocation breakpoint disrupts a gene(s) that result in a phenotype(s). Such patients with a balanced translocation and an associated disease phenotype are extremely rare, but potentially enable the identification of a disease gene. Identification of the *DMD* gene is one such example. Translocation may also cause a single-gene disease through a position effect by disturbing the normal regulation of a gene close to the breakpoint.[16] Translocations with breakpoints at a 15- to 250-kb distance from the sonic hedgehog (*SHH*) gene may suppress *SHH* transcription by a *position effect* and result in holoprosencephaly (MIM #142945).

Individuals with balanced translocations are at a high risk of transmitting a chromosome with missing or excess genetic information and conceiving a child with an unbalanced karyotype. Balanced translocation carriers are frequent in the population, occurring in about 1:550 to 1:625 individuals. This mechanism should be clinically considered when a couple has had three or more spontaneous abortions or a history of infertility.

Deletion, Duplication, and Inversion

Deletion, duplication, and inversion are intrachromosomal rearrangements of particular segments within a single chromosome, resulting from strand exchange between either two homologous chromosomes or two sister chromatids.

Deletions can be terminal (at the end of the chromosome) or interstitial. Large deletions are usually lethal; only microdeletions are clinically relevant. Well-recognized terminal deletion syndromes include monosomy 1p (del(1)(p36.3), Wolf-Hirschhorn syndrome (MIM #194190, del(4)(p16), Cri-du-chat syndrome (MIM #123450, del(5)(p15), Jacobsen syndrome (MIM #147791, del(11)(q23), and Miller-Dieker lissencephaly syndrome (MIM #247200, del(17)(p13.3). Moreover, as mentioned earlier, microdeletions of telomeric termini appear to play a role in the etiology of idiopathic mental retardation. Terminal deletions have been identified for each chromosome. The size of each deletion appears to vary in different individuals. Some terminal deletions occur more frequently than others. This may reflect the relative viability of monosomy for the region or may result from the underlying genomic structure that leads to rearrangement susceptibility.

In contrast, interstitial deletions and their reciprocal duplications appear to occur recurrently in specific segments of human chromosomes and have been associated with a number of syndromes presenting behavioral and neurologic phenotypes (Table 3–1). Common disorders associated with interstitial deletion include Williams-Beuren syndrome (MIM #194050, del(7) (q11.23q 11.23)), PWS (pat del(15)(q11.2q13)), AS (mat del(15) (q11.2q13)), Smith-Magenis syndrome (MIM #182290, del(17)(p11.2p11.2)), hereditary neuropathy with liability to pressure palsy (MIM #162500, del(17)(p12p12)), and DiGeorge syndrome/velocardiofacial syndrome (MIM #188400, del(22)(q11.2q11.2)). Interstitial duplications, some of which have recently been recognized as the reciprocal to the deletions, have been observed in disorders such as Russell Silver syndrome (dup(7)(p12p13)), autistic syndrome (mat inv dup(15)(q11.2q13)), dup 17p11.2 syndrome (dup(17) (p11.2p11.2)), Charcot-Marie-Tooth disease type 1A (MIM #118220, dup(17)(p12p12)), Pelizaeus-Merzbacher disease (MIM #312080, dup(X)

TABLE 3–1. Behavioral Phenotypes in Genomic Disorders

Syndromes	Deletion/Duplication	Behavioral Phenotype
Williams-Beuren	del(7)(q11.23 q11.23)	gregarious and loquacious behavior, impaired visuospatial recognition
Prader-Willi	pat del(15)(q11.2 q13)	hyperphagia, oppositional, mood instability, skin picking, puzzle solving
Angelman	mat del(15)(q11.2 q13)	hyperactivity, agressive behavior, paroxysmal laughter, "happy" faces
Smith-Magenis	del(17)(p11.2 p11.2)	self-injurious and aggressive behavior, self-hugging, attention seeking, onychotillomania, polyembolokoilamania
DiGeorge/VCFS	del(22)(q11.2 q11.2)	obsessive behavior and schizophreniform disorders
Autistic disorder	mat inv dup(15) (q11.2 q13)	motor coordination deficit, intellectual impairment, atypical autistic disorder
Anxiety neurosis	dup(15)(q24 q26)	panic disorder, agoraphobia, social phobia, joint laxity

VCFS = velocardiofacial syndrome, del = deletion, dup = duplication, pat = paternal, mat = maternal, inv = inversion.
Adapted from Shaffer LG, Ledbetter DH, Lupski JR: Molecular cytogenetics of contiguous gene syndromes: Mechanisms and consequences of gene dosage imbalance. In Scriver CR, Beaudet AL, Sly WS, Vallel (eds): The Metabolic and Molecular Basis of Inherited Diseases. New York, McGraw-Hill, 2001, pp 1291–1324.

(q22.2q22.2), and panic and phobic disorder with joint laxity (MIM #167870; dup(15)(q24q26). The abnormal karyotype due to deletions and duplications are also called segmental aneuploidy, or partial monosomy and partial trisomy, respectively.

The genomic segments that are deleted or duplicated appear to contain multiple genes. Phenotypic consequences for deletions may result from monoallelic gene deficiencies (haploinsufficiency), whereas those for duplications result from excess gene copies. Based on the fact that the phenotype observed in disorders caused by chromosomal deletion or duplication was thought to result from the effects of several genes that happen to be contiguous in the genome, these conditions have been called contiguous gene syndromes. However, recent studies have revealed that the disease-specific phenotypes are associated with a small number of genes, or even a single gene, that are sensitive to dosage alterations (dosage-sensitive genes).[17]

In general, chromosome microdeletion of a genomic segment has more profound phenotypic consequences than duplication of the same segment. One exception to this trend is CMT1A and HNPP. Increased gene dosage of the *PMP22* gene by CMT1A duplication results in a progressive demyelinating neuropathy, whereas haploinsufficiency of *PMP22* by HNPP deletion results in an episodic milder neuropathy. Similarly, a more severe phenotype is observed in Pelizaeus-Merzbacher disease patients with *PLP1* duplications than those with *PLP1* deletions.

Inversion is an intrachromosomal rearrangement generated by chromosomal breaks at two locations and "flipping" of the internal chromosomal segment. Inversions that involve the centromere are termed *pericentric inversions,* whereas those occurring within single chromosomal arms are termed *paracentric inversions.* Both types of inversions are usually balanced and thus result in no phenotypic manifestation. Homologous pairs

of chromosomes with an inversion may have a greater chance of generating a gamete with an unbalanced chromosome by misalignment at the inverted segment in meiosis followed by recombination within the inverted segments.

Isochromosomes

An isochromosome is a mirror-image abnormal chromosome consisting of two copies of either a short arm or a long arm, often observed for X and acrocentric chromosomes. Isochromosome X is the most common (approximately 1:13,000) and accounts for more than 15% of Turner syndrome patients. Isochromosome 21 can result in a trisomy 21 and Down syndrome. Both dicentric (two centromeres) and monocentric (one centromere) formations have been found. A U-type strand exchange between sister chromatids at the short arm (dicentric) or misdivision of centromere (monocentric) is likely the mechanism for the formation of isochromosomes.

Mechanism Underlying Chromosomal and Genomic Rearrangements

At least three general mechanisms have been identified that may result in chromosomal and genomic rearrangements; many other mechanisms to explain various chromosomal rearrangements remain to be elucidated.

Aneuploidy. Most chromosome aneuploidy results from nondisjunction of allelic chromosomes in maternal meiosis.[18] Meiosis consists of one chromosome replication ($2n$ to $4n$) and two contiguous cell divisions ($4n$ to $2n$, then $2n$ to $1n$). The first division separates homologous chromosomes from each other (meiosis I), followed by the second division that separates sister chromatids (meiosis II), resulting in a haploid set of 23 chromosomes. Most aneuploidy formation occurs in meiosis I with complete nondisjunction of both homologous chromosomes, resulting in a 4:0 segregation. Genetic examination of maternal meiosis revealed that a reduced recombination is associated with susceptibility to trisomy formation.[19] Chromosomes with a low recombination frequency typically possess no recombination (achiasmate bivalent) or contain only one strand exchange (chiasma formation) with disproportionate localization at the distal end. Evidence in model organisms such as yeast and the fruit fly support that these two factors, absent or reduced recombination and suboptimally positioned chiasma formation, appear to increase the susceptibility to nondisjunction.[18]

Maternal age is a significant risk factor for trisomies, but the underlying mechanisms have been a mystery. One hypothesis favors relaxed selection in the uterine environment in older-age mothers, which may allow nondisjunction zygotes to be conceived and to escape abortion. Alternatively, recent studies revealed that the increased risk of nondisjunction in advanced-age pregnancies was associated only with chromosome of maternal origin, but no such effect was seen in paternal nondisjunction.[18] These findings suggest that the egg is the source of the age effect. Indeed, human female gametes are arrested in the dictyotene stage of meiosis since before birth, and nondisjunction has been postulated to result from breakdown of meiotic processes over prolonged time periods.

Translocations. Molecular mechanisms for interchromosomal translocations remain largely unknown. Most of these constitutional chromosomal translocations are unique to each individual and, therefore, it is difficult to investigate the mechanism for the recombination at the molecular level. In contrast, some recurrent translocations, including robertsonian translocations between chromosomes 13 and 14 (rob(13q14q)), as well as those between chromosome 14 and 21 (rob(14q21q)), and the reciprocal translocation between chromosome 11 and 22 (t(11;22)(q23;q11.2)), are likely associated with certain genomic architectural features that predispose to frequent chromosome rearrangements.[20]

The presence of homologous repeat sequences has been proposed as a mechanism underlying the preferential formation of the two most common Robertsonian translocations. Detailed molecular analyses of t(11;22) revealed that breakpoints on chromosomes 11 and 22 are located in the center of palindromic AT-rich repeats on both chromosomes. Palindromic AT-rich repeats may form a DNA hairpin structure that may predispose these regions to DNA double-strand breaks and increase the susceptibility to DNA end-joining of chromosomes 11 and 22.

Interstitial Deletions, Duplications, and Inversions. Molecular mechanisms for interstitial chromosomal rearrangements are perhaps the best characterized inherited chromosomal disorders to date. Molecular studies of such DNA rearrangements have revealed the presence of a common mechanism underlying the susceptibility to the specific genomic rearrangements and solidified the concept of *genomic disorders.*

Genomic disorders refer to a group of genetic diseases caused by genomic rearrangements that result from unique genome architectural features.[21] De novo genomic rearrangements often observed in patients with genomic disorders are highly recurrent and frequent (approximately 1×10^{-4}). An identical rearrangement occurs independently in different individuals. In addition, each of these genomic abnormalities is recurrent in distinct world populations with no particular bias in ethnic background.

Each locus for a given genomic disorder has a characteristic genome architecture that influences the recombination events. Low-copy repeats (LCRs) are often present flanking the deleted or duplicated unique genomic segments. LCRs range from a few to several hundred kb in size and contain homologous sequences with high identity (usually higher than 97%). When two copies of LCRs (paralogues) are present in a tandem orientation in a chromosome, the high sequence homology between these paralogous LCRs may allow nonallelic copies to align during meiosis. Homologous recombination between these nonallelic paralogues may lead to an unequal crossing over that results in recombinant chromosomes with loss or gain of a unique genomic segment flanked by the LCRs (Fig. 3–3A). This recombination mechanism is referred to as *nonallelic homologous recombination* (NAHR).[22] Changes in the dosage of the genes located within these rearranged genomic segments are directly associated with the disease phenotype observed in genomic disorders.[17]

If paralogous LCRs are present in an inverted orientation, NAHR results in an inversion of the unique sequence genomic segment flanked by these LCRs (see Fig. 3–3B). An inversion does not alter the copy number of the rearranged genomic segment, but it may disrupt a gene that spans the recombination breakpoints. Some LCRs found in the human genome show a complex structure. They contain multiple modules with some units in a direct orientation and other units in an inverted orientation. Depending on which modules are used as substrates for NAHR, deletion/duplication (between tandem modules) or inversion (between inverted modules) may occur (see Fig. 3–3C).

Molecular studies of LCRs revealed further evidence to explain the mechanisms for genomic disorders. In addition to the fact that the LCRs associated with genomic disorders reveal extremely high sequence similarity, studies of recombination breakpoints within a few LCRs revealed clustering of the strand exchange to a small region of perfect sequence identity (>300 bp). These observations suggest not only that substantial regions of homology are required to facilitate NAHR, but also that

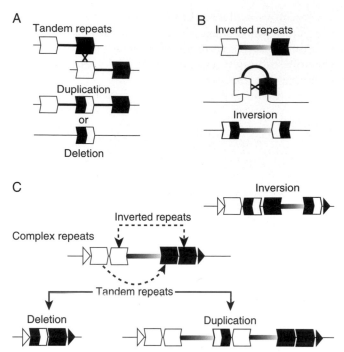

FIGURE 3–3. Schematic models of molecular mechanisms for meiotic nonallelic homologous recombination (NAHR) mediated by low-copy repeats (LCRs). *A,* Crossing over between aligned paralogous LCRs *(filled and open boxes)* in direct orientation result in reciprocal deletion and duplication. Resulting recombinant products reveal a loss or gain of unique genomic fragment flanked by LCRs *(thick line).* *B,* Recombination between inverted LCRs results in an inversion of the flanked genomic segment *(thick line with gradient for orientation),* but no gain or loss of the genomic segment is observed. *C,* A combination of direct and inverted modules constitutes a composite LCR. In such cases, recombination product may vary, depending on which portion of the unit is used in the strand exchange. Deletion/duplication may result from recombination between tandem modules, whereas inversion may occur if inverted modules are used for recombination.

a certain length of perfect sequence match is necessary for efficient NAHR. Moreover, nucleotide sequence spanning the recombination junctions revealed that DNA double-strand breaks likely initiate the NAHR.[17] Thus, molecular investigations indicate that common architectural features of the human genome predispose to genomic rearrangements that lead to genomic disorders.

LCRs are abundantly present in the human genome, and account for at least 5% to 10% of genome sequence. Significant sequence identity (>97%) throughout the LCRs, regardless of exons, introns, or nongenic regions, indicates that the LCRs evolved recently during primate speciation. In addition, LCRs appear to be enriched in humans compared with lower organisms such as yeast or fruit flies. Consequently, primate genome evolution appears to contribute to the formation of the genome architecture that provides the underlying basis for the pathogenesis of genomic disorders.[23]

Terminal Deletions. Most terminal deletions occur randomly, at least at the chromosomal level, and the underlying molecular mechanisms are largely unknown except for a few disorders. One such example is del(11)(q23) associated with Jacobsen syndrome in which chromosomal fragile-sites play a role in the terminal deletions. Two Jacobsen syndrome breakpoints were exactly mapped at the CCG repeat–associated folate-sensitive fragile site *FRA11B,* and other breakpoints appeared to colocalize with other regions containing CCG repeats clustered on chromosomes 11q23.3–q24. These findings suggest the potential role of genome instability at CCG repeats as a mechanism for chromosome breakage.[24]

REPEAT EXPANSION DISORDERS

We assume that with mendelian traits a mutation in a gene is stable during the transmission to succeeding generations and the resulting phenotype is similar in offspring. Inheritance observed in the repeat expansion disorders, in which unstable expansion of tandem nucleotide repeats results in different disease phenotypes, is a challenge to this principle. To date, 19 such disorders have been identified. Most of them are associated with expansion of trinucleotide repeats, except for a few that are caused by expansion of tetra-, penta- and dodecanucleotide repeats (see Chapters 1 and 12 for details of each disorder). Although pedigrees with repeat expansion disorders reveal a monogenic inheritance pattern, some features are present that do not correspond to classic mendelian inheritance.

Anticipation

In some families, affected individuals in successive generations may present with a more severe disease phenotype at an earlier age of onset compared to their affected predecessors. This phenomenon is termed *anticipation.* Anticipation is associated with the instability of repeat length accompanying repeat expansion. The repeats tend to increase in number through the transmission from parent to offspring. The longer repeats usually correlate with a more severe disease phenotype and earlier age of onset. Anticipation is also associated with expressivity in a family. Phenotypic manifestations may dramatically change between generations with anticipation, as observed in myotonic dystrophy type 1 (MIM #160900) and Huntington disease (MIM #143100).

Unstable Repeats in Normal and Disease Populations

Normal-sized alleles of these disease-causing repeats are polymorphic in the general population and are stably transmitted in both meiosis and mitosis. However, in some clinically unaffected individuals, the number of repeats appears to exceed beyond the normal range of the general population in a state called *premutation*. Premutations show both somatic and germline instability and often can be found in the phenotypically normal antecedent of patients in a pedigree. Premutations often develop into full mutations that contain larger repeat expansions and cause disease phenotypes. For example, in Fragile X syndrome (MIM #309550), a CGG repeat in the 5′ untranslated region of the *FMR1* gene on Xq27.3 ranges in size from approximately 5 to 44 repeat units in the normal population. There is a gray zone or inconclusive range of approximately 45 to 54 repeats, which may correspond to large normal alleles or to unstable premutations in some families. The premutation range for *FMR1* is between approximately 55 and 200 repeats, while full mutations exceed 230 repeats, often expanding from hundreds to thousands of repeats with hypermethylation typically present. The large expansion of the CGG repeats is chromosomally expressed as a folate-sensitive fragile site, *FRAXA*, on the X chromosome. Of note, a subset of individuals with premutations displays unique phenotypes, including late-onset progressive intention tremor, ataxia, and cognitive decline.

Repeat expansions can be found in untranslated regions (UTR) of genes (3′ distal UTR, 5′ proximal UTR, introns, and antisense sequence). These may also occur within the coding sequences, such as CAG polyglutamine repeats in autosomal dominant spinocerebellar ataxias.[25] Disorders in the former group usually reveal multisystemic involvement and greater repeat instability. For example, the autosomal recessive disorder Friedreich ataxia (MIM #229300) is caused mostly by homozygous expansions of an intronic GAA triplet repeat in the *FRDA* gene. Premutations usually consist of approximately 34 to 65 repeats, and expansions typically number in the hundreds of repeats. Expansion to full mutations with 300 to 650 repeats has been observed in a single transmission. Expanded CTG repeats in *DMPK*, the causative gene for DM1, reveal extreme somatic variability in repeat length. The tetranucleotide CCTG repeat expansion in an intron of the *ZNF9* gene for myotonic dystrophy type 2 (MIM #602668) can increase 500 repeats over 3 years in a single individual.[26] In contrast, diseases resulting from repeat expansions in the coding regions are characterized by progressive neurodegeneration and by a smaller magnitude of repeat instability, probably owing to the selective pressure against very large expansion that is likely to become embryonically lethal.

Parent-of-origin effects on anticipation are often obvious and associated with a sex difference in the repeat instability. Paternal intergenerational instability is more common, whereas Fragile X syndrome, Friedreich ataxia, and myotonic dystrophy type 1 usually reveal greater repeat instability on maternal transmission. Although the exact molecular basis of this parental origin effect is unknown, rare observations of large expansions from opposite parents suggest the presence of mitotic large expansions in the germline of both sexes and negative selection of longer repeats in either sperms or oocytes that result in the gender effect of preferential repeat expansion.

Linkage Disequilibrium and Founder Mutations in Repeat Expansion Disorders

In some repeat expansion disorders, expanded repeat alleles often associate with certain haplotypes of nearby genetic markers on the disease chromosome more frequently than expected by chance, indicating the presence of *linkage disequilibrium* (LD). LD results from one (or more) chromosome(s) with ancestral mutations that were distributed in the particular population as a common disease allele. This condition is referred to as a *founder effect*. Myotonic dystrophy type 1 shows complete LD both in white and Japanese individuals, suggesting a common Eurasian founder mutation. Huntington disease also reveals multiple founder alleles that result in strong LD in different populations. Machado-Joseph disease (MIM #109150), the most frequent spinocerebellar ataxia, appeared to originate from the Azorean islands in Portugal and spread throughout the world. In fact, many sporadic cases of repeat expansion diseases are not new mutations. Rather, they are likely new full mutations expanded from inherited founder chromosomes that carry premutations. This represents a sharp contrast to genomic disorders wherein many sporadic cases are de novo mutations and no founder mutations exist.

MULTIGENIC INHERITANCE

Mendelian traits segregate with mutations in one or both alleles of a single gene that in itself is sufficient to express the disease phenotype. In contrast, complex traits appear to result from multifactorial interaction of various susceptibility genes and environmental exposures; thus the role of a single gene may not be fundamental. The concept of multigenic inheritance was solidified when it appeared that some diseases have primarily a genetic etiology, but involve two or more genes in their pathophysiology.

Dilemmas in Genotype-Phenotype Correlations in Mendelian Traits

Following the identification of mendelian disease genes, enormous efforts of mutation analyses have been carried out in search of genotype-phenotype correlations enabling prognostic information and potentially influencing management decisions. Except for a limited number of disease alleles, the vast majority of mendelian diseases have failed to establish robust and reproducible precise genotype-phenotype correlations. These findings have suggested that, even in a disease that is inherited as a simple mendelian trait, phenotypic manifestations are likely modified by other factors.

Phenylketonuria (MIM #261600) is a classic example of genotype-phenotype discordance in a monogenic mendelian autosomal recessive disorder.[27] In patients with phenylketonuria, homozygous mutations in the phenylalanine hydroxylase gene *(PAH)* result in a deficient enzyme activity of liver PAH. This leads to hyperphenylalaninemia, which has a toxic effect on brain development and function, therefore causing mental retardation. Thus, phenylketonuria is composed of genotype (mutations), enzymatic phenotype (PAH activity), metabolic phenotype (blood phenylalanine level), and cognitive phenotype (IQ). At each level, various cofactors that modulate the phenotype are likely present and may result in the inconsistency of genotype-phenotype correlations.

Intrafamilial variability (same genotype but different phenotype within a family) and interfamilial variability (same genotype but different phenotype among different families) have been observed in many other diseases, including Gaucher disease (MIM #231005), Charcot-Marie-Tooth disease, and Wolfram syndrome (MIM #222300).[28]

Modifier Genes in Mendelian and Nonmedelian Diseases

In some cases, genetic factors that modify the phenotype have been isolated by recent molecular and genetic approaches.[29] Cystic fibrosis (MIM #219700) demonstrated an insufficient correlation between *CFTR* mutations and clinical phenotype. A genetic approach was used to isolate some modifier loci or genes. These modifier loci include the *CFM1* locus on 19q13 for meconium ileus susceptibility, low-expressing mannose-binding lectin gene *(MBL)*, HLA class II polymorphisms, tumor necrosis factor alpha gene *(TNFA)*, transforming growth factor B1 gene *(TGFB1)* for the pulmonary phenotype, nitric oxide synthase 1 *(NOS1)* for microbial infection, and mucin for gastrointestinal aspects.[29]

Familial amyotrophic lateral sclerosis accounts for approximately 15% to 20% of amyotrophic lateral sclerosis. Of those, approximately 20% of patients are associated with mutations in the superoxide dismutase 1 gene *(SOD1)* as an autosomal dominant trait with almost complete penetrance. In a family with *SOD1* mutation, a patient who also has homozygous mutation in the ciliary neurotrophic factor gene *(CNTF)* revealed an early onset with rapid disease course.[30] Moreover, transgenic mice with the human *SOD1*-G93A mutation crossed with *Cntf*-deficient mice had an earlier onset than wild-type mice. Also, human patients with sporadic amyotrophic lateral sclerosis who are homozygous for *CNTF* mutations likely show earlier onset than those with wild-type *CNTF*. Each of these observations suggests that CNTF is likely a modifier for age of onset of familial amyotrophic

lateral sclerosis and possibly of sporadic amyotrophic lateral sclerosis.[30] Independently, copy number of either survival motor neuron gene *SMN1* or *SMN2* (the former is responsible for spinal muscular atrophy and the latter modifies the severity of spinal muscular atrophy) were suggested as modifiers for sporadic amyotrophic lateral sclerosis.[31,32] Furthermore, a modifier locus for the amyotrophic lateral sclerosis phenotype in the G86R *SOD1* transgenic mouse was mapped to spinal muscular atrophy syntenic region on chromosomes 13, supporting the hypothesis of modifying effect of two motor neuron diseases.[33]

Digenic Inheritance

In addition to these modifier genes for mendelian traits, extensive mutational studies have identified examples in which coexistence of mutations in two independent genes was required to manifest a phenotype. In such families, the mode of inheritance is referred to as *digenic inheritance* (see Fig. 3–1J).

The first such example was found in families with retinitis pigmentosa (DFNB1, MIM #268000), a genetically and clinically heterogeneous disease. In three unrelated families, a combination of heterozygous mutations in two photoreceptor-specific genes *RDS* and *ROM1* appeared to result in retinitis pigmentosa, but either of the two mutations by itself did not result in symptoms.[34] Subsequent studies have found that *RDS* and *ROM1* proteins actually physically interact in the rod photoreceptor outer segment.[35]

A subset of patients with mutations of the most common locus for recessive nonsyndromic deafness (MIM #220290) have one mutation in the gap-junction protein connexin 26 gene *(GJB2)* and heterozygous genomic deletion containing the connexin 30 gene *(GJB6)*. This deletion maps within the DFNB1 locus adjacent to *GJB2* but leaves *GJB2* intact. Either the *GJB2* mutation or the *GJB6* deletion acts as a monogenic autosomal recessive trait, but digenic compound heterozygous mutations of *GJB2* and *GJB6* also play a major role in the etiology of DFNB1.[36]

Digenic inheritance was also observed in a family with severe insulin resistance and diabetes mellitus type 2. Individuals with hyperinsulinemia and severe insulin resistance appeared to carry compound heterozygous mutations for peroxisome proliferative activated receptor γ *(PPARG)* and protein phosphatase 1 regulatory subunit 3A *(PPP1R3A)*, whereas individuals with single heterozygous mutation of either gene revealed no phenotype or only a partial phenotype.[37]

A variation of digenic inheritance was recently described in Bardet-Biedl syndrome (MIM #209900), a genetically heterogeneous (7 loci identified to date) multisystemic disorder associated with retinitis pigmentosa, obesity, polydactyly, and mental retardation. In some families, mutations in three alleles at two loci are apparently necessary and sufficient to manifest a BBS phenotype. The term *triallelic inheritance* was proposed to describe this mode of inheritance.[38]

COMPLEX TRAITS

In common diseases such as multiple sclerosis, Alzheimer disease (AD), amyotrophic lateral sclerosis, Parkinson disease, ischemic stroke, migraine, epilepsy, autism, schizophrenia, and bipolar disorder, the contribution of heredity or genetic factors to disease etiology is apparent to a different degree. The role of hereditary influence is suggested by observations in increased disease coincidence in monozygotic twins and presence of familial aggregation of disease. However, the mode of inheritance is unclear and distinct from mendelian traits.

Common diseases have been thought to involve multiple environmental and genetic factors that influence the risk of an individual being affected. Environmental factors may exhibit a mixture of exogenous and endogenous aspects such as diet, body weight, habits, sex difference, drug exposure, pollution, climate, infection history, and other life events and circumstances. Genetic factors may include causative genes that provide a major impact on the expression of the disease phenotype, and susceptibility or protective genes that may confer or reduce different risks of developing disease.

Genetic Features of Complex Traits

Common diseases with complex traits present some features that are distinct from mendelian traits.[39] First, the genetic model of inheritance is often unknown and a certain inheritance mode cannot be specified. Parameters in penetrance, allele frequency, and mode of transmission may be variable for both causative and susceptibility genes. In addition, environmental factors may independently influence these parameters, making the estimation of genetic models in common complex traits extremely challenging.

A second confounding factor is that genetic heterogeneity is present in complex disease traits. Each disease phenotype may result from the contribution of multiple loci in the genome, which all act independently to increase (or decrease) susceptibility to disease. The degree of such effects may vary in different families or populations. Thus, in one family gene X may play a major role, while in another family with the same disease gene Y is the major contributor. These variations appear as "noise" in the genetic analyses, especially when analyzing a mixed population. One way to reduce such variables is to use isolated populations.[40]

Third, phenotypic heterogeneity may confound the genetic analyses of complex traits. The degree of phenotypic manifestation is often variable between individuals and is represented as a continuous fraction from normal to disease state. Influence from environmental factors

may interact with genetic factors, giving rise to further complication. In many common diseases, the definition of affected individuals by consensus diagnostic standards is relatively simple, but identification of unaffected family members is often impractical.

Fourth, disease parameters in mendelian and complex traits are often qualitative, as revealed in the classification of individuals (affected or unaffected), while quantitative measurement of physiologic factors (body weight, height, body mass index, blood pressure, lipoprotein level, IQ, and some psychological evaluation) is also crucial to the analysis of disease with complex traits. These quantitative values may represent biologic markers or intermediate disease states. Genetic loci that are tightly related to these quantitative values are termed *quantitative trait loci*. The analysis of quantitative trait loci has undergone significant technological progress, and practical applications in human genetics have been promoting the identification of susceptibility genes.

Fifth, it is likely that complex traits have complex genetics as well as complex phenotypes. The presence or absence of disease may reflect a final common injury pathway with multiple underlying biochemical/phenotypic inputs, each in turn affected by multiple genes. One way proposed to dissect complex trait diseases is to investigate the genetics of the component subphenotypes (referred to as endophenotypes). Often the component phenotypes are quantitative. An example would be HDL cholesterol levels (as a risk factor in atherosclerosis) in which major loci have been mapped.

Basic Concepts of Methods to Analyze Complex Disease Loci

Unraveling the genetic nature of complex disease traits is challenging and requires distinct strategies and methods of genetic analyses. Two general strategies include candidate-gene studies, wherein an association between disease phenotype and variations at each candidate locus predicted by other biologic information is tested, and a genome-scan approach, in which association between the disease phenotype and the location of a specific genetic marker from a marker set representing the entire genome is examined. Discrete methods are currently present for each strategy.[41]

The examination of affected sib pairs is one of the most common methodologies for linkage analysis of complex traits. A collection of pairs of siblings who are both affected by a disease, along with available parents, is subjected to haplotype analysis either at loci of interest predicted by the candidate gene approach or throughout the entire genome by a genome-scan approach. If a susceptibility gene is linked to a particular locus, one would expect more affected sib pairs to share alleles that are inherited from the same allele in a parent, a condition termed *identical by descent*. In such analyses, no parameters for an inheritance pattern are required; thus these are referred to as nonparametric analysis or model-free analysis. Short tandem repeat (STR) markers, which are highly polymorphic and are distributed throughout the genome, have been utilized for haplotyping of each locus. Affected sib-pair analysis may be performed on either qualitative traits or quantitative trait loci.

An alternative approach is an association analysis by searching genotypes for particular variants of polymorphic alleles that increase the risk of disease in patients versus unaffected controls matched for ethnicity (case-control samples). In this approach, the frequency of alleles at given loci are compared in populations of cases and controls. Higher frequency of a particular allele in cases than in controls would be considered an association between this allele and susceptibility to a disease. This method has been used mainly in the candidate gene approach. The given allelic variations can be directly associated with disease susceptibility, as depicted in the APOE4 allele for AD (MIM #104300). Alternatively, the variations may not have pathophysiologic significance, but represent linkage disequilibrium to disease-associated alleles.

The possibility of applying association analyses in genome scan studies has received a great deal of attention lately. In order to detect small founder genomic segments that represent linkage disequilibrium, high-resolution high-throughput association studies using markers with significant density is necessary. The recent discovery of a large number of single nucleotide polymorphisms and the development of single nucleotide polymorphism databases has been proposed for genome-scan linkage disequilibrium analysis because of their density and enrichment within functional genes.

Examples of Susceptibility Genes for Complex Traits

Contribution of Mendelian Alleles as Susceptibility Loci for Common Diseases

Rare mendelian diseases often display a phenotype similar to a common disease. Thus, genes for such mendelian traits can be strong candidates for susceptibility genes for the complex trait. Wolfram syndrome is a rare autosomal recessive disorder characterized with juvenile diabetes mellitus and progressive optic atrophy caused by mutation in the WFS1 gene. Patients with Wolfram syndrome often present with severe psychiatric manifestations. Heterozygous carriers for WLF1 mutations have a 26-fold increased risk for hospitalization due to psychiatric illness, especially for depression. Ataxia-telangiectasia (MIM #208900) is an autosomal recessive disorder characterized by cerebellar ataxia, telangiectases, immune defects, and a predisposition to malignancy of different types caused by mutations in the ATM gene. Heterozygous carriers for ATM mutations have an estimate of relative risk of 5:1 to develop breast cancer.

Common Disease with Major Contribution of Heredity

Inheritance of Hirschsprung disease (MIM #142623), also known as congenital intestinal aganglionosis, apparently reveals a nonmendelian inheritance pattern with low penetrance and a gender effect for recurrence risk. Phenotypic heterogeneity with long-segment and short-segment forms, each with distinct genetic characteristics, is present. In addition, Hirschsprung disease is also genetically heterogeneous. The receptor tyrosine kinase gene (RET) is likely a major contributor for both forms, but the penetrance of mutations is far from complete. Several other genes, including GDNF, EDNRB, EDN3, and SOX10, likely contribute to the expression of the disease along with RET or independently. Moreover, nonparametric genome-scan analyses reveal an unknown gene on 9q31 that increases susceptibility of long-segment Hirschsprung disease and two other modifier loci in the more common short-segment form.[42] A current model best supports the hypothesis that certain alleles of RET and two loci on 3p21 and 19q12 work together to increase the susceptibility to the disease.

Common Diseases with Multiple Susceptibility Loci

Genetic studies of AD have been challenging because of the complex nature of the disease.[43] Three fully penetrant genes, APP, PSEN1, and PSEN2, have been identified to cause diseases in rare families with dominantly inherited AD, but they are not likely to confer major susceptibility to common sporadic AD. In contrast, the ε4 allele of apolipoprotein E gene (APOE4) appears to increase the risk of common late-onset AD approximately threefold. Over 30 genes have been selected based on the physiologic role in the AD pathogenesis and tested for association with common late-onset AD, but overall the results have been controversial. Recently, linkage analyses using a quantitative trait loci model have identified at least three additional susceptibility loci for AD on chromosomes 9, 10, and 12.

CONCLUSIONS

Recognizing the mode of inheritance in a family with a genetic disease is not only crucial for accurate diagnosis but also essential to provide appropriate counseling for the recurrent risk, prognosis, medical management, and possible therapeutic choices to the family. Human disease traits display many different patterns of inheritance. Because the mode of inheritance is recognized as observed traits in pedigrees, obtaining a thorough family history is important and should be performed in great detail in all patients.[1] At the same time, genetics may play an important role in the etiology of diseases that present as sporadic cases. Thus, because of new mutation and

TABLE 3–2. Selected available databases on the Internet for medical genetics

Database	Web Address
Online Mendelian Inheritance in Man	www.ncbi.nlm.nih.gov:80/entrez/query.fcgi? db=OMIM
GeneTests/GeneClinics	www.genetests.org
The Human Gene Mutation Database	http://archive.uwcm.ac.uk/uwcm/mg/hgmd0.html
HUGO, The Human Genome Organization (including mutation database)	www.gene.ucl.ac.uk/hugo/
GenBank/Blast	www.ncbi.nlm.nih.gov/Genbank/index.html
	www.ncbi.nlm.nih.gov/BLAST
Ensembl	www.ensembl.org/
The UCSC Genome Database	http://genome.ucsc.edu/

penetrance issues, transmission or inheritance is not always observed in genetic disorders.

Since the last edition of this book, one of the most dramatic changes in practical and basic medical genetics is the increasing availability of on-line electronic databases that provide updated information about human genetic disorders, the availability of a multitude of genetic tests, and collections of mutations found in disease-causing genes (Table 3–2). Furthermore, a number of databases and analysis tools for human genetic and genomic information have been integrated into powerful and convenient on-line packages, which can be utilized in further investigations of human genes responsible for inherited diseases (see Table 3–2).

Undoubtedly, the rapid advances in human and medical genetics in combination with the Human Genome Project have promoted major progress in the discovery of genes and genetic mechanisms responsible for neurologic and psychiatric diseases. Clearly, this trend will continue. One can anticipate that this progress will provide the practitioner with novel tools for diagnosis, management, and treatment of neuropsychiatric disorders.

REFERENCES

1. Beaudet AL, Scriver CR, Sly WS, Valle D: Genetics, biochemistry, and molecular bases of variant human phenotypes. In Scriver CR, Beaudet AL, Sly WS, Valle D (eds): The Metabolic and Molecular Basis of Inherited Diseases. New York, McGraw-Hill, 2001, pp 3–125.

2. Vogel F, Motulsky AG: Human Genetics: Problems and Approaches. Berlin, Springer, 1996.

3. Ott J: Analysis of Human Genetic Linkage. Baltimore, Johns Hopkins University Press, 1999.

4. Willard HF: The sex chromosomes and X chromosome inactivation. In Scriver CR, Beaudet AL, Sly WS, Valle D (eds): The Metabolic and Molecular Basis of Inherited Diseases. New York, McGraw-Hill, 2001, pp 1191–1211.

5. Muller HJ: Further studies on the nature and causes of gene mutations. Proceedings of the 6th International Congress of Genetics 1932;1:213–255.

6. Gabellini D, Green M, Tupler R: Inappropriate gene activation in FSHD: A repressor complex binds a chromosomal repeat deleted in dystrophic muscle. Cell 2002;110:339–348.

7. Knudson AG Jr: Mutation and cancer: Statistical study of retinoblastoma. Proc Natl Acad Sci U S A 1971;68:820–823.

8. Schwartz M, Vissing J: Paternal inheritance of mitochondrial DNA. N Engl J Med 2002;347:576–580.

9. Hall JG: Genomic imprinting: Review and relevance to human diseases. Am J Hum Genet 1990;46: 857–873.

10. Sapienza C, Hall JG: Genome imprinting in human disease. In Scriver CR, Beaudet AL, Sly WS, Valle D (eds): The Metabolic and Molecular Basis of Inherited Diseases. New York, McGraw-Hill, 2001, pp 417–431.

11. Li E, Bestor TH, Jaenisch R: Targeted mutation of the DNA methyltransferase gene results in embryonic lethality. Cell 1992;69:915–926.

12. Brannan CI, Bartolomei MS: Mechanisms of genomic imprinting. Curr Opin Genet Dev 1999;9: 164–170.

13. Engel E: A new genetic concept: Uniparental disomy and its potential effect, isodisomy. Am J Med Genet 1980;6:137–143.

14. Spence JE, Perciaccante RG, Greig GM, et al: Uniparental disomy as a mechanism for human genetic disease. Am J Hum Genet 1988;42:217–226.

15. Engel E, Antonarakis SE: Genomic Imprinting and Uniparental Disomy in Medicine: Clinical and Molecular Aspects. New York, Wiley-Liss, 2002.

16. Kleinjan DJ, van Heyningen V: Position effect in human genetic disease. Hum Mol Genet 1998;7: 1611–1618.

17. Inoue K, Lupski JR: Molecular mechanisms for genomic disorders. Annu Rev Genomics Hum Genet 2002;3:199–242.

18. Hassold T, Hunt P: To err (meiotically) is human: The genesis of human aneuploidy. Nat Rev Genet 2001;2:280–291.

19. Sherman SL, Takaesu N, Freeman SB, et al: Trisomy 21: Association between reduced recombination and nondisjunction. Am J Hum Genet 1991;49:608–620.

20. Shaffer LG, Lupski JR: Molecular mechanisms for constitutional chromosomal rearrangements in humans. Annu Rev Genet 2000;34:297–329.

21. Lupski JR: Genomic disorders: Structural features of the genome can lead to DNA rearrangements and human disease traits. Trends Genet 1998;14:417–422.

22. Stankiewicz P, Lupski JR: Genome architecture, rearrangements and genomic disorders. Trends Genet 2002;18:74–82.

23. Stankiewicz P, Lupski JR: Molecular-evolutionary mechanisms for genomic disorders. Curr Opin Genet Dev 2002;12:312–319.

24. Jones C, Mullenbach R, Grossfeld P, et al: Colocalisation of CCG repeats and chromosome deletion breakpoints in Jacobsen syndrome: Evidence for a common mechanism of chromosome breakage. Hum Mol Genet 2000;9:1201–1208.

25. Cummings CJ, Zoghbi HY: Trinucleotide repeats: Mechanisms and pathophysiology. Annu Rev Genomics Hum Genet 2000;1:281–328.

26. Ranum LP, Day JW: Dominantly inherited, noncoding microsatellite expansion disorders. Curr Opin Genet Dev 2002;12:266–271.

27. Scriver CR, Waters PJ: Monogenic traits are not simple: Lessons from phenylketonuria. Trends Genet 1999;15:267–272.

28. Dipple KM, McCabe ER: Phenotypes of patients with "simple" Mendelian disorders are complex traits: Thresholds, modifiers, and systems dynamics. Am J Hum Genet 2000;66:1729–1735.

29. Dipple KM, McCabe ER: Modifier genes convert "simple" Mendelian disorders to complex traits. Mol Genet Metab 2000;71:43–50.

30. Giess R, Holtmann B, Braga M, et al: Early onset of severe familial amyotrophic lateral sclerosis with a SOD-1 mutation: Potential impact of CNTF as a candidate modifier gene. Am J Hum Genet 2002;70:1277–1286.

31. Corcia P, Mayeux-Portas V, Khoris J, et al: Abnormal SMN1 gene copy number is a susceptibility factor for amyotrophic lateral sclerosis. Ann Neurol 2002;51:243–246.

32. Veldink JH, van den Berg LH, Cobben JM, et al: Homozygous deletion of the survival motor neuron 2 gene is a prognostic factor in sporadic ALS. Neurology 2001;56:749–752.

33. Kunst CB, Messer L, Gordon J, et al: Genetic mapping of a mouse modifier gene that can prevent ALS onset. Genomics 2000;70:181–189.

34. Kajiwara K, Berson EL, Dryja TP: Digenic retinitis pigmentosa due to mutations at the unlinked peripherin/RDS and ROM1 loci. Science 1994;264:1604–1608.

35. Goldberg AF, Molday RS: Defective subunit assembly underlies a digenic form of retinitis pigmentosa linked to mutations in peripherin/rds and rom-1. Proc Natl Acad Sci U S A 1996;93:13726–13730.

36. del Castillo I, Villamar M, Moreno-Pelayo MA, et al: A deletion involving the connexin 30 gene in nonsyndromic hearing impairment. N Engl J Med 2002;346:243–249.

37. Savage DB, Agostini M, Barroso I, et al: Digenic inheritance of severe insulin resistance in a human pedigree. Nat Genet 2002;31:379–384.

38. Katsanis N, Ansley SJ, Badano JL, et al: Triallelic inheritance in Bardet-Biedl syndrome, a Mendelian recessive disorder. Science 2001;293:2256–2259.

39. Hauser ER, Pericak-Vance MA: Genetic analysis for common complex disease. Am Heart J 2000;140:36–44.

40. Peltonen L, Palotie A, Lange K: Use of population isolates for mapping complex traits. Nat Rev Genet 2000;1:182–190.

41. Anderson NH, Dominiczak AN: Genetic analysis of complex traits. In Rimoin DL, Connor JM, Pyeritz RE, Korf BR (eds): Principles and Practice of Medical Genetics, vol. 1. London, Churchhill Livingstone, 2002, pp 410–424.

42. Bork Gabriel S, Salomon R, Pelet A, et al: Segregation at three loci explains familial and population risk in Hirschsprung disease. Nat Genet 2002;31:89–93.

43. Tanzi RE, Bertram L: New frontiers in Alzheimer's disease genetics. Neuron 2001;32:181–184.

4

Degenerative Diseases and Protein Processing

Stanley B. Prusiner

The discovery of prions, as well as many other findings, permits a molecular definition and classification of the neurodegenerative diseases. Alzheimer and Parkinson diseases, as well as amyotrophic lateral sclerosis (ALS), frontotemporal dementia (FTD), and the prion diseases are all disorders of protein processing, as are Huntington disease and the spinocerebellar ataxias. Clinical signs and neuropathologic lesions were once the primary means of describing these disorders. Although these characteristics remain useful in diagnosis, the etiologies can now be attributed to the misprocessing of particular proteins. In each of the neurodegenerative disorders, the particular protein that undergoes misprocessing determines the disease-specific phenotype, which results from the malfunction of distinct sets of neurons. Studies on the molecular pathogenesis of neurodegeneration are beginning to identify targets for therapeutic intervention, but difficulties in developing effective drugs should not be underestimated.

Previously, there was little understanding of the causes of neurodegeneration. In fact, the term *degenerative disease* was used as a catch-all phrase for illnesses of unknown etiology. Progress since the early 1970s in research focused on degenerative disorders of the central nervous system (CNS) has been impressive. It is now clear that neurodegenerative diseases are caused by the misprocessing of proteins. In each disease, one or more specific proteins that are misprocessed have been identified; this results in the accumulation of one or more particular proteins.

The proteins that accumulate in the CNS of patients with neurodegenerative diseases were initially identified by purifying these polypeptides from the brains of animals or humans with these diseases.[1-3] Subsequently, molecular genetics was used to identify the genes respon-

sible for the familial forms of Alzheimer and Parkinson diseases as well as ALS and FTD. Similarly, molecular genetic investigations of Huntington disease and the spinocerebellar ataxias led to the identification of the genes responsible for the pathogenesis of these illnesses.

Of all the studies on neurodegenerative diseases, the discovery of prions has been the most unexpected. The finding that a protein can act as an infectious pathogen and cause degeneration of the CNS was unprecedented.[4] In fact, the prion concept was so novel that achieving acceptance required a long and arduous battle.[5] The prion concept not only explained how a disease can be both infectious and genetic, but it has also created new disease paradigms and revolutionized thinking in biology.

Although progress in the study of neurodegeneration has been impressive, there are still no curative treatments. Only for patients with Parkinson disease is there a palliative drug with reasonable efficacy.[6] L-dopa and related drugs do not stop the underlying degeneration, which often renders patients refractory to pharmacologic treatment in the later stages of Parkinson disease.[7] Stereotactic surgery has produced limited success in ameliorating the symptoms of Parkinson disease when L-dopa becomes ineffective. Transplantation of cells secreting dopamine into the brains of patients with advanced Parkinson disease is the subject of much research. It is noteworthy that many patients with Parkinson disease develop dementia in the later stages of this disorder.

This chapter is not intended as an exhaustive review of neurodegenerative diseases and, as such, the bibliography is limited. Rather, it is an attempt to view the many common features of these degenerative illnesses from the perspective of the prion diseases.[8,9] Progress in deciphering the etiologies of many neurodegenerative diseases has greatly strengthened the unifying concepts reviewed here.

Aging and Neurodegeneration

Age is the single most important risk factor for degenerative diseases of the CNS.[10–12] Many, but not all, cases of neurodegenerative diseases are sporadic in that no heritable, toxic, or infectious etiology can be discerned. These disorders are often characterized by a chronic, progressive deterioration of the CNS lasting from several months to more than a decade. Although the disease process is relentless, the immune system seems to remain quiescent. Patients are afebrile and exhibit neither leukocytosis in blood nor pleocytosis in the cerebrospinal fluid (CSF).

Although a complete compendium of neurodegenerative diseases is quite long, a brief list composed of the more common disorders and a few less common maladies, which have been particularly amenable to investigation, are discussed here (Table 4–1). Alzheimer and Parkinson diseases are the most common neurodegenerative diseases. Over four million people suffer from Alzheimer disease in the United States and another million have Parkinson disease.[10,12,13] Far less common are ALS, FTD, prion diseases, Huntington disease, and spinocerebellar ataxias. The vast majority of the first five neurodegenerative diseases are sporadic, with 10% or less of cases being inherited (Table 4–2). In contrast, virtually all cases of Huntington disease and the spinocerebellar ataxias are inherited disorders.

Because people are living longer, there is now considerable concern about the increasing numbers of individuals who are developing Alzheimer and Parkinson diseases. At 60 years of age, the risk of developing Alzheimer disease is approximately 1 in 10,000, but by 85 years of age, the risk is greater than 1 in 3.[14] Such statistics argue that, by the year 2025, more than 10 million people will suffer from Alzheimer disease in the United States, and by the year 2050, the number of afflicted individuals will approach 20 million.[12] Just as staggering as the number of people with Alzheimer disease is the cost of caring for these patients. It is estimated that Alzheimer disease costs the United States as much as $200 billion annually for the care of these people as well as in lost productivity of both the patients and caregivers.

Like Alzheimer disease, age is the most important risk factor for parkinson disease. By age 85 years, nearly 50% of people exhibit at least one symptom or sign of parkinsonism.[15]

Common Themes Define Neurodegeneration

With the recognition that a common feature of all well studied neurodegenerative diseases is the misprocessing of proteins, it was reasonable to propose a definition of neurodegenerative disease based on this unifying etiologic characteristic: "Neurodegenerative diseases are progressive nervous system disorders of protein processing. Aberrant protein processing includes misfolding, altered post-translational modification, aberrant proteolytic cleavage, anomalous gene splicing, improper expression, and diminished clearance. The misprocessed proteins often accumulate because the cellular mechanisms for removing these proteins are ineffective. Neurodegenerative diseases typically present with sporadic and genetic maladies of delayed onset, but they can also be infectious illnesses with prolonged incubation times. The particular protein that undergoes misprocessing determines the disease-specific phenotype, which results from the malfunction of distinct sets of neurons."[9]

In the past, degenerative diseases of the CNS have often been defined as idiopathic disorders accompanied by mental deterioration. Neuropathologically, they have been defined in terms of region-specific retrogressive changes in cells resulting in impaired function. Such pathologic changes have also been equated with the death of specific neuronal populations.[16]

TABLE 4–1. Epidemiology of Neurodegenerative Diseases

Disease	Number of U.S. patients	U.S. prevalence per 100,000*
Prion diseases	400	0.1
Alzheimer disease	4,000,000	1,450
Parkinson disease	1,000,000	360
FTD	40,000	14
Pick disease	5,000	2
PSP	15,000	5
ALS	20,000	7
Huntington disease	30,000	11
Spinocerebellar ataxias	12,000	4

*Population of United States is approximately 275 million in the year 2000.
ALS, amyotrophic lateral sclerosis; FTD, frontotemporal dementia; PSP, progressive supranuclear palsy.

TABLE 4–2. Sporadic, Genetic, and Infectious Etiologies of Neurodegenerative Diseases

Disease	Etiologic frequency (%)		
	Sporadic	*Genetic*	*Infectious*
Prion diseases	85	>10	<1
Alzheimer disease	90	10	–
Parkinson disease	95	<5	–
FTD	90	10	–
Pick disease	95	<5	–
PSP	95	<5	–
ALS	90	10	–
Huntington disease	–	100	–
Spinocerebellar ataxias	–	100	–

ALS, amyotrophic lateral sclerosis; FTD, frontotemporal dementia; PSP, progressive supranuclear palsy.

The broad spectrum of presenting clinical deficits in the prion diseases illustrates how ineffective a clinical classification scheme can be: patients with these diseases can present with dementia, ataxia, insomnia, paraplegia, paresthesias, and deviant behavior.[17]

Although none of the clinical presentations of prion diseases is diagnostic, patients who present with a rapidly progressive dementia accompanied by myoclonus often have Creutzfeldt-Jakob disease (CJD). The spectrum of neuropathologic changes in prion diseases ranges from none to widespread atrophy, from rare to frequent neuronal loss, from sparse to severe vacuolation or spongiform change, from mild to intense reactive astrocytic gliosis, and from none to abundant PrP amyloid plaques.[18] None of these neuropathologic changes, except the presence of PrP amyloid plaques, is unequivocally diagnostic. Past attempts to classify and character-

ize other neurodegenerative diseases (see Table 4–1) based on the clinical presentations or neuropathologic manifestations have been equally unsatisfying.

The discovery of amyloid in brain fractions enriched for prion infectivity was completely unexpected.[19] The amyloid plaques in prion diseases and Alzheimer disease, as well as large intracellular structures such as Lewy and Pick bodies, were not considered to be of etiologic importance. Once anti-PrP 27–30 antibodies were raised, the amyloid plaques in prion diseases were found to stain readily.[20,21]

It seems likely that the mechanisms by which misprocessed proteins disrupt cellular functions, such as signal transduction and gene transcription, are diverse. The secondary responses to misprocessed proteins may amplify the damage done by these macromolecules by activation of cytokine release, reactive gliosis, apoptosis,

TABLE 4–3. Protein Deposition in Neurodegenerative Diseases

Disease	Protein	Aggregate
Prion diseases	PrP^{Sc}	PrP amyloid
Alzheimer disease	Aβ	Aβ amyloid
	tau	PHF in NFT
Parkinson disease	α-synuclein	Lewy bodies
FTD	tau	Straight filaments and PHF
Pick disease	tau	Pick bodies
PSP	tau	Straight filaments in NFT
ALS	neurofilament	Bunina bodies
Huntington disease	huntingtin	Nuclear inclusions
Spinocerebellar ataxia 1	ataxin 1	Nuclear inclusions
Spinocerebellar ataxia 2	ataxin 2	Cytoplasmic inclusions
Machado-Joseph disease	ataxin 3	Nuclear inclusions

ALS, amyotrophic lateral sclerosis; FTD, frontotemporal dementia; PSP, progressive supranuclear palsy.

and oxidative injury.[22,23] In some neurodegenerative diseases, the misprocessed proteins might cause CNS dysfunction when they are monomers or oligomers, whereas in other disorders larger aggregates may prove to be the culprits.[24] In the case of the disease-causing isoform of the prion protein (PrP^{Sc}), it accumulates and fragments sometimes polymerize to form amyloid fibrils that are deposited in the extracellular space as plaques. With α-synuclein, tau and mutant huntingtin proteins, ubiquitinated deposits are found as Lewy bodies, Pick bodies, and nuclear aggregates, respectively (Table 4–3). As discussed subsequently, the aggregates may not cause cellular dysfunction but simply represent the attempt of cells to sequester these misprocessed proteins in a form that is less deleterious. Finding ubiquitinated deposits of α-synuclein, tau, and mutant huntingtin argues that these proteins were destined for clearance but the process was incomplete. The covalent attachment of ubiquitin, which is a highly conserved 76-residue polypeptide, to particular proteins targets them for degradation.[25]

In sporadic cases of prion disease, which account for more than 85% of occurrences (see Table 4–2), the prion concept explains how the wild-type (wt), normal cellular isoform of the prion protein (PrP^C) is progressively converted into PrP^{Sc}. Although the mechanism of prion replication is unclear, the stimulation of this process by PrP^{Sc} provides the driving force for the misfolding of PrP^C into PrP^{Sc}. No similar formulation exists to explain the progressive deterioration of the nervous system that follows the misprocessing of proteins in sporadic cases of Alzheimer disease, FTD, Parkinson disease, and ALS. For example, factors driving the accumulation of the Aβ-peptide in the CNS of people destined to develop sporadic Alzheimer disease are unknown except for the allelic variants of apolipoprotein E (ApoE). Likewise, factors driving the accumulation of α-synuclein to form Lewy bodies within neurons of the substantia nigra of people destined to develop sporadic Parkinson disease are unknown.

In the inherited neurodegenerative diseases, the same problem attends in the sense that these diseases are usually of late onset although the mutations are present from conception. With few exceptions, the inherited neurodegenerative diseases are autosomal dominant disorders, so the mutations are unlikely to produce disease through loss of function. Instead, such dominant mutations are likely to act as gain of dysfunction or as dominant negatives. Although the mutant protein is expressed in the CNS early in life, no damage is detected clinically for decades in the inherited cases of Alzheimer disease, Parkinson disease, FTD, ALS, and the prion diseases. Only in the triplet repeat diseases, such as Huntington disease, do children manifest neurologic disease when the repeat expansions become very large.

How the aging process features in these diseases is unclear. Is the misprocessing of a particular protein simply a stochastic process, which happens with a much higher probability when it is mutated? In such a model,

prolonged periods of time are required for either the mutant or wt protein to be misprocessed into a disease-causing form. But perhaps, the milieu of the aging brain provides a more permissive environment for the misprocessing of proteins. The accumulation of proteins modified by oxidation has been suggested as a possible factor in virtually every degenerative disease.[22] Clearance of misprocessed proteins may diminish with age and thus may be responsible for their accumulation.

The neurodegenerative diseases elude detection by the immune and interferon defense systems: patients remain afebrile throughout the courses of their illnesses and show no leukocytosis in blood or pleocytosis in the CSF. Grossly, the brain can be atrophic with enlarged ventricles as in many cases of Alzheimer disease; alternatively, the basal ganglia may show selective atrophy as in Huntington disease. The degree of neuronal loss and the extent of reactive astrocytic gliosis can be quite variable for a particular disease. Although microglia often accumulate and cytokines are released late in the various neurodegenerative diseases, no inflammatory response characterized by accumulation of antigen-antibody complexes, lymphocytic infiltration, or the perivascular accumulation of monocytes is generally seen.

Sporadic and Genetic Neurodegenerative Diseases

Prion Diseases. The mechanism by which sporadic prion disease is initiated is unknown. Three different hypotheses have been offered to explain the etiology of sporadic CJD. One mechanism may be a somatic mutation, in which a spontaneous mutation occurs in a cell capable of transforming PrP^C into PrP^{Sc}. The spontaneous formation of prions would then evolve in a manner similar to that for germline mutations in inherited disease (Table 4–4). In a second scenario, the activation barrier separating wt PrP^C from PrP^{Sc} could be crossed on rare occasions when viewed in the context of a large population of molecules.[26] A third scenario can be envisioned in which PrP^{Sc} is formed physiologically but at sufficiently low levels that it cannot be detected by bioassay in laboratory rodents. Studies with recombinant antibody fragments (recFabs) show that PrP^{Sc} is cleared from scrapie-infected neuroblastoma (ScN2a) cells with a $t_{1/2}$ of approximately 30 hours.[27] These findings argue that PrP^{Sc} might be made constantly at low levels and only becomes deleterious when the rate of formation exceeds the rate of clearance. Once this happens, PrP^{Sc} begins to accumulate and eventually the level of PrP^{Sc} is sufficiently high to cause disease.

More than 30 different mutations in the human *PRNP* gene resulting in nonconservative substitutions have been found to segregate with inherited human prion diseases, to date.[28] Missense mutations and expansions in the octapeptide repeat region of the gene are responsible for familial forms of prion disease. Five different

TABLE 4–4. Mutant Genes in Familial Neurodegenerative Diseases

Inherited Disease	Gene	Mutation
Prion diseases	*PRNP*	Point mutations and octarepeat expansions
Alzheimer disease	*APP*	Point mutations
	PS1	
	PS2	
Parkinson disease	*SCNA*	Point mutations
	Parkin[*]	
FTD	*tau*	Point mutations, deletions
Pick disease	*tau*	Point mutations
ALS	*SOD1*	Point mutations
	ALS2[*]	
Huntington disease	*HD*	Polyglutamine expansions
Spinocerebellar ataxia 1	SCA1	Polyglutamine expansions
Spinocerebellar ataxia 2	SCA2	Polyglutamine expansions
Machado-Joseph disease	SCA3	Polyglutamine expansions

[*]Familial diseases caused by mutations in these genes are autosomal recessive disorders. All other familial neurodegenerative diseases in this table are autosomal dominant disorders.
ALS, Amyotrophic lateral sclerosis; FTD, Frontotemporal dementia.

mutations of the *PRNP* gene have been linked genetically to heritable prion disease.[29–33]

Alzheimer Disease. In Alzheimer disease, Aβ-amyloid plaques and neurofibrillary tangles (NFT) are found whether the disease is sporadic or inherited (see Table 4–3). Like the familial prion diseases, the inheritance of familial Alzheimer disease is autosomal dominant. In contrast to the prion diseases, in which only mutations in the *PRNP* gene have been identified to cause familial prion disease, familial Alzheimer disease can be caused by a mutation in one of at least three different genes: amyloid precursor protein (*APP*), presenilin 1 (*PS1*), and presenilin 2 (*PS2*) (see Table 4–4).[34] Cleavage of APP at residue 671 by β-secretase and at either residue 711 or 713 by γ-secretase produces Aβ(1–40) or Aβ(1–42), respectively. Aβ(1–40) is soluble and its levels do not correlate with Alzheimer disease whereas Aβ(1–42) readily forms fibrils and is thought to cause CNS dysfunction before being deposited in plaques.[35–37] The cleavage of APP by γ-secretase within the plasma membrane is a highly regulated, complex process.[37,38] Cleavage at residue 687 by α-secretase prevents Aβ-peptide formation. Six different mutations of the *APP* gene have been implicated in familial Alzheimer disease. More than 30 mutations of the *PS1* gene and two of the *PS2* gene in familial Alzheimer disease have been found.[34] PS1 and PS2 are thought to form complexes with at least one other protein, nicastrin, and these complexes have γ-secretase activity.[39] Mutations in *PS1* have been shown to increase the amount of Aβ-peptide(1–42).

NFTs in Alzheimer disease are composed of paired helical filaments (PHF) that are composed of hyperphosphorylated tau.[40–42] The tau protein binds to microtubules and facilitates assembly of these polymers but hyperphosphorylated tau isolated from Alzheimer-diseased brains does not bind to microtubules. Six different isoforms of tau are produced by alternative splicing of a single copy gene expressed in brain. Although mutations of the *tau* gene cause neurodegeneration as described later, they do not cause Alzheimer disease.

The age of onset of both the sporadic and familial Alzheimer disease is modulated by the allelic variants of ApoE.[43] Three alternative allelic products of ApoE, denoted ε2, ε3 and ε4, differ at residues 112 and 158. Many people with two E4 alleles can expect to develop Alzheimer disease at least a decade before those with two copies of E2, whereas those with E3 exhibit an intermediate age of onset.[44] How ApoE modulates the onset of Alzheimer disease is unknown but one hypothesis suggests that ApoE features in the clearance of Aβ(1–42). A less compelling hypothesis argues that ApoE modulates the formation of NFTs that are composed of PHF.[45]

Frontotemporal Dementia. Mutations in the *tau* gene are responsible for inherited cases of FTD and Pick disease.[46–48] Like Alzheimer disease, about 90% of FTD cases are sporadic and approximately 10% are familial (see Table 4–2). In familial FTD, straight filaments composed of hyperphosphorylated mutant tau have been found (see Table 4–3).[49] In patients from some families with FTD, NFT composed of PHF have been found; the formation of PHF seems to depend on the specific *tau* mutation and the expression of specific isoforms that are determined by alternative splicing.[50] In sporadic FTD, aggregates of *tau* are rarely found.

Approximately 15% of FTD cases coming to autopsy were found to have Pick bodies,[51] which are the neuropathologic hallmark of Pick disease. Pick bodies are intracellular collections of ubiquitinated tau fibrils.[52] Like FTD, most cases of Pick disease are sporadic.

In some familial cases of FTD that are caused by *tau* mutations, Parkinson disease and disinhibition have been found.[53] Additional disorders caused by the misprocessing of *tau* include progressive supranuclear palsy (PSP), progressive subcortical gliosis, and corticobasal degeneration.[50,52,54,55]

Parkinson Disease. In Parkinson disease, the same theme of protein deposits in the CNS of patients with sporadic and familial forms of the disease has been discovered. Although most patients with Parkinson disease have a sporadic form of the disease,[56,57] mutations have been discovered in the α-synuclein gene of patients with familial Parkinson disease.[58] When antibodies were raised to α-synuclein, they were found to stain intracellular aggregates of protein, called Lewy bodies, in malfunctioning neurons of the substantia nigra.[59] Lewy bodies are present in both the sporadic and familial forms of Parkinson disease. Although the inheritance of Parkinson disease caused by mutations in the α-synuclein gene is autosomal dominant, a childhood form of Parkinson disease caused by mutations in the ubiquitin-protein ligase gene (*Parkin*) is a recessive disorder (see Table 4–4).[60] Whether people carrying mutations in the *Parkin* gene develop Parkinson disease due to decreased ubiquitination of α-synuclein is unknown, but the ubiquitin pathway is known to participate in the degradation of α-synuclein. There is considerable interest in the possible role of oxidative metabolism in the etiology of Parkinson disease and selective nitration of α-synuclein in Lewy bodies has been found.[61]

The onset of Parkinson disease in people age 70 years or older is associated with a high incidence of dementia.[62] At autopsy, the brains of these people often display the neuropathologic hallmarks of both Alzheimer and Parkinson diseases. Ubiquitin and α-synuclein immunostaining to identify cortical Lewy bodies has helped resolve the conundrum of how a patient could have insufficient numbers of plaques and NFTs for diagnosis of Alzheimer disease but still be demented. It is estimated that α-synuclein deposition as Lewy bodies in cortical neurons may by itself, or in combination with Alzheimer disease changes, be the second most common form of neurodegeneration, accounting for 20% to 30% of dementia cases in people older than 60 years.[63,64] A small group of younger people with Parkinson disease become demented because of diffuse Lewy body disease, in which Lewy bodies are found throughout the cerebral cortex.[65]

For nearly two decades, some investigators have argued that Parkinson disease is acquired by the accumulation of toxic molecules in neurons of the substantia nigra.[57] The dramatic ability of the synthetic heroin derivative MPTP to produce the symptoms and signs of Parkinson disease in humans and apes provided seductive evidence in favor of the toxin hypothesis, as did the possibility that a molecule in cycad plants causes an ALS-Parkinson disease complex in the indigenous people of Guam.[66,67] Studies of the etiology of Parkinson disease have also been complicated by parkinsonism (or the symptoms of Parkinson disease) that is seen in a variety of neurologic disorders, including postencephalitis lethargica (following the influenza pandemic of 1916 to 1926) and posthypoxic encephalopathy.

Amyotrophic Lateral Sclerosis. Although most cases of ALS are sporadic, familial cases have been identified (see Table 4–2).[68–70] Approximately 20% of all familial ALS cases have been shown to be due to mutations in the cytoplasmic superoxide dismutase gene (*SOD1*) (see Table 4–4).[71] Deposits of SOD have been found in the CNS of some patients with sporadic and familial forms of ALS.[72] Of note, some mutant SOD molecules exhibit increased SOD activity compared with wt SOD, whereas others display activities that are similar or decreased compared with wt SOD.[73] In some cases of ALS, abnormal collections of neurofilaments have been seen in degenerating motor neurons, but no familial cases of ALS have been shown to be due to mutations in any of the neurofilament genes.[72] In a few cases of sporadic ALS and in one family with ALS, deletions in the tail domain of the large neurofilament subunit (NF-H) have been reported. Besides familial cases of ALS being caused by *SOD1* mutations, familial ALS has also been shown to be caused by mutations in *ALS2*, or the alsin gene. This disease is an autosomal recessive disorder, which is manifest in children.[74,75] In ALS, Bunina bodies are often found. These intraneuronal inclusions contain cystatin C as well as neurofilaments. Attempts to demonstrate SOD or phosphorylated neurofilaments by immunostaining have been negative.[76,77]

Huntington Disease and Spinocerebellar Ataxias. Huntington disease (HD) and the spinocerebellar ataxias (SCAs) provide important contrasts and similarities to the foregoing neurodegenerative diseases. In contrast to Alzheimer disease, FTD, Parkinson disease, ALS, and the prion diseases, in which most of the cases are sporadic, both HD and the SCAs are exclusively genetic diseases (see Table 4–2)[78] caused by expanded polyglutamine repeats (see Table 4–4).[16,79,80] But as in the inherited forms of Alzheimer disease, FTD, Parkinson disease, ALS, and the prion diseases, most patients with HD and the SCAs present with neurologic deficits in adulthood, despite the mutant gene products being expressed in the CNS from early in life. Childhood forms of HD and the

SCAs are known to be due to enlarged expansions of the triplet repeats that cause these diseases.[79,81,82]

In both HD and the SCAs, the mutant gene products appear to be deposited in the CNS of patients. These misprocessed mutant proteins seem to accumulate in malfunctioning neurons and to be responsible for the neurologic deficits that these patients exhibit. In HD, SCA1, and Machado-Joseph disease (SCA3), as well as in some cases of SCA2, nuclear inclusions of the mutant proteins, which are ubiquitinated, have been found.[79,83]

Additional disorders caused by the misprocessing of proteins with expanded polyglutamine repeats include spinobulbar muscular atrophy (SBMA), also called Kennedy syndrome, in which the androgen receptor carries the expanded repeat,[84] as well as dentatorubropallidoluysian atrophy (DRPLA), and the spinocerebellar ataxias 6 and 7.[16,80]

The neurodegenerative diseases described here represent only a small fraction of the total number of neurologic maladies given this label. Undoubtedly, many of these disorders will require reclassification as the molecular basis of each is elucidated.

TRANSGENIC MODELS OF NEURODEGENERATION

Prion Diseases. Transgenic (Tg) mouse models that reproduce virtually every aspect of the naturally occurring prion diseases have created a firm foundation on which to decipher the molecular pathogenesis of these diseases. Many studies employing Tg mice expressing wt or mutant PrP are summarized elsewhere (see Chapters 2 and 13).

Alzheimer Disease. Tg mice expressing mutant APP have been found to develop amyloid plaques filled with the Aβ-peptide.[85,86] In some cases, these mice show behavioral abnormalities, whereas in others, such changes have not been reported. The development of Aβ plaques was accelerated when extracts from the brains of patients with Alzheimer disease were injected into Tg mice expressing mutant APP.[87] In earlier studies, Alzheimer disease brain fractions were enriched for tau-induced deposits of Aβ in the brains of rats.[88] In uninjected bigenic mice, development of Aβ plaques was hastened by expression of mutant *APP* and *PS1* transgenes.[89] (The term *bigenic mice* denotes Tg mice expressing two transgenes.) In other bigenic mice expressing human mutant APP and human ApoEε4 but not ε3, cognitive deficits were identified at age 6 months, although no Aβ plaques could be found.[90] These findings argue that the neuronal dysfunction in Alzheimer disease may not be due to the Aβ plaques, but to events occurring before the sequestration of Aβ and other molecules into the plaques.[91] Such a scenario would be in accord with the findings for prion diseases, in which PrP amyloid plaques are not obligatory for disease pathogenesis. In fruit flies, disruption of the APP-like gene or presenilin causes nervous system dysfunction, and overexpression of wt presenilin causes cell death. In worms, suppression of nicastrin expression induces a phenotype similar to that seen with disruption of the presenilin-like genes.[39]

Nicastrin and the presenilins are thought to form complexes that have γ-secretase activity, which may function in regulated intramembrane proteolysis (Rip) to produce the Aβ-peptide from APP.[92] Several other examples of intramembrane proteases acting in diverse metabolic processes have been discovered.[37,38]

Frontotemporal Dementia. Expression of human tau with the P301L mutation in Tg mice produced neurofibrillary tangles and Pick bodies in neurons throughout the CNS.[93] By age 10 months, about 90% of these Tg mice developed progressive neurologic dysfunction resulting in death within 1 month.

Parkinson Disease. The expression of either wt or mutant human α-synuclein in fruit flies produced adult-onset loss of dopaminergic neurons and locomotor dysfunction.[94] Additionally, filamentous, intraneuronal inclusions of α-synuclein were found. In Tg mice expressing mutant and wt human α-synuclein, intraneuronal inclusions of human α-synuclein were found in the neocortex and hippocampus, as well as in the substantia nigra, where a significant loss of dopaminergic neurons was observed.[95,96]

Amyotrophic Lateral Sclerosis. In Tg mice expressing mutant SOD1, vacuolation, neuronal death, and reactive gliosis in the spinal cord, as well as cytoplasmic inclusions of SOD1 in motor neurons, have been found.[72] Tg mice overexpressing human NF-H produced altered function in large myelinated motor neurons.[97] Of particular interest are bigenic mice in which wt NF-H and mutant SOD1(G37R) have been expressed. The overexpression of NF-H extended the life span of mice expressing mutant SOD1 by approximately 6 months.[98] The results of these experiments suggest that much of the neurofilament protein was trapped in cell bodies and thus was prevented from being transported into the axons where altered neurofilaments would cause dysfunction. Less striking is the increase in survival by about 40 days in Tg mice expressing mutant SOD1(G37R) because of disruption of the neurofilament genes.[99]

Huntington Disease. Tg mice expressing the mutant huntingtin protein with 48 or 89 repeating Gln residues develop neurologic dysfunction and striatal degeneration.[100] In attempts to reproduce all aspects of HD, a large number of Tg mice have been produced using different vectors and varying numbers of CAG repeats.[101] Notably, YAC clones of the huntingtin gene with 46 or 72 repeating Gln residues have been used to produce selective striatal degeneration.[102] Using the tetracycline-inducible transgene system, regulated expression of exon 1 of the huntingtin gene with 94 polyglutamine residues produced an HD model with reversible neurodegeneration.[103] Using exon 1 with 92 and 111 repeating Gln residues, gene targeting produced knock-in mice that show accumulation of mutant huntingtin in the nuclei of spiny neurons of the striatum.[104] In *Drosophila*, expression of the huntingtin protein carrying a polyglutamine repeat of 75 amino acids produced striking neuronal degeneration.[105]

Using cultured neurons from the striatum and hippocampus of the rat, expression of a fragment of the huntingtin protein with 68 repeating Gln residues produced nuclear inclusions of the mutant protein and apoptosis.[106] When the nuclear inclusions were diminished by inhibiting ubiquitination, apoptosis increased, arguing that aggregation of the mutant protein helps protect cells. Although some investigators argue that aggregation is an essential feature of the polyglutamine repeat diseases,[107] these results and those discussed later for Tg mice expressing mutant ataxin 1 argue that the misfolding of monomers or oligomers of proteins with Gln expansions is responsible for disease and that nuclear inclusions, which are often seen in humans and Tg models, may reflect sequestration of potentially pathogenic proteins.

Spinocerebellar Ataxias. Expanded Gln repeats in ataxin 1 causing SCA1 have been expressed in Tg mice and shown to cause ataxia and Purkinje cell degeneration. Mutation of the nuclear localization signal in ataxin 1 with 82 repeating Gln residues prevented disease in Tg mice.[79,108] In contrast, deletion of 122 amino acids comprising the self-aggregation domain in ataxin 1 with 77 repeating Gln residues caused disease when expressed in Tg mice. These results argue that nuclear localization is required for disease pathogenesis but aggregation is not. In Tg mice, ataxin 2 expression with an expanded glutamine repeat of 58 residues resulted in impaired motor skills and cytoplasmic, but not nuclear, aggregates of the protein in Purkinje cells.[109] Tg mice expressing ataxin 3 with an expanded glutamine repeat of 79 residues failed to develop neurologic dysfunction, as well as degeneration of cerebellar dentate neurons and the basal ganglia that is seen in Machado-Joseph disease, also known as SCA3.[110] When 79 Gln residues were expressed with adjacent 42 amino acids that are found at the C-terminus of the repeat, Tg mice developed ataxia by 4 weeks of age and showed widespread degeneration of the cerebellum by 8 weeks of age. In *Drosophila*, expression of ataxin 3 carrying a polyglutamine repeat of 78 amino acids resulted in degeneration of the eye.[111]

The ability to reproduce virtually every aspect of the human prion diseases in Tg mice has proved to be a useful goal for studies of other neurodegenerative diseases. The progress in modeling other neurodegenerative disorders in Tg mice, flies, and worms is impressive. When CNS dysfunction accompanied by region-specific neuropathology mimicking the human disease is produced in organisms expressing mutant transgenes, it is reasonable to assume that significant progress in understanding the disease process is being made.

Oligomers versus Large Aggregates

In a cell culture model of HD and in Tg mice expressing mutant ataxin 1, formation of nuclear aggregates was separated from cell death as described earlier. The issue of whether large aggregates of misprocessed proteins or misfolded monomers (or oligomers) cause CNS degeneration has been addressed in studies summarized elsewhere (see Chapter 13). Although intracellular collections of misprocessed proteins, such as Lewy bodies, nuclear inclusions, and Pick bodies may represent a mechanism whereby cells sequester proteins that cannot be readily degraded, PrP and Aβ-amyloid plaques may play a similar role in the extracellular space of the CNS (see Table 4–3).

Prevention and Therapeutics

There is no known effective therapy for treating or preventing CJD or any of the other neurodegenerative diseases. Only in Parkinson disease does an effective treatment exist that ameliorates the symptoms,[6,7] but it does not halt the underlying degeneration. Because the prion diseases progress more rapidly than the other neurodegenerative disorders, fatalities from these maladies are more readily measured. There are no well-documented cases of patients with CJD showing recovery either spontaneously or after therapy, with one possible exception[112] for which there is no confirmatory example. In the highlands of New Guinea, individuals who were thought to have recovered from kuru were eventually shown to have hysterical illnesses.

The difficulty of developing effective drugs for the prevention and treatment of the neurodegenerative diseases should not be underestimated. New principles of pharmacotherapeutics will undoubtedly emerge from development of drugs for treating neurodegeneration. The history of successful therapeutics for preventing or reversing protein misprocessing is extremely limited. As more is learned about the molecular pathogenesis of the neurodegenerative diseases, more opportunities for drug targets will emerge.[113] Directing these new drugs to specific regions of the CNS will also be challenging.

Preventing Misprocessing. Structure-based drug design predicated on dominant-negative inhibition of prion formation has produced several lead compounds.[114] Prion replication depends on protein-to-protein interactions and a subset of these interactions gives rise to dominant-negative phenotypes produced by single residue substitutions.[115,116] The task of exchanging polypeptide scaffolds for small heterocyclic structures without loss of biologic activity remains difficult. Whether this approach designed to prevent the misfolding and aberrant processing of proteins will provide general methods for developing novel therapeutics for Alzheimer and Parkinson diseases, as well as ALS and other neurodegenerative diseases, remains to be established.

The γ-secretase, which catalyzes the hydrolytic cleavage of APP in the production of the Aβ-peptide, continues to be a focus with respect to possible therapeutics for Alzheimer disease.[36] Inhibitors of γ-secretase have been identified and are being evaluated for their efficacy in slowing the ravages of Alzheimer disease. Studies suggest that anti-inflammatory and cholesterol-reducing drugs can significantly reduce the risk of Alzheimer disease.[117]

Enhanced Clearance. Several compounds have been demonstrated to eliminate prions from prion-infected cultured cells. A class of compounds known as *dendrimers* seems particularly efficacious in this regard.[118] Numerous drugs have been demonstrated to delay the onset of disease in animals inoculated with prions, if the drugs are given around the time of the inoculation.[119] The scenario in which one would want to treat humans is either patients showing signs of disease or presymptomatic patients carrying mutations predisposing them to develop prion disease. No treatment has shown any efficacy in animal models of these two scenarios.

A novel approach to treating Alzheimer disease has been developed using Tg mice overexpressing a mutant *APP* gene. Immunization of these Tg mice with the Aβ-peptide resulted in a profound decrease in the Aβ-amyloid in the CNS, presumably by accelerating the clearance of Aβ-peptides.[120] Whether this approach will prove to be fruitful in patients suffering from Alzheimer disease or applicable to other neurodegenerative disorders is unknown.[121]

Replacement Therapy. Because the neurodegeneration in Parkinson disease is confined largely to the substantia nigra, especially early in the disease process, replacement therapy has proved to be useful; however, many patients eventually become refractory to L-dopa[7] as discussed earlier.

Similar approaches to Alzheimer disease have been disappointing in large part because the disease process is so widespread. The widespread neuropathology in ALS, FTD, and prion diseases also makes replacement therapy an approach that is unlikely to be successful.

Speculation on the Spectrum of Degenerative Diseases

In addition to the neurodegenerative diseases that were discussed previously, it is tempting to speculate that protein misprocessing occurs in other common diseases of the CNS, such as schizophrenia, bipolar disorders, and autism. Most cases of schizophrenia, bipolar disorders, and autism are sporadic but a substantial minority of cases appear to be familial. The lack of consistent neuropathologic changes in the brains of people with these diseases has impeded studies and complicated phenotypic analysis. Not unlike these diseases are alcoholism and other forms of addiction in which most cases are sporadic but a minority of them are familial. In one group of patients with inherited FTD, alcoholism and Parkinson disease are prominent features; these people carry a mutation in the *tau* gene.[53]

Whether diseases that are frequently classified as neurodegenerative diseases, such as multiple sclerosis (MS), are caused by protein misprocessing is unknown.[122] In MS, the immune system features prominently in the pathogenesis of the disease, and thus it is often argued that MS should be classified as a T cell–mediated autoimmune disorder. In some MS cases, antibody-mediated demyelination has been found[123] and in other cases, degeneration of oligodendrocytes has been observed with little or no evidence of immune-mediated damage.[124]

Whether the misprocessing of proteins occurs in neurodegeneration that is independent of the inflammatory process in MS or initiates an aberrant immune response is unknown. Like the neurodegenerative diseases discussed earlier, most cases of MS are sporadic, whereas a minority are familial. The inheritance of MS is polygenic, but to date no single mutant gene causing MS has been identified.[125] Molecular mimicry has been suggested as the mechanism that initiates the immune-mediated demyelination of the CNS in MS, in which an antigenic site on the protein of an infectious pathogen, such as a virus, provokes an immune response directed at an epitope of a myelin protein.[126,127] The participation of an infectious pathogen in MS remains an attractive hypothesis that could explain how the risk for MS is acquired during childhood, as well as the geographically isolated clusters.

When reflecting on MS, perhaps illnesses such as ulcerative colitis, Crohn disease, rheumatoid arthritis, and lupus ought to be considered as possible disorders of protein misprocessing in which misfolded proteins might evoke an autoimmune response. Like the neurodegenerative disorders (see Table 4–2), a minority of these autoimmune diseases are familial, whereas the majority are sporadic.

Systemic diseases such as juvenile type I and adult-onset type II diabetes mellitus are likely to be caused by protein misprocessing. Juvenile diabetes seems to be an autoimmune disease; despite control of the insulin deficiency, progressive degeneration of peripheral nerves, the retinas, and kidneys often proceeds.[128] In the β-islet cells of patients with type II diabetes, the protein amylin frequently accumulates as amyloid fibrils. Like the juvenile form of diabetes, control of the insulin deficiency does not prevent the development of polyneuropathy, retinopathy, and renal disease in adult-onset diabetes.

The systemic amyloidoses share important features with the neurodegenerative diseases. In primary amyloidosis, immunoglobulin light chains form amyloid deposits that can cause cardiomyopathy, renal failure, and polyneuropathy.[129] In response to chronic inflammatory diseases, the serum amyloid A protein is cleaved to form the amyloid A protein, which is deposited as fibrils in the kidney, liver, and spleen. The most common systemic hereditary amyloidosis is caused by the deposition of mutant transthyretin. More than 40 mutations of the transthyretin gene have been found to result in proteins causing familial amyloidotic polyneuropathy.

Although speculation about the possible role of protein misprocessing in many diseases presents a series of attractive and, in some instances, provocative hypotheses, other mechanisms that compromise cell function need to be entertained. For example, apoptosis can be initiated by a variety of pathways in which protein misprocessing is likely to play little or no role.

The Future

As the life span of humans continues to increase through the efforts of modern medical science, an increasing burden of degenerative diseases is emerging. Developing effective means of preventing these disorders and treating them when they do occur are paramount to the personal, political, and economic future of our planet. The problems caused by Alzheimer and Parkinson diseases are already so large that if these maladies continue to increase in accord with the changing demographics of the world population, they will bankrupt both the developed and developing nations over the next 50 years. It is remarkable to think that by the year 2025, more than 65% of people over the age of 65 will be living in countries that are now designated as developing nations.[130] Without effective treatments and methods of prevention, this immense group of people will be subject to the same risk for Alzheimer and Parkinson diseases, as well as other neurodegenerative disorders, as people who are currently living in the most affluent of nations.

In summary, the discovery of prions and many other findings now permit a molecular definition and classification of the neurodegenerative diseases. Alzheimer and Parkinson diseases, as well as ALS, FTD, and the prion diseases are all disorders of protein processing, as are Huntington disease and the spinocerebellar ataxias. Clinical signs and neuropathologic lesions were once the primary means of describing these disorders. Although these characteristics remain useful in diagnosis, the etiologies can now be attributed to the misprocessing of particular proteins. In each of the neurodegenerative disorders, the particular protein that undergoes misprocessing determines the disease-specific phenotype, which results from the malfunction of distinct sets of neurons.

The remarkable progress in elucidating the etiologies of the major neurodegenerative diseases since the 1980s argues that the time has come to intensify the search for drug targets and develop compounds that interrupt the disease processes. In some of the neurodegenerative diseases, it may be most efficacious to design drugs that specifically block the misprocessing of a particular protein, whereas in other cases drugs that enhance the clearance of an aberrant protein or fragment may prove to be more useful. Regardless of the therapeutic approach, the need for accurate, early detection of neurodegeneration will be extremely important so that drugs can be given before significant damage to the CNS has occurred.

The task of developing useful diagnostic tests and effective therapeutics for neurodegenerative diseases should not be underestimated. Past experience with cardiovascular disease and cancer should be a bellwether of the difficult paths that lie ahead. Nevertheless, the remarkable progress in deciphering the etiologies of the neurodegenerative diseases and the urgency to prevent these age-dependent disorders should provide vigorous encouragement.

Acknowledgments

This work was supported by grants from the National Institutes of Health. I thank Drs. Fred Cohen, Stephen DeArmond, Kirk Wilhelmsen, Robert Edwards, Warren Olanow, Steve Finkbiener, and Steve Hauser for their important criticisms and valuable suggestions.

REFERENCES

1. Prusiner SB, Bolton DC, Groth DF, et al: Further purification and characterization of scrapie prions. Biochemistry 1982;21:6942–6950.

2. Glenner GG, Wong CW: Alzheimer's disease: Initial report of the purification and characterization of a novel cerebrovascular amyloid protein. Biochem Biophys Res Commun 1984;120:885–890.

3. Masters CL, Simms G, Weinman NA, et al: Amyloid plaque core protein in Alzheimer disease and Down syndrome. Proc Natl Acad Sci U S A 1985;82: 4245–4249.

4. Prusiner SB: Prions. Proc Natl Acad Sci U S A 1998;95:13363–13383.

5. Prusiner SB: Development of the prion concept. In Prion Biology and Diseases. Cold Spring Harbor, NY, Cold Spring Harbor Laboratory Press, 1999, pp 67–112.

6. Cotzias GC, Van Woert MH, Schiffer LM: Aromatic amino acids and modification of parkinsonism. N Engl J Med 1967;276:374–379.

7. Marsden CD, Parkes JD: Success and problems of long-term levodopa therapy in Parkinson's disease. Lancet 1977;1:345–349.

8. Prusiner SB: Some speculations about prions, amyloid, and Alzheimer's disease. N Engl J Med 1984; 310:661–663.

9. Prusiner SB: Shattuck lecture—neurodegenerative diseases and prions. N Engl J Med 2001;344: 1516–1526.

10. Lilienfield DE: An epidemiological overview of amyotrophic lateral sclerosis, Parkinson's disease, and dementia of the Alzheimer's type. In Calne DB (ed): Neurodegenerative Diseases. Philadelphia, WB Saunders, 1993, pp 399–425.

11. Holman RC, Khan AS, Belay ED, Schonberger LB: Creutzfeldt-Jakob disease in the United States, 1979–1994: Using national mortality data to assess the possible occurrence of variant cases. Emerg Infect Dis 1996;2:333–337.

12. Kawas CH, Katzman R: Epidemiology of dementia and Alzheimer disease. In Terry RD, Katzman R, Bick KL, Sisodia SS (eds): Alzheimer Disease, 2nd ed. Philadelphia, Lippincott Williams & Wilkins, 1999, pp 95–116.

13. Tanner CM, Goldman SM: Epidemiology of Parkinson's disease. Neuroepidemiology 1996;14: 317–335.

14. Evans DA, Funkenstein HH, Albert MS, et al: Prevalence of Alzheimer's disease in a community population of older persons—higher than previously reported. J Am Med Assoc 1989;10:2551–2556.

15. Bennett DA, Beckett LA, Murray AM, et al: Prevalence of parkinsonian signs and associated mortality in a community population of older people. N Engl J Med 1996;334:71–76.

16. Martin JB: Molecular basis of the neurodegenerative disorders. N Engl J Med 1999;340:1970–1980.

17. Will RG, Alpers MP, Dormont D, et al: Infectious and sporadic prion diseases. In Prusiner SB (ed): Prion Biology and Diseases. Cold Spring Harbor, NY, Cold Spring Harbor Laboratory Press, 1999, pp 465–507.

18. DeArmond SJ, Prusiner SB: Prion diseases. In Lantos P, Graham D (eds): Greenfield's Neuropathology, 6th ed. London, Edward Arnold, 1997, pp 235–280.

19. Prusiner SB, McKinley MP, Bowman KA, et al: Scrapie prions aggregate to form amyloid-like birefringent rods. Cell 1983;35:349–358.

20. Bendheim PE, Barry RA, DeArmond SJ, et al: Antibodies to a scrapie prion protein. Nature 1984;310: 418–421.

21. DeArmond SJ, McKinley MP, Barry RA, et al: Identification of prion amyloid filaments in scrapie-infected brain. Cell 1985;41:221–235.

22. Markesbery WR, Ehmann WD: Oxidative stress in Alzheimer disease. In Terry RD, Katzman R, Bick KL, Sisodia SS (eds): Alzheimer Disease, 2nd ed. Philadelphia, Lippincott Williams & Wilkins, 1999, pp 401–414.

23. Cotman CW, Ivins KJ, Anderson AJ: Apoptosis in Alzheimer disease. In Terry RD, Katzman R, Bick KL, Sisodia SS (eds): Alzheimer Disease, 2nd ed. Philadelphia, Lippincott Williams & Wilkins, 1999, pp 347–357.

24. Chiti F, Webster P, Taddei N, et al: Designing conditions for *in vitro* formation of amyloid protofilaments and fibrils. Proc Natl Acad Sci U S A 1999;96: 3590–3594.

25. Hershko A, Ciechanover A: The ubiquitin system. Annu Rev Biochem 1998;67:425–479.

26. Cohen FE, Prusiner SB: Pathologic conformations of prion proteins. Annu Rev Biochem 1998;67: 793–819.

27. Peretz D, Williamson RA, Kaneko K, et al: Antibodies inhibit prion propagation and clear cell cultures of prion infectivity. Nature 2001;412:739–743.

28. Gambetti P, Peterson RB, Parchi P, et al: Inherited prion diseases. In Prusiner SB (ed): Prion Biology and Diseases. Cold Spring Harbor, NY, Cold Spring Harbor Laboratory Press, 1999:509–583.

29. Hsiao K, Baker HF, Crow TJ, et al: Linkage of a prion protein missense variant to Gerstmann-Sträussler syndrome. Nature 1989;338:342–345.

30. Dlouhy SR, Hsiao K, Farlow MR, et al: Linkage of the Indiana kindred of Gerstmann-Sträussler-Scheinker disease to the prion protein gene. Nat Genet 1992;1:64–67.

31. Petersen RB, Tabaton M, Berg L, et al: Analysis of the prion protein gene in thalamic dementia. Neurology 1992;42:1859–1863.

32. Poulter M, Baker HF, Frith CD, et al: Inherited prion disease with 144 base pair gene insertion. 1. Genealogical and molecular studies. Brain 1992;115: 675–685.

33. Gabizon R, Rosenmann H, Meiner Z, et al: Mutation and polymorphism of the prion protein gene in Libyan Jews with Creutzfeldt-Jakob disease (CJD). Am J Hum Genet 1993;53:828–835.

34. St George-Hyslop PH: Molecular genetics of Alzheimer disease. In Terry RD, Katzman R, Bick KL, Sisodia SS (eds): Alzheimer Disease, 2nd ed. Philadelphia, Lippincott Williams & Wilkins, 1999, pp 311–326.

35. Wilson CA, Doms RW, Lee VMY: Intracellular APP processing and Aβ production in Alzheimer disease. J Neuropathol Exp Neurol 1999;58:787–794.

36. Selkoe DJ: Translating cell biology into therapeutic advances in Alzheimer's disease. Nature 1999; 399:A23–A31.

37. De Strooper B, Annaert W: Proteolytic processing and cell biological functions of the amyloid precursor protein. J Cell Sci 2000;113:1857–1870.

38. Brown MS, Ye J, Rawson RB, Goldstein JL: Regulated intramembrane proteolysis: A control mechanism conserved from bacteria to humans. Cell 2000;100: 391–398.

39. Yu G, Nishimura M, Arawaka S, et al: Nicastrin modulates presenilin-mediated *notch/glp-1* signal transduction and βAPP processing. Nature 2000;407:48–54.

40. Wolozin BL, Pruchniki A, Dickson D, Davies P: A neuronal antigen in the brain of Alzheimer's disease. Science 1986;232:648–650.

41. Goedert M, Wischik CM, Crowther RA, et al: Cloning and sequencing of the cDNA encoding a core protein of the paired helical filament of Alzheimer disease: Identification as the microtubule-associated protein tau. Proc Natl Acad Sci U S A 1988;85:4051–4055.

42. Lee VMY, Balin BJ, Orvos IJ, Trojanowksi JQ: A68: A major subunit of paired helical filaments and derivatized forms of normal tau. Science 1991;251: 645–678.

43. Saunders AM, Strittmatter WJ, Schmechel D, et al: Association of apolipoprotein E allele ε4 with late-onset familial and sporadic Alzheimer's disease. Neurology 1993;43:1467–1472.

44. Farrer LA, Cupples LA, Haines JL, et al: Effects of age, sex, and ethnicity on the association between apolipoprotein E genotype and Alzheimer disease. JAMA 1997;278:1349–1356.

45. Roses AD: Apolipoprotein E affects the rate of Alzheimer disease expression: β-amyloid burden is a secondary consequence dependent on APOE genotype and duration of disease. J Neuropathol Exp Neurol 1994;53: 429–437.

46. Clark LN, Poorkaj P, Wszolek Z, et al: Pathogenic implications of mutations in the tau gene in pallido-ponto-nigral degeneration and related neurodegenerative disorders linked to chromosome 17. Proc Natl Acad Sci U S A 1998;95:13103–13107.

47. Hutton M, Lendon CL, Rizzu P, et al: Association of missense and 5′ß-splice-site mutations in tau with the inherited dementia FTDP-17. Nature 1998;393:702–705.

48. Spillantini MG, Murrell JR, Goedert M, et al: Mutation in the tau gene in familial multiple system tauopathy with presenile dementia. Proc Natl Acad Sci U S A 1998;95:7737–7741.

49. Hong M, Zhukareva V, Vogelsberg-Ragaglia V, et al: Mutation-specific functional impairments in distinct tau isoforms of hereditary FTDP-17. Science 1998;282:1914–1917.

50. Buée L, Bussière T, Buée-Scherrer V, et al: Tau protein isoforms, phosphorylation and role in neurodegenerative disorders. Brain Res Brain Res Rev 2000;33: 95–130.

51. Brun A: Frontal lobe degeneration of non-Alzheimer type revisited. Dementia 1993;4:126–131.

52. Kertesz A, Munoz DG: Pick's Disease and Pick Complex. New York, Wiley-Liss, 1998, p 301.

53. Wilhelmsen KC, Lynch T, Pavlou E, et al: Localization of disinhibition-dementia-parkinsonism-amyotrophy complex to 17q21-22. Am J Hum Genet 1994;55:1159–1165.

54. Conrad C, Andreadis A, Trojanowski JQ, et al: Genetic evidence for the involvement of tau in progressive supranuclear palsy. Ann Neurol 1997;41:277–281.

55. Goedert M, Spillantini MG, Crowther RA, et al: Tau gene mutation in familial progressive subcortical gliosis. Nat Med 1999;5:454–457.

56. Nussbaum RL, Polymeropoulos MH: Genetics of Parkinson's disease. Hum Mol Genet 1997;6: 1687–1691.

57. Tanner CM, Ottman R, Goldman SM, et al: Parkinson disease in twins: An etiologic study. JAMA 1999;281:341–346.

58. Polymeropoulos MH, Lavedan C, Leroy E, et al: Mutation in the α-synuclein gene identified in families with Parkinson's disease. Science 1997;276:2045–2047.

59. Spillantini MG, Schmidt ML, Lee VMY, et al: α-Synuclein in Lewy bodies. Nature 1997;388:839–840.

60. Shimura H, Hattori N, Kubo SI, et al: Familial Parkinson disease gene product, parkin, is a ubiquitin-protein ligase. Nat Genet 2000;25:302–305.

61. Giasson BI, Duda JE, Murray IVJ, et al: Oxidative damage linked to neurodegeneration by selective α-synuclein nitration in synucleinopathy lesions. Science 2000;290:985–989.

62. Hughes TA, Ross HF, Musa S, et al: A 10-year study of the incidence of and factors predicting dementia in Parkinson's disease. Neurology 2000;54:1596–1624.

63. Hansen L, Salmon D, Galasko D, et al: The Lewy body variant of Alzheimer's disease: A clinical and pathologic entity. Neurology 1990;40:1–8.

64. Hashimoto M, Masliah E: α-Synuclein in Lewy body disease and Alzheimer's disease. Brain Pathol 1999;9:707–720.

65. Spillantini MG, Crowther RA, Jakes R, et al: α-Synuclein in filamentous inclusions of Lewy bodies from Parkinson's disease and dementia with Lewy bodies. Proc Natl Acad Sci U S A 1998;95:6469–6473.

66. Langston JW, Quik M, Petzinger G, et al: Investigating Levodopa-induced dyskinesias in the Parkinsonian primate. Ann Neurol 2000;47:S79–S89.

67. Spencer PS, Allen RG, Kisby GE, Ludolph AC: Excitotoxic disorders. Science 1990;248:144.

68. Hudson AJ: Amyotrophic lateral sclerosis and its association with dementia, parkinsonism and other neurological disorders: A review. Brain 1981;104: 217–247.

69. Swash M: Clinical features and diagnosis of amyotrophic lateral sclerosis. In Brown RH Jr, Meininger V, Swash M (eds): Amyotrophic Lateral Sclerosis. London, Martin Dunitz, 2000, pp 3–30.

70. Bobowick AR, Brody JA: Epidemiology of motor-neuron diseases. N Engl J Med 1973;288: 1047–1055.

71. Rosen DR, Siddique T, Patterson D, et al: Mutations in Cu/Zn superoxide dismutase gene are associated with familial amyotrophic lateral sclerosis. Nature 1993;362:59–62.

72. Cleveland DW, Liu J: Oxidation versus aggregation—how do SOD1 mutants cause ALS? Nat Med 2000;6:1320–1321.

73. Wong PC, Pardo CA, Borchelt DR, et al: An adverse property of a familial ALS-linked SOD1 mutation causes motor neuron disease characterized by vacuo-

lar degeneration of mitochondria. Neuron 1995;14: 1105–1116.

74. Hadano S, Hand CK, Osuga H, et al: A gene encoding a putative GTPase regulator is mutated in familial amyotrophic lateral sclerosis 2. Nat Genet 2001;29: 166–173.

75. Yang Y, Hentati A, Deng HX, et al: The gene encoding alsin, a protein with three guanine-nucleotide exchange factor domains, is mutated in a form of recessive amyotrophic lateral sclerosis. Nat Genet 2001;29: 160–165.

76. Uchihara T, Sato T, Suzuki H, et al: Bunina body in frontal lobe dementia without clinical manifestations of motor neuron disease. Acta Neuropathol 2001;101: 281–284.

77. Wada M, Uchihara T, Nakamura A, et al: Bunina bodies in amyotrophic lateral sclerosis on Guam: A histochemical, immunohistochemical and ultrastructural investigation. Acta Neuropathol 1999;98: 150–156.

78. Reed TE, Neel JV: Huntington's chorea in Michigan. Am J Hum Genet 1959;11:107–136.

79. Lin X, Cummings CJ, Zoghbi HY: Expanding our understanding of polyglutamine diseases through mouse models. Neuron 1999;24:499–502.

80. Paulson HL: Protein fate in neurodegenerative proteinopathies: Polyglutamine diseases join the (mis)fold. Am J Hum Genet 1999;64:339–345.

81. The Huntington's Disease Collaborative Research Group: A novel gene containing a trinucleotide repeat that is expanded and unstable on Huntington's disease chromosomes. Cell 1993;72:971–983.

82. Zoghbi HY, Orr HT: Glutamine repeats and neurodegeneration. Annu Rev Neurosci 2000;23:217–247.

83. Koyano S, Uchihara T, Fujigasaki H, et al: Neuronal intranuclear inclusions in spinocerebellar ataxia type 2: Triple-labeling immunofluorescent study. Neurosci Lett 1999;273:117–120.

84. LaSpada AR, Wilson EM, Lubahn DB, et al: Androgen receptor gene mutations in X-linked spinal and bulbar muscular atrophy. Nature 1991;352:377.

85. Games D, Adams D, Alessandrini R, et al: Alzheimer-type neuropathology in transgenic mice overexpressing V717F β-amyloid precursor protein. Nature 1995;373:523–527.

86. Hsiao K, Chapman P, Nilsen S, et al: Correlative memory deficits, Aβ elevation, and amyloid plaques in transgenic mice. Science 1996;274:99–102.

87. Kane MD, Lipinski WJ, Callahan MJ, et al: Evidence for seeding of beta-amyloid by intracerebral infusion of Alzheimer brain extracts in beta-amyloid precursor protein-transgenic mice. J Neurosci 2000;20: 3606–3611.

88. Shin R-W, Bramblett GT, Lee VMY, Trojanowski JQ: Alzheimer disease A68 proteins injected into rat brain induce codeposits of β-amyloid, ubiquitin, and α1-antichymotrypsin. Proc Natl Acad Sci U S A 1993; 90:6825–6828.

89. Borchelt DR, Ratovitski T, van Lare J, et al: Accelerated amyloid deposition in the brains of transgenic mice coexpressing mutant presenilin 1 and amyloid precursor proteins. Neuron 1997;19:939–945.

90. Raber J, Wong D, Yu GQ, et al: Apolipoprotein E and cognitive performance. Nature 2000;404:352–354.

91. Mucke L, Masliah E, Yu GQ, et al: High-level neuronal expression of Aβ$_{1-42}$ in wild-type human amyloid protein precursor transgenic mice: Synaptotoxicity without plaque formation. J Neurosci 2000;20: 4050–4058.

92. De Strooper B, Annaert W, Cupers P, et al: A presenilin-1-dependent γ-secretase-like protease mediates release of Notch intracellular domain. Nature 1999;398:518–522.

93. Lewis J, McGowan E, Rockwood J, et al: Neurofibrillary tangles, amyotrophy and progressive motor disturbance in mice expressing mutant (P301L) tau protein. Nat Genet 2000;25:402–405.

94. Feany MB, Bender WW: A *Drosophila* model of Parkinson's disease. Nature 2000;404:394–398.

95. van der Putten H, Wiederhold KH, Probst A, et al: Neuropathology in mice expressing human α-synuclein. J Neurosci 2000;20:6021–6029.

96. Masliah E, Rockenstein E, Veinbergs I, et al: Dopaminergic loss and inclusion body formation in α-synuclein mice: Implications for neurodegenerative disorders. Science 2000;287:1265–1269.

97. Kriz J, Meier J, Julien JP, Padjen AL: Altered ionic conductances in axons of transgenic mouse expressing the human neurofilament heavy gene: A mouse model of amyotrophic lateral sclerosis. Exp Neurol 2000; 163:414–421.

98. Couillard-Després S, Zhu Q, Wong PC, et al: Protective effect of neurofilament heavy gene overexpression in motor neuron disease induced by mutant superoxide dismutase. Proc Natl Acad Sci U S A 1998;95:9626–9630.

99. Williamson TL, Bruijn LI, Zhu Q, et al: Absence of neurofilaments reduces the selective vulnerability of motor neurons and slows disease caused by a familial amyotrophic lateral sclerosis-linked superoxide dismutase 1 mutant. Proc Natl Acad Sci U S A 1998;95:9631–9636.

100. Reddy PH, Williams M, Charles V, et al: Behavioural abnormalities and selective neuronal loss in HD transgenic mice expressing mutated full-length HD cDNA. Nat Genet 1998;20:198–202.

101. Shelbourne PF, Killeen N, Hevner RF, et al: A Huntington's disease CAG expansion at the murine Hdh locus is unstable and associated with behavioural abnormalities in mice. Hum Mol Genet 1999;8:763–774.

102. Hodgson JG, Agopyan N, Gutekunst C, et al: A YAC mouse model for Huntington's disease with full-length mutant huntingtin, cytoplasmic toxicity, and selective striatal neurodegeneration. Neuron 1999;23: 181–192.

103. Yamamoto A, Lucas JJ, Hen R: Reversal of neuropathology and motor dysfunction in a conditional model of Huntington's disease. Cell 2000;101:57–66.

104. Wheeler VC, White JK, Gutekunst CA, et al: Long glutamine tracts cause nuclear localization of a novel form of huntingtin in medium spiny striatal neurons in Hdh^{Q92} and Hdh^{Q111} knock-in mice. Hum Mol Genet 2000;9:503–513.

105. Jackson GR, Salecker I, Dong X, et al: Polyglutamine-expanded human huntingtin transgenes induce degeneration of *Drosophila* photoreceptor neurons. Neuron 1998;21:633–642.

106. Saudou F, Finkbeiner S, Devys D, Greenberg M: Huntingtin acts in the nucleus to induce apoptosis but death does not correlate with the formation of intranuclear inclusions. Cell 1998;95:55–66.

107. Perutz MF: Glutamine repeats and inherited neurodegenerative diseases: Molecular aspects. Curr Opin Struct Biol 1996;6:848–858.

108. Klement IA, Skinner PJ, Kaytor MD, et al: Ataxin-1 nuclear localization and aggregation: Role in polyglutamine-induced disease in SCA1 transgenic mice. Cell 1998;95:41–53.

109. Huynh DP, Figueroa K, Hoang N, Pulst SM: Nuclear localization or inclusion body formation of ataxin-2 are not necessary for SCA2 pathogenesis in mouse or human. Nat Genet 2000;26:44–50.

110. Ikeda H, Yamaguchi M, Sugai S, et al: Expanded polyglutamine in the Machado-Joseph disease protein induces cell death *in vitro* and *in vivo*. Nat Genet 1996;13:196–202.

111. Warrick JM, Chan HYE, Gray-Board Gl, et al: Suppression of polyglutamine-mediated neurodegeneration in *Drosophila* by the molecular chaperone HSP70. Nat Genet 1999;23:425–428.

112. Manuelidis E, Kim J, Angelo J, Manuelidis L: Serial propagation of Creutzfeldt-Jakob disease in guinea pigs. Proc Natl Acad Sci U S A 1976;73:223–227.

113. Orr HT, Zoghbi HY: Reversing neurodegeneration: A promise unfolds. Cell 2000;101:1–4.

114. Perrier V, Wallace AC, Kaneko K, et al: Mimicking dominant negative inhibition of prion replication through structure-based drug design. Proc Natl Acad Sci U S A 2000;97:6073–6078.

115. Kaneko K, Zulianello L, Scott M, et al: Evidence for protein X binding to a discontinuous epitope on the cellular prion protein during scrapie prion propagation. Proc Natl Acad Sci U S A 1997;94:10069–10074.

116. Zulianello L, Kaneko K, Scott M, et al: Dominant-negative inhibition of prion formation diminished by deletion mutagenesis of the prion protein. J Virol 2000;74:4351–4360.

117. Jick H, Zornberg GL, Jick SS, et al: Statins and the risk of dementia. Lancet 2000;356:1627–1631.

118. Supattapone S, Nguyen H-OB, Cohen FE, et al: Elimination of prions by branched polyamines and implications for therapeutics. Proc Natl Acad Sci U S A 1999;96:14529–14534.

119. Priola SA, Raines A, Caughey WS: Porphyrin and phthalocyanine antiscrapie compounds. Science 2000;287:1503–1506.

120. Schenk D, Barbour R, Dunn W, et al: Immunization with amyloid-beta attenuates Alzheimer-disease-like pathology in the PDAPP mouse. Nature 1999;400:173–177.

121. Birmingham K, Frantz S: Set back to Alzheimer vaccine studies. Nat Med 2002;8:199–200.

122. Seboun E, Oksenberg JR, Hauser SL: Molecular and genetic aspects of multiple sclerosis. In Rosenberg RN, Prusiner SB, DiMauro S, Barchi RL (eds): The Molecular and Genetic Basis of Neurological Disease, 2nd ed. Boston, Butterworth-Heinemann, 1997, pp 631–660.

123. Genain CP, Cannella B, Hauser SL, Raine CS: Identification of autoantibodies associated with myelin damage in multiple sclerosis. Nat Med 1999;5:170–175.

124. Lucchinetti C, Brück W, Parisi J, et al: Heterogeneity of multiple sclerosis lesions: Implications for the pathogenesis of demyelination. Ann Neurol 2000;47:707–717.

125. Haines JL, Terwedow HA, Burgess K, et al: Linkage of the MHC to familial multiple sclerosis suggests genetic heterogeneity. Hum Mol Genet 1998; 7:1229–1234.

126. Fujinami RS, Oldstone MBA: Amino acid homology between the encephalitogenic site of myelin basic protein and virus: Mechanism for autoimmunity. Science 1985;230:1043–1045.

127. Wucherpfennig KW, Strominger JL: Molecular mimicry in T cell-mediated autoimmunity: Viral peptides activate human T-cell clones specific for myelin basic protein. Cell 1995;80:695–705.

128. Taylor SI: Diabetes mellitus. In Scriver CR, Beaudet AL, Sly WS, Valle D (eds): The Metabolic and Molecular Bases of Inherited Disease, 7th ed, vol 1. New York, McGraw-Hill, 1995, pp 843–896.

129. Benson MD: Amyloidosis. In Scriver CR, Beaudet AL, Sly WS, Valle D (eds): The Metabolic and Molecular Bases of Inherited Disease, 7th ed, vol 1. New York, McGraw-Hill, 1995, pp 4159–4191.

130. United Nations: World population prospects the 1998 revision: The Sex and Age Distribution of the World Population, vol. 2. New York, United Nations Department of Economic and Social Affairs Population Division, 1999, pp 1–833.

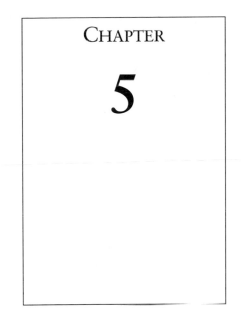

CHAPTER 5

Selected Genetically Engineered Models Relevant to Human Neurodegenerative Disease

Donald L. Price, David R. Borchelt
Michael K. Lee, Philip C. Wong

This review, which focuses on selected neurodegenerative diseases (Table 5–1), including Alzheimer's disease (AD), amyotrophic lateral sclerosis (ALS), and Parkinson's disease (PD), is designed to demonstrate how genetically engineered models have provided new insights into the mechanisms of these disorders and have identified new targets for therapy. These illnesses are among the most challenging diseases in medicine because of their overall prevalence, cost, lack of mechanism-based treatments, and impact on individuals and caregivers.[1,2] They are characterized by distinct clinical phenotypes reflecting dysfunction and death of specific populations of neurons and by the presence of intracellular or extracellular peptides/aggregates, which appear to be critical contributors to neurotoxicity. Genetic risk factors influence these age-associated, chronic illnesses. In rare instances, cases are inherited in mendelian fashion, but more commonly, susceptibility genes, environmental risks, or other factors that remain to be defined influence the diseases. Information from genetics has allowed investigators to express or to target genes in efforts to model these diseases and to study the molecular participants critical in pathogenic pathways. Although symptomatic treatments exist, at present, mechanism-based therapies are not available.

In this review, we emphasize the value of genetically engineered mouse models (Table 5–2) for studies of mechanisms and for experimental therapeutics, but we also briefly describe the extraordinary utility of non-mammalian genetic models. Similar animal modeling approaches have illuminated the mechanisms of other neurodegenerative diseases, including the tauopathies, the trinucleotide repeat diseases, and the prion disorders (see Table 5–2).[3–7] We focus on models of familial vari-

ants of AD, ALS, and PD—autosomal dominant FAD, FALS, and FPD. The identification of mutations in specific genes causing each of these illnesses has provided new opportunities for scientists to investigate the molecular participants in pathologic processes and to explore disease mechanisms using transgenic approaches. In these autosomal dominant disorders, the mutant proteins often do not exhibit reductions in normal functions, but instead, malfolded mutant peptides acquire toxic properties that have a direct or indirect impact on the structures, functions, and viabilities of neural cells. Introducing mutant genes into mice reproduces some features of these diseases. Moreover, targeting the genes that influence pathogenic pathways has provided new insights into disease mechanisms and has led to identification of potential therapeutic targets. We anticipate that additional targets will be identified and that novel treatments will be tested in these model systems and eventually examined in clinical trials. Because of limitations on citations, our references are predominantly reviews.[1–4,8–24]

ALZHEIMER'S DISEASE

Clinical Features, Pathology, and Genetics

Affected individuals usually develop clinical manifestations (difficulty in memory and cognitive functions followed by progressive dementia) during the seventh decade (earlier in familial cases).[1,2,17,24,25] These signs result from selective degeneration of population neurons in the central nervous system (CNS), including those in the basal forebrain cholinergic system, hippocampus, and cortex (Figs. 5–1 and 5–2). Dysfunction and death of

TABLE 5–1. Neurodegenerative Diseases

Chronic and progressive

Sporadic and/or familial

Autosomal dominant, recessive, X-linked, allele-associated

Clinical manifestations reflecting selective vulnerability of subsets of cells

Associated with intracellular or extracellular protein aggregates, degeneration of synapses and axons, and evidence of cell dysfunction/death

Significant causes of morbidity and mortality

Enormous costs to society

With rare exceptions, no effective therapies

From model systems, new opportunities for identifying therapeutic targets and testing mechanism-based treatments

these neurons disrupts synaptic communication in these systems, which are critical for the memories, cognitive abilities, and brain functions that make each person unique. These alterations are reflected by decrements in synaptic markers in target fields of these neurons. The pathologic hallmarks of AD are neurofibrillary tangles (NFT), dystrophic neurites, deposition of Aβ, and local glial reactions; the latter three pathologies are components of plaques (see Fig. 5–1). The principal structural elements in NFT (fibrillar intracytoplasmic inclusions in cell bodies/proximal dendrites of affected neurons) and in swollen neurites (filament-containing distal axons and terminals) are poorly soluble paired helical filaments (PHF) composed of hyperphosphorylated isoforms of tau, a microtubule-associated protein. Aβ, a 4-kD amyloid peptide derived by cleavages of the amyloid precursor protein (APP), appears in the brain extracellular space (neuropil) as monomers, oligomers, and multimers,

which, in β-pleated sheet conformations, assemble into protofilaments and then fibrils. Extracellular Aβ fibrils are present in the cores of neuritic plaques (see Fig. 5–1), which preferentially localize to the cortex, hippocampus, and amygdala.[2,17,24,25]

In some individuals with autosomal dominant AD, mutations have been identified in three different genes: amyloid precursor protein (APP), PS1, and PS2 (see Fig. 5–1). APP, a type I transmembrane protein existing as several isoforms, is expressed in many different cell types. Significantly, APP is particularly abundant in neurons. It is synthesized in cell bodies and is transported rapidly anterograde in axons by interacting with a kinesin motor, and possibly serves as a cargo receptor. Cleavages of APP generate Aβ peptides via the activities of BACE1 (β-site APP cleaving enzyme 1) and the γ-secretase complex,[20,24,26,27] which generate the N- and C-termini of Aβ peptides, respectively (Fig. 5–3A, B). The γ-secretase cleavage liberates the APP intracellular domain (AICD) which, on translocation to the nucleus, appears to play a role in transcription.[24,28] It is hypothesized that the levels and distributions of APP and the neuronal pro-amyloidogenic cleavage enzymes, particularly BACE1, are principal determinants of high levels of Aβ in the brain.[27,29] In contrast, formation of Aβ is precluded by cleavage of APP within the Aβ domain by α-secretase and by BACE2, which are either expressed at low or nondetectable levels, respectively, in the brain, but at variably higher levels in other organs.[2]

Several FAD links of APP mutations are located in proximity to the pro-amyloidogenic cleavage sites.[19,24] For example, the APPswe mutation, a double mutation at the N-terminus of Aβ, enhances BACE1 cleavage manyfold and is associated with elevated levels of all Aβ peptides, including Aβ42. The APP 717 mutation, located near the C-terminus of Aβ, promotes γ-secretase activity, leading to increased secretion of Aβ42, the longer and more toxic Aβ peptide.

TABLE 5–2. Dominant Neurodegenerative Diseases and Models

Disease	Mutant Gene	Intracellular or Extracellular Aggregates	Components of Aggregates	Transgene in Models
FAD	APP	Extracellular amyloid	Aβ	Mutant APP and APP/PS1
	PS1			
	PS2			
FALS	SOD1	Cytoplasmic inclusions	SOD1	Mutant SOD1
FTDP-17	Tau	Tangle-like structures	Tau	Wt/mutant tau
PD	α-syn	Lewy bodies	α-syn/peptide fragments	Wt (or mutant) α-syn
		Lewy neurites		
Prion	PrP	Amyloid-like material	PRP^sc	Mutant PrP
SCA-1	ataxin-1	Intranuclear Inclusions	ataxin-1	ataxin-1 (expanded repeat)
SCA-3	ataxin-3	Intranuclear inclusions	ataxin-3	ataxin-3 (expanded repeat)

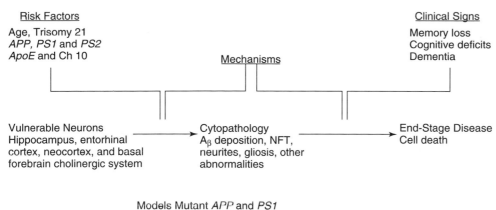

Risk Factors

Age, Trisomy 21
APP, PS1 and *PS2*
ApoE and Ch 10

Mechanisms

Clinical Signs

Memory loss
Cognitive deficits
Dementia

Vulnerable Neurons
Hippocampus, entorhinal
cortex, neocortex, and basal
forebrain cholinergic system

Cytopathology
Aβ deposition, NFT,
neurites, gliosis, other
abnormalities

End-Stage Disease
Cell death

Models Mutant *APP* and *PS1*
BACE1, PS1, and *Nicastrin* targeted mice

FIGURE 5–1. Experimental therapeutics in Alzheimer's disease.

PS1 and *PS2*, which encode two highly homologous 43-kD to 50-kD multipass transmembrane proteins that are processed to stable N-terminal and C-terminal fragments, are conserved from invertebrates to humans and are involved in Notch 1 signaling critical for cell fate decisions.[16,24] They are widely expressed at low abundance in the CNS. *PS1* and *PS2* influence APP processing and are recognized as components of the γ-secretase complex along with Nicastrin, a type I transmembrane glycoprotein,[16,24] as well as Aph1 and Pen2, two multipass transmembrane proteins.[30] The *PS1* gene has been reported to harbor more than 80 different FAD mutations, whereas only a small number of mutations have been found in *PS2*-linked families.[19,24,31] The majority of abnormalities in *PS* genes are missense mutations that result in single amino acid substitutions, which enhance γ-secretase activity and increase the levels of the Aβ42 peptides. See the section on gene targeting relevant to Alzheimer's disease for discussion of the results of gene targeting studies. These studies have begun to clarify some of the properties of APP, BACE1, and components of the δ-secretase complex.

Mouse Models of Aβ Amyloidosis

In mice, expression of *swe* or *717* minigenes encoding FAD-linked mutations in *APP* (with or without mutant *PS1*) leads to Aβ amyloidosis in the CNS. Levels of Aβ are elevated, and diffuse Aβ deposits and neuritic plaques appear in the hippocampus and cortex.[1,2,17,32] Classical neurofibrillary tangles are not present in a region of the brain. The pathology evolves in stages: elevated levels of Aβ; synaptic alterations; formation of neurites; axon degeneration; and diffuse amyloid evolving to plaques (see Fig. 5–2). The nature and levels of the expressed transgene and the specific mutation influence the severity of the pathology. Mice expressing both mutant *PS1* and mutant *APP* develop accelerated disease.[32] Learning deficits, problems in object-recognition memory, and difficulties performing tasks assessing spatial reference and working memory have been identified in some of the lines of mutant mice.[33] Thus, these animals have an Aβ amyloidosis in the CNS. Although the mutant mice do not fully recapitulate the full phenotypes of AD, they are very useful subjects for research designed to examine mechanisms and to test therapies for this type of disease.

In attempts to obtain mice with both plaques and tangles, mutant *APP* transgenic mice have been mated to mice expressing the *P301L Tau* mutant, a mutation linked to familial frontotemporal dementia with parkinsonism (FTDP). These mice appear to have a greater number of tangles and an apparent shift in distribution of NFT.[6] Moreover, tau pathology appears to be induced by introducing Aβ fibrils into the brains of *P301L tau* mutant mice. However, mice bearing both mutant *tau* and *APP* or mutant *tau* mice injected with Aβ are problematic as models of FAD because the FTDP mutation alone is associated with the presence of tangles.

Vulnerability Transmitter System in AD

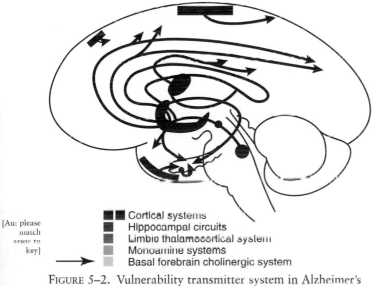

[Au: please match areas to key]

■■ Cortical systems
■ Hippocampal circuits
■ Limbic thalamocortical system
■ Monoamine systems
■ Basal forebrain cholinergic system
→

FIGURE 5–2. Vulnerability transmitter system in Alzheimer's disease.

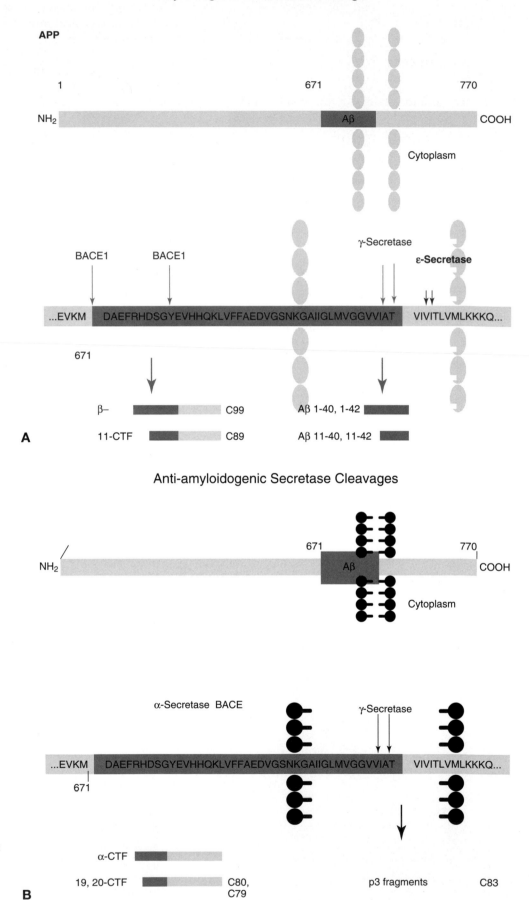

FIGURE 5–3. *A*, Amyloidogenic secretase cleavages. *B*, anti-amyloidogenic secretase cleavages.

Coexpression of mutant FAD-linked genes and all six iso-forms of wild-type human Tau may achieve a more appropriate model of AD.

Gene Targeting Relevant to Alzheimer's Disease

In an effort to understand the functions of some of the genes thought to play roles in AD, investigators have targeted a variety of genes, including *APP, APLPs, BACE1,* and *PS1*.

Homozygous *APP*[-/-] mice are viable and fertile, but supports to have subtle decreases in locomotor activity and forelimb grip strength.[34] The absence of substantial phenotypes in *APP*[-/-] mice is thought to be related to functional redundancy of two amyloid precursor-like proteins, APLP1 and APLP2, homologous to APP. Consistent with this idea, *APLP2*[-/-] mice appear normal, but *APP* and *APLP2* null mice and *APLP1* and *APLP2* null mice do not survive the perinatal period.[35]

BACE1, a type 1 transmembrane aspartyl protease, is relatively abundant in brain, is enriched in neurons versus glia, and is transported to axons to terminals. *BACE1* null mice are viable and healthy, have no obvious phenotype or pathology, and can mate successfully.[20,27,36] Importantly, cortical neurons cultured from *BACE1*[-/-] embryos do not show cleavages at the +1 and +11 sites of Aβ, and the secretion of Aβ peptides is abolished even in the presence of elevated levels of exogenous wt or mutant APP.[27] In brains of *BACE1* null mice, Aβ peptides are not produced. These results establish that BACE1 is the neuronal β-secretase required to cleave APP to generate the N-termini of Aβ.[27] At present, there is no consensus on other substrates cleaved by BACE1. Behavioral studies of the null mice, in vitro and in vivo challenges of *BACE1* neural cells, and two-dimensional gels of organs from

BACE[+/+], *BACE*[+/-], and *BACE*[-/-] mice will be critical in determining the consequences of the absence of BACE1 on behavior, susceptibility to challenge, and other substrates that may be cleaved by the enzyme. Results thus far indicate that BACE1 is an excellent therapeutic target for development of an anti-amyloidogenic drug.

The source of APP giving rise to Aβ has been debated.[29] Significantly, key participants in Aβ amyloidosis (APP, PS1, and BACE1) are synthesized by neurons, transported to terminals, and colocalized with neurites in immediate proximity to sites of Aβ deposition in brain. This provides circumstantial evidence consistent with a neuronal origin for Aβ. Moreover, APP is cleaved by BACE in distal axons terminal to generate C-terminal amyloidogenic peptides (see Fig. 5–3A, B). More compelling is the demonstration that lesions of specific neuronal populations or their axonal projections (i.e., entorhinal cortex or perforant pathway) reduce the levels of Aβ and the number of plaques in terminal fields of these neurons (Figs. 5–4 and 5–5).[37]

Because BACE1 is the principal β-secretase in neurons and BACE2, and α-secretase may serve to limit the secretion of Aβ peptides in other organs, we have hypothesized that the relative levels of BACE1 and BACE2 activities, in conjunction with high levels of APP in neurons, are major determinants of Aβ amyloidosis in the CNS (Fig. 5–6).[27,29] This hypothesis predicts that the secretion of Aβ peptides will be the highest in neurons and brain as compared to other cell types or tissues because neurons express high levels of APP and BACE1 coupled with low-level expression of BACE2 *and* α-secretase. Seemingly inconsistent with this hypothesis is a study showing high levels of BACE1 mRNA in the pancreas. *BACE1* is critical for Aβ amyloidosis, and both BACE1 and APP are expressed in β cells of the pancreas. Then why do AD and diabetes mellitus not occur together? It appears that

Evolution of Pathology in *APPswe x PS1 δE9* Mice

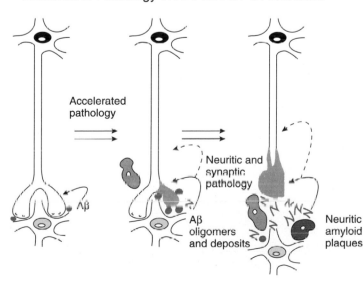

FIGURE 5–4. Evolution of pathology in *APPswe × PS1δE9* mice.

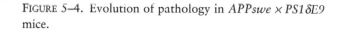

Reduction in Aβ Burden After Damage to ERC or
Transection of Perforant Pathway of *APP*swe Mice

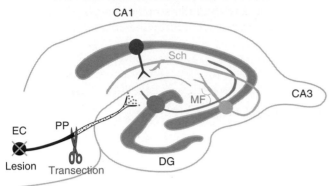

FIGURE 5–5. Reduction in Aβ burden after damage to ERC or transection of perforant pathway of *APPswe* mice.

BACE1 mRNAs in the pancreas are alternatively spliced to generate a BACE1 isoform that is incapable of cleaving APP. Taken together with the observations that pancreas possesses low levels of normal BACE1 protein and activity, these results are consistent with the view that a high ratio of BACE1 to BACE2 activity leads to the selective vulnerability of neurons to Aβ amyloidosis, and the cells of the pancreas are spared.

In contrast to *BACE* null mice, *PS1*⁻/⁻ mice do not survive beyond the early postnatal period and show severe developmental abnormalities of the axial skeleton, ribs, and spinal ganglia, features resembling a partial *Notch1*⁻/⁻ phenotype.[38] These abnormalities occur because PS1 along with Nicastrin, APH1, PEN2, and perhaps other proteins, are components of the ψ-*secretase* complex that carries out the S3 intramembranous cleavage of Notch1, a receptor protein involved in critical cell-fate decisions during development. Without this cleavage, the Notch1 intracellular domain (NICD) is not released from the plasma membrane and does not reach the nucleus to initiate transcriptional processes essential for cell fate decisions. In cell culture, absence of *PS1* or substitution of particular aspartate residues leads to reduced levels of ψ-secretase cleavage products and levels of Aβ. *PS2* null mice are viable and fertile, though they develop age-associated mild pulmonary fibrosis and hemorrhage. Mice lacking *PS1* and heterozygous for *PS2* die midway through gestation with full *Notch1* null-like phenotype. To study the role of PS1 in vivo in adult mice, two groups generated conditional *PS1*-targeted mice lacking PS1 expression in the forebrain after embryonic development. As expected, the absence of PS1 resulted in decreased generation of Aβ, further establishing that PS1 is critical for γ-secretase activity in the brain. As discussed, more recent work has established that Nicastrin, APH1, and PEN2 are also components of the δ-secretase complex and are critical for stabilizing PS and for generation of Aβ.[30] In concert, these findings suggest that γ-secretase inhibitors may be useful as therapeutic agents for Aβ amyloidosis.

Potential Therapeutics for Alzheimer's Disease

Although these mutant transgenic mice do not recapitulate the full phenotype of AD, they represent excellent models of Aβ amyloidosis and are highly suitable for identification of therapeutic targets and for testing new treatments (see Fig. 5–6). Both β- and γ-secretase activities represent therapeutic targets for the development of novel protease inhibitors for AD. However, the demonstration that BACE1 is the principal β-secretase in cultured neurons and that (in contrast to *PS1*⁻/⁻ mice) the *BACE1*⁻/⁻ mice seem to be normal, provides an excellent rationale for focusing on the design of novel therapeutics to inhibit BACE1 activity in brain. Significantly, BACE1-deficient neurons fail to secrete Aβ even when coexpressing the *APPswe* and mutant *PS1* genes, and these *BACE-1* coexpressing mutant *APP/PS* gene mice do not exhibit Aβ plaques in the brain (H Cai, DL Price, PC Wong: unpublished data). PS, Nicastrin, APH1, and PEN2 are necessary for α-secretase activity. With the latter, these proteins stabilize PS. Research suggests that PS1 is essential for activity, but it is not the protease performing γ cleavage (at least for Notch1).[39] Because of the role of the γ-secretase complex in Notch processing, it may be valuable to try to design therapeutics that inhibit selectively the γ-secretase activity with regard to APP without allowing the activity involved in Notch1 processing. This approach is being pursued because several populations of cells, hematopoietic stem cells in particular, use Notch 1 signaling for cell-fate decisions even in adults.

A variety of other treatments have been tested in mouse models (Table 5–3), but space constraints limit

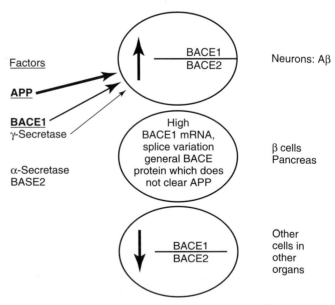

FIGURE 5–6. Distribution of BACE 1 and 2 in different cell populations influence generation of Aβ.

TABLE 5–3. Selected Experimental Treatment Strategies

1. Inhibitors of BACE1 and γ-secretase
2. Active or passive Aβ immunotherapy
3. NSAIDS—preferentially decrease Aβ42 (increase Aβ1-38)
4. Cu/Zn chelator (Clioquinol) solubilizes/decreases Aβ
5. Inhibition of Acyl-coA:cholesterol acyltransferase (catalyzes formation of cholesterol esters)
6. Disruption of aggregates (Congo red, rifampicin, anthracycline, short peptides)
7. Block binding of glycosoaminoglycans to Aβ (destabilize deposits)
8. Deplete SAP (which binds to amyloid) using competitive inhibitor of binding of SAP (promotes clearance of SAP and of amyloid by making latter accessible)
9. COX inhibition (suppress inflammation/oxidative injury)

discussion. However, to illustrate the challenges of extrapolating outcomes in mice to trials with humans, it is useful to briefly discuss recent problems with Aβ immunotherapy. In prevention and treatment trials, both Aβ immunization (with Freund's adjuvant) and passive transfer of Aβ antibodies reduce levels of Aβ and plaque burden in mutant APP transgenic mice. Efficacy seems to be related to antibody titer. The mechanisms of enhanced clearance are not certain, but two not mutually exclusive hypotheses have been suggested: (1) a small amount of Aβ antibody reaches the brain, binds to Aβ peptides, promotes the disassembly of fibrils, and via the Fc antibody domain attracts activated microglia that remove Aβ[40], and (2) serum antibodies serve as a sink to draw the amyloid peptides from the brain into the circulation, thus changing the equilibrium of Aβ in different compartments and promoting removal from the brain.[41] Immunotherapy in transgenic mice was successful in clearing Aβ and attenuates learning and behavioral deficits in at least two cohorts of mutant APP mice. Although phase 1 trials with Aβ peptide and adjuvant were not associated with any adverse events, phase 2 trials of this strategy have been suspended because of severe adverse reactions (encephalomyelitis) in a subset of patients.

AMYOTROPHIC LATERAL SCLEROSIS

Clinical Features, Pathology, and Genetics

Individuals with this motor neuron disease have muscle weakness and atrophy, as well as spastic paralysis (Fig. 5–7)[9,13,15] These signs result from selective degeneration of spinal and corticospinal motor neurons, respectively. In motor neurons (Fig. 5–8), proximal axonal segments are swollen with accumulations of neurofilaments, and cell bodies show ubiquitin-positive protein aggregates. Distal motor axons degenerate, and terminals become disconnected from the denervated muscles. Presumably, as trophic support is compromised, cell bodies shrink and then dendrites are attenuated. Clinical signs appear to be most closely linked to the disconnection of the motor terminals from their targets. Ultimately, neurons degenerate, exhibiting several features consistent with oxidative damage and programmed cell death (Table 5–4). Ultimately, the numbers of motor neurons in the spinal cord and brain stem nuclei are reduced.

Approximately 10% of cases of ALS are familial, and, in most of these individuals, the disease is inherited in an autosomal dominant pattern. Approximately 15% to 20% of patients with autosomal dominant FALS (less than –2% of all ALS cases) have mutations in the gene that encodes cytosolic Cu/Zn superoxide dismutase (SOD1), a widely expressed and abundant antioxidant enzyme that catalyzes the conversion of $?O_2^-$ to O_2 and H_2O_2. To date, more than 90 different missense mutations have been identified in the *SOD1* gene. Although some FALS *SOD1* mutants show reduced enzymatic

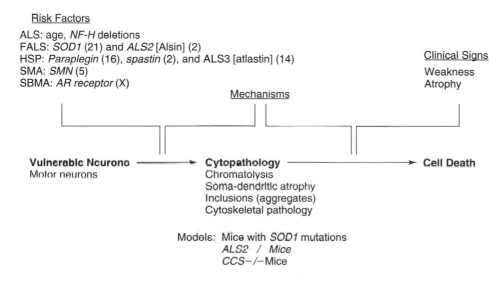

Risk Factors

ALS: age, *NF-H* deletions
FALS: *SOD1* (21) and *ALS2* [Alsin] (2)
HSP: *Paraplegin* (16), *spastin* (2), and ALS3 [atlastin] (14)
SMA: *SMN* (5)
SBMA: *AR receptor* (X)

Clinical Signs

Weakness
Atrophy

Mechanisms

Vulnerable Neurons ⟶ **Cytopathology** ⟶ **Cell Death**
Motor neurons   Chromatolysis
                             Soma-dendritic atrophy
                             Inclusions (aggregates)
                             Cytoskeletal pathology

Models: Mice with *SOD1* mutations
        ALS2 / Mice
        CCS–/–Mice

FIGURE 5–7. Motor neuron diseases/models.

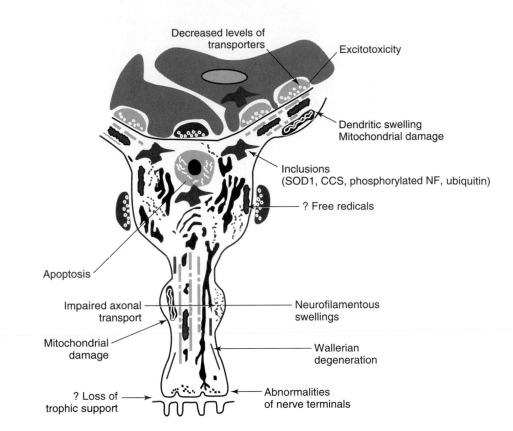

FIGURE 5–8. Abnormalities in ALS.

activities, many variants retain full activity as occurs with the G37R *SOD1* mutation.[42] These mutations are scattered throughout the protein and are not preferentially localized near the active site or the dimer interface. It is puzzling how these mutations lead to a common phenotype. Thus, it is hypothesized that the mutant enzyme causes selective neuronal degeneration through a gain of toxic property (Table 5–5), a concept consistent with autosomal dominant inheritance.[43] It has been suggested

TABLE 5–4. PCD in Motor Neurons of/Cases ALS

Stages of degeneration:

    Chromatolysis

    Atrophy of dendrites and soma (accompanied by condensation of cytoplasm and nucleus)

    Apoptosis

TUNEL-positive cells visualized when atrophy is present

Internucleosomal patterns of DNA fragmentation

DFF-40 (CAD) present at high levels in cytosolic fractions

Caspase-3 and caspase-1 activity increased

Bcl-2 decreased in mitochondrial fraction, but increased in cytosol; Bax and Bak show patterns opposite to Bcl-2

that the misfolded mutant SOD1 could catalyze aberrant reactions, including enhanced peroxidase activity, increased reactions with peroxinitrite, and mutation-induced conformational changes that result in aberrant activity catalyzed by Cu bound to mutant SOD1 (see section on potential therapies for amyotrophic lateral sclerosis for discussion of potential aberrant copper chemistry in mutant SOD-mediated disease).[44] The presence of ubiquitin aggregates containing mutant SOD1 protein raises the possibility that aggregated mutant proteins, which may exhibit conformational changes, are toxic, that the protein aggregates sequester molecules that are critical for cell viability, or the malfolded mutant proteins damage proteosomal degradative machinery.[13]

SOD1 Mutant Mice

Although there are a variety of other extraordinarily interesting models of motor neuron disease,[13,15] this review focuses on mice expressing FALS-linked mutant *SOD1*. The mice harboring mutations develop progressive weakness and muscle atrophy, and cellular pathology closely resembling that occurring in ALS. For example, the *G37R SOD1* mice accumulate to 3 to 12 times the endogenous levels in the spinal cord, and the levels of the mutant protein influence the age of onset.[43] High molecular weight complexes of mutant SOD

TABLE 5–5. Mutant SOD1 Gains a Toxic Property

- Some mutant *SOD1* genes do not show loss of activity, and some are quite stable
- No dominant-negative effects of mutant *SOD1*
- *SOD1* –/– mice do not develop FALS-like syndrome
- Mutant *SOD1* mice develop impaired extension of hind limbs; tremor; altered gait; progressive weakness/slowness of movement; muscle wasting
- Increasing or decreasing level of SOD1 has no effect on phenotype of mutant mice

accumulate in neural tissues but not in non-nervous system organs.[45] Some neuronal cell bodies show SOD1, ubiquitin, and phosphorylated NF-H immunoreactive inclusions; in some lines of mutant mice, vacuolization and swelling of mitochondria appear early in some motor neurons. Toxic SOD1 is transported anterograde in axons, and early on, SOD1 accumulates in axons, where it is associated with structural pathology, occurring approximately two to three months before the appearance of clinical signs. Thus, SOD1, neurofilaments, and degenerating mitochondria appear in irregular, swollen, intraparenchymal portions of motor axons, and axonal transport is abnormal. Wallerian degeneration of axons occurs, and the mice become weak.[2,43,46] In mutant mice (and in cases of ALS), it has been reported that caspase 1 and 3 activities increase (early and late, respectively), followed by evidence of action of caspase 9.[13,47] Eventually, the number of motor neurons is decreased and glial proliferation is present in the anterior horns.

Potential Therapies for Amyotrophic Lateral Sclerosis

Mutant *SOD1* mice have been used to test pharmacologic and gene-based therapies.[13] Several potential treatments have been tested, including administration of vitamin E, selenium, riluzole, gabapentin, and d-penicillamine (a copper chelator), but the results have not been encouraging. Treatments with creatine, caspase inhibitors, and minocycline (which inhibits release of cytochrome C from mitochondria) have had modest influences on onset of disease and survival.

Treatment strategies would be more effectively targeted if the molecular mechanisms whereby mutant *SOD1* causes selective degeneration of motor neurons was better understood. It was initially speculated that loss of enzyme activity might be a factor in disease. However, this idea is not compatible with the following observations: Some mutants show full activity; SOD1 null mice do not develop motor neuron phenotypes; and elevations or reductions in mutant SOD1 by mating *SOD1* overexpressors or *SOD1* null mice, respectively, to animals with

mutations, does not influence phenotype.[13,48] It has been proposed that the toxic property of mutant *SOD1* involves mutation-induced conformational changes in SOD1 that result in aberrant oxidative activities. In this scenario, cell dysfunction and death can be initiated by chemistries catalyzed by Cu bound in the active site of mutant SOD1.[49] To test this hypothesis, we took advantage of the discovery in yeast of Ly7 T+HL and its mammalian homologue Cu chaperone SOD1 (CCS); generated mice lacking *CCS* showed what is required for Cu loading of mammalian SOD1.[50] Inactivation of the *CCS* gene in mice demonstrates that CCS is required for efficient Cu incorporation into SOD1 in mammals, and the phenotypes of the *CCS* null mice resemble those of the *SOD1* null mice. These mice were crossed with multiple lines of mutant SOD1 mice. Metabolic Cu labeling studies in mutant *SOD1* mice lacking CCS show that copper incorporation into wild-type and mutant SOD1 is significantly diminished. Thus, CCS is necessary for efficient copper incorporation into SOD1 of motor neurons. However, although the absence of the CCS results in a significant reduction in the level of Cu-loaded mutant SOD1, the *CCS*[–/–] genotype has no effect on the onset, progression, or pathology of the motor neuron disease occurring in mutant *SOD1* mice.[49] This result (Table 5–6) is inconsistent with the concept that aberrant, Cu-dependent activity of mutant SOD1 is involved in the pathogenesis of FALS.

A pathologic hallmark of ALS is the accumulation of neurofilaments in swollen proximal axons (and cell bodies) of motor neurons; whether primary or secondary, these abnormalities are associated with axonal transport, a process important for the long-term viability of neurons.[9,13,15] To test the role of neurofilaments in mutant *SOD1*-induced motor neuron disease, mutant *SOD1*

TABLE 5–6. Mutant *SOD1* Causes Disease Independent of Copper

- Hypothesis: Copper-mediated toxicity plays essential role in mutant *SOD1*-linked FALS
- CCS required to incorporate copper into SOD1
- *CCS* +/– mice bred to wild-type or G37R, G93A, G85R *SOD1* mice to generate cohort of either wild-type or mutant *SOD1* mice with or without CCS
- Levels of mutant *SOD1* similar in all groups (CCS +/+, +/–, –/–)
- Copper labeled SOD1 not present in spinal cord of mice lacking CCS, and enzyme activity markedly reduced
- Following facial nerve axotomy, neurons of CCS –/– mice show increased cell death (like *SOD1* nulls)
- Onset and progression of clinical signs/pathology (including aggregates) in mutant *SOD1* mice not influenced by presence or absence of CCS

mice were crossbred to several lines of mice with altered levels or distributions of neurofilament proteins. When mice expressing NF-H-β-galactosidase fusion protein NF-H-lacZ (which cross-links neurofilaments and prevents their export into axons) are crossed with mutant *SOD1* mice, the progeny show no changes in progression of disease. Mutant *SOD1* mice lacking *NF-L* (neurofilament light chain) have a moderate increase in life span, while mutant *SOD1* mice overexpressing wild-type *NF-L* exhibit attenuation of disease progression and an increased life span. A more significant protection of motor neurons was achieved by introducing the *NF-H* gene into lines of mutant *SOD1* mice. However, it is possible that some of the influences on phenotype described with genetic mutations may be related to the introduction of new strain backgrounds into mutant mice rather than the presence or absence of specific genes.

Although the molecular mechanisms underlying mutant *SOD1*-linked familial ALS remain unclear, several pathogenic mechanisms[1,13] other than the copper hypothesis have been proposed. These mechanisms include roles for toxicity or sequestration of mutant SOD1-containing aggregates; excitotoxicity related to reduction in levels of GLT1 or activity of this glial transporter important in glutamate uptake in the spinal cord; reduced chaperone activity; damage to the proteosomal degradative machinery by malfolded or aggregated mutant SOD1; and activation of caspases. These hypotheses are being explored. For example, overexpression of *BcL2* in mutant *SOD1* mice has a modest impact on onset and survival.

At present, riluzole is the only drug approved for therapy in human ALS, but the benefits are modest. Investigators are examining other ways to ameliorate excitotoxicity, possibly by influencing the levels or activity of the glial glutamate transporter. Trials with growth factors were stopped because of complications. To date, there have been no trials of inhibitors of apoptosis nor have engineered cells or stem cells been implanted, although these areas of research are promising.

PARKINSON'S DISEASE

Clinical Features, Pathology and Genetics

Usually appearing in the sixth or seventh decade, classical parkinsonism is characterized by resting tremor, rigidity, slowness of voluntary movement (bradykinesia), stooped posture, impaired postural stability, and shuffling gate (Fig. 5–9).[14,21–23,23,51–54] PD is the record most common neurodegenerative disease (to AD) and affects approximately 1% of individuals over 65 years of age. Both sexes are equally affected. Motor deficits are related to degeneration of pigmented dopaminergic neurons in the substantia nigra pars compacta (SNpc).[55–60] These neurons often exhibit Lewy Bodies (LB), which are spherical, intracytoplasmic, usually ubiquitin-immunoreactive inclusions with a filamentous core often surrounded by clear halo; and Lewy neurites LN), which are LB-like, smaller inclusions in processes of nigral neurons and several other affected neuronal populations.[57,61–63] A major fibrillar component of these two types of inclusions is α-synuclein (α-syn)[64] (see *α-Syn* Transgenic Mice section), but other proteins, including synphilin,[65] are associated with these inclusions. The abnormalities in the nigral neurons are associated with reductions (80% to 95%) in dopaminergic markers and the number of dopamine receptors in striatum.[66] In the basal ganglia, the loss of dopaminergic influences on striatal cells[23,67] leads to overactivity of the indirect pathway and decreased activity of the direct pathway. Because of different actions of D1 and D2 receptors in these two pathways, the result of dopaminergic deafferentation of the striatum leads to increased activity of nerve cells in the globus palas interna. This, in turn, leads to enhanced inhibition of

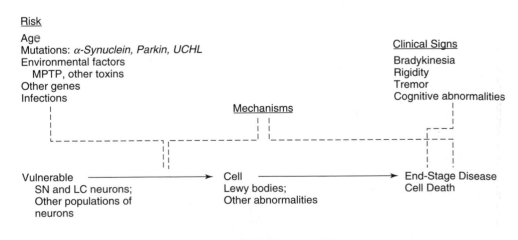

FIGURE 5–9. Parkinsonism.

thalamocortical neurons; the clinical outcome is brady-kinesia.

The disease may be familial in approximately 10% of cases, and mutations have been identified in *α-syn*, ubiquitin carboxy terminal hydrolase l1 (*UCH-L1*), and *parkin*.[10,21,68,69] The first disease-specific mutation (A53Tα) was located within the exon 4 of *α-syn* (chromosome 4aq21–q23).[70,71] A sequence is normally present in α-syn (of rodents) and in synelfin, an avian α-syn homologue (of zebra finches) (Fig. 5–10).[72] The same mutation was found in several Greek kindreds. More recently, a second *α-syn* mutation (A30P) was discovered in two affected members of a small German pedigree.[70,71] α-syn, comprised of 140 amino acids, is a highly conserved protein found in mammals, fish, and birds (95% to 86% identity).[73,74–76] In mammals, *α-syn* is a member of a multigene family consisting of at least two other *synuclein* genes (*β-Syn* and *γ-Syn*).[77,78] The synucleins, small cytosolic proteins of unknown function enriched at the synaptic terminals of neurons, show a conserved N-terminal repeat region (100 amino acids) consisting of seven imperfect repeats of 11 amino acid residues (KTKEGV), a hydrophobic sequence in the middle of the protein, and a less-well-conserved, negatively charged C-terminal domain (see Fig. 5–10).

Mutations (I93M) in the *UCH-L1* gene have been identified in two members of kindred with autosomal dominant PD. However, it is not certain that this mutation is truly causative of disease.

An autosomal recessive form of juvenile parkinsonism (AR-JP) has been linked to truncations, frameshifts, and missense/nonsense mutations in *parkin* (chromosome 6q27).[68,69,79] Parkin,[79] a protein that shows some features common with ubiquitin at the amino terminus and has a cysteine ring-finger motive at the carboxy-terminus, acts as an E3-ubiquitin ligase, and as such provides for substrate specificity of ubiquitination.[10,80,81] Parkin may participate in ubiquitination and metabolism of α-syn and synphilin, an α-syn-interacting protein implicated in α-syn aggregation. It is generally believed that *parkin* mutations lead to PD without LBs and that other substrates of parkin, such as Pae1 receptor, may be toxic to neurons if not degraded. It has been suggested that reduced parkin activity may result in the accumulation of proteins/peptides (α-syn and Pae1 receptor)

that are toxic to dopaminergic neurons leading to parkinsonian phenotype in vivo.[10]

α-Syn Transgenic Mice

To understand the mechanisms whereby mutant *α-syn* leads to motoric abnormalities and neurodegeneration, investigators have produced multiple lines of transgenic mice.[82–85] For example, we have expressed high levels of either wild-type or FPD-linked A30P or A53T human *α-syn* in mice.[82] To achieve high levels of transgene expression in mice, the transgene expression (cDNAs encoding human wild-type *A30P* or *A53T α-syn*) was controlled by the murine prion promotor MoPrP-*Hu α-syn*. Analysis of transgene-derived mRNA and protein show high levels of *Hu α-syn* expression in the brains of these mice. The levels of total α-syn protein (human and mouse combined) in the brains of MoPrP-*Hu α-syn* mice are 4 to 15 times higher than in the nontransgenic mice. In situ hybridization discloses widespread expression of transgene-derived Hu α-syn mRNA in all brain regions, particularly the brain stem. The *A53T Hu α-syn* mice, but not mice with wild-type or *A30P* variants, develop adult-onset, progressive motoric dysfunction leading to death. Affected mice accumulate α-syn and ubiquitin in neuronal perikarya and neurites, and brain regions with pathology show detergent-insoluble α-syn and α-syn aggregates. Immunoblot analyses of total SDS-soluble proteins disclose three α-syn polypeptides and peptide fragments corresponding to the full-length α-syn polypeptide (α-syn16) and two truncated α-syn polypeptides (α-syn12 and α-syn10) (see Fig. 5–10). The majority of α-syn fractionates with the S1 fraction, an observation consistent with α-syn being a cytosolic protein. However, α-syn in the P2 fractions from the brain stems of clinically affected A53T *Hu α-syn* mice are different quantitatively and qualitatively from α-syn polypeptides in the other P2 fractions. Specifically, the brain stem P2 fraction from the affected *A53T* Hu α-syn mice contain significantly more detergent-insoluble full-length (≈16-kDa) α-syn. Moreover, the P2 fraction is also enriched for α-syn species with a lower molecular mass α-syn (α-syn 10 and α-syn 12) and a series of higher molecular mass aggregates of α-syn. Parallel analysis of (wt) Hu α-syn and A30P Hu α-syn mice show that the α-syn species enriched in the P2

Proteolytic Processing of

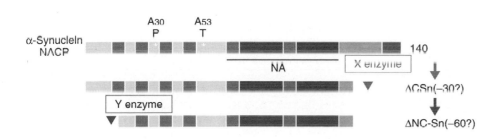

FIGURE 5–10. Proteolytic processing of α-synuclein NACP.

fraction is specific of A53T Hu α-syn or the expression. These results suggest that mutant α-syn can be cleaved (by "synucleinases") in both the N- and C-terminal regions (see Fig. 5–10), generating peptides that aggregate, gain a toxic property, and track with the disease. Moreover, the A53T α-syn and derived peptides are associated with significantly greater in vivo neurotoxicity as compared with other α-syn variants, and α-syn-dependent neurodegeneration is associated with abnormal accumulation of detergent-insoluble α-syn. In a similar study,[84] mice were generated expressing either wild-type or *A53T Hu α-syn*. Only the mice expressing the mutant protein developed motor impairments, paralysis, premature death, and age-dependent intracytoplasmic α-syn fibrillary inclusions in neurons. α-Syn was present in the detergent-insoluble fraction, but there were no comments on α-syn peptide fragments. A major research question in this field is whether these α-syn segments are present in FPD and in sporadic PD. If such is the case, it will be critical to identify the enzymes carrying out these cleavages, which may be targets for therapy.

Although the expression of wild-type or mutant *α-Syn* has been associated with neuropathology in several lines of transgenic mice and in flies, these studies of *A53Tα-syn* document that the expression of this mutant gene leads to formation of truncated α-syn peptide high molecular aggregates in vivo neurotoxicity compared with either *A30P* or *WT Hu α-syn* variants associated with progressive neurodegeneration and death (but not classic PD). Although increased in vivo toxicity of the *A53T* mutation is consistent with a more aggressive disease course in humans than the *A30P* mutation, the lack of significant neuropathology in mice expressing A30P Hu *α-Syn* is unexpected. Although the *A30P* mutation is found in a small pedigree with only two affected members, the potential for toxicity was assumed to be greater than with *A53T* mutation. This is because *A30P* is a highly nonconservative substitution, whereas the *A53T* mutation is actually a normal sequence in rodents. It remains possible that the two mutations in Hu *α-syn* initiate disease in different ways, or that the *A30P* variant could be a rare polymorphism.

α-Syn Gene Targeted Mice

Initial studies of *α-syn^{-/-}* mice indicate that α-syn is not essential for the viability of the mice. Knockout mice are viable and fertile; neural development appears normal; the complement of dopaminergic cell bodies, fibers, and synapses is normal; and the pattern of dopamine discharge and reuptake in response to electrical stimulation is unremarkable. However, dopaminergic terminals in *α-syn^{-/-}* mice exhibit faster recovery from paired pulse stimuli.[86] Shortened recovery from the prepulse can be mimicked in the wild-type mice by elevations of extracellular calcium. Significantly, *α-syn^{-/-}* mice exhibit reductions in total striatal dopamine levels and

in the dopamine-dependent locomotor response to amphetamines. These results are consistent with the concept that α-syn is a presynaptic, activity-dependent, negative regulator of dopaminergic neurotransmission. It is possible that both β-syn and γ-syn can compensate for the loss of α-synuclein expression, and it will be useful to study mice with other syn isotypes to determine the importance of various syn proteins regarding normal synaptic activity.

CONCLUSION

The identification of genes mutated or deleted in the inherited forms of many neurodegenerative diseases has allowed investigators to create in vivo and in vitro model systems relevant to a wide variety of human neurologic disorders.

In this review, we emphasized the value of transgenic and gene-targeted models and the lessons they provided for understanding mechanisms of their neurodegenerative diseases (see Tables 5–1 and 5–2). For example, the study of *BACE1^{-/-}* mice and mutant *APP/PS1* transgenic models has provided extraordinary new insights into the mechanisms of Aβ amyloidogenesis, the reasons AD is a brain amyloidosis, and potential therapeutic targets. In contrast, our studies of mutant SOD1 mice lacking CCS demonstrate that aberrant activities dependent on copper-loaded SOD1 are unlikely to be involved with pathogenic mechanisms and that other mechanisms/targets should be explored. Finally, with regard to mutant α-syn–linked FPD, results from studies of mouse models suggest that α-syn may undergo C- and N-terminal cleavages, generating toxic peptides. Strategies designed to delineate the participants in these cleavage processes, discover separate synucleinases, and determine the consequence of deleting or inhibiting these enzymes will need to be explored. If these cleavages occur in humans with PD, it will be essential to understand the mechanisms of cell injury and to design inhibitors that block cleavages of α-syn.

Invertebrate organisms, such as *Caenorhabditis elegans* or *Drosophila melanogaster,* provide excellent genetically manipulatable model systems for examining many aspects of neurodegenerative diseases.[3,87–90] Invertebrates harboring mutant transgenes can be generated rapidly, and their nervous systems are relatively simple. Moreover, behavior can be scored with flies having the ability to carry out more complex behaviors and having a longer life span than worms. Significant new information has come from transgenic technologies, which have allowed mutant genes to be introduced into or ablated in flies and worms. For example, when wild-type or mutant human α-syn is expressed in the nervous system of flies, dopaminergic neurons degenerate in adult life, nerve cells show accumulations of γ-syn and filamentous inclusions, and animals develop progressive motor dysfunction.[87] Similar experiments have been carried out in models of the CAG repeat diseases that encode expansions of polyglutamine.[88–90] When expanded ataxin-3 is expressed in the retina of *Drosophila*, the retina degenerates, but the disease can be attenuated by manipulations of P35 or Hsp70. Similarly, introductions of wild-type or mutant human tau into flies, models of tau-related neurodegenerative disease, can be performed. Flies carrying these transgenes exhibit adult-onset progressive neurodegeneration, evidence of enhanced toxicity of mutant tau, accumulations of abnormal tau in cells (but without neurofibrillary tangles), and early lethality.[90] Because these invertebrate models reproduce aspects of pathology variety occurring in human neurodegenerative diseases, studies of these systems should prove very useful in delineating disease pathways, identifying suppressors and enhancers of these processes, and testing the influences of drugs on phenotypes in flies and worms.

These new models allow investigators to examine the molecular mechanisms by which mutant proteins cause selective dysfunction and death of neurons and to determine possible pathogenic pathways that can be tested by crossing animals with either mutated or deleted alleles of other molecular players in the pathogenic process. The use of RNAi methods will accelerate the validation of molecules involved in pathogenic pathways. The results of these approaches will provide a better understanding of the mechanisms that lead to disease.

In summary, investigations of genetically engineered (transgenic or gene-targeted) mice have disclosed participants in pathogenic pathways, reproduced some features of human neurodegenerative disorders, supplied important new information about the disease mechanisms, and allowed identification of new therapeutic targets. Moreover, the models can be used for testing novel treatments. These lines of research have made spectacular progress over the past few years, and we anticipate that discoveries will lead to design of more promising therapies that can be tested in models of these devastating diseases.

REFERENCES

1. Wong PC, Cai H, Borchelt DR, Price DL: Genetically engineered mouse models of neurodegenerative diseases. Nat Neurosci 2002;5:633–639.

2. Lipp HP, Wolfer DP: Genetically modified mice and cognition. Curr Opin Neurobiol 1998;8:272–280.

3. Lin X, Cummings CJ, Zoghbi HY: Expanding our understanding of polyglutamine diseases through mouse models. Neuron 1999;24:499–502.

4. Lee VMY, Trojanowski JQ: Neurodegenerative tauopathics: Human disease and transgenic mouse models. Neuron 1999;24:507–510.

5. Lewis J, McGowan E, Rockwood J, et al: Neurofibrillary tangles, amyotrophy and progressive disturbance in mice expressing mutant (P301L) tau protein. Nat Genet 2000;25:402–405.

6. Lewis J, Dickson DW, Lin W-L, et al: Enhanced neurofibrillary degeneration in transgenic mice expressing mutant tau and APP. Science 2001;293:1487–1491.

7. Yamamoto A, Lucas JJ, Hen R: Reversal of neuropathology and motor dysfunction in a conditional model of Huntington's disease. Cell 2000;101:57–66.

8. Lee MK, Price DL: Advances in genetic models of Parkinson's disease. Clin Neurosci Res 2001;1:456–466.

9. Wong PC, Rothstein JD, Price DL: The genetic and molecular mechanisms of motor neuron disease. Curr Opin Neurobiol 1998;8:791–799.

10. Dawson TM, Mandir AS, Lee MK: Animal Models of PD: Pieces of the Same Puzzle? Neuron 2002;35:219–222.

11. Goedert M: Alpha-synuclein and neurodegenerative diseases. Nature 2001;2:492.

12. Sherman MY, Goldberg AL: Cellular defenses against unfolded proteins: A cell biologist thinks about neurodegenerative diseases. Neuron 2001;29:15–32.

13. Cleveland DW, Rothstein JD: From Charcot to Lou Gehrig: Deciphering selective motor neurons death in ALS. Nature 2001;2:806–819.

14. Dunnett SB, Bjorklund A: Prospects for new restorative and neuroprotective treatments in Parkinson's Disease. Nature 1999;399:A32–A39.

15. Julien J-P: Amyotrophic lateral sclerosis: Unfolding the toxicity of the misfolded. Cell 2001;104:581–591.

16. Kopan R, Goate A: Aph-2/Nicastrin: An essential component of gamma-secretase and regulator of notch signaling and presenilin localization. Neuron 2002;33:321–324.

17. Price DL, Tanzi RE, Borchelt DR, Sisodia SS: Alzheimer's disease: Genetic studies and transgenic models. Annu Rev Genet 1998;32:461–493.

18. Selkoe DJ: Clearing the brain's amyloid cobwebs. Neuron 2001;32:177–180.

19. Tanzi RE: New frontiers in Alzheimer's disease genetics. Neuron 2001;32:181–184.

20. Vassar R, Citron M: Aβ-generating enzymes: Recent advances in β- and γ-secretase research. Neuron 2000;27:419–422.

21. Goedert M: The significance of tau and α-synuclein inclusions in neurodegenerative diseases. Curr Opin Genet Dev 2001;11:343–351.

22. Olanow CW, Tatton WG: Etiology and pathogenesis of Parkinson's disease. Annu Rev Neurosci 1999;22:123–144.

23. Wichmann T, DeLong MR: Functional and pathophysiological models of the basal ganglia. Curr Opin Neurobiol 1996;6:752–758.

24. Sisodia SS, George Hyslop PH: Gamma-secretase, Notch, Abeta and Alzheimer's disease: Where do the presenilins fit in? Nat Rev Neurosci 2002;3:281–290.

25. Selkoe DJ: Alzheimer's Disease: Genes, proteins, and therapy. Psychol Rev 2001;81:741–766.

26. Vassar R, Bennett BD, Babu-Khan S, et al: β-secretase cleavage of Alzheimer's amyloid precursor protein by the transmembrane aspartic protease BACE. Science 1999;286:735–741.

27. Cai H, Wang Y, McCarthy D, et al: BACE1 is the major β-secretase for generation of Aβ peptides by neurons. Nat Neurosci 2001;4:233–234.

28. Cao X, Sdhof TC: A transcriptively active complex of APP with Fe65 and histone acetyltransferase Tip60. Science 2001;293:115–120.

29. Wong PC, Price DL, Cai H: The brain's susceptibility to amyloid plaques. Science 2001;293:1434–1435.

30. Francis R, McGrath G, Zhang J, et al: aph-1 and pen-2 are required for notch pathway signaling, gamma-secretase cleavage of betaAPP, and presenilin protein accumulation. Dev Cell 2002;3:85–97.

31. Sherrington R, Rogaev EI, Liang Y, et al: Cloning of a gene bearing missense mutations in early-onset familial Alzheimer's disease. Nature 1995;375: 754–760.

32. Benoist C, Mathis D: Cell death mediators in autoimmune diabetes—no shortage of suspects. Cell 1997;89:1–3.

33. Chen G, Chen KS, Knox J, et al: A learning deficit related to age and β-amyloid plaques in a mouse model of Alzheimer's disease. Nature 2000;408:975–979.

34. Zheng H, Jiang M-H, Trumbauer ME, et al: β-amyloid precursor protein-deficient mice show reactive gliosis and decreased locomotor activity. Cell 1995;81:525–531.

35. Heber S, Herms J, Gajic V, et al: Mice with combined gene knock-outs reveal essential and partially redundant functions of amyloid precursor protein family members. J Neurosci 2000;20:7951–7963.

36. Luo Y, Bolon B, Kahn S, et al: Mice deficient in BACE1, the Alzheimer's β-secretase, have normal phenotype and abolished β-amyloid generation. Nature 2001;4:231–232.

37. Sheng JG, Price DL, Koliatsos VE: Disruption of corticocortical connections ameliorates amyloid burden in terminal fields in a transgenic model of Abeta amyloidosis. J Neurosci 2002;22:9794–9799.

38. Wong PC, Zheng H, Chen H, et al: Presenilin 1 is required for Notch1 and Dll1 expression in the paraxial mesoderm. Nature 1997;387:288–292.

39. Taniguchi Y, Karlstrom H, Lundkvist J, et al: Notch receptor cleavage depends on but is not directly executed by presenilins. Proc Natl Acad Sci U S A 2002; 99:4014–4019.

40. Schenk D, Barbour R, Dunn W, et al: Immunization with amyloid-attenuates Alzheimer-disease-like pathology in the PDAPP mouse. Nature 1999;400:173–177.

41. DeMattos RB, Bales KR, Cummins DJ, et al: Peripheral anti-Aβ antibody alters CNS and plasma Aβ clearance and decreases brain Aβ burden in a mouse model of Alzheimer's disease. Proc Natl Acad Sci U S A 2001;98:8850–8855.

42. Borchelt DR, Guarnieri M, Wong PC, et al: Superoxide dismutase 1 subunits with mutations linked to familial amyotrophic lateral sclerosis do not affect wild-type subunit function. J Biol Chem 1995;270: 3234–3238.

43. Wong PC, Pardo CA, Borchelt DR, et al: An adverse property of a familial ALS-linked SOD1 mutation causes motor neuron disease characterized by vacuolar degeneration of mitochondria. Neuron 1995;14: 1105–1116.

44. Ichas F, Jouaville LS, Mazat JP: Mitochondria are excitable organelles capable of generating and conveying electrical and calcium signals. Cell 1997;89: 1145–1153.

45. Wang J, Xu G, and Borchelt DR: High molecular weight complexes of mutant superoxide dismutase 1: Age-dependent and tissue-specific accumulation. Neurobiol Dis 2002;9:139–148.

46. Bruijn LI, Becher MW, Lee MK, et al: ALS-linked SOD1 mutant G85R mediates damage to astrocytes and promotes rapidly progressive disease with SOD1-containing inclusions. Neuron 1997;18: 327–338.

47. Li M, Ona VO, Gugan C, et al: Functional role of caspase-1 and caspase-3 in an ALS transgenic mouse model. Science 2000;288:335–339.

48. Bruijn LI, Houseweart MK, Kato S, et al: Aggregation and motor neuron toxicity of an ALS-linked SOD1 mutant independent from wild-type SOD1. Science 1998;281:1851–1854.

49. Subramaniam JR, Lyons WE, Liu J, et al: Mutant SOD1 causes motor neuron disease independent of copper chaperone-mediated copper loading. Nat Neurosci 2002;5:301–307.

50. Wong PC, Waggoner D, Subramaniam JR, et al: Proc Natl Acad Sci U S A 2000;97:2886–2891.

51. Lozano AM, Lang AE, Hutchison WD, Dostrovsky JO: New developments in understanding the etiology of Parkinson's disease and in its treatment. Curr Opin Neurobiol 1998;8:783–790.

52. Baron MS, Vitek JL, Bakay RAE: Treatment of advanced Parkinson's disease by posterior GPi pallidotomy: 1-year results of a pilot study. Ann Neurol 1996; 40:355–366.

53. Vázques J, Fernández-Shaw C, Marina A, et al: Antibodies to human brain spectrin in Alzheimer's disease. J Neuroimmunol 1996;68:39–44.

54. Markham CH, Diamond SG: Clinical overview of Parkinson's disease. Clin Neurosci 1993;1: 5–11.

55. Foix MC: Les lesions anatomiques de la maladie de Parkinson. Rev Neurol 1921;28:595–600.

56. Hassler R: Zur Pathologie der Paralysis agitans und des postencephalitischen Parkinsonismus. J Psychol Neurol (Lpz) 1938;48:367–476.

57. Greenfield JG, Bosanquet FD: The brain-stem lesions in Parkinsonism. J Neurol Neurosurg Psychiatr 1953;16:213–226.

58. Oppenheimer DR, Esiri MM: Diseases of the basal ganglia, cerebellum and motor neurons. In Adams JH, Duchen LW (eds): Greenfield's Neuropathology. New York, Oxford University Press, 1992, pp 988–1045.

59. Sima AAF, Defendini R, Keohane C, et al: The neuropathology of chromosome 17-linked dementia. Ann Neurol 1996;39:734–743.

60. Forno LS, Langston JW, DeLanney LE, et al: Locus ceruleus lesions and eosinophilic inclusions in MPTP-treated monkeys. Ann Neurol 1986;20:449–455.

61. Forno LS: Pathology of parkinsonism. A preliminary report of 24 cases. J Neurosurg 1966;24:266–271.

62. Braak H, Sandmann-Keil D, Gai W, Braak E: Extensive axonal Lewy neurites in Parkinson's disease: A novel pathological feature revealed by alpha-synuclein immunocytochemistry. Neurosci Lett 1999;265:67–69.

63. Braak H, Rub U, Sandmann-Keil D, et al: Parkinson's disease: Affection of brain stem nuclei controlling premotor and motor neurons of the somatomotor system. Acta Neuropathol (Berl) 2000;99:489–495.

64. Spillantini MG, Schmidt ML, Lee VM, et al: Alpha-synuclein in Lewy bodies. Nature 1997;388:839–840.

65. Chung KKK, Zhang Y, Lim KL, et al: Parkin ubiquitinates the α-synuclein-interacting protein, synphilin-1: Implications for Lewy body formation in Parkinson's disease. Nature Med 2001;7:1144–1150.

66. Langlais PJ, Thal L, Hansen L, et al: Neurotransmitters in basal ganglia and cortex of Alzheimer's disease with and without Lewy bodies. Neurology 1993;43:1927–1934.

67. Lozano AM, Lang AE, Hutchinson WD, Dostrovsky JO: New developments in understanding the etiology of Parkinson's Disease and in its treatments. Curr Opin Neurobiol 1998;8:783–790.

68. Kitada T, Asakawa S, Hattori N, et al: Mutations in the parkin gene cause autosomal recessive juvenile parkinsonism. Nature 1998;392:605–608.

69. Armstrong RA, Cairns NJ, Myers D, et al: A comparison of β-amyloid deposition in the medial temporal lobe in sporadic Alzheimer's disease, Down's syndrome and normal elderly brains. Neurodegeneration 1996;5:35–41.

70. Kruger R, Kuhn W, Muller T, et al: Ala30Pro mutation in the gene encoding alpha-synuclein in Parkinson's disease. Nat Genet 1998;18:106–108.

71. Polymeropoulos MH, Lavedan C, Leroy E, et al: Mutation in the α-synuclein gene identified in families with Parkinson's disease. Science 1997;276:2045–2047.

72. Polymeropoulos MH: Autosomal dominant Parkinson's disease and à-synuclein. Ann Neurol 1998;44:63–64.

73. Ueda K, Fukushima H, Masliah E, et al: Molecular cloning of cDNA encoding an unrecognized component of amyloid in Alzheimer disease. Proc Natl Acad Sci U S A 1993;90:11282–11286.

74. George JM, Jin H, Woods WS, Clayton DF: Characterization of a novel protein regulated during the critical period for song learning in the zebra finch. Neuron 1995;15:361–372.

75. Südhof TC: The synaptic vesicle cycle: A cascade of protein-protein interactions. Nature 1995;375:645–653.

76. Irizarry MC, Kim TW, McNamara M, et al: Characterization of the precursor protein of the non-A beta component of senile plaques (NACP) in the human central nervous system. J Neuropathol Exp Neurol 1996;55:889–895.

77. Maroteaux L, Campanelli JT, and Scheller RH: Synuclein: A neuron-specific protein localized to the nucleus and presynaptic nerve terminal. J Neurosci 1988;8:2804–2815.

78. Goedert M: The awakening of α-synuclein. Nature 1997;388:232–233.

79. Lucking CB, Durr A, Bonifati V, et al: Association between early-onset Parkinson's disease and mutations in the parkin gene. N Engl J Med 2000;342:1560–1567.

80. Zhang Y, Gao J, Chung KK, et al: Parkin functions as an E2-dependent ubiquitin-protein ligase and promotes the degradation of the synaptic vesicle-associated protein, CDCrel-1. Proc Natl Acad Sci U S A 2000;97:13354–13359.

81. Imai Y, Soda M, Takahashi R: Parkin suppresses unfolded protein stress-induced cell death through its E3 ubiquitin-protein ligase activity. J Biol Chem 2000;275:35661–35664.

82. Laptook AR, Corbett RJT, Arencibia-Mireles O, et al: The effects of systemic glucose concentration on brain metabolism following repeated brain ischemia. Brain Res 1994;638:78–84.

83. Masliah E, Rockenstein E, Veinbergs I, et al: Dopaminergic loss and inclusion body formation in alpha-synuclein mice: Implications for neurodegenerative disorders. Science 2000;287:1265–1269.

84. Giasson BI, Duda JE, Quinn SM, et al: Neuronal alpha-synucleinopathy with severe movement disorder in mice expressing A53T human alpha-synuclein. Neuron 2002;34:521–533.

85. Van der Putten H, Wiederhold KH, Probst A, et al: Neuropathology in mice expressing human à-synuclein. J Neurosci 2000;20:6021–6029.

86. Abeliovich A, Schmitz Y, Farinas I, et al: Mice lacking alpha-synuclein display functional deficits in the nigrostriatal dopamine system. Neuron 2000;25:239–252.

87. Feany MB: Studying human neurodegenerative diseases in flies and worms. J Neuropath Exp Neurol 2000;59:847–856.

88. Warrick JM, Chan HYE, Board G, et al: Suppression of polyglutamine-mediated neurodegeneration in *Drosophila* by the molecular chaperone HSP70. Nat Genet 1999;23:425–428.

89. Warrick JM, Paulson HL, Board G, et al: Expanded polyglutamine protein forms nuclear inclusions and causes neural degeneration in *Drosophila*. Cell 1998;93:939–949.

90. Wittmann CW, Wszolek MF, Shulman JM, et al: Tauopathy in Drosophila: Neurodegeneration without neurofibrillary tangles. Science 2001;293: 711–714.

CHAPTER 6

Gene Mapping to Gene Targeting: Application of Mouse Genetics to Human Disease

George A. Carlson

The availability of a complete nucleotide sequence for the human species has dramatically changed many aspects of identification of genes underlying neurologic and psychiatric disease. While the basic principles of mapping have remained unchanged for decades, the density of markers and development of new technologies provide unprecedented opportunities to effectively pursue polygenic disease susceptibility and the interplay between environment and heredity. On the other hand, even given the complete code for every protein expressed throughout life and the nucleotide sequences involved in regulating temporal and spatial expression of every protein, current computational approaches cannot accurately identify all exons, let alone predict protein function based on nucleotide sequence. Added to this are the Lamarckian complexities of brain development and function under the control of a genome whose plasticity, with few exceptions, is manifest only on an evolutionary time scale. Only a small fraction of nucleotide sequence has been annotated with function. While the processes of linking a disease gene to a particular chromosomal interval and identifying the underlying nucleotide sequence have been greatly accelerated, difficulties remain. The goal of this chapter is to present some of these difficulties and to discuss the role that mouse genetics and manipulation of the mouse genome can play in identifying human disease loci and confirming the identity of human disease genes.

GENETIC MAPPING IN THE POST-GENOMIC ERA

Gene mapping changed dramatically with the application of neutral variations in human DNA sequence as genetic markers in linkage analysis. Restriction fragment length polymorphisms[1] and later microsatellite repeat polymorphisms[2,3] allowed localization of mendelian traits to specific chromosomes and subchromosomal regions without prior prejudice to the identity of the underlying gene. Positional cloning, though arduous, led to identification of numerous genes causing disease.[4] The need for identification of overlapping bacterial artificial chromosome (BAC) clones (contigs), marker development, and extensive nucleotide sequencing has been made obsolete by the availability of nearly complete genomic sequence. Positional cloning has been replaced by positional gene identification.

Mendelian disease gene mapping is based on non-random association of genetic markers in affected, compared to unaffected, individuals.[5,6] Family studies and affected sib-pair analysis are the most common approaches. Nonallelic heterogeneity in which distinct genes cause an indistinguishable phenotype is illustrated below, using familial Alzheimer's disease as an example. If any one of the distinct genes causing the same disease affects only a small proportion of families, analysis of individual large families may be helpful in obtaining significant evidence for linkage. Even for nonmendelian inheritance, linkage analysis can reveal individual genes contributing to risk of disease; late onset or sporadic Alzheimer's disease serves as an illustration of this. Candidate gene approaches that search for overrepresentation of an allele in unrelated affected individuals also may be useful.

FAMILIAL ALZHEIMER'S DISEASE: ONE DISEASE, THREE GENES

Mutations in any one of three genes, *APP*, *PSEN1*, and *PSEN2*, cause early-onset familial Alzheimer's disease (FAD). Since the amyloid precursor protein *(APP)* gene was cloned based on the sequence of the Aβ peptide that is found in AD plaques, it was an immediate suspect when it was cloned in 1987; however, initial studies showed no linkage between *APP* and disease.[7] This failure, entirely understandable in retrospect, was due to the assumption that since early-onset FAD appeared to be a single clinical entity it was probably caused by mutations in a single gene. Linkage to *APP* was not demonstrated until 1991 using a large pedigree in England.[8] For the purposes of this presentation, the important considerations are the criteria for concluding that *APP*, statistically linked to a FAD gene, actually was responsible for the disease—a conclusion that required no evidence or support from experimental results using the mouse (the last such example in this chapter). In addition to highly significant linkage and the fact that APP is the precursor for amyloidogenic Aβ peptide, other evidence also supported APP mutations as causal. There are multiple distinct mutations flanking the sequence encoding Aβ peptide in different families, and these mutations in *APP* lead to elevation of Aß peptide, arguing strongly that *APP* was indeed a FAD gene. Interestingly, despite numerous attempts, creation of APP transgenic mice that developed amyloid plaques was not successful until 1995.[9] Although plaque formation and learning deficits have been documented in APP transgenic mice, none of these transgenic models fully recapitulate the neuronal loss and neurofibrillary tangles seen in the human disease.[10]

The subsequent finding of multiple mutations in the presenilin-1 *(PSEN1)* and presenilin-2 *(PSEN2)* genes that were tightly linked to FAD loci on chromosomes 14 and 1 strongly implicated these genes as FAD loci.[11,12] Mutation carriers were found to have an elevated proportion of the longer, more amyloidogenic Aβ42 peptide in their plasma, providing a biochemical marker and potential pathogenic mechanism for these FAD loci.[13] Transgenic mice and transformed fibroblasts expressing mutant human presenilin transgenes fully recapitulated the elevation of Aβ42 seen in human mutation carriers, firmly tying the biochemical change to *PSEN* mutations. Were it not for this biochemical marker, PSEN transgenic mice would not have provided any suggestion for involvement of *PSEN* in AD; no pathologic changes occur in these transgenic animals, and the existence of behavioral abnormalities in PSEN transgenic mice is controversial.[10]

The lessons from identification of early-onset FAD genes are the importance of not assuming that the same gene is responsible for disease in all families (nonalleleic heterogeneity) and the value of biochemical markers for validation in the mouse. Other seemingly homogeneous familial human diseases, such as amyotrophic lateral sclerosis, also show heterogeneity in genetic etiology.

POLYGENIC DISEASE AND DISEASE MODIFIERS: THE SEARCH FOR LATE-ONSET ALZHEIMER'S DISEASE GENES

Autosomal dominant, early-onset FAD represents a small fraction of the total number of AD cases, the majority of which occur later than age 65 years and do not show a simple mendelian pattern of inheritance. This complex pattern of inheritance results from interplay among environmental factors (head injury, for example), genetic susceptibility genes, and disease modifier genes. The effect of disease modifiers can be seen in early-onset FAD families. Variability in age of onset within large AD families is well documented. For example, age of onset in a very large kindred segregating the E280A *PS1* mutation ranged from 34 to 62 years.[14]

In contrast to the three highly penetrant early-onset FAD loci, all individuals carrying a disease susceptibility allele do not develop dementia while some individuals lacking the susceptibility allele become demented. In spite of this complexity, the apolipoprotein E gene, *APOE*, has been unequivocally associated with late-onset AD. Early studies that suggested weak linkage to the *APOE*-containing region on chromosome 19q spurred application of association studies that have greater power than linkage for detecting genes with small effects. Association studies compare the frequencies of candidate gene alleles in unrelated affected individuals with those in age-matched controls.[15] A significantly increased frequency of the ε4 allele of *APOE* was found in AD cases[16]; this association is robust and has been replicated in numerous studies. Although each additional ε4 allele increases risk of late-onset AD approximately threefold, it is important to stress that *APOE*-ε4 is neither necessary nor sufficient for development of Alzheimer's dementia.[17] Only 50% at most of late-onset AD can be accounted for by the ε4 allele of *APOE*. This indicates that other susceptibility genes and environmental factors play a role.

At least one of these additional susceptibility genes may be located on chromosome 10. This region was implicated in a full genome scan of affected sib pairs to identify regions of suggestive linkage to disease genes.[18] Sixteen regions showed suggestive but nonsignificant linkage, one of which was on chromosome 10. Three independent approaches were used to follow up on the chromosome 10 candidate region, which was quite broad.[19] The first was to expand the affected sib-pair analysis with additional markers and sib pairs. Significance increased dramatically. The second approach was a linkage analysis of families selected on the basis of elevated plasma Aß peptide levels. A gene controlling this quantitative trait mapped to the same interval as that for frank disease. Although not yet certain that the two genes are identical, the importance of dissecting a phenotype to its component parts is stressed. A third approach involved testing disease linkage and linkage disequilibrium to the chromosome 10 gene encoding insulin-degrading enzyme (IDE), which was selected based on the enzyme's ability to degrade Aβ. Although this gene was approximately 40 cM distal from the Lod score peak determined from sib-pair analysis and from linkage to plasma Aβ levels, genetic evidence in support of its proximity to a late-onset disease gene was presented. Allelic differences in IDE activity, localization, or concentration may provide a more attractive marker. Breaking down a complex phenotype (disease) into biochemical markers provides a means to progress from multiple regions influencing a complex or quantitative trait to identification of the underlying gene. The better understood a complex disease is, the more powerful a genetic approach becomes.

Identification of genes underlying diseases with a strong phenotype-genotype association has progressed phenomenally in the past decade. As noted previously, even multigenic diseases such as late-onset Alzheimer's disease are susceptible to existing methodologies. The next challenge will be true polygenic diseases such as psychiatric disorders and schizophrenia that likely have high phenotypic and genetic heterogeneity. The full exploitation of complete nucleotide sequence to dissect complex diseases, behavior, and cognition will be driven by new technologies and expanded computational power. The density of single nucleotide polymorphisms is sufficient to perform high-density genome scans on large numbers of individuals, but cost and time considerations currently limit human quantitative trait (QT) studies to hundreds of individuals using hundreds of markers.[20] The importance of extensive genotyping can be illustrated by the QT analysis in the mouse—a much more tractable system for dissecting complex traits than human population analysis. Given the advantages of using pairs of inbred strains, identification of chromosomal regions containing genes that contain QT loci (QTL) is relatively straightforward. However, identification of the sequence underlying the modifier genes is difficult and there are few examples of success. A common approach is to isolate the QTL-containing regions on a uniform genetic background by producing congenic strains through repeated backcrossing. This, in theory, allows the effects of the gene in the differential segment to be studied in isolation from other QTL. It is not an uncommon occurrence, however, that individual QTL show no effect or influence on the trait following their genetic isolation through selective breeding. In addition to the small effect size of individual genes in complex traits, interactions among unlinked QTL may be essential to see an effect. Computational approaches to stratify analysis to analyze the effects of each locus in the presence or absence of every other modifier are available, but large population numbers and high marker density are required. The high marker density now provided by single nucleotide polymorphisms will facilitate assessment of linkage disequilibrium to deduce ancestral disease gene haplotype and aid in stratification of mixed populations.[21]

FROM LOCATION TO GENE: COMBINING OBSERVATIONAL AND EXPERIMENTAL APPROACHES

Determining the locations of genes causing or modifying disease is not an end in itself. The goal is to determine the identity of these genes, to unravel the functions of their gene products in disease and in normal physiology, and to use this knowledge to prevent or treat disease. Once a chromosomal location for a phenotype has been established, a wealth of information is available. Complete sequence information for any genetic interval now is likely to be available. The relative completeness of nucleotide sequence is in stark contrast to the paucity of functional information. Prediction of exons based on nucleotide sequence is inexact, and there may be many unannotated genes within an interval. Computational gene prediction is improving as genome sequence from additional species becomes available for identification of conserved sequence. New expressed sequence tags and full-length cDNAs are readily assigned a location in the genome and help determine intron-exon structure. However, unrepresented alternative splice variants can lead to unidentified exons and missed functions. Even assuming identification of every complete gene in an interval, the ability to predict function based on protein primary structure is in its infancy. Even identifying a gene product as a member of a gene family (e.g., tyrosine kinases) does not reveal the role of the protein in disease susceptibility.

Prioritizing candidate disease genes or disease modifiers is essential, particularly when the chromosomal interval containing the gene is large. Information on temporal and spatial patterns of gene expression also are important in prioritizing candidate genes; generally, a candidate gene should be expressed in the organ or tissue affected by the disease. For autosomal recessive or X-linked monogenic diseases, the presence of premature stop codons, altered splice donor or acceptor sites, deletions, or other major changes that reduce or eliminate gene expression in affected individuals can be sufficient evidence that a particular gene underlies a disease. Autosomal dominant disorders also can be due to similar catastrophic mutations with the observed phenotype due to haploinsufficiency or reduction in the concentration of the functional allele. Nonconservative changes in protein sequence in affected and unaffected individuals can cause altered protein function, but to attribute disease to any particular point mutation in a gene requires functional information. Fine genetic mapping can be helpful in distinguishing harmless polymorphisms from disease-causing mutations by recombination or haplotype analysis, but production of transgenic or gene-targeted mice can be definitive, in addition to the potential for providing an animal model for the disease. The ability of mutant presenilins to elevate Aß peptides in cell culture and in transgenic mice illustrates the value of this approach.

Disease modifiers or genes controlling quantitative traits may not be due to gain or loss of function, but more likely represent natural polymorphisms that only slightly alter gene function or expression. The possibilities are many: changes in regulatory sequences may alter level or timing of expression, changes in the active site of an enzyme may alter its kinetics or specificity, or receptor-ligand affinity may be altered. Thus, functional information will be paramount in dissecting complex disorders. The mouse provides an experimentally tractable, genetically defined organism that will play a major role in functional annotation of the human genome sequence and offers a resource that can speed gene identification.

CONSERVATION OF CHROMOSOMAL SEGMENTS

In addition to evolutionary conservation indicated by homologous genes in mouse and humans reflecting their common origin, chromosomal segments containing multiple genes and long-range sequence organization have been conserved.[22] Thus, localization of a gene to a chromosomal region in one species can simultaneously indicate its location in the other. The human genome sequence was used as the substrate to align mouse contigs and markers to accelerate construction of a physical map of the mouse genome.[23] This framework will greatly accelerate completion of the mouse's nucleotide sequence, as well as provide the ability to identify at least one mouse BAC clone corresponding to almost any chromosomal position in the human. These clones can be used to create targeting vectors or transgenes to test disease candidate genes and to determine gene function. The conserved segments (gene order is the same in both species) and conserved synteny (conservation of chromosomal location but not necessarily gene order) between mouse and human also provide the opportunity to exploit the expanding resource of induced mutations scattered across the mouse genome.

PHENOTYPE-DRIVEN GENETICS: LARGE-SCALE MUTAGENESIS PROGRAMS

The ability of chemicals and radiation to cause mutations has been appreciated and exploited for many years. Until relatively recently, the majority of mouse mutants exhibited phenotypes that were obvious during routine animal care, and variations in coat color or overt behavioral abnormalities such as circling were overrepresented. Improvements in the efficiency of chemical mutagenesis, coupled with the availability of high-density genetic markers, has lead to directed screens for less obvious mutants and rapid molecular identification of the mutant genes. An exciting early example of success in screening for obscure phenotypes is the identification of the mouse *Clock* gene that was detected in a screen for dominant mutations affecting circadian rhythm.[24] The completion of a mouse physical map and nearly complete sequence of the mouse genome has spurred an increased emphasis on the phenotype-driven approach to gene function and identification of many new mutants.

Estimation of mutation frequencies is based on the pioneering work of Russell and colleagues by screening for easily scored new recessive mutations of known genes (such as albino) in G1 offspring of mutagen-treated males and tester mice.[25] N-nitroso-N-ethylurea (ENU) is the most efficient and commonly used chemical mutagen. The ENU-induced mutation frequency per locus per gamete ranges from approximately 60×10^{-5} to 150×10^{-5}. This high frequency is of an order of magnitude to make a mammalian saturation mutagenesis project a realistic proposition. To be able to identify at least one mutation in every locus (saturation mutagenesis), it is estimated that approximately 3000 F1 offspring need to be screened, assuming accurate detection of each mutation capable of producing a phenotype. The key to success is development of phenotyping screens that can detect as broad a spectrum of mutations as possible since individual genes can have effects on a many systems and at different stages of life.

Exploitation of deletions and inversions allows mutation screens to be heavily biased to specific chromosomal regions. By screening over a deletion, loss of function mutations can be detected without breeding to homozygosity. Gene targeting technologies based on Cre/loxP recombination are used to engineer deletions, inversions, and markers at any desired chromosomal interval in the mouse, and efforts to saturate the genome with mutations are under way using this approach.[26]

Large-scale mutagenesis programs under way in England; Germany; Oak Ridge, Tennessee; Toronto, Canada; Houston, Texas; and several other centers have identified, mapped, and determined the underlying lesion for scores of new mutations over the past few years. These mouse mutant libraries are rapidly providing functional annotation of nucleotide sequence and are becoming an increasingly valuable resource for human disease gene identification.[27,28]

MUTATION BANKS: GENE-BASED SCREENING

Advances in cryopreservation of mouse sperm facilitate the creation of banks of sperm from first generation (G1) offspring of ENU-treated males. Each G1 male may contain hundreds of point mutations, and each bank may contain sperm from thousands of mice. This resource can be scanned for individuals with mutation in any desired sequence. Since the mutations are random, this approach is particularly valuable for genes whose functions are incompletely understood. In vitro fertilization is used to obtain a set of animals with different mutations in the same gene. In contrast, creation of a set of mice with various point mutations in a gene using embryonic stem cells and gene targeting is more arduous. An additional effort under way in several laboratories is the generation of randomly generated mouse embryonic stem (ES) cell clones with loss of function mutation tagged with reporters for gene expression.[29] These and other publicly available mouse mutant resources will increase the fraction of genes (currently 15% at best) for which at least one function is known.

GENE TARGETING

The ability to manipulate the germ line of mice through use of homologous recombination in embryonic stem (ES) cells has revolutionized mammalian genetics.[30,31] ES cells are totipotent cells derived in culture from the inner cell mass of blastocysts and are capable of contributing to every cell type and tissue, including the germ-line, when injected into blastocysts that are transferred into foster mothers. The basic procedure involves introducing a recombinant DNA targeting vector containing drug selectable markers into ES cells and screening for homologous integrants. The targeting vector generally contains the bacterial neomycin (neo) transposon that confers resistance to the antibiotic G418. The *neo* gene is flanked by mouse genomic sequence that directly flanks the sequence to be replaced or disrupted. Some investigators include at one end of the construct a marker whose expression can be selected against; homologous integrants are somewhat more likely than nonhomologous integrants to have lost the nonhomologous end sequences. In general, the greater the extent of homology the greater the efficiency of gene targeting. At least for targeting constructs up to 10 kb, homologous recombination frequency is much higher when the genomic sequence is from the same mouse strain as the ES cells. ES cells surviving drug selection are tested to determine that the desired homologous recombination event occurred. Cells from targeted clones are then injected into the inner cell mass of blastocysts from mice that differ in color from the ES cell donor strain. Most ES cell lines are derived from agouti sublines of 129 mice, and nonagouti (black in color) C57BL/6J (B6) mice serve as blastocyst donors. Chimerism in the offspring is assessed by coat color, and chimeric animals are bred to select ES-cell–derived offspring based on coat color. Detailed information on the development of gene targeting using ES cells is available elsewhere.[30,31]

GENE ABLATION BY NEO INSERTION: STRATEGIES, GENETIC BACKGROUND EFFECTS, AND PITFALLS

Targeting strategies designed to ablate gene expression by disruption of an early exon have been the most common, though this approach is being supplanted by more powerful and flexible technologies. Careful consideration of targeting vector design should include the possibility of incomplete ablation owing to exon skipping and other effects. A revealing example comparing the effects of different targeting strategies is provided by ablation of the prion protein gene (*Prnp*).[32] The first *Prnp* knockout that was produced developed normally, showed no obvious behavioral abnormalities, and had a normal life span.

Although shedding no light on prion protein (PrP) function, the viability of *Prnp*-null mice made them extremely valuable for prion research, and they were used to demonstrate the necessity of PrP for prion replication. Subsequently, additional laboratories constructed *Prnp* knockouts. Two dramatically different results were observed. One new line recapitulated the initial observation that *Prnp*-null mice lack of any obvious phenotype, while two other lines developed late-onset ataxia and cerebellar degeneration. *Prnp* ablated lines that were constructed without deleting the splice acceptor of the open reading frame–containing third exon had no phenotype. Those null mutants that deleted the exon 3-splice acceptor developed the neurologic deficits. A previously unknown PrP-related gene downstream of *Prnp*, called *Prnd*, is normally not expressed in the brain. Destruction of the splice acceptor site by insertion of the neo cassette allowed exon skipping and production of chimeric *Prnp/Prnd* mRNAs that expressed *Prnd*-encoded doppel (Dpl) at high levels in the brain. The hypothesis that Dpl expression in the brain, rather than lack of PrP, was responsible for cerebellar neurodegeneration was supported by the finding that expression of Dpl-encoding transgenes in the brain recapitulated the phenotype.[33] Thus, careful construct preparation and analysis of gene expression is essential for interpretation of results from gene knockouts.

Often, after considerable effort in producing a knockout mouse, there is no obvious phenotype in null homozygotes. This can be due to redundancy in gene function, which can include compensatory changes in expression of other genes during development. It also is important to appreciate the fact the laboratory mice live in a sheltered environment, and gene function may be obvious only in specific situations or when the animal is stressed. Genetic background also plays a role in determining whether a phenotype is observed.[34] An effect of the null allele may be obvious only in combination with particular alleles of other genes. Traditionally, chimeric mice have been crossed with C57BL/6J (B6) mice to identify offspring of ES-cell–derived gametes by coat color; thus, targeted mice are heterozygous for the desired null allele as well as the 129- and B6-derived alleles at every locus. In subsequent intercrosses to produce mice homozygous for the null allele, each individual is unique. It is common to produce congenic mice carrying the 129-derived null allele on a uniform genetic background by repeated backcrossing to B6. An alternative is to maintain the null allele on the ES-cell donor inbred mouse strain from the start. Rather than outcrossing, chimeric offspring are mated to the ES cell donor strain, most often a 129-strain subline. While avoiding genetic heterogeneity, the effect of gene ablation is sampled in only a single genetic environment, and most 129 sublines are poor breeders. In short, there is no one solution to the problem of genetic background effects. The effect of background on the phenotype induced by gene ablation also can offer a tremendous opportunity to study complex interactions and phenotype penetrance.

Gene ablation frequently causes embryonic lethality, an undesirable result if the goal of constructing the knockout was to determine its function in adults or in human disease. Genetic background also can affect whether the consequence of gene ablation is embryonic lethality. Homozygosity for a null mutation may cause embryonic death on one genetic background but not on another. Embryonic lethality caused by homozygosity for a null allele reveals the earliest nonredundant function of a gene, but is unhelpful in determining the functions of a gene in the adult. For this reason, strategies have been developed to allow conditional control of gene expression in specific tissues and at the time desired.

The potential value of mice heterozygous for an ablated allele should not be underestimated. In anticipation of potential embryonic lethality or lack of an obvious phenotype in null mutant homozygotes, a reporter for gene expression such as *lacZ* may be incorporated into the targeting construct. In heterozygotes, the reporter provides an indication of temporal and spatial expression of the target locus, which is valuable information for determining gene function and for design of future experiments. In the case of modifier or quantitative trait loci, null mutant heterozygous mice may mimic effects of naturally occurring allelic differences in expression level, binding affinity, or enzyme activity and be useful in assessing candidate genes. Comparison of mice heterozygous for a null allele with mice carrying two wild-type alleles can be used to identify modifier genes whose effects reflect differences in the effective concentration of the encoded protein.

RECOMBINEERING: EASING THE PRODUCTION OF COMPLEX TARGETING CONSTRUCTS

The limitations of gene ablation by simple disruption of an exon call for more complex constructs, even if the complexity is limited to addition of a reporter gene. A major limitation in the ability to produce targeting constructs for some of the applications discussed later is the lack of appropriate unique restriction sites, and the requirement for several cloning steps to overcome this difficulty. These problems are particularly acute when using large BAC and P1 artificial chromosome (PAC) clones that are seeing increasing use in gene modification by homologous recombination. The development of phage-based homologous recombination systems has simplified the generation of knockout constructs and facilitated engineering of large segments of DNA.[35] The use of phage recombination for genetic engineering has been termed *recombineering*.

Recombineering takes advantage of the fact that bacteria, including *Escherichia coli,* encode their own homologous recombination systems. Phage also can carry their own recombination functions that can interact with those of the bacteria. A number of elegantly designed protocols and bacterial clone-phage combinations have been developed and are under constant improvement. RecET/lambda Red homologous recombination can now be used to engineer DNA in *E. coli* without use of restriction endonucleases or DNA ligases. Segments of homology of only 40 to 50 bp are needed, so insertions or specific mutations can be rapidly inserted into BAC clones. The high rate of recombination efficiency permits screening, rather than drug selection, for recombinants. Thus, a single step is required to create a modification without introduction of selectable markers that can alter function of a nearby sequence. One example of an innovative application of recombineering is the introduction of a *cre*-expressing targeting cassette into the 3′ end of a large 250 kb BAC containing the neuron-specific enolase-2 gene (*Eno2*).[36] Shorter subclones were similarly modified. Using a reporter for Cre activity, only mice that carried the large BAC produced Cre in all *Eno2* positive neurons indicating that important regulatory sequences can be located hundreds of kb away from a gene. Such large engineered BACs are useful for production of *cre*-expressing transgenic lines that faithfully recapitulate expression of a gene for use in conditional ablation of gene expression.

Recombineering may be the most important technical advance to result from the imminent completion of the mouse genome sequence. The ability to rapidly engineer targeting constructs makes possible formerly unthinkable projects, such as the production of an ES cell library to create conditional knockouts for every gene in the mouse. Construction of complex vectors should no longer be a deterrent to implementing advanced gene-targeting techniques. The rate-limiting steps for construction of conditional knockouts now become those inherent in reproductive biology for production of mice from clones of ES cells.

CONDITIONAL CONTROL OF GENE EXPRESSION

The shortcomings of simple gene ablation for annotating genomic sequence with biologic function can be overcome by the ability to turn genes on or off at will. It is now possible to switch genes on or off using binary systems for gene regulation or ablation.[37] Two different types of systems are in use. The first exploits site-specific recombination where an effector transgene encodes recombinases that catalyze recombination between recognition sites introduced into a target locus by homologous recombination. The second, most often using two different transgenes rather than gene targeting, employs an effector transgene encoding a transactivator that induces transcription of the target transgene. These two distinct binary systems can be combined with one another and with traditional knockout approaches in ingenious ways to precisely control gene expression for the analysis of complex biologic processes.

Site-specific recombinases from bacteriophage P1 (Cre) or from the yeast *Saccharomyces cerevisiae* (Flp) currently are used as effectors of site-specific recombination. Cre recombinase catalyzes recombination between 34 bp *loxP* recognition sites, while Flp recombinase acts on identically sized *FRT* sites. Both systems operate by similar mechanisms, and their efficiencies are comparable. For historical reasons and because an ever-increasing arsenal of tissue-specific Cre expressing transgenic mice is available, academic laboratories favor use of the Cre-*loxP* system. Patent and royalty issues attached to the use of Cre/*loxP* lead commercial ventures to favor use of the Flp/*FRT* system. This discussion will use Cre/*loxP* as the model, though Flp/*FRT* could equally well have served as the example.

If a sequence is flanked by directly repeated *loxP* sites, that sequence is excised when Cre recombinase is present, leaving behind a single *loxP* site. Sequenced flanked by *loxP* sites is said to be floxed. Recombination between *loxP* sites can be over a long distance, and megabase size deletions have been created by targeting *loxP* sites to distant sites on the same chromosome.[26]

Cre/loxP offers the capability of deleting an entire gene, avoiding problems of exon skipping and novel splice variants that can arise with conventional gene targeting. Recombineering to engineer larger constructs can avoid the need for two sequential rounds of homologous recombination and selection in creating floxed sequence in the ES cells. Floxed genes avoid the problem of embryonic lethality induced by gene ablation. Floxing a locus does not preclude production of null mutant embryos by either crossing to a Cre deletor strain or by transiently introducing a Cre expression cassette into the ES cells. Constructs also can be engineered to activate reporter loci after the target sequence is excised. Thus, there is little justification for producing simple null mutants by traditional gene targeting.

The key to producing faithful tissue-specific gene deletion is the Cre-expressing mice that are crossed to the ES cell-derived mice with the floxed target sequence. Transgene tissue-specific promoters are used to drive Cre expression, and multiple lines often need to be screened to assure accurate spatial and temporal expression. Larger constructs are more likely to operate independently of the site of integration, and the ability to readily engineer BAC or PAC clones should facilitate production of tissue-specific Cre expressors. An early example of the use of Cre/*loxP* for dissection of a complex neurologic phenotype is the use of a transgenic line expressing Cre under the control of the alpha-calcium-calmodulin dependent kinase II (*Camk2a*) promoter, which restricts Cre expression to the CA1 region of the hippocampus in adults.[38] Cre activity was assessed by using a lacZ reporter transgene in which a floxed sequence containing a stop codon was between an actin promoter and the lacZ reporter

gene. In cells expressing Cre, the stop signal was excised, allowing expression of the reporter. A Cre transgenic line was selected in which lacZ was expressed only in the CA1 pyramidal cell layer. Two *loxP* sites were introduced into the N-methyl-D-aspartate receptor gene *Nmdar1* in ES cells, and targeted clones were used to generate germ-line chimeras that transmitted the floxed gene. A requirement for successful use of conditional deletions is that the flanking *loxP* sites do not interfere with gene expression; this appeared to be the case in this instance. The Cre transgenic mice were mated to mice homozygous for floxed *Nmdar1* alleles to produce Cre transgene positive (Cre/+), floxed *Nmdar1* heterozygous (fNR1/+) mice. Crossing (Cre/+, fNR1/+) and (+/+, fNR1/+) mice gave Cre-positive mice homozygous for the floxed *Nmdar1* gene and control animals. The mice lacking *Nmdar1* in their CA1 pyramidal cells did not have any obvious abnormalities but exhibited impaired spatial memory with no deficits in nonspatial learning.[39] The mice failed to exhibit long-term potentiation in CA1 synapses, presumably owing to lack of NMDA receptor-mediated synaptic currents. This example illustrates the power of tissue-specific gene ablation to dissect complex neurologic phenotypes.

Another important use of site-specific recombination is to discriminate between polymorphisms and causal mutations in a candidate disease susceptibility gene. Although mutations can be introduced into an exon simply by including the selectable neo marker in an adjacent intron, the neo gene can interfere with gene expression. By flanking the neo cassette with *loxP* sites, only a 34-bp site remains after Cre catalyzed recombination.

Transcriptional transactivation, the second binary system for conditional control of gene expression, can be combined with Cre/*loxP* site-specific recombination to provide temporal control of gene deletion. The most widely used system is tetracycline dependent transcriptional transactivation.[40] The inducible effectors were constructed by fusing sequences encoding the VP16 transactivation domain and the *E. coli* tetracycline repressor protein. These transactivators specifically bind tetracycline (or the less toxic doxycycline) and the *tet* operon (*tetO*) that controls the transcription of the target transgenes. There are tet-on and tet-off versions of the transactivator. The tTA tetracycline transactivator fails to bind *tetO* when doxycycline is present; thus the target gene is on until doxycycline is given. The reverse transactivator, rtTA, binds *tetO* sequences only when doxycycline is present; thus doxycycline turns on the gene. Generally, the transactivator is under control of the desired promoter while the target transgene is regulated by *tetO*, which activates transcription from a minimal promoter. Gene-ablated mice provide the environment for avoiding the effects of endogenous gene expression. Although there can be problems with leakiness of gene expression, this is a powerful system. Combining transactivation with Cre-mediated recombination allows temporal control of gene ablation by expressing Cre under the control of the tet operon.

MICE IN SERVICE OF HUMAN GENETICS

The importance of mice for the understanding and experimental analysis of human disease has increased as completion of entire genomic sequence for humans, mice, and other vertebrates nears. The challenge of understanding the genetic basis for complex, polygenic disease susceptibility requires annotation of nucleotide sequence with function. Large-scale phenotype-driven mutagenesis programs are providing such annotation as well as a resource for disease modeling. Targeted gene modification by homologous recombination is benefiting from new approaches for conditional gene ablation and for more rapid construction of targeting constructs. Creating a library of ES cells with every gene flanked by *loxP* sites is a formidable task, but one that is no longer considered fantasy.

REFERENCES

1. Botstein D, White RL, Skolnick M, Davis RW: Construction of a genetic linkage map in man using restriction fragment length polymorphisms. Am J Hum Genet 1980;32:314–331.

2. Weber JL, May PE: Abundant class of human DNA polymorphisms which can be typed using the polymerase chain reaction. Am J Hum Genet 1989;44:388–396.

3. Litt M, Luty JA: A hypervariable microsatellite revealed by in vitro amplification of a dinucleotide repeat within the cardiac muscle actin gene. Am J Hum Genet 1989;44:397–401.

4. Collins FS: Positional cloning moves from perditional to traditional. Nat Genet 1995;9:347–350.

5. Risch NJ: Searching for genetic determinants in the new millennium. Nature 2000;405:847–856.

6. Strachan T, Read AP: Human Molecular Genetics, New York, Wiley-Liss, 1999.

7. Kang J, et al: The precursor of Alzheimer's disease amyloid A4 protein resembles a cell-surface receptor. Nature 1987;325:733–736.

8. Goate A, et al: Segregation of a missense mutation in the amyloid precursor protein gene with familial Alzheimer's disease. Nature 1991;349:704–706.

9. Games D, et al: Alzheimer-type neuropathology in transgenic mice overexpressing V717F β-amyloid precursor protein. Nature 1995;373:523–527.

10. Price DL, Tanzi RE, Borchelt DR, Sisodia SS: Alzheimer's disease: Genetic studies and transgenic models. Annu Rev Genet 1998;32:461–493.

11. Rogaev EI, et al: Familial Alzheimer's disease in kindreds with missense mutations in a gene on chromosome 1 related to the Alzheimer's disease type 3 gene. Nature 1995;376:775–778.

12. Levy-Lahad E, et al: Candidate gene for the chromosome 1 familial Alzheimer's disease locus. Science 1995;269,973–976.

13. Scheuner D, et al: Secreted amyloid β-protein similar to that in the senile plaques of Alzheimer's disease is increased in vivo by the presenilin 1 and 2 and APP mutations linked to familial Alzheimer's disease. Nat Med 1996;2:864–870.

14. Lopera F, et al: Clinical features of early-onset Alzheimer disease in a large kindred with an E280A presenilin-1 mutation. J Am Med Assoc 1997;227:793–799.

15. Liu L, et al: Allelic association but only weak evidence for linkage to the apolipoprotein E locus in late-onset Swedish Alzheimer families. Am J Med Genet 1996;67:306–311.

16. Strittmatter WJ, et al: Apolipoprotein E: High-avidity binding to beta-amyloid and increased frequency of type 4 allele in late-onset familial Alzheimer disease. Proc Natl Acad Sci U S A 1993;90:1977–1981.

17. Corder EH, et al: Gene dose of apolipoprotein E type 4 allele and the risk of Alzheimer's disease in late onset families. Science 1993;261:921–923.

18. Kehoe P, et al: A full genome scan for late onset Alzheimer's disease. Hum Mol Genet 1993;8:237–245.

19. Lendon C, Craddock N: Susceptibility gene(s) for Alzheimer's disease on chromosome 10. Trends Neurosci 2001;24:557–559.

20. Wang DG, et al: Large-scale identification, mapping, and genotyping of single-nucleotide polymorphisms in the human genome. Science 1998;280:1077–1082.

21. Dawson E, et al: A first-generation linkage disequilibrium map of human chromosome 22. Nature 2002;418:544–548.

22. Nadeau JH, Taylor BA: Lengths of chromosomal segments conserved since divergence of man and mouse. Proc Nat Acad Sci U S A 1984;81:814–818.

23. Gregory SG, et al: A physical map of the mouse genome. Nature 2002;418:743–750.

24. Vitaterna MH, et al: Mutagenesis and mapping of a mouse gene, *clock,* essential for circadian behavior. Science 1994;264:719–725.

25. Rinchik EM: Chemical mutagenesis and fine-structure functional analysis of the mouse genome. Trends Genet 1991;7:15–21.

26. Yu Y, Bradley A: Engineering chromosomal rearrangements in mice. Nat Rev Genet 2001;2:780–790.

27. Nolan PM, et al: A systematic, genome-wide, phenotype-driven mutagenesis programme for gene function studies in the mouse. Nat Genet 2000;25:440–443.

28. Hrabe de Angelis, MH, et al: Genome-wide, large-scale production of mutant mice by ENU mutagenesis. Nat Genet 2000;25:444–447.

29. Stanford WL, Cohn, JB, Cordes SP: Gene-trap mutagenesis: Past, present and beyond. Nat Rev Genet 2001;2:756–768.

30. Capecchi MR: Altering the genome by homologous recombination. Science 1989;244:1288–1292.

31. Smithies O: Animal models of human genetic diseases. Trends Genet 1993;9:112–116.

32. Moore RC, et al: Ataxia in prion protein (PrP)-deficient mice is associated with upregulation of the novel PrP-like protein doppel. J Mol Biol 1999;292:797–817.

33. Moore RC, et al: Doppel-induced cerebellar degeneration in transgenic mice. Proc Natl Acad Sci U S A 2001;98:15288–15293.

34. Threadgill DW, et al: Targeted disruption of mouse EGF receptor: Effect of genetic background on mutant phenotype. Science 1995;269:230–234.

35. Copeland NG, Jenkins NA, Court DL: Recombineering: A powerful new tool for mouse functional genomics. Nat Rev Genet 2001;2:769–779.

36. Lee EC, et al: A highly efficient *Escherichia coli*-based chromosome engineering system adapted for recombinogenic targeting and subcloning of BAC DNA. Genomics 2001;73:56–65.

37. Lewandoski M: Conditional control of gene expression in the mouse. Nat Rev Genet 2001;2:743–755.

38. Tsien JZ, et al: Subregion- and cell type-restricted gene knockout in mouse brain. Cell 1996;87:1317–1326.

39. Tsien JZ, Huerta PT, Tonegawa S: The essential role of hippocampal CA1 NMDA receptor-dependent synaptic plasticity in spatial memory. Cell 1996;87:1327–1338.

40. Baron U, Gossen M, Bujard H: Tetracycline-controlled transcription in eukaryotes: Novel transactivators with graded transactivation potential. Nucleic Acids Res 1997;25:2723–2729.

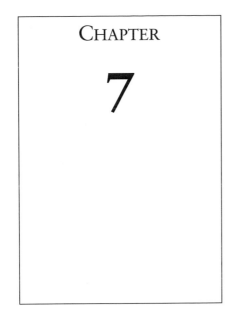

CHAPTER 7

The Human Genome Project

Robert L. Nussbaum

The Human Genome Project (HGP) is an international cooperative effort to determine the complete sequence of the approximately 3.2 billion base pairs of DNA containing all the genetic information within a haploid human cell, and to make the data freely available. The project was put forward in the 1980s by scientists who concluded that elucidating the role of mutation in causing cancer would require knowing the complete sequence of human DNA to identify even very subtle mutations responsible for the disease.[1] The United States launched its efforts in the HGP in the late 1980s at the Department of Energy and the National Institutes of Health, with the goal of determining the entire human sequence within 15 years.[2] The HGP quickly developed into a worldwide effort involving universities, private foundations, and government laboratories in the United States, Great Britain, France, Germany, China, and Japan.

The initial plan called for the creation of genetic and physical maps containing landmarks around which to anchor the sequence. These maps were largely completed by the mid-1990s.[3] One immediate benefit was that a detailed genetic map of the human genome, based on polymorphic short-tandem repeat DNA markers that could be genotyped by the polymerase chain reaction (PCR), made mapping human disease genes by linkage analysis (discussed later) far more rapid and efficient than it had been previously. The late 1990s saw a massive scale-up in sequencing capacity and throughput in order to accomplish the goal of completing the sequence within 15 years. A major milestone was reached in February 2001 when two "draft" versions consisting of over 90% of the human DNA sequence was published, one that was freely available from the public HGP[4] and the other accessible by paid subscription from a private biotech-

nology company that had independently sequenced human DNA and pooled the publicly available HGP data with its own.[5] The sequences was considered in draft form because it consisted of sequences from thousands of segments of DNA, varying in size from a few thousand to many million base pairs, separated by gaps in the sequence. Closing the gaps and aligning all the individual segments of DNA sequence remains a massive undertaking that the public HGP expects to complete in 2003, to coincide with the 50th anniversary of the publication of the double-helix structure of DNA by Watson and Crick.[6]

In addition to the sequencing of entire genomes, the 1990s also saw the expansion of efforts aimed at developing catalogs of sequence from mRNAs, the transcribed portions of genes. These first efforts, occurring both in the private sector and in the public HGP, involved determining the sequence of a few hundred base pairs from the ends of cDNA copies of mRNAs isolated from a wide range of tissues. Although a few hundred base pairs is usually too short to encompass the entire sequence of most mRNAs, it was still more than sufficient to specify a transcript uniquely and, therefore, was referred to as an expressed sequence tag or EST.[7] More recently, both publicly funded and public–private industry partnerships in the United States and elsewhere have expanded their EST sequencing to include the entire sequence of as complete a collection of mRNAs from as large a number of normal and neoplastic tissues as possible.[8] These full-length mRNA sequencing projects provide researchers with the primary amino acid sequence of tens of thousands of proteins and contain a wealth of information on what is transcribed from the genome. EST databases are proving themselves to be critically important to the efforts to identify all the genes encoded in human DNA.[9]

An essential element of the public international HGP was the commitment to make all the data immediately and freely available for scientific study and analysis. Computer scientists in the field of bioinformatics have developed software tools to deal with how to store large volumes of sequence and other types of molecular genetic information in a readily searchable form, how to query and cross-reference the databases, and how to analyze the data and extract important information and insights. Currently, the National Center for Biotechnology Information in the United States, the DNA Databank of Japan, and the Sanger Center in Great Britain support web-based databases open to anyone with access to a computer and the Internet.[10,11]

APPLICATIONS OF THE HUMAN GENOME PROJECT

Long-Range Topography of the Human Genome

The complete sequence of the human genome affords scientists a detailed map of the "topographical features" of the genome. Characteristics such as the frequency of cytosine-guanine (GC) base pairs, the complement of genes, the identity and density of repetitive DNA sequence, and sex-specific meiotic recombination (crossing-over) rates versus physical distance, to name a few, are known to vary among different regions of a chromosome. With the complete genome sequence, we have the highest-resolution map possible, the sequence of individual nucleotides, on which to place these topographical features.[4] Thus, for example, the distribution of the GC base pair, which makes up 41% of base pairs overall in the genome, is clearly not homogeneous and ranges from as low as 33% to as high as 65% in certain regions of the genome. GC content correlates directly with Giemsa-banding of chromosomes. Light areas have higher GC content; Giemsa-dark staining regions have lower GC content. Gene density varies similarly, with GC-rich regions having the highest density of genes and GC-poor regions showing the lowest gene density.

Complete genome sequence has revealed that nearly 45% of all human DNA is made up of repetitive DNA sequences present in hundreds of thousands to millions of copies. Three-quarters of these repeat sequences are derived from elements that can act as retroposons (i.e., sequences that can be transcribed into an RNA that is reverse-transcribed into DNA and inserted elsewhere in the genome). Repetitive sequences such as short interspersed elements (SINEs), including the Alu repeat, and long interspersed elements (LINEs), including LINEs 1, 2, and 3, seem to have spread through the human genome by retroposition. However, they show nonrandom distribution, with SINES clustered in gene-rich regions and LINES clustered in gene-poor regions.

Large-scale analysis of meiotic recombination has also allowed for interesting comparisons of physical dis-

tance, measured in base pairs, and genetic distance, measured in centiMorgans (cM), which correspond over short distances to approximately 1% recombination frequency in meiosis. Over the entire genome in a female, 3.2 billion base pairs (3200 megabases) of DNA have an average genetic length of 3200 cM, yielding a ratio of 1 cM per megabase (Mb). The length of the male genome in genetic units of distance is less, approximately 2700 cM, for an average of 0.83 cM per Mb. At a level of resolution of a few megabases, the ratio of cM to Mb is variable. It can be as high as 2.5 cM per Mb at the telomeric ends of chromosomes of females, and even higher in males, up to 5 cM per Mb, at the ends of some chromosomes.[4]

The topographical features of the human genome are beginning to be described and explored. Such information will be applied to understanding the evolution of complex genomes, the structure of chromosomes and their behavior in meiosis, and the mechanisms of long-range regulation of gene expression by chromatin structure and accessibility.

Comparative Genomics

From the beginning of the project, scientists in the HGP recognized the importance of having the complete genomic sequence of organisms other than *Homo sapiens*. The genomes of yeast, the *Caenorhabditis elegans* worm, the fruit fly, honeybee, zebra fish, puffer fish, chicken, mouse, rat, dog, and chimpanzee, as well as other organisms and plants of biological and agricultural interest, have either been completely sequenced, or the sequencing is in progress or in advanced planning stage. Some of these organisms are considered model organisms because naturally occurring genetic variants and/or artificially induced mutant strains demonstrate alterations in a wide range of developmental and physiological processes that are of interest to human biology and importance to medicine. Complete genome sequence allows a thorough investigation of the relationship between genotype and phenotype in these model organisms. More generally, the complete sequence of many organisms provides crucial raw material for studies in evolutionary biology. The field of comparative genomics endeavors to use comparisons between the DNA sequence of organisms of varying degrees of evolutionary closeness or divergence to gain important biological insights critical to understanding evolution.[12] Determining how the coding regions of individual genes, the organization of gene complexes and gene families, and the structure of chromosomes have changed along various evolutionary lineages adds a molecular dimension to the more classical studies of structure and function used in evolutionary analyses.

Comparative genomics is also being applied in biomedical research to learning how to extract the information contained within DNA sequence, particularly the molecular landmarks that specify a gene and the signals in the DNA that are used to regulate gene expression.[13]

Although reading the triplet code that specifies the amino acids in a protein has been a straightforward practice since the 1960s, we still lack highly sensitive and specific software tools for scanning genomic DNA sequence and finding all the landmarks, exons, introns, regulatory sequences, that together constitute a gene.[14] For example, despite having a nearly complete sequence of human DNA and millions of partial and complete sequences from transcribed genes in various databases of ESTs, estimates of the number of transcribed genes in the human genome still range from as few as 30,000 to greater than 70,000.[4] By matching transcribed EST sequences to genomic DNA and comparing human genomic sequence to that of other organisms, our best estimate at present is that there are 30,000 to 40,000 genes in the human genome. Approximately one third of human DNA is transcribed into RNA; of that, approximately 4.5%, or 1.5% of the entire human genome, is coding sequence.

An even more difficult task is to extract regulatory information located outside the coding regions of genes.

Comparing the sequence in and around genes from many different species, to identify segments of DNA outside the coding region that have been conserved, is a powerful way to identify regions of possible functional importance (Fig. 7–1).[15,16] Such comparisons have to be done carefully, however. If organisms are too closely related evolutionarily, then noncoding regions of DNA may be conserved not because of evolutionary pressure to protect regulatory information content but because the two organisms have a common ancestor that is too recent to have allowed nonessential DNA to accumulate mutations and diverge.[14]

Genetic Variation

The product of the HGP is a prototypical DNA sequence derived from a small number of humans. For biomedical science, the next step is to catalog the variations in DNA sequence from many individuals and ethnic groups and to correlate these differences with phenotypic differences

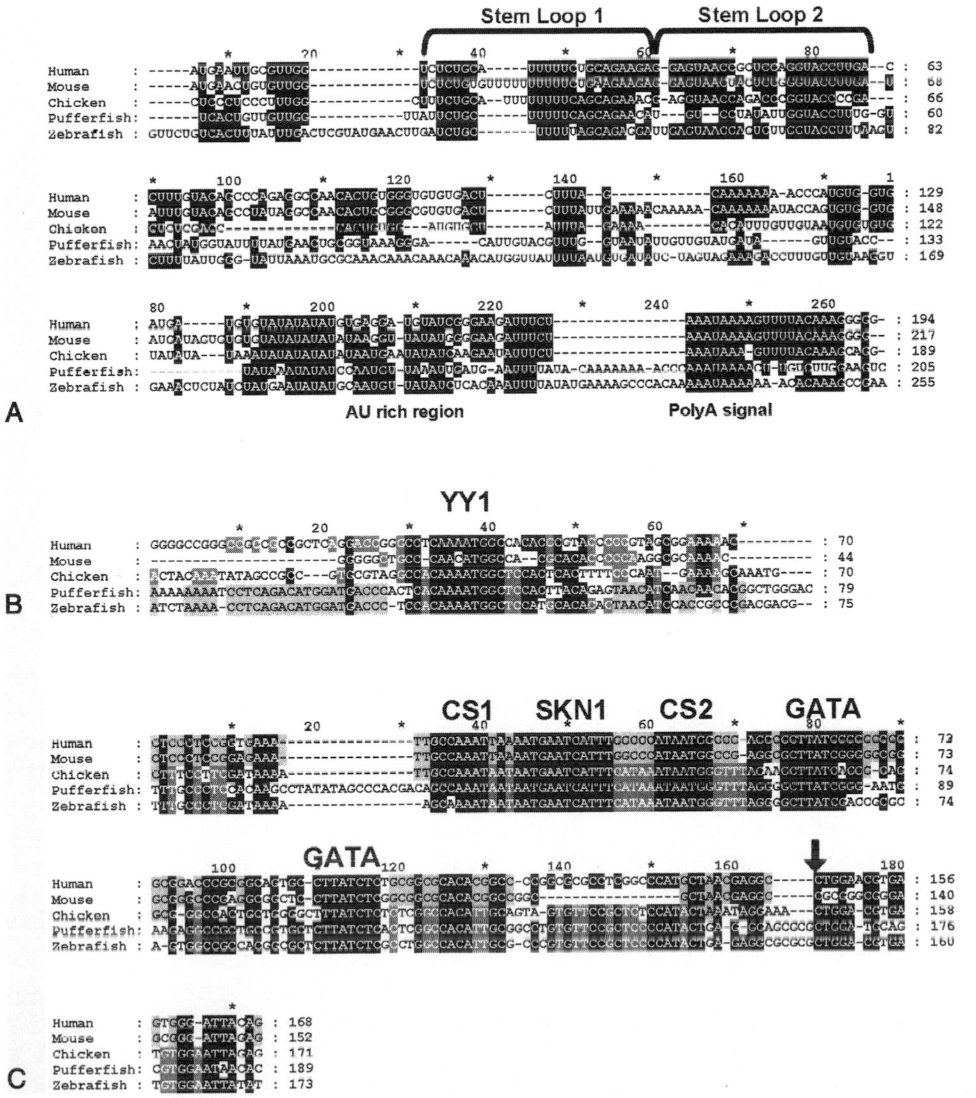

FIGURE 7–1. Alignment of noncoding regions of the same gene, stem cell leukemia factor *(SCL)*, in five different vertebrate species.[15] Alignments demonstrate highly conserved regions outside the coding region that are known or suspected of being involved in gene regulation, either as transcription-factor–binding sites or as sites involved in determining mRNA stability. (From Gottgens B, Barton LM, Chapman MA, et al: Transcriptional regulation of the stem cell leukemia gene (SCL)—comparative analysis of five vertebrate SCL loci. Genome Res 2002;12:749–759.)

among individuals. Variants in a gene are called alleles; common alleles present in 2% or more of a population are called polymorphic alleles or polymorphisms. The most frequent type of variation between human DNA sequences in different individuals is the single nucleotide change known as a single nucleotide polymorphism or SNP (pronounced "snip"). On average, one chromosome in a pair of human homologous chromosomes differs from the other chromosome of the pair at one in every 1000 base pairs; between any two individuals, there are at least 3,000,000 differences.[17] Not all alleles are present in any two individuals, and estimates are that there are likely to be, in the aggregate, more than 10,000,000 differences among all the individuals in a population. Some of these changes may be in coding regions and may or may not alter the amino acid encoded at that position, while others will be in introns or in regions of DNA between genes. Although only approximately 1.5% of human DNA is contained within the coding region of genes, variation in regulatory regions may also be functionally important. As one of the important next phases of the HGP, a consortium of academic and industry scientists have set out to find, map, and catalog human SNPs, and to determine their allele frequency in various human populations. To date, millions of such SNPs have been identified and put into publicly available databases.[18,19]

Linkage Disequilibrium

The availability of high-resolution maps of SNPs has made possible a very detailed analysis of the genetic structure of human chromosomes. A set of alleles in a region of a single chromosome is called a haplotype. Given a set of n SNPs, each with two alleles, the number of different haplotypes that could be formed by these alleles is 2^n if all possible combinations were possible. In fact, over varying distances of the genome, ranging from 1 to over 20 kilobases (kb), many fewer combinations of alleles are seen.[20] This phenomenon, known as linkage disequilibrium (LD), describes a situation in which certain alleles are found preferentially with other alleles close by on a chromosome.[21] In its simplest form, when only two SNPs are involved, one with alleles A,a and the other with alleles B,b, the frequency of finding a particular haplotype consisting of allele A and allele B on the same chromosome, f (AB), is not what one would predict from simply taking the product of the frequency of each allele alone in the population, f (A) × f (B). LD need not be absolute; f (AB) may diverge significantly from f (A) × f (B) without all chromosomes that carry an A allele exclusively carrying the B allele as well. The usual interpretation of LD is that it is a founder effect in which one allele arose on a chromosome carrying alleles already in LD with each other. The ancestral haplotype persists at a disproportionately high frequency because the alleles are located too close together for recombination to have shuffled them onto other chromosomes and disrupted their close

association. The physical extent in base pairs of some degree of LD measurable above an arbitrary threshold on either side of a polymorphic marker in the genome has come to be referred to as an LD block.[20]

The size of an LD block is likely to be a reflection of unknown biological properties of meiosis that govern the choice of sites of recombination along a chromosome, filtered through such population genetic processes such as genetic drift and population bottlenecks and expansions.[17] For example, at the resolution of the entire genome or of individual chromosomes, recombination averages 1 cM per Mb, with some variability between sexes and at telomeric versus centromeric portions of chromosomes. Even at a level of resolution of less than a megabase, one study of recombination between SNPs within a 200-kb segment of the major histocompatibility complex revealed an average ratio of genetic to physical distance of 2 cM:Mb as measured by genotyping individual sperm.[22] At an even higher level of resolution, inhomogeneity in the ratio of genetic to physical distance begins to appear. A 40-kb segment of DNA was found to contain three LD blocks, ranging in size from 3 to 15 kb, separated by short segments of a few kb with no detectable LD where the ratio of genetic to physical distance was much higher than the genome average, including one segment with a ratio of >150 cM:Mb (Fig. 7–2). In contrast, little or no recombination was measurable in regions of complete LD while regions of high, but not complete, LD had ratios of genetic to physical distance of 0.1 to 0.4 cM:Mb, substantially lower than the genome average. Short DNA segments of very high recombination frequency may very well serve as boundaries of regions of low recombination that then develop as LD blocks. However, the precise length and location of LD blocks are not identical between every human's genome. Individuals from Africa have more numerous and shorter LD blocks than do European whites, probably reflecting their much older population structure and greater opportunity for recombination.[20]

Finding Disease Genes
Linkage Analysis

MENDELIAN DISORDERS
Geneticists have had great success in understanding the genetic basis of many *rare* hereditary diseases because they are caused by relatively infrequent mutations that have a major effect on the expression of a particular gene, resulting in a typical mendelian pattern of inheritance with high penetrance.[23] These include disorders such as Duchenne muscular dystrophy, triplet repeat disorders (Huntington's disease and the spinocerebellar ataxias), early-onset familial Alzheimer's disease, sodium and potassium channelopathies, and some forms of epilepsy. If the inheritance pattern of a disease is clearly evident in a pedigree, one can use linkage analysis to simply identify

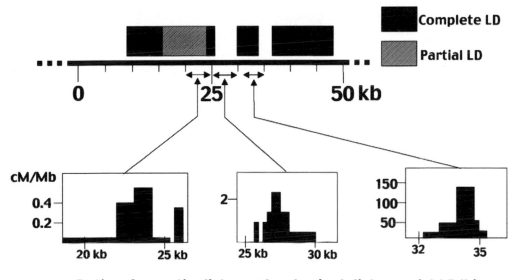

Ratio of genetic distance to physical distance (cM/Mb)

FIGURE 7–2. High-resolution mapping of genetic distance versus physical distance within the human histocompatibility complex on chromosome 6p. Blocks of complete or partial linkage disequilibrium along a 50-kb segment of the complex are shown *(rectangles at top)*. The ratio of genetic to physical distance in cM per Mb are shown at various points along the 50-kb segment of the MHC locus *(bar graphs)*. The distance ratio was measured by genotyping SNPs in single sperm. (From Jeffreys AJ, Kauppi L, Neumann R: Intensely punctate meiotic recombination in the class II region of the major histocompatibility complex. Nat Genet 2001;29:217–222.)

which region of which chromosome is harboring the responsible mutant gene.[24] With linkage analysis, one compares the inheritance of polymorphic markers located throughout the genome with the inheritance of the disease gene itself in order to find a region (marked by one or more polymorphic alleles) that is nonrandomly passed from parent to child when the disease gene is transmitted (Fig. 7–3A). Cotransmission of the markers in a particular region with a disease gene indicates that the gene is likely to be "close" in genetic distance (cM) to the markers; otherwise, meiotic crossing over during gametogenesis in parents carrying the disease gene would shuffle the link between the markers and the disease gene as the disease gene is passed on to children. In linkage analysis, one makes the best statistical estimate of the frequency of recombination (as a measure of genetic distance) between a marker and a disease. How good an estimate it is depends on the size and completeness of the family data and how close the disease gene is to the markers; the quality of the estimate is given as a lod score. By convention, a lod score over 3 at a particular genetic distance between the disease gene and a marker is considered strong evidence that the disease is indeed linked to that particular marker (Fig. 7–3B). Finding disease genes by linkage analysis always requires family studies because all linkage methods involve tracking the inheritance of particular chromosomal segments from one generation to the next in a family affected with a particular disease.

COMPLEX DISORDERS

Genetic influences on health extend far beyond the predominantly rare disorders with mendelian inheritance. Twin and family studies suggest that an individual's genetic makeup is likely to contribute to the development of many common diseases as well, including such disorders as multiple sclerosis, schizophrenia, hypertension, Parkinson's disease, and Alzheimer's disease. The contribution of genetic variation to these diseases is far subtler than in rare disorders with clear mendelian inheritance patterns. They are thought to result from multiple interacting predisposing genetic variants as well as environmental and random factors and are, therefore, frequently referred to as complex traits.[25] Diseases inherited as complex traits may show familial aggregation because relatives of an affected individual are more likely than unrelated individuals to have alleles, including those that predispose to disease, in common with the affected person. The closer these relatives are to the affected person, the greater the incidence of disease, because the more closely related two people are genetically, the more likely they are to share predisposing alleles. The genes involved in complex traits are, however, hard to identify through family studies because many different genes of low penetrance may be involved and gene-gene and gene-environment interactions are likely to be required for disease to occur. One of the greatest challenges facing modern medical genetics today is to develop methods for

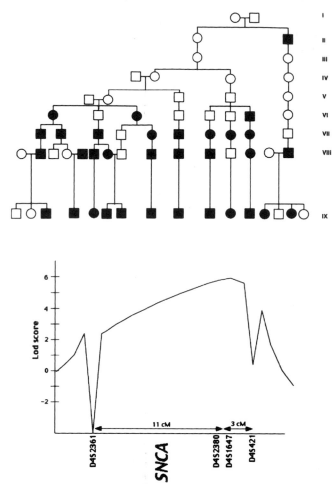

FIGURE 7–3. *A,* Partial pedigree of family with autosomal dominant, early-onset, Lewy body–positive Parkinson's disease. *B,* Multipoint lod score analysis indicating linkage of familial Parkinson's disease in the family in panel A to a region on chromosome 4q of approximately 14 cM, bounded by short-tandem repeat polymorphic markers D4S2361 and D4S421. Lod scores of 6 are found with markers D4S2380 and D4S1647. This region contained the *SNCA* gene encoding the protein α-synuclein. This gene was later shown to carry pathogenic mutations responsible for Parkinson's disease in this and other families.(*A,* From Polymeropoulos MH, Higgins JJ, Golbe LI, et al: Mapping of a gene for Parkinson's disease to chromosome 4q21–q23. Science 1996;274:1197–1199; *B,* from Polymeropoulos MH, Lavedan C, Leroy E, et al: Mutation in the alpha-synuclein gene identified in families with Parkinson's disease. Science 1997;276:2045–2047 and from Kruger R, Kuhn W, Muller T, et al: Ala30Pro mutation in the gene encoding alpha-synuclein in Parkinson's disease. Nat Genet 1998;18:106–108.)

dissecting the multiple genetic and environmental contributions to common disease and identifying those particular alleles that either predispose to or protect from disease.

Linkage analysis can be applied to locating the genes involved in complex diseases, where the exact mode of inheritance is not known, by restricting one's attention to affected individuals only. Such affected pedigree member methods avoid the problems posed by lack of penetrance of the disease gene and simply focus on whether multiple affected relatives in a family share certain segments of chromosomes inherited from a common ancestor more frequently than by chance alone.[26] Multiple genes located in many parts of the genome may be involved and may interact with each other as well as with the environment. Unfortunately, this can obscure the signal from any one particular region of the genome in affected pedigree member linkage analysis and, therefore, reduce the power to detect the contribution of any one gene and its alleles to a complex trait. For these reasons, linkage analysis in complex traits has so far met with far less success than in mendelian disorders.[27] In complex disorders such as late-onset Alzheimer's disease,[28] late-onset Parkinson's disease,[29] and bipolar disorder and schizophrenia,[30] linkage analysis has suggested that certain regions of the genome harbor alleles that predispose to these disorders. Although linkage analysis occasionally implicates the same regions repeatedly in multiple studies, it is unfortunately all too often the case that the same region does not show significant linkage to the disease in follow-up studies, either because the original study was a false-positive, different genes in different populations cause the disease, or the replication study was insufficient to avoid a false-negative result.

Association Studies

Another approach to finding alleles predisposing to disease is by finding a disease association with a particular allele.[24] Association methods are not family-based. They are population-based and derive their power by comparing the frequency of a particular allele in affected versus unaffected individuals who are otherwise matched by ethnic background, environmental exposure, and other variables of potential importance. As opposed to linkage analysis, where a region of the genome harboring a gene with a presumed, but unidentified, predisposition allele is responsible for inheritance of a disease, association studies look for a significant increase or decrease in the frequency of a particular allele of a gene among individuals with the disease. A significantly different frequency of the allele in affected individuals versus normal controls would indicate a correlation between carrying a particular allele with having increased or decreased disease susceptibility. Association studies can be done in a cohort, although, most frequently, they rely on a case-control study design. The degree of association is measured by the relative risk, where a relative risk of 1 indicates no difference in allele frequency between affected individuals and control. The number of individuals needed to be sure that a disease association, if present, will be detected depends on the strength of the association. Detecting small increases in relative risk (1.1, for example) may require studying many thousands of cases and controls.

An association between a disease and a particular allele of a gene is simply a correlation and does not mean that the allele necessarily contributes etiologically to the disease. There are a number of explanations for a statistically significant association between a hypothetical disease and an allele, A, of a gene, G:

1. Allele A does actually contribute directly to disease susceptibility or resistance.
2. Allele A is not etiologically involved but is in linkage disequilibrium with another allele, B, located close to allele A (either in gene G or in a neighboring gene). If the B allele is etiologically involved in the disease, a difference in the frequency of B between affected and control individuals will make the frequency of allele A also look to be different in affected individuals versus controls because of LD between alleles A and B.
3. The association is spurious and results from inhomogeneity in allele frequencies in the study population. If a disease happens to be more frequent in one ethnic group as compared to another, any allele that happens to be significantly more or less frequent in that ethnic group as compared to the population at large will appear to be associated with the disease. The extent to which this phenomenon, known as population stratification, exists and confounds association studies is a subject of current debate. Genotyping a large number of polymorphisms sprinkled throughout the genome would allow an investigator to determine whether the allele frequencies are different between affected and control groups (suggesting stratification is present) or whether they are very similar (suggesting it is not).[31] New association methods have also been developed that are insensitive to stratification because they test for whether a specific allele is inherited nonrandomly by an affected individual from a parent.[32]

Association studies are more sensitive than linkage analysis for finding genes involved in complex traits, if the correct allele in the relevant gene is tested for association with the disease.[24] It is also much simpler and cheaper to collect very large populations for a case-control study than to ascertain and collect data from families. Association studies to date have been performed primarily by analyzing a limited number of alleles, those that happen to be known, in a small set of genes, generally chosen because the genes encode proteins considered to be physiologically relevant in some way to the disease in

question. A number of important associations have been discovered and confirmed, such as the association between the ε4 allele of the apolipoprotein ε gene, and late-onset Alzheimer's disease.[33] However, large numbers of association studies have failed to be replicated, either because the original report was a false positive or the replication studies were underpowered and gave false-negative results.[34]

Avoiding the insensitivity and bias of doing association studies that are limited by which alleles and genes are chosen for study requires that we carry out complete association studies on a genomewide scale. To accomplish this goal, we need a complete catalog of all SNPs with any functional significance.[35] Although there may be only 30,000 to 40,000 genes, there are multiple alleles in each gene. Also, it is estimated that there may be more than 1,000,000 common alleles within genes and another 9,000,000 in introns and between genes that could have functional significance and, therefore, contribute to disease susceptibility or resistance. Genomewide association studies with such a large number of alleles would be extremely expensive and labor-intensive, but they may ultimately be required to find the genetic contributions to complex diseases.[25] One approach for doing a cost-effective genomewide association study using fewer markers has been proposed. The process involves searching for association between a disease and a set of haplotypes throughout the genome when each haplotype has been defined by a minimum number of alleles that are in LD and sit on a single LD block.[36,37] The creation of a map of such haplotypes is under way.[38] If an allele that contributes to a complex disease sits on an LD block, it may be possible to see a positive association between the disease and the haplotype if there is sufficient LD between the alleles that make up the haplotype and the disease-predisposing allele. The expectation would be that a much smaller number of genotypes would need to be done to find an association with a haplotype than with every possible functional SNP in the genome. However, this approach to whole-genome association assumes that the alleles that predispose to disease are common and are in LD with the alleles forming a haplotype, a situation commonly referred to as the common variant:common disease hypothesis (Fig. 7–4A). If, however, alleles associated with the disease have occurred multiple times in human history on different haplotype blocks, then the association with any particular haplotype will be obscured (Fig. 7–4B). Finally, if the allele associated with the disease is relatively rare, too many individuals will have the haplotype without the disease-causing allele and the association with any particular haplotype will also be obscured (Fig. 7–4C). The use of a haplotype map for genomewide association studies, and the common variant:common disease hypothesis that provides the rational underpinning for this approach, are controversial and will be rigorously tested over the next few years.

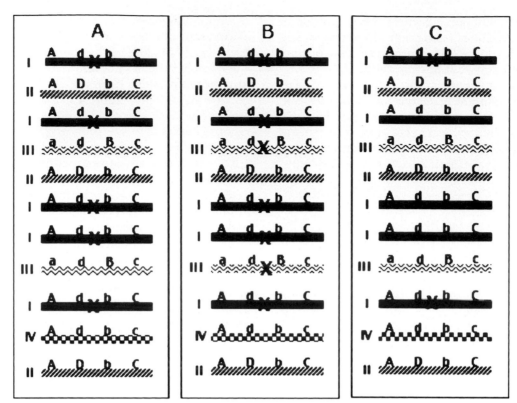

FIGURE 7–4. Models for genomewide association analysis using haplotypes contained on LD blocks. Horizontal bar represents a single LD block. Although there are four loci, each with two alleles, giving potentially $2^4 = 16$ possible haplotypes, LD has resulted in only four haplotypes defined by the alleles at these four loci: haplotype I is defined by alleles AdbC, haplotype II is defined by alleles ADbC, haplotype III is defined by alleles adBc, and haplotype IV is defined by alleles Adbc. *Panel A,* Disease susceptibility allele X is in linkage disequilibrium with haplotype I. An association study done with haplotype I is likely to demonstrate a positive association with the disease allele without having to test for association directly with the disease susceptibility allele itself. *Panel B,* Disease susceptibility allele X is in linkage disequilibrium with haplotypes I and III. An association study may have difficulty detecting an association with either haplotype. *Panel C,* Disease susceptibility allele X is rare and is found on only a small fraction of chromosomes carrying haplotype I. An association with haplotype I may be difficult to detect because too many chromosomes carrying haplotype I do not have the disease allele.

THE HGP AND SOCIETY

The sequence of the human genome has made powerful new tools available to basic scientists from a broad range of disciplines including evolutionary biology, chromosome structure and function, molecular biology, population genetics, and developmental biology. Scientists in these fields are rapidly incorporating this information into their research endeavors. However, it is the medical applications of the HGP that have garnered the most interest and concern for society. First, genome information, particularly the databases of human variation, will be used to answer questions concerning the role of genetic variation in a broad range of medical and public health applications. In the near future, genetic factors will be investigated and perhaps defined in important phenotypes such as susceptibility to degenerative disease, longevity, responsiveness to drug therapy and sensitivity to adverse drug reactions, immune competence against infections or in developing immunity through vaccina-

tion, and the metabolism of various dietary nutrients or environmental toxins. Some success has already been seen in the discovery of gene variants in asthma[39] and type 2 diabetes[40] that employed a combined strategy of linkage and association methods. The discovery of an allele that increases risk for disease may provide critical information on metabolic pathways or physiological processes and, thus, serve as the basis for the development of prevention or treatment strategies. For the pharmaceutical industry in particular, the field of pharmacogenomics is concerned with the role of genetic variation in therapeutic response and adverse drug reactions.

It is important, however, to remember that the HGP is not being conducted in a societal vacuum. From the very inception of the public HGP in the United States, funding has been mandated for the study of the ethical, legal, and social implications (ELSI) of the project.[41,42] The ELSI arm of the public HGP has made the societal impact of human genome research its chief concern and has supported a growing body of research on how genome information should and can be used.[43] For example, information as to an individual's genetic makeup and any disease susceptibilities conferred by an individual's genotype must be used for the benefit of that individual, with full respect for personal privacy and protection from discrimination. Equally important is that the discovery of genetic contributions to diseases that also have significant environmental and societal influences not be used to stigmatize individuals and serve as a pretext for placing blame for an individual's health problems solely on that individual's genotype instead of addressing social inequities that contribute to poor health outcomes. Finally, there is the possibility that a detailed investigation of human genetic diversity may result in the identification of the genetic contribution to complex traits that are of little or no medical importance, but of great personal or financial interest to some in society. Scientists and physicians who generate and use the tools of the HGP are committed to addressing these issues so as to ensure that the results of the HGP are used effectively, wisely, and fairly, for the benefit of society and its individual members.[3]

REFERENCES

1. Dulbecco R: A turning point in cancer research: Sequencing the human genome. Science 1986;231:1055–1056.

2. Collins F, Galas D: A new five-year plan for the U.S. Human Genome Project. Science 1993;262:43–46.

3. Collins FS, Patrinos A, Jordan E, et al: New goals for the U.S. Human Genome Project: 1998–2003. Science 1998;282:682–689.

4. Lander ES, Linton LM, Birren B, et al: Initial sequencing and analysis of the human genome. Nature 2001;409:860–921.

5. Venter JC, Adams MD, Myers EW, et al: The sequence of the human genome. Science 2001;291:1304–1351.

6. Watson JD, Crick FH: Molecular structure of nucleic acids. A structure for deoxyribose nucleic acid. Nature 1953;171:737–738.

7. Adams MD, Soares MB, Kerlavage AR, et al: Rapid cDNA sequencing (expressed sequence tags) from a directionally cloned human infant brain cDNA library. Nat Genet 1993;4:373–380.

8. Riggins GJ, Strausberg RL: Genome and genetic resources from the Cancer Genome Anatomy Project. Hum Mol Genet 2001;10:663–667.

9. Birney E, Bateman A, Clamp ME, et al: Mining the draft human genome. Nature 2001;409:827–828.

10. Baxevanis AD: Information retrieval from biological databases. Methods Biochem Anal 2001;43:155–185.

11. Baxevanis AD: The Molecular Biology Database Collection: An updated compilation of biological database resources. Nucleic Acids Res 2001;29:1–10.

12. Li WH, Gu Z, Wang H, et al: Evolutionary analyses of the human genome. Nature 2001;409:847–849.

13. Rubin GM: The draft sequences. Comparing species. Nature 2001;409:820–821.

14. Miller W: So many genomes, so little time. Nat Biotechnol 2000;18:148–149.

15. Gottgens B, Barton LM, Chapman MA, et al: Transcriptional regulation of the stem cell leukemia gene (SCL)—comparative analysis of five vertebrate SCL loci. Genome Res 2002;12:749–759.

16. Pennacchio LA, Rubin EM: Genomic strategies to identify mammalian regulatory sequences. Nat Rev Genet 2001;2:100–109.

17. Stoneking M. Single nucleotide polymorphisms. From the evolutionary past. Nature 2001;409:821–822.

18. Sachidanandam R, Weissman D, Schmidt SC, et al: A map of human genome sequence variation containing 1.42 million single nucleotide polymorphisms. Nature 2001;409:928–933.

19. Holden AL: The SNP consortium: Summary of a private consortium effort to develop an applied map of the human genome. Biotechniques 2002;(Suppl):S22–S24, S26.

20. Gabriel SB, Schaffner SF, Nguyen H, et al: The structure of haplotype blocks in the human genome. Science 2002;296:2225–2229.

21. Daly MJ, Rioux JD, Schaffner SF, et al: High-resolution haplotype structure in the human genome. Nat Genet 2001;29:229–232.

22. Jeffreys AJ, Kauppi L, Neumann R: Intensely punctate meiotic recombination in the class II region of the major histocompatibility complex. Nat Genet 2001;29:217–222.

23. McKusick VA: Online Mendelian Inheritance in Man, OMIM, 2002. http://www.ncbi.nlm.nih.gov/omim/

24. Borecki IB, Suarez BK: Linkage and association: Basic concepts. Adv Genet 2001;42:45–66.

25. Risch N, Merikangas K: The future of genetic studies of complex human diseases. Science 1996;273:1516–1517.

26. Brown DL, Gorin MB, Weeks DE: Efficient strategies for genomic searching using the affected-pedigree-member method of linkage analysis. Am J Hum Genet 1994;54:544–552.

27. Xu J, Wiesch DG, Taylor EW, et al: Evaluation of replication studies, combined data analysis, and analytical methods in complex diseases. Genet Epidemiol 1999;17(Suppl):S773–S778.

28. Myers AJ, Goate AM: The genetics of late-onset Alzheimer's disease. Curr Opin Neurol 2001;14:433–440.

29. Scott WK, Nance MA, Watts RL, et al: Complete genomic screen in Parkinson disease: Evidence for multiple genes. JAMA 2001;286:2239–2244.

30. Sklar P: Linkage analysis in psychiatric disorders: The emerging picture. Annu Rev Genomics Hum Genet 2002;3:371–413.

31. Pritchard JK, Rosenberg NA: Use of unlinked genetic markers to detect population stratification in association studies. Am J Hum Genet 1999;65:220–228.

32. Spielman RS, McGinnis RE, Ewens WJ: Transmission test for linkage disequilibrium: The insulin gene region and insulin-dependent diabetes mellitus (IDDM). Am J Hum Genet 1993;52:506–516.

33. Strittmatter WJ, Roses AD: Apolipoprotein E and Alzheimer's Disease. Annu Rev Neurosci 1996; 19:53–77.

34. Hirschhorn JN, Lohmueller K, Byrne E, et al: A comprehensive review of genetic association studies. Genet Med 2002;4:45–61.

35. Chakravarti A: To a future of genetic medicine. Nature 2001;409:822–823.

36. Jorde LB: Linkage disequilibrium and the search for complex disease genes. Genome Res 2000;10: 1435–1444.

37. Johnson GC, Esposito L, Barratt BJ, et al: Haplotype tagging for the identification of common disease genes. Nat Genet 2001;29:233–237.

38. Dawson E, Abecasis GR, Bumpstead S, et al: A first-generation linkage disequilibrium map of human chromosome 22. Nature 2002;418:544–548.

39. Van Eerdewegh P, Little RD, Dupuis J, et al: Association of the ADAM33 gene with asthma and bronchial hyperresponsiveness. Nature 2002;418: 426–430.

40. Horikawa Y, Oda N, Cox NJ, et al: Genetic variation in the gene encoding calpain-10 is associated with type 2 diabetes mellitus. Nat Genet 2000;26:163–175.

41. Juengst ET, Watson JD. Human genome research and the responsible use of new genetic knowledge. J Int Bioethique 1991;2:99–102.

42. Meslin EM, Thomson EJ, Boyer JT: The Ethical, Legal, and Social Implications Research Program at the National Human Genome Research Institute. Kennedy Inst Ethics J 1997;7:291–298.

43. A decade of ELSI research: A celebration of the first ten years of the Ethical, Legal, and Social Implications (ELSI) programs. January 16–18, 2001. Abstracts. J Law Med Ethics 2001;29:1–65.

44. Polymeropoulos MH, Higgins JJ, Golbe LI, et al: Mapping of a gene for Parkinson's disease to chromosome 4q21–q23. Science 1996;274:1197–1199.

45. Polymeropoulos MH, Lavedan C, Leroy E, et al: Mutation in the alpha-synuclein gene identified in families with Parkinson's disease. Science 1997;276: 2045–2047.

46. Kruger R, Kuhn W, Muller T, et al: Ala30Pro mutation in the gene encoding alpha-synuclein in Parkinson's disease. Nat Genet 1998;18:106–108.

8

Gene Therapy for Central Nervous System Disorders

Theodore Friedmann

After several decades of anticipation and promise, the field of human gene therapy has now achieved its first likely success. Children with an X-linked form of severe combined immunodeficiency disease are demonstrating what seems to be a full immunologic reconstitution after retrovirus-mediated gene transfer into CD34+ bone marrow stem cells followed by grafting of the corrected cells into patients.[1] Human gene therapy is no longer an area of mere theoretical promise, but rather one in which patients with serious disease are benefiting. Additional examples of clinical success are being achieved or are imminent in disorders such as hemophilia,[2,3] coronary artery and peripheral artery disease,[4] some forms of cancer,[5] and slowly but surely, other disorders among the more than 400 clinical studies so far undertaken.[6]

Just as is true for these disorders and for most somatic tissues and organs, progress has also been made in the past several years toward the goal of gene therapy for human neurologic disease. Although it is fair to say that progress toward gene therapy for neurologic disease has been slow, it is equally true that major advances and real therapeutic efficacy are likely in the coming several years.

TECHNICAL CONSIDERATIONS AND OBSTACLES TO GENE THERAPY IN THE NERVOUS SYSTEM

Nature of Target Tissue

The central nervous system (CNS) poses a number of difficult problems to gene-based therapy.[7] One of the potentially more soluble problems is that target cells in the fully developed CNS (in most cases, neurons) are generally thought to be largely postmitotic and fully differentiated at the time of disease development and detection and therefore refractory to some of the most useful and efficient methods for gene transfer. Fortunately, a number of gene transfer methods have recently become available for such nonreplicating cells, particularly through the use of virus vectors derived from lentiviruses and adeno-associated virus (discussed later). More of a problem, however, is the fact that cell-cell interactions in the CNS, unlike all other organs, are staggeringly complex and often may be irreversibly fixed into aberrant pathways before any aspect of the disease phenotype is evident and before therapy can generally begin. By the time expression of an aberrant phenotype becomes overt, the CNS may not be plastic enough to allow structural or functional remodeling and correction of at least many forms of CNS disease. The implication of lack of plasticity may be that effective therapy for some kinds of CNS disease, whether genetic or more traditional, must be instituted early in life, possibly even at a fetal stage. In other disorders, such as those characterized by major elements of environmental toxicity or slow accumulative damage as in the case of the lysosomal storage diseases, treatments begun later in life may be more feasible. Finally, the well-known difficulty posed by the existence of the protective function of the blood-brain barrier makes the development of efficient humoral delivery of therapeutic agents more of a challenge in the CNS than is true of many other organs.

Gene Delivery

As is true of approaches to gene therapy for other organs, the approach for CNS disease takes the form of ex vivo gene transfer or direct in vivo gene delivery (Fig. 8-1).[8]

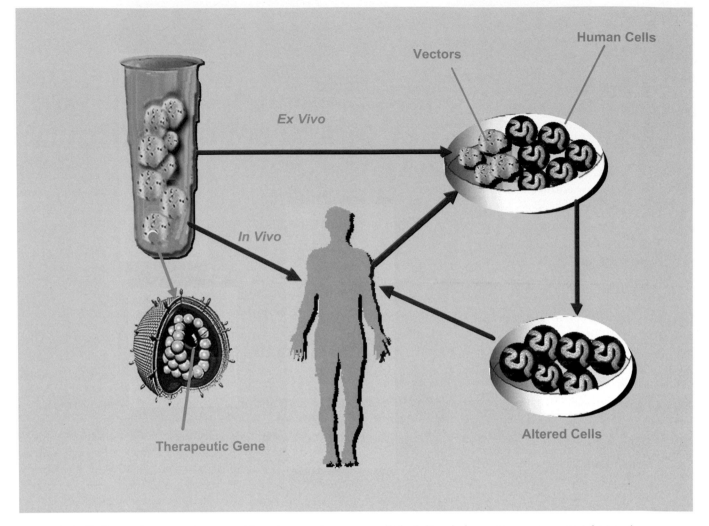

FIGURE 8–1. Delivery of genes to human subjects is sometimes accomplished directly by putting vectors straight into large tissue (in vivo). More often, the ex vivo approach is used. Physicians remove cells from a patient, add the desired gene in the laboratory, and return the genetically corrected cells to the patient. An in vivo approach still in development would rely on "smart" vectors that could be injected into the bloodstream or elsewhere and would home to specific cell types anywhere in the body.

The ex vivo strategy involves the introduction of a therapeutic gene into cells that can then be grafted to the CNS into a site that provides a local source of a needed neurotransmitter, a neuro-protective factor, an inducer of repair mechanisms, or other structural components. The in vivo approach involves the administration of the genetic element directly to the diseased tissues or cells in the CNS. With advances in our understanding of disease pathogenesis and improvements in the design of both viral and nonviral gene transfer vectors, both approaches are being applied to preclinical animal studies and to human clinical studies in CNS disease. The approaches are still quite inexact and crude, but continuing technical advances and, particularly, the eventual development of techniques for specific, targeted, and efficient in vivo delivery of foreign genes to the CNS will greatly facilitate gene therapies for CNS disease.

TARGET DISEASES

Single Gene Inborn Errors of Metabolism

From the beginnings of gene therapy, the simplest target diseases seemed to be the single gene inborn errors of metabolism,[8] many of which produce a neurologic phenotype such as Lesch-Nyhan disease, Tay-Sachs and other lysosomal storage diseases, Huntington's disease, and the mucopolysaccharidoses. Because the complex neurologic disorder in those cases is ultimately caused by a simple genetic change, reconstitution of those single functions would seem to provide an opportunity for a definitive gene-based cure. However, while such diseases represent useful model systems for demonstrations of proof of principle, effective correction of full neurologic phenotypes has proven just as elusive as it has in nonneurologic disorders. The reason for this unexpected level of complexity of single gene defects is the likelihood that neurologic presentations of even such straightforward genetic defects result from pleiotropic gene effects and aberrations of complex neurophysiologic networks that affect the expression of a number of secondary downstream gene functions. In turn, these functions may irreversibly affect aspects of neural development and function in ways not predictable by the nature of the primary genetic and metabolic defect. Nevertheless, this class of disease remains a popular target for basic and preclinical studies toward gene therapy and for a number of active clinical studies in single gene neurologic diseases.

Lysosomal Storage Diseases: Mucopolysaccharidosis

The CNS damage resulting from lysosomal storage disease may lend itself particularly well to gene-based therapy. The disease related enzymes can be provided to defective cells from donor cells by virtue of their mechanisms of secretion from wild-type or genetically engineered cells and functional re-uptake into other cells. Genetically defective recipient cells, although not genetically corrected, are able to take up and express the functional enzyme because of their proximity to genetically modified cells or, in some cases, through hematogenous delivery of a functional transgenic product. Enzyme-deficient cells are thereby able to pick up functional enzymes from their environment and clear stored lysosomal products and thus correct disease phenotypes of lysosomal storage disease. Some initial gene therapy studies centered around Gaucher's disease, and while preclinical results were often promising,[9] delivery to clinical efficacy in humans has not been convincing. More recently, there have been a number of impressive animal studies in the mucopolysaccharidosis VII model. These studies have demonstrated that local injections into the brain of adeno-associated virus (AAV) or lentivirus vectors expressing the wild type β-glucuronidase enzyme can lead to prolonged expression of enzyme and improvement of the neuropathologic changes in affected brain.[10-15] Similarly, even the systemic administration of adenovirus and AAV vectors has led to the appearance of enzyme activity in a variety of organs and some degree of correction of the neuropathologic defects in the brain.[16]

Canavan's Disease

Canavan's disease is an inborn error of metabolism that produces severe, early, and untreatable gray matter vacuolization and extensive demyelination. The underlying defect is in the expression of the gene encoding the enzyme aspartoacylase (ASPA) with resulting brain accumulation of the proximal metabolite proximal to the block, N-acetyl aspartic acid (NAA).[17] Studies with wild-type rodents have demonstrated prolonged expression of the enzyme from liposomes containing an ASPA plasmid after intraventricular or intraparenchymal injection with resulting reduction of NAA accumulation. The recent development of a faithful mouse knockout model for the disease will facilitate additional preclinical studies, but even in the absence of results in the ASPA-deficient mouse, a human phase I clinical trial of liposome-mediated gene transfer into the brain has been approved and undertaken. Definitive results are not yet available, but it has been reported anecdotally that treated patients are said to have shown ASPA gene expression and some degree of reduced levels of NAA. An alternative approach involving the use of an adeno-associated virus vector instead of the liposome vectors is also being developed for clinical evaluation in patients with Canavan's disease.

Complex, Multigenic, and Multifactorial Neurodegenerative Diseases: Parkinson's Disease

Even before clinical success has been achieved with the presumably simpler single gene defects, interest has shifted toward the more complex, multigenic, and multifactorial neurodegenerative diseases such as Parkinson's disease, Alzheimer's disease, amyotrophic lateral sclerosis, multiple sclerosis, and others. The surge of interest in these complex and largely untreatable disorders stems from the fact that they are common and represent enormous medical and social burdens on our society. Furthermore, identification of the many genes associated with the primary neurophysiologic defects, clarification of the role of additional neurotrophic factors in the function of the relevant CNS cells, and development of suitable transgenic, knockout, or neurotoxicity animal models have made these diseases very alluring targets for genetic intervention. One of the most attractive model diseases for the study of gene-based therapy for complex CNS disease is Parkinson's disease, known to be associated with strong environmental influences as well as with mutations in a number of genes such as *PARK 1–6*, α-*synuclein*, the protease *parkin*, and other genes.[18] For instance, in the case of Parkinson's disease, it is known that loss of dopaminergic neurons in the substantia nigra is primarily responsible for the movement disorder and that the development of this disease is also associated with the appearance of extracellular inclusion bodies termed Lewy bodies that consist of accumulated proteins and lipids in the affected brains.

The biochemical pathways of dopamine biosynthesis are well understood. This understanding has been augmented recently by extensive new understanding of the role of neurotrophic factors such as glial-derived growth factor (GDNF), brain-derived growth factor (BDNF), and others in promoting the survival and function of dopaminergic neurons.[19,20] These advances have led to studies of the effects of genetic reconstitution in Parkinson's animal models with vectors expressing genes encoding functions of the dopamine biosynthetic pathway (tyrosine hydroxylase, aromatic amino acid decarboxylase, GTP cyclohydrolase), genes encoding neuroprotective functions (GDNF, BDNF, β-fibroblast growth factors) to prevent neuronal degeneration, or genes encoding glutamate decarboxylase (the enzyme that catalyzes decarboxylation to form γ-aminobutyric acid).[7] Genetic reconstitution of these systems has included both ex vivo and in vivo approaches. In the ex vivo approach, foreign genes are introduced into cells in vitro, then genetically modified cells are grafted into affected portions of the CNS. In the in vivo gene delivery method, gene transfer vectors are introduced directly into the brain. These gene transfer approaches have shown a variety of encouraging results in animal models, including reduced neuronal degeneration in the nigrostriatum and even regeneration, restored dopamine production, improvements in apomorphine-induced rotational behavior, and improvements in other parameters of impaired neural function.[21–23]

Other Degenerative Diseases

The potentially protective role of neurotrophic factors and anti-apoptosis functions has been examined in animal models for a number of other neurodegenerative disorders, including most notably Alzheimer's disease, Huntington's disease and amyotrophic lateral sclerosis (ALS). In the case of Alzheimer's disease,[24] it has been recognized for more than a decade that the ex vivo approach of grafting cells genetically modified to express neurotrophic growth factor (NGF) protects a variety of neurons from degeneration after toxic damage or CNS injury.[25] This early study demonstrated that grafts of fibroblasts genetically modified by retrovirus-mediated transduction to produce NGF had protected cholinergic neurons from degeneration caused by fimbria fornix lesioning. Based on this model and on many subsequent animal studies, an approach to the prevention of neurodegeneration in Alzheimer's disease has been carried to a human clinical trial. In this trial, a patient's fibroblasts infected with a retrovirus expressing NGF are injected into the brain of patients in the early stages of Alzheimer's disease. Because of the global or at least the very diffuse nature of the neuropathology in Alzheimer's disease and the limited efficacy of untargeted local vector delivery, it will be difficult for this approach to achieve major improvement in this difficult disease. Nevertheless, helpful information is likely to come from these early clinical studies.

Additional neurodegenerative diseases are also becoming attractive targets for attempts at gene-based therapy. ALS is a degenerative disorder characterized by loss of motor neurons in the brain, brainstem, and spinal cord. In animal studies, the introduction by AAV-mediated gene transfer of the anti-apoptotic function bcl-2 directly into the spinal cord was reported to increase the survival of motor neurons in the mouse model of ALS that is produced by overexpression of a mutant superoxide dismutase 1 *(SOD1)*. However, there was no effect on survival of affected animals. An alternative approach in this disease involves the use of vectors that transfer a gene encoding ciliary neurotrophic factor (CNTF).[26] Nonhuman cells genetically modified to produce and secrete human CNTF have been encapsulated and introduced intrathecally into the spinal cord of ALS patients. The CNTF secreted by the cells is able to pass through the capsules into the CSF and, in principle, protect some of the motor neurons from further degeneration. Studies have indeed demonstrated detectable levels of CNTF in the patient's CSF, but clinical benefit was not apparent in this early phase I study. A technical difficulty of such a study lies in the unproved long-term stability of the capsules holding the xenogeneic cells and in the possible induction of host immune responses that cause immune destruction of the genetically modified cells. Conceptually similar neuroprotective approaches to an eventual gene-based treatment of Huntington's disease have also been suggested.[29] One such strategy, for instance, is based on the demonstration of reduced levels of the neurotrophic factor BDNF in cells expressing a mutant huntingtin gene product. However, the specific role of BDNF in the development and function of cells at risk in this disorder has not been fully defined. Its potential role as a neuroprotective agent has not reached the level of convincing demonstration of efficacy in animal model studies, and it is certainly not ready for human clinical trials.

CELLULAR DELIVERY VEHICLES: NEURAL STEM CELLS

A combined gene vector-cell grafting approach to the introduction of therapeutic genes into the CNS has recently become feasible through the use of genetically modified neural stem cells (NSC). During the past decade, cells with properties of neural stem or early progenitor cells have been discovered in the CNS. That is, under the appropriate neuroanatomic conditions and with the appropriate biochemical signal, they are able to differentiate into a variety of specialized cells, including specific classes of neurons, and take part in normal and restorative cyto-architectural development of the brain. Neural stem and early progenitor cells exist in the developing as well as the adult nervous system. They are characterized by a number of properties that make them good candidates for therapy in the CNS, both in their native state and after genetic manipulation. These properties include facile engraftability and potential for integration into normal cytoarchitectural structure and circuitry of the CNS; ability to differentiate along all CNS lineages; propensity to seek out areas of some forms of CNS damage and degeneration; susceptibility to genetic manipulation; and plasticity and ability to accommodate to regional signals and possibly a state of some degree of immunotolerance. They have been used to provide potentially therapeutic transgenes in a variety of disease and CNS injury models.[30–33] This includes correction of global CNS defects in mucopolysaccharidosis type VII in the mouse after grafting with NSC transduced to overexpress wild-type β-glucuronidase (GUSB) to complement the underlying defect. Similarly, it has been reported that regional grafting of NSC genetically modified to produce and secrete therapeutic gene products has also succeeded in reversing or preventing other disease phenotypes. For instance, grafting of genetically modified NSC expressing the neuroprotective NGF has been reported to reverse age-related cognitive defects in rats.[34] Similarly, genetically modified NSC corrected aspects of the Parkinson's disease phenotype[31] and other CNS defects. Therefore, since unmodified and genetically modified NSC can distribute themselves widely throughout the brain and integrate after focal grafting, it seems very likely that such cells will increasingly provide potential approaches to therapy for a variety of CNS diseases, both global and multifocal.

Furthermore, NSC may also allow an important additional approach to gene transfer into the CNS. Lynch et al[35] have reported that NSC can be converted into virus-producing cells that permit infection of cells in situ in the CNS. In this preliminary study of that approach to in vivo gene transfer, NSCs producing an MLV-based retrovirus vector were shown to allow efficient infection of microglia in vivo. However, the study was not designed to determine whether a similar approach with an appropriate vector able to infect postmitotic cells (unlike MLV) would also allow transduction of neurons in vivo. Nevertheless, the general method with appropriately modified NSC seems suitable for stably expressing a virus vector as a local source of large amounts of transducing vectors for efficient infection and gene transfer into neighboring cells in vivo after grafting to the CNS. Such an approach could avert some of the problems associated with direct in vivo vector delivery and thereby provide an efficient and cyto-architecturally appropriate means of delivering therapeutic genes to the CNS. Similarly, neural precursor cells have been used as platforms to generate producer cells for herpes-virus–based vectors.

NEOPLASTIC DISEASE

Malignancies of the brain, such as glioblastoma multiforme, have been appealing targets for gene therapy approaches because current methods of therapy are so ineffective. Most initial approaches to gene-based therapy have been based on an ex vivo model in which cells that produce large amounts of a retrovirus vector expressing a "suicide" gene, such as the herpes simplex thymidine kinase (TK) gene, are grafted into a tumor bed in the brain.[7,36,37] The approach is based on the expectation that a locally produced vector will diffuse throughout the tumor and infect replicating tumor cells but spare normal postmitotic neurons in the target area. After several days, patients are treated with a drug, such as ganciclovir, that becomes toxic only in cells expressing the TK transgene. Ganclivoir is a specific substrate of the viral TK enzyme and is converted to a toxic, DNA-replication inhibitor. Even though the transduction efficiency can be quite low, the efficacy of this approach is thought to be augmented by the phenomenon of the "bystander effect" through which relatively small numbers of cells expressing the TK gene can induce ganciclovir sensitivity in many nontransduced cells in their vicinity. This kind of "prodrug" or suicide approach can also involve alternative genes, such as cytosine deaminase.

An alternative approach to gene-based treatment of CNS malignancies features the selective use of replication-competent lytic viruses such as herpesviruses to infect and destroy malignant cells.[38] While the approach has theoretical advantages, major safety and efficiency obstacles remain in the development of methods selective enough for tumor cells to permit widespread clinical application of this approach in human patients.

CONCLUSION

There is very good reason to think that conceptually new approaches to the development of gene-based treatments for central and peripheral nervous system disorders are imminent. Powerful new approaches to gene transfer technology coupled with an increasingly profound understanding of the genetic mechanisms underlying nervous system disease make this new approach to more effective and possibly even definitive therapy inevitable. Many technical and conceptual hurdles remain in achieving this goal, but the correctness of the approach with the rapid maturation of the technology combine to ensure that patients with these devastating and otherwise poorly treated diseases will have new hope for improved quality of life.

REFERENCES

1. Cavazzana-Calvo M, Hacein-Bey S, de Saint Basile G, et al: Gene therapy of human severe combined immunodeficiency (SCID)-X1 disease. Science 2000; 288:669–672.

2. Kay MA, Manno CS, Ragni MV, et al: Evidence for gene transfer and expression of factor IX in haemophilia B patients treated with an AAV vector. Nat Genet 2000;24:257–261.

3. Kay MA, High K: Gene therapy for the hemophilias. Proc Natl Acad Sci U S A 1999;96:9973–9975.

4. Isner JM: Myocardial gene therapy. Nature 2002;10;234–239.

5. Curiel DT, Gerritsen WR, Krul MR: Progress in cancer gene therapy. Cancer Gene Ther 2000;7: 1197–1199.

6. Friedmann, T: The Development of Human Gene Therapy. Cold Spring Harbor, New York, Cold Spring Harbor Press, 1999.

7. Hsich G, Sena-Esteves M, Breakefield XO: Critical issues in gene therapy for neurologic disease. Hum Gene Ther 2002;13:579–604.

8. Friedmann T: Overcoming the obstacles to gene therapy. Sci Am 1997;276:95–101.

9. Dunbar CE, Kohn DB, Schiffmann R, et al: Retroviral transfer of the glucocerebrosidase gene into CD34+ cells from patients with Gaucher disease: In vivo detection of transduced cells without myeloablation. Hum Gene Ther 1998;9:2629–2640.

10. Bosch A, Perret E, Desmaris N, Heard JM. Long-term and significant correction of brain lesions in adult mucopolysaccharidosis type VII mice using recombinant AAV vectors. Mol Ther 2000;1:63–70.

11. Bosch A, Perret E, Desmaris N, et al: Reversal of pathology in the entire brain of mucopolysaccharidosis type VII mice after lentivirus-mediated gene transfer. Hum Gene Ther 2000;11:1139–1150.

12. Daly TM, Ohlemiller KK, Roberts MS, et al: Prevention of systemic clinical disease in MPS VII mice following AAV-mediated neonatal gene transfer. Gene Ther 2001;8:1291–1298.

13. Frisella WA, O'Connor LH, Vogler CA, et al: Intracranial injection of recombinant adeno-associated virus improves cognitive function in a murine model of mucopolysaccharidosis type VII. Mol Ther 2001;3:351–358.

14. Daly TM, Vogler C, Levy B, et al: Neonatal gene transfer leads to widespread correction of pathology in a murine model of lysosomal storage disease. Proc Natl Acad Sci U S A 1999;96:2296–2300.

15. Daly TM, Okuyama T, Vogler C, et al: Neonatal intramuscular injection with recombinant adeno-associated virus results in prolonged beta-glucuronidase expression in situ and correction of liver pathology in mucopolysaccharidosis type VII mice. Hum Gene Ther 1999;10:85–94.

16. Stein CS, Ghodsi A, Derksen T, Davidson BL: Systemic and central nervous system correction of lysosomal storage in mucopolysaccharidosis type VII mice. J Virol 1999;73:3424–3429.

17. Leone P, Janson CG, Bilaniuk L, et al: Aspartoacylase gene transfer to the mammalian central nervous system with therapeutic implications for Canavan disease. Ann Neurol 2000;48:27–38.

18. Kitada T, Asakawa S, Matsumine H, et al: Related articles progress in the clinical and molecular genetics of familial parkinsonism. Neurogenetics 2000;2:207–218.

19. Mizuno Y, Hattori N, Kitada T, et al: Familial Parkinson's disease. Alpha-synuclein and parkin. Adv Neurol 2001;86:13–21.

20. Valente EM, Bentivoglio AR, Dixon PH, et al: Localization of a novel locus for autosomal recessive early-onset parkinsonism, PARK6, on human chromosome 1p35–p36. Am J Hum Genet 2001;68:895–900.

21. Zurn AD, Widmer HR, Aebischer P: Sustained delivery of GDNF: Towards a treatment for Parkinson's disease. Brain Res Brain Res Rev 2001;36:222–229.

22. Wolff JA, Fisher LJ, et al: Grafting fibroblasts genetically modified to produce L-DOPA in a rat model of Parkinson's disease. Proc Natl Acad Sci U S A 1989;86:9011–9014.

23. Raymon HK, Thode S, Gage FH: Application of ex vivo gene therapy in the treatment of Parkinson's disease. Exp Neurol 1997;144:82–91.

24. Rosenberg RN: The molecular and genetic basis of AD: The end of the beginning: The 2000 Wartenberg lecture. Neurology 2000;54:2045–2054.

25. Rosenberg MB, Friedmann T, Robertson RC, et al: Grafting of genetically modified cells to the damaged brain: Restorative effects of NGF gene expression. Science 1988;242:1575–1578.

26. Bachoud-Levi AC, Deglon N, Nguyen JP, et al: Neuroprotective gene therapy for Huntington's disease using a polymer encapsulated BHK cell line engineered to secrete human CNTF. Hum Gene Ther 2000;11:1723–1729.

27. Lacroix S, Tuszynski MH: Neurotrophic factors and gene therapy in spinal cord injury. Neurorehabil Neural Repair 2000;14:265–275.

28. Mittoux V, Joseph JM, Conde F, et al: Restoration of cognitive and motor functions by ciliary neurotrophic factor in a primate model of Huntington's disease. Hum Gene Ther 2000;11:1177–1187.

29. Mittoux V, Joseph JM, Conde F, et al: Restoration of cognitive and motor functions by ciliary neurotrophic factor in a primate model of Huntington's disease. Hum Gene Ther 2000;11:1177–1187.

30. Philips MF, Mattiasson G, Wieloch T, et al: Neuroprotective and behavioral efficacy of nerve growth factor transfected hippocampal progenitor cell transplants after experimental traumatic brain injury. J Neurosurg 2001;94:765–774.

31. Anton R, Kordower JH, Maidment NT, et al: Neural targeted gene therapy for rodent and primate hemiparkinsonism. Exp Neurol 1994;127:207–218.

32. Akerud P, Canals JM, Snyder EY, Arenas E: Neuroprotection through delivery of glial cell line-derived neurotrophic factor by neural stem cells in a mouse model of Parkinson's disease. J Neurosci 2001;21:8108–8118.

33. Himes BT, Liu Y, Solowska JM, et al: Transplants of cells genetically modified to express neurotrophin-3 rescue axotomized Clarke's nucleus neurons after spinal cord hemisection in adult rats. J Neurosci Res 2001;65:549–564.

34. Martinez-Serrano A, Bjorklund A: Ex vivo nerve growth factor gene transfer to the basal forebrain in pre-symptomatic middle-aged rats prevents the development of cholinergic neuron atrophy and cognitive impair-

ment during aging. Proc Natl Acad Sci U S A 1998;95: 1858–1863.

35. Lynch WP, Sharpe AH, Snyder EY: Neural stem cells as engraftable packaging lines can mediate gene delivery to microglia: Evidence from studying retroviral env-related neurodegeneration. J Virol 1999;73: 6841–6851.

36. Jacobs A, Breakefield XO, Fraefel C: HSV-1-based vectors for gene therapy of neurological diseases and brain tumors: Part II. Vector systems and applications. Neoplasia 1999;1:402–416.

37. Ma HI, Guo P, Li J, et al: Suppression of intracranial human glioma growth after intramuscular administration of an adeno-associated viral vector expressing angiostatin. Cancer Res 2002;62:756–763.

38. Sandmair AM, Loimas S, Puranen P, et al: Thymidine kinase gene therapy for human malignant glioma, using replication-deficient retroviruses or adenoviruses. Hum Gene Ther 2000;11:2197–2205.

39. Markert JM, Gillespie GY, Weichselbaum RR, et al: Genetically engineered HSV in the treatment of glioma: A review. Rev Med Virol 2000;10:17–30.

CHAPTER

9

Emerging Ethical Issues in Neurology, Psychiatry, and the Neurosciences

Arthur L. Caplan

Martha J. Farah

The U.S. Congress declared the 1990s to be "the decade of the brain." This was certainly appropriate since huge advances were made in understanding the structure and function of animal and human brains. The ability to ascertain the structure and function of many components of the human brain has led to a dramatic increase in the ability to ascertain and diagnose a variety of states and conditions of medical interest. There is every reason to presume that significant advances in diagnosis will continue to occur as techniques for imaging the brain continue to evolve. It is becoming much less costly and burdensome for researchers to utilize human subjects in pursuit of knowledge about the brain, neurologic illness, and mental illness.

However, rapid progress in neurology and the neurosciences presents a new type of ethical problem. Equivalent advances in therapy have not accompanied new diagnostic information. The explosion of new knowledge about the brain's structure, chemistry, wiring, and pharmacokinetics has not resulted in many significant new therapies for neurologic or psychiatric disorders and ailments. The asymmetry between diagnosis and treatment, while not entirely new in neurology and the neurosciences,[1] is growing and is likely to persist for some time. This gap is likely to be the basis for most of the ethical challenges that will confront neuroscience and clinical neurology for the next decade.

There are, however, some lessons to be learned from a similar situation that has prevailed in genetics for a number of years.[2] Knowing more about factors that predispose a person or a family to disease or the ways in which persons differ in their biologic makeup is not an unalloyed good. While knowledge is desirable (and most patients would prefer knowledge over ignorance concerning their diagnosis, risk factors, or medical problems that can be passed on to their offspring), the ethical challenges facing neuroscience when diagnosis is possible but therapy is not readily at hand will be central to the ethics of the field.

There are, however, areas that raise unique ethical challenges. These are areas in which treatments have emerged or are close to being available. The use of pharmacologic agents to treat mood and cognitive disorders, implants to assist in the treatment of parkinsonism, and microsurgical techniques (e.g., stents to prevent aneurysms in the brain) raises questions about what is acceptable research risk, the adequacy of informed consent, and what constitutes equitable access.

Perhaps the most intriguing ethical challenge facing those in neurology and clinical neurosciences involves whether and how to set limits on clinical application. What may work to treat clear-cut instances of disease or disorder, such as autism, epilepsy, parkinsonism, or severe depression, may also be used to enhance, improve, or increase neurologic capabilities. Although restoration of function and amelioration of symptoms remain uncontroversial goals for clinicians, researchers, third-party payers, and the general public, this is not true when the possibility exists of enhancement or improvement.[3] A drug that can be used to help persons with sleep disorders, such as Cephelon's Provigil®, can also be used to help those without dysfunction go without sleep for prolonged periods of time. An implant that can control the symptoms of parkinsonism or epilepsy can also be used to enhance or improve motor skills and abilities. A drug that can be used to help slow memory loss can be used prophylactically to prevent the onset of disease when no symptoms or risk factors are present. The ethical issue of which goals advances in diagnosis and therapy are to serve and where improvement and enhancement fit into the purveyance of clinical neurology, neurosurgery, and neuroscience will be the subject of debate in years to come.

ETHICS OF DIAGNOSIS

Functional brain imaging has advanced greatly from the highly invasive methods and poor spatial and temporal resolution of single photon emission computed tomography (SPECT) and positron emission tomography (PET) in the 1970s and 1980s. Safety concerns that limited the use of scanning technology and raised difficult ethical questions about acceptable risks to present to patients or subjects are no longer an issue. An array of scanning methods are available that can image the brain with a spatial resolution of millimeters and allow processes to be tracked over intervals as brief as 5 seconds.

The ability to explore, map, and diagnose the brain and nervous system permits the correlation of slight anatomical variations with sensations, psychological traits and dispositions, risk factors, or presymptomatic stages of disease. However, there are no standards in place as to what constitutes the requisite specificity or sensitivity for this type of testing before it is made available clinically. Nor are there agreed-upon standards about who should perform testing or what type of counseling for patients should accompany it.

The lack of standards is a major ethical challenge facing neurology and neuroscience. Professionally determined standards should govern how diagnostic technologies are used, what training is required to use them, and what counseling should accompany the disclosure of findings and results. Before the technology is applied to patients or in patient care, it is morally required that agreement exist concerning the nature of patient consent to testing, storing, and accessing findings, images, and data and concerning what type of permission is required to allow third parties access to large sets of stored information or to patient records.[4]

In general, in western societies, a person's right to control information about himself or herself dominates all other normative considerations with respect to testing. While considerations of public health or even national security might overcome this presumption, it is still the basic moral presumption that sets the framework for all testing.[4] Without standards, the possibility for abuse of diagnostic technology by third parties or of misunderstanding on the part of the general public about the confidentiality of identifiable information is enormous.

Not all patients will want to have information collected and kept. This is especially true if there are no effective treatments that reduce risk or the onset of disease or if the results of such tests can be used by third parties to restrict access to insurance, employment, or educational opportunities.[4-6] This has proven to be a major obstacle for those who may avail themselves of genetic testing for incurable neurologic disorders.[4-7] Those in neurology and the neurosciences must advocate for public policies that reduce the risks of persons being discriminated against or harmed by the intentional and inadvertent disclosure of sensitive information. The ability to diagnose the brain or nervous system without being able to treat it makes it morally incumbent on practitioners to conscientiously seek to do no harm to those in their care, including social and psychological harm.[6-9]

In some cases, diagnostic information can be acquired without a person's knowledge, cooperation, or consent. Testing done for one purpose might be used to acquire information for other purposes. In some situations, a person may consent to neurologic testing for personal health reasons but not realize that this information could be used by third parties in ways that could adversely affect employment, insurance, immigration rights, or even criminal liability. In other cases, employers may ask that various tests be done without making it clear to subjects that the information is only for the benefit of the company, organization, or payer.[8-12] Persons or their surrogates must always be fully informed about all risks and benefits associated with diagnostic testing, including social, psychological, and economic harms.[8,11] No testing should be undertaken without the express consent of the person being tested or a reasonable surrogate.[2,3]

IMAGING MENTAL TRAITS AND CHARACTERISTICS

A number of personal traits have neural correlates detectable with PET or magnetic resonance imaging (MRI).[1,13] For most traits, the sensitivity of these techniques is sufficient to distinguish small groups of individuals on the basis of the trait, but a single individual's mental state cannot yet be reliably described. However, the discriminating power of single-subject scans has steadily increased due to technical advances in scanning. Also, new knowledge of the brain areas and behavioral tasks most likely to reveal diagnostic information are being identified. There is no reason to expect this progress to stop short of the accurate description of individuals.

A history of severe depression, even when successfully treated and in remission, leaves a mark on the brain that may be detectable in a resting PET scan. Even structural scans may discriminate previously severely depressed from never-depressed subjects. A phobic who stoically suppresses any behavioral response will nevertheless activate specific anxiety-related brain circuits, even when unaware of the presence of a fear-inducing object. It has been shown that those who have or have had severe addictions to drugs have manifested a pattern of brain activation indicative of craving when confronted with photos of drugs and drug paraphernalia.[13] Imaging research on these and other psychiatric disorders will make mental health status increasingly transparent to anyone with the right instruments.[14]

These abilities raise profound ethical questions. Mental illness carries enormous stigma in modern society. Moreover, mental abilities and competency are crucial in determining a person's right to act as an autonomous agent. The temptation to intervene prophylactically with children or even in utero will be enormous even if the information available is only probabilistic. Current social policy presumes the existence of disease as relevant in making decisions about employment or insurability. There is no consensus on how to handle probabilistic information of the sort that genetic testing now provides and neurologic testing soon will provide.

Even normal personality traits, such as conscientiousness, curiosity, and empathy are in principle correlated with characteristic patterns of brain activity. Early research in this area shows that at least some such differences are reflected in functional brain scans.[15] Studies of the brain also reveal associations and correlations between individual differences in normal psychological traits and the size of specific anatomical structures.[14]

Neuroimaging is capable of revealing more transient mental state information as well as information about specific traits. Research on the neural correlates of mood in normal subjects shows certain reliable PET correlates of sadness, happiness, and anxiety.[16] It is even possible to detect activity in these circuits when evoked by subliminal cues. This creates a situation in which a third party observer may believe he or she knows more about a person's true state of mind then the person actually knows or remembers.[17,18]

The ability to analyze information that may or may not be present in a person's brain has obvious implications for the legal system. The ability to ascertain reliable memories from false memories, even if only done with a high degree of probability, would have immediate impact in determinations of guilt, punishment, and parole.[19]

The main problems posed by these developments are loss of privacy and loss of a sense of personal autonomy. Techniques that can assess the state of a person's mind or offer probabilistic interpretations of that state of mind greatly threaten the individual's right to control what is known about his or her emotional, cognitive, and motivational states as well as the independence necessary to act as a free agent. Employers, juries, military officials, and various government agencies will certainly want access to this sort of information. It is unclear that current protections of confidentiality and privacy adequately protect individual human rights to keep such information private. It is also unclear how constitutional safeguards against self-incrimination will be applied to this emerging area of clinical neurology.

ETHICS AND THERAPY

In the 1990s, much has been learned about the neural systems that control anger and depression. Impulsive violence has been linked to abnormalities in serotonergic systems spanning orbital prefrontal cortex and the amygdala, on the basis of studies in psychiatric patients and prison inmates.[19] Accordingly, selective serotonin reuptake inhibitors (SSRIs) have been found to be helpful in many cases. Sex drive can be regulated hormonally as well as by using SSRIs. It is likely that new generations of drugs will prove effective in helping to control other mental states and behavior. Moreover, it is also likely that in the future psychosurgery, implants, or various forms of virtual reality equipment may prove effective in treating and rehabilitating criminals or in preventing crime in at-risk populations of adults or children.[2]

Unfortunately, the track record of medicine in utilizing various interventions to control unwanted behavior is far from stellar. The history of psychiatry and early neurology is replete with examples such as clitorectomies, castration, or lobotomies where interventions were used without consent, or upon children or incompetent adults.[20] There are also numerous examples in which governments have used "mind control" and behavior modification to modify or punish unpopular or seditious behavior such as in the former Soviet Union's policy of detention for political dissidents using a diagnosis of sluggish schizophrenia or during the Cambodian genocide with its torture-laden reprogramming camps.

The line between beneficial therapy and forced compliance is a very fine one. Since no competent person is under any obligation to be a patient, the imposition of a treatment or therapy in the name of their best interests must always be viewed with caution and skepticism. Because efforts to use drugs or other technologies to modify behavior in children may involve permanent and irreversible change in developing human beings or a loss of autonomy in adults,[21] there is again an ethical duty to always seek the least invasive intervention in trying to forestall unwanted behavior to redirect dangerous or violent behavior.

Insisting on the informed consent of every patient before the provision of therapy is the best ethical shield against abuse—well-meaning or otherwise. One may defend the use of highly invasive or risky therapies on prisoners, especially if those convicted of crime are given a choice between therapy and incarceration. However, for most people such a choice amounts to no choice since the alternative is simply unacceptable. A choice cannot be a choice if it is the result of coercion. By offering an option that is completely unacceptable to any reasonable person, it is still possible to create a coercive environment while providing a choice. So, in most cases, prisoners fall into the category of those who cannot give consent and for whom special provisions such as the appointment of guardians or surrogates must be undertaken before the use of any therapy.

THE ETHICS OF ENHANCEMENT

Thanks to the molecular revolution in neurochemistry, it is certain that new and more powerful types of antidepressants and anxiolytics with fewer side effects will emerge. Functions as varied as sleep, sex, fear, aggression, and empathy may yield to pharmacologic interventions. As concerns about side effects and safety drop away, the question of whether healthy people should take these or other drugs to enhance their quality of life will become the subject of much discussion within clinical medicine and among policy makers.

The treatment of sexual dysfunction is illustrative. The drug Viagra was introduced as an effective treatment for impotency. But as its safety became evident and as dosage rates were established for efficacy, the manufacturers of the drug and consumers began to press to make the drug available to those not suffering from chronic impotency. Although the early drug advertising campaign for Viagra used a respected retired politician, marketing campaigns for the drug quickly evolved into using baseball players and race car drivers to attract customer interest. What began as a treatment for a physiologic disorder evolved into something that individuals could use to prevent or ensure against an unexpected failure or even to try to enhance their sexual performance.

Numerous arguments have been advanced against the ethical acceptability of using technology to enhance or increase brain function or capacity.[2] While many of these seem plausible on further inspection, the moral case against enhancement as a legitimate aspect of neuroscience and clinical neurologic intervention may not be so clear.

Many people hold the belief that one cannot experience the beauty and joy of life unless one is also acquainted with life's pain. One fear of pharmacologic or technological enhancement of our behavior, moods, or cognitive capabilities is that we would not have to suffer in order to achieve them or that we would not appreciate them as much without being exposed to the experience of pain and suffering historically requisite to attain them.

But the view that there is "no gain without pain" may not be true. It may be possible to use technology to gain as when we substitute electronic calculators for memorizing multiplication tables or have computers figure out the correct change in daily business transactions rather than trying to do the computations. It is not clear that enhancing the brain will remove all aspects of pain or suffering from an individual's life, so that the ability to see the difference between pleasure and pain or to profit from hard work and the struggle to succeed is not incompatible with using drugs or implants to enhance brain capacities or behavioral traits.

Another social problem with at least some forms of enhancement is that widespread enhancement will raise our standards of normalcy. This, in turn, can put individuals who choose not to enhance at a disadvantage, and amount to indirect coercion. Some parents have already felt this coercion when their nonmedicated child attends school where a majority of children take Ritalin. Something similar to this seems to have happened in

organized sports at the professional and advanced amateur levels. Many athletes involved in cycling, baseball, football, weightlifting, and long-distance running think that in order to remain competitive they must utilize drugs or technologies such as blood doping even if they would rather not do so.

The desire to gain an edge can create situations in which all must try to enhance themselves to secure a reasonable chance of success. However, this situation is not as ethically troubling if it affects only behavior where people are free to choose whether to compete. There may be real ethical issues raised by the prospect of enhancement if enhancement became a prerequisite for obtaining a job, securing necessary resources for daily life, or access to valued social goods and services.

Many people believe that enhancement or improvement would simply be unfair. Some people would get an improved brain and some people would not.[22]

It is certainly possible—in fact, likely—that if nothing is done to ensure fair access, then inequities will exist with respect to the ability to use technology to improve the brain. Stanley Kaplan courses, music camps, and fancy private high schools remind us that there is already unfair access to things that are known to advantage the brain. It does not make inequity right, but the solution to the problem is to provide fair access to drugs or technologies that can enhance our minds—whether they are teachers or implantable chips.

Ensuring equal access to the rich and the poor is a huge problem that has never been solved in the health care systems in America and many other nations. But inequity is not an argument that shows that improvement in itself is wrong. Nor is the reality of unequal access an argument against improvement; it is an argument against inequity.

Another objection to trying to improve or enhance the brain is that the equality of human beings may be threatened if some people become advantaged. However, the equality of human beings does not presuppose biologic equality. It is instead a claim about moral worth that goes beyond particular attributes, properties, and behaviors. It is a normative stance about how every human being should be treated. It is simply fallacious to argue that our notion of human equality depends on biologic equality. The United Nations Convention on Human Rights and the constitutions of the United States, France, and other nations do not ground the notion of human equality in any particular view of human capability. Some maintain that it is wrong to improve our minds because it would further disadvantage those who are the least well off. People with mental retardation or mental illness do not fare well today in most societies, and opening bigger gaps between them and the rest of the population may lead to even more problems.

There is always a risk of discrimination and stigma with respect to mental illness and mental differences. However, disability and difference confront us now, and there is no reason people who are different should be foreclosed from using interventions to improve or enhance brain function. It is arguable that disadvantaged people should have first claim on enhancement resources. They would still retain the right, central to the provision of therapy, to choose or not to choose to utilize drugs or technology that could ameliorate or enhance their abilities. Whether people choose to try and improve their functional or affective abilities should not be a reason to think that trying to have a better memory, for example, is going to make others feel less tolerant of people with Alzheimer's disease. We can do what is wrong in dealing with people with Alzheimer's disease, but it is not an argument against allowing someone to seek to improve their memory by drugs or devices.

A last objection is that brain engineering is unnatural. If we change or engineer ourselves to modify our brains for any purpose other than therapy, then we risk becoming inhuman.[2]

The main flaw with this argument is that it is made by people who wear eyeglasses; use insulin; have artificial hips or heart valves; benefit from cell, tissue, or organ transplants; ride on airplanes; dye their hair; talk on phones; sit under electric lights; and take vitamins. In other words, we have already taken steps to reengineer ourselves in ways that our distant ancestors would find frightening and perhaps even unnatural. But is there any reason to think that the use of laser surgery to improve one's vision beyond normalcy somehow makes us less than human? Are we less than human if we ride but do not walk? We may be less healthy, but does reliance on technology to get around cast doubt on our humanity? Is there an argument for a natural boundary or limit, beyond which our nature is defiled by technology? If there is, it is unclear exactly where to draw it in the long history of our attempts to improve and enhance our environment and our bodies.

CONCLUSION

Neurology and neuroscience are on the cusp of a revolution at least as dramatic as that sweeping through genetics as a result of advances in genomics. In the short run, the major ethical challenges will turn on how well increases in diagnosis of mental traits and characteristics are managed. Privacy is the overarching value that must be protected in order to use diagnostic technology responsibly. Sooner or later, therapies will follow in the wake of diagnostic advances. There will be tremendous pressure from the marketplace and from social institutions to utilize these therapies. The core value in protecting individual dignity when new and powerful therapies emerge is informed choice on the part of the patient. As these therapies emerge, it is likely that an enormous controversy will follow about the ethical legitimacy of using technologies that alter or modify the brain for the purposes of enhancement or improvement. Those who propose limits on such use must present convincing arguments as to why the benefits carry either too great a risk to justify the benefit or create too negative an impact upon others.

REFERENCES

1. Bernat JL: Ethical Issues in Neurology, 2nd ed. Boston, Butterworth, 2002.

2. Caplan AL: Genetics and the human genome: Implications for access to tests and therapy. In Evans CH, Osterweis M (eds): Insurance and Beyond. Washington, AHC, 2001, pp 81–92.

3. Fukuyama F: Our Posthuman Future. New York, Farrar, Strauss & Giroux, 2002.

4. Bartels D, LeRoy B, Caplan AL (eds): Prescribing Our Future: Ethical Challenges in Genetic Counseling. New York, Aldine, 1993.

5. Post SG, Whitehouse PJ, Binstock RH, et al: The clinical introduction of genetic testing for Alzheimer disease: An ethical perspective. JAMA 1997;277:832–836.

6. Rothenberg KH, Terry SF: Before it's too late: Addressing fear of genetic information. Science 2002;297:196–197.

7. Smith RA: Effects of the early diagnosis of amyotrophic lateral sclerosis on the patient: Disadvantages. Amyotrophic Lateral Sclerosis Other Motor Neuron Disorders 2000;1(suppl 1):75–77.

8. Hedera P: Ethical principles and pitfalls of genetic testing for dementia. J Geriatr Psychiatry Neurol 2001;14:213–221.

9. Grodin MA, Laurie GT: Susceptibility genes and neurological disorders: Learning the right lessons from the human genome project. Arch Neurol 2000;57:1569–1574.

10. Burgess MM, d'Agincourt-Canning L: Genetic testing for hereditary disease: Attending to relational responsibility. J Clin Ethics 2001;12:361–372.

11. Kapp MB: Physicians' legal duties regarding the use of genetic tests to predict and diagnose Alzheimer disease. J Leg Med 2000;21:445–475.

12. Nowlan W: A rational view of insurance and genetic discrimination. Science 2002;297:195–196.

13. Gazzaniga MS, Ivry RB, Mangun GR: Cognitive Neuroscience. New York, WW Norton, 1999.

14. Castellanos FX, Lee PP, Sharp W, et al: Developmental trajectories of brain volume abnormalities in children and adolescents with attention-deficit/hyperactivity disorder. JAMA 2002;288:1740–1748.

15. Malhi GS, Valenzuela M, Wen W, Sachdev P: Magnetic resonance spectroscopy and its applications in psychiatry Aust N Z J Psychiatry 2002;36.31–43.

16. Grady CL, Keightley ML: Studies of altered social cognition in neuropsychiatric disorders using functional neuroimaging. Can J Psychiatry 2002;48:327–336.

17. Allen JJB: The role of psychophysiology in clinical assessment: ERPs in the evaluation of memory. Psychophysiology 2002;39:261–280.

18. Langleben DD, Schroeder L, Maldjian JA: Brain activity during simulated deception: An event-related functional magnetic resonance study. Neuroimage 2002;15:727–732.

19. Winslade WJ: Confronting Traumatic Brain Injury. New Haven, Yale University Press, 1998.

20. Gaylin WM, Meisner JS, Neville RC (eds): Operating on the Mind: The Psychosurgery Conflict. New York, Basic Books, 1975.

21. Wolpaw JR, Birbaumer N, McFarland DJ, et al: Brain-computer interfaces for communication and control. Clin Neurophysiol 2002;113:767–791.

22. Rose S: The future of the brain. Biologist 2000;47:96–99.

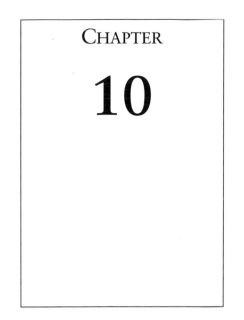

CHAPTER

10

Genotype-Phenotype Correlations

Thomas D. Bird

Gerard Schellenberg

In neurogenetics, the present era is experiencing a fascinating interplay between the fields of molecular biology and clinical neurology. The clinical description of diseases leads to the discovery of underlying genes which, in turn, leads to a more accurate classification of the diseases, which then allows the discovery of additional genes. This circle of understanding has really just begun and will continue for many years. This also has led to a tremendous effort to tease out the mechanisms at the biochemical and physiologic levels connecting gene mutations to disease manifestation. This field of genotype-phenotype correlations, although only in its infancy, is already an area of widespread investigation that cannot possibly be fully documented here. Instead, our aim is to highlight a few models that are likely to generate new knowledge in the near future and will serve as a common ground for communication and collaboration between bench and clinical scientists.

SINGLE PHENOTYPE: MULTIPLE GENES

Many relatively common neurological phenotypes have proved to have multiple genetic etiologies. This is the phenomenon of nonallelic genetic heterogeneity. Figure 10–1 indicates six neurogenetic phenotypes and the diverse array of genes thus far discovered to underlie them.

The most impressive examples of this phenomenon are the autosomal dominant spinocerebellar ataxias (SCAs).[1] The common characteristics of this syndrome are progressive cerebellar atrophy associated with unsteady gait and poor coordination. Mutations in no less than 16 different genes have been associated with this general phenotype. The genes discovered to date probably represent about 70% of the affected families.[2] Thus, there are additional genes that remain to be discovered.

This situation reflects the complexity of cerebellar circuits involving several different types of neurons and their connections. The number of proteins that must be involved in these neuronal circuits should suggest the large number of genes that could potentially produce this phenotype. It is of interest that many of the known mutations producing cerebellar ataxia are trinucleotide repeat expansions. The association of this particular type of mutation with diseases of the nervous system represents a fruitful field for further investigation. In general, the ataxia phenotype does not predict the genotype. A careful examination of the ataxia phenotype, however, leads to some consistent clinical differences among these diseases, such as the association of retinopathy with SCA 7, peripheral neuropathy with SCA 4, and dementia or mental retardation with several of the others.[3]

A similar story occurs with the various genetic forms of epilepsy.[4] The common phenotype is recurrent seizures associated with abnormalities in the electroencephalogram (EEG). The phenotypes sometimes can be subdivided on the bases of age of onset (infantile vs. childhood), location of seizure focus (frontal, temporal, or occipital lobes) or other features (nocturnal or febrile). Several of the identified genes encode ion channel proteins. Many genes remain to be discovered and are indicated only by regional chromosomal location.

Alzheimer disease (AD) is of special interest because there is both a pathologic and clinical phenotype. The clinical disease is progressive dementia and the neuropathologic characteristics are diffuse cerebral cortical atrophy with neuronal loss, neuritic amyloid plaques, amyloid angiopathy, and neuronal neurofibrillary tangles. Mutations in three distinct genes (amyloid precursor protein [APP], presenilin 1 [PS1], presenilin 2 [PS2]) all produce essentially an identical clinical and pathologic

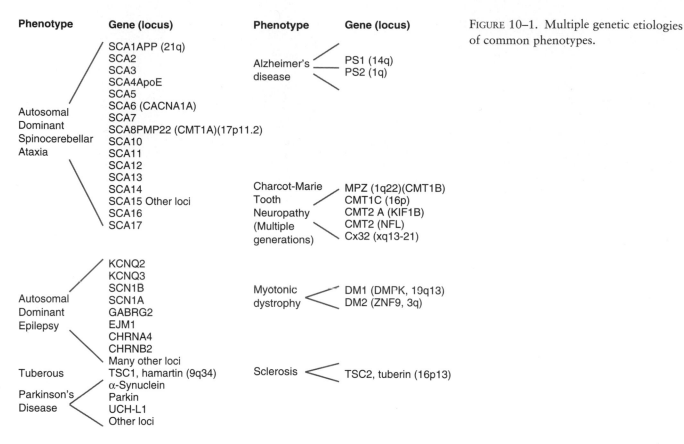

Figure 10–1. Multiple genetic etiologies of common phenotypes.

SINGLE GENE: MULTIPLE PHENOTYPES

phenotype.[5] The phenotypes are so similar that neither an astute clinician nor an experienced neuropathologist can accurately predict the underlying genotype in any single case. The three genes all influence the same biochemical pathway: the production of Aβ amyloid. Apolipoprotein E also seems to influence this amyloid system. This knowledge has led to an intense investigation of how this accumulation results in the disease phenotype and how the presenilin proteins may be involved in amyloid metabolism.

The phenotype of Parkinson disease is caused by mutations in three identified genes (α-synuclein, parkin, and UCH-L1) and unknown genes at several other loci.[6] The three known genes are all involved with the ubiquitin-proteosome complex. Persons with parkin mutations are characterized by earlier age of onset and lack of Lewy body pathology.

The multigenerational Charcot-Marie-Tooth (CMT) hereditary neuropathy syndrome can be caused by mutations in at least five different genes.[7,8] Myotonic muscular dystrophy (DM) and tuberous sclerosis (TS) have each been associated with mutations in two separate genes.[9,10] The phenotypes within each of these three categories are so similar and overlapping that the genotype cannot be predicted consistently from the individual clinical presentation. Just as in the cerebellar ataxias and the epilepsies, this indicates multiple mechanisms affecting a final common pathway such as peripheral nerve function in CMT and loss of tumor suppression in TS.

Conversely, there are many examples of mutations in a single gene producing different and sometimes quite distinct phenotypes (Fig. 10–2). A voltage-dependent calcium channel gene (CACNA1A) on chromosome 19p13 is associated with three different phenotypes.[11,12] A small CAG trinucleotide repeat expansion in the coding region of this gene produces an autosomal dominant, slowly progressive, late-onset cerebellar ataxia (SCA 6). Point mutations resulting in protein truncation produce an episodic ataxia (EA 2) in which individuals are clinically normal between episodes. Missense mutations are associated with familial hemiplegic migraine (FHM). Some persons with FHM eventually develop cerebellar atrophy and ataxia. Although different, each of these three phenotypes involves a cerebellar theme. This genotype-phenotype association has stimulated investigations into the involvement of ion channels in more common forms of migraine and cerebellar physiology.

Mutations in the peripheral myelin protein 22 gene (PMP22) can produce three different forms of familial neuropathy.[7,8,13] Duplication of this gene causes autosomal dominant CMT with slow nerve conductions (CMT1A), whereas deletion of PMP22 results in hereditary neuropathy with liability to pressure palsy (HNPP). Thus, there is a dosage effect in which too much or too little of the protein produces peripheral nerve dysfunction. Also, missense point mutations in this gene have been

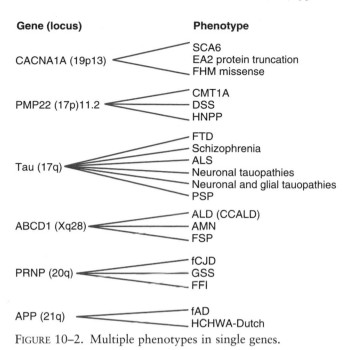

Gene (locus)	Phenotype
CACNA1A (19p13)	SCA6 EA2 protein truncation FHM missense
PMP22 (17p)11.2	CMT1A DSS HNPP
Tau (17q)	FTD Schizophrenia ALS Neuronal tauopathies Neuronal and glial tauopathies PSP
ABCD1 (Xq28)	ALD (CCALD) AMN FSP
PRNP (20q)	fCJD GSS FFI
APP (21q)	fAD HCHWA-Dutch

FIGURE 10–2. Multiple phenotypes in single genes.

associated with severe, early onset neuropathy of infancy or childhood called the Dejerine-Sottas syndrome (DSS).

Mutations in the microtubule-associated protein tau can produce a variety of phenotypes including frontotemporal dementia (FTD), atypical schizophrenia, and motor neuron disease.[14] At the neuropathologic level, mutations in exon 10 of tau are associated with an accumulation of tau proteins in neurons and glial cells, whereas mutations in exons 12 and 13 produce tau accumulation only in neurons. Some mutations in this gene cause tau to abnormally interact with microtubules, whereas others cause a change in the proportions of two tau isoforms (three-repeat and four-repeat tau). A specific haplotype of tau is also a risk factor for progressive supranuclear palsy (PSP), another degenerative neurological phenotype with abnormal neuronal tau inclusions.

Mutations in the *ABCD1* gene on the X chromosome affect a peroxisomal ABC half transporter involved in the import of very long chain fatty acids.[15,16] For reasons that remain obscure, different mutations in this gene can result in severe, early onset adrenoleukodystrophy or milder, later onset adrenomyeloneuropathy, or a relatively uncomplicated spastic paraplegia.

Mutations in the prion protein gene (*PRNP*) on chromosome 20 produce the severe, rapidly progressive, dementing syndrome of familial Creutzfeldt-Jakob disease (fCJD).[17] Some mutations in the same gene produce a somewhat less rapidly progressive disorder often associated with ataxia and cerebral cortical prion-containing plaques known as Gerstmann-Sträussler-Scheinker (GSS) disease. A missense mutation at codon 178 may produce the unusual phenotype of familial fatal insomnia (FFI). Whether the mutation at codon 178 results in CJD or FFI depends on the presence or absence of methionine at codon 129. Thus the interaction between a mutation and

a normal polymorphism in the same gene can alter the resulting phenotype through mechanisms that are not understood.

Missense mutations in the *APP* gene usually result in familial, early onset Alzheimer disease. However, a specific mutation at codon 693 occurring in a large Dutch family produces primarily an amyloid angiopathy associated with severe hemorrhagic stroke (HCHWA-D).[18] Both phenotypes have the common phenomenon of amyloid accumulation, but it is unclear why the Dutch mutation primarily directs the accumulation to cerebral blood vessels.

NEURONAL/CELLULAR SELECTIVE VULNERABILITY

An important issue in moving from genotype to phenotype is why only certain cell types become dysfunctional, degenerate, and die, while thousands of others remain healthy. The vulnerable cell type will obviously direct the clinical phenotype. Factors determining cellular vulnerability must vary from disease to disease and are not well understood for many disorders. A few are obvious and fairly straightforward. For example, PMP22 and MPZ are proteins associated with myelin in the peripheral nervous system. Mutations disrupting these proteins result in abnormal myelin function, peripheral nerve disease, and the syndrome of hereditary neuropathy (CMT).

Examples of several other neurogenetic diseases and their relatively specific cell type targets are listed in Figure 10–3. For each disease, there are ongoing investigations attempting to determine precisely how each mutation is directed to disrupt function in only selected neurons. For example, normal ataxin 7, the protein relevant to SCA 7, has been found to be widely expressed in brain, retina, and other peripheral tissues and even in the central nervous system (CNS), it is not limited to areas in which neurons degenerate.[19,20] In general, differential cellular expression of genes rarely seems to explain the selective phenotypic effects on specific cell populations. Ataxin 7 has been shown to have a functional nuclear localization signal at codons 378 to 393 and localizes preferentially to the nuclear compartment of cells in the cerebellum, pons, inferior olive, and retinal photoreceptor cells.[21] LaSpada and coworkers have further demonstrated in transgenic mice that polyglutamine-expanded ataxin 7 can suppress the transactivation of CRX, a cone-rod homeobox protein.[22] This interference seems to account for the retinal degeneration observed in the phenotype in SCA 7 and provides an explanation for how cell type specificity is achieved in this polyglutamine-repeat disease. Similar approaches are being taken for the other diseases. For example, it needs to be explained why the mutation in chorea acanthocytosis is limited to certain neurons as well as red blood cell membranes.[23,24] These two very different cell types must have a common protein that makes them both vulnerable to mutations in this

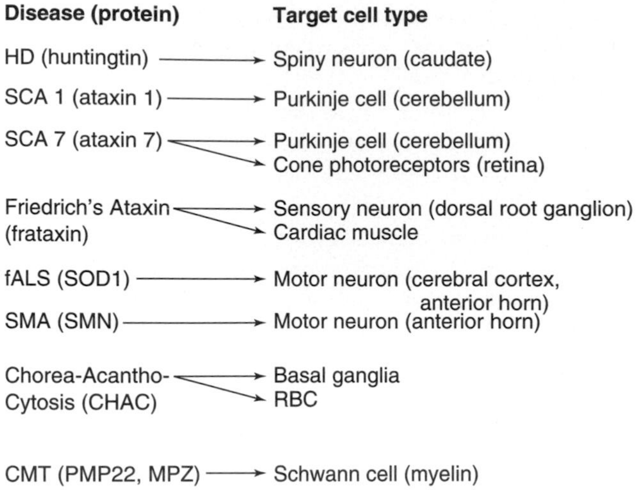

Disease (protein)   **Target cell type**

HD (huntingtin) ⟶ Spiny neuron (caudate)

SCA 1 (ataxin 1) ⟶ Purkinje cell (cerebellum)

SCA 7 (ataxin 7) ⟶ Purkinje cell (cerebellum)
⟶ Cone photoreceptors (retina)

Friedrich's Ataxin ⟶ Sensory neuron (dorsal root ganglion)
(frataxin) ⟶ Cardiac muscle

fALS (SOD1) ⟶ Motor neuron (cerebral cortex, anterior horn)
SMA (SMN) ⟶ Motor neuron (anterior horn)

Chorea-Acantho- ⟶ Basal ganglia
Cytosis (CHAC) ⟶ RBC

CMT (PMP22, MPZ) ⟶ Schwann cell (myelin)

FIGURE 10–3. Neurogenetic diseases and their specific cell type targets.

gene. Likewise, the special vulnerability of dorsal root ganglia sensory neurons and cardiac muscle in Friedreich ataxia must be related to the involvement of iron transport in mitochondria in this disease.[25]

HIGHLY VARIABLE SYSTEMIC PHENOTYPES

Although mutations in some genes result in abnormal function in only single or a limited number of cell types, mutations in other genes produce a remarkable variety of abnormalities in many different organs and cell types. Three examples are shown in Table 10–1, namely myotonic muscular dystrophy (DM1), tuberous sclerosis (TS), and neurofibromatosis type 1 (NF1). DM1 is associated with a CTG repeat expansion in the 3′ untranslated region (UTR) of the *DMPK* gene on chromosome 19q. The disease affects skeletal, smooth and cardiac muscle, skin, ocular lens, endocrine glands, skull, and brain. The molecular mechanism appears to include expanded CUG repeats in RNA having a toxic gain of function effect on cell metabolism in a variety of organs.[26–28]

The two types of TS and NF1 have many phenotypic characteristics in common. Both are neurocutaneous syndromes affecting the nervous system and skin. They are associated with a wide variety of tumors and cancers.[29,30] They also have genetic molecular similarities in that they are caused by mutations in various documented or presumed tumor suppressor genes.[31] The highly variable expression fits the Knudson two hit hypothesis.[32] Affected persons are heterozygotes who have inherited a single tumor suppressor gene mutation from one parent. Over a lifetime, random environmentally acquired mutations in the homologous gene on the other chromosome (the second hit) produce a loss of heterozygosity, loss of tumor suppression, and unregulated cell growth. Furthermore, early somatic mutations in these genes may produce individuals who are mosaics

TABLE 10–1. Single Genes with Wide Ranging Systemic Phenotypes

Myotonic Muscular Dystrophy (DM1)

Muscle weakness

Myotonia

Cataract

Cardiac arrhythmia

Diabetes

Intestinal dysmotility

Baldness

Gall bladder disease

Thick skull/large sinuses

Cognitive deficits

Cerebral white matter changes

Sleep apnea

Testicular atrophy

Pilomatrixomas

Tuberous Sclerosis (TSC1/TSC2)

Mental retardation

Epilepsy

Cutaneous changes (angiofibroma, hypomelanotic macules, shagreen patches, ungual fibroma)

Brain tumors/nodules

Kidney tumors

Cardiac rhabdomyomas

Pulmonary lymphangiomyomatosis

Retinal nodules

Neurofibromatosis (NF1)

Neurofibromas

Café au lait spots

Lisch nodules (iris)

Skeletal anomalies

Brain gliomas

Mental retardation/learning disabilities

Seizures

Vascular dysplasia

Malignant tumors

Axillary freckling

Optic glioma

Hypertension

Leukemia

and have only partial or anatomically restricted phenotypes.[33,34] The two different TS genes (hamartin and tuberin) affect the same molecular pathway through direct interaction with each other.[35]

PENETRANCE AND AGE OF ONSET

Penetrance refers to the proportion of gene mutation carriers who express any aspect of the phenotype. Penetrance is age- and test-dependent. That is, at a young age, only a small proportion of mutation carriers may manifest the phenotype, whereas at a later age, a much larger proportion will do so. An example of test dependence would be a person carrying an epilepsy gene mutation who may never have a clinical seizure but may have an abnormal EEG with electrical seizure discharges. The penetrance is only revealed by the more sensitive test. Likewise, some persons with the DM1 mutation may have only subclinical cataract on slit lamp examination or persons with a TS mutation may have no symptoms or signs other than intracranial calcification on imaging studies. The genetic factors influencing age of onset and incomplete penetrance are poorly understood. Several possible mechanisms are presented in Tables 10–2 and 10–3.

The rate at which a cell or organ accumulates a toxic substance certainly correlates with the age at onset of symptoms. The best examples are the genetic lipid storage diseases. Mutations result in defective enzymatic metabolism of a substance that is toxic to the cell, such as the toxic accumulation of sulfatide in metachromatic leukodystrophy, glucocerebroside in Krabbe leukodystrophy and nonesterified cholesterol in Niemann-Pick type C disease. Some mutations result in a complete absence of enzyme activity, relatively rapid toxin accumulation, and early onset. Other mutations allow partial, very low enzyme activity, slower toxin accumulation, and later onset. Some storage disorders such as Niemann-Pick type C have a wide range in age of onset without a clear-

TABLE 10–2. Examples of Factors Affecting Penetrance and Age of Onset

Accumulation of a toxin or protein

Lipid storage diseases

polyglutamine disorders

Alzheimer disease

Partial v. complete absence of a protein/enzyme

Duchenne muscular dystrophy vs. Becker's muscular dystrophy

Infantile vs. juvenile metachromatic leukodystrophy

Infantile vs. adult Tay-Sachs disease

Gene/environment interactions

Acute intermittent porphyria

Knudson two hit phenomenon/tumor suppression

Unknown mechanisms

Alzheimer disease/apolipoprotein E

Torsion dystonia (DYT1)

Adrenoleukodystrophy (ALD)

TABLE 10–3. Correlation of Trinucleotide Repeat Expansion Size with Disease Penetrance and Severity in Huntington's Disease and Myotonic Dystrophy

	HD (CAG)	DM1 (CTG)
Normal	2–27	5–37
Premutation	28–35	38–49
Decreased penetrance	36–39	50–100
Full penetrance	40+	100+
Severe early onset	70+	1000+

cut genotype-phenotype correlation.[36] Slow accumulation of a toxic protein may play a role in many other neurodegenerative diseases such as AD (Aß amyloid), FTD (tau), Huntington disease (HD), and other CAG repeat (polyglutamine) expansion disorders.

Duchenne and Becker muscular dystrophies are overlapping clinical syndromes caused by a variety of mutations in the same dystrophin gene.[37] The earlier onset Duchenne muscular dystrophy (DMD) phenotype is associated with mutations that result in the absence of the dystrophin protein. In the Becker syndrome, the less severe phenotype, other mutations allow a small amount of protein to be produced, enable partial functional integrity of dystrophin, and result in a later onset.

Alzheimer disease has a very wide range in age of onset. Many of the early-onset familial types are caused by single gene mutation in *APP*, *PS1*, and *PS2*. Nevertheless, the sporadic, late-onset variety of AD has an at least 40-year range of onset (60 to 100 years). Apolipoprotein E (ApoE) influences this age of onset variability.[38,39] Through unclear mechanisms, the ApoE 4 allele is a risk factor for AD that lowers the average age of onset in a dose-dependent manner for persons carrying one or two copies of the E4 allele. The E2 allele may have a protective influence and delay the age of onset. Other unidentified genetic factors must also play a role in AD. For example, in the Volga German fAD kindreds carrying the same *PS2* mutation, there is a 35-year difference in the age of onset (40 to 75 years). Therefore, the ApoE genotype is responsible for only a fraction of this difference.

The trinucleotide-repeat expansion disorders have provided additional insights into the phenomena of age of onset and penetrance.[40] Both onset age and severity of disease correlate with the size of the repeat expansion. This is especially well illustrated with the CAG repeat in HD and the CTG repeat in DM1 (see Table 10–3). The CAG expansion in HD has a normal size seen in the general population that is not associated with disease, a premutation range that is also never associated with clinical disease but may expand to a larger size in the next generation, a decreased penetrance range in which persons may or may not show clinical signs during a normal life span, and a full penetrance range in which persons always develop clinical signs during a normal life span.[41] The expansion size is also correlated with age of onset. HD individuals with 70 or greater CAG expansions often have both early onset and severe, more rapidly progressive disease.

A similar phenomenon occurs in DM1. Small CTG expansions may fall into a clearly abnormal range, but be associated with minimal clinical expression (only cataracts), whereas expansions of 1000 or greater may be associated with severe, infantile onset (congenital myotonic dystrophy).[42]

Type 1 torsion dystonia (DYT1) is associated with a GAG deletion in codon 302 of the torsin A gene.[43] For unknown reasons, only 30% to 40% of mutation carriers ever manifest symptoms (30% to 40% penetrance). Other genetic or environmental factors, or both, must play a role.

We have seen an unpublished family with a mutation in the TSC1 (hamartin) gene. Two persons in this family have had severe classic signs of tuberous sclerosis. However, another person in the family carrying the identical mutation displays no symptoms, signs, or manifestations of the phenotype on extensive imaging studies. Perhaps this family represents the wide range in random occurrence of second mutation hits in the relevant tumor suppressor gene.

There has been an interesting report of monozygotic twins carrying the same mutation for X-linked ALD,[44] with a surprising and dramatic difference in disease severity between the two twins.

Certainly some of the differences in penetrance, age of onset, and expression of neurogenetic disease must be related to an extensive variety of environmental influences. It is easy to speculate on the nature of these environmental factors (smoking, alcohol, bacteria, viruses, chemicals, and so on), but it is much more difficult to document and establish their impact. Clearly, various drugs and medications may unmask the phenotype in a previously unrecognized gene mutation carrier. A well known example is acute intermittent porphyria (AIP) in which the medical use of barbiturates or sulfa drugs may result in serious neurological symptoms in otherwise asymptomatic carriers of mutations in the gene encoding hydroxymethylbilane (HMB) synthase.[45] These drugs inhibit activity in the porphyrin-heme pathway that is already compromised by reduced activity of the HMB synthase. Genetic and environmental interactions such as these represent yet another area for extensive investigation into the mechanisms of genotype-phenotype correlations.

CONCLUSION AND FUTURE DIRECTIONS

The relationships between mutations in genes (genotype) and the associated clinical characteristics (phenotype) represent a fascinating, complicated, and developing area of investigation. In this chapter, we have given a brief overview of several aspects of this area, including: (1) single phenotypes caused by multiple genes; (2) single genes associated with multiple phenotypes; (3) neuronal and cellular selective vulnerability; (4) genes related to highly variable systemic phenotypes; and (5) issues concerning penetrance and age of onset. The next decade will experience an increased understanding of these phenomena and how our genetic constitution initiates and modifies both common and rare diseases of the nervous system.

REFERENCES

1. Subramony SH, Filla A: Autosomal dominant spinocerebellar ataxias ad infinitum? Neurology 2001;56:287–289.

2. Moseley ML, Benzow KA, Schut LJ, et al: Incidence of dominant spinocerebellar and Friedreich triplet repeats among 361 ataxia families. Neurology 1998;51:1666–1671.

3. Schols L, Amoiridis G, Buttner T, et al: Autosomal dominant cerebellar ataxia: Phenotype differences in genetically defined subtypes? Ann Neurol 1997;42:924–932.

4. Prasad AN, Prasad C, Stafstrom CE: Recent advances in the genetics of epilepsy: Insights from human and animal studies. Epilepsia 1999;40:1329–1352.

5. Levy-Lahad E, Tsuang D, Bird TD: Recent advances in the genetics of Alzheimer's disease. J Geriatr Psychiatry Neurol 1998;11:42–54.

6. Mouradian M: Recent advances in the genetics and pathogenesis of Parkinson disease. Neurology 2002;58:179–185.

7. Nelis E, Timmerman V, De Jonghe P, et al: Molecular genetics and biology of inherited peripheral neuropathies: A fast-moving field. Neurogenetics 1999;2;137–148.

8. Kamholz J, Menichella D, Jani A, et al: Charcot-Marie-Tooth disease type 1 molecular pathogenesis to gene therapy. Brain 2000;123:222–233.

9. Liquori CL, Ricker K, Moseley M, et al: Myotonic dystrophy type 2 caused by a CCTG expansion in intron 1 of ZNF9. Science 2001;293:864–867.

10. Jones AC, Shyamsundar MM, Thomas MW, et al: Comprehensive mutation analysis of TSC1 and TSC2 and phenotypic correlations in 150 families with tuberous sclerosis. Am J Hum Genet 1999;64:1305–1315.

11. Sinke RJ, Ippel EF, Diepstraten CM, et al: Clinical and molecular correlations in spinocerebellar ataxia type 6. Arch Neurol 2001;58:1839–1844.

12. Toru S, Murakoshi T, Ishikawa K, et al: Spinocerebellar ataxia type 6 mutation alters P-type calcium channel function. J Biol Chem 2000;275:10893–10898.

13. Schenone A, Mancardi GL: Molecular basis of inherited neuropathies. Curr Opin Neurol 1999;12:603–616.

14. Reed LA, Wszolek ZK, Hutton M: Phenotypic correlations in FTDP-17. Neurobiol Aging 2001;22:89–107.

15. Kemp S, Pujol A, Waterham HR, et al: ABCD1 mutations and the X-linked adrenoleukodystrophy mutation database: Role in diagnosis and clinical correlations. Hum Mutat 2001;18:499–515.

16. Wichers M, Kohler W, Brennemann W, et al: X-linked adrenomyeloneuropathy associated with 14 novel ALD-gene mutations: No correlation between type of mutation and age of onset. Hum Genet 1999;105: 116–119.

17. Mastrianni JA: The prion diseases: Creutzfeldt-Jakob, Gerstmann-Straussler-Scheinker, and related disorders. J Geriatr Psychiatry Neurol 1998;11:78–97.

18. Natte R, Maat-Schieman MLC, Haan J, et al: Dementia in hereditary cerebral hemorrhage with amyloidosis-Dutch type is associated with cerebral amyloid angiopathy but is independent of plaques and neurofibrillary tangles. Ann Neurol 2001;50:765–771.

19. Cancel G, Duyckaerts C, Holmberg M, et al: Distribution of ataxin-7 in normal human brain and retina. Brain 2000;123:2519–2530.

20. Lindenberg KS, Yvert G, Muller K, Landwehrmeyer GB: Expression analysis of ataxin-7 mRNA and protein in human brain: Evidence for a widespread distribution and focal protein accumulation. Brain Pathol 2000;10:385–394.

21. Kaytor MD, Duvick LA, Skinner PJ, et al: Nuclear localization of the spinocerebellar ataxia type 7 protein, ataxina-7. Hum Mol Genet 1999;8:1657–1664.

22. LaSpada AR, Fu Y-H, Sopher BL, et al: Polyglutamine-expanded ataxin-7 antagonizes CRX function and induces cone-rod dystrophy in a mouse model of SCA7. Neuron 2001;31:1–15.

23. Ueno S, Maruki Y, Nakamura M, et al: The gene encoding a newly discovered protein, chorein, is mutated in chorea-acanthocytosis. Nat Genet 2001;28:121–122.

24. Rampoldi L, Dobson-Stone C, Rubio JP, et al: A conserved sorting-associated protein is mutant in chorea-acanthocytosis. Nat Genet 2001;28:119–120.

25. Patel PI, Isaya G: Friedreich ataxia: From GAA triplet-repeat expansion to Frataxin deficiency. Am J Hum Genet 2001;69:15–24.

26. Savkur RS, Philips AV, Cooper TA: Aberrant regulation of insulin receptor alternative splicing is associated with insulin resistance in myotonic dystrophy. Nat Genet 2001;29:40–47.

27. Mankodi A, Logigian E, Callahan L, et al: Myotonic dystrophy in transgenic mice expressing an expanded CUG repeat. Science 2000;289:1769–1772.

28. Tapscott SJ: Deconstructing myotonic dystrophy. Science 2000;289:1701–1702.

29. Dabora SL, Jozwiak S, Franz DN, et al: Mutational analysis in a cohort of 224 tuberous sclerosis patients indicates increased severity of TSC2, compared with TSC1, disease in multiple organs. Am J Hum Genet 2001;68:64–80.

30. Creange A, Zellar J, Rostaing-Rigattieri S, et al: Neurological complications of neurofibromatosis type 1 in adulthood. Brain 1999;122:473–481.

31. Miloloza A, Rosner M, Nellist M, et al: The TSC1 gene product, hamartin, negatively regulates cell proliferation. Hum Molec Genet 2000;9:1721–1727.

32. Serra E, Puig S, Otero D, et al: Confirmation of a double-hit model for the NF1 gene in benign neurofibromas. Am J Hum Genet 1997;61:512–519.

33. Niida Y, Stemmer-Rachamimov AO, Logrip M, et al: Survey of somatic mutations in tuberous sclerosis complex (TSC) hamartomas suggests different genetic mechanisms for pathogenesis of TSC lesions. Am J Hum Genet 2001;69:493–503.

34. Ruggieri M, Huson SM: The clinical and diagnostic implications of mosaicism in the neurofibromatoses. Neurology 2001;56:1433–1443.

35. Hodges AK, Li S, Maynard J, et al: Pathological mutations in TSC1 and TSC2 disrupt the interaction between hamartin and tuberin. Hum Molec Genet 2001;25:2899–2905.

36. Lossos A, Schlesinger I, Okon E, et al: Adult-onset Niemann-Pick type C disease. Arch Neurol 1997; 54:1536–1541.

37. Beggs AH, Hoffman EP, Snyder JR, et al: Exploring the molecular basis for variability among patients with Becker muscular dystrophy: Dystrophin gene and protein studies. Am J Hum Genet 1991; 49:54–67.

38. Corder EH, Saunders AM, Strittmatter WJ, et al: Gene dose of apolipoprotein E type 4 allele and the risk of Alzheimer's disease in late onset families. Science 1993;261:921–923.

39. Breitner JCS, Wysc BW, Anthony JC, et al: APOE-epsilon4 count predicts age when prevalence of AD increases, then declines. Neurology 1999,53: 321–331.

40. Lindblad K, Schalling M: Expanded repeat sequences and disease. Semin Neurol 1999;19:289–299.

41. Brinkman RR, Mezei MM, Theilmann J, et al: The likelihood of being affected with Huntington disease by a particular age, for a specific CAG size. Am J Hum Genet 1997;60:1202–1210.

42. Harley HG, Rundle SA, MacMillan JC, et al: Size of the unstable CTG repeat sequence in relation to phenotype and parental transmission in myotonic dystrophy. Am J Hum Genet 1993;52:1164–1174.

43. Klein C, Breakefield XO, Ozelius LJ: Genetics of primary dystonia. Semin Neurol 1999;19:271–280.

44. Sobue G, Ueno-Natsukari I, Okamoto H, et al: Phenotypic heterogeneity of an adult form of adrenoleukodystrophy in monozygotic twins. Ann Neurol 1994;36:912–915.

45. Suarez JI, Cohen ML, Larkin J, et al: Acute intermittent porphyria: Clinicopathologic correlation. Neurology 1997;48:1678–1683.

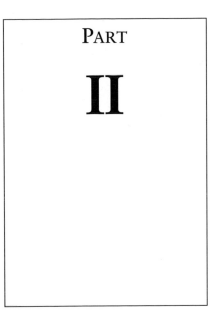

PART

II

NEUROLOGIC DISEASES

CHAPTER 11

Down Syndrome

Charles J. Epstein

Down syndrome (DS) is the prototype of all chromosome abnormality syndromes. It is the phenotypic manifestation of trisomy 21 and occurs when an extra copy of chromosome 21 is present in the genome. In contrast to monogenic disorders, which result from the effects of mutant genes, chromosomal disorders are the result of abnormalities in the numbers of otherwise normal genes. In the case of the autosomal trisomies, such as trisomy 21, there are three rather than two copies of each gene carried by the unbalanced chromosome. Therefore, DS can be considered a condition that results from the combined effects of an increase in number of many or all of the genes present on the chromosome. However, despite the fact that a large number of genes may be involved in the causation of DS, the overall pattern of abnormalities that results is quite specific and easily recognized. This chapter is principally concerned with the genetic and neurologic aspects of DS. A comprehensive review of all aspects of DS is provided in reference 1, and a recent review of the neurologic and neuroscience aspects is provided in reference 2. Bibliographic citations for many of the statements in this chapter may be found in references 1 and 3.

CLINICAL FEATURES AND DIAGNOSTIC EVALUATION

The most immediately apparent, if not the most serious, manifestations of DS are the minor dysmorphic features that collectively constitute its distinctive physical phenotype. These include brachycephaly, oblique (up-slanting) palpebral fissures, Brushfield spots, epicanthic folds, flat nasal bridge, folded or dysplastic ears, open mouth, narrow palate, protruding and furrowed tongue, abnormal teeth, short neck with loose skin on nape, short and broad hands, short and incurved fifth finger (clinodactyly), transverse palmar crease, gap between first and second toes, and hyperflexibility. Although any person with DS will have many of the characteristic features and be easily recognized as having the syndrome, it would be very rare for any person with DS to have all of these features. None of the features in the list is unique either to DS or to chromosome abnormalities in general, and the presence of one or a few minor dysmorphic features in an otherwise normal person does not in itself signify the existence of a chromosomal abnormality. Major malformations are few in DS, with the exception of congenital heart disease, most typically an atrioventricular canal or related anomaly in about 40%, and duodenal atresia or stenosis in about 2.5% to 5% of cases.

Early Development

The most characteristic feature of DS in newborns and infants is hypotonia, often profound. It persists, although somewhat less markedly, throughout childhood and adolescence and is accompanied by a decrease in strength. The basis for the decreased muscle tone is unknown, but it is assumed to be central in origin. With the exception of the hypotonia, the behavior of infants with DS is generally normal at birth. However, developmental retardation usually becomes obvious during the first several months of life, and the mean age at which developmental landmarks are attained becomes increasingly more delayed. Although the average delay may be 2 months for very early landmarks (e.g., rolling over, transferring objects, reaching), it gradually lengthens and may reach 1 to 2 years for functions such as imitative drawing and using three-word sentences that ordinarily appear at about age 2 years. However, because of the great variability in attainment of landmarks in both normal infants and infants with DS, this delay may or may not be obvious for any single child with DS.

In addition to hypotonia, there is a delayed dissolution of early reflexes and automatisms such as grasp reflexes, the Moro response, and automatic stepping. Abnormal or deficient responses have included the traction response, position in ventral suspension, and the patellar jerk. In later years, atlantoaxial/atlanto-occipital instability may be present in about 15% to 20% of children with DS, but symptomatic manifestations appear to be rare. A decreased visual acuity unrelated to ocular disorders or refractive errors and believed to be neurologic in origin has also been observed in infants and children with DS. When exposed to a cold stimulus, there is an increased time before pain is reported and a reduced ability to localize the site of the pain precisely.

Cognitive Function

Many studies of development during the first decade of life have suggested that there is a progressive decline in the mean developmental quotient (DQ) or IQ and the social quotient (SQ), but this may not always be true. Furthermore, environmental factors such as poor or inadequate motivation, rather than biologic factors, may play a role.[4] Nevertheless, even in a stimulating environment, once a child with DS reaches school age, the cognitive delays lead to serious learning problems that require major attention. Relative to other mentally retarded individuals, persons with DS have selective deficits in rule based systems such as number and grammar, specific deficits in linguistic structure such as syntax and phonology, greater difficulty in recalling sequences of verbal information presented auditorially, and a slower rate of vocabulary acquisition.[5] Personality stereotypes attributed to persons with DS have also been seriously questioned and probably have little validity.

Although DS is usually associated with moderate mental retardation, there are rare instances in which persons with DS without known mosaicism have attained IQs above 80 and have performed in the low-average range. Such cases illustrate the variability of the syndrome and raise the question of what factors influence mental development. One possible factor is the intrinsic genetic differences among individuals. Examination of the relationship between parental education levels or IQs and the IQs of their children with DS has produced evidence both for and against the existence of correlations that would suggest a genetic component. The social and intellectual environment in which the person with DS is raised is another factor, although parental IQ and education may influence environment. Evidence for the potential impact of environmental factors on intellectual development stems from the outcomes of both early intervention programs and studies of home-reared versus

institutionalized persons with DS that have shown a positive benefit by as much as 20 IQ points. (See later section on therapy.)

Neurologic Problems in Adult Life

Although a variety of nonspecific abnormalities may be noted, there are relatively few neurologic abnormalities specifically associated with DS in adults. Seizures of various types, which can begin either in infancy or as late as the third decade, have been reported. The prevalence of seizures increases with age, reaching close to 50% in persons older than 50 years. Seizures beginning after age 35 years are considered indicative of the development of dementia.

The brains of older persons with DS exhibit a pathology characteristic of Alzheimer's disease (AD). However, a significant proportion of adults with DS does not appear to have dementia by any criterion. Furthermore, some persons with DS who are thought to be demented are, in fact, suffering from major depression. Estimates of the frequency of dementia in DS range from 25% to 75%, depending on age. In one study, 84% of demented persons had seizures, 20% had Parkinsonian features, and all showed loss of brain tissue by computed tomography, especially in the temporal lobes.[6] In institutionalized populations, the mean age of onset of dementia was between 51 and 54 years, and the mean duration of dementia in patients who died was about 5 years.[6] However, regardless of whether frank dementia occurs, there appears to be a progressive loss of a variety of intellectual functions, such as the formation of long-term memories and visuospatial construction. There also appears to be a progressive loss of receptive language not attributable simply to mental retardation in many older persons with DS.

The ability to identify odors is impaired in persons with DS in comparison to age- and IQ-matched mentally retarded persons and to normal controls. The deficit is greater in older persons with DS, and it has been suggested that this increasing impairment with age could represent a manifestation of developing AD.

Electrophysiology

There are no specific electroencephalographic (EEG) patterns associated with DS, and the abnormalities that have been observed are not well correlated with specific behavioral or neurologic signs and symptoms. It has been suggested, however, that there is an incomplete postnatal development of neuronal interconnections or an immaturity of cerebral development, and the development of EEG coherence is abnormal. Somewhat closer to the issue of neuronal function in DS are the studies of visual, olfactory, and auditory evoked potentials. Significant differences in patterns are found between DS and other retarded and nonretarded subjects. These differences have been interpreted as indicative of abnormal neural activity in numerous neural systems. These neural systems range from sensory to cognitive in DS, with reduced inhibitory control, reduced selectivity and specificity of responsiveness, increased neural responsiveness, abnormalities in the timing of neural responses, and abnormal mechanisms involved in temporal integration and information storage.

In addition to in vivo studies of neuronal function, functional studies have found several physiologic parameters of cultured fetal trisomy 21 dorsal root ganglion neurons to be altered.[7] In the presence of nerve growth factor (NGF), these neurons display a shortened action potential with accelerated rates of depolarization and repolarization resulting from shorter time constants for the fast tetrodotoxin-sensitive inward Na current and two outward K currents. Removal of NGF lengthens the action potential, but the difference from normal still persists. It has been speculated that these abnormal neuronal electrical properties could lead to abnormal development of synapses and neural networks and thereby contribute to the development of mental retardation.[7]

Imaging of the Brain

Magnetic resonance imaging (MRI) has been used to evaluate the brains of living persons with DS. After adjustment for differences in body size, the brains of healthy adults with DS ranging in age from 22 to 50 years displayed smaller than normal cerebral and cerebellar hemispheres, ventral pons, mammillary bodies, and hippocampal formations, and larger than normal parahippocampal gyri. General intelligence and mastery of linguistic concepts appear to have a negative correlation with the size of the parahippocampal gyrus. In children and young adults, the mean brain volume is also smaller, and the cerebellar and hippocampal volumes were disproportionately even smaller (33% and 30%, respectively).[8] By contrast, the temporal and parietal lobes are relatively less reduced in volume, and there is preservation of subcortical structures.

Computed tomography has shown increased cerebrospinal fluid volume and accelerated rates of lateral ventricle and suprasellar cistern dilatation in demented adults with DS. Likewise, positron emission tomography has shown reductions of glucose metabolic rates in the parietal and temporal motor areas in demented adults with DS. These rate reductions are not seen in nondemented adults with DS.

PATHOLOGY

Development of the Brain

There has been considerable disagreement about the frequency and nature of anatomic abnormalities of the brain in DS. Although the histologic findings have been inconsistent, brain weight is in the low-normal range, and the size of the cerebellum and brainstem may be reduced to an even greater extent. There is foreshortening of the fronto-occipital diameter of the forebrain and narrowing of the superior temporal gyrus. Among the semispecific findings in DS are nerve cell heterotopias in the white layers of the cerebellum and vermis, which are found in 16% of infantile and fetal DS brains. These heterotopias are attributed to a disturbance or retardation of embryonic cell migration. A delay in myelination has been noted in about one fourth of DS brains. The anterior commissure in adults with DS is reduced in the cross-sectional area.

Detailed neuronal architecture, studied with Golgi-type preparations, has been analyzed in a handful of cases. Because of the limitations in numbers, all reports must be viewed with caution. Nevertheless, there appear to be abnormalities in the numbers and morphology of dendritic spines in infants and children with DS,[9] with atrophy of the dendritic tree. Other evidence for defects in brain histogenesis has also been reported. Quantitative studies of neuron migration to the superior temporal neocortex during fetal development have demonstrated a delay and disorganization of maturation and lamination along with a normal or increased density of neurons.[10] This aberrant pattern of cortical maturation is believed to reflect abnormal axonal and dendritic arborization that can lead to disrupted organization of local circuits and neural system connections. A poverty of granule cells, possibly the aspinous stellate cells, throughout the cortex has also been described, as have decreased neuronal densities in layer II and IV of the occipital cortex (area 17). Synaptic density in the neocortex has been reported as normal, although presynaptic and postsynaptic width and length may be reduced. Similarly, the surface area of synaptic contact may be lower than normal in the occipital cortex.

From this discussion, it is obvious that a clear picture of the state of the *wiring* of the brain in DS does not emerge. Although there is accumulating evidence for abnormalities of neuronal differentiation and migration in fetal and infant brains, it is not certain how many changes are permanent or functionally significant if the developmental plasticity of the young brain is taken into account.

Alzheimer's Disease

The possibility of a relationship between DS and dementia has been recognized for more than 100 years and between DS and AD (as defined pathologically) for more than 50 years. This relationship is now well established, and the consensus of a large number of reports is that the brains of adults with DS possess all of the pathologic and neurochemical hallmarks of AD. However, detailed analyses suggest that the pathologic changes found in adult DS brains may differ quantitatively in some areas from those found in AD and that the density of amyloid deposition is greater and the distribution more wide-spread in DS. However, the relationship between numbers of tangles and plaques and the degree of dementia in DS is not known.

The time of appearance and the frequency of the lesions characteristic of AD in DS have been of particular concern. Interest in the relationship between the two conditions has been as much a function of the early and generalized appearance of the lesions as of the nature of the lesions themselves. It is generally believed that the neuropathologic changes of AD are almost universal in persons with DS older than 35 years. The earliest pathologic change indicative of developing AD appears to be an enlargement of early endosomes within pyramidal neurons, even during fetal life.[11] Another early manifestation is the preplaque, a diffuse deposition of amyloid (β/A4) protein adjacent to the cell bodies of morphologically normal neurons. It has been proposed, therefore, that amyloid progressively accumulates around the cell body until the enclosed neuron degenerates, with the appearance of neurofibrillary tangles, and the typical senile plaque develops. Based on immunocytochemical analyses, it is claimed that the deposition of the β/A4 amyloid protein in the brains of persons with DS begins 50 years earlier than it does in normal brains, possibly as the result of overexpression of the amyloid precursor protein (APP) gene.[12]

BIOCHEMICAL AND ENZYMATIC FINDINGS

In older persons with DS, there is a 20% reduction in total phospholipids in the frontal cortex and cerebellum and an even greater reduction in phosphatidylinositol and ethanolamine plasmalogen. These reductions have been attributed to a loss of dendrites and dendritic spines or to a generalized alteration of phospholipid metabolism. Changes in the proportions of monounsaturated and polyunsaturated fatty acids in myelin have also been described, but it is not clear whether they result in or are from other developmental and functional abnormalities of the nervous system.

Considerable interest has focused on peripheral neurotransmitter function in DS. Hypersensitivity to the mydriatic effect of atropine and tropicamide has been repeatedly confirmed, but there is still debate about its cardioacceleratory effects. The activity of the enzyme, dopamine-ß hydroxylase, which converts dopamine to norepinephrine, is significantly decreased in the plasma of persons with DS, but plasma concentrations of both epinephrine and norepinephrine were normal. Studies of cerebrospinal fluid monoamine metabolism in young adults with DS showing increased concentrations of cerebrospinal fluid 5-hydroxyindoleacetic acid (5-HIAA) and norepinephrine were interpreted as indicating an increased turnover of monoamines. It was believed, however, that this alteration was not related to a cognitive decline with age.

Abnormalities of platelet serotonin (5-hydroxytryptamine) in DS have been of interest because of their possible relevance to central nervous system (CNS) neurotransmitter function. The principal observation has been that the concentration of serotonin is decreased in whole blood to about 65% of normal. Studies of serotonin uptake by platelets have demonstrated a reduced rate of influx, which has been attributed to a reduction in Na^+, K^+-ATPase activity, with concomitant abnormalities of sodium, potassium, or calcium fluxes. Although it has been suggested that the platelet, with its uptake and storage of amines, can serve as a model for synaptosomes in the CNS, this remains to be shown. A trial with 5-hydroxytryptamine had no beneficial effect on the development of intelligence.

A vast number of studies have been carried out to search for biochemical abnormalities in the brains of fetuses and persons with DS. In more recent years, newer analytical techniques such as subtractive hybridization, differential display, and two dimensional gel electrophoresis coupled with mass spectrometry have been employed to look at changes in gene expression. Changes, both increases and decreases, have been observed for a variety of genes that are not on chromosome 21, but their significance remains to be determined.

MOLECULAR AND GENETIC DATA

Cytogenetics

The extra chromosome 21 that causes DS can be present in the genome either as a free whole chromosome (93% to 96% of the time), as part of a Robertsonian fusion chromosome carrying the long arm of chromosome 21 in combination with the long arm of another acrocentric chromosome (2% to 5%), or in rare instances as part of a reciprocal translocation (<1%). Of the cases associated with Robertsonian fusions between chromosome 21 and one of chromosomes 13, 14, or 15, approximately 40% to 45% are familial in that they are inherited from a cytogenetically balanced parent; for fusions between chromosome 21 and either chromosome 21 or 22, only about 4% are familial.

In 2% to 4% of cases of DS, there is mosaicism with two populations of cells, one diploid and one trisomic, being present. Trisomy 21 mosaicism is generally recognized in one of three ways: during cytogenetic investigation of typical cases of DS, during evaluation of mild or possible cases of DS or of mildly retarded or dysmorphic children without obvious diagnosis, and during studies of parents who have had more than one child with trisomy 21. It has been estimated that parental mosaicism is present in 3% to 4% of families.

There does not appear to be any correlation between mental development and the proportion of trisomic cells present in either peripheral blood lymphocytes or fibroblasts in mosaic cases ascertained because of presumed or suspected DS or because of mental retardation, although such a correlation had been claimed for fibroblasts. No data are available that would permit an assessment of the degree of mosaicism in other tissues of the body, particularly the brain. Nevertheless, when considered as a group, the mean IQs and DQs for mosaic cases do appear to be somewhat higher, perhaps 10 to 20 points, than for matched individuals with nonmosaic trisomy 21. Because of the wide variability, the existence of mosaicism per se is not of great prognostic value. The physical phenotype can be quite variable, ranging from typical DS to only mental retardation and subtle dysmorphic features. Congenital heart disease appears to occur infrequently, if at all.

It has long been recognized that the risk of having a child with DS increases with maternal age and that the distribution of maternal age in the population of women having children is the primary determinant of the overall incidence of DS. A variety of estimates of the incidence of DS in the newborn population have been made, and most recent figures are in the vicinity of 1 per 1000. The figures can be broken down to provide maternal age specific rates per thousand live births: 0.6 at 20 years, 1.0 at 30 years, 2.6 at 35 years, 9.1 at 40 years, 24.9 at 44 years, 41.2 at 46 years. A population-based analysis using DNA markers has shown that maternal nondisjunction accounts for 86% of all cases of trisomy 21, with 75% of cases occurring at meiosis I (MI) and 25% at meiosis II (MII). The maternal age effect is greater for MII than MI errors. Nine percent of cases are paternally derived (50% MI, 50% MII), and 5% are somatic in origin.

Genomics

Chromosome 21 is the smallest of the human autosomes, constituting approximately 1% to 1.5% of the length of the haploid genome. The long arm of the chromosome is estimated to contain about 33.65 Mb of DNA[13] and has a characteristic banding pattern consisting of 3 or 4 bands at low resolution and as many as 11 dark and light bands resolvable by prometaphase banding. All genes of known function (other than for ribosomal RNA) are located on this arm of chromosome 21, and only this arm is essential for normal development and function. The presence of a Robertsonian fusion chromosome in which the short arms of two acrocentric chromosomes (sometimes both chromosomes 21) are deleted does not cause detectable abnormalities if the genome is otherwise balanced.

The virtually complete DNA sequence of chromosome 21 was reported in 2000.[13] A total of 225 genes were identified, 127 of which were known and 95 predicted. Although these numbers are continually changing as annotation of the genome proceeds, the total is still considerably lower than had been expected. The centromere-proximal half of 21q, with half of the DNA, contains only 25% of the mapped genes, and the overall gene density of the chromosome appears to be relatively low.

This may account for the ability of humans with trisomy 21 to survive while those with trisomy 22, which involves twice as many genes, do not.

Phenotypic Mapping

Cases in which only part of chromosome 21 is triplicated have been intensively studied to arrive at a phenotypic map that will permit a correlation of particular phenotypic features of DS with specific regions or loci on the chromosome. The consensus of studies carried out before molecular markers became available is that the full DS phenotype (as manifested by mental retardation, congenital heart disease, characteristic facial appearance, hand anomalies, and dermatoglyphic changes) appears when band 21q22 is duplicated, and of this, subbands 21q22.1 and probably 21q22.2 are required. Molecular analysis has been used to define the extent of triplication in the regions of chromosome 21, and the results have been used to generate phenotypic maps.[14] Although interpretations vary, it seems clear that many of the phenotypic features appear to be associated with imbalance in the region surrounding and distal to *D21S55*. However, there is also evidence for contributions of genes outside the *D21S55* region, especially in the proximal part of 21q, although the region responsible for congenital heart disease seems to be confined to the distal part of 21q. The genes that, when present in extra copies, contribute to impaired cognition appear to be located in several regions of the chromosome.

Pathogenesis of the Down Syndrome Phenotype

The immediate consequence of an aneuploid state is a gene dosage effect for each of the loci present on the unbalanced chromosome or chromosome segment. Such gene dosage effects have been reported for several chromosome 21 loci. With the exception of APP in the brains of fetuses with DS, the measured increases in activities or concentrations in trisomic cells are close to the theoretically expected value of 1.5. Taken in the aggregate, these results confirm the existence of precise dosage effects in cells that are aneuploid for chromosome 21.

Much attention has been devoted to the pathogenesis of the cognitive deficits and AD in DS. The effects of increased expression of several loci on chromosome 21 have been considered, and it is possible to construct plausible explanations for how overexpression of each locus can affect the development, function, and integrity of the CNS.[2,15] A recent case in point is the gene for cystathionine synthase, the overexpression of which in DS results in depressed levels of plasma homocysteine. It has been suggested that altered homocysteine metabolism could compromise the folate-dependent resynthesis of methionine and create a functional folate deficiency, with numerous consequences on CNS function. In considering such possibilities, it is important to keep in mind that whereas imbalance of an individual locus could have significant effects on the CNS, it is unlikely that it will provide a unitary explanation for the entire range of deficits found in DS.

Numerous proposals have been put forward to explain the development of AD in adults with DS,[15] and they can be summarized by two hypotheses. The first hypothesis is that genetic imbalance present in trisomy 21 indirectly causes AD by (1) causing the nervous system to be intrinsically defective from early in life and thereby enhancing susceptibility of the brain to exogenous agents that cause AD or (2) causing premature aging. With regard to these two possibilities, there is no hard evidence that premature aging is a consequence of trisomy 21[15]; in fact, the major point in favor of such an assumption is the existence of AD itself. The nervous system, as has already been described, is abnormal from early in life. It is not obvious, however, how the observed deficiencies and defects would predispose to degenerative changes later in life, particularly since no exogenous agents have yet been shown to cause AD.

The second hypothesis is that genetic imbalance in trisomy 21 directly causes AD because the increased dosage of one or more chromosome 21 loci results in increased activities or concentrations of one or more gene products that, in turn, produce injury to the brain. Thus, even though the phenotypic mapping results presented earlier indicate that the visible phenotype of DS along with mental retardation can occur in the absence of triplication of *SOD1*, the locus for the enzyme CuZn-superoxide dismutase (CuZnSOD), virtually all persons with DS have an extra copy of this locus. Because the H_2O_2 generated as a result of CuZnSOD action is toxic and may, in combination with O_2^-, give rise to the even more dangerous hydroxyl radical (OH·), it has been argued that increased CuZnSOD activity may under certain circumstances have a deleterious effect, particularly in the brain. Increases in 8-hydroxyguanine/8-hydroxydeoxyguanine and nitrotyrosine, markers of oxidative stress, have been detected in the brains of persons with DS prior to the accumulation of β-amyloid. The cortex of the fetal brain has also been reported to show evidence of increased lipid peroxidation and of protein oxidation (carbonyls and glycated products).

Of greater potential importance, insofar as the development of AD in persons with DS is concerned, is the evidence for a significant overproduction of APP mRNA in the brains of fetuses with DS and mouse fetuses (discussed later) with trisomy 16. It may be postulated that such overproduction, if sustained, could lead to the early accumulation of APP that has been observed in the brains of young persons with DS and that this accumulation may have toxic effects on neurons that are already impaired. A relevant observation is the absence of clinical or pathologic evidence of AD in a 78-year-old woman with DS resulting from segmental trisomy 21 with only two copies of *APP*.

Because of the discovery that the presence of the apolipoprotein E allele ε4 is a risk factor for the development of both sporadic and familial AD unrelated to DS, numerous studies have been carried out to determine whether the same is true in DS. Presence of the ε4 allele has been reported to be associated with a higher frequency of clinical AD, a tendency to an earlier age of onset of dementia, poorer language ability, more rapid cognitive decline, and earlier age of death. Conversely, presence of the ε2 allele appears to decrease the risk of dementia in DS, similar to its effect in the non-DS population.

ANIMAL MODELS

The fact that many consequences of aneuploidy in humans arise during morphogenesis and affect the development and function of the CNS places special stumbling blocks in the way of their investigation. Research on events occurring during gestation, especially early gestation, is both technically impractical and, at the present time and for the foreseeable future, ethically and legally impossible. Similarly, there are severe limitations to the study of CNS function in living individuals, and experimental genetic alterations are impossible. It is for this reason that interest has turned to the development of animal models for DS.

Since ultimate concern is with humans and human disease, we require models that will duplicate the human condition in developmental and functional terms as closely as possible. No model can be exact, since no other organism duplicates the human with respect to all biologic and genetic attributes. Nevertheless, models based on mammals that share numerous biologic similarities with humans seem most appropriate. Primates with the genetic and clinical equivalent of trisomy 21 and DS have been observed, but do not offer significant advantages over humans for investigational purposes. Therefore, the mouse has been the model animal of choice for reasons including ease of manipulation and genetic control and similarities to humans in morphogenesis and probably CNS function, in neurobiologic if not psychological terms. Furthermore, despite considerable rearrangement of the mammalian genome, sizable chromosomal regions carrying many genes remain intact and structurally similar in both humans and mice.

There are still problems with models based on the mouse. It is not always easy or possible to obtain postnatally viable animals when sizable regions of the genome are unbalanced.[15] Furthermore, if it was possible, mice will never be able to duplicate higher CNS functions such as cognition, which are vulnerable to the effects of aneuploidy in humans. As difficult as it is to define mental retardation in an aneuploid human, it is even more difficult to specify the proper functional homology in an aneuploid mouse. Nevertheless, elementary forms of learning are common to all animals with an evolved nervous system, and there appears to be a conservation of relevant biochemical mechanisms.[16] Therefore, the mouse can be considered to be a legitimate model for learning and memory in humans.

Modeling of human trisomy 21 in the mouse started at two ends of the possible spectrum of such models. At one end is the trisomic mouse with an extra copy of mouse chromosome 16, which most closely resembles human chromosome 21. At the other end is the transgenic mouse with an extra copy or copies of human chromosome 21 gene. Several intermediate possibilities, with duplications of only parts of mouse chromosome 16 or the insertion of mouse or human yeast artificial chromosome (YAC) transgenes, have been developed recently. (A general review of mouse models of DS is presented in reference 17.)

Trisomy 16 Mice

With perhaps one exception, all loci in human 21q from the centromere to the *MX1* locus in the distal part of band 21q22.3 (approximately 150) map to the distal part of mouse chromosome 16 (see http://www.informatics.jax.org). The remaining 75 or so loci not on mouse chromosome 16 have been mapped to mouse chromosomes 10 and 17. These loci are outside the region shown by phenotypic mapping to be responsible for the facial features of DS. Furthermore, there are genes present on mouse chromosome 16 that map to other human chromosomes (3, 8, 16, and 22). Therefore, trisomy for all of mouse chromosome 16, while reproducing much of the genetic imbalance associated with human trisomy 21, results in an overall degree of imbalance that is more extensive than in the human trisomy and an overall phenotype that is more severe. Therefore, the results of studies with mouse trisomy 16 (Ts16) must be viewed with concern insofar as modeling DS is concerned.

Nevertheless, three findings are of particular interest: (1) There is a tissue-dependent dysregulation of APP mRNA synthesis, with a greater than 1.5-fold increase. This may be related to (a) the increased number of copies of the *App* gene, (b) a more general effect on the expression of certain genes in the trisomic cells, or (c) most likely a combination of both; (2) Fetal Ts16 basal forebrain cells transplanted into or abutting the dentate gyrus of the hippocampus of a normal host underwent a striking atrophy (by 25% in cross-sectional area) 6 months after transplant. This atrophy could be prevented by a fimbria fornix lesion, which causes the release of trophic factors such as NGF; (3) When inoculated intracerebrally with the scrapie prion, Ts16↔2n chimeras had an accelerated incubation period, a more fulminant course, and an earlier time of death than did 2n↔2n chimeric controls.

Segmentally Trisomic Mice

Because of genetic discrepancies between mouse chromosome 16 and human chromosome 21, segmentally trisomic mice (designated Ts65Dn) in which only the human chromosome 21 orthologous region is triplicated were produced.[18] In these animals, approximately 115 of 225 genes on human chromosome 21q are represented. The trisomic animals do not have the major anomalies present in Ts16. Their salient phenotypic abnormalities are confined to the craniofacial structures and the CNS, although they exhibit male sterility. As in persons with DS, there is a reduction in the size and granule cell density of the cerebellum, a reduced sensitivity to pain, elevation of brain myo-inositol, and abnormalities of dendritic spines. Although motor learning is normal, Ts65Dn mice have major deficits in learning and behavior and show abnormalities in long-term potentiation (LTP) and depression and in hippocampal (cAMP) generation. The pattern of behavioral and learning deficits suggests impairment of hippocampal spatial learning and prefrontal functions.[19] LTP and cAMP abnormalities are also indicative of hippocampal dysfunction. There is an age-dependent loss of function and atrophy of cholinergic neurons in the medial septum of the basal forebrain, which correlates with the loss of cognitive function and appears to be related to an abnormality of NGF transport. This finding is also consistent with hippocampal dysfunction.[20] It is of note, in this regard, that a reduction in TRK-A immunoreactive cholinergic neurons has been observed in the nucleus basalis of persons with DS.

A second segmentally trisomic mouse, Ts1Cje, is functionally trisomic for the region of mouse chromosome 16 distal to *Sod1*.[21] This trisomy involves approximately 87 chromosome 21-orthologous genes and still includes the region responsible for major phenotypic abnormalities in DS. Ts1Cje mice have learning deficits that are similar to but somewhat less severe than those of Ts65Dn animals. Similarly, they show a reduction in the volume of the cerebellum, but granule cell density is much less affected. However, they do not appear to exhibit degeneration of the cholinergic neurons. A third segmentally trisomic mouse, designated Ms1Ts65, represents a triplication of the region of difference between Ts65Dn and Ts1Cje and involves about 30 chromosome 21-orthologous genes.[21] These animals have only minimal learning deficits, but they are still not normal.

Taken together with the comparison of Ts65Dn and Ts1Cje, the results with Ms1Ts65 indicate that the major genes responsible for behavioral and learning abnormalities of Ts65Dn mice are located distal to *Sod1*. These studies constitute the first step in phenotypic mapping of segmental trisomy DS models by a subtractive approach in which a known phenotype (Ts65Dn) is compared with the phenotype obtained after reduction of the region of trisomy (Ts1Cje). The same approach has been used to compare alterations in craniofacial morphogenesis produced by Ts65Dn and Ts1Cje. Both trisomies demonstrate alterations in craniofacial skeletal formation that are similar to those observed in DS, with changes in Ts1Cje being largely the same as those in Ts65Dn.[22] This again demonstrates that the major genes responsible for these skeletal abnormalities in Ts65Dn mice are located distal to *Sod1*. The ability to generate these various segmental trisomies and to compare their phenotypes directly provides a precedent for the systematic creation of smaller and smaller segmental trisomies and the dissection of the trisomic phenotype.

Transgenic Mice

In contrast to the formation of trisomic animals, the construction of transgenic mice is an approach that permits analysis of the effects of an increased dosage of individual human chromosome 21 genes. Several strains of such transgenic mice carrying *SOD1*, the gene for human CuZnSOD, have been made and shown to have a 1.6- to 6-fold increase in activity of CuZnSOD in the brain and other tissues. Several effects of increased activity of CuZnSOD that resemble changes in persons with DS have been found[23]: (1) Transgenic mouse platelets have diminished levels of serotonin and decreased rates of serotonin accumulation that are attributed to a diminished pH gradient across the granule membrane. However, the content of serotonin in the striatum is normal; (2) There is a reduction in prostaglandin E_2 and prostaglandin D_2 biosynthesis in transgenic primary fetal cells and in the cerebellum and hippocampus; (3) The neuromuscular junctions of the transgenic tongue muscles are abnormal, with atrophy, degeneration, withdrawal and destruction of terminal axons, development of multiple small terminals, decreased ratio of terminal axon area to postsynaptic membrane, and hyperplastic secondary folds; (4) Transgenic mice also have anatomical abnormalities of the thymus and premature thymic involution. Impairment of LTP has also been reported.

Many of the abnormalities in transgenic tissues discussed previously are presumed to be mediated by alterations in the metabolism of oxygen-free radicals resulting from increased CuZnSOD activity (this enzyme mediating the first step in the ultimate conversion of superoxide anions to water). In these instances, the outcome was a deleterious one in that the transgenic tissues were structurally or functionally abnormal. However, there is considerable evidence that increased CuZnSOD activity can have beneficial effects under conditions of acute oxidative stress.

Limited work has been done with other types of transgenic mice carrying individual human chromosome 21 genes or their murine orthologues. Although they do not develop the full pathology of AD, mice expressing the human APP-751 isoform gene have diffuse and amorphous extracellular deposits of β-amyloid that resemble those of early AD, and they manifest deficits in spatial learning. Transgenic mice overexpressing the Ets2 transcription factor develop craniofacial and other skeletal anomalies, with brachycephaly and short necks, thought to resemble anomalies found in DS and mouse Ts16. However, similar anomalies are not found in the segmental trisomics of chromosome 16, even though *Ets2* is present in three copies. Overexpression of *HMG14* results in abnormalities of the thymus and epithelial cysts, and mice transgenic for the mouse *single-minded* gene, *mSim2*, have impaired spatial learning.

The transgenes just described all involve loci present on mouse chromosome 16 as well as human chromosome 21. Therefore, the absence of similar findings in trisomic mice involving the same regions is of concern. The following two loci, however, are represented on mouse chromosome 10, and the trisomy 16 models are therefore not relevant. Transgenic mice overexpressing the gene for the protein subunit S100β were reported to be hyperactive, to have learning impairments, and to manifest astrocytosis, axonal proliferation, and a significant loss of dendrites in the hippocampus. Mice overexpressing liver-type phosphofructokinase had elevated activity during fetal life but not during adult life.

Another approach to the generation of transgenic models for DS has been the insertion of genomic segments larger than individual genes in the form of yeast artificial chromosomes. A mouse produced in this manner had abnormalities of learning and behavior similar to but less severe than were observed with the segmental trisomies Ts1Cje and Ts65Dn. Since the major and possibly only gene in the integrated segment of human DNA was the human minibrain gene (*Dyrk*), it was suggested that imbalance of this locus is responsible for the observed abnormalities. Mice that are transgenic for the *Dyrk1A* gene support this inference. These animals display delayed neuromotor development and impairment in spatial learning with defective reference memory, which are considered indicative of hippocampal and prefrontal cortex dysfunction.[24]

THERAPY

Therapy for DS is presently symptomatic in nature and addresses treatment of the various medical and surgical conditions that may be associated with it. There is no specific form of pharmacologic or other therapy known to have reproducibly beneficial effects on neurologic and cognitive function in DS. In addition to unsuccessful trials with 5-hydroxytryptophan and vitamin B_6 used in an attempt to raise central serotonin levels, numerous other agents have been used in an attempt to improve the development of children with DS. Orthomolecular approaches based on administration of mixtures of vitamins, minerals, thyroid hormone, and other substances have been prominent among these attempts. Despite claims for remarkable successes, with IQs reported to increase between 10 and 25 points over a 4- to 8-month period, these results have not been replicated in carefully controlled trials. Another approach has been sicca cell therapy, in which lyophilized embryonic animal cells are injected at frequent intervals. Again, contrary to the claims of its proponents, this therapy has not been shown in controlled trials to have efficacy. In fact, there is considerable concern that it may be dangerous. The most recent agent to be tested, the nootropic drug piracetam, had no beneficial effect on cognition. In addition, piracetam had undesirable stimulatory effects.

Although short-term benefits have been claimed for early intervention programs, the existence of long-term effects remains to be proved. Evidence exists that early intervention can have a positive effect on early development, particularly in the domains of fine coordination, self-help skills, and DQ/IQ scores.[25] Research in this area is difficult for a variety of reasons, and definitive conclusions are difficult to obtain. A recent evaluation of 21 early intervention demonstration studies, however, indicated that IQ gains recede over time to levels of the control group or comparison database, and that although primary school performance is critically lacking in many subjects, social acceptance in school is relatively good.[25]

CONCLUSIONS AND FUTURE DIRECTIONS

The sequencing of human chromosome 21 has led new impetus to research on DS. There appears to be a far fewer number of genes present on the chromosome than had previously been thought. Even though the evaluation of the functional consequences of genetic imbalance for somewhat over 200 genes is still a formidable challenge, it is still within the realm of reality within a reasonable period of time.

Despite the many studies that have been carried out with humans with DS and with cells and tissues obtained from them, we still know relatively little about the alterations of structure and function in the brain that lead to cognitive deficits and age-dependent neuronal degeneration. Obtaining information in this domain is limited by restrictions on what types of research are ethically and practically feasible with humans. However, progress should occur as newer noninvasive methods for evaluating neuronal function in humans are developed.

Developing and manipulating segmentally trisomic mice and working out the genomic structure of mouse chromosomes provide powerful tools for investigating the developmental and functional consequences of genetic imbalance affecting individual genes and groups of genes. Identification of these consequences will, in turn, make it possible to test the potential benefits of new therapeutic modalities in correcting the alterations in neuronal function. However, as these systems are exploited, the need to correlate the abnormalities in trisomic mice with those found in persons with DS becomes more pressing. As good a model as the mouse may be, the human situation is the subject of ultimate concern.

Although I have placed emphasis on the roles of genetics and neuroscience in gaining an understanding of the mechanisms at work in DS and, thereby, formulating new therapeutic strategies, this is not meant to diminish the importance of social, educational, and medical approaches. There seems to be little question that there are positive effects from a warm and stimulating environment, well-considered educational interventions, attention to medical problems, and increasing acceptance of persons with DS into general society. Despite controversy about long-term effects of early stimulation programs and approaches targeting increased cognitive capacity, it is likely that in the absence of therapies specifically targeted to correct known functional abnormalities, they are bringing affected persons closer to the maximum level of achievement of which they are capable. In making this assertion, for which definitive proof is lacking, I hasten to point out that approaches must have a rational basis. The unfortunate fact is that many supposed therapies have been promoted with little scientific basis to support their use and no evidence, even when sought, that they have any benefit.

REFERENCES

1. Epstein CJ: Down syndrome (trisomy 21). In Scriver CR, Beaudet AL, Sly WS, Valle D (eds): The Metabolic and Molecular Bases of Inherited Disease (8th ed). New York, McGraw-Hill, 2001, pp 1223–1256.

2. Capone GT: Down syndrome: Advances in molecular biology and the neurosciences. Dev Behav Pediatr 2001;22:40–59.

3. Epstein CJ: Down syndrome. In Rosenberg RN, Prusiner SB, DiMauro J, Barchi RL (eds): The Molecular and Genetic Basis of Neurological Disease (2nd ed). Boston, Butterworth-Heinemann, 1997, pp 51–79.

4. Wishart JG: Cognitive abilities in children with Down syndrome: Developmental instability and motivational deficits. In Epstein CJ, Hassold T, Lott IT, et al (eds): Etiology and Pathogenesis of Down Syndrome. New York, Wiley-Liss, 1995, 57–91.

5. Nadel L: Down syndrome in psychobiological profile. In Nadel L (ed): The Psychobiology of Down Syndrome. Cambridge, MA, MIT Press, 1988, 369–374.

6. Lai F, Williams RS: A prospective study of Alzheimer disease in Down syndrome. Arch Neurol 1989;46:849–853.

7. Galdzicki Z, Siarey R, Pearce R, et al: On the cause of mental retardation in Down syndrome: Extrapolation from full and segmental trisomy 16 models. Brain Res Rev 2001;35:115–145.

8. Pinter JD, Eliez S, Schmitt JE, et al: Neuroanatomy of Down's syndrome: A high resolution MRI study. Am J Psychiatry 2001;158:1659–1665.

9. Takashima S, Iida K, Mito T, Arima M: Dendritic and histochemical development and ageing in patients with Down's syndrome. J Intellect Disabil Res 1994;38:265–273.

10. Golden JA, Hyman BT: Development of the superior temporal neocortex is anomalous in trisomy 21. J Neuropathol Exp Neurol 1994;53:513–520.

11. Cataldo AM, Peterhoff CM, Troncoso JC, et al: Endocytic pathway abnormalities precede amyloid β deposition in sporadic Alzheimer's disease and Down syndrome: Differential effects of APOE genotype and presenilin mutations. Am J Pathol 2000;157:277–286.

12. Rumble B, Retallack R, Hilbich C, et al: Amyloid A4 protein and its precursor in Down's syndrome and Alzheimer's disease. N Engl J Med 1989;320:1446–1452.

13. Hattori M, Fujiyama A, Taylor TD, et al: The DNA sequence of human chromosome 21. Nature 2000;405:311–319.

14. Korenberg JR, Chen XN, Schipper R, et al: Down syndrome phenotypes: The consequences of chromosome imbalance. Proc Natl Acad Sci USA 1994;91:4997–5001.

15. Epstein CJ: The Consequences of Chromosome Imbalance: Principles, Mechanisms, and Models. New York, Cambridge University Press, 1986.

16. Kandel ER: The molecular biology of memory storage: A dialogue between genes and synapses. Science 2001;294:1030–1038.

17. Dierssen M, Fillat C, Crnic L, et al: Murine models for Down syndrome. Physiol Behav 2001;73:859–871.

18. Reeves RH, Irving NG, Moran TH, et al: A mouse model for Down syndrome exhibits learning and behaviour deficits. Nat Genet 1995;11:177–184.

19. Hyde LA, Frisone DF, Crnic LS: Ts65Dn mice, a model for Down syndrome, have deficits in context discrimination learning suggesting impaired hippocampal function. Behav Brain Res 2001;118:53–60.

20. Cooper J, Salehi A, Delcroix JD, et al: Failed retrograde transport of NGF in a mouse model of Down's syndrome: Reversal of cholinergic neurodegenerative phenotypes following NGF infusion. Proc Natl Acad Sci U S A 2001;98:10439–10444.

21. Sago H, Carlson EJ, Smith DJ, et al: Genetic dissection of the region associated with behavioral abnormalities in mouse models of Down syndrome. Pediatr Res 2000;48:606–613.

22. Richtsmeier JT, Zumwalt A, Carlson EJ, et al: Craniofacial anomalies in segmentally trisomic mouse models for Down syndrome. Am J Med Genet 2002;107:317–324.

23. Groner Y: Transgenic models for chromosome 21 gene dosage effects. In Epstein CJ, Hassold T, Lott IT, et al (eds): Etiology and Pathogenesis of Down Syndrome. New York, Wiley-Liss, 1995, 193–212.

24. Altafaj X, Dierssen M, Baamonde C, et al: Neurodevelopmental delay, motor abnormalities and cognitive deficits in transgenic mice overexpressing Dyrk1A (minibrain), a murine model of Down's syndrome. Hum Mol Genet 2001;10:1915–1923.

25. Gibson D, Harris A: Aggregated early intervention effects for Down's syndrome persons: Patterning and longevity of benefits. J Ment Defic Res 1988;32:1–17.

Triplet Repeats: Genetics, Clinical Features, and Pathogenesis

Vicky L. Brandt

Huda Y. Zoghbi

Since the discovery of dynamic mutations in 1991, unstable triplet repeats have been revealed as the underlying pathogenic mechanism in 15 neurologic diseases. The importance of understanding this group of diseases, several of which are rare, stems from two facts: (1) triplet repeats will likely keep appearing as we uncover the molecular genetic basis of other neurologic diseases and (2) research on this circumscribed group of disorders has already illuminated fundamental processes involved in several major neurodegenerative diseases.

This chapter begins with the polyglutamine diseases, in which a coding CAG repeat expansion produces an expanded polyglutamine tract in the resulting protein. We will then consider two ataxias that are caused by a different mechanism—a repeat expansion in a noncoding region—since they are phenotypically very similar to the first group. We will close the chapter by discussing three multisystem disorders also caused by noncoding repeats: Friedreich's ataxia, fragile X syndrome, and fragile XE mental retardation. (Myotonic dystrophy, the other disease caused by noncoding triplets, is discussed in detail in Chapter 47.)

THE POLYGLUTAMINE DISEASES

The polyglutamine neurodegenerative diseases include spinobulbar muscular atrophy (SBMA), Huntington's disease (HD), dentatorubropallidoluysian atrophy (DRPLA), and the spinocerebellar ataxias (SCA1, 2, 3, 6, 7, and 17). These diseases result from the expansion of an unstable CAG trinucleotide repeat coding for polyglutamine tracts in the respective proteins (Table 12–1). The CAG repeat tracts are polymorphic and vary in their instability: the SCA7 repeat, for example, may expand by hundreds in one intergenerational transmission, whereas

the SCA6 CAG tract is relatively stable, with only a three-repeat difference in length between wild-type and the shortest mutant allele. But in all of these diseases, triplet repeats exceeding their normal range cause progressive neuronal dysfunction and death within 10 to 20 years after onset of symptoms, with longer repeat tracts causing earlier age of onset and more severe disease. Thus, the genetically distinguishing effect of a dynamic mutation is anticipation: intergenerational repeat instability produces a more severe form of the disease and earlier onset in affected members of each successive generation. Anticipation can be so extreme that children may die of disease complications before an affected parent is symptomatic; such an apparently negative family history is a chief cause of misdiagnosis. (We should note that the length of the CAG tract accounts for only part of the variability in age of onset; other genetic and environmental factors are also involved.)

Despite the ubiquitous expression of the disease genes, the phenotypes of all the polyglutamine disorders are neurologic; moreover, in typical adult-onset cases, only certain subsets of neurons are vulnerable to degeneration. HD primarily afflicts the striatum, for example, whereas the SCAs show a predilection for the cerebellum and a few other neuronal groups. Nonetheless, with the exception of SBMA and HD, these diseases can be terribly difficult to differentiate on the basis of clinical features alone. The small phenotypic and neuropathologic differences that exist among these disorders almost disappears when the expansions are very large and lead to severe, juvenile- or infantile-onset disease. This loss of cell specificity with large expansions is intriguing, and hints that toxicity may affect even nonneuronal cells if the expansions are large enough. Given the fact that 100 to 200 repeats is sufficient to cause infantile disease in most of

TABLE 12–1. Autosomal-Dominant Ataxias with an Identified Genetic Defect

Disease	Inheritance	Normal and Disease-Causing Repeat Lengths	Most Common Presenting Features	Principal Regions Affected
SBMA	X-linked recessive	11–33 38–66	Muscle cramps, weakness, gynecomastia	Lower motor neurons, anterior horn cells
HD	AD	6–39* 36–121	Cognitive impairment, depression, irritability, chorea	Striatum, cortex
DRPLA	AD	6–35 49–88	Dementia, ataxia, choreoathetosis	Dentate nucleus, red nucleus, globus pallidus, subthalamic nucleus, cerebellar cortex, cortex
SCA1	AD	6–44* 36–81	Hypermetric saccades, ataxia, dysarthria, ophthalmoparesis	Purkinje cells, dentate nucleus, inferior olive
SCA2	AD	14–31 35–64	Ataxia, hyporeflexia, slow saccades	Purkinje cells, granule cells, inferior olive
SCA3	AD	12–41* 40–84	Ataxia, gaze-evoked nystagmus, bulging eyes, dystonia, spasticity	Dentate nucleus, pontine neurons, substantia nigra, anterior horn cells
SCA6	AD	4–18 21–33	Ataxia, late onset (>50), sometimes sporadic	Purkinje cells, granule cells
SCA7	AD	4–35 37–306	Ataxia and/or visual loss due to retinal degeneration; hearing loss	Purkinje cells, retina (cone-rod degeneration)
SCA8	AD	15–37 80–250**	Scanning dysarthria, ataxia	Purkinje cells
SCA10	AD	10–20 500–4500	Ataxia, seizures	Purkinje cells
SCA12	AD	7–28 66–78	Early arm tremor, hyperreflexia, ataxia	Purkinje cells, cortical and cerebellar atrophy
SCA17	AD	29–42 47–63	Dysphagia, intellectual deterioration, ataxia, absence seizures	Purkinje cells, granule layer, upper motor neurons

*Alleles with 21 or more repeats are interrupted by 1–3 (CAT) units; disease alleles contain pure CAG tracts.
**Pathogenic range varies among families.

the polyglutamine diseases, however, it is likely that very large expansions, such as those seen in the coding repeat diseases, would be embryonic-lethal.

Although the disease-causing proteins share no homology aside from the polyglutamine tract, their pathogenic processes are strikingly similar. Most notably, each of the mutant polyglutamine-containing proteins accumulates in one or more components of the cell. The roles protein accumulation and nuclear localization play in disease will be discussed in greater detail after a brief presentation of the clinical features and molecular genetics of each disease.

Spinobulbar Muscular Atrophy: Kennedy Disease

Clinical Features

Spinobulbar muscular atrophy (SBMA), or Kennedy disease, is unique among the polyglutamine diseases in showing an X-linked recessive pattern of inheritance. Affected males may suffer muscle cramps for years before seeking medical attention for proximal muscle weakness in the fourth or fifth decade. Tendon reflexes are usually absent, and sensation is normal. Weakness, wasting, and fasciculations involve the face and distal musculature; gynecomastia is common, and late hypogonadism, progressive loss of libido, difficulty in maintaining an erection, and late sterility have been reported. Female carriers can display mild muscle weakness, frequent muscle cramps, slightly elevated serum creatinine kinase levels, and neurogenic changes on the electromyogram.[1] SBMA causes anterior horn cell, bulbar neuron, and dorsal root ganglion cell degeneration. EMG studies on SBMA patients indicate a neurogenic basis of atrophy with the presence of fibrillations and fasciculations. Muscle biopsies show evidence of chronic denervation, often with collateral reinnervation.

Differential Diagnosis

SBMA is most often confused with amyotrophic lateral sclerosis (ALS), although a thorough history and physical examination can usually distinguish these disorders. ALS affects a wider range of muscle groups and induces much more rapid deterioration than SBMA. Furthermore, ALS involves upper motor neurons as well as lower motor neurons, so patients will display upper motor neuron signs such as hyperreflexia and spasticity. Androgen insensitivity is a hallmark of SBMA and often causes gynecomastia. Finally, X-linked transmission has not been reported for ALS.

Molecular Genetics

The expanded polymorphic CAG repeat tract in SBMA patients lies in the coding region of the androgen receptor *(AR)* gene. Wild-type alleles of the *AR* gene have 9 to 36 CAG repeats; disease-causing alleles have 38 to 62 CAGs.

The *AR* is a member of the steroid hormone receptor family. Like other members of this protein family, it contains domains for hormone and DNA binding. Upon binding of androgen in the cytoplasm, the receptor/ligand complex is transported to the nucleus, where it activates the transcription of hormone-responsive genes. An *AR* lacking the polyglutamine tract is still able to transactivate hormone-responsive genes; expansion of the glutamine repeat has no effect on hormone binding and only slightly reduces the receptor's ability to transactivate responsive genes. The expansion may cause partial loss of receptor function that could be responsible for some signs of androgen insensitivity in affected males, but complete absence of *AR* leads to testicular feminization rather than a motor neuron disease. The predominant effect of CAG expansion is probably a toxic gain of function, as in the other polyglutamine diseases.

Nuclear inclusions (NIs) containing mutant *AR* have been reported in motor neurons within the pons, medulla, and spinal cord. Although NIs are absent in unaffected neural tissues, they are present in a select group of unaffected nonneuronal tissues (scrotal skin, dermis, kidney, and, less frequently, heart and testis).

Several attempts were made to create a transgenic mouse model of SBMA using full-length *AR* constructs with as many as 65 CAG repeats. Although expressed under promoters that produced two to five times the normal endogenous protein levels, and despite bearing a longer repeat tract than any that had been reported in humans, these constructs failed to produce a phenotype in the mice. Success was finally met when Abel and colleagues[2] generated transgenic mice using a truncated *AR* (only the 5' portion of the gene) and 112 CAGs under the same promoters as used previously. The subtle neurologic phenotype displayed by these mice at about 8 months of age worsened to spasticity and muscle weakness of the hind limbs and hips. Neuropathologic studies revealed NIs in the brain stem, cortex, and spinal cord motor neurons; these NIs were ubiquitinated and contained proteasomal components, several molecular chaperones, and the transcriptional activator CREB-binding protein. These findings suggest that the expanded *AR* is misfolded and targeted for proteasomal degradation—a model that is gaining support from many polyglutamine studies.

Therapy

No specific treatment is available for SBMA patients.

Huntington's Disease

Clinical Features

Chorea, the most well-known motor symptom in adult patients, may actually not appear until memory deficits, affective disturbance, and changes in personality have made themselves manifest. Parkinsonism, dystonia, and involuntary motor impairments develop over time, as do oculomotor disturbances. All patients suffer a global decline in cognition that impairs memory, slows thought processes, and interferes with their ability to manipulate acquired knowledge. Juvenile-onset patients show marked bradykinesia and rigidity, epilepsy, severe dementia, and rapid decline.

Diffuse, severe atrophy of the neostriatum, sometimes worse in the caudate than the putamen, is the pathologic hallmark of HD. The globus pallidus can show a volume loss comparable to that seen in the striatum, in part because of the loss of striatopallidal projection fibers. Early-onset cases of HD show loss of cerebellar Purkinje cells along with generalized brain atrophy.

Differential Diagnosis

A number of sporadic conditions are associated with chorea, but most of these (e.g., tardive dyskinesia, thyrotoxicosis, cerebrovascular disease, cerebral lupus, polycythemia) can be excluded based on history, associated findings, and disease course. Benign hereditary chorea, an autosomal dominant condition, is usually nonprogressive and does not produce cognitive decline or psychiatric features. One should consider neuroacanthocytosis, another autosomal dominant condition that causes chorea, if the patient also displays muscle wasting, absent lower-limb tendon reflexes, and signs of neuropathy; it can be differentiated from HD by testing for acanthocytes in a thick, wet blood smear. There is one disease that is particularly likely to be confused with HD, and that is Huntington disease-like 2, discovered in some patients with apparent HD who do not bear CAG repeat expansions. HD-like 2 is also caused by a dynamic mutation, a triplet repeat in an alternatively spliced exon of the gene encoding junctophilin-3 (JPH3). Depending on which splice acceptor site is used, this repeat is either in frame or in a 3′ untranslated region.

Molecular Genetics

The CAG tract in the first exon of the HD gene varies from 6 to 34 repeats on unaffected chromosomes and from 36 to 121 repeats on disease alleles. Adult onset typically occurs when the repeat contains 40 to 50 units; more than 70 repeats results in the more severe juvenile form of the disease. HD-homozygous patients have phenotypes similar in severity to those of their heterozygote siblings, suggesting HD is a true dominant disorder.

There have been many mouse and fly models of HD, too numerous to mention here, but all helpful in piecing together clues about polyglutamine pathogenesis.[3] We will make two summary observations regarding the toxicity of the polyglutamine tract: (1) Mice expressing a truncated huntingtin protein with an expanded CAG tract suffer worse neurologic dysfunction than those bearing full-length huntingtin proteins, and (2) the greater the proportion of the protein taken up by the CAG tract, the more severe the resulting phenotype. This recalls the SBMA experience. HD research has also, however, produced knockin mouse models that bear the full-length protein at endogenous levels, and in this case even 150 CAGs, a greater expansion than any reported in humans, is able to elicit only some mild features of HD when the mice are quite mature. We will return to this point in the section on polyglutamine pathogenesis and future directions for therapies.

Abnormal nuclear and neuropil aggregation of mutant huntingtin has been reported in postmortem HD brain. Neuropil aggregates, occurring in dendrites and dendritic spines, are similar in structure but are more common in HD brains than NIs. Moreover, the progressive appearance of the neuropil aggregates correlates with neurologic symptoms in patients and HD mice, suggesting they may play a role in HD pathogenesis by affecting nerve terminal function. In contrast, NIs form primarily in the cortex but are rarely detected in the striatum, which is the region most vulnerable to degeneration in HD. All huntingtin aggregates are recognized only with antibodies specific for the N-terminus of huntingtin; these and other data indicate that proteolytic or caspase cleavage and release of a toxic expanded polyglutamine protein may be an important step in pathogenesis.

Some of the most important insights gained from HD animal model studies regard huntingtin's function. Accumulating evidence indicates that deregulation of transcriptional programs is key to HD pathogenesis (e.g., inhibiting expression of the dopamine D2 receptor), and several specific transcriptional activators and coactivators that interact with huntingtin have been found.[4] It is interesting to note that one of these is a multiprotein complex that contains the TATA-box binding protein (TBP), which is mutated in SCA17 (discussed later). Given HD's wide expression throughout the brain and its association with dendritic microtubules and synaptic vesicles in axon terminals, it is easy to understand why both cognition and motor control are compromised.

Therapy

Pharmacologic therapy is limited to symptomatic treatment. Neuroleptics may prove somewhat useful in suppressing choreic movements, and anti-Parkinsonian agents may be able to mitigate hypokinesia and rigidity. Psychotropic drugs can help control depression, psychosis, and outbursts of aggression. Cognitive impairment does not respond to pharmacotherapy, but an increasing body of evidence suggests that exposure to a stimulating environment (preferably before disease onset) helps prevent loss of cerebral volume and delays the onset of motor disorders. Minocycline has been shown to delay disease progression in HD mice by inhibiting caspase upregulation and decreasing inducible nitric oxide synthetase activity; lithium has been effective in reducing cell death in HD cell lines by allowing upregulation of molecular chaperones. Both these possible interventions are currently under investigation.

Dentatorubropallidoluysian Atrophy

Clinical Features

Age of onset and clinical features are quite variable in dentatorubropallidoluysian atrophy (DRPLA). Symptoms may begin in childhood or as late as the seventh decade, but most patients present with choreoathetosis, cerebellar symptoms, and tremors. Psychiatric disturbances can also present early in the disease course; in some patients involuntary movements and dementia mask the presence of ataxia. Pyramidal signs, opsoclonus, dystonia, ballismus, and myoclonus are common. The majority of patients develop epilepsy, and dementia occurs in the later stages of the disease. Patients with juvenile onset often present with myoclonus and invariably suffer seizures that can be induced by photic, tactile, or auditory stimuli and variable degrees of mental retardation or dementia.

The neuropathology of DRPLA is quite extensive, with marked neuronal loss in the cerebral cortex, cerebellar cortex, globus pallidus, striatum, and the dentate, subthalamic (Luys body), and red nuclei. There is intense gliosis and severe demyelination at the sites of neuronal degeneration. DRPLA patients with late-onset disease often have symmetrical high-signal lesions on MRI in the cerebral white matter and brain stem that are suggestive of leukodystrophic changes, and some have calcifications of the basal ganglia.

Differential Diagnosis

Adult-onset DRPLA with dementia and choreoathetosis resembles Huntington's disease and other dominantly inherited ataxias. The presence of ataxia can differentiate HD and DRPLA, but when involuntary movements and dementia mask it, imaging studies can be used to look for DRPLA's characteristic atrophy of the cerebellum and the pontine tegmentum. Atrophy of the caudate nucleus favors HD. However, when DRPLA patients have only mildly expanded CAG repeats (49 to 55), they may present simply with pure cerebellar symptoms, which necessitates a full SCA panel to establish the diagnosis.

The symptoms of early-onset DRPLA (ataxia, progressive intellectual deterioration, myoclonus, and epilepsy) may also bring to mind Unverricht-Lundborg disease, neuronal ceroid-lipofuscinosis, sialidosis, galactosialidosis, Gaucher disease, neuroaxonal dystrophy, pantothenate kinase associated neurodegeneration, and benign adult familial myoclonus epilepsy.

Molecular Genetics

The glutamine repeat in DRPLA is found near the C-terminus of the DRPLA gene product, atrophin-1. The normal repeat range is 6 to 35; expanded alleles have 49 to 88 repeats. Atrophin-1 is widely expressed and localizes primarily to the cytoplasm in neurons and peripheral cells, but nuclear localization has been reported.

Transgenic mice expressing full-length human atrophin-1 with 65 glutamines exhibit ataxia, tremors, abnormal movements, seizures, and premature death. These mice accumulate atrophin-1 nuclear inclusions in multiple populations of neurons. As is the case with HD, subcellular fractionation reveals nuclear fragments of mutant atrophin-1, whose abundance increases with age and phenotypic severity. Brains of DRPLA patients show apparently identical nuclear fragments. The evolution of neuropathology in DRPLA, as in HD, thus seems to involve proteolytic processing of mutant atrophin-1 and nuclear accumulation of truncated fragments.

The precise function of atrophin-1 is not yet known, although many protein interactors have been found in vitro. The *Drosophila melanogaster* atrophin homolog is required in numerous developmental processes, including embryonic patterning. Interestingly, both atrophin-1 and huntingtin interfere with CREB-binding-protein–mediated transcription. The *Drosophila* atrophin homolog is also required for the in vivo function of the transcriptional repressor even-skipped, and the transcriptional repression activity of both the human and fly proteins is reduced by polyglutamine expansion.[5] As with HD, transcriptional deregulation seems to contribute to DRPLA pathogenesis.

Spinocerebellar Ataxia Type 1

Clinical Features

The primary clinical features in all the spinocerebellar ataxias (SCAs) are progressive cerebellar ataxia, dysarthria, and eventual bulbar dysfunction. Early symptoms of SCA1 include gait ataxia, slurred speech, brisk deep tendon reflexes, and mild limb ataxia. Hypermetric saccades and nystagmus can also be noted in early stages as well as mild dysphagia. Patients may also present with pyramidal signs and peripheral neuropathy.

As the disease progresses, patients develop oculomotor deficits, including slow saccadic velocity and upgaze palsy. Nystagmus often disappears with evolving saccadic abnormalities. As dysarthria and ataxia worsen, patients develop hyperreflexia and other cerebellar signs such as dysmetria, dysdiadochokinesia, hypotonia, and the rebound phenomenon. Optic nerve atrophy and various degrees of ophthalmoparesis can occur. Muscle atrophy, decreased or absent deep-tendon reflexes, and loss of proprioception or vibration sense occur in the middle or late stages of disease. Cognition may become impaired. Extrapyramidal signs show up as chorea and dystonia in advanced disease. In the final stages, bulbar signs (atrophy of facial and masticatory muscles, perioral fasciculations, and severe dysphagia) become quite problematic. The most common causes of death are respiratory failure and pneumonia.

SCA1 is characterized pathologically by cerebellar atrophy with severe loss of Purkinje cells, dentate nucleus neurons, and neurons in the inferior olive and cranial nerve nuclei III, IV, IX, X, and XII. Neuropathologic studies also reveal gliosis of the cerebellar molecular layer and, within the internal granular layer, eosinophilic spheres or "torpedoes" are present in axons of degenerating Purkinje cells. Demyelination is marked in the dorsal and ventral spinocerebellar tracts and is present to a lesser degree in the posterior columns.

Molecular Genetics

The highly polymorphic CAG repeat in the *SCA1* gene results in a polyglutamine tract in the amino terminal half of its protein product, ataxin-1. Normal alleles contain 6 to 44 repeats, and tracts with more than 20 CAGs are stabilized by interruptions of 1 to 4 CAT repeat units encoding histidine. Disease alleles contain a pure stretch of uninterrupted CAG trinucleotides that range from 39 to 82 repeats.

Ataxin-1 is a novel protein of unknown function and ubiquitous expression, although it is expressed in the central nervous system at two to four times the levels found in peripheral tissues. In SCA1 patients, mutant ataxin-1 localizes to a single ubiquitin-positive nuclear inclusion in brain stem neurons but not in the cerebellum, which is the primary region affected by disease. This and similar observations in HD brains were the first suggestion that NI are formed in those neurons that are more likely to resist neurodegeneration. Studies in transgenic mice revealed that ataxin-1 must localize to the nucleus in order to exert toxic effects, and recent in vitro work suggests that ataxin-1 may bind RNA (see the section on polyglutamine pathogenesis and future directions for therapies).

Spinocerebellar Ataxia Type 2

Clinical Features

Ataxia, dysarthria, and tremor characterize SCA2. The earliest presenting symptom is typically gait ataxia accompanied by leg cramps, although some families present with apparent parkinsonism.[6] Most patients exhibit nystagmus before developing markedly slow saccades; ophthalmoparesis occurs in over half of the patients. Retinal pigmentary degeneration has recently been reported, undermining the supposedly unique association of this feature with SCA7. Pyramidal signs are very frequent; deep tendon reflexes are brisk early on but disappear later in the disease course. Cognitive impairment can occur with or without dementia, and dysphagia and bulbar failure characterize end-stage disease. The infantile phenotype is broadly devastating; one SCA2 infant with more than 200 CAG repeats showed neonatal hypotonia, developmental delay, dysphagia, and postnatal retinitis pigmentosa.[7]

Neuropathology corresponds to symptomatology. The cerebellum and brain stem show degeneration with marked reduction in the number of Purkinje and granule cells. Atrophy of the fronto-temporal lobes, degeneration of the substantia nigra, and gliosis in the inferior olive and pons have all been reported.

Molecular Genetics

The CAG repeat located in the N-terminal coding region of SCA2 is less polymorphic than the repeats in other polyglutamine diseases: 95% of alleles contain 22 or 23 repeats. Normal alleles may contain 14 to 31 repeats and are normally interrupted by two CAA sequences. Disease alleles contain a perfectly uninterrupted CAG tract that ranges from 33 to 200 repeats. The phenotype produced by 33 repeats can be extremely late-onset; one patient manifested mild balance problems at the age of 86, but her daughter developed mild ataxia in her 70s with the same 33 repeat expansion. As in other polyglutamine diseases, variability in age of onset is not solely a function of CAG repeat size.

The SCA2 gene product, ataxin-2, is a novel cytoplasmic protein of unknown function, but it contains Sm1 and Sm2 motifs previously found in proteins that are involved in RNA splicing and protein-protein interaction. SCA2 is widely expressed throughout the body and brain, with high levels in cerebellar Purkinje cells. Ataxin-2 immunoreactivity is more intense in SCA2 brains than

in normal brains, suggesting that the mutant protein undergoes altered catabolism. Recently, mutant ataxin-2 was shown to aggregate in ubiquitin-positive nuclear inclusions, but only 1% to 2% of the surviving neurons were NI-positive. As with SCA1, the cerebellum was completely devoid of NIs despite extensive neuronal degeneration.

Spinocerebellar Ataxia Type 3: Machado-Joseph Disease

Clinical Features

SCA3, or Machado-Joseph disease (MJD), is one of the most common hereditary spinocerebellar ataxias. Ataxia and its history illustrate the diagnostic challenges posed by these diseases. The disease was first described in (and named after) two families of Portuguese-Azorean origin afflicted with ataxia, amyotrophy, external ophthalmoplegia, bulging eyes, muscle weakness, facial and lingual fasciculations, neuropathy, Parkinsonism, and spasticity. Takiyama and colleagues mapped the MJD gene in Japanese families to human chromosome 14q24.3–q32, and additional mapping studies in Portuguese-Azorean kindreds confirmed the mapping of MJD to 14q. At this point, some attempts were made to divide MJD into clinical subtypes based on different combinations of clinical findings and age of onset. Unfortunately, considerable phenotypic variability produced different "subtypes" within the same family, with affected individuals often evolving from one "subtype" to another, thereby rendering such clinical subclassifications problematic.

In the meantime, Stevanin and colleagues studied a different family with a dominantly inherited ataxia, mapping the disease gene to chromosome 14q24.3–qter. The new locus was designated SCA3 because the clinical features of this family resembled SCA1 more than MJD: increased reflexes, nystagmus, and decreased vibration sense in addition to ataxia and dysarthria, amyotrophy, and supranuclear ophthalmoplegia. Dementia, dystonia, and extrapyramidal rigidity were found in less than 20% of the patients, and optic atrophy was rare. As the disease progressed, sphincter abnormalities and swallowing difficulties developed. Although several studies subsequently demonstrated that MJD and SCA3 are caused by the same mutation within the MJD1 gene, MJD persists in the nomenclature.

Degeneration is most prominent in the basal ganglia, brain stem, spinal cord, and dentate neurons of the cerebellum. Purkinje cell loss is mild, and the inferior olive is typically spared.

Molecular Genetics

The polyglutamine repeat in the SCA3/MJD1 gene product is near the C-terminus. Normal individuals have between 12 and 40 glutamines, and in disease the repeat expands to a length of 55 to 84 glutamines. The *MJD1* gene encodes a ubiquitously expressed protein that has no known function or any known homology with other proteins. Ataxin-3 is a predominantly cytoplasmic protein, but in SCA3 patient neurons, expanded ataxin-3 accumulates in ubiquitinated nuclear inclusions that also contain proteasomal components. Chaperone overexpression has been able to reduce this aggregation in cell culture studies (see the section on polyglutamine pathogenesis and future directions for therapies).[8]

Spinocerebellar Ataxia Type 6

Clinical Features

Patients with SCA6 first present with mild, slowly progressive ataxia and dysarthria. As the disease worsens, patients suffer from upper-limb incoordination and intention tremor. Dysphagia is a frequent problem in patients who have had the disease more than 5 years. Very mild neuropathy (minimal distal wasting and decreased ankle jerks) is seen in some patients. About half of the patients develop diplopia, hyperreflexia, and extensor plantar responses. Some patients exhibit horizontal gaze-evoked and vertical nystagmus. Approximately 25% of patients show basal ganglia signs such as dystonia and blepharospasm; about 10% of older patients have dementia.

Neuropathologic findings in SCA6 include marked cerebellar atrophy and mild atrophy of the brain stem. There is severe loss of cerebellar Purkinje cells with moderate loss of cerebellar granule cells, dentate nucleus neurons, and neurons of the inferior olive.

Molecular Genetics

SCA6 is caused by a CAG repeat expansion in the α_{1A}-voltage–dependent calcium channel (*CACNA1A*). Voltage-sensitive calcium channels are multimeric complexes made of the pore-forming α_{1A} subunit and several regulatory subunits. These channels mediate calcium entry into excitable cells and thereby play roles in a variety of neuronal functions that include neurotransmitter release and gene expression. The α_{1A} subunit gene is abundantly expressed in the CNS, with highest levels in cerebellar Purkinje cells. Interestingly, mutant α_{1A} calcium channels aggregate in the cytoplasm of SCA6 Purkinje cells. These inclusions occur in the peripheral perikaryal cytoplasm and in the proximal dendrites but not in the nucleus. The inclusions are ubiquitin-negative but can be identified with both amino- and carboxy-terminal antibodies, suggesting that the full-length protein is present.

The CAG repeat in *CACNA1A* is relatively stable and exceptionally small, with fewer than 18 repeats on normal chromosomes. Disease-causing repeats are also small and range from 20 to 33 CAGs. These small expansions, however, are sufficient to increase alpha 1A protein

expression at the cellular surface and thus Ca^{2+} current.[9] (Interestingly, there is a gene dosage effect in SCA6, with homozygosity leading to retinitis pigmentosa.) Missense, splice, and protein truncating mutations in *CACNA1A* have been reported in episodic ataxia type 2 (EA 2) and familial hemiplegic migraine. Furthermore, the tottering and tottering-leaner mice bear nonexpansion mutations in this subunit. The fact that some patients with SCA6 experience episodic ataxia in the early stages of the disease raises the possibility that SCA6 and EA 2 represent different points along a phenotypic continuum of the same disease.

Spinocerebellar Ataxia Type 7

Clinical Features

Approximately half of SCA7 patients develop cerebellar ataxia and visual deficits simultaneously; among the remaining half, most present with cerebellar ataxia and may maintain normal vision for decades. The minority who first present with visual deficits usually develop ataxia within a few years. Decreased visual acuity is secondary to progressive pigmentary macular degeneration; the earliest finding is dyschromatopsia in the blue-yellow axis. Patients complain of progressive loss of central vision but note that peripheral and night vision are intact. Funduscopic exam reveals loss of foveal reflex and increased macular pigmentation. Secondary optic atrophy occurs in the later stages of the disease. Visual loss usually progresses to bilateral blindness. Additional features of SCA7 include increased reflexes and spasticity, slow saccades, ophthalmoplegia, and hearing deficits. Extrapyramidal signs such as oro-facial dyskinesias, choreoathetosis, dystonia, limb rigidity, and tremors occur in some patients. Behavioral disturbances such as auditory hallucinations, progressive psychosis, and delusions have been reported. Depression and emotional lability can be prominent in juvenile-onset cases.[10] Infantile SCA7 produces somatic features in addition to the visual and neuronal deficits: severe hypotonia, patent ductus arteriosus, congestive heart failure, and death in the first year of life.[7]

Neuronal loss occurs primarily in the cerebellum, inferior olive, and some cranial nerve nuclei. Hypomyelination of the optic tract and gliosis of the lateral geniculate body and visual cortex are also characteristic of SCA7. Electron microscopy studies of skeletal muscles of SCA7 patients reveal mitochondrial abnormalities (uneven distribution, subsarcolemmal accumulations, autophagic vacuoles, and paracrystalline inclusions).

Molecular Genetics

The polyglutamine tract is near the amino terminus of the SCA7 gene product, ataxin-7. All normal alleles contain pure CAG tracts without any evidence of interruption (typically 4 to 35 repeats), whereas adult-onset disease occurs when the repeats exceed 37. The SCA7 mutation is the most unstable in the polyglutamine disease family and manifests the most extreme intergenerational CAG repeat instability, with an enlargement of 263 repeats reported in one father-to-son transmission. As with most other triplet repeat diseases, larger expansions are more frequently associated with paternal transmission. Disease, however, is more frequently observed upon maternal transmission, suggesting that the very large expansions in paternally transmitted alleles are embryonic-lethal.

The function of ataxin-7 is unknown, and it shares no significant homology with other proteins. SCA7 shows ubiquitous expression, with the high levels in the heart, placenta, skeletal muscle, pancreas, and brain. Within the CNS, the SCA7 transcript is most abundant in the cerebellum. In SCA7 patients, ataxin-7 nuclear aggregates were identified in affected brain regions (brain stem, especially pons and inferior olive). In one juvenile-onset patient, they were also found in brain regions not associated with disease (cerebral cortex). Studies in several transgenic models of SCA7 and a knockin model of the disease demonstrate that mutant ataxin-7 alters transcription of at least photoreceptor-specific genes, making SCA7 yet another polyglutamine disease in which transcriptional dysregulation is a prime component of pathogenesis.

Spinocerebellar Ataxia Type 17

Clinical Features

SCA17 has been documented in only a few kindreds thus far, and the phenotype varies by family.[11] SCA17 tends to manifest itself in the third decade with ataxia, dementia, or parkinsonism, depending on the patient. Truncal dystonia, dysmetria, dysdiadochokinesia, hyperreflexia, and paucity of movement usually follow. Parkinsonism in these cases consisted mainly of bradykinesia, accelerated gait, marche á petits pas, and postural reflex disturbance (retropulsion); tremor and muscle rigidity are less prominent. Epilepsy was the first neurologic symptom in one patient but a very late feature in other patients. No abnormal eye movements were noted. Initial clinical diagnoses varied from dementia-related atypical Holmes'-like spinocerebellar degeneration to DRPLA-like spinocerebellar degeneration, atypical HD, and atypical Parkinsonism with progressive dementia.

MRI or CT findings for all the patients indicated diffuse cortical and cerebellar atrophy. Neuropathologic examination reveals shrinkage and loss of small neurons with gliosis in the caudate nucleus and putamen; large neurons are relatively preserved. Similar changes are detected in the thalamus, frontal cortex, and temporal cortex. The cerebellum shows moderate Purkinje cell loss and an increase of Bergmann glia.

Molecular Genetics

SCA17 is caused by a CAG repeat expansion in the TATA-binding protein (TBP) gene, which encodes a general transcription initiation factor. Normal repeat tracts range from 29 to 42 CAGs, and disease alleles bear 47 to 55 repeats. TBP is the DNA-binding subunit of RNA polymerase II transcription factor D (TFIID), a multi-subunit complex crucial for the expression of most genes. The long polyglutamine domain is located in the N-terminus, which regulates the DNA-binding activity of the C-terminus of the protein.

ATAXIAS WITH NONCODING REPEATS

Spinocerebellar Ataxia Type 8

Clinical Features

SCA8 is a slowly progressive ataxia that typically manifests in adulthood, although the reported age of onset ranges from 1 to 65 years.[12] The most common presenting symptoms are ataxia and scanning dysarthria with a very drawn-out quality; some patients present with nystagmus, dysmetric saccades, and, rarely, ophthalmoplegia. In the early stages of the disease, speech is disproportionally worse than other cerebellar signs, and ataxic symptoms of the lower extremities appear to be more pronounced than in upper extremities. Marked truncal titubation worsens over decades, along with other symptoms, regardless of the age of onset. In very advanced disease, some patients develop hyperactive tendon reflexes and extensor plantar responses. Life span is typically not shortened.

MRI shows mild atrophy of the cerebellar vermis and hemispheres.

Molecular Genetics

Like myotonic dystrophy, SCA8 is caused by an untranslated CTG expansion. In this case, the repeat lies near the 3' end of a processed, noncoding mRNA. The CTG repeat is located in the antisense transcript of KLHL1, a protein of unknown function, which suggests that the SCA8 transcript may be an endogenous antisense RNA that regulates KLHL1 expression.

The SCA8 expansion is unique among triplet repeats in that a specific range of repeats rather than just an increase over the normal tract length causes the disease. Intriguingly, very large expansions between 250 and 800 repeats can leave an individual entirely unaffected, just like the 20 to 30 repeats present in the normal population: only repeats between 100 and 250 seem to be pathogenic. Very large repeats may interfere with SCA8 expression or alter RNA processing or stability so that there is no toxic gain of function when the CUG tract is >250. Disease-causing repeats tend to be transmitted maternally, whereas paternal transmissions have a strong tendency to contract.

Spinocerebellar Ataxia Type 12

Clinical Features

SCA12 has been described in only a few pedigrees of German, American, and Indian descent. The disease typically presents with tremor in the fourth decade, progressing to include ataxia, dysmetria, dysdiadokinesis, hyperreflexia, paucity of movement, abnormal eye movements, and, in the oldest subjects, dementia. Reported ages of onset have ranged from 8 to 55 years. MRI or CT scans of five cases indicated both cortical and cerebellar atrophy.

Molecular Genetics

SCA12 is caused by a noncoding CAG trinucleotide repeat expansion in the 5′ untranslated region of the PPP2R2B gene,[13] which encodes a brain-specific regulatory subunit of protein phosphatase 2A (PP2A PR55). The function of this particular subunit is unknown, as is the effect of the repeat expansion. Normal alleles contain 7 to 28 repeats, whereas expanded alleles have 66 to 78 repeats. Given this limited range of expanded alleles, it is not possible yet to say whether there is a correlation between repeat size and age of onset or disease severity. Furthermore, the precise age of onset of tremor, typically the first symptom, is often difficult to determine.

Differential Diagnosis

Table 12–1 lists the polyglutaminopathies, the features most commonly noted when the disease first presents itself, and the principal brain regions affected by each disease. SCA10 bears special mention here, as it is not a polyglutamine disease but is caused by an expansion of a pentanucleotide (ATTCT) repeat in intron 9 of the *SCA10* gene (for which a test is available). SCA10 patients often show complex partial seizures in addition to ataxia, dysarthria, and nystagmus. As we have tried to emphasize, the inter- and intrafamilial phenotypic variability of the SCAs will vex even the most astute clinician. Molecular genetic testing provides the only definitive diagnosis. For the sake of thoroughness, Table 12–2 lists the autosomal-dominant ataxias for which the causative gene has been mapped but not yet cloned. Pediatric neurologists may benefit from more detailed information on the presentation of juvenile-onset cases.[7]

Therapy

Therapy for all the ataxias discussed in this chapter is supportive at best. Some of the motor abnormalities, such as the dystonia, bradykinesia, and rigidity in SCA3 respond to levodopa, but no drugs have been consistently found to mitigate cerebellar symptoms. Vitamin supplements are recommended, however, particularly if caloric intake is reduced. Exercise should be maintained as long as possible. Recent work points to an interesting coincidence of gluten sensitivity and both hereditary and sporadic ataxias; it may be prudent to screen patients for IgG and IgA antigliadin antibodies (AGA) or encourage patients to test whether eliminating gluten from their diet brings any

TABLE 12–2. Autosomal Dominant Ataxias That Have Been Mapped but Not Cloned

Disease	Locus	Principal Features
SCA4	16q22.1	Slowly progressive ataxia, prominent axonal sensory neuropathy and extensor plantar reflexes, late areflexia
SCA5	11p11–11q11	Slowly progressive mild ataxia, increased reflexes, gazed-evoked nystagmus, facial myokymia, decreased vibration sense Juvenile-onset: pyramidal and bulbar dysfunction
SCA9		No clinical disorder assigned
SCA11	15q14–q21.3	Benign, slowly progressive pure cerebellar syndrome; occasional noncerebellar signs, e.g., mild hyperreflexia; vertical nystagmus
SCA13	19q13.3–13.4	Usual onset in childhood of slowly progressive ataxia with dysarthria, moderate mental retardation, and mild developmental delay in motor acquisition; possible seizures
SCA14	19q13.14	Late-onset (≥39 years old): pure cerebellar ataxia Early-onset (≤27 years old): present intermittent axial myoclonus followed by ataxia
SCA16	8q22.1–24.1	Ataxia and head tremor

relief of symptoms. In the authors' experience, a significant proportion of autosomal dominant ataxia patients also had thyroid disease. Although it has not been established that thyroid dysfunction occurs more frequently in SCA patients than in other populations, thyroid disorders are themselves common and tend to be undertreated. Some patients may benefit in overall health from careful attention to thyroid function and maintenance of thyroid-stimulating hormone levels at the low end of the range.

Polyglutamine Pathogenesis and Future Directions for Therapies

As the attentive reader will realize, there is one conspicuous feature common to the polyglutaminopathies: accumulation of mutant protein. Abnormal protein aggregates are also hallmarks of Alzheimer's disease, Parkinson's disease, prion diseases, frontotemporal dementia, and motor neuron disease. Transgenic mouse models have recapitulated the major neurologic features of these disorders, as well as this particular pathologic feature.[14] The discovery that nuclear aggregates stain positive for ubiquitin, the molecular chaperone HDJ-2/HSDJ, and the proteasome has led to the hypothesis that the expanded polyglutamine tract alters the native conformation of the protein, causing it to misfold. These observations have been made for SCA1, HD, SCA3, and the other polyglutamine diseases.

The failure of proteins to adopt their proper conformation is a significant threat to cell function and viability. Cells have several pathways by which to deal with misfolded proteins. Molecular chaperones usher nascent polypeptides from the ribosome and promote their proper folding while protecting them from aberrant interactions. If the chaperones fail in this task, the improperly folded protein is tagged for proteolytic degradation by ubiquitin. (This ubiquitin-proteasome pathway also degrades normal proteins when they have served their function.) If the misfolded protein evades this second system and accumulates in sufficient quantities, aggregates will form.

The formation of NIs is often conceived as a passive process, with misfolded proteins floating by a site of aggregation and getting drawn in to the inclusion, but increasing evidence suggests that the cell quite deliberately sequesters mutant protein into NIs to contain their toxic effects. Some misfolded proteins, for example, are delivered to NIs by microtubule transport.[15] More direct evidence, however, comes from animal models of polyglutamine disease. SCA1 mice that are deficient in *Ube3a*, a component of the ubiquitin-proteasome pathway, have dramatically worse pathology than their *Sca1* littermates—and they cannot form NIs.[14] Also recall that in patient material, NIs are often not observed in the neurons that are vulnerable to disease. It is as if the neurons that can form inclusions are able to survive the insult of

polyglutamine toxicity longer. Indeed, a knockin model of SCA1 recently provided confirmation of this model. Mice bearing 154 CAG repeats in the endogenous mouse *Sca1* locus develop a neurodegenerative disorder that closely resembles human SCA1: deteriorating motor coordination, cognitive deficits, wasting, and premature death accompanied by Purkinje cell loss and age-related hippocampal synaptic dysfunction.[16] The most interesting finding in these mice was that mutant ataxin-1 solubility varied by brain region, being most soluble in those neurons most vulnerable to degeneration. Mutant protein solubility decreased overall with advancing age, but the Purkinje cells, which are most affected in SCA1, were unable to form inclusions until a very late stage of disease. The paucity of NIs in vulnerable neurons in both humans and knockin mice suggests that the selective neuropathology in polyglutamine diseases reflects a combination of mutant protein levels, protein solubility, and the presence of factors that help process the mutant proteins for ubiquitin-proteasome pathway clearance or sequester the mutant proteins into protective NIs. This hypothesis has received further support from studies of a knockin model for SCA7.

Several studies provide more indirect support for the impaired protein clearance hypothesis. Overexpression of chaperones such as Hsp70 and dHDJ1 suppresses the phenotype of MJD/SCA3 flies and flies overexpressing expanded CAG repeats, respectively.[14] Chaperone overexpression also improves motor function in SCA1 mice.[16] Several groups have also reported suppression of mutant huntingtin-induced cell death by overexpressing chaperones such as GroEL, Hsp104, Hsp40, and Hsp70.[14] Since nuclear accumulation of mutant protein is observed in most polyglutamine diseases (SCA1, SCA3/MJD, SCA7, HD, SBMA, and DRPLA), protein misfolding and alteration of turnover rate seems to be a shared pathogenetic mechanism.[17,18] Downstream pathogenetic mechanisms may differ from one disease to the next, however, particularly in SCA2 and SCA6, in which mutant protein accumulates in the cytoplasm instead of the nucleus. For example, *Drosophila* screens for modifiers of polyglutamine disease phenotypes pull out genes involved in RNA processing, transcriptional regulation, and cellular detoxification.[19] Therefore, there are undoubtedly multiple pathways involved in pathogenesis.

Transcriptional dysregulation is another leitmotif in the triplet repeat diseases. Lin and colleagues reported that several neuronal genes were downregulated during the early pathogenesis of a SCA1 transgenic mouse model.[14,17] Expanded polyglutamine proteins have been found to cause the redistribution of many key transcription factors, such as nuclear receptor corepressor and CREB-binding protein, in mouse models, cellular models, and human tissues.[4] The sequestration of such factors might have detrimental effects on transcription. Moreover, several polyglutamine-containing proteins seem to be directly involved in transcription.[4] This pathway provides another opening for research into pharmacologic interventions.[17] For example, the histone deacetylase inhibitors suberoylamide hydroxamic acid and sodium butyrate suppress neuronal degeneration and improve viability of flies bearing exon 1 of huntingtin with 93 CAG repeats.

Will it be possible to slow down or halt neurodegeneration in polyglutamine disorders after symptoms appear? Yamamoto and colleagues[20] show that it is possible for neurons to recover if the production of mutant protein is arrested. They generated a conditional HD transgenic mouse model using a tetracycline-regulatable system that controls transgene expression by feeding mice tetracycline or its analogue, doxycycline. When the transgene is turned on, these mice develop nuclear inclusions, characteristic HD neuropathology, and progressive motor dysfunction. Once this gene is turned off in symptomatic mice, however, nuclear inclusions disappear and the behavioral phenotype improves, demonstrating that a continuous flux of mutant protein is required to maintain the disease state. This result raises the possibility that HD, and perhaps other neurodegenerative diseases, may be reversible. The challenge will be finding a method for slowing or stopping the expression of mutant proteins that is feasible for human therapy.

MULTISYSTEM DISORDERS CAUSED BY NONCODING TRIPLET REPEATS

Friedreich's Ataxia

Clinical Features

Friedreich's ataxia (FRDA) is the most common autosomal recessive ataxia, afflicting 1 in 30,000 individuals. FRDA usually manifests between 5 and 10 years of age, but onset can sometimes be detected as early as 2 years or well into the second decade of life. The first sign is a progressive gait ataxia, with widening of the base and wavering, that seems to be due to a loss of proprioception. (The poor balance is accentuated when visual input is removed, as in the Romberg test.) The gait can be grossly disorganized, with such a marked reeling or lurching quality that it appears contrived. The upper extremities soon become uncoordinated, distal muscles begin to waste, and tremor or choreiform movements may develop in the face and arms. Irregular ocular pursuit is often prominent; dysmetric saccades, square wave jerks, and failure of fixation suppression of the vestibulo-ocular reflex are common. Cataracts, retinitis pigmentosa, and optic atrophy can also occur. Dysarthria typically develops early in the disease course, and the slurring and staccato volume changes are severe enough to quickly render speech ineffectual. Auditory dysfunction is common and may be accompanied by vertigo. After several years, kyphoscoliosis develops and, by shifting the patient's center of gravity, makes walking nearly impossible.

Deep tendon reflexes are lost early on in the disease course, unless the patient had adult onset (usually beyond age 25 years). Position and vibration senses are grossly impaired, and pain and temperature sensations are lost in the distal extremities. Clubfoot and pes cavus are nearly always present. Cardiomyopathy occurs in 66% of FRDA patients, and is progressive and occasionally documented by EKG abnormalities even before ataxia manifests itself. In advanced stages of the disease, patients may experience exertional dyspnea, palpitations, and anginal pain; later in the disease course, arrhythmias (especially atrial fibrillation) and congestive heart failure are frequent. Diabetes mellitus develops in 10% of FRDA patients. Even in its absence another 20% of patients show an abnormal glucose tolerance curve owing to insulin resistance (which may also affect relatives). Thermal dysregulation, intermittent emesis, and respiratory dysfunction have been reported. Life span is inevitably shortened, with a mean age of death in the mid-thirties.

In the minority of patients with shorter GAA expansions (<500) the age of onset is between 26 years and 40 years or older, with the smaller repeats producing later onset and milder symptoms. Disease progression is slower in these patients, and they have a lower incidence of secondary skeletal abnormalities. Very rarely, patients homozygous for GAA expansions may present with spastic paraparesis and hyperreflexia but not ataxia.

Pathology

FRDA is characterized pathologically by fiber loss, demyelination, and gliosis of the posterior columns, spinocerebellar tracts, corticospinal tracts, and the posterior rootlets. Although both axons and myelin are involved, the medullary gray matter masses are usually spared. There is invariable loss of large primary sensory neurons of the dorsal root ganglia and atrophy of the lumbar spinal nerves. The cerebellar cortex shows varying, late-stage degeneration; the inferior olive, vestibular nuclei, and pontine nuclei are involved to different degrees.

Differential Diagnosis

Diagnostic criteria put forth before the discovery of the GAA repeat expansion in FRDA include autosomal recessive inheritance (which prevents the anticipation common to other triplet repeat disorders), gait ataxia, dysarthria, absent deep tendon reflexes (although late-onset patients may retain these), dorsal column signs, weakness, and abnormal 5-hour glucose tolerance curve. Spinal fluid may show elevated protein content and mild pleocytosis. As many as 25% of FRDA patients display atypical clinical signs, however, so DNA testing is the only means to a definitive diagnosis. FRDA is most frequently confused with demyelinating hereditary motor and sensory neuropathy type I

(HMSN 1 or CMT 1), which can present in childhood with clumsiness, areflexia, and minimal distal muscle weakness. Children with FRDA who have not yet developed dysarthria or extensor plantar responses may be difficult to distinguish on clinical criteria alone, so again, molecular genetic testing is recommended. Autosomal recessive spastic ataxia of Charlevoix-Saguenay, caused by deletions or point mutations in the *sacsin* gene, is another consideration: patients are characterized by spasticity, dysarthria, distal muscle wasting, foot deformities, truncal ataxia, absence of sensory potentials in the lower limbs, retinal striations similar to those in Leber's optic atrophy, and frequent mitral valve prolapse. Vitamin E deficiency causes ataxia with areflexia, and indeed can fulfill the diagnostic criteria for FRDA, but is usually distinguishable from FRDA by the greater likelihood of hyperkinesia and titubation. It is obviously important to test for both abetalipoproteinemia and α-tocopherol deficiency, since these ataxias can be cured by large doses of vitamin E.

Molecular Genetics

Friedreich's ataxia is most often caused by a large intronic GAA repeat expansion in the center of an Alu repeat in the *X25* gene, also known as *frataxin*. This expansion interferes with transcription and causes a severe deficiency of frataxin protein. FRDA is unique among the triplet repeat disorders because of the repeat location (intronic) and nucleotide sequence (AT-rich unlike GC-rich triplets) and because affected individuals carry two mutant alleles. Also remarkable is that the GAA repeat expansion is the most common to date, which explains the high carrier frequency of 1 in 85. Normal alleles contain 7 to 34 repeats, and disease-causing alleles contain more than 100. Intermediate premutation alleles containing 34 to 65 pure GAA repeats have been found to expand to 300 to 650 repeats in a single generation. The unstable GAA repeat undergoes both expansions and contractions following maternal transmission but predominantly contracts when passed through the father.

As with most other triplet repeat disorders, a direct correlation exists between the GAA repeat size and disease severity; the longer the expansion, the less frataxin produced, and the more severe the symptoms. In FRDA, however, since most patients are homozygous for expansions, the correlation between severity and repeat length is based on the shorter of the two alleles. Given the severe deficiency associated with very long repeats, the total residual FRDA mRNA in those homozygous for the GAA expansion is determined by the lesser repeat. Patients who carry only one expanded allele and one truncating point mutation on the second allele have all the clinical features of typical FRDA, further supporting the notion that FRDA is caused by a loss of frataxin function.

Pathogenesis

Studies have found that the generation of reactive oxygen species and mitochondrial dysfunction[21] play a significant part in FRDA pathogenesis. This is consistent with two long-standing observations. First, vitamin E deficiency and FRDA produce almost identical phenotypes. Second, the cell types most vulnerable to dysfunction in FRDA (neurons and cardiomyocytes) have limited antioxidant defenses, despite the fact that brain cells consume 20% of the oxygen utilized by the body and therefore generate reactive oxygen species at an enormous rate. Increased oxidative stress has been demonstrated recently in FRDA patients by the presence of plasma malondialdehyde (a product of lipid peroxidation), elevated urinary concentrations of 8-hydroxy-2′-deoxyguanosine (a marker of oxidative DNA damage), or decreased concentrations of glutathione in the blood. Glutathione is the most abundant intracellular antioxidant in normal individuals, and its depletion has been proposed to contribute to the pathogenesis of Parkinson's disease and other major neurodegenerative disorders.

Early yeast studies had led researchers to suspect that mitochondrial iron accumulation was the primary defect in FRDA, because yeast deficient for the frataxin homolog *(Yfh1)* lose mitochondrial DNA and develop abnormal accumulation of mitochondrial iron and respiratory deficiency. A deficiency of iron sulfur cluster enzymes mediated by oxidative damage was considered to be a secondary effect. More recent research in mice, however, presents a different picture. Inactivation of the mouse homologue causes early embryonic lethality without iron accumulation; a conditional, tissue-specific knockout mouse developed respiratory deficiency and tissue pathology prior to intramitochondrial iron deposition. Key data from FRDA fibroblasts showed that they are unable to upregulate mitochondrial superoxide dismutase or increase iron import in response to endogenously produced superoxides, and conditional mouse models of FRDA show abnormally low superoxide dismutase activity in heart muscle. Interestingly, in vitro studies on cultured cardiomyocytes have shown that superoxide production leads to cellular hypertrophy, which provides a ready explanation for the cardiac hypertrophy seen in FRDA patients and mouse models. The mechanism by which frataxin may help induce the proper oxidative stress response remains to be determined.

Therapy

Diabetes, heart failure, and arrhythmias are treated by the usual means. The cerebellar symptoms have been found in several studies to respond to 5-hydroxytryptophan; another study found 5-hydroxytryptophan to relieve breathing dysrhythmias and apnea. A preliminary study evaluating the effects of idebenone, a short-chain analogue of coenzyme Q10, on FRDA cardiomyopathy yielded promising results, although the neurologic consequences need to be evaluated. Treatment of FRDA patients with vitamin E and CoQ10 for six months increased the cardiac phosphocreatine-to-ATP ratios and improved muscle mitochondrial ATP production, although it is not yet clear how much clinical benefit resulted during this brief period. Recent work on the efficacy of glutathione in protecting against oxidative stress may prove beneficial for future interventions.[22]

Fragile X Syndrome

Fragile X syndrome (FRAXA), also sometimes referred to as Martin-Bell or Marker X syndrome, is an X-linked disorder with prevalence estimated to be as high as 1:4000. This figure does not, however, take into account the milder phenotypes caused by smaller expansions of the CGG repeat in the 5'-untranslated region of the fragile X gene, *FMR1*. Indeed, while mental retardation is the most well-known feature of FRAXA, the full range of phenotypes is considerable. The prevalence of the subtler phenotypes is unknown, but some studies indicate there are as many as 1:100 female (and 1:255 male) "premutation carriers" (those who bear slight expansions that are likely to expand into disease-causing range but do not themselves cause overt phenotypes).

Clinical Features

Males with full mutations of over 230 methylated repeats are always affected. The three physical hallmarks of FRAXA in the adult male are a long narrow face, prominent ears (more common in whites than other racial groups), and large testicles. (There are two variant physical phenotypes that produce either a Soto-like appearance with general overgrowth or a Prader-Willi–like obesity with a full, round face, small hands and feet, and regional hyperpigmentation.) The growth pattern appears to be disturbed, perhaps because of hypothalmic dysfunction; compared to controls, males are tall before their (early) puberty but usually achieve a relatively short stature in adulthood. The prominence of the ears is likely related to a generalized connective tissue dysplasia that also manifests itself in hyperextensible finger joints, velvety skin, mitral valve prolapse, and flat feet. Speech tends to be perseverative, and boys' voices have a low-pitched, harsh quality. Seizures afflict perhaps 25% of affected males, usually in the first 15 years of life. In childhood, fully affected males are delayed in reaching developmental milestones (but sometimes only after the first year), and show hyperactivity, hand-flapping or other motor stereotypies, temper tantrums, and autistic features (tactile withdrawal and poor social interaction, communication, and eye contact). Most males have moderate to severe mental retardation by the time they reach adulthood. It is interesting to note that nearly half of FRAXA preschool children test in the borderline to average IQ range but experience a decline after the first decade of life. The reason for this longitudinal decline is unknown.

Approximately 50% of females with the same mutation will be affected by similar features, but more mildly than their male counterparts. Males and females with a full mutation that is not methylated will show slight dysfunction; males are usually affected but highly functional, even having a low-normal intellect, and females may display only slight cognitive deficits or have normal intellectual capacity.

The effects of a premutation (55 to 230 repeats) on males and females have only recently begun to be appreciated. Premature ovarian failure is common among females with alleles in this repeat range. In female premutation carriers with more than 100 repeats, several studies have noted a tendency toward depression, interpersonal sensitivity, withdrawal behaviors, and schizotypal features. Male premutation carriers offer an intriguingly different profile. They can suffer anxiety and emotional lability, but they can also develop an intention tremor in the sixth decade of life that worsens until it interferes with quotidian tasks; these males subsequently develop gait ataxia and parkinsonian features.[23] Imaging studies of these male patients show global brain atrophy with dilated ventricles and signs of deep brain white matter disease.

There have been very few studies on the neuropathology of FRAXA patients. Neuroanatomical examination reveals abnormal dendritic spines that are immature and exceptionally long and tortuous. MRI studies are somewhat inconsistent, but show decreased size of the posterior vermis of the cerebellum, enlarged fourth ventricle, decreased hippocampal volumes, and increased volume of the caudate nucleus.

Differential Diagnosis

Any male or female child with delay in speech or motor development should be considered for fragile X testing, especially when there is a positive family history of mental retardation and absence of structural abnormalities of the brain. Other disorders that can produce similar early phenotypes are Soto syndrome, Prader-Willi syndrome, attention deficit hyperactivity disorder, and autism. DNA testing is usually necessary to establish the diagnosis, because the early features of FRAXA are nonspecific.

Molecular Genetics

Nearly all cases of FRAXA are caused by the expansion of an unstable CGG repeat in the 5' untranslated region of *FMR1*. There are occasional point mutations or deletions in this gene that produce a typical FRAXA phenotype (though without the manifestation of the fragile site), offering evidence that no other genes near *FMR1* contribute to the phenotype. The dynamic nature of the mutation explains why the risk for FRAXA increases with each generation, but the location of the gene on the X chromosome adds a certain measure of complexity to the inheritance pattern. A female premutation carrier has a 50% chance of passing on the unstable expansion to her offspring, as is true for any X-linked gene. The risk of the premutation becoming a full mutation is high, becoming greater with increasing repeat number; less than 5% of alleles with fewer than 60 repeats will expand to a full mutation, but half of those alleles with 60 to 80 repeats will expand to a full mutation, and nearly all expansions with 90 repeats will become a full mutation. As would be expected for X-linked inheritance, a male premutation carrier will pass the mutation on to his daughters but not to his sons. Interestingly, the premutation does not change dramatically when transmitted to his daughters; indeed, it may even contract. Even more strangely, the greater the premutation allele size of the father, the greater the likelihood the expansion will contract.

The severity of clinical features correlates inversely with the amount of *FMR1* protein (FMRP) produced. In the full mutation range, low protein levels (or complete absence of protein) results from hypermethylation and thus silencing of *FMR1*. Clinical involvement in premutation carriers thus presents something of a puzzle, since premutation alleles are usually not methylated. Low-repeat alleles do result in reduced FMRP levels, but the reduction is not due to impaired transcription of the gene; rather, reduced efficiency of translation seems to account for the protein deficit. Premutation carriers have quite elevated mRNA levels, perhaps reflecting a compensatory effort to stimulate transcription. Precisely how translation is impaired remains unknown. It may be that the CGG repeat forms a higher-order structure that blocks translation.

The functions of FMRP are just beginning to be elucidated. FRAXA patients display neurite morphology defects in the brain, which may be the basis of their mental retardation. The *Drosophila* homolog of *FMR1*, dfmr1, is required for normal neurite extension, guidance, and branching; dfmr1 mutants display strong eclosion failure and circadian rhythm defects. Interestingly, distinct neuronal cell types show different phenotypes, suggesting that dfmr differentially regulates diverse targets in the brain.[24] There has been, in fact, biochemical evidence that FMRP binds a subset of mRNAs and acts as a regulator of translation. More recently, it was discovered that a form of protein-synthesis–dependent synaptic plasticity (long-term depression triggered by activation of metabotropic glutamate receptors) is selectively enhanced in the hippocampus of mutant mice lacking FMRP. This finding indicates that FMRP plays an important role in regulating activity-dependent synaptic plasticity in the brain and suggests new therapeutic approaches for FRAXA.[25] The knockout mice exhibit immature dendritic spine morphology, behavioral deficits, and macro-orchidism reminiscent of the human

disease, and should provide an excellent model for interventional studies.

Therapy

Although there is no cure for FRAXA, supportive therapy, enriched environments, and special education are important for enhancing social interactions and targeting specific learning difficulties. Because children with FRAXA can have an increased incidence of recurrent ear infections, sinusitis, and strabismus, care should be taken to evaluate and treat these conditions (along with mitral valve prolapse and seizures) so that they do not hinder a child's ability to benefit from educational and behavioral therapies.

Fragile XE Mental Retardation

Clinical Features

Fragile XE (FRAXE) patients present a much milder clinical picture than FRAXA patients; they display none of the physical features of FRAXA and usually have mild mental retardation, learning deficits, and developmental delay. Some FRAXE individuals present with behavioral abnormalities, which may include attention deficit and hyperactivity. The prevalence of FRAXE is 1% to 4% that of FRAXA, and the cognitive deficits are milder in females, as expected for an X-linked trait.

Molecular Genetics

FRAXE is caused by an expansion of a CGG repeat in a folate-sensitive fragile site immediately adjacent to a CpG island, 600 kb distal to the FRAXA locus. The repeat size varies from 6 to 35 copies on normal alleles that are relatively stable on transmission, whereas repeat sizes in the premutation range (61 to 200) may expand to the full mutation (>200). Parent-of-origin effects are similar to those described above with FRAXA, except that reductions in repeat number are more frequently observed in FRAXE upon germline transmission, and males with the full mutation have affected daughters with full mutations.

The FRAXE CGG repeat resides in the promoter region of a gene termed *FMR2*. As with FRAXA, the expanded repeats are abnormally methylated, silencing transcription of *FMR2*. The *FMR2* gene product shows nuclear localization, DNA-binding capacity, and transcription transactivation potential; *FMR2* transcripts have been detected in multiple tissues. Within the brain, the hippocampus and the amygdala have the highest expression levels.

The cognitive and behavioral deficits in FRAXE likely result from transcriptional silencing of *FMR2* and subsequent loss of FMR2 protein function. Patients with deletions in *FMR2* resulting in loss-of-function mutations have phenotypes very similar to FRAXE individuals carrying an expanded repeat. FMR2 is a member of a family of proteins that have been associated with transcriptional activation; its high level of expression in areas of the brain involved in learning, memory, and emotion suggest that the pathogenic mechanism in FRAXE alters neuronal gene regulation. Mice lacking Fmr2 show a delay-dependent conditioned fear impairment. Interestingly, long-term potentiation is enhanced in hippocampal slices of Fmr2 knockout mice. Although a number of studies have suggested that diminished long-term potentiation is associated with memory impairment, these data suggest that increased long-term potentiation may lead to impaired cognitive processing as well.

FURTHER READING

We regret that space constraints preclude citing all the work that has contributed to our understanding of the clinical phenotypes of these diseases and their pathogenesis. We offer the following abbreviated list as a guide for further exploration, following the order of discussion in this chapter.

REFERENCES

1. Ishihara H, Kanda F, Nishio H, et al: Clinical features and skewed X-chromosome inactivation in female carriers of X-linked recessive spinal and bulbar muscular atrophy. J Neurol 2001;248:856–860.

2. Abel A, Walcott J, Woods J, et al: Expression of expanded repeat androgen receptor produces neurologic disease in transgenic mice. Hum Mol Genet 2001; 10:107–116.

3. Tobin AJ, Signer ER: Huntington's disease: The challenge for cell biologists. Trends Cell Biol 2000; 10: 531–536.

4. Dunah AW, Jeong H, Griffin A, et al: Sp1 and TAFII130 transcriptional activity disrupted in early Huntington's disease. Science 2002;296: 2238–2243. (See comment, pp 2149–2150.)

5. Zhang S, Xu L, Lee J, Xu T: Drosophila atrophin homolog functions as a transcriptional corepressor in multiple developmental processes. Cell 2002;108:45–56.

6. Shan DE, Soong BW, Sun CM, et al: Spinocerebellar ataxia type 2 presenting as familial levodopa-responsive parkinsonism. Ann Neurol 2001;50: 812–815.

7. Yoo, S-Y, Zoghbi HY: Dominantly inherited spinocerebellar syndromes. In Jones HR, De Vivo DC, Darras BT (eds): Neuromuscular Disorders of Infancy and Childhood: A Clinician's Approach. Woburn, MA, Butterworth-Heinemann, 2002, pp 1165–1183.

8. Yoshida H, Yoshizawa T, Shibasaki F, et al: Chemical chaperones reduce aggregate formation and cell death caused by the truncated Machado-Joseph disease gene product with an expanded polyglutamine stretch. Neurobiol Dis 2002;10:88–99.

9. Piedras-Renteria ES, Watase K, Harata N, et al: Increased expression of alpha 1A Ca^{2+} channel currents arising from expanded trinucleotide repeats in spinocerebellar ataxia type 6. J Neurosci 2001;21: 9185–9193.

10. Woodworth JA, Conn M, Beckett RS, et al: A composite of hereditary ataxias: A familiar disorder with features of olivopontocerebellar atrophy, Leber's optic atrophy and Friedreich's ataxia. Arch Intern Med 1959;104:594–606.

11. Nakamura K, Jeong SY, Uchihara T, et al: SCA17, a novel autosomal dominant cerebellar ataxia caused by an expanded polyglutamine in TATA-binding protein. Hum Mol Genet 2001;10:1441–1448.

12. Koob MD, Moseley ML, Schut LJ, et al: An untranslated CTG expansion causes a novel form of spinocerebellar ataxia (SCA8). Nat Genet 1999;21: 379–384.

13. Holmes SE, O'Hearn EE, McInnis MG, et al: Expansion of a novel CAG trinucleotide repeat in the 5′ region of PPP2R2B is associated with SCA12. Nat Genet 1999;23:391–392.

14. Zoghbi H, Botas J: Mouse and fly models of neurodegeneration. Trends Genet 2002;18:463–471.

15. Kopito RR: Aggresomes, inclusion bodies and protein aggregation. Trends Cell Biol 2000;10: 524–530.

16. Watase K, Weeber EJ, Xu B, et al: A long CAG repeat in the mouse Sca1 locus replicates SCA1 features and reveals the impact of protein solubility on selective neurodegeneration. Neuron 2002;34:905–919.

17. Hughes RE, Olson JM: Therapeutic opportunities in polyglutamine disease. Nat Med 2001;7:419–423.

18. Orr HT: Beyond the Qs in the polyglutamine diseases. Genes Dev 2001;15:925–932.

19. Fernandez-Funez P, Nino-Rosales ML, de Gouyon B, et al: Identification of genes that modify ataxin-1-induced neurodegeneration. Nature 2000;408. 101–106.

20. Yamamoto A, Lucas JJ, Hen R: Reversal of neuropathology and motor dysfunction in a conditional model of Huntington's disease. Cell 2000;101: 57–66.

21. Puccio H, Koenig M: Friedreich ataxia: A paradigm for mitochondrial diseases. Curr Opin Genet Dev 2002;3:272–277.

22. Lynch DR, Farmer JM, Balcer LJ, Wilson RB: Friedreich ataxia: Effects of genetic understanding on clinical evaluation and therapy. Arch Neurol 2002;59: 743–747.

23. Greco CM, Hagerman RJ, Tassone F, et al: Neuronal intranuclear inclusions in a new cerebellar tremor/ataxia syndrome among fragile X carriers. Brain 2002;125:1760–1771.

24. Moine H, Mandel JL: Do G quartets orchestrate fragile X pathology? Science 2001;294:2487–2488.

25. Gu Y, McIlwain KL, Weeber EJ, et al: Impaired conditioned fear and enhanced long-term potentiation in Fmr2 knock-out mice. J Neurosci 2002;22: 2753–2763.

Prion Diseases

Stephen J. DeArmond

Stanley B. Prusiner

Prions cause neurodegeneration. Diseases caused by prions are unusual in that they can be manifest as genetic, sporadic, and infectious disorders of the central nervous system (CNS). The human prion diseases are frequently referred to as Creutzfeldt-Jakob disease (CJD), Gerstmann-Sträussler-Scheinker disease (GSS), fatal familial insomnia (FFI), and kuru (Table 13–1). The prion diseases of animals include scrapie of sheep and goats, bovine spongiform encephalopathy (BSE), chronic wasting disease (CWD), and transmissible mink encephalopathy (TME).

Because prions and the mechanism of disease pathogenesis are unprecedented, the classification of the prion diseases has been quite varied. For many years, the human prion diseases were classified as neurodegenerative disorders of unknown etiology based upon pathologic changes confined to the CNS. With the transmission of kuru and CJD to apes, investigators began to view these diseases as CNS infectious illnesses caused by "slow viruses."[1] Although the familial nature of a subset of CJD cases was well described, the significance of this observation became more obscure with the transmission of CJD to animals.[2,3] Eventually, the meaning of heritable CJD became clear with the discovery of mutations in the PrP gene (*PRNP*).[4,5]

Neurodegenerative diseases were previously defined in terms of the neuropathology that each produced. The selected sets of neurons afflicted in neurodegenerative diseases have been used as a basis for classifying these diseases.[6] Based on studies over the past 20 years, we can now classify neurodegenerative diseases in terms of the proteins that are misprocessed in these disorders (see also Chapter 4, reference 7). Prion diseases are all caused by the misprocessing of the prion protein (PrP). The details of this misprocessing are described here and in Chapter 2.

The history of prion diseases is a fascinating saga in the annals of biomedical science. For nearly five decades with no clue as to the cause, physicians watched patients with CJD die, often within a few months of its onset.[8–10] CJD prions destroy the brain while the body remains unaware of this process. No febrile response, no leukocytosis or pleocytosis, and no humoral immune response are mounted in response to this devastating disease. Despite its recognition as a distinct clinical entity, CJD remained a rare disease; first, it was the province of neuropsychiatrists and later, neurologists and neuropathologists. Although multiple cases of CJD were recognized in families quite early,[2,11–19] this observation did little to advance understanding of the disorder.

The unraveling of the etiology of CJD is a wonderful story that has many threads, each representing a distinct piece of the puzzle. An important observation was made by Igor Klatzo in 1959, when he recognized that the neuropathology of kuru resembled that of CJD[20]; the same year, William Hadlow suggested that kuru, a disease of New Guinea highlanders, was similar to scrapie, a hypothesis also based on light microscopic similarities of brain sections.[21] But Hadlow's insight was much more profound because he suggested that kuru is a transmissible disease like scrapie and that demonstration of the infectivity of kuru could be accomplished using chimpanzees because they are so closely related to humans. He also noted that many months or years might be required before clinically recognizable disease would be seen in these inoculated non human primates. Moreover, he argued that brain tissue from patients dying of kuru should be homogenized and injected intracerebrally into the chimpanzees, as was often done in studies of sheep scrapie.

TABLE 13–1. The Prion Diseases

Disease	Host	Mechanism of pathogenesis
A. Kuru	Fore people	Infection through ritualistic cannibalism
iCJD*	Humans	Infection from prion-contaminated HGH, dura mater grafts, etc.
vCJD	Humans	Infection from bovine prions?
fCJD	Humans	Germline mutations in PrP gene
GSS	Humans	Germline mutations in PrP gene
FFI	Humans	Germline mutation in PrP gene (D178N, M129)
sCJD	Humans	Somatic mutation or spontaneous conversion of PrP^{PC} into PrP^{Sc}?
sFI	Humans	Somatic mutation or spontaneous conversion of PrP^{PC} into PrP^{Sc}?
B. Scrapie	Sheep	Infection in genetically susceptible sheep
BSE	Cattle	Infection with prion-contaminated MBM
TME	Mink	Infection with prions from sheep or cattle
CWD	Deer, elk	Unknown
FSE	Cats	Infection with prion-contaminated beef
exotic ungulate encephalopathy	Greater kudu, nyala, oryx	Infection with prion-contaminated MBM

*Abbreviations: BSE, bovine spongiform encephalopathy; CJD, Creutzfeldt-Jakob disease; sCJD, sporadic CJD; fCJD, familial CJD; iCJD, iatrogenic CJD; vCJD, variant CJD; CWD, chronic wasting disease; FFI, fatal familial insomnia; FSE, feline spongiform encephalopathy; GSS, Gerstmann-Sträussler-Scheinker disease; HGH, human growth hormone; MBM, meat and bone meal; sFI, sporadic fatal insomnia; TME, transmissible mink encephalopathy.

At the time Hadlow's hypothesis was set forth, scrapie was considered to be caused by a slow virus. The term *slow virus* had been coined by Bjorn Sigurdsson in 1954 based on his studies in Iceland on scrapie and visna of sheep.[22] Although Hadlow suggested that kuru, like scrapie, was caused by a slow virus, he did not perform the experiments required to demonstrate this phenomenon.[21,23] In fact, seven years were to pass before the transmissibility of kuru was established by passaging the disease to chimpanzees,[24] and in 1968, the transmission of CJD to chimpanzees after intracerebral inoculation was reported.[1]

An early clue to the unusual properties of the scrapie agent emerged from studies of 18,000 sheep that were inadvertently inoculated with the scrapie agent or slow virus. These animals had been vaccinated against louping ill virus with a formalin-treated suspension of ovine brain and spleen that, as was subsequently shown, had been contaminated with the scrapie agent.[25] Three different batches of vaccines were administered, and two years later, 1500 sheep developed scrapie. These findings demonstrated that the scrapie agent is resistant to inactivation by formalin, unlike most viruses, which are readily inactivated by such treatment.

The unusual biologic properties of the scrapie agent were no less puzzling than the disease process itself, for the infectious agent caused devastating degeneration of the CNS in the absence of an inflammatory response.[26,27] Although the immune system remained intact, its surveillance system was unaware of a raging infection. The infectious agent that causes scrapie, now generally referred to as a prion, achieved status as a scientific curiosity when its extreme resistance to ionizing and ultraviolet (UV) irradiation was discovered.[28–30] Later, similar resistance to inactivation by UV and ionizing radiation was reported for the CJD agent.[31] Tikvah Alper's radiation-resistance data on the scrapie agent evoked a torrent of hypotheses concerning its composition. Suggestions as to the nature of the scrapie agent ranged from small DNA viruses to membrane fragments to polysaccharides to proteins, the last of which eventually proved to be correct.[32–38]

Because the scrapie agent had been passaged from sheep into mice,[39] scrapie was the most amenable of these diseases to study experimentally. While the agents causing scrapie, CJD, and kuru were for many years thought to be different slow viruses, we now know that prions cause all these disorders and that this distinction was artificial.

Studies of prions have wide implications, ranging from basic principles of protein conformation to the development of effective therapies for prion diseases.[40] In this chapter, we review the naturally occurring human and animal prion diseases; in addition, we describe some of the molecular genetic studies performed in experimental animals.

PRION BIOLOGY AND DISEASES

The sporadic form of CJD is the most common prion disorder in humans and typically presents with dementia and myoclonus. Sporadic CJD (sCJD) accounts for approximately 85% of all cases of human prion disease while inherited prion diseases account for 10% to 15% of all cases. Familial CJD (fCJD), GSS, and FFI are all dominantly inherited prion diseases caused by mutations in the PrP gene.[4,41–44]

Even though the familial nature of a subset of CJD cases had been well described,[10] the significance of this observation became more obscure with the transmission of CJD to animals.[1] The conundrum that faced investigators reporting transmission of familial cases of CJD and GSS to apes and monkeys[3,18] is of considerable interest. They offered three hypotheses to explain fCJD and GSS. First, the "CJD virus" was transmitted to family members living in close proximity. Second, patients with fCJD or GSS carried a genetic predisposition to the ubiquitous CJD virus. Third, the CJD virus was transmitted from parent to offspring either *in utero* or during birth as was later seen with HIV. All three explanations proved to be incorrect: The CJD virus does not exist and the familial prion diseases are caused by mutations in the PrP gene.[45]

The prion concept readily explains how a disease can be manifest as a heritable or sporadic disorder as well as an infectious illness. Moreover, the hallmark common to all of the prion diseases, whether sporadic, dominantly inherited, or acquired by infection, is that they involve the aberrant metabolism of PrP.

In both the sporadic and inherited prion diseases, infectious prions are generated *de novo* within the host. The infectious prion is composed of an abnormal isoform of PrP, designated PrP^{Sc} (Table 13–2). PrP^{Sc} is derived from the normal, cellular PrP isoform, designated PrP^C. In the sporadic prion diseases, wild-type (wt) PrP^C is converted into wt PrP^{Sc}, which is infectious. In the inherited prion diseases, mutant PrP^C is converted into mutant PrP^{Sc}, which in some cases appears to be able to stimulate the conversion of wt PrP^C into wt PrP^{Sc}. In these diseases, the process of prion formation begins endogenously. The accumulation of sufficient wt PrP^{Sc} to establish a slow infection and ultimately disease is a rare event and is presumably governed by both the frequency of PrP^{Sc} formation and the rate of PrP^{Sc} clearance. In contrast, the accumulation of sufficient mutant PrP^{Sc} to establish a slow infection and ultimately disease is a much more frequent event since all people carrying a PrP mutation will develop disease if they live long enough.[46,47] Whether some pathologic PrP mutations act primarily by increasing the frequency of PrP^{Sc} formation and others by decreasing the rate of PrP^{Sc} clearance remains to be established.

Six diseases of animals are caused by prions (see Table 13–1). Scrapie of sheep and goats is the prototypic prion disease. TME, CWD, BSE, feline spongiform encephalopathy (FSE), and exotic ungulate encephalopathy are all thought to occur after the consumption of prion-infected foodstuffs.

Epidemiology

Prions cause CJD in humans throughout the world. The incidence of sCJD is approximately 1 case per million people,[48] but is nearly 5 per million people between ages 60 and 74 years (Fig. 13–1).[49] Patients as young as 17 years and as old as 83 years have been recorded.[48,50] CJD is a relentlessly progressive malady that results in death usually within a year of onset. Each geographic cluster of prion disease was initially thought to be a

TABLE 13–2. Glossary of Prion Terminology

Term	Description
Prion	A proteinaceous infectious particle that lacks nucleic acid. Prions are composed largely, if not entirely, of PrP^{Sc} molecules.
PrP^{Sc}	Abnormal, pathogenic isoform of the prion protein that causes illness. This protein is the only identifiable macromolecule in purified preparations of prions.
PrP^C	Normal, cellular isoform of the prion protein.
PrP 27–30	Fragment of PrP^{Sc} after digestion with proteinase K, generated by hydrolysis of the N-terminus.
PRNP	Human PrP gene located on chromosome 20.
Prnp	Mouse PrP gene located on syntenic chromosome 2. *Prnp* controls the length of the prion incubation time and is congruent with the incubation time genes *Sinc* and *Prn-i*. PrP-deficient (*Prnp$^{0/0}$*) mice are resistant to prions.
PrP amyloid	Fibril of PrP fragments derived from PrP^{Sc} by proteolysis. Plaques containing PrP amyloid are found in the brains of some mammals with prion disease.
Prion rod	An amyloid polymer composed of PrP 27–30 molecules. Created by detergent extraction and limited proteolysis of PrP^{Sc}.
Protein X	A hypothetical macromolecule that is thought to act like a molecular chaperone in facilitating the conversion of PrP^C into PrP^{Sc}.

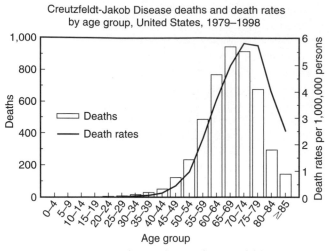

FIGURE 13–1. Age-specific incidence of Creutzfeldt-Jakob disease in the United States. Total numbers of deaths for the period 1979 to 1998 are shown by the open bars and the death rates per million population are depicted by the solid line. (Graph prepared by Lawrence Schonberger.)

manifestation of the communicability of the CJD virus,[51] but each was later shown to be due to a *PRNP* gene mutation, which results in a nonconservative substitution. Although infectious prion diseases account for less than 1% of all cases, and infection does not seem to play an important role in the natural history of these illnesses, the transmissibility of prions is an important biologic feature. Attempts to identify common exposure to some etiologic agent have been unsuccessful for both the sporadic and familial cases.[52] Ingestion of scrapie-infected sheep or goat meat as a cause of CJD in humans has not been demonstrated by epidemiologic studies although speculation about this potential route of infection continues.[53] Studies with Syrian hamsters demonstrated that oral infection by prions can occur, but the process is quite inefficient compared to intracerebral inoculation.[54]

Why the human prion diseases are so rare compared to the more common disorders of Alzheimer disease and Parkinson disease is unknown. Indeed, Alzheimer disease is about four times more common than Parkinson disease and approximately 10,000 times more common than CJD. Deciphering the mechanism of these remarkable differences in prevalence may help elucidate the factors underlying the etiologies and pathogeneses of these maladies.

Neuropathology

Frequently, the brains of patients with CJD show no recognizable abnormalities upon gross examination. In patients surviving several years, variable degrees of cerebral atrophy are likely to result in brain weights as low as 850 g.

The pathologic hallmarks of CJD at the light microscopic level are spongiform degeneration and astrogliosis

(Fig. 13–2*A*, *B*).[55] The lack of an inflammatory response in CJD and other prion diseases is an important feature of these degenerative disorders. Generally, the spongiform changes occur in the cerebral cortex, putamen, caudate nucleus, thalamus, and molecular layer of the cerebellum. Spongiform degeneration is characterized by many 5-μm to 20-μm vacuoles in the neuropil between nerve cell bodies. Astrocytic gliosis is a constant but nonspecific feature of prion diseases.[56] Widespread proliferation of fibrous astrocytes is found throughout the gray matter of brains infected with CJD prions. Astrocytic processes filled with glial filaments form extensive networks.

Amyloid plaques have been found in approximately 10% of CJD cases. Purified CJD prions from humans and animals exhibit the ultrastructural and histochemical characteristics of amyloid.[57] In first passage from some Japanese CJD cases, amyloid plaques were found in mouse brains.[58] These plaques stained with antiserum raised against PrP.

The amyloid plaques of GSS are distinct from those seen in kuru, Alzheimer disease, or scrapie. GSS plaques consist of a central dense core of amyloid surrounded by smaller globules of amyloid (Fig. 13–2*C,D*). Ultrastructurally, they consist of a radiating network of amyloid fibrils with scant or no neuritic degeneration. The plaques can be distributed throughout the brain but are most frequently found in the cerebellum. They are often located adjacent to blood vessels. Congophilic angiopathy has been noted in some cases of GSS. In addition to the multicentric plaques of GSS, unicentric kuru plaques may also be seen.[18] In GSS caused by the F198S mutation, neurofibrillary tangles (NFT) composed of paired helical filaments (PHF) are frequently seen surrounding PrP amyloid plaques.[41,59]

In variant CJD (vCJD), a characteristic feature is the presence of "florid plaques." These are composed of a central core of PrP amyloid surrounded by vacuoles in a pattern suggesting petals on a flower (Fig. 13–2*E, F*).

MOLECULAR PATHOGENESIS OF PRION DISEASE

Pathogenesis of PrP Amyloid

The first evidence that PrP^{Sc} participates in the pathogenesis of prion diseases was the finding that the amyloid plaques in human and animal prion diseases react specifically with PrP antibodies (see Fig. 13–2).[60–65] However, amyloid plaques are not a constant feature of prion diseases. They are detected by standard hematoxylin and eosin (H&E) stain, periodic acid–Schiff (PAS) reaction, or Congo red dye stain in only 5% to 10% of CJD and 50% to 70% of kuru cases.[18] By definition, all patients with GSS have amyloid plaques because the diagnosis requires the triad of cerebellar and/or corticospinal tract degeneration, dementia, and cerebral amyloidosis.[66]

In experimental scrapie of rodents, amyloid plaques are found in some but not all instances. Amyloid deposi-

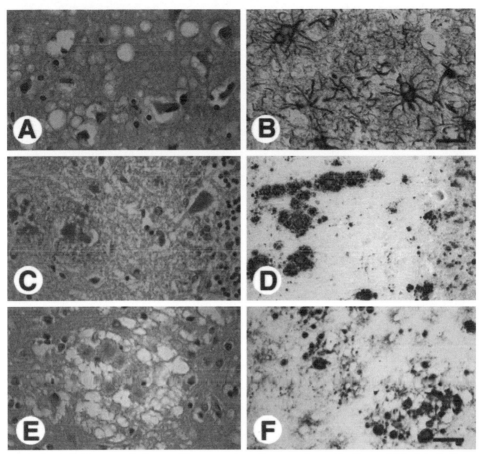

FIGURE 13–2. (See Color Plate III) Neuropathology of human prion diseases. Sporadic Creutzfeldt-Jakob disease (sCJD) is characterized by vacuolation of the neuropil of the gray matter, by exuberant reactive astrocytic gliosis, the intensity of which is proportional to the degree of nerve cell loss, and rarely by PrP amyloid plaque formation (not shown). The neuropathology of familial CJD is similar. GSS(P102L), as well as other inherited forms of Gerstmann-Straussler-Scheinker disease (not shown), is characterized by numerous deposits of PrP amyloid throughout the central nervous system. Variant CJD (vCJD) has clinical and epidemiological features that suggest it was acquired by infection with bovine spongiform encephalopathy (BSE) prions. The neuropathological features of vCJD are unique among CJD cases because of the abundance of PrP amyloid plaques that are often surrounded by a halo of intense vacuolation. *A*, sCJD, cerebral cortex stained with hematoxylin and eosin showing widespread spongiform degeneration; *B*, sCJD, cerebral cortex immunostained with anti-GFAP antibodies demonstrating the widespread reactive astrocytic gliosis; *C*, GSS, cerebellum with most of the GSS-plaques in the molecular layer (left 80% of micrograph) and many but not all stained positively for the periodic acid–Schiff (PAS) reaction. Granule cells and a single Purkinje cell are seen in the right 20% of the panel; *D*, GSS, cerebellum at the same location as *C* with PrP immunohistochemistry after hydrolytic autoclaving reveals more PrP plaques than seen with the PAS reaction; *E*, vCJD, cerebral cortex stained with hematoxylin and eosin shows that the plaque deposits are uniquely located within vacuoles. With this histology, these amyloid deposits have been referred to as "florid plaques"; *F*, vCJD, cerebral cortex stained with PrP immunohistochemistry after hydrolytic autoclaving reveals numerous PrP plaques often occurring in clusters as well as minute PrP deposits surrounding many cortical neurons and their proximal processes. Bar in *B* represents 50 μm and applies also to panels *A, C,* and *E*. Bar in *F* represents 100 μm and applies also to panel *D*.

tion depends on the prion isolate or "strain" used to inoculate the animal and on the sequence of the PrP gene. In fact, amyloidogenicity has been one characteristic used to define differences among prion isolates.[67] For example, the 87V prion isolate leads to the formation of well-defined PrP amyloid plaques in several inbred mouse strains, but 22A prions do not. Because the amino acid sequence of PrP in a particular murine host is the same regardless of the prion isolate, we are forced to postulate

that the amyloidogenic properties of 87V prions are the result of a specific conformation of PrP^{Sc} in contrast to the conformation of PrP^{Sc} in 22A prions, which do not give rise to PrP amyloid plaques.

The inherited prion diseases of humans show that formation of PrP amyloid is also related to the amino acid sequence of PrP. For example, in patients with GSS(P102L), PrP amyloid plaques containing the mutant protein always develop, as determined by amino acid sequencing.[4,68] In contrast, patients with fCJD(E200K) exhibit profound spongiform degeneration but do not show PrP amyloid accumulation.[44,69] Although PrP amyloid plaques always develop in patients with GSS, amyloidosis occurs in only those transgenic (Tg) mice that express a mouse PrP transgene mimicking the codon 102 mutation of GSS.[70,71] The deposition of PrP in these mice, designated Tg(MoPrP,P101L) mice, was greatly increased when the animals were crossed with PrP-deficient ($Prnp^{0/0}$) mice, in which the expression of wt PrP^C was eliminated. Based on these findings, it will be of interest to learn whether or not PrP amyloid plaques develop in patients homozygous for the E200K mutation through intermarriage.[44,69]

The amyloidogenic potential of PrP^{Sc} is probably inherent in its high content of β-sheet in that all amyloids are composed of proteins with a pleated β-sheet conformation.[72,73] PrP^{Sc} extracted from the brains of scrapie-infected Syrian hamsters has a high β-sheet content,[74,75] but this protein does not spontaneously polymerize into amyloid rods *in vitro*. After limited digestion of PrP^{Sc} by proteinase K (PK) in the presence of detergents, the resulting PrP 27–30 polymerizes into rods that bind Congo red dye and show green birefringence in polarized light.[57,76] The isolation of prion rods from human brains has been used to identify and verify cases of CJD.[77]

PrP^{Sc} Accumulation Causes CNS Dysfunction

Multiple lines of evidence indicate that accumulation of PrP^{Sc} in the gray matter causes spongiform degeneration and nerve cell loss. PrP^{Sc} is found in human and animal prion diseases.[63,77-80] Second, there is a temporal relationship between the accumulation of PrP^{Sc} and the development of neuropathology because spongiform degeneration and reactive astrocytic gliosis follow PrP^{Sc} accumulation.[81] Third, PrP^{Sc} accumulation, spongiform degeneration, and reactive astrocytic gliosis colocalize in the brains of mice and Syrian hamsters with scrapie.[63,82-84] Fourth, Tg mice that express MoPrP with the P102L mutation of GSS spontaneously develop a neurodegenerative disorder characterized by spongiform degeneration of gray matter and PrP amyloid plaque formation (see Fig. 13–2).[71,85]

Mechanisms of Prion Accumulation

Neurons appear to be the main source for PrP^{Sc} in the brain in that they express by far the highest levels of PrP mRNA[86,87]; in addition, neurons contain the highest levels of PrP^C.[63] The mechanisms of prion accumulation in the brain after inoculation of scrapie prions were examined in Syrian hamsters and in Tg mice expressing different PrP constructs. Two mechanisms were identified based on patterns of PrP^{Sc} accumulation.[88] Prions

spread along neuroanatomic pathways that interconnect neuronal populations. Presumably, PrP^{Sc} is carried by axonal transport mechanisms to synapses, where it is released and can infect the postsynaptic neurons, if they are susceptible. Axonal transport of PrP^C has been described.[89] Prions can also spread between regions not neuroanatomically interconnected through the CNS extracellular space where PrP diffuses rapidly to susceptible neuronal populations. That extracellular deposits of PrP accumulate in amyloid plaques in some of the prion diseases suggests that a proportion of PrP^{Sc} is released from sites of synthesis into the extracellular space of the CNS.

Selective Vulnerability of Neuronal Populations

CJD in humans and scrapie in animals are characterized by a diversity of clinical features. The concept that there are "strains" of scrapie agent (e.g., different prion isolates) to account for clinical diversity arose when a set of clinical features that could be transmitted faithfully among goats of the same genotype was found.[90] Furthermore, the early studies of scrapie in inbred mouse strains showed that clinical diversity was associated with distinct distributions of spongiform degeneration in the brain.[91] Thus, each prion isolate appeared to cause degeneration of different nerve cell populations. More recently, selective targeting of neuronal populations by prion isolates was clearly demonstrated by the histoblot method for localizing PrP^{Sc}.[88]

The best examples of selective targeting of neuronal populations by prion isolates for the synthesis and accumulation of PrP^{Sc} are found in Tg mice that express high levels of Syrian hamster (SHa) PrP^C. In these Tg(SHaPrP) mice, incubation times for the Sc237 and 139H prion isolates after intrathalamic inoculation were the same (50 days); however, fewer brain regions accumulated SHaPrP^{Sc} with Sc237 than with 139H prions.[82] The neuroanatomic distribution of SHaPrP^{Sc} was even more restricted with the Me7H isolate than with Sc237 prions in Tg(SHaPrP) mice.[84] Even though all of the prion isolates were inoculated into the thalamus, the thalamus was only minimally affected by the Me7H isolate. The most intense SHaPrP^{Sc} signals were found in the hypothalamus, limbic lobe, and periaqueductal gray matter of the midbrain. The highly restricted distribution of PrP^{Sc} with the Me7H isolate could not be attributed to insufficient time for prions to spread in the brain because the incubation time for this isolate was approximately 185 days. Prion isolates passaged in an inbred mouse line showed a similar targeting of neurons.[92] Two mouse prion isolates, 87V and 22A, resulted in markedly different distributions of MoPrP^{Sc}; however, Rocky Mountain Laboratory (RML) prions inoculated into the same mouse line resulted in PrP^{Sc} distribution similar to that from 22A prions.

These findings argue that prion isolates target different nerve cell populations for conversion of PrP^C to nascent PrP^{Sc} and that the final distribution of PrP^{Sc} is independent of incubation time. Because the local accumulation of PrP^{Sc} appears to cause neuronal degeneration, the distribution of PrP^{Sc} is the main determinant of the clinical and neuropathologic differences that distinguish prion isolates. Although the selectivity of prion isolates for different neuronal populations was evident from these studies, the results also showed that the same brain regions were often targeted by more than one prion isolate. Whether this overlap is due to infection of different subpopulations of neurons in a brain region or if a specific nerve cell type can synthesize different prion isolates is unknown. Our current understanding of the molecular mechanisms underlying prion isolate diversity and neuronal targeting is incomplete. A more extended discussion of prion diversity can be found in Chapter 2 of this textbook.

EXPERIMENTAL PRION DISEASE

Once a PrP cDNA probe became available, molecular genetic studies were undertaken to determine whether the PrP gene controls scrapie incubation times in mice. Independent of the enriching of brain fractions for scrapie infectivity that led to the discovery of PrP^{Sc}, the PrP gene was shown to be genetically linked to a locus controlling the incubation time for experimental scrapie in mice.[93,94] Subsequently, mutation of the PrP gene was shown to be genetically linked to the development of familial prion disease.[4]

Tg Mice

The development of Tg mouse models that reproduce virtually every aspect of naturally occurring prion disease created a firm foundation upon which to decipher the molecular pathogenesis of prion disease. Tg mice expressing mutant PrP develop CNS degeneration spontaneously and transmit disease to inoculated recipients.[71] Tg(SHaPrP) mice were shown to render the animals highly susceptible to SHa prions, which demonstrated that expression of a foreign PrP gene could abrogate the "species barrier."[95,96] The species barrier is manifest as a prolongation of the incubation time upon first passage in a foreign host with shortening on the second passage in the new host.[32] As the level of PrP transgene expression was increased, the incubation time decreased.[96] The species barrier was reproduced in Tg mice expressing a mouse PrP molecule of 106 amino acids with two large deletions accounting for almost 50% of the residues. In these mice, a transmission barrier was observed after inoculation with prions from wt mice, but was abolished once miniprions composed of PrP^{Sc} with 106 residues were used as the inoculum.[97] In other studies, *Prnp*$^{0/0}$ mice were found to be resistant to prion infection and

failed to replicate prions, as expected.[98,99] The results of these studies indicated that PrP must play a central role in the transmission and pathogenesis of prion disease, but equally important, they helped establish that the abnormal isoform is an essential component of the prion particle.[100]

PrP Gene Control of Incubation Time

Scrapie incubation times in mice were used to distinguish prion strains and to identify a gene controlling its length.[101,102] This gene was initially called *Sinc* based on genetic crosses between inbred C57Bl and VM mice that exhibited short and long incubation times, respectively.[101] Because the distribution of VM mice was restricted, we searched for another mouse with long incubation times. Inbred (Iln) mice proved to be a suitable substitute for VM mice; eventually, ILn and VM mice were found to be derived from a common ancestor. Using first genetic linkage and later Tg mice, the PrP gene was shown to control the length of the scrapie incubation time in mice.[92–94]

Overexpression of Wild-Type PrP Transgenes

Mice were constructed expressing different levels of the wt SHaPrP transgene.[95] Inoculation of these Tg(SHaPrP) mice with SHa prions demonstrated abrogation of the species barrier, resulting in abbreviated incubation times due to a nonstochastic process.[96] The length of the incubation time after inoculation with SHa prions was inversely proportional to the level of SHaPrP^C in the brains of Tg(SHaPrP) mice.[96] Bioassays of brain extracts from clinically ill Tg(SHaPrP) mice inoculated with mouse (Mo) prions revealed that Mo prions but no SHa prions were produced. Conversely, inoculation of Tg(SHaPrP) mice with SHa prions led only to the synthesis of SHa prions. These studies demonstrated that the rate of PrP^{Sc} formation is directly proportional to the level of PrP^C expression in Tg mice but the level to which PrP^{Sc} accumulates is independent of PrP^C concentration.[96]

Prnp$^{0/0}$ Mice

The development and lifespan of two lines of *Prnp*$^{0/0}$ mice were indistinguishable from controls.[103,104] In these two *Prnp*$^{0/0}$ lines with normal development, altered sleep-wake cycles[105] and synaptic behavior in brain slices have been reported,[106,107] but the synaptic changes could not be confirmed by others.[108,109]

Resistance to Prions

Prnp$^{0/0}$ mice are resistant to prions.[98,99] *Prnp*$^{0/0}$ mice were sacrificed 5 days, 60 days, 120 days, and 315 days after inoculation with RML prions and brain extracts were bioassayed in CD-1 Swiss mice. Except for residual infectivity from the inoculum detected at 5 days after inoculation, no infectivity was detected in the brains of $Prnp^{0/0}$ mice.[99] One group of investigators found that $Prnp^{0/0}$ mice inoculated with RML prions and sacrificed 20 weeks later had $10^{3.6}$ infectious (ID_{50}) units/ml of homogenate by bioassay.[98] Others have used this report to argue that prion infectivity replicates in the absence of PrP.[110, 111] Neither we nor the authors of the initial report could confirm the finding of prion replication in $Prnp^{0/0}$ mice.[9,112]

DOPPEL AND *PRN* GENE FAMILY

Studies on a third line of $Prnp^{0/0}$ mice found that these animals developed ataxia and Purkinje cell degeneration at ~70 weeks of age.[113] The ataxia and Purkinje cell degeneration exhibited by this line of $Prnp^{0/0}$ mice and by another line of $Prnp^{0/0}$ mice was found to be due to the overexpression of an adjacent gene, *Prnd*, which encodes the protein doppel (Dpl).[114] The Dpl and PrP genes form the *Prn* gene family; the Dpl gene lies approximately 18 kb downstream from the PrP allele. PrP and Dpl represent ancient gene duplication with considerable sequence divergence but structural conservation.[115]

Dpl Protein

The mouse Dpl gene encodes a protein of 179 residues, which is approximately 25% homologous with mouse PrP. Like PrP, Dpl is a sialoglycoprotein that is anchored to the surface of cells by a glycosyl phosphatidyl-inositol (GPI) anchor.[116] Dpl is expressed at high levels only in the testis[114] in contrast to PrP, which is expressed in many tissues with the levels in the brain being the highest. Dpl-deficient male mice are sterile.[117] The function of neither Dpl nor PrP is known.

In mice developing cerebellar degeneration, high levels of an intergenic mRNA were found in which the two untranslated exons of *Prnp* were spliced to the *Prnd* exon containing the open reading frame (ORF) or protein-coding region.[114,118] High levels of Dpl protein expression were found to be toxic for Purkinje cells, but overexpression of PrP rescued the ataxic phenotype.[119]

Tg Mice Expressing Dpl

When $Prnp^{0/0}$ mice overexpressing Dpl were crossed with mice expressing PrP^C, Purkinje cell degeneration was prevented. In other studies, Tg(Dpl)$Prnp^{0/0}$ mice developed ataxia due to Purkinje cell degeneration, demonstrating that Dpl overexpression, as suggested by earlier studies on $Prnp^{0/0}$ mice, is responsible for cerebellar degeneration.[120] Crossing Tg(Dpl)$Prnp^{0/0}$ mice with $Prnp^{+/+}$ mice

prevented Purkinje cell degeneration, as found earlier with one line of $Prnp^{0/0}$ mice.[119]

Inducible PrP Transgenes

To control the expression of PrP^C in Tg mice, a tetracycline transactivator (tTA) driven by the PrP gene control elements and a tTA-responsive operator linked to a PrP gene were used.[121] Adult Tg mice showed no deleterious effects upon repression of PrP^C expression greater than 90% by doxycycline administered orally, but the mice developed progressive ataxia at approximately 50 days after inoculation with prions unless maintained on doxycycline.[122] Although Tg mice on doxycycline accumulated low levels of PrP^{Sc}, they showed no neurologic dysfunction, indicating that low levels of PrP^{Sc} can be tolerated. Use of the tTA system to control PrP expression allowed production of Tg mice with high levels of PrP that otherwise cause many embryonic and neonatal deaths. Measurement of PrP^{Sc} clearance in Tg mice should be possible, facilitating the development of pharmacotherapeutics.

STRAINS OF PRIONS

The biological properties of prion strains are enciphered in the conformation of PrP^{Sc}. The mechanism by which the conformation of PrP^{Sc} is transferred to PrP^C as nascent prions are formed is unknown. Moreover, the code used to encipher the biological properties of a particular prion strain in the tertiary structure of PrP^{Sc} is also unknown, as described elsewhere.[123]

Mechanism of Selective Neuronal Targeting

In addition to incubation times, neuropathologic profiles of spongiform change have been used to characterize prion strains.[124] However, studies with PrP transgenes argue that such profiles are not an intrinsic feature of strains.[125,126] The mechanism by which prion strains modify the pattern of spongiform degeneration was perplexing since earlier investigations had shown that PrP^{Sc} deposition precedes neuronal vacuolation and reactive gliosis.[63] When FFI prions were inoculated into mice expressing chimeric mouse-human transgenes [Tg(MHu2M)], PrP^{Sc} was confined largely to the thalamus (Fig. 13–3A), as is the case for FFI in humans.[127] In contrast, fCJD(E200K) prions inoculated into Tg(MHu2M) mice produced widespread deposition of PrP^{Sc} throughout the cortical mantle and many of the deep structures of the CNS (Fig. 13–3B), as is seen in fCJD(E200K) of humans. To examine whether the diverse patterns of PrP^{Sc} deposition are influenced by Asn-linked glycosylation of PrP^C, we constructed Tg mice expressing PrPs mutated at one or both of the Asn-linked glycosylation consensus sites.[126] These mutations

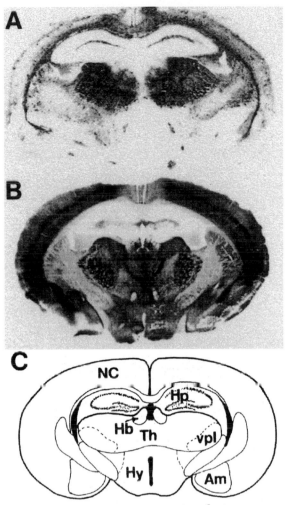

FIGURE 13–3. Regional distribution of PrP^{Sc} deposition in Tg(MHu2M)$Prnp^{0/0}$ mice inoculated with prions from humans who died of inherited prion diseases. Histoblot of PrP^{Sc} deposition in a coronal section of a Tg(MHu2M)$Prnp^{0/0}$ mouse through the hippocampus and thalamus.[127] *A,* A Tg mouse was inoculated with a brain extract prepared from a patient who died of FFI. *B,* A Tg mouse was inoculated with an extract from a patient with familial Creutzfeldt-Jakob disease (fCJD)(E200K). Cryostat sections were mounted on nitrocellulose and treated with proteinase K to eliminate PrP^{C}.[217] To enhance the antigenicity of PrP^{Sc}, the histoblots were exposed to 3 M guanidinium isothiocyanate before immunostaining using α-PrP 3F4 mAb.[283] *C,* Labelled diagram of a coronal section of the hippocampus/thalamus region. NC, neocortex; Hp, hippocampus; Hb, habenula; Th, thalamus; vpl, ventral posterior lateral thalamic nucleus; Hy, hypothalamus; Am, amygdala. (Reprinted with permission from Almqvist & Wiksell International, copyright 1998 by The Nobel Foundation.)

resulted in aberrant neuroanatomic topologies of PrP^{C} within the CNS, whereas pathologic point mutations adjacent to the consensus sites did not alter the distribution of PrP^{C}. Tg mice with a mutation of the second PrP

glycosylation site exhibited prion incubation times of greater than 500 days and unusual patterns of PrP^{Sc} deposition. As noted earlier, glycosylation can modify the conformation of PrP and affect either the turnover of PrP^{C} or the clearance of PrP^{Sc}. Regional differences in the rate of deposition or clearance might result in specific patterns of PrP^{Sc} accumulation.

HUMAN PRION DISEASES

The human prion diseases present as infectious, genetic, and sporadic disorders.[128] This unprecedented spectrum of disease presentations demanded a new mechanism; prions provide a conceptual framework within which this remarkably diverse spectrum of etiologies can be accommodated.

Human prion disease should be considered in any patient who develops a progressive subacute or chronic decline in cognitive or motor function.[129] Most cases of human prion disease present with rapidly progressive dementia, but some manifest cerebellar ataxia. Although the brains of patients appear grossly normal upon postmortem examination, they usually show spongiform degeneration and astrocytic gliosis under the light microscope (see Fig. 13–2). In all cases of GSS and vCJD, PrP amyloid plaques are found.[130] Before PrP immunostaining was available, histochemical staining was used to examine brains from kuru patients in which approximately 70% of cases were thought to have amyloid plaques.[20] The presence or absence of PrP amyloid plaques in sporadic and inherited CJD is quite variable.[56]

SPORADIC PRION DISEASES

In humans, more than 85% of all prion disease is sporadic. Yet sporadic prion disease, generally referred to as sCJD, is relatively infrequent. The incidence of sCJD is generally thought to be 1 to 2 cases per 1 million people worldwide.[48] Despite numerous attempts to find an infectious or genetic etiology for sCJD, none has been identified. In people with sporadic prion disease, no mutation of the PrP gene has been found and no exogenous source of prions can be identified.

Most people with sCJD present with rapidly progressive dementia, but some manifest cerebellar ataxia initially.[3,131] Patients with sCJD usually have an onset of symptoms between ages 40 and 80 years. The highest rates of sCJD are found between the ages of 65 and 75 (see Fig. 13–1).[49,132] A small number of patients with fatal insomnia (FI) has also been identified with no family history of the disease. Patients with sporadic FI (sFI) do not carry a mutation in their PrP genes.[133–136]

In animals, there is no information on the frequency of sporadic prion disease. It seems likely that scrapie presents as a sporadic disease in some sheep and then spreads to others as an infectious illness.[137] It has been hypothesized that a case of sporadic prion disease was responsible for an outbreak of TME in Stetsonville, Wisconsin.[138] It has also been suggested that BSE might have started with a sporadic case of prion disease in a cow in southern England.[139]

Etiology of sCJD

The mechanism by which sporadic prion disease is initiated in humans and animals is unknown. One mechanism may be a somatic mutation. In this scenario, a spontaneous mutation would occur in a cell capable of transforming PrP^C into PrP^{Sc}. The spontaneous formation of prions would then evolve in a manner similar to that for germline mutations in inherited disease. In this situation, the mutant PrP^{Sc} must be capable of recruiting wt PrP^C, a process known to be possible for some mutations (e.g., E200K, D178N) but less likely for others (e.g., P102L).[140]

In a second scenario, the activation barrier separating wt PrP^C from PrP^{Sc} could be crossed on rare occasions when viewed in the context of a large population of molecules (Fig. 13–4).[141] PrP^C is constantly being synthesized and degraded. Over a 70-year period (the typical age of onset for sCJD), a large population of PrP^C molecules will have been produced, any one of which could spontaneously transform into PrP^{Sc} to initiate the propagation of prions.

A third scenario can be envisioned, in which PrP^{Sc} is formed physiologically but at sufficiently low levels that it cannot be detected by bioassay in laboratory rodents. In other words, normal brains contain fewer than 10^6 PrP^{Sc} molecules per ml of 10% (w/v) homogenate because such brains do not transmit prion disease (one ID$_{50}$ unit of prions is thought to contain approximately 10^6 PrP^{Sc} molecules).[57] Studies with recombinant antibody fragments (recFabs) show that PrP^{Sc} is cleared from scrapie-infected neuroblastoma (ScN2a) cells with a $t_{1/2}$ of approximately 30 hours.[142] These findings argue that PrP^{Sc} might be made at low levels constantly and becomes deleterious only when the rate of formation exceeds the rate of clearance. Once this happens, PrP^{Sc} begins to accumulate and eventually the level of PrP^{Sc} is sufficiently high to cause disease. Which, if any, of the foregoing three scenarios is correct remains to be established.

PRP GENE POLYMORPHISMS

Codon 129 Polymorphism

At PrP codon 129, an amino acid polymorphism encoding Met or Val was identified (Fig. 13–5).[143] This polymorphism appears able to influence prion disease expression in not only the sporadic form, but also in the iatrogenic and inherited forms of prion disease.[144–146]

Studies of Caucasian patients with sCJD have shown that most are homozygous for Met or Val at codon 129.[144] This contrasts with the general

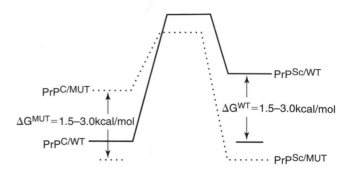

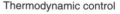

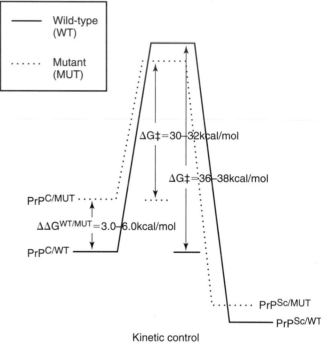

Thermodynamic control

Kinetic control

FIGURE 13–4. An illustration of the distinction between thermodynamic and kinetic models for the energetics of the conversion of PrP^C carrying the wild-type (WT) and mutant (MUT) sequences into PrP^{Sc}. ΔG is the free energy difference between the PrP^C and PrP^{Sc} states and ΔG is the activation energy barrier separating these two states. ΔΔG$^{WT/MUT}$ is the difference between ΔG^{WT} and ΔG^{MUT}. The free energy diagrams for the wild-type sequences (solid lines), and the mutant sequences (broken lines) are shown. (Reprinted with permission from Annu Rev Biochem, copyright 1998 Annual Reviews.)

Caucasian population, in which frequencies for the codon 129 polymorphism are 12% Val/Val, 37% Met/Met, and 51% Met/Val.[147] In contrast, the frequency of the Val allele in the Japanese population is much lower[148,149]; heterozygosity (Met/Val) at codon 129 is more frequent (18%) in Japanese CJD patients than in the general Japanese population, in which the

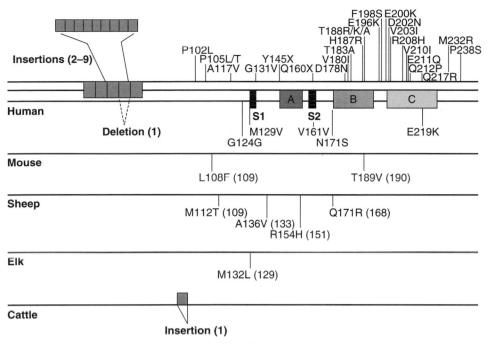

FIGURE 13–5. Mutations causing inherited prion disease and polymorphisms in human, mouse, sheep, elk, and cattle. Above the line of the human sequence are mutations that cause inherited prion disease. Below the lines are polymorphisms, some but not all of which are known to influence the onset as well as the phenotype of disease. Residue numbers in parentheses correspond to the human codons.

polymorphism frequencies are 0% Val/Val, 92% Met/Met, and 8% Met/Val.[150]

While no specific mutations have been identified in the PrP gene of patients with sCJD,[151] homozygosity at codon 129[144] is consistent with the results of Tg mouse studies. The finding that homozygosity at codon 129 predisposes to sCJD supports a model of prion production that favors PrP interactions between homologous proteins, as appears to occur in Tg mice expressing SHaPrP inoculated with either hamster prions or mouse prions,[95,96,100] as well as Tg mice expressing a chimeric SHa/Mo PrP transgene inoculated with "artificial" prions.[83]

Other Polymorphisms

A second polymorphism results in an amino acid substitution at codon 171 (Asn to Ser)[152], which lies adjacent to the binding site for a putative conversion cofactor, provisionally designated "protein X." This polymorphism has been found in Caucasians but it has not been studied extensively and it is not known to influence the frequency of prion disease. A third polymorphism is the deletion of a single octarepeat (24 bp), which has been found in 2.5% of whites.[153–155] In another study of more than 700 individuals, this single octarepeat deletion was found in 1.0% of the population.[156]

Dominant Negative Inhibition

A polymorphism resulting in an amino acid substitution at codon 219 (Glu/Lys) has been reported to occur with a frequency of about 12% in the Japanese population but not in whites (see Fig. 13–5).[144,157] Lys at 219 appears to protect against sCJD.[159] In ScN2a cells and Tg mice, substitution of lysine at position 218 of MoPrP produced dominant-negative inhibition of prion replication by preventing wt PrP^C from being converted into PrP^{Sc} (see also references 160 to 162). In addition, MoPrP^C(Q218K) could not be converted into PrP^{Sc} in either ScN2a cells or Tg(MoPrP, Q218K) *Prnp*$^{0/0}$ mice.

Dominant-negative inhibition of prion replication has been found in sheep with the substitution of the basic residue arginine at position 171. These sheep are resistant to naturally occurring scrapie.[163,164] Both the inability to support prion replication and the demonstration of dominant-negative inhibition by MoPrP(Q167R) have been demonstrated in ScN2a cells and Tg mice.[160–162] Codon 171 in sheep PrP corresponds to codon 167 in MoPrP. Like the Q218K polymorphism, MoPrP^C(Q167R) could not be converted into PrP^{Sc} in either ScN2a cells or Tg(MoPrP,Q167R)*Prnp*$^{0/0}$ mice.

Tg Mice Expressing Chimeric Human-Mouse PrP

Sporadic CJD transmits into Tg(MHu2M)22372/*Prnp*$^{0/0}$ mice with an incubation time of approximately 200 days.[165] Individual human residues in the chimeric MHu2M transgene were reverted to mouse residues to test whether these might improve susceptibility to human prions. Mutations were made at the N-terminal end of the human insert, at positions 96 (Ser to Asn), 108 (Met to Leu), and 111 (Met to Val), and at the C-terminal end of the human insert, at positions 165 (Met to Val) and 167 (Glu to Gln).[166] Additionally, residues M165 and E167 were mutated together to produce Tg(MHu2M,M165V, E167Q)22372/$Prnp^{0/0}$ mice, which express chimeric PrP at a level one to two times that of SHaPrP^C. Uninoculated mice from this line remain healthy at greater than 620 days. These mice were inoculated with brain homogenates from 10 different sCJD cases, one case of fCJD (E200K), one case of FFI(MV,D178N), and one case of sFI.[134] MV refers to the amino acids encoded at position 129 of HuPrP for each of the two alleles; MM or VV indicates homozygosity at codon 129. The mean incubation times after inoculation with sCJD(MM1) prions ranged from 106 to 114 days. No sCJD(VV2) cases have efficiently transmitted disease yet at greater than 450 days after inoculation. MM1 indicates that the deglycosylated PrP 27–30 molecule has an apparent molecular mass of 21 kDa that is denoted "type 1," whereas VV2 indicates a mass of 19 dKa, denoted "type 2." The fCJD(E200K) prions transmitted in 109 days (repassage: 100 days), similar to sCJD(MM1) prions, whereas FFI and sFI prions transmitted inefficiently, with mice becoming ill after an average incubation time of 263 ± 15 days ($n/n_0=5/6$; repassage 97 days) and 303 ± 20 days ($n/n_0=4/6$), respectively.

These strain-specific patterns of incubation times from different inocula are similar to those in Tg(MHu2M)5378/$Prnp^{0/0}$ mice. Tg(MHu2M)5378/$Prnp^{0/0}$ mice inoculated with brain homogenates from patients with fCJD(E200K) showed an incubation time of 170 ± 2 days ($n/n_0=10/10$) and no further shortening of incubation time on second passage. Inoculation of Tg(MHu2M)5378/$Prnp^{0/0}$ mice with brain homogenates from three patients with FFI(M129,D178N) led to incubation times on first passage of 247 ± 6 days ($n/n_0=7/7$), 206 ± 7 days (7/7), and 193 ± 5 days (9/9), whereas second passage yielded shorter incubation times of 123 ± 3 days (7/7), 132 ± 5 days (9/9), and 136 ± 1 days (6/6), respectively. The shortening of incubation times on second passage demonstrates a transmission barrier for FFI prions in Tg(MHu2M)5378/$Prnp^{0/0}$ mice.

Preliminary studies with Tg(MHu2M,M165V) 17030/$Prnp^{0/0}$ mice expressing MHu2MPrP(M165V) suggest that the M165V mutation alone might be sufficient to give shortened incubation times, since inoculation of these mice with sCJD(MM1) (RG) prions resulted in incubation times of 105 ± 2 days ($n/n_0=10/10$). This line expresses the transgene product at two to four times the PrP^C found in Syrian hamsters.

INHERITED PRION DISEASES

Familial CJD cases suggested that genetic factors might influence disease pathogenesis,[2,12,16] but this was difficult to reconcile with the transmissibility of fCJD and GSS.[18] The discovery of genetic linkage between the PrP gene and scrapie incubation times in mice[93] raised the possibility that mutations might feature in the hereditary human prion diseases. The P102L mutation was the first

PrP mutation to be genetically linked to CNS dysfunction in GSS (see Fig. 13–5).[4]

GSS and Genetic Linkage

The discovery that GSS, which was known to be a familial disease, could be transmitted to apes and monkeys was first reported when many still thought that scrapie, CJD, and related disorders were caused by viruses.[18] The discovery that the P102L mutation is genetically linked to GSS permitted the unprecedented conclusion that prion disease can have both genetic and infectious etiologies.[4,128] In that study, the codon 102 mutation was linked to development of GSS with a logarithm of the odds (LOD) score exceeding 3, demonstrating a tight association between the altered genotype and the disease phenotype (Table 13–3). This mutation may be caused by the deamination of a methylated CpG in a germline PrP gene, which results in the substitution of a thymine (T) for cytosine (C). This mutation has been found in many GSS families throughout the world,[167,168] including the original family described by Gerstmann, Sträussler, and Scheinker.[169]

To date, more than 30 different mutations in *PRNP* resulting in non-conservative substitutions have been found in the inherited human prion diseases (see Fig. 13–5).[59,170–175] Missense mutations and expansions in the octapeptide repeat region of the gene are responsible for familial forms of prion disease. Five different mutations of the PrP gene have been linked genetically to heritable prion disease.[4,41–44]

GSS in Tg Mice

The P102L mutation causing GSS in humans was engineered into mouse PrP at the corresponding position to produce a mutant transgene product designated PrP(P101L). Five different Tg lines expressing high levels

TABLE 13–3. Examples of Human PrP Gene Mutations Found in the Inherited Prion Diseases

Inherited Prion disease	PrP gene mutation
GSS	P102L*
GSS	A117V
fCJD	D178N, V129
FFI	D178N, M129*
GSS	F198S*
fCJD	E200K*
GSS	Q217R
fCJD	octarepeat insert*

* Signifies genetic linkage between the mutation and the inherited prion disease. 4, 41–44
Abbreviations: fCJD, familial Creutzfeldt-Jakob disease; FFI, fatal familial insomnia; GSS, Gerstmann-Sträussler-Scheinker disease.

of mouse PrP(P101L) developed signs of spontaneous CNS dysfunction from 50 to 200 days of age.[70,71,176] On neuropathologic examination, widespread vacuolation of the neuropil, astrocytic gliosis, and numerous PrP amyloid plaques similar to those seen in the brains of humans who die from GSS(P102L) were found. Although protease-resistant PrP^{Sc} was virtually undetectable by limited digestion of brain homogenates at 37°C with proteinase K, a protease-resistant mouse PrP^{Sc}(P101L) was detected by performing the digestion at 4°C, as previously reported for other mutant PrPs.[177]

Extracts from the brains of Tg mice expressing high levels of mouse PrP(P101L) transmitted disease to Tg mice, designated Tg196, expressing the same mutant transgene product at a low level. The inoculated Tg196 mice developed neurologic signs of disease approximately 240 days after receiving the brain extract, demonstrating that the disease could be serially transmitted. Uninoculated Tg196 mice infrequently develop spontaneous disease. A synthetic peptide of 55 residues carrying the P102L mutation produced disease in Tg196 mice approximately 360 days after inoculation and the illness could be serially transmitted.[178] Only the mutant peptide in a β sheet conformation induced by exposure to acetonitrile produced neurologic disease. These studies, combined with the transmission of prions from patients who died of GSS to apes and monkeys[18] or to Tg(MHu2M,P101L) mice,[140] offer compelling evidence that prions are generated *de novo* by mutations in PrP.

An artificial set of mutations in a PrP transgene consisting of A113V, A115V, and A118V produced neurodegeneration in neonatal mice; these Val substitutions were selected for their propensity to form β-sheet.[177-179] Brain extracts from these mice failed to transmit disease to inoculated rodents.

Phenotypic Variation among the Inherited Prion Diseases

Although phenotypes may vary dramatically within families, there is a tendency for certain phenotypes to associate with specific mutations.[59] A clinical phenotype indistinguishable from typical sCJD is usually seen with substitutions at codons 180, 183, 200, 208, 210, or 232. Substitutions at codons 117, 102, 105, 198, or 217 generally produce GSS disease. The normal human PrP sequence contains five repeats of an octapeptide sequence. Insertions of an additional two to nine extra octapeptide repeats are associated with variable phenotypes ranging from a condition indistinguishable from CJD to a slowly progressive dementing illness of many years' duration. A mutation at codon 178 resulting in substitution of Asn for Asp produces FFI if a Met is encoded at the polymorphic 129 residue on the same allele.[145] Typical CJD is seen if a Val is encoded at position 129 of the mutant allele.

Particularly puzzling are the factors that determine the disease phenotype. As noted earlier, there is excellent evidence that the tertiary structure of PrP^{Sc} determines whether this disease-causing protein is deposited in subsets of thalamic neurons to produce FI, or deposited more widely, resulting in CJD. As more cases of inherited prion disease have been studied, multiple exceptions have been recorded, including a mutation that produces GSS with ataxia and also results in a dementing illness.[180,181] Within a single family carrying a PrP mutation, some patients develop peripheral neuropathies while others do not.[4,16] Elucidating all of the factors that govern the clinical and neuropathologic phenotypes will be challenging.

fCJD Caused by Octarepeat Inserts

An insert of 144 bp containing six octarepeats at codon 53, in addition to the five that are normally present, was described in patients with CJD from four families residing in southern England.[5,43] Genealogic investigations have shown that all four families are related, arguing for a single founder born more than two centuries ago. The LOD score for this extended pedigree exceeds 11. Studies from several laboratories have demonstrated that inserts of two, four, five, six, seven, eight, or nine octarepeats in addition to the normal five are found in individuals with inherited CJD (see Fig. 13–5).[5,182]

fCJD in Libyan Jews

The unusually high incidence of CJD among Israeli Jews of Libyan origin was thought to be due to the consumption of lightly cooked sheep brain or eyeballs.[51] Molecular genetic investigations revealed that Libyan and Tunisian Jews with fCJD have a PrP gene point mutation at codon 200 resulting in a Glu-to-Lys substitution (see Fig. 13–5).[69,183] The E200K mutation has been genetically linked to fCJD with an LOD score exceeding 3 (see also reference 44) and the same mutation has also been found in patients from Orava in North Central Slovakia,[183] in a cluster of familial cases in Chile,[184] and in a large German family living in the United States.[185]

Most patients are heterozygous for the mutation and thus express both mutant and wt PrP^C. In the brains of patients who die of fCJD(E200K), the mutant PrP^{Sc} is both insoluble and protease-resistant while much of wt PrP^{Sc} differs from both PrP^C and PrP^{Sc} in that it is insoluble but readily digested by proteases. Whether this form of PrP is an intermediate in the conversion of PrP^C into PrP^{Sc} remains to be established.[186]

As described earlier, prions from patients with fCJD(E200K) have been transmitted to Tg mice expressing chimeric mouse-human transgenes as well as other Tg mice expressing HuPrP (see Chapter 2).

Penetrance of fCJD

Life-table analyses of carriers harboring the E200K mutation exhibit complete penetrance.[46,47] In other words, if the carriers live long enough, they will all eventually develop prion disease. Some investigators have argued that the inherited prion diseases are not fully penetrant and thus an environmental factor such as the ubiquitous "scrapie virus" is required for illness to be manifest, but as reviewed earlier, no viral pathogen has been found in prion disease.[184,187]

FFI

Studies of inherited human prion diseases demonstrate that changing a single polymorphic residue at position 129 in addition to the D178N pathogenic mutation alters the clinical and neuropathologic phenotype. The D178N mutation combined with a Met encoded at position 129 results in FFI (see also references 145, 188). In this disease, adults generally older than age 50 years present with a progressive sleep disorder and usually die within approximately one year.[189] In their brains, deposition of PrP^{Sc} is confined largely within the anteroventral and the dorsal medial nuclei of the thalamus. The D178N mutation has been linked to the development of FFI with an LOD score exceeding 5 (see also reference 42). More than 30 families worldwide with FFI have been recorded.[190] In contrast, the same D178N mutation with a Val encoded at position 129 produces fCJD in which the patients present with dementia, and widespread deposition of PrP^{Sc} is found postmortem.[191] The first family to be recognized with CJD was found to carry the D178N mutation.[2,192]

As described earlier, prions from patients with inherited and sporadic FI have been transmitted to Tg mice expressing chimeric mouse-human transgenes as well as to other Tg mice expressing HuPrP.

INFECTIOUS PRION DISEASES

Although infectious prion diseases constitute less than 1% of all cases, the circumstances surrounding these infectious illnesses are often dramatic.[129] The ritualistic cannibalism involved the transmission of kuru among the Fore people of New Guinea, the industrial cannibalism responsible for "mad cow disease" in Europe, and the growing group of patients with vCJD contracted from prion-tainted beef products are all examples of infectious prion diseases.

Kuru

Kuru has disappeared, but the impact of this illness on medical science remains immense. Kuru was the first human prion disease to be transmitted to experimental animals.[24] Based on the similarities of the neuropathologic lesions of scrapie and kuru,[21] transmission studies to apes were performed and similar investigations followed with CJD.[1,20] The transmissibility of kuru suggested that the disease resulted from ritualistic cannibalism among the Fore people living in the high-

lands of New Guinea.[193] Presumably, kuru began with a person who had developed a sporadic case of prion disease; at death, the brain was removed and ingested by relatives in order to immortalize the spirit of the deceased. Since cannibalism ceased more than 40 years ago in the highlands of New Guinea, those cases of kuru recorded over the last two decades are thought to have incubation periods of 20 to 40 years.[194,195] No one born since the cessation of cannibalism has developed kuru, and over the last five years fewer than two cases per year have been recorded (M. Alpers, personal communication).

Iatrogenic Prion Disease

Accidental transmission of CJD to humans appears to have occurred with corneal transplantation[196] and contaminated electroencephalogram (EEG) electrode implantation.[197] Corneas were removed from donors who unknowingly had CJD and were transplanted to apparently healthy recipients who developed CJD after prolonged incubation periods. Improperly decontaminated EEG electrodes that caused CJD in two young patients with intractable epilepsy were experimentally implanted in a chimpanzee and were found to cause CJD 18 months later.[198]

Surgical procedures may have resulted in accidental prion infection in patients,[199–201] presumably because some instrument or apparatus in the operating theater became contaminated when a CJD patient underwent surgery. Although the epidemiology of these studies is highly suggestive, no proof for such episodes exists.

Dura Mater Grafts

More than 100 cases of CJD after implantation of dura mater grafts have been recorded.[202] All of the grafts were thought to have been acquired from a single manufacturer whose preparative procedures were inadequate to inactivate human prions. One case of CJD occurred after repair of an eardrum perforation with a pericardium graft.[203]

Human Growth Hormone Therapy

The possibility of transmission of CJD from contaminated human growth hormone (HGH) preparations derived from human pituitaries has been raised by the occurrence of fatal cerebellar disorders with dementia in more than 100 patients ranging from age 10 to 41 years.[129,204] These patients received injections of HGH every 2 to 4 days for 4 to 12 years.[205] Assuming these patients developed CJD from injections of prion-contaminated HGH preparations, the possible incubation periods range from 4 to 30 years. Even though several investigations argue for the efficacy of inactivating prions in HGH fractions prepared from human pituitaries using 6 M urea, it seems doubtful that such protocols will be used for purifying HGH because recombinant HGH is available. Four cases of CJD have occurred in women receiving human pituitary gonadotropin.[206]

vCJD

The restricted geographical occurrence and chronology of vCJD have raised the possibility that BSE prions have been transmitted to humans. More than 100 vCJD cases have been recorded, but the incidence has been too low to be useful in establishing the origin of the disease.[207,208] No set of dietary habits distinguishes vCJD patients from apparently healthy people. Moreover, there is no explanation for the predilection of vCJD for teenagers and young adults. It is noteworthy that epidemiologic studies over the past three decades have failed to find evidence for transmission of sheep prions to humans.[52] Attempts to predict the future number of cases of vCJD, assuming exposure to bovine prions before the offal ban, have been questioned because so few cases of vCJD have occurred.[209] Are we at the beginning of a prion disease epidemic in Great Britain like those seen for BSE and kuru, or will the number of vCJD cases remain small as seen with iCJD caused by cadaveric HGH?

Although the mechanism of infection of vCJD has not been established yet, mounting evidence argues for transmission of bovine prions to humans. This conclusion is based on multiple lines of inquiry, including (1) the spatial-temporal clustering of vCJD (reference 130,210); (2) the successful transmission of BSE to macaques with the induction of PrP plaques similar to those seen in vCJD (reference 211) ; (3) the similarity of the glycoform pattern of PrP^{Sc} in brain but not in tonsil in vCJD patients to that in cattle, mice, domestic cats, and macaques infected with BSE prions[212,213]; and (4) transmission studies in non-Tg mice suggesting that vCJD and BSE represent the same prion strain.[214] The prolonged incubation periods and inefficient transmission of prions that are seen after inoculation of foreign prions into non-Tg mice can readily confuse the interpretation of the findings.[111,215]

The most compelling evidence that vCJD is caused by BSE prions has come from experiments using mice expressing the bovine (Bo) PrP transgene.[216] The incubation times, neuropathologic profiles, and patterns of PrP^{Sc} deposition in these Tg(BoPrP) mice were indistinguishable whether the inoculum originated from the brains of cattle with BSE or of humans with vCJD (reference 216). Neither sCJD nor fCJD(E200K) prions have transmitted disease to Tg(BoPrP) mice after more than 500 days. In contrast, sCJD and fCJD(E200K) prions transmit disease efficiently to Tg(MHu2M)5378/*Prnp*$^{0/0}$ mice expressing a chimeric mouse-human PrP transgene, whereas vCJD prions do not.

When vCJD prions were inoculated into Tg(MHu2M)5378/*Prnp*$^{0/0}$ mice, a few mice developed prion disease after about 350 days.[166] By 500 days,

approximately 25% of the mice were ill (Fig. 13–6) and by 700 days, all the mice had succumbed to disease. On second passage of prions from some of the ill mice, the incubation times showed a biphasic distribution; on third passage, at least two distinct strains of prions could be demonstrated: one strain with a 200-day incubation time and the other with a 350-day period. Interestingly, none of the Tg mice inoculated with BSE prions from cattle developed disease after more than 600 days. The results of these studies question the assumption that BSE and vCJD prions represent a single strain.

DIAGNOSTIC TESTS

The need for accurate, sensitive diagnostic tests for prion diseases, preferably blood or urine based, is extreme. Advances in imaging the CNS may also aid in the early diagnosis of prion disease. When effective treatments for prion diseases are eventually developed, as discussed later, early and accurate detection of the disease will be critical to institute therapies before CNS function is substantially compromised.

With the exception of brain biopsy, there are no diagnostic tests for CJD. If the constellation of pathologic changes frequently found in CJD is seen in a brain biopsy, then the diagnosis is reasonably secure (see Fig. 13–2A, B). The rapid and reliable diagnosis of CJD postmortem can be accomplished by using antisera to PrP. Numerous

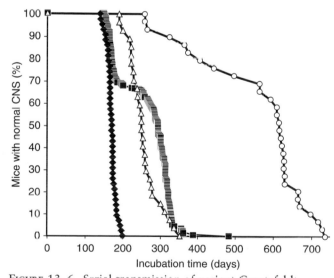

FIGURE 13–6. Serial transmission of variant Creutzfeldt-Jakob disease (vCJD) in Tg(MHu2M)5378/*Prnp*$^{0/0}$ mice. The solid line with the open circles represents the first passage of vCJD prions into Tg(MHu2M)5378/*Prnp*$^{0/0}$ mice; filled squares depict the second passage; open triangles show the third passage of the strain with the long incubation time; and the filled diamonds illustrate the third passage of the strain with the short incubation time.

Western blotting studies have consistently demonstrated PrP-immunoreactive proteins that are proteinase K-resistant in the brains of patients with CJD. It is noteworthy that PrP^Sc is not uniformly distributed throughout the CNS so that the apparent absence of PrP^Sc in a limited sample, such as a biopsy, does not rule out prion disease.[80,217]

If a patient has a family history suggestive of inherited CJD, sequencing the PrP gene may facilitate the diagnosis. Sometimes, PrP sequencing is helpful in even seemingly non-familial cases. Obviously, DNA sequencing is a crucial diagnostic tool in all of the inherited neurodegenerative diseases as well as in the familial forms of prion disease.

Magnetic resonance imaging has become increasingly useful in confirming the diagnosis of CJD. Both T2 and proton-density weighted images of CJD cases show hyperintensities of the basal ganglia. Diffusion-weighted images of the cortex and basal ganglia show increased signals in the brains of both sCJD and vCJD patients. In vCJD but not sCJD patients, hyperintensity of the pulvinar of the thalamus is seen in most cases.[218]

In contrast to most neurodegenerative diseases, the EEG is often useful in the diagnosis of CJD. During the early phase of CJD, the EEG is usually normal or shows only scattered theta activity. In most advanced cases, repetitive, high-voltage, triphasic, and polyphasic sharp discharges are seen, but in many cases, their presence is transient. The presence of these stereotyped periodic bursts of less than 200-msec duration, occurring every 1 to 2 sec, makes the diagnosis of CJD very likely.[10,50,53,219] These discharges are frequently but not always symmetrical; there may be a one-sided predominance in amplitude. As CJD progresses, normal background rhythms become fragmentary and slower.

In all of the neurodegenerative diseases, the cerebrospinal fluid (CSF) is nearly always normal but may show minimal protein elevation.[50] Although the protein 14-3-3 is elevated in the CSF of many CJD patients, similar elevations of 14-3-3 are found in patients with herpes simplex virus encephalitis, multi-infarct dementia, and stroke.[53,220] In Alzheimer disease, 14-3-3 is generally not elevated. In the serum of some patients with CJD, the S-100 protein is elevated, but like 14-3-3, this elevation is not specific.[220]

The possibility of Hashimoto's thyroiditis should always be considered in the differential diagnosis of CJD (reference 221) since this autoimmune disease is treatable and CJD is not. That the clinical and neuropathologic findings can be so similar in Hashimoto's thyroiditis and CJD is striking; moreover, it raises the possibility that protein misprocessing may underlie both degenerative and autoimmune diseases.

A highly sensitive and quantitative immunoassay was developed based upon epitopes that are exposed in PrP^C but buried in PrP^Sc (Fig. 13–7). Unlike all other immunoassays for PrP^Sc, this conformation-dependent

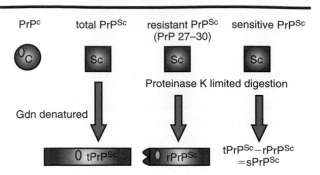

Conformation dependent immunoassay (CDI) for PrP^Sc

FIGURE 13–7. The conformation-dependent immunoassay (CDI) permits measurement of PrP^Sc without limited digestion by protease to eliminate PrP^C; instead, antibodies binding to epitopes that are exposed in PrP^C but buried in PrP^Sc are used to distinguish between the two isoforms. Using the CDI, it became possible to detect two different forms of PrP^Sc: one that is resistant to limited protease digestion (r) and the other that is readily digested (s). Using one fraction of a sample, total (t) PrP^Sc was measured while another aliquot was digested before determining the rPrP^Sc level. rPrP^Sc is equivalent to PrP 27–30. By subtracting rPrP^Sc from tPrP^Sc, the amount of sPrP^Sc can be determined.

immunoassay (CDI) does not require limited proteolysis to hydrolyze PrP^C before measuring the protease-resistant core of PrP^Sc (PrP 27–30).[222] Using the CDI, a new form of PrP^Sc, which is protease-sensitive (s), was identified. The levels of sPrP^Sc are proportional to the length of the incubation time and are often much higher than those of protease-resistant PrP^Sc. Why levels of sPrP^Sc should be directly proportional to the length of the incubation time is unclear but this might indicate a relationship between sPrP^Sc and the development of pathologic changes. Whether or not measurements of sPrP^Sc will become the basis of diagnostic tests for prion diseases remains to be established.

PRION DISEASES OF ANIMALS

The prion diseases of animals include scrapie of sheep and goats, BSE, TME, CWD of deer and elk, feline spongiform encephalopathy (FSE), and exotic ungulate encephalopathy (see Table 13–1).

PrP Gene Polymorphisms in Sheep and Cattle

Parry argued that host genes were responsible for the development of scrapie in sheep. He was convinced that natural scrapie is a genetic disease that could be eradicated by proper breeding protocols.[137,223] He considered its transmission by inoculation of importance primarily for laboratory studies and its communicable infection of little consequence in nature. Other investigators viewed natural scrapie as an infectious disease and argued that host genetics only modulate susceptibility to an endemic infectious agent.[224]

In sheep, polymorphisms at codons 136, 154, and 171 of the PrP gene that produce amino acid substitutions have been studied with respect to the occurrence of scrapie (see Fig. 13–5).[225–228] Studies of natural scrapie in the United States have shown that ~85% of the afflicted sheep are of the Suffolk breed. Only those Suffolk sheep homozygous for Gln (Q) at codon 171 developed scrapie, although healthy controls with QQ, QR, and RR genotypes were also found.[163,164,228–234] These results argue that susceptibility in Suffolk sheep is governed by the PrP codon 171 polymorphism. In Cheviot sheep, the PrP codon 171 polymorphism has a profound influence on susceptibility to scrapie, as in the Suffolk breed, and codon 136 seems to play a less pronounced role.[235,236]

In contrast to sheep, different breeds of cattle have no specific PrP polymorphisms. The only polymorphism recorded in cattle is a variation in the number of octarepeats; most cattle, like humans, have five octarepeats but some have six.[237,238] However, the presence of six octarepeats does not seem to be overrepresented in BSE.[237–239]

BSE

BSE is a massive common-source epidemic caused by meat and bone meal (MBM) fed primarily to dairy cows.[240,241] Prion strains and the species barrier are of paramount importance in understanding the BSE epidemic in Great Britain, in which it is estimated that almost 1 million cattle were infected with prions.[241,242] MBM was prepared from the offal of sheep, cattle, pigs, and chickens as a high-protein nutritional supplement. In the late 1970s, the hydrocarbon-solvent extraction method used in the rendering of offal began to be abandoned, resulting in MBM with a much higher fat content.[240] It is now thought that this change in the rendering process allowed scrapie prions from sheep to survive rendering and to be passed into cattle. Alternatively, bovine prions may have been present at low levels before modification of the rendering process and, with the processing change, survived in sufficient numbers to initiate the BSE epidemic when reintroduced back into cattle orally through MBM. Against the latter hypothesis is the widespread geographical distribution of the initial 17 cases of BSE throughout England, which occurred almost simultaneously.[241,243,244] Furthermore, there is no evidence of a preexisting prion disease of cattle, in Great Britain or elsewhere. The mean incubation time for BSE is approximately five years. Therefore, most cattle did not manifest disease symptoms because they were slaughtered between ages two and three years.[245] Nevertheless, more

than 180,000 cattle, primarily dairy cows, have died of BSE over the past decade.[242]

Origin of BSE Prions?

The origin of the bovine prions causing BSE cannot be determined by examining the amino acid sequence of PrP^{Sc} because the PrP^{Sc} in these diseased animals has the bovine sequence whether the initial prions came from cattle or sheep. The bovine PrP sequence differs from that of sheep at seven or eight positions.[226,237,238]

Brain extracts from cattle with BSE cause disease in cattle, sheep, mice, pigs, and mink after intracerebral inoculation,[214,246–249] but prions in brain extracts from sheep with scrapie fed to cattle produced an illness substantially different from BSE.[250] However, no exhaustive effort has been made to test different strains of sheep prions or to examine the disease following bovine-to-bovine passage. The annual incidence of sheep with scrapie in Great Britain over the past two decades has remained relatively low (J Wilesmith, unpublished data). In July 1988, the practice of feeding MBM to sheep and cattle was banned. Recent statistical analysis argues that the epidemic is now disappearing as a result of this ruminant feed ban,[242] reminiscent of the disappearance of kuru in the Fore people of New Guinea.[199,251]

Because Tg(BoPrP) mice were found to be excellent hosts for transmission of natural sheep scrapie,[216] this raises the possibility that sheep carry several strains of prions, including the BSE strain (M Scott and SB Prusiner, in preparation). But the BSE strain might replicate more slowly than many scrapie strains in sheep and, thus, is present at low levels. If the scrapie strains were more heatlabile than the BSE strain, then the rendering process used in the late 1970s and most of the next decade might have selected for the BSE strain. This BSE strain might have then been re-selected multiple times as cattle were infected by ingesting prion-contaminated MBM. In this situation, the infected cattle were slaughtered and their offal rendered into more MBM, which was subsequently fed to more cattle. The foregoing scenario suggests that the BSE strain may be widely distributed in sheep and that those prions composed of sheep PrP^{Sc} are non-pathogenic to humans. Once BSE prions are passaged through cattle, they acquire bovine PrP^{Sc} and become pathogenic to humans.

Two other hypotheses have been offered with respect to the origin of BSE. One hypothesis suggests that the BSE strain of prions was produced by the altered rendering process adopted in the late 1970s and the second hypothesis suggests that the BSE strain arose spontaneously in a cow with a sporadic case of BSE in southern England.[139]

Monitoring Cattle for BSE Prions

Although many plans have been offered for the culling of older cattle in order to minimize the spread of BSE,[242] it seems more important to monitor the frequency of prion disease in cattle as they are slaughtered for human consumption. No reliable, specific test for prion disease in live animals is available, but immunoassays for PrP^Sc in the brain stems of cattle might provide a reasonable approach to establishing the incidence of subclinical BSE in cattle entering the human food chain.[80,217,238,252–254] Determining how early in the incubation period PrP^Sc can be detected by immunological methods is now possible since a reliable bioassay has been created by expressing the BoPrP gene in Tg mice.[255] Before development of Tg(BoPrP)*Prnp*^0/0 mice, non-Tg mice inoculated intracerebrally with BSE brain extracts required more than 300 days to develop disease.[111,214,256,257] Depending on the titer of the inoculum and the structures of PrP^C, PrP^Sc, and the putative binding partner protein X, the number of inoculated animals developing disease can vary over a wide range. Some investigators have stated that transmission of BSE to mice is quite variable, with incubation periods exceeding one year.[111] Other investigators report low prion titers in brain homogenates from BSE-infected cattle[256,257] compared to brain homogenates from scrapie-infected rodents.[258–261]

CWD

More than 15% of deer and elk in the Rocky Mountain area of the United States are thought to have CWD.[262,263] CWD has been found in both wild and domesticated herds. In the brains of deer and elk with CWD, numerous amyloid plaques that readily immunostain for PrP have been found.[264,265]

The etiology of CWD is uncertain. Feed contaminated with prions from sheep was once hypothesized to be the cause. It seems more likely that, like scrapie, some animals develop the disease spontaneously while others become infected through horizontal transmission. While there is no evidence for transmission of prions from deer or elk to humans, a small number of deer hunters with CJD as well as cases of CJD in young people who consumed venison have been recorded.[266]

THERAPEUTICS FOR PRION DISEASES

Defining the pathogenesis of prion disease is an important issue with respect to developing an effective therapy. The issue of whether large aggregates of misprocessed proteins or misfolded monomers (or oligomers) cause CNS degeneration has been addressed in several studies of prion diseases in humans as well as in Tg mice. In humans, the frequency of PrP amyloid plaques varies from 100% in GSS and vCJD (reference 130) to approximately 70% in kuru[20] and approximately 10% in sCJD, arguing that these plaques are a nonobligatory feature of disease.[56] In Tg mice expressing both MoPrP and SHaPrP, animals inoculated with hamster prions produced hamster prions and developed amyloid plaques

composed of ShaPrP.[96] In contrast, Tg mice inoculated with mouse prions did not develop plaques even though they produced mouse prions and died of scrapie.

Prion Therapeutics

Various compounds have been proposed as potential therapeutics for treatment of prion diseases; these include polysulfated anions, dextrans, and cyclic tetrapyrroles, all of which have been shown to increase survival time when given before prion infection in rodents, but not when given after infection has been initiated.[267–271]

Besides studies in rodents, ScN2a cells chronically infected with scrapie prions have been used to identify several candidate antiprion drugs,[272–277] but none of these drugs have been shown to be effective in halting prion diseases in either animals or humans. Structure-based drug design based on dominant-negative inhibition of prion formation has produced several lead compounds.[276] Prion replication depends on protein-protein interactions and a subset of these interactions gives rise to dominant-negative phenotypes produced by single residue substitutions.[160,161]

Quinacrine and Other Acridine Derivatives

Tricyclic derivatives of acridine exhibit half maximal inhibition of PrP^Sc formation at effective concentrations (IC$_{50}$) between 0.3 μM and 3 μM in cultured ScN2a cells.[277,278] The IC$_{50}$ for chlorpromazine was 3 μM while quinacrine was 10 times more potent. A variety of nine-substituted, acridine-based analogues of quinacrine were synthesized, which demonstrated variable potencies similar to chlorpromazine and emphasized the importance of the side-chain in mediating the inhibition of PrP^Sc formation.[278] These studies showed that tricyclic compounds with an aliphatic side-chain at the middle ring moiety constitute a new class of antiprion agents. Because quinacrine and chlorpromazine have been used in humans as antimalarial and antipsychotic drugs, respectively, for many years and are known to pass the blood-brain barrier (BBB), these drugs became immediate candidates for the treatment of CJD and other prion diseases.

An asymmetric carbon in the side-chain of quinacrine creates two stereoisomers (Fig. 13–8A). The (S)-quinacrine enantiomer is two to three times more potent than the (R)-isomer (Fig. 13–8B). Whether the use of (S)-quinacrine enantiomer in place of the racemic mixture will allow significantly more drug to be given remains to be established. Studies performed almost six decades ago in humans demonstrated that (S)-quinacrine is selectively metabolized and that (R)-quinacrine remains intact.[279] Whether (R)-quinacrine or the metabolites of (S)-quinacrine are responsible for the side effects recorded in patients receiving the racemic mixture

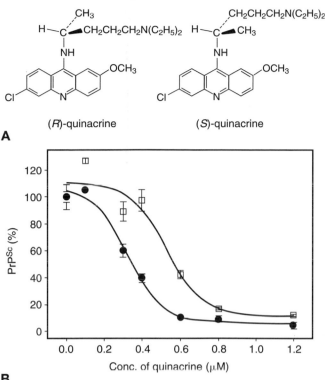

A

B

FIGURE 13–8. Quinacrine isomers and inhibition of PrP^Sc formation in cultured ScN2a cells. *A*, Structures of (*S*)-quinacrine and (*R*)-quinacrine; *B*, Differential accumulation of proteinase K-resistant PrP^Sc in ScN2a cells treated with two stereoisomers of quinacrine. ELISA determinations of proteinase K-digested ScN2a cell lysates incubated with (*S*)-quinacrine (filled circles) and (*R*)-quinacrine (open squares) are shown (Ryou et al., in preparation). ScN2a cells were cultivated in minimal essential medium (MEM) with 10% fetal calf serum and GlutaMax. For treatments, ScN2a cells were plated to about 2% to 3% confluency. Indicated concentrations (0 to 1.2 μM) of quinacrine stereoisomers were added to the cell cultures. Culture media including quinacrine were changed on alternate days during the six-day treatment.

is unknown. Side effects of quinacrine include liver toxicity, cardiomyopathy, and toxic psychoses.[280]

recFabs

A panel of recFabs recognizing different epitope regions on PrP was studied with respect to inhibition of prion propagation in cultured ScN2a cells.[142] Recombinant Fabs binding to PrP^C on the cell surface inhibited PrP^Sc formation in a dose-dependent manner. In ScN2a cells treated with the most potent recFab, D18, prion replication was completely abolished and pre-existing PrP^Sc was rapidly cleared, suggesting that this antibody may cure established infection. The activity of recFab D18 is associated with its ability to recognize more completely the total population

of PrP^C molecules on the cell surface than other recFabs. In other studies, a monoclonal antibody, 6H4, which is thought to bind to the same region of PrP as the D18 recFab, was found to inhibit prion accumulation in ScN2a cells.[281] Whether such antibodies or Fabs can be effectively administered for prevention and treatment of prion diseases in humans is unclear. Neither antibodies nor Fabs cross the BBB in high concentration, so that delivery of these proteins to the CNS remains a critical issue.

CONCLUDING REMARKS

As the life span of humans continues to increase through the efforts of modern medical science, an increasing burden of degenerative diseases is emerging. Developing effective means of preventing these disorders and treating them when they do occur is paramount to the personal, political, and economic future of our planet. The problems caused by Alzheimer and Parkinson diseases are already so large that if these maladies continue to increase in accordance with the changing demographics of the world population, they will bankrupt both developed and underdeveloped nations over the next 50 years. It is remarkable to think that by the year 2025, more than 65% of people older than 65 years will be living in countries that are now designated as developing nations.[282] Unless effective treatments and methods of prevention are developed, this immense group of people will be subject to the same risk for Alzheimer disease, Parkinson disease, and other neurodegenerative disorders as people who are currently living in the most affluent nations.

Acknowledgments

We thank Drs. Fred Cohen, Jiri Safar, and Michael Scott for helpful discussions. This research was supported by grants from the National Institutes of Health.

REFERENCES

1. Gibbs CJ Jr, Gajdusek DC, Asher DM, et al: Creutzfeldt-Jakob disease (spongiform encephalopathy): Transmission to the chimpanzee. Science 1968;161: 388–389.

2. Meggendorfer F: Klinische und genealogische Beobachtungen bei einem Fall von spastischer Pseudosklerose Jakobs. Z Gesamte Neurol Psychiatrie 1930; 128:337–341.

3. Roos R, Gajdusek DC, Gibbs CJ Jr: The clinical characteristics of transmissible Creutzfeldt-Jakob disease. Brain 1973;96:1–20.

4. Hsiao K, Baker HF, Crow TJ, et al: Linkage of a prion protein missense variant to Gerstmann-Sträussler syndrome. Nature 1989;338:342–345.

5. Owen F, Poulter M, Lofthouse R, et al: Insertion in prion protein gene in familial Creutzfeldt-Jakob disease. Lancet 1989;1:51–52.

6. Martin JB: Molecular basis of the neurodegenerative disorders. N Engl J Med 1999;340:1970–1980.

7. Prusiner SB: Shattuck Lecture—Neurodegenerative diseases and prions. N Engl J Med 2001; 344:1516–1526.

8. Creutzfeldt HG: Über eine eigenartige herdförmige Erkrankung des Zentralnervensystems. Z Gesamte Neurol Psychiatrie 1920;57:1–18.

9. Jakob A: Über eigenartige Erkrankungen des Zentralnervensystems mit bemerkenswertem anatomischen Befunde (spastische Pseudosklerose-Encephalomyelopathie mit disseminierten Degenerationsherden). Z Gesamte Neurol Psychiatrie 1921;64:147–228.

10. Kirschbaum WR: Jakob-Creutzfeldt Disease. Amsterdam, Elsevier, 1968.

11. Kirschbaum WR: Zwei eigenartige Erkrankungen des Zentralnervensystems nach Art der spastischen Pseudosklerose (Jakob). Z Gesamte Neurol Psychiatrie 1924;92:175–220.

12. Stender A: Weitere Beiträge zum Kapitel "Spastische Pseudosklerose Jakobs." Z Gesamte Neurol Psychiatrie 1930;128:528–543.

13. Davison C, Rabiner AM: Spastic pseudosclerosis (disseminated encephalomyelopathy; corticopallidospinal degeneration). Familial and nonfamilial incidence (a clinico-pathologic study). Arch Neurol Psychiatry 1940;44:578–598.

14. Jacob H, Pyrkosch W, Strube H: Die erbliche Form der Creutzfeldt-Jakobschen Krankheit. Arch Psychiatr Zeitsch Neurol 1950;184:653–674.

15. Friede RL, DeJong RN: Neuronal enzymatic failure in Creutzfeldt-Jakob disease. A familial study. Arch Neurol 1964;10:181–195.

16. Rosenthal NP, Keesey J, Crandall B, Brown WJ: Familial neurological disease associated with spongiform encephalopathy. Arch Neurol 1976;33:252–259.

17. Masters CL, Gajdusek DC, Gibbs CJ Jr, et al: Familial Creutzfeldt-Jakob disease and other familial dementias: An inquiry into possible models of virus-induced familial diseases. In Prusiner SB, Hadlow WJ (eds): Slow Transmissible Diseases of the Nervous System, vol 1. New York, Academic Press, 1979, pp 143–194.

18. Masters CL, Gajdusek DC, Gibbs CJ Jr: Creutzfeldt-Jakob disease virus isolations from the Gerstmann-Sträussler syndrome. Brain 1981;104:559–588.

19. Masters CL, Gajdusek DC, Gibbs CJ Jr: The familial occurrence of Creutzfeldt-Jakob disease and Alzheimer's disease. Brain 1981;104:535–558.

20. Klatzo I, Gajdusek DC, Zigas V: Pathology of kuru. Lab Invest 1959;8:799–847.

21. Hadlow WJ: Scrapie and kuru. Lancet 1959; 2:289–290.

22. Sigurdsson B: Rida, a chronic encephalitis of sheep with general remarks on infections which develop slowly and some of their special characteristics. Br Vet J 1954;110:341–354.

23. Hadlow WJ: Neuropathology and the scrapie-kuru connection. Brain Pathol 1959;5:27–31.

24. Gajdusek DC, Gibbs CJ Jr, Alpers M: Experimental transmission of a kuru-like syndrome to chimpanzees. Nature 1966;209:794–796.

25. Gordon WS: Advances in veterinary research. Vet Res 1946;58:516–520.

26. Zlotnik I: The pathology of scrapie: A comparative study of lesions in the brain of sheep and goats. Acta Neuropathol (Berl) [suppl] 1962;1:61–70.

27. Beck E, Daniel PM, Parry HB: Degeneration of the cerebellar and hypothalamo-neurohypophysial systems in sheep with scrapie, and its relationship to human system degenerations. Brain 1964;87:153–176.

28. Alper T, Haig DA, Clarke MC: The exceptionally small size of the scrapie agent. Biochem Biophys Res Commun 1966;22:278–284.

29. Alper T, Cramp WA, Haig DA, Clarke MC: Does the agent of scrapie replicate without nucleic acid? Nature 1967;214:764–766.

30. Latarjet R, Muel B, Haig DA, et al: Inactivation of the scrapie agent by near monochromatic ultraviolet light. Nature 1970;227:1341–1343.

31. Gibbs CJ Jr, Gajdusek DC, Latarjet R: Unusual resistance to ionizing radiation of the viruses of kuru, Creutzfeldt-Jakob disease. Proc Natl Acad Sci U S A 1978;75:6268–6270.

32. Pattison IH: Experiments with scrapie with special reference to the nature of the agent and the pathology of the disease. In Gajdusek DC, Gibbs CJ Jr, Alpers MP (eds): Slow, Latent and Temperate Virus Infections, NINDB Monograph 2. Washington, DC, US Government Printing, 1965, pp 249–257.

33. Gibbons RA, Hunter GD: Nature of the scrapie agent. Nature 1967;215:1041–1043.

34. Griffith JS: Self-replication and scrapie. Nature 1967;215:1043–1044.

35. Pattison IH, Jones KM: The possible nature of the transmissible agent of scrapie. Vet Rec 1967;80:1–8.

36. Hunter GD, Kimberlin RH, Gibbons RA: Scrapie: A modified membrane hypothesis. J Theor Biol 1968;20:355–357.

37. Field EJ, Farmer F, Caspary EA, Joyce G: Susceptibility of scrapie agent to ionizing radiation. Nature 1969;222:90–91.

38. Hunter GD: Scrapie: A prototype slow infection. J Infect Dis 1972;125:427–440.

39. Chandler RL: Encephalopathy in mice produced by inoculation with scrapie brain material. Lancet 1961;1:1378–1379.

40. Prusiner SB: Prions (Les Prix Nobel Lecture). In Frängsmyr T (ed): Les Prix Nobel. Stockholm, Almqvist & Wiksell International, 1998, pp 268–323.

41. Dlouhy SR, Hsiao K, Farlow MR, et al: Linkage of the Indiana kindred of Gerstmann-Sträussler-Scheinker disease to the prion protein gene. Nat Genet 1992;1:64–67.

42. Petersen RB, Tabaton M, Berg L, et al: Analysis of the prion protein gene in thalamic dementia. Neurology 1992;42:1859–1863.

43. Poulter M, Baker HF, Frith CD, et al: Inherited prion disease with 144 base pair gene insertion. 1. Genealogical and molecular studies. Brain 1992;115:675–685.

44. Gabizon R, Rosenmann H, Meiner Z, et al: Mutation and polymorphism of the prion protein gene in Libyan Jews with Creutzfeldt-Jakob disease (CJD). Am J Hum Genet 1993;53:828–835.

45. Hsiao KK, Doh-ura K, Kitamoto T, et al: A prion protein amino acid substitution in ataxic Gerstmann-Sträussler syndrome. Ann Neurol 1989;26:137.

46. Chapman J, Ben-Israel J, Goldhammer Y, Korczyn AD: The risk of developing Creutzfeldt-Jakob disease in subjects with the PRNP gene codon 200 point mutation. Neurology 1994;44:1683–1686.

47. Spudich S, Mastrianni JA, Wrensch M, et al: Complete penetrance of Creutzfeldt-Jakob disease in Libyan Jews carrying the E200K mutation in the prion protein gene. Mol Med 1995;1:607–613.

48. Masters CL, Harris JO, Gajdusek DC, et al: Creutzfeldt-Jakob disease: Patterns of worldwide occurrence and the significance of familial and sporadic clustering. Ann Neurol 1978;5:177–188.

49. Holman RC, Khan AS, Belay ED, Schonberger LB: Creutzfeldt-Jakob disease in the United States, 1979–1994: Using national mortality data to assess the possible occurrence of variant cases. Emerg Infect Dis 1996;2:333–337.

50. Cathala F, Baron H: Clinical aspects of Creutzfeldt-Jakob disease. In Prusiner SB, McKinley MP (eds): Prions—Novel Infectious Pathogens Causing Scrapie and Creutzfeldt-Jakob Disease. Orlando, Academic Press, 1987, pp 467–509.

51. Kahana E, Milton A, Braham J, Sofer D: Creutzfeldt-Jakob disease: Focus among Libyan Jews in Israel. Science 1974;183:90–91.

52. Cousens SN, Harries-Jones R, Knight R, et al: Geographical distribution of cases of Creutzfeldt-Jakob disease in England and Wales 1970–84. J Neurol Neurosurg Psychiatry 1990;53:459–465.

53. Johnson RT, Gibbs CJ Jr: Creutzfeldt-Jakob disease and related transmissible spongiform encephalopathies. N Engl J Med 1998;339:1994–2004.

54. Prusiner SB, Cochran SP, Alpers MP: Transmission of scrapie in hamsters. J Infect Dis 1985;152:971–978.

55. DeArmond SJ, Ironside JW: Neuropathology of prion diseases. In Prusiner SB (ed): Prion Biology and Diseases. Cold Spring Harbor, NY: Cold Spring Harbor Laboratory Press, 1999, pp 585–652.

56. DeArmond SJ, Prusiner SB: Prion diseases. In Lantos P, Graham D (eds): Greenfield's Neuropathology, 6th ed. London, Edward Arnold, 1997, pp 235–280.

57. Prusiner SB, McKinley MP, Bowman KA, et al: Scrapie prions aggregate to form amyloid-like birefringent rods. Cell 1983;35:349–358.

58. Tateishi J, Kitamoto T, Hoque MZ, Furukawa H: Experimental transmission of Creutzfeldt-Jakob disease and related diseases to rodents. Neurology 1996;46:532–537.

59. Gambetti P, Peterson RB, Parchi P, et al: Inherited prion diseases. In Prusiner SB (ed): Prion Biology and Diseases. Cold Spring Harbor, NY: Cold Spring Harbor Laboratory Press, 1999, pp 509–583.

60. Bendheim PE, Barry RA, DeArmond SJ, et al: Antibodies to a scrapie prion protein. Nature 1984;310:418–421.

61. DeArmond SJ, McKinley MP, Barry RA, et al: Identification of prion amyloid filaments in scrapie-infected brain. Cell 1985;41:221–235.

62. Kitamoto T, Tateishi J, Tashima I, et al: Amyloid plaques in Creutzfeldt-Jakob disease stain with prion protein antibodies. Ann Neurol 1986;20:204–208.

63. DeArmond SJ, Mobley WC, DeMott DL, et al: Changes in the localization of brain prion proteins during scrapie infection. Neurology 1987;37:1271–1280.

64. Roberts GW, Lofthouse R, Allsop D, et al: CNS amyloid proteins in neurodegenerative diseases. Neurology 1988;38:1534–1540.

65. Snow AD, Kisilevsky R, Willmer J, et al: Sulfated glycosaminoglycans in amyloid plaques of prion diseases. Acta Neuropathol (Berl) 1989;77:337–342.

66. Gerstmann J, Sträussler E, Scheinker I: Über eine eigenartige hereditär-familiäre Erkrankung des Zentralnervensystems zugleich ein Beitrag zur Frage des vorzeitigen lokalen Alterns. Z Neurol 1936;154:736–762.

67. Bruce ME, Dickinson AG, Fraser H: Cerebral amyloidosis in scrapie in the mouse: Effect of agent strain and mouse genotype. Neuropathol Appl Neurobiol 1976;2:471–478.

68. Kitamoto T, Yamaguchi K, Doh-ura K, Tateishi J: A prion protein missense variant is integrated in kuru plaque cores in patients with Gerstmann-Sträussler syndrome. Neurology 1991;41:306–310.

69. Hsiao K, Meiner Z, Kahana E, et al: Mutation of the prion protein in Libyan Jews with Creutzfeldt-Jakob disease. N Engl J Med 1991;324:1091–1097.

70. Hsiao KK, Scott M, Foster D, et al: Spontaneous neurodegeneration in transgenic mice with mutant prion protein. Science 1990;250:1587–1590.

71. Hsiao KK, Groth D, Scott M, et al: Serial transmission in rodents of neurodegeneration from transgenic mice expressing mutant prion protein. Proc Natl Acad Sci U S A 1994;91:9126–9130.

72. Glenner GG, Eanes ED, Bladen HA, et al: Beta-pleated sheet fibrils—A comparison of native amyloid with synthetic protein fibrils. J Histochem Cytochem 1974;22:1141–1158.

73. Glenner GG: Amyloid deposits and amyloidosis. N Engl J Med 1980;302:1283–1292.

74. Pan K-M, Baldwin M, Nguyen J, et al: Conversion of α-helices into β-sheets features in the formation of the scrapie prion proteins. Proc Natl Acad Sci U S A 1993;90:10962–10966.

75. Safar J, Roller PP, Gajdusek DC, Gibbs CJ Jr: Conformational transitions, dissociation, and unfolding of scrapie amyloid (prion) protein. J Biol Chem 1993; 268:20276–20284.

76. McKinley MP, Meyer RK, Kenaga L, et al: Scrapie prion rod formation in vitro requires both detergent extraction and limited proteolysis. J Virol 1991; 65:1340–1351.

77. Bockman JM, Kingsbury DT, McKinley MP, et al: Creutzfeldt-Jakob disease prion proteins in human brains. N Engl J Med 1985;312:73–78.

78. Brown P, Coker-Vann M, Pomeroy K, et al: Diagnosis of Creutzfeldt-Jakob disease by Western blot identification of marker protein in human brain tissue. N Engl J Med 1986;314:547–551.

79. Prusiner SB, DeArmond SJ: Biology of disease: Prions causing nervous system degeneration. Lab Invest 1987;56:349–363.

80. Serban D, Taraboulos A, DeArmond SJ, Prusiner SB: Rapid detection of Creutzfeldt-Jakob disease and scrapie prion proteins. Neurology 1990;40:110–117.

81. Jendroska K, Heinzel FP, Torchia M, et al: Proteinase-resistant prion protein accumulation in Syrian hamster brain correlates with regional pathology and scrapie infectivity. Neurology 1991;41:1482–1490.

82. Hecker R, Taraboulos A, Scott M, et al: Replication of distinct scrapie prion isolates is region-specific in brains of transgenic mice and hamsters. Genes Dev 1992;6:1213–1228.

83. Scott M, Groth D, Foster D, et al: Propagation of prions with artificial properties in transgenic mice expressing chimeric PrP genes. Cell 1993;73:979–988.

84. DeArmond SJ, Yang S-L, Lee A, et al: Three scrapie prion isolates exhibit different accumulation patterns of the prion protein scrapie isoform. Proc Natl Acad Sci U S A 1993;90:6449–6453.

85. Hsiao K, Scott M, Foster D, et al: Spontaneous neurodegeneration in transgenic mice with prion protein codon 101 proline→leucine substitution. Ann N Y Acad Sci 1991;640:166–170.

86. Oesch B, Westaway D, Wälchli M, et al: A cellular gene encodes scrapie PrP 27–30 protein. Cell 1985;40:735–746.

87. Kretzschmar HA, Prusiner SB, Stowring LE, DeArmond SJ: Scrapie prion proteins are synthesized in neurons. Am J Pathol 1986;122:1–5.

88. DeArmond SJ, Prusiner SB: The neurochemistry of prion diseases. J Neurochem 1993;61:1589–1601.

89. Borchelt DR, Koliatsis VE, Guarnieri M, et al: Rapid anterograde axonal transport of the cellular prion glycoprotein in the peripheral and central nervous systems. J Biol Chem 1994;269:14711–14714.

90. Pattison IH, Millson GC: Scrapie produced experimentally in goats with special reference to the clinical syndrome. J Comp Pathol 1961;71:101–108.

91. Fraser H, Dickinson AG: Scrapie in mice. Agent-strain differences in the distribution and intensity of grey matter vacuolation. J Comp Pathol 1973; 83:29–40.

92. Carlson GA, Ebeling C, Yang S-L, et al: Prion isolate specified allotypic interactions between the cellular and scrapie prion proteins in congenic and transgenic mice. Proc Natl Acad Sci U S A 1994;91:5690–5694.

93. Carlson GA, Kingsbury DT, Goodman PA, et al: Linkage of prion protein and scrapie incubation time genes. Cell 1986;46:503–511.

94. Moore RC, Hope J, McBride PA, et al: Mice with gene targetted prion protein alterations show that Prn-p, Sinc and Prni are congruent. Nat Genet 1998; 18:118–125.

95. Scott M, Foster D, Mirenda C, et al: Transgenic mice expressing hamster prion protein produce species-specific scrapie infectivity and amyloid plaques. Cell 1989;59:847–857.

96. Prusiner SB, Scott M, Foster D, et al: Transgenetic studies implicate interactions between homologous PrP isoforms in scrapie prion replication. Cell 1990;63:673–686.

97. Supattapone S, Bosque P, Muramoto T, et al: Prion protein of 106 residues creates an artificial transmission barrier for prion replication in transgenic mice. Cell 1999;96:869–878.

98. Büeler H, Aguzzi A, Sailer A, et al: Mice devoid of PrP are resistant to scrapie. Cell 1993;73:1339–1347.

99. Prusiner SB, Groth D, Serban A, et al: Ablation of the prion protein (PrP) gene in mice prevents scrapie and facilitates production of anti-PrP antibodies. Proc Natl Acad Sci U S A 1993;90:10608–10612.

100. Prusiner SB: Molecular biology of prion diseases. Science 1991;252:1515–1522.

101. Dickinson AG, Meikle VMH, Fraser H: Identification of a gene which controls the incubation period of some strains of scrapie agent in mice. J Comp Pathol 1968;78:293–299.

102. Scott MR, Groth D, Tatzelt J, et al: Propagation of prion strains through specific conformers of the prion protein. J Virol 1997;71:9032–9044.

103. Büeler H, Fisher M, Lang Y, et al: Normal development and behaviour of mice lacking the neuronal cell-surface PrP protein. Nature 1992;356:577–582.

104. Manson JC, Clarke AR, Hooper ML, et al: 129/Ola mice carrying a null mutation in PrP that abolishes mRNA production are developmentally normal. Mol Neurobiol 1994;8:121–127.

105. Tobler I, Gaus SE, Deboer T, et al: Altered circadian activity rhythms and sleep in mice devoid of prion protein. Nature 1996;380:639–642.

106. Collinge J, Whittington MA, Sidle KC, et al: Prion protein is necessary for normal synaptic function. Nature 1994;370:295–297.

107. Whittington MA, Sidle KCL, Gowland I, et al: Rescue of neurophysiological phenotype seen in PrP null mice by transgene encoding human prion protein. Nat Genet 1995;9:197–201.

108. Herms JW, Kretzschmar HA, Titz S, Keller BU: Patch-clamp analysis of synaptic transmission to cerebellar Purkinje cells of prion protein knockout mice. Eur J Neurosci 1995;7:2508–2512.

109. Lledo P-M, Tremblay P, DeArmond SJ, et al: Mice deficient for prion protein exhibit normal neuronal excitability and synaptic transmission in the hippocampus. Proc Natl Acad Sci U S A 1996;93:2403–2407.

110. Chesebro B, Caughey B: Scrapie agent replication without the prion protein? Curr Biol 1993;3:696–698.

111. Lasmézas CI, Deslys J-P, Robain O, et al: Transmission of the BSE agent to mice in the absence of detectable abnormal prion protein. Science 1997;275:402–405.

112. Sailer A, Büeler H, Fischer M, et al: No propagation of prions in mice devoid of PrP. Cell 1994;77:967–968.

113. Sakaguchi S, Katamine S, Nishida N, et al: Loss of cerebellar Purkinje cells in aged mice homozygous for a disrupted PrP gene. Nature 1996;380:528–531.

114. Moore RC, Lee IY, Silverman GL, et al: Ataxia in prion protein (PrP) deficient mice is associated with upregulation of the novel PrP-like protein doppel. J Mol Biol 1999;292:797–817.

115. Mo H, Moore RC, Cohen FE, et al: Two different neurodegenerative diseases caused by proteins with similar structures. Proc Natl Acad Sci U S A 2001;98:2352–2357.

116. Silverman GL, Qin K, Moore RC, et al: Doppel is an N-glycosylated, glycosylphosphatidylinositol-anchored protein. J Biol Chem 2000;275:26834–26841.

117. Behrens A, Genoud N, Naumann H, et al: Absence of the prion protein homologue Doppel causes male sterility. EMBO J 2002;21:3652–3658.

118. Rossi D, Cozzio A, Flechsig E, et al: Onset of ataxia and Purkinje cell loss in PrP null mice inversely correlated with Dpl level in brain. EMBO J 2001;20:694–702.

119. Nishida N, Tremblay P, Sugimoto T, et al: A mouse prion protein transgene rescues mice deficient for the prion protein gene from Purkinje cell degeneration and demyelination. Lab Invest 1999;79:689–697.

120. Moore RC, Mastrangelo P, Bouzamondo E, et al: Doppel-induced cerebellar degeneration in transgenic mice. Proc Natl Acad Sci U S A 2001;98:15288–15293.

121. Gossen M, Bujard H: Tight control of gene expression in mammalian cells by tetracycline-responsive promoters. Proc Natl Acad Sci U S A 1992;89:5547–5551.

122. Tremblay P, Meiner Z, Galou M, et al: Doxycyline control of prion protein transgene expression modulates prion disease in mice. Proc Natl Acad Sci U S A 1998;95:12580–12585.

123. Prusiner SB: Biology of prions. In Rosenberg RN, Prusiner SB, DiMauro S, Barchi RL (eds): The Molecular and Genetic Basis of Neurological Disease, 2nd ed. Stoneham, Mass.: Butterworth-Heinneman, 1997, pp 103–143.

124. Fraser H, Dickinson AG: The sequential development of the brain lesions of scrapie in three strains of mice. J Comp Pathol 1968;78:301–311.

125. Carp RI, Meeker H, Sersen E: Scrapie strains retain their distinctive characteristics following passages of homogenates from different brain regions and spleen. J Gen Virol 1997;78:283–290.

126. DeArmond SJ, Sánchez H, Yehiely F, et al: Selective neuronal targeting in prion disease. Neuron 1997;19:1337–1348.

127. Telling GC, Parchi P, DeArmond SJ, et al: Evidence for the conformation of the pathologic isoform of the prion protein enciphering and propagating prion diversity. Science 1996;274:2079–2082.

128. Prusiner SB: Scrapie prions. Annu Rev Microbiol 1989;43:345–374.

129. Will RG, Alpers MP, Dormont D, et al: Infectious and sporadic prion diseases. In Prusiner SB (ed.): Prion Biology and Diseases. Cold Spring Harbor, NY: Cold Spring Harbor Laboratory Press, 1999, pp 465–507.

130. Will RG, Ironside JW, Zeidler M, et al: A new variant of Creutzfeldt-Jakob disease in the UK. Lancet 1996;347:921–925.

131. Brown P, Gibbs CJ Jr, Rodgers-Johnson P, et al: Human spongiform encephalopathy: The National Institutes of Health series of 300 cases of experimentally transmitted disease. Ann Neurol 1994;35:513–529.

132. Holman RC, Khan AS, Kent J, et al: Epidemiology of Creutzfeldt-Jakob disease in the United States, 1979–1990: Analysis of national mortality data. Neuroepidemiology 1995;14:174–181.

133. Mastrianni J, Nixon F, Layzer R, et al: Fatal sporadic insomnia: Fatal familial insomnia phenotype without a mutation of the prion protein gene. Neurology 1997;48 [suppl]:A296.

134. Mastrianni JA, Nixon R, Layzer R, et al: Prion protein conformation in a patient with sporadic fatal insomnia. N Engl J Med 1999;340:1630–1638.

135. Parchi P, Capellari S, Chin S, et al: A subtype of sporadic prion disease mimicking fatal familial insomnia. Neurology 1999;52:1757–1763.

136. Gambetti P, Parchi P: Insomnia in prion diseases: Sporadic and familial. N Engl J Med 1999;340:1675–1677.

137. Parry HB (edited by DR Oppenheimer): Scrapie Disease in Sheep: Historical, Clinical, Epidemiological,

Pathological, and Practical Aspects of the Natural Diseases. New York, Academic Press, 1983.

138. Marsh RF, Bessen RA, Lehmann S, Hartsough GR: Epidemiological and experimental studies on a new incident of transmissible mink encephalopathy. J Gen Virol 1991;72:589–594.

139. Phillips NA, Bridgeman J, Ferguson-Smith M: Findings and Conclusions. The BSE Inquiry, vol 1. London, Stationery Office, 2000.

140. Telling GC, Scott M, Mastrianni J, et al: Prion propagation in mice expressing human and chimeric PrP transgenes implicates the interaction of cellular PrP with another protein. Cell 1995;83:79–90.

141. Cohen FE, Prusiner SB: Pathologic conformations of prion proteins. Annu Rev Biochem 1998;67:793–819.

142. Peretz D, Williamson RA, Kaneko K, et al: Antibodies inhibit prion propagation and clear cell cultures of prion infectivity. Nature 2001;412:739–743.

143. Owen F, Poulter M, Collinge J, Crow TJ: Codon 129 changes in the prion protein gene in Caucasians. Am J Hum Genet 1990;46:1215–1216.

144. Palmer MS, Dryden AJ, Hughes JT, Collinge J: Homozygous prion protein genotype predisposes to sporadic Creutzfeldt-Jakob disease. Nature 1991;352:340–342.

145. Goldfarb LG, Petersen RB, Tabaton M, et al: Fatal familial insomnia and familial Creutzfeldt-Jakob disease: Disease phenotype determined by a DNA polymorphism. Science 1992;258:806–808.

146. Collinge J, Palmer MS: Human prion diseases. In Collinge J, Palmer MS (eds): Prion Diseases. Oxford, Oxford University Press, 1997:18–56.

147. Collinge J, Palmer MS, Dryden AJ: Genetic predisposition to iatrogenic Creutzfeldt-Jakob disease. Lancet 1991;337:1441–1442.

148. Doh-ura K, Kitamoto T, Sakaki Y, Tateishi J: CJD discrepancy. Nature 1991;353:801–802.

149. Miyazono M, Kitamoto T, Doh-ura K, et al: Creutzfeldt-Jakob disease with codon 129 polymorphism (valine): A comparative study of patients with codon 102 point mutation or without mutations. Acta Neuropathol (Berl) 1992;84:349–354.

150. Tateishi J, Kitamoto T: Developments in diagnosis for prion diseases. Br Med Bull 1993;49:971–979.

151. Goldfarb LG, Brown P, Goldgaber D, et al: Creutzfeldt-Jakob disease and kuru patients lack a mutation consistently found in the Gerstmann-Sträussler-Scheinker syndrome. Exp Neurol 1990;108:247–250.

152. Fink JK, Peacock ML, Warren JT, et al: Detecting prion protein gene mutations by denaturing gradient gel electrophoresis. Hum Mutat 1994;4:42–50.

153. Laplanche J-L, Chatelain J, Launay J-M, et al: Deletion in prion protein gene in a Moroccan family. Nucleic Acids Res 1990;18:6745.

154. Vnencak-Jones CL, Phillips JA: Identification of heterogeneous PrP gene deletions in controls by detection of allele-specific heteroduplexes (DASH). Am J Hum Genet 1992;50:871–872.

155. Cervenáková L, Brown P, Piccardo P, et al: 24-nucleotide deletion in the PRNP gene: Analysis of associated phenotypes. In Court L, Dodet B (eds): Transmissible Subacute Spongiform Encephalopathies: Prion Diseases. Paris, Elsevier, 1996, pp 433–444.

156. Palmer MS, Mahal SP, Campbell TA, et al: Deletions in the prion protein gene are not associated with CJD. Hum Mol Genet 1993;2:541–544.

157. Kitamoto T, Tateishi J: Human prion diseases with variant prion protein. Philos Trans R Soc Lond B Biol Sci 1994;343:391–398.

158. Furukawa H, Kitamoto T, Tanaka Y, Tateishi J: New variant prion protein in a Japanese family with Gerstmann-Sträussler syndrome. Mol Brain Res 1995;30:385–388.

159. Shibuya S, Higuchi J, Shin R-W, et al: Codon 219 Lys allele of PRNP is not found in sporadic Creutzfeldt-Jakob disease. Ann Neurol 1998;43:826–828.

160. Kaneko K, Zulianello L, Scott M, et al: Evidence for protein X binding to a discontinuous epitope on the cellular prion protein during scrapie prion propagation. Proc Natl Acad Sci U S A 1997;94:10069–10074.

161. Zulianello L, Kaneko K, Scott M, et al: Dominant-negative inhibition of prion formation diminished by deletion mutagenesis of the prion protein. J Virol 2000;74:4351–4360.

162. Perrier V, Kaneko K, Safar J, et al: Dominant-negative inhibition of prion replication in transgenic mice. Proc Natl Acad Sci U S A 2002;99:13079–13084.

163. Westaway D, Zuliani V, Cooper CM, et al: Homozygosity for prion protein alleles encoding glutamine-171 renders sheep susceptible to natural scrapie. Genes Dev 1994;8:959–969.

164. Hunter N, Moore L, Hosie BD, et al: Association between natural scrapie and PrP genotype in a flock of Suffolk sheep in Scotland. Vet Rec 1997;140:59–63.

165. Telling GC, Scott M, Hsiao KK, et al: Transmission of Creutzfeldt-Jakob disease from humans to transgenic mice expressing chimeric human-mouse prion protein. Proc Natl Acad Sci U S A 1994;91:9936–9940.

166. Korth C, Kaneko K, Groth D, et al: Abbreviated incubation times for human prions in mice expressing a chimeric mouse-human prion protein transgene. Proc Natl Acad Sci U S A 2003 (in press).

167. Doh-ura K, Tateishi J, Sasaki H, et al: Pro→Leu change at position 102 of prion protein is the most common but not the sole mutation related to Gerstmann-Sträussler syndrome. Biochem Biophys Res Commun 1989;163:974–979.

168. Goldgaber D, Goldfarb LG, Brown P, et al: Mutations in familial Creutzfeldt-Jakob disease and Gerstmann-Sträussler-Scheinker's syndrome. Exp Neurol 1989;106:204–206.

169. Kretzschmar HA, Honold G, Seitelberger F, et al: Prion protein mutation in family first reported by Gerstmann, Sträussler, and Scheinker. Lancet 1991;337:1160.

170. Cervenakova L, Buetefisch C, Lee HS, et al: Novel PRNP sequence variant associated with familial encephalopathy. Am J Med Genet 1999;88:653–656.

171. Windl O, Giese A, Schulz-Schaeffer W, et al: Molecular genetics of human prion diseases in Germany. Hum Genet 1999;105:244–252.

172. Collins S, Boyd A, Fletcher A, et al: Novel prion protein gene mutation in an octogenarian with Creutzfeldt-Jakob disease. Arch Neurol 2000;57:1058–1063.

173. Peoc'h K, Manivet P, Beaudry P, et al: Identification of three novel mutations (E196K, V203I, E211Q) in the prion protein gene (PRNP) in inherited prion diseases with Creutzfeldt-Jakob disease phenotype. Hum Mutat 2000;15:482.

174. Finckh U, Muller-Thomsen T, Mann U, et al: High prevalence of pathogenic mutations in patients with early-onset dementia detected by sequence analyses of four different genes. Am J Hum Genet 2000;66:110–117.

175. Panegyres PK, Toufexis K, Kakulas BA, et al: A new PRNP mutation (G131V) associated with Gerstmann-Sträussler-Scheinker disease. Arch Neurol 2001;58:1899–1902.

176. Telling GC, Haga T, Torchia M, et al: Interactions between wild-type and mutant prion proteins modulate neurodegeneration in transgenic mice. Genes Dev 1996;10:1736–1750.

177. Hegde RS, Tremblay P, Groth D, et al: Transmissible and genetic prion diseases share a common pathway of neurodegeneration. Nature 1999;402:822–826.

178. Kaneko K, Ball HL, Wille H, et al: A synthetic peptide initiates Gerstmann-Sträussler-Scheinker (GSS) disease in transgenic mice. J Mol Biol 2000;295:997–1007.

179. Scott MR, Nguyen O, Stöckel J, et al: Designer mutations in the prion protein promote β-sheet formation in vitro and cause neurodegeneration in transgenic mice (Abstr). Protein Sci 1997;6 [suppl 1]:84.

180. Hsiao KK, Cass C, Schellenberg G, et al: Correlation of specific prion protein mutations with different forms of prion diseases. Neurology 1990;40:388.

181. Mastrianni JA, Curtis MT, Oberholtzer JC, et al: Prion disease (PrP-A117V) presenting with ataxia instead of dementia. Neurology 1995;45:2042–2050.

182. Goldfarb LG, Brown P, McCombie WR, et al: Transmissible familial Creutzfeldt-Jakob disease associated with five, seven, and eight extra octapeptide coding repeats in the PRNP gene. Proc Natl Acad Sci U S A 1991;88:10926–10930.

183. Goldfarb LG, Mitrova E, Brown P, et al: Mutation in codon 200 of scrapie amyloid protein gene in two clusters of Creutzfeldt-Jakob disease in Slovakia. Lancet 1990;336:514–515.

184. Goldfarb LG, Brown P, Mitrova E, et al: Creutzfeldt-Jacob disease associated with the PRNP codon 200^{Lys} mutation: An analysis of 45 families. Eur J Epidemiol 1991;7:477–486.

185. Bertoni JM, Brown P, Goldfarb L, et al: Familial Creutzfeldt-Jakob disease with the PRNP codon 200^{Lys} mutation and supranuclear palsy but without myoclonus or periodic EEG complexes. Neurology 1992;42 [no 4, suppl 3]:350 [abstr].

186. Gabizon R, Telling G, Meiner Z, et al: Insoluble wild-type and protease-resistant mutant prion protein in brains of patients with inherited prion disease. Nat Med 1996;2:59–64.

187. Goldfarb L, Brown P, Goldgaber D, et al: Identical mutation in unrelated patients with Creutzfeldt-Jakob disease. Lancet 1990;336:174–175.

188. Medori R, Montagna P, Tritschler HJ, et al: Fatal familial insomnia: A second kindred with mutation of prion protein gene at codon 178. Neurology 1992;42:669–670.

189. Lugaresi E, Medori R, Montagna P, et al: Fatal familial insomnia and dysautonomia with selective degeneration of thalamic nuclei. N Engl J Med 1986;315:997–1003.

190. Gambetti P, Parchi P, Petersen RB, et al: Fatal familial insomnia and familial Creutzfeldt-Jakob disease: Clinical, pathological and molecular features. Brain Pathol 1995;5:43–51.

191. Goldfarb LG, Haltia M, Brown P, et al: New mutation in scrapie amyloid precursor gene (at codon 178) in Finnish Creutzfeldt-Jakob kindred. Lancet 1991;337:425.

192. Kretzschmar HA, Neumann M, Stavrou D: Codon 178 mutation of the human prion protein gene in a German family (Backer family): Sequencing data from 72-year-old celloidin-embedded brain tissue. Acta Neuropathol (Berl) 1995;89:96–98.

193. Alpers MP: Kuru: Implications of its transmissibility for the interpretation of its changing epidemiological pattern. In Bailey OT, Smith DE (eds): The Central Nervous System: Some Experimental Models of Neurological Diseases. Baltimore, Williams & Wilkins, 1968:234–251.

194. Gajdusek DC, Gibbs CJ Jr, Asher DM, et al: Precautions in medical care of, and in handling materials from, patients with transmissible virus dementia (Creutzfeldt-Jakob disease). N Engl J Med 1977;297:1253–1258.

195. Klitzman RL, Alpers MP, Gajdusek DC: The natural incubation period of kuru and the episodes of transmission in three clusters of patients. Neuroepidemiology 1984;3:3–20.

196. Duffy P, Wolf J, Collins G, et al: Possible person to person transmission of Creutzfeldt-Jakob disease. N Engl J Med 1974;290:692–693.

197. Bernouilli C, Siegfried J, Baumgartner G, et al: Danger of accidental person to person transmission of

Creutzfeldt-Jakob disease by surgery. Lancet 1977;1: 478–479.

198. Gibbs CJ Jr, Asher DM, Kobrine A, et al: Transmission of Creutzfeldt-Jakob disease to a chimpanzee by electrodes contaminated during neurosurgery. J Neurol Neurosurg Psychiatry 1994;57:757–758.

199. Gajdusek DC: Unconventional viruses and the origin and disappearance of kuru. Science 1977;197: 943–960.

200. Will RG, Matthews WB: Evidence for case-to-case transmission of Creutzfeldt-Jakob disease. J Neurol Neurosurg Psychiatry 1982;45:235–238.

201. Collins S, Law MG, Fletcher A, et al: Surgical treatment and risk of sporadic Creutzfeldt-Jakob disease: A case-control study. Lancet 1999;353:693–697.

202. Centers for Disease Control: Creutzfeldt-Jakob disease associated with cadaveric dura mater grafts—Japan, January 1979–May 1996. MMWR Morb Mortal Wkly Rep 1997;46:1066–1069.

203. Tange RA, Troost D, Limburg M: Progressive fatal dementia (Creutzfeldt-Jakob disease) in a patient who received homograft tissue for tympanic membrane closure. Eur Arch Otorhinolaryngol 1989;247:199–201.

204. Fradkin JE, Schonberger LB, Mills JL, et al: Creutzfeldt-Jakob disease in pituitary growth hormone recipients in the United States. JAMA 1991;265: 880–884.

205. PHS: Report on Human Growth Hormone and Creutzfeldt-Jakob Disease, vol. 14. Public Health Service Interagency Coordinating Committee, 1997:1–11.

206. Cochius JI, Mack K, Burns RJ, et al: Creutzfeldt-Jakob disease in a recipient of human pituitary-derived gonadotropin. Aust N Z J Med 1990;20: 592–593.

207. Will RG, Cousens SN, Farrington CP, et al: Deaths from variant Creutzfeldt-Jakob disease. Lancet 1999;353:979.

208. Balter M: Tracking the human fallout from "mad cow disease." Science 2000;289:1452–1454.

209. Ghani AC, Ferguson NM, Donnelly CA, Anderson RM: Predicted vCJD mortality in Great Britain. Nature 2000;406:583–584.

210. Zeidler M, Stewart GE, Barraclough CR, et al: New variant Creutzfeldt-Jakob disease: Neurological features and diagnostic tests. Lancet 1997;350:903–907.

211. Lasmézas CI, Deslys J-P, Demaimay R, et al: BSE transmission to macaques. Nature 1996;381:743–744.

212. Hill AF, Desbruslais M, Joiner S, et al: The same prion strain causes vCJD and BSE. Nature 1997;389: 448–450.

213. Hill AF, Butterworth RJ, Joiner S, et al: Investigation of variant Creutzfeldt-Jakob disease and other human prion diseases with tonsil biopsy samples. Lancet 1999;353:183–189.

214. Bruce ME, Will RG, Ironside JW, et al: Transmissions to mice indicate that "new variant" CJD is caused by the BSE agent. Nature 1997;389:498–501.

215. Prusiner SB: Molecular neurology of prion diseases. In Martin JB (ed): Molecular Neurology. New York, Scientific American, 1998.

216. Scott MR, Will R, Ironside J, et al: Compelling transgenetic evidence for transmission of bovine spongiform encephalopathy prions to humans. Proc Natl Acad Sci U S A 1999;96:15137–15142.

217. Taraboulos A, Jendroska K, Serban D, et al: Regional mapping of prion proteins in brains. Proc Natl Acad Sci U S A 1992;89:7620–7624.

218. Collie DA, Sellar RJ, Zeidler M, et al: MRI of Creutzfeldt-Jakob disease: Imaging features and recommended MRI protocol. Clin Radiol 2001;56:726–739.

219. Nevin S, McMenemy WH, Behrman S, Jones DP: Subacute spongiform encephalopathy—A subacute form of encephalopathy attributable to vascular dysfunction (spongiform cerebral atrophy). Brain 1960;83: 519–564.

220. Zerr I, Bodemer M, Gefeller O, et al: Detection of 14-3-3 protein in the cerebrospinal fluid supports the diagnosis of Creutzfeldt-Jakob disease. Ann Neurol 1998;43:32–40.

221. Seipelt M, Zerr I, Nau R, et al: Hashimoto's encephalitis as a differential diagnosis of Creutzfeldt-Jakob disease. J Neurol Neurosurg Psychiatry 1999;66: 172–176.

222. Safar J, Wille H, Itri V, et al: Eight prion strains have PrPSc molecules with different conformations. Nat Med 1998;4:1157–1165.

223. Parry HB: Scrapie: A transmissible and hereditary disease of sheep. Heredity 1962;17:75–105.

224. Dickinson AG, Young GB, Stamp JT, Renwick CC: An analysis of natural scrapie in Suffolk sheep. Heredity 1965;20:485–503.

225. Goldmann W, Hunter N, Foster JD, et al: Two alleles of a neural protein gene linked to scrapie in sheep. Proc Natl Acad Sci U S A 1990;87:2476–2480.

226. Goldmann W, Hunter N, Manson J, Hope J: The PrP gene of the sheep, a natural host of scrapie. Proceedings of the Eighth International Congress of Virology, Aug 26, 1990, Berlin.

227. Laplanche J-L, Chatelain J, Beaudry P, et al: French autochthonous scrapied sheep without the 136Val PrP polymorphism. Mamm Genome 1993;4: 463–464.

228. Clousard C, Beaudry P, Elsen JM, et al: Different allelic effects of the codons 136 and 171 of the prion protein gene in sheep with natural scrapie. J Gen Virol 1995;76:2097–2101.

229. Hunter N, Goldmann W, Benson G, et al: Swaledale sheep affected by natural scrapie differ significantly in PrP genotype frequencies from healthy sheep and those selected for reduced incidence of scrapie. J Gen Virol 1993;74:1025–1031.

230. Goldmann W, Hunter N, Smith G, et al: PrP genotype and agent effects in scrapie: Change in allelic interaction with different isolates of agent in sheep, a natural host of scrapie. J Gen Virol 1994;75:989–995.

231. Belt PBGM, Muileman IH, Schreuder BEC, et al: Identification of five allelic variants of the sheep PrP gene and their association with natural scrapie. J Gen Virol 1995;76:509–517.

232. Ikeda T, Horiuchi M, Ishiguro N, et al: Amino acid polymorphisms of PrP with reference to onset of scrapie in Suffolk and Corriedale sheep in Japan. J Gen Virol 1995;76:2577–2581.

233. Hunter N, Cairns D, Foster JD, et al: Is scrapie solely a genetic disease? Nature 1997;386:137.

234. O'Rourke KI, Holyoak GR, Clark WW, et al: PrP genotypes and experimental scrapie in orally inoculated Suffolk sheep in the United States. J Gen Virol 1997;78:975–978.

235. Goldmann W, Hunter N, Benson G, et al: Different scrapie-associated fibril proteins (PrP) are encoded by lines of sheep selected for different alleles of the Sip gene. J Gen Virol 1991;72:2411–2417.

236. Hunter N, Foster JD, Benson G, Hope J: Restriction fragment length polymorphisms of the scrapie-associated fibril protein (PrP) gene and their association with susceptibility to natural scrapie in British sheep. J Gen Virol 1991;72:1287–1292.

237. Goldmann W, Hunter N, Martin T, et al: Different forms of the bovine PrP gene have five or six copies of a short, G-C-rich element within the protein-coding exon. J Gen Virol 1991;72:201–204.

238. Prusiner SB, Fuzi M, Scott M, et al: Immunologic and molecular biological studies of prion proteins in bovine spongiform encephalopathy. J Infect Dis 1993;167:602–613.

239. Hunter N, Goldmann W, Smith G, Hope J: Frequencies of PrP gene variants in healthy cattle and cattle with BSE in Scotland. Vet Rec 1994;135:400–403.

240. Wilesmith JW, Ryan JBM, Atkinson MJ: Bovine spongiform encephalopathy—Epidemiologic studies on the origin. Vet Rec 1991;128:199–203.

241. Nathanson N, Wilesmith J, Griot C: Bovine spongiform encephalopathy (BSE): Cause and consequences of a common source epidemic. Am J Epidemiol 1997;145:959–969.

242. Anderson RM, Donnelly CA, Ferguson NM, et al: Transmission dynamics and epidemiology of BSE in British cattle. Nature 1996;382:779–788.

243. Wilesmith JW: The epidemiology of bovine spongiform encephalopathy. Semin Virol 1991;2:239–245.

244. Kimberlin RH: Speculations on the origin of BSE and the epidemiology of CJD. In Gibbs CJ Jr (ed): Bovine Spongiform Encephalopathy: The BSE Dilemma. New York, Springer, 1996, pp 155–175.

245. Stekel DJ, Nowak MA, Southwood TRE: Prediction of future BSE spread. Nature 1996;381:119.

246. Fraser H, McConnell I, Wells GAH, Dawson M: Transmission of bovine spongiform encephalopathy to mice. Vet Rec 1988;123:472.

247. Dawson M, Wells GAH, Parker BNJ: Preliminary evidence of the experimental transmissibility of bovine spongiform encephalopathy to cattle. Vet Rec 1990;126:112–113.

248. Dawson M, Wells GAH, Parker BNJ, Scott AC: Primary parenteral transmission of bovine spongiform encephalopathy to the pig. Vet Rec 1990;127:338.

249. Bruce M, Chree A, McConnell I, et al: Transmissions of BSE, scrapie and related diseases to mice [abstract]. Proceedings of the Ninth International Congress of Virology, Aug 9, 1993, Glasgow, Scotland.

250. Robinson MM, Hadlow WJ, Knowles DP, et al: Experimental infection of cattle with the agents of transmissible mink encephalopathy and scrapie. J Comp Path 1995;113:241–251.

251. Alpers M: Epidemiology and clinical aspects of kuru. In Prusiner SB, McKinley MP (eds): Prions—Novel Infectious Pathogens Causing Scrapie and Creutzfeldt-Jakob Disease. Orlando, FL, Academic Press, 1987, pp 451–465.

252. Hope J, Reekie LJD, Hunter N, et al: Fibrils from brains of cows with new cattle disease contain scrapie-associated protein. Nature 1988;336:390–392.

253. Grathwohl K-UD, Horiuchi M, Ishiguro N, Shinagawa M: Sensitive enzyme-linked immunosorbent assay for detection of PrP^{Sc} in crude tissue extracts from scrapie-affected mice. J Virol Methods 1997;64:205–216.

254. Korth C, Stierli B, Streit P, et al: Prion (PrP^{Sc})-specific epitope defined by a monoclonal antibody. Nature 1997;389:74–77.

255. Scott MR, Safar J, Telling G, et al: Identification of a prion protein epitope modulating transmission of bovine spongiform encephalopathy prions to transgenic mice. Proc Natl Acad Sci U S A 1997;94:14279–14284.

256. Taylor KC: The control of bovine spongiform encephalopathy in Great Britain. Vet Rec 1991;129:522–526.

257. Fraser H, Bruce ME, Chree A, et al: Transmission of bovine spongiform encephalopathy and scrapie to mice. J Gen Virol 1992;73:1891–1897.

258. Hunter GD, Millson GC, Chandler RL: Observations on the comparative infectivity of cellular fractions derived from homogenates of mouse-scrapie brain. Res Vet Sci 1963;4:543–549.

259. Eklund CM, Kennedy RC, Hadlow WJ: Pathogenesis of scrapie virus infection in the mouse. J Infect Dis 1967;117:15–22.

260. Kimberlin R, Walker C: Characteristics of a short incubation model of scrapie in the golden hamster. J Gen Virol 1977;34:295–304.

261. Prusiner SB, Cochran SP, Groth DF, et al: Measurement of the scrapie agent using an incubation time interval assay. Ann Neurol 1982;11:353–358.

262. Spraker TR, Miller MW, Williams ES, et al: Spongiform encephalopathy in free-ranging mule deer (*Odocoileus hemionus*), white tailed deer (*Odocoileus virginianus*), and Rocky Mountain elk (*Cervus elaphus*

nelsoni) in north central Colorado. J Wildl Dis 1997; 33:1–6.

263. Miller MW, Wild MA, Williams ES: Epidemiology of chronic wasting disease in captive Rocky Mountain elk. J Wildl Dis 1998;34:532–538.

264. Bahmanyar S, Williams ES, Johnson FB, et al: Amyloid plaques in spongiform encephalopathy of mule deer. J Comp Pathol 1985;95:1–5.

265. Williams ES, Young S: Neuropathology of chronic wasting disease of mule deer (*Odocoileus hemionus*) and elk (*Cervus elaphus nelsoni*). Vet Pathol 1993;30:36–45.

266. Belay ED, Gambetti P, Schonberger LB, et al: Creutzfeldt-Jakob disease in unusually young patients who consumed venison. Arch Neurol 2001;58:1673–1678.

267. Kimberlin RH, Walker CA: The antiviral compound HPA-23 can prevent scrapie when administered at the time of infection. Arch Virol 1983;78:9–18.

268. Ehlers B, Diringer H: Dextran sulphate 500 delays and prevents mouse scrapie by impairment of agent replication in spleen. J Gen Virol 1984;65:1325–1330.

269. Diringer H: Transmissible spongiform encephalopathies (TSE) virus-induced amyloidoses of the central nervous system (CNS). Eur J Epidemiol 1991;7: 562–566.

270. Dickinson AG, Fraser H, Outram GW: Scrapie incubation time can exceed natural lifespan. Nature 1975;256:732–733.

271. Priola SA, Raines A, Caughey WS: Porphyrin and phthalocyanine antiscrapie compounds. Science 2000;287:1503–1506.

272. Caughey B, Race RE: Potent inhibition of scrapie-associated PrP accumulation by Congo red. J Neurochem 1992;59:768–771.

273. Gorodinsky A, Harris DA: Glycolipid-anchored proteins in neuroblastoma cells form detergent-resistant complexes without caveolin. J Cell Biol 1995;129: 619–627.

274. Taraboulos A, Scott M, Semenov A, et al: Cholesterol depletion and modification of COOH-terminal targeting sequence of the prion protein inhibits formation of the scrapie isoform. J Cell Biol 1995;129:121–132.

275. Supattapone S, Nguyen H-OB, Cohen FE, et al: Elimination of prions by branched polyamines and impli-cations for therapeutics. Proc Natl Acad Sci USA 1999; 96:14529–14534.

276. Perrier V, Wallace AC, Kaneko K, et al: Mimicking dominant negative inhibition of prion replication through structure-based drug design. Proc Natl Acad Sci USA 2000;97:6073–6078.

277. Doh-ura K, Iwaki T, Caughey B: Lysosomotropic agents and cysteine protease inhibitors inhibit scrapie-associated prion protein accumulation. J Virol 2000;74:4894–4897.

278. Korth C, May BCH, Cohen FE, Prusiner SB: Acridine and phenothiazine derivatives as pharmacotherapeutics for prion disease. Proc Natl Acad Sci U S A 2001;98:9836–9841.

279. Hammick DL, Chambers WE: Optical activity of excreted mepacrine. Nature 1945;155:141.

280. Goodman LS, Gilman A: The Pharmacological Basis of Therapeutics; a Textbook of Pharmacology, Toxicology, and Therapeutics for Physicians and Medical Students. New York, Macmillan, 1970.

281. Enari M, Flechsig E, Weissmann C: Scrapie prion protein accumulation by scrapie-infected neuroblastoma cells abrogated by exposure to a prion protein antibody. Proc Natl Acad Sci U S A 2001;98:9295–9299.

282. United Nations: World population prospects, the 1998 revision volume II: The sex and age distribution of the world population, vol 2. New York, United Nations Department of Economic and Social Affairs Population Division, 1999.

283. Kascsak RJ, Rubenstein R, Merz PA, et al: Mouse polyclonal and monoclonal antibody to scrapie-associated fibril proteins. J Virol 1987;61:3688–3693.

284. Laplanche J-L, Hunter N, Shinagawa M, Williams E: Scrapie, chronic wasting disease, and transmissible mink encephalopathy. In Prusiner SB (ed): Prion Biology and Diseases. Cold Spring Harbor, NY: Cold Spring Harbor Laboratory Press, 1999, pp 393–429.

285. O'Rourke KI, Besser TE, Miller MW, et al: PrP genotypes of captive and free-ranging Rocky Mountain elk (*Cervus elaphus nelsoni*) with chronic wasting disease. J Gen Virol 1999;80:2765–2769.

CHAPTER

14

The Mitochondrial Genome

Eric A. Schon

MITOCHONDRIAL ORIGINS

Mitochondria are tiny organelles located in the cytoplasm of almost all mammalian cells. Vitally important functions take place in the mitochondria, such as the citric acid cycle, amino acid biosynthesis, fatty acid oxidation, apoptosis, and oxidative phosphorylation. Their small size reflects their evolutionary origin. The widely accepted endosymbiont hypothesis states that mitochondria were once bacteria. These bacteria were "captured" by a proto-eukaryote early in evolution.[1] Due, in part, to the action of primitive photosynthetic organisms, the earth's atmosphere began to shift from a reducing one (rich in ammonia, methane, carbon monoxide, and hydrogen) to an oxidizing one (rich in nitrogen and oxygen). Bacteria were among the first organisms to evolve systems to deal with a new environmental toxin—oxygen—and convert it into nontoxic or less toxic forms, such as carbon dioxide, nitrate, and water. A bonus that resulted from this evolutionary leap was the increased efficiency of energy utilization afforded by the oxidation of reduced substrates.

It has been hypothesized that at some point an early single-celled eukaryote ingested these more energy-efficient, oxygen-detoxifying, autonomously-replicating bacteria (possibly from the prokaryotic group called the purple photosynthetic bacteria, but even mycoplasma have been proposed as the ancestor of mitochondria). Over time, the relationship between the two organisms became a symbiotic one, in which the eukaryotic host provided food and shelter, while the bacterium detoxified the oxygen that threatened the host's survival and, at the same time, provided extra oxidative energy. Two events cemented this symbiotic relationship and eventually converted the bacterium into the mitochondrion we see today: the bacterium lost 99% of its genes (many of which entered the nucleus and became incorporated into nuclear DNA), and the bacterium's translation apparatus evolved so that it could only utilize a modified form of the "universal" genetic code to translate the few remaining messenger RNAs specified by its DNA (now called mitochondrial DNA, or mtDNA).

There are a number of structural and functional features of mitochondria that are still reminiscent of its bacterial origin. The most obvious one is morphology: mitochondria are about 1 μ in length, thus approximating the size of most bacteria. Their shapes vary from spherical to rodlike, and can have a network-like appearance with many "arms." Like many bacteria, they have a two-membrane structure: an *outer mitochondrial membrane* surrounds an *inner mitochondrial membrane*, which is itself invaginated at numerous points to form *cristae*. The *intermembrane space* is located between the outer and inner membranes, while the latter encloses the *matrix* in the organelle's interior. Other similarities to bacteria will become evident as we discuss the unique biochemical and genetic features of mitochondria.

GENOME ORGANIZATION

There is huge diversity in the mitochondrial genomes from different organisms. The malarial parasite *Plasmodium falciparum* contains a small linear mtDNA about 6 kilobase pairs (kb) long. The mtDNA in maize is a huge circular genome about 700 kb long, and the mtDNA in some plants can be up to 2500 kb long (about half the size of the circular bacterial genome of *Escherichia coli*). Most fungi (e.g., *Saccharomyces cerevisiae*, or baker's yeast) have mtDNA about 85 kb long. Among eukaryotes, the mitochondrial genomes of insects and mammals are only 15 to 20 kb long, which is an example of genetic economy.

The human mitochondrial genome (Fig. 14–1) is a double-stranded circle of 16,569 base pairs (bp).[2] It is highly asymmetric in its base composition, with one strand rich in nucleotides G and T (called the heavy strand) and the other correspondingly rich in C and A (called the light strand). The "heavy" and "light" nomenclature refers to the differential mobility of the separated strands in alkaline cesium chloride gradients. Of the approximately 4000 genes presumably present in the protomitochondrion, only 37 remain in the modern human mitochondrial genome. About 850 of the lost genes now reside in the nuclear DNA and encode proteins that are synthesized in the cytoplasm and are then imported into mitochondria. Most of these lost genes have "housekeeping" functions, such as specifying the gene products necessary for protein import, nucleic acid metabolism, protein translation, β-oxidation, the citric acid cycle, the urea cycle, amino acid metabolism, steroid metabolism, and oxidative metabolism.

Of the 37 genes on human mtDNA, only 13 specify polypeptides, and like bacterial DNA, none of them contain introns. Remarkably, all 13 encode related functions, as they are all components of the respiratory chain/oxidative phosphorylation system (Fig. 14–2). This system is a set of five biochemically-related complexes located in the mitochondrial inner membrane. Complexes I, III, IV, and V are composed of polypeptides encoded by both nuclear and mitochondrial genes. Nucleus-encoded genes (some of

which are tissue-specific, such as the two muscle-specific subunits VIa and VIIa of cytochrome c oxidase) are imported into mitochondria, and are co-assembled with mtDNA-encoded genes into the respective enzyme complexes in the mitochondrial inner membrane. Complex II has two noteworthy features. First, unlike the other four complexes, complex II contains no mtDNA-encoded subunits, and is therefore often used as an "internal control" for the presence, amount, and viability of mitochondria in situations where mutations in mtDNA render some or all of the other four respiratory complexes inactive. Second, two of its four subunits comprise the activity of succinate dehydrogenase (SDH); because SDH is also a key enzyme in the citric acid cycle, complex II enables the respiratory chain to monitor CoA utilization and reducing equivalents (NADH; FADH2) in the organelle.

The other 24 genes on human mtDNA are required for translation inside of the organelle. Two genes specify ribosomal RNAs (called 12S and 16S rRNA). These rRNAs are more closely related to bacterial rRNAs than to nucleus-encoded cytoplasmic rRNAs. Twenty-two genes specify transfer RNAs (tRNAs), which are required for incorporation of amino acids into the growing polypeptide chain as the mtDNA-encoded mRNAs are translated on mitochondrial ribosomes. These tRNA genes are located strategically around the circle, precisely at the borders between the rRNA and most of the polypeptide-coding genes. This "punctuation" is believed to be crucial to the precise maturation of the tRNAs, rRNA, and mRNAs (see the section on transcription).

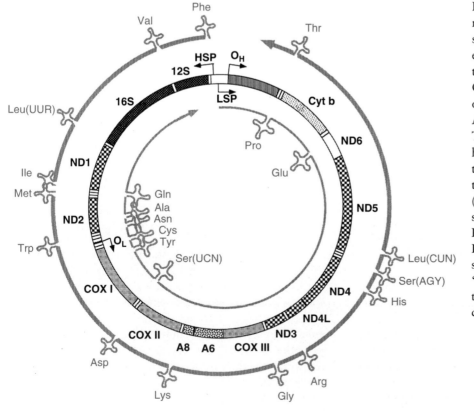

FIGURE 14–1. Map of the human mitochondrial genome, showing the structural genes for the mtDNA-encoded 12S and 16S ribosomal RNAs, the subunits of NADH-coenzyme Q oxidoreductase (ND), cytochrome c oxidase (COX), cytochrome b (Cyt b), ATP synthetase (A), and 22 tRNAs. The origins of light-strand (O_L) and heavy-strand (O_H) replication, and of the promoters for initiation of transcription from the light-strand (LSP) and heavy-strand (HSP), are shown (arrows). Transcription of the H-strand (outer gray circle) and L-strand (inner gray circle) is shown schematically, with the tRNAs "punctuating" the polycistronic transcripts. (See text for further description).

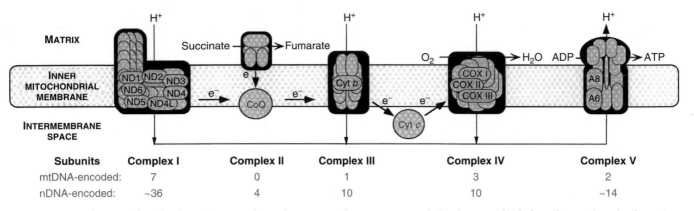

FIGURE 14–2. The mitochondrial respiratory chain showing nuclear DNA-encoded subunits *(shaded)* and mitochondrial DNA-encoded subunits *(labeled as in Figure 14-1)*. Protons (H^+) are pumped from the matrix to the intermembrane space through Complexes I, III, and IV. They are then transported back to the matrix through Complex V, with the concomitant production of ATP. Ubiquinone (Coenzyme Q, or CoQ) and cytochrome c (Cyt c) are nucleus-encoded electron transfer proteins.

Because respiratory chain complexes are derived from both mitochondrial and nuclear genes, mitochondrial respiratory-chain disorders are both mendelian-inherited (e.g., mutations in nDNA-encoded subunits) and maternally inherited (e.g., mutations in mtDNA-encoded subunits). Enormous progress has been made to uncover the molecular bases of maternally-inherited disorders, many of which are associated with qualitative and quantitative defects in mtDNA-encoded respiratory chain subunits. Progress on the etiology of the mendelian-inherited gene errors is well under way.

MITOCHONDRIAL INHERITANCE

Mammalian mitochondria, and therefore mammalian mtDNAs, are maternally inherited. This means that a mother transmits mitochondria to all of her children, both boys and girls, but only her daughters will transmit their mitochondria to their children. There are at least two competing hypotheses that might explain the limitation of mitochondrial transmission to females. The first hypothesis is based simply on numbers. The typical mammalian sperm contains relatively few mitochondria (albeit large ones, wrapped around the "neck" of the sperm midpiece), whereas the oocyte contains about 100,000 mitochondria. Since only 1% of the mitochondria present at fertilization will eventually repopulate the embryo (those in the inner cell mass; the remainder become part of the extraembryonic tissues), the chances that a paternal mitochondrion will enter the fetus is extremely low. Even if it entered the fetus, it would be extremely hard to detect amid the vast majority of maternal mitochondria.

The second hypothesis is based on the finding that during fertilization the sperm enters the ovum in its entirety.[3] The widely-held view that only the head of the sperm (which contains the nucleus but no mitochondria) enters the ovum, while the tail (which contains the paternal mitochondria) falls away and never enters the egg, is erroneous. Although paternal mitochondria enter the ovum at fertilization, they are selectively destroyed by an unknown mechanism, as if the paternal mitochondrion were a foreign "antigen." Although paternal mitochondria are not inherited in the offspring of matings between mice of the same strains, they can be inherited at high frequency in matings between mice of two different strains.[4] This finding strengthens the "foreign-body" hypotheses. An explanation consistent with this finding is that unknown factors in the ovum recognize and then destroy mitochondria derived from sperm of the same species (the usual situation), but these factors are incapable of recognizing or destroying mitochondria from a different species.

SEGREGATION AND HETEROPLASMY

One of the most important concepts in mitochondrial genetics is that it is *population* genetics. This key feature distinguishes it from mendelian genetics. Depending on the energy requirements of a particular tissue, there may be hundreds or even thousands of mitochondria in a cell, with multiple mtDNAs in each organelle. The timing of organellar division and of mtDNA replication are apparently stochastic events unrelated to the cell cycle. Thus, the numbers of mitochondria present in a cell vary both in space (among cells and tissues) and in time (during development and aging). The numbers can also increase or decrease based on the oxidative energy requirements of the moment (e.g., after prolonged training in athletes, after acclimation at high altitude). This dynamic aspect of mitochondrial transmission from cell to cell is termed *mitotic segregation*.

In mendelian genetics, a person's nuclear DNA can contain, at most, only two alleles for any particular autosomal gene, one paternally-derived (e.g., allele "A") and the other maternally derived (e.g., allele "B"). Thus, an individual may be homozygous (A/A or B/B), heterozygous (A/B), or even hemizygous (A/null or B/null) at a particular gene locus. In mitochondrial genetics, on the other hand, there are theoretically as many alleles for a particular gene in a cell as there are mtDNAs in that cell. To all intents and purposes, however, the mitochondrial genotypes of all mtDNAs are identical in a normal person. On the other hand, of the 16,569 bp that form the mtDNA genotype, the mtDNA sequence typically differs between two unrelated individuals at approximately 50 positions. These differences are presumably neutral polymorphisms, at least in the normal population. Note that mating does not alter these differences: if a man with mtDNA genotype A marries a woman with mtDNA genotype B, their children will have only genotype B, owing to the effect of exclusive maternal inheritance. Thus, in the normal course of events, individuals have *homoplasmic* mitochondrial genotypes (all mtDNAs are identical).

The presence of different mitochondrial genotypes begs the question as to why different genotypes exist at all. As with nuclear DNA, mtDNA mutations arise in single molecules spontaneously, probably during DNA replication. In mtDNA, these mutations are usually transitions: purines (A or G) replace purines, and pyrimidines (C or T) replace pyrimidines; transversions (purines replacing pyrimidines or vice versa) are relatively rare. Once a mutation is fixed, the cell is considered to be *heteroplasmic* (with coexistence of different mtDNA genotypes). If the mutation arises in the female germline, it can be transmitted to the next generation. However, the *bottleneck hypothesis* states that the number of mtDNAs transmitted from mother to child is quite small (estimated at between 5 and 200 segregating units[5]), so even if the germline is heteroplasmic, purification to homoplasmy can take place within a few generations. This would explain why mtDNA genotypes vary among individuals, and yet those individuals are homoplasmic for their particular genotype.

Obviously, a child can be born with heteroplasmic mtDNA if there were heteroplasmy among the few mtDNAs that pass through the mitochondrial bottleneck between mother and child. This is most clearly seen in the maternal inheritance of rare pathogenic mtDNA mutations, in which both the clinical phenotype and the associated mtDNA genotype can be tracked in the maternal lineage of a pedigree. In the vast majority of situations, those pathogenic mutations are heteroplasmic (there is a coexistence of normal and mutated mtDNAs). Presumably, homoplasmic pathogenic mtDNA mutations are rarely seen because they would result either in oocyte failure or in embryonic lethality. The combination of heteroplasmy and mitotic segregation can result in mitochondrial disorders with variable presentation of the pathogenic phenotype among affected members of a pedigree, among different tissues in an affected individual, and during the life span of that individual.

MITOCHONDRIAL DNA REPLICATION

The replication of circular human mtDNA is somewhat "prokaryote-like," but has a number of features that make it unusual. In a typical bacterium, such as *E. coli*, the circular genome has a single origin of replication that initiates bidirectional replication from a fixed position on the genome. Thus, daughter-strand DNA synthesis in *E. coli*, controlled by the combined action of RNA polymerase that synthesizes short RNA primers, and DNA polymerases that use the RNA primers to extend the newly-forming daughter DNA using the parental strand as the template, proceeds simultaneously in opposite directions. It proceeds clockwise from the top strand and counterclockwise from the bottom strand. Replication on both strands creates a pair of catenated circles. Each circle is a double helix consisting of one "old" parental strand and one "new" daughter strand. The circles are then separated into two free-standing, or *de-catenated* circles by the action of an enzyme called topoisomerase II. (This mode of replication is quite distinct from that of eukaryotic nuclear DNA, in which thousands of origins of replication, or "eyes," are spaced along the length of the linear chromosomal DNA.)

Human mtDNA also has a single origin of replication, except for one crucial difference: the mtDNA origin has been physically separated into two halves, each controlling synthesis of one of the two daughter DNA strands (Fig. 14–3). Synthesis of one strand begins at the *origin of heavy-strand replication* (O_H), which is located at the top of the circle, around map position 200 (nomenclature of Reference 2; see Fig. 14–3), within the 1123-bp "control region" between the tRNA^{Phe} gene (at map position 577) and the tRNA^{Pro} gene (at map position 16023), and proceeds in a clockwise direction. Synthesis of the other strand begins at the *origin of light-strand replication* (O_L), which is located at about "8 o'clock" on the circle (near position 5750), and proceeds in a counterclockwise direction.

This separation of the two origins results in a rather baroque mechanism for overall replication[6] and requires a number of nucleus-encoded polypeptides (and RNAs) that are imported into the organelle. As with bacterial DNA, there is a requirement for the synthesis of an RNA primer for initiating DNA synthesis. This RNA primer is synthesized by mitochondrial RNA polymerase as a relatively large precursor molecule starting near one of the three upstream *conserved sequence blocks* (CSB I, II, and III) located between O_H and tRNA^{Phe}. This RNA hybridizes to the L-strand and displaces a portion of the H-strand in the control region, thereby exposing the so-called "D- loop" (D is for "displacement"). DNA replication does not commence until the precursor RNA is cleaved at a precise location on the RNA by mitochon-

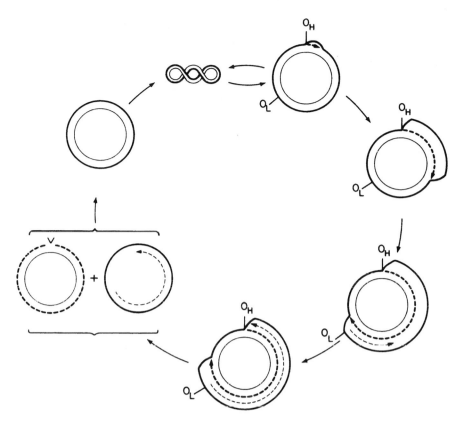

FIGURE 14–3. Replication of human mtDNA *(clockwise from circle located at "1 o'clock")*. Replication of the parental mtDNA *(thick solid lines are heavy H strands; thin solid lines are light L strands)* proceeds from O_H in the D-loop region until daughter strand synthesis *(heavy dashed line)* reaches O_L, at which point daughter light-strand synthesis *(light dashed line)* initiates in a counterclockwise direction. Following completion of synthesis of the two daughter strands, the two progeny molecules, which are initially catenated circles (not shown), are unlinked; the "relaxed" circles are then supercoiled by topoisomerase. See text for further description. (Adapted from Clayton DA: Replication of animal mitochondrial DNA. Cell 1982;28:693. Reproduced with permission from Cell Press, Cambridge, Mass.)

drial RNA-processing ribonuclease. RNase MRP is a polypeptide associated with a nucleus-encoded RNA (i.e., a ribonucleoprotein) that is imported into mitochondria to form the primer required by the mitochondrial DNA polymerase (called polymerase γ, to distinguish it from polymerases α, β, δ, and ε, which control replication of nuclear DNA).

The nascent daughter H-strand is synthesized from "1 o'clock" toward "8 o'clock," all the while extending the parental D-loop forward as daughter H-strand DNA is laid down on parental L-strand DNA. As the polymerase (and the displaced DNA) passes "8 o'clock," a specific segment of single-stranded parental H-strand O_L is "revealed." Owing to the presence of an inverted repeat sequence in this region, the single-stranded DNA around O_L forms a "hairpin" or "stem-loop" structure containing a repeat of Ts in the loop of the hairpin. A second RNA primer, containing a complementary repeat of As, binds to the loop, and becomes a primer for synthesis of daughter L-strand DNA in the opposite (counterclockwise) direction, with the assistance of an O_L-specific "primase." The two opposite-growing strands continue until they both have traversed their respective circles completely.

A second mode of replication has been described, which appears to operate under special circumstances (e.g., when cells are increasing their mtDNA copy number rapidly). This mode of replication is similar to the classic "theta replication" mechanism by which circular bacterial genomes divide, as previously described. In this model, replication initiates from a single origin and pro-

ceeds symmetrically in both a clockwise and counterclockwise direction (intermediates in such a mode of replication look like the Greek letter theta). Because all DNA polymerases synthesize daughter strand DNA only in the 5′ → 3′ direction, in this mode of replication one strand (the "leading" strand) is extended in a continuous fashion, whereas the other (the "lagging" strand) is not. In particular, in order for the lagging strand to grow in the 3′ → 5′ direction, it is made as a series of fragments that are actually synthesized in the 5′ → 3′ direction, albeit discontinuously, with each segment ligated to its adjacent partners.

In both mechanisms, replication terminates with the creation of a pair of catenated circles (each circle is a double helix containing one "old" parental strand and one "new" daughter strand). Mitochondrial DNA topoisomerase now decatenates the circles, releasing the two daughter molecules. The entire process takes a remarkably long time—approximately two hours to replicate the 16,569 bp of mitochondrial DNA. (Compare this to the 40 minutes required to replicate about 4 million bp of *E. coli* DNA.)

There are a number of mendelian-inherited mitochondrial disorders that are due to errors in the components of the replication machinery or in the regulation of the organellar nucleotide pools. One such disorder is mtDNA depletion, in which infants are born with a severe deficiency in the number of mitochondrial genomes present in specific tissues.[8] Another group of disorders are the mendelian-inherited mtDNA multiple deletion disorders. In these diseases, patients inherit a defective gene that appears to increase the frequency of mtDNA rearrangements, thereby causing pathologic consequences, and are manifested as both autosomal-dominant and autosomal-recessive inherited forms. Mutations causing depletion and multiple deletion syndromes have now been found in genes encoding DNA polymerase γ, mitochondrial thymidine kinase, mitochondrial deoxyguanosine kinase, the adenine nucleotide translocator, and cytosolic thymidine phosphorylase. It should be noted that mtDNA rearrangements can also be inherited in a maternal fashion, and can even be sporadic, but the mechanisms responsible for these latter conditions almost certainly do not involve intrinsic defects in the replicative machinery.

TRANSCRIPTION

Like mtDNA replication, transcription of human mtDNA has a prokaryotic "look" about it. In broad view, all of the 37 genes encoded by human mtDNA are initially synthesized on two huge polycistronic precursor transcripts, one encoded by the L-strand and the other by the H-strand (see Fig. 14–1). Of the 37 genes, 28 (2 rRNAs, 14 tRNAs, and 12 polypeptide-coding genes) are encoded by the H-strand (note that these RNAs are *encoded* by the H-strand, meaning that they have the *same sequence* as the L-strand). Only 8 tRNAs and 1 mRNA (ND6) are encoded by the L-strand. Since the precursor RNAs are single-stranded, the tRNA genes that "punctuate" the circle at strategic positions[9] can now adopt their typical "cloverleaf" conformation (see Fig. 14–1). It is thought that these tRNAs become targets for the action of two enzymes, called RNase P (another imported ribonucleoprotein) and 3′-tRNase.[10] These enzymes excise the tRNAs by cleaving them precisely at their 5′ and 3′ edges in the precursor transcript, respectively, thereby releasing not only the tRNAs, but the flanking rRNAs and mRNAs as well. However, there is no tRNA separating ATPase 6 from COX III, and it is not clear how these two messages are processed.

Many details of mitochondrial transcription have been elucidated.[6] Human mtDNA contains only two promoters for RNA transcription, both located within the 150-bp region in the D-loop containing the CSBs. One promoter controls transcription of the H-strand (the heavy-strand promoter, or HSP), while the other controls L-strand transcription (the LSP). The LSP is also important because it is required for synthesis of the RNA primer required for replication at O_H. Two *trans*-acting transcription factors, called mtTFA and mtTFB, bind to specific sequences upstream of both the HSP and LSP transcription start sites to promote transcription in the presence of mt-RNA polymerase.[11, 12]

Because transcription is polycistronic, an interesting arithmetic problem presents itself. Polycistronic transcription means that all of the mature RNAs ultimately generated off the H-strand (or the L-strand) are produced in equimolar amounts. Since each mRNA requires large numbers of rRNAs and tRNAs for its translation, there must be mechanisms whereby the steady-state levels of tRNAs and rRNAs are sufficient to satisfy the translational demands of the mRNAs specifying all 13 polypeptides. One such regulatory mechanism is likely to be differential turnover of classes of RNAs, especially mRNAs as compared to tRNAs.[13]

For rRNAs, however, mitochondria have also evolved at least one elegant solution to the problem. Besides the long 16-kb polycistronic transcript generated off the HSP and encompassing all the H-strand genes, a shorter 3-kb transcript is also synthesized. This transcript, which encompasses only the two rRNA genes and their flanking tRNAs, is synthesized at approximately 25 times the abundance of the long transcript,[14] thereby enabling a sufficient amount of 12S and 16S rRNA to be made for all the ribosomes that the organelle needs for translation. This, of course, raises a new question: how does the transcriptional machinery produce both long and short H-strand transcripts off the same promoter, and in vastly different amounts? It turns out that there is a protein that binds to the tRNA$^{Leu(UUR)}$ gene located immediately downstream of the 16S rRNA gene.[15] When this protein, called mitochondrial transcription termination factor (mtTERF), binds to a specific sequence located in the middle of the tRNA$^{Leu(UUR)}$ gene, it blocks the advance of the RNA polymerase, and the short form of the H-strand transcript is released. When mtTERF does not bind (either because it is not present in sufficient amounts, or because it is prevented from binding by another factor), the polymerase advances unhindered and the long form of the transcript is made.

Following cleavage of the precursor polycistronic RNAs, other processing events are required for maturation of the RNAs before translation can proceed. The 3′ termini of the mRNAs are polyadenylated (polyadenylation is absent in prokaryotes; thus it is one of the rare instances where a mammalian mitochondrial function is more similar to a process that occurs in eukaryotic, nuclear DNA). The trinucleotide CCA is added to the 3′ termini of the tRNAs (CCA addition is required for aminoacylation of the tRNAs by their cognate aminoacyl synthetases), and specific tRNA bases are chemically modified (e.g., conversion of uridine to pseudouridine).

TRANSLATION

Translation of mitochondrial mRNAs takes place on mitochondrial ribosomes, which consist of mtDNA-encoded 12S and 16S rRNAs together with imported ribosomal proteins. Translation of mRNAs has features unique to mitochondria. The first has to do with the structure of the mRNA. Like bacterial messages, the upstream end of the message (the "5′ end") contains no added "recognition" structure ("cap") for translation initiation. The 5′ end, however, poses a conceptual problem for translation initiation. Ordinarily, the ribosome binds to a specific position in the 5′-untranslated region (the ribosome binding site). The ribosome then travels along the message until it finds the first appropriate initiation codon (usually AUG, specifying methionine). At this point, reading of the codon triplets produces the translated message until the ribosome encounters a "stop" codon (UAA, UAG, or UGA) at the other end of the message. In mammalian mitochondria, however, the initiation codon is located at the very beginning of the mature message (there is little or no 5′-untranslated region). In this case, it is unclear how the ribosome recognizes and binds to the message. It is known that the initiation codon is sequestered in a stem structure to which the mitochondrial ribosome binds, but this may not be obligatory. Also, factors similar to those required for translation initiation on prokaryotic and eukaryotic messages are present in mammalian mitochondria.

The downstream end of the message (called the "3′ end") contains its own quirks. Except for COX II, none of the mRNAs has a 3′-untranslated region (a feature present in both bacterial and eukaryotic nuclear mRNAs). The last amino acid–specifying codon is thus located within one or two nucleotides of the end of the message, and the messages often end with a U or a UA. Interestingly, addition of the poly(A) tail to the mRNA converts these "supernumerary" nucleotides to UAA, which is a translational stop codon.

Two of the mRNAs contain overlapping messages, that is, one contiguous piece of mRNA specifies two different polypeptides. In both cases, the pair of overlapping polypeptides belong to the same respiratory complex: one message encodes both ND4L and ND4 of Complex I, while the other encodes both ATPase 8 and ATPase 6 of Complex V; both overlaps are out of frame with each other.

Finally, as noted earlier, human mitochondria have their own genetic code, which differs from the universal code at four of the 64 triplet positions (AUA specifies Met instead of Ile; UGA specifies Trp instead of Stop; and AGA and AGG specify Stop instead of Arg). This alteration ensures that only mtDNA-encoded messages can be translated faithfully, even if a "stray" piece of cytoplasmic RNA were to enter the organelle. Conversely, mitochondrial sequences that stray into the nucleus and integrate into nuclear DNA (rare but documented events) would not be translated correctly on cytoplasmic ribosomes even if transcribed, and these polypeptides would likely be degraded rapidly.

Errors in mitochondrial translation have been associated with a number of mitochondrial diseases. The most notable diseases are sporadic Kearns-Sayre syndrome and sporadic progressive external ophthalmoplegia (mtDNA-encoded mRNAs are not translated) and maternally-inherited MELAS (the amount of translation products is reduced) and MERRF (the amount of translation and aberrant translation products is reduced).

IMPORTATION

As noted earlier, the vast majority of mitochondrial proteins is nucleus-encoded and imported into mitochondria from the cytosol. The elucidation of the mechanism of importation of cytosolic proteins into mitochondria has been a major achievement. The process is surprisingly complex, as there are different pathways for the importation and sorting of mitochondrially-targeted polypeptides to the various organellar compartments (outer and inner membranes, intermembrane space, and matrix).[16] Among the more interesting aspects of this process is the fact that components of the import machinery are members of the family of "heat shock proteins." These "molecular chaperones" are ATP-dependent proteins that unfold and then refold the mitochondrial-targeted polypeptides as they are inserted through the import receptors and are sorted to the appropriate compartments.

A mitochondrial targeting signal, which is located at the N-terminus of most mitochondrially-imported polypeptides, must be present to address mitochondrial-imported proteins to the correct target (the mitochondria).[17] This "leader peptide," which is cleaved inside the organelle to release the mature polypeptide, is usually highly basic, with many arginine and lysine residues and few or no aspartate or glutamate residues. The leader peptide often contains consensus sequence elements that determine the precise point of cleavage of the presequence inside the organelle (Fig. 14–4).

Mutations in leader sequences should result in mendelian-inherited mitochondrial disorders.[18] A number of such mutations have been identified to date, such as those in the leader peptides of methylmalonyl-CoA mutase (an enzyme of β-oxidation) causing methylmalonic acidemia, and in ornithine transcarbamoylase (an enzyme required in the urea cycle and in arginine biosynthesis). Surprisingly, importation errors can result from mutations in the *mature* portion of the protein, implying that the import machinery recognizes elements downstream of the leader and precursor cleavage site. Mutations in the mature portion of ornithine aminotransferase (OAT) prevent the entry of the OAT precursor into mitochondria, causing gyrate atrophy[19, 20] and deletion of a segment of mature isovaleryl-CoA dehydrogenase (another β-oxidation enzyme) inhibit import, thereby causing isovaleryl acidemia.[21]

Of the nuclear genes encoding mitochondrial-imported polypeptides, a subset of perhaps 50 to 100 genes appears to contain regulatory transcriptional elements that are held in common. This subset includes nuclear genes required for the synthesis of many respiratory chain subunits and some genes required for mtDNA replication. The best two examples of such elements are

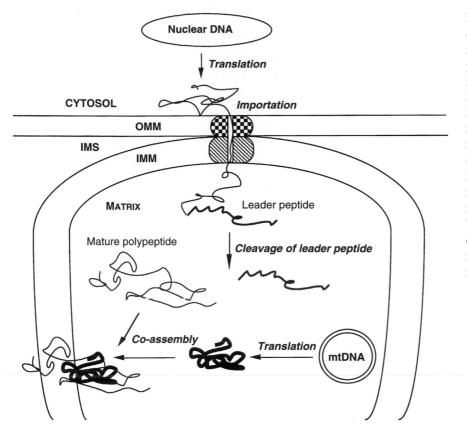

FIGURE 14–4. Targeting and importation of cytoplasmic polypeptides to mitochondria. Nucleus-encoded polypeptides are imported into mitochondria through a complex importation machinery (*hatched boxes*) at import sites where the outer mitochondrial membrane (OMM) and inner mitochondrial membrane (IMM) are apposed. The leader peptide is removed by specific proteases after importation into mitochondria. For respiratory-chain complexes I, III, IV, and V, imported nucleus-encoded subunits are co-assembled with the appropriate mtDNA-encoded polypeptides and inserted into the IMM, as shown.

called nuclear respiratory factors 1 and 2 (NRF-1 and NRF-2). These factors have been identified in the promoter region or first intron of a number of such genes.[22] More recently, an entirely new class of regulators of mitochondrial biogenesis has been found, which is associated with the coactivator of the peroxisome proliferate-activated receptor gamma subunit (PPAR-γ). Three such genes have been found, called PGC-1α (PPAR-γ coactivator-1α), PGC-1β (PPAR-γ coactivator-1β), and PRC (PGC1-related coactivator).[23] Thus, these regulatory elements may be one of the ways in which the nuclear and mitochondrial genomes "communicate" with each other.

REFERENCES

1. Margulis LS: On the origin of mitosing cells. J Theoret Biol 1967;14:225.

2. Anderson S, Bankier AT, Barrel BG, et al: Sequence and organization of the human mitochondrial genome. Nature 1981;290:457.

3. Shalgi R, Magnus A, Jones R, et al: Fate of sperm organelles during early embryogenesis in the rat. Mol Reprod Dev 1994;37:264.

4. Kaneda H, Hayashi JI, Takahama S, et al: Elimination of paternal mitochondrial DNA in intraspecific crosses during early mouse embryogenesis. Proc Natl Acad Sci U S A 1995;92:4542.

5. Jenuth JP, Peterson AC, Fu K, et al: Random genetic drift in the female germline explains the rapid segregation of mammalian mitochondrial DNA. Nat Genet 1996;13:146.

6. Clayton DA: Transcription and replication of animal mitochondrial DNAs. Int Rev Cytol 1992; 141:217.

7. Holt IJ, Lorimer HE, Jacobs HT: Coupled leading- and lagging-strand synthesis of mammalian mitochondrial DNA. Cell 2000;100:515.

8. Vu TH, Sciacco M, Tanji K, et al: Clinical manifestations of mitochondrial DNA depletion. Neurology 1998;50:1783.

9. Ojala D, Montoya J, Attardi G: tRNA punctuation model of RNA processing in human mitochondria. Nature 1981;290:470.

10. Rossmanith W, Tullo A, Potuschak T, et al: Human mitochondrial tRNA processing. J Biol Chem 1995;270:12885.

11. McCulloch V, Seidel-Rogol BL, Shadel GS: A human mitochondrial transcription factor is related to RNA adenine methyltransferase and binds S-adenosylmethionine. Mol Cell Biol 2002;22:1116.

12. Parisi MA, Clayton DA: Similarity of human mitochondrial transcription factor 1 to high mobility group proteins. Science 1991;252:965.

13. King MP, Attardi G: Post-transcriptional regulation of the steady-state levels of mitochondrial tRNAs in HeLa cells. J Biol Chem 1993;268:10228.

14. Gelfand R, Attardi G: Synthesis and turnover of mitochondrial ribonucleic acid in HeLa cells: The mature ribosomal and messenger ribonucleic acid

species are metabolically unstable. Mol Cell Biol 1981;1:497.

15. Kruse B, Narasimhan N, Attardi G: Termination of transcription in human mitochondria: Identification and purification of a DNA binding protein factor that promotes termination. Cell 1989;58:391.

16. Paschen SA, Neupert W: Protein import into mitochondria. IUBMB Life 2001;52:101.

17. Emanuelsson O, von Heijne G: Prediction of organellar targeting signals. Biochim Biophys Acta 2001;1541:114.

18. Fenton WA: Mitochondrial protein transport: A system in search of mutations. Am J Hum Genet 1995;57:235.

19. Inana G, Chambers C, Hotta Y, et al: Point mutation affecting processing of the ornithine aminotransferase precursor protein in gyrate atrophy. J Biol Chem 1989;264:17432.

20. Kobayashi T, Ogawa H, Kasahara M, et al: A single amino acid substitution within the mature sequence of ornithine aminotransferase obstructs mitochondrial entry of the precursor. Am J Hum Genet 1995;57:284.

21. Vockley J, Nagao M, Parimoo B, et al: The variant human isovaleryl-CoA dehydrogenase gene responsible for type II isovaleric acidemia determines an RNA splicing error, leading to the deletion of the entire second coding exon and the production of truncated precursor protein that interacts poorly with mitochondrial import receptors. J Biol Chem 1992;267:2494.

22. Scarpulla RC: Nuclear control of respiratory chain expression in mammalian cells. J Bioenerg Biomembr 1997;29:109.

23. Scarpulla RC: Nuclear activators and coactivators in mammalian mitochondrial biogenesis. Biochim Biophys Acta 2002;1576:1.

24. Clayton DA: Replication of animal mitochondrial DNA. Cell 1982;28:693.

Mitochondrial Disorders Due to Mutations in the Mitochondrial Genome

Salvatore DiMauro

Eduardo Bonilla

Although mitochondrial DNA (mtDNA) was discovered almost 40 years ago and its biology has been extensively studied,[1] pathogenic mutations in the mitochondrial genome were not reported until 1988. In that year, Holt et al described large-scale deletions in patients with mitochondrial myopathies,[2] and Wallace et al described a point mutation in the gene encoding subunit 4 of complex I (ND4) in a family with Leber's hereditary optic neuropathy (LHON).[3] However, these two papers opened up a veritable Pandora's box: the "morbidity map" of mtDNA has gone from the one-point mutation of 1988 to 118 point mutations listed in the January 2002 issue of *Neuromuscular Disorders* (Fig. 15–1).[4]

CLINICAL FEATURES

Mitochondria and mtDNA are ubiquitous, which explains why every tissue in the body can be affected by mtDNA mutations. This is illustrated in Table 15–1, a compilation of all symptoms and signs reported in patients with three different types of mtDNA mutations, including single deletions, point mutations in two distinct tRNA genes, and point mutations in a protein-coding gene. As shown by the boxes, certain constellations of symptoms and signs are so characteristic as to make the diagnosis in typical patients relatively easy. On the other hand, because of the peculiar rules of mitochondrial genetics, different tissues harboring the same mtDNA mutation may be affected to different degrees or not at all, which explains the sometimes-puzzling variety of syndromes associated with mtDNA mutations, even within a single pedigree.

Among the maternally inherited encephalomyopathies, four syndromes are more common. The first is MELAS (mitochondrial encephalomyopathy, lactic acidosis, and stroke-like episodes), which usually presents in children or young adults after normal early development. Symptoms include recurrent vomiting, migraine-like headache, and stroke-like episodes causing cortical blindness, hemiparesis, or hemianopia. MRI of the brain shows "infarcts" that do not correspond to the distribution of major vessels, raising the question of whether the strokes are vascular or metabolic in nature. The most common mtDNA mutation is $A3243G$ in the $tRNA^{Leu(UUR)}$ gene, but about a dozen other mutations have been associated with MELAS.[5]

The second syndrome is MERRF (myoclonus epilepsy with ragged red fibers), characterized by myoclonus, seizures, mitochondrial myopathy, and cerebellar ataxia. Less common signs include dementia, hearing loss, peripheral neuropathy, and multiple lipomas. The typical mtDNA mutation in MERRF is $A8344G$ in the $tRNA^{Lys}$ gene, but other mutations in the same gene have been reported.[6]

The third syndrome has two types: (1) NARP (neuropathy, ataxia, retinitis pigmentosa) usually affects young adults and causes retinitis pigmentosa, dementia, seizures, ataxia, proximal weakness, and sensory neuropathy and (2) maternally inherited Leigh syndrome (MILS) is a more severe infantile encephalopathy with characteristic symmetrical lesions in the basal ganglia and the brainstem.[5]

The fourth syndrome, LHON, is characterized by acute or subacute loss of vision in young adults, more frequently males, due to bilateral optic atrophy. Mutations in three genes of complex I (ND genes) have been associated with LHON, $G11778A$ in ND4, $G3460A$ in ND1, and $T14484C$ in ND6.[7]

Three sporadic conditions are associated with mtDNA single deletions, Kearns-Sayre syndrome (KSS), chronic progressive external ophthalmoplegia (CPEO), and Pearson syndrome (PS). KSS is a multisystem

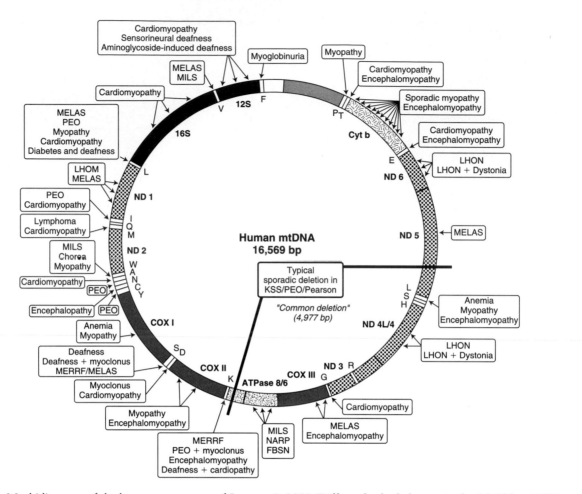

FIGURE 15–1. Morbidity map of the human genome as of January 1, 2002. Differently shaded areas in the 15.5 kb mtDNA map represent the protein-coding genes for the seven subunits of complex I (ND), three subunits of complex IV (COX), cytochrome *b* (Cyt b), two subunits of ATP synthetase (ATPase 6 and 8), 12S and 16S rRNA, and the 22 trNAs. *(One-letter codes represent the corresponding amino acids. The two mutations described in 1988 [LHON] are shown in boldface.)* FBSN, familial bilateral striatal necrosis; KSS, Kearns-Sayre syndrome; LHON, Leber's hereditary optic neuropathy; MELAS, mitochondrial encephalomyopathy, lactic acidosis, and strokelike episodes; MERRF, myoclonic epilepsy with ragged-red fibers; MILS, maternally inherited Leigh syndrome; NARP, neuropathy, ataxia, retinitis pigmentosa; PEO, progressive external ophthalmoplegia.

disorder with onset before age 20 of impaired eye movements (progressive external ophthalmoplegia [PEO]), pigmentary retinopathy, and heart block. Frequent additional signs include ataxia, dementia, and endocrine problems (diabetes mellitus, short stature, hypoparathyroidism). Lactic acidosis and markedly elevated cerebrospinal fluid (CSF) protein (over 100 mg/dL) are typical laboratory abnormalities.[5]

CPEO is a relatively benign disorder characterized by ptosis, PEO, and proximal myopathy.

Sideroblastic anemia and exocrine pancreatic dysfunction characterize Pearson syndrome, a usually fatal disorder of infancy.

It is often stated that any patient having multiple organ involvement and evidence of maternal inheritance

should be suspected of harboring a pathogenic mtDNA mutation until proven otherwise. While this rule of thumb has some practical value, it is also important to keep in mind that the reverse is not true. That is, patients with involvement of a single tissue and no evidence of maternal inheritance can still have pathogenic mutations of mtDNA. This is especially true for skeletal muscle. We have seen how isolated myopathy with PEO can be due to single large-scale mtDNA deletions. Isolated myopathy without PEO has been associated with point mutations in several tRNA genes.[8]

In addition, we have come to appreciate that exercise intolerance, myalgia, and myoglobinuria can be the sole presentation of respiratory chain defects due to mutations in protein-coding genes (discussed later).[8]

TABLE 15–1. Clinical Features in Mitochondrial Diseases due to mtDNA Mutations

Tissue	Symptom/Sign	Δ-mtDNA		tRNA		ATPase	
		KSS	Pearson	MERRF	MELAS	NARP	MILS
CNS	Seizures	-	-	+	+	-	+
	Ataxia	+	-	+	+	+	±
	Myoclonus	-	-	+	±	-	-
	Psychomotor retardation	-	-	-	-	-	+
	Psychomotor regression	+	-	±	+	-	-
	Hemiparesis/hemianopia	-	-	-	+	-	-
	Cortical blindness	-	-	-	+	-	-
	Migraine-like headaches	-	-	-	+	-	-
	Dystonia	-	-	-	+	-	+
PNS	Peripheral neuropathy	±	-	±	±	+	-
Muscle	Weakness/exercise intolerance	+	-	+	+	+	+
	Ophthalmoplegia	+	±	-	-	-	-
	Ptosis	+	-	-	-	-	-
Eye	Pigmentary retinopathy	+	-	-	-	+	±
	Optic atrophy	-	-	-	-	±	±
	Cataracts	-	-	-	-	-	-
Blood	Sideroblastic anemia	±	+	-	-	-	-
Endocrine	Diabetes mellitus	±	-	-	±	-	-
	Short stature	+	-	+	+	-	-
	Hypoparathyroidism	±	-	-	-	-	-
Heart	Conduction block	+	-	-	±	-	-
	Cardiomyopathy	±	-	-	±	-	±
GI	Exocrine pancreatic dysfunction	±	+	-	-	-	-
	Intestinal pseudo-obstruction	-	-	-	-	-	-
ENT	Sensorineural hearing loss	-	-	+	+	±	-
Kidney	Fanconi's syndrome	±	±	-	±	-	-
Laboratory	Lactic acidosis	+	+	+	+	-	+
	Muscle biopsy: RRFs	+	±	+	+	-	-
Inheritance	Maternal	-	-	+	+	+	+
	Sporadic	+	+	-	-	-	-

DIAGNOSTIC EVALUATION

The striking clinical heterogeneity of mtDNA-related disorders poses a diagnostic challenge. The following five criteria may be of some help.[9]

Clinical Presentation

As mentioned earlier, the very complexity of the clinical presentation can direct attention to mutations in mtDNA, especially when certain telltale symptoms coexist: short stature, neurosensory hearing loss, PEO, axonal neuropathy, diabetes mellitus, hypertrophic cardiomyopathy, or renal tubular acidosis. On the other hand, it is equally important not to exclude mtDNA mutations in patients with involvement of a single tissue, such as myopathy, cardiomyopathy, or renal disease.

Inheritance

Because most mtDNA-related disorders are maternally inherited but clinical expression is extremely variable, it is crucially important to collect a meticulous family history, with special attention to soft signs in maternal relatives, such as short stature, migraine, deafness, and diabetes. Lack of maternal inheritance, however, does not exclude the diagnosis (such as in cases of KSS and myopathy, discussed previously).

Laboratory

Lactic acidosis is a common finding in defects of the respiratory chain, and the lactate to pyruvate ratio is usually elevated (50:1 to 200:1, compared to a normal ratio of 25:1). Information about CSF lactate and pyruvate is important because CSF values can be increased in children with encephalopathy and normal blood lactate. However, lack of lactic acidosis does not exclude the diagnosis. For example, in patients with NARP or MILS, blood lactate and pyruvate can be normal or only mildly elevated. Serum creatine kinase (CK) levels are usually normal or modestly increased except, of course, in patients with myopathy during episodes of myoglobinuria.

Neuroradiology

Bilateral MRI signals hyperintensities in basal ganglia are typical of Leigh syndrome (LS). Strokelike lesions in the posterior cerebral hemispheres are typically seen in patients with MELAS. Diffuse signal abnormality of the central white matter is characteristic of KSS, whereas basal ganglia calcifications are common in both MELAS and KSS syndrome. Proton magnetic resonance spectroscopy reveals lactate accumulation in the CSF and in specific areas of the brain, where lactate concentration can be compared to the concentration of N-acetyl-L-aspartate (NAA), an indicator of cell viability.[6]

Exercise Physiology

Impaired oxygen extraction by exercising muscle can be detected by near-infrared spectroscopy, which measures the degree of deoxygenation of hemoglobin. A simpler test is based on the measurement of the partial pressure of oxygen (Po_2) in cubital venous blood after forearm aerobic exercise. Po_2 rises paradoxically in patients with mitochondrial myopathy or PEO, and the degree of rise reflects the severity of oxidative impairment.[10] By ^{31}P-magnetic resonance spectroscopy, the ratio of phosphocreatine to inorganic phosphate (PCr to Pi) can be measured in muscle at rest, during exercise, and during recovery. In patients with mitochondrial dysfunction, PCr to Pi ratios are lower than normal at rest, decrease excessively during exercise, and return to baseline more slowly than normal.

PATHOLOGY

Skeletal Muscle

Muscle biopsy has a central role in the diagnosis of mtDNA-related disorders. Abnormal mitochondrial proliferation, a hallmark of mitochondrial dysfunction, can be revealed with the modified Gomori trichrome stain ("ragged-red fibers" [RRF])[11] or better, with the succinate dehydrogenase (SDH) reaction ("ragged blue fibers"). RRF are present in muscle biopsies from patients with most disorders due to mtDNA mutations. Rare exceptions to this rule include NARP/MILS and LHON.

The cytochrome c oxidase (COX) histochemical reaction typically reveals scattered COX-negative fibers, which usually correspond to—but are not confined to—RRF. RRF are COX-positive in two main conditions: (1) typical MELAS syndrome and (2) mutations in mtDNA genes encoding cytochrome b or complex I subunits.[8,12] To confirm the pathogenicity of an mtDNA mutation, single fibers can be dissected out of thick cross-sections of muscle and used to determine the levels of a given mutation by polymerase chain reaction (PCR). Finding higher levels of the mutation in affected (ragged-red or COX-negative fibers) than in unaffected (non-ragged-red, COX-positive fibers) is strong evidence that the mutation in question is pathogenic.[12]

Electron microscopy has lost much of its historical diagnostic value, but it can reveal focal accumulations of mitochondria in cases in which histochemical results are equivocal.

Neuropathology

The basic neuropathology in mitochondrial encephalomyopathies consists of four histologic lesions: spongy degeneration, neuronal loss, gliosis, and demyelination.[13] While these lesions are nonspecific, they are expressed in different topographic patterns in patients with different mtDNA-related disorders. Thus, the neuropathology of KSS is characterized by spongiform degeneration, which is usually generalized and affects both gray and white matter. In MELAS, multifocal necrosis predominates, affecting the cerebral cortex or the subcortical white matter, but also the cerebellum, thalamus, and basal ganglia. Calcification of basal ganglia is common. In MERRF, neuronal degeneration, astrocytosis, and demyelination affect preferentially the cerebellum (especially the dentate nucleus), the brainstem (especially the olivary nucleus), and the spinal cord. In LS, there are symmetrical, bilateral foci of necrosis in the basal ganglia, thalamus, midbrain, and pons. Microscopically, the lesions show vascular proliferation, gliosis, neuronal loss, demyelination, and cystic cavitation.

BIOCHEMICAL FINDINGS

All 13 proteins encoded by mtDNA are components of the mitochondrial respiratory chain. Seven (ND1-ND5, ND5L, ND6) are subunits of complex I, one (cytochrome b) is part of complex III, three (COX I, COX II, and COX III) are subunits of complex IV, and two (ATPase 6 and ATPase 8) are subunits of complex V (Fig. 15-2). Therefore, disorders owing to mutations of mtDNA are usually associated with biochemical defects of oxidative phosphorylation. Skeletal muscle is the preferred tissue for biochemical analysis, because it is rich in

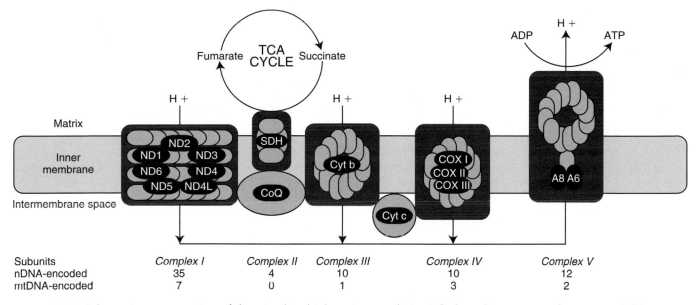

Subunits	Complex I	Complex II	Complex III	Complex IV	Complex V
nDNA-encoded	35	4	10	10	12
mtDNA-encoded	7	0	1	3	2

FIGURE 15-2. Schematic representation of the mitochondrial respiratory chain. *(Black ovals represent subunits encoded by mtDNA.)* CoQ, coenzyme Q10 (ubiquinone); Cyt c, cytochrome *c;* SDH, succinate dehydrogenase; TCA, tricarboxylic acid. (Other abbreviations as in Fig. 15–1.)

mitochondria, it is invariably affected in multisystem disorders (mitochondrial encephalomyopathies), and it is the most common tissue affected in isolation (mitochondrial myopathies). There is some controversy about whether fresh muscle tissue is needed or frozen tissue suffices. It is our view that—except for the rare cases in which freshly isolated mitochondria for polarographic analyses are required—frozen specimens provide adequate biochemical information. Because mitochondrial proliferation in muscle (RRF) is a common occurrence, activities of respiratory chain complexes should be referred to the activity of citrate synthase, a nuclear encoded enzyme of the mitochondrial matrix that is a good marker of mitochondrial abundance.

Biochemical studies in muscle extract from patients with mtDNA-related disorders yield two main types of results. The first pattern consists of partial defects in the activities of multiple complexes containing mtDNA-encoded subunits (I, III, and IV) contrasting with normal or increased activities of SDH (complex II) and citrate synthase. The second pattern is a severe deficiency in the activity of one specific respiratory complex. As a rule, the first pattern is found in patients with single mtDNA deletions (e.g., KSS), or mutations in tRNA genes (e.g., MELAS, MERRF) because these genetic errors impair mitochondrial protein synthesis in toto. The second pattern is typical of mutations in mtDNA protein-coding genes. For example, mutations in the cytochrome *b* gene cause isolated complex III deficiency.[12]

MOLECULAR GENETIC FINDINGS

Human mtDNA is a 16,569-bp circle of double-stranded DNA. It is highly compact, and contains only 37 genes

(see Fig. 15–1): 2 genes encode ribosomal RNAs (rRNAs), 22 encode transfer RNAs (tRNAs), and 13 encode polypeptides. All 13 polypeptides are components of the respiratory chain (discussed previously). Mitochondrial genetics differs from mendelian genetics in three major aspects.

Maternal Inheritance

At fertilization, all mitochondria (and all mtDNAs) in the zygote derive from the oöcyte. Therefore, a mother carrying an mtDNA mutation is expected to pass it on to all her children, but only her daughters may transmit it to their progeny.

Heteroplasmy/Threshold Effect

In contrast to nuclear genes, each consisting of one maternal and one paternal allele, there are hundreds or thousands of mtDNA molecules in each cell. Deleterious mutations of mtDNA usually affect some but not all genomes, such that cells, tissues, or whole individuals, will harbor two populations of mtDNA: normal (wild-type) and mutant, a situation known as heteroplasmy. The situation of normal subjects, in whom all mtDNAs are identical, is called homoplasmy. Nondeleterious mutations of mtDNA (neutral polymorphisms) are homoplasmic, whereas pathogenic mutations are usually, but not invariably, heteroplasmic.

Not surprisingly, a minimum critical number of mutant mtDNAs must be present before oxidative dysfunction and clinical signs become apparent (threshold effect). Also not surprisingly, the pathogenic threshold will be lower in tissues that are highly dependent on oxidative metabolism than in tissues with higher capacity for anaerobic metabolism.

Mitotic Segregation

At cell division, the proportion of mutant mtDNAs in daughter cells can shift: if and when the pathogenic threshold for a given tissue is surpassed, the phenotype can also change. This explains the time-related variability of clinical features frequently observed in mtDNA-related disorders.

As already mentioned above, mtDNA mutations fall into two main groups: those affecting mitochondrial protein synthesis and those affecting specific proteins.

Mutations Affecting Mitochondrial Protein Synthesis

Mutations affecting protein synthesis include single deletions (which always encompass one or more tRNA genes), and point mutations in rRNA or in tRNA genes. Clinical experience suggests that these mutations are usually associated with multisystem disorders, lactic acidosis, and massive mitochondrial proliferation in muscle, resulting in the "ragged-red" appearance of fibers in the muscle biopsy. Examples include KSS, MELAS, and MERRF. As far as inheritance is concerned, conditions associated with point mutations, such as MELAS and MERRF, are transmitted maternally, whereas single mtDNA deletions are sporadic events in almost all cases.

While mutations in tRNA genes are usually associated with multisystem disorders, in some cases there is involvement of a single tissue, most commonly skeletal muscle. Family history is negative in some of the patients with pure myopathy, suggesting that the mutations occurred ex novo. However, in most patients the mutation was also present in blood or cultured skin fibroblasts, implying "skewed heteroplasmy," with preferential accumulation of the pathogenic mutation in skeletal muscle.[8]

Mutations in Protein-Coding Genes

The two most common maternally inherited, multisystemic syndromes associated with mutations in mtDNA protein-coding genes are LHON and NARP/MILS. Recently, however, we have come to appreciate that sporadic patients with exercise intolerance, myalgia, and myoglobinuria often harbor mutations in protein-coding genes causing defects of complex I, complex III, or complex IV.[8] The sporadic nature and the tissue specificity of these disorders suggests that the underlying mutations are somatic—that is, spontaneous events that occur in muscle and do not affect germ-line cells.

However, numerous mutations in protein-coding genes have been associated with encephalomyopathies other than LHON and NARP/MILS, including typical MELAS, LS, and a phenocopy of amyotrophic lateral sclerosis (ALS). Other phenotypes varied greatly, from predominantly myopathic syndromes to severe encephalopathies.[8]

ANIMAL MODELS

A formidable obstacle to the generation of the so-called "mito-mice" was our inability to introduce mutant mtDNA into mitochondria of a mammalian cell. To solve this problem, Inoue et al[14] first prepared synaptosomes from the brain of aging mice, which contained a certain percentage of deleted mtDNAs. They then fused the synaptosomes with mtDNA-less rho[0] cells, thus obtaining hybrid cell lines. One such cell line harboring mtDNA deletions was enucleated, fused with donor embryos, and implanted in pseudopregnant females. Heteroplasmic founder females were bred and mtDNA deletions were transmitted through three generations. Although there are significant differences between these mito-mice and human patients with mtDNA deletions, the fact remains that the animals show mitochondrial dysfunction in various organs.[15]

A slightly more complicated strategy was employed by Sligh et al[16] to generate mice harboring a point mutation for chloramphenicol resistance (CAP[R]). The mutation in homoplasmic or heteroplasmic CAP[R] mutants was severe enough to cause death in utero or within 11 days of birth, and affected animals showed dilated cardiomyopathy and abnormal mitochondria in both cardiac and skeletal muscle, features often observed in human mtDNA diseases. At the very least, the papers by Inoue et al and Sligh et al prove the principle that heteroplasmic mtDNA mutations can be transmitted through germlines and will produce phenotypic abnormalities.

THERAPY

Therapy of mtDNA-related diseases is still woefully inadequate. Besides palliative pharmacologic and surgical interventions directed at alleviating symptoms, approaches to therapy include (1) removing toxic products, especially lactic acid; (2) administering artificial electron acceptors, such as vitamin K3 and vitamin C; (3) administering metabolites and cofactors, such as L-carnitine and coenzyme Q10 (CoQ10); and (4) administering oxygen radical scavengers, such as CoQ10.[17]

Gene therapy is daunting in these conditions for much the same reasons that made creation of animal models such a challenge. However, if we could cause even a small shift in the relative proportion of mutant and normal mtDNAs, thus lowering the mutant load below the pathogenic threshold, we probably would improve the clinical expression dramatically. Various strategies are being considered, including the use of peptide nucleic acids (PNAs) to inhibit the replication of complementary mutant mtDNAs,[17] or pharmacologic approaches directed to eliminate mitochondria with high proportions of mutations. The observation that myoblasts often contain lesser amounts of pathogenic mtDNA mutations than mature muscle fibers has led to the use of myotoxic agents or isometric exercise to induce limited muscle damage, which would be followed by regeneration of muscle fibers harboring lower mutational loads.[17] Although these therapies have met with mixed results, they show our ability of affecting mutational loads, at least in skeletal muscle.

CONCLUSION

Although the mtDNA circle is crowded with pathogenic mutations (see Fig. 15–1), there is room for more, and new mutations are still being described, especially in protein-coding genes. In addition, we still do not fully understand the pathophysiology of mtDNA-related diseases, although the advent of "mitomice" and of knockout mice for nuclear genes will undoubtedly help us in this endeavor.[18] Finally, our therapeutic armamentarium is still totally inadequate, although some interesting novel approaches are being considered.[17] Here, again, the availability of animal models will be of great help.

Acknowledgments

Part of the work presented here was supported by National Institutes of Health grants NS11766 and PO1HD32062, and by a grant from the Muscular Dystrophy Association.

REFERENCES

1. Smeitink J, van den Heuvel L, DiMauro S: The genetics and pathology of oxidative phosphorylation. Nature Rev Genet 2001;2:342–352.
2. Holt IJ, Harding AE, Morgan Hughes JA: Deletions of muscle mitochondrial DNA in patients with mitochondrial myopathies. Nature 1988;331:717–719.
3. Wallace DC, Singh G, Lott MT, et al: Mitochondrial DNA mutation associated with Leber's hereditary optic neuropathy. Science 1988;242:1427–1430.
4. Servidei S: Mitochondrial encephalomyopathies: Gene mutation. Neuromusc Disord 2002;12:101–110.
5. Schon EA, Hirano M, DiMauro S: Molecular genetic basis of the mitochondrial encephalomyopathies. In Schapira AHV, DiMauro S (eds):

Mitochondrial Disorders in Neurology. Boston, Butterworth-Heinemann, 2002, pp 69–113.
6. DiMauro S, Hirano M, Kaufmann P, et al: Clinical features and genetics of myoclonic epilepsy with ragged red fibers. In Fahn S, Frucht SJ (eds): Myoclonus and Paroxysmal Dyskinesia. Philadelphia, Lippincott Williams & Wilkins, 2002, pp 217–229.
7. Carelli V: Leber's hereditary optic neuropathy. In Schapira AHV, DiMauro S (eds): Mitochondrial Disorders in Neurology. Boston, Butterworth-Heinemann, 2002, pp 115–142.
8. DiMauro S, Schon EA: Mitochondrial DNA mutations in human disease. Am J Med Genet 2001;106:18–26.
9. DiMauro S, Bonilla E, De Vivo DC: Does the patient have a mitochondrial encephalomyopathy? J Child Neurol 1999;14:23–35.
10. Taivassalo T, Abbott A, Wyrick P, Haller RG: Venous oxygen levels during aerobic forearm exercise: An index of impaired oxidative metabolism in mitochondrial myopathy. Ann Neurol 2002;51:38–44.
11. Engel WK, Cunningham G: Rapid examination of muscle tissue: An improved trichome stain method for fresh-frozen biopsy sections. Neurology 1963;13:919–923.
12. Andreu AL, Hanna MG, Reichmann H, et al: Exercise intolerance due to mutations in the cytochrome b gene of mitochondrial DNA. N Engl J Med 1999;341:1037–1044.
13. Tanji K, Kunimatsu T, Vu TH, Bonilla E: Neuropathological features of mitochondrial disorders. Cell Develop Biol 2001;12:429–439.
14. Inoue K, Nakada K, Ogura A, et al: Generation of mice with mitochondrial dysfunction by introducing mouse mtDNA carrying a deletion into zygotes. Nat Genet 2000;26:176–181.
15. Shoubridge EA: A debut for mito-mouse. Nat Genet 2000;26:132–134.
16. Sligh JE, Levy SE, Waymire KG, et al: Maternal germ-line transmission of mutant mtDNAs from embryonic stem cell-derived chimeric mice. Proc Nat Acad Sci U S A 2000;97:14461–14466.
17. Taylor RW, Turnbull DM: Current and future prospects for the treatment of mitochondrial disorders. In Schapira AHV, DiMauro S (eds): Mitochondrial Disorders in Neurology. Boston, Butterworth-Heinemann, 2002, pp 213–228.
18. Wallace DC: Pathophysiology of mitochondrial disease as illuminated by animal models. In Schapira AHV, DiMauro S (eds): Mitochondrial Disorders in Neurology. Boston, Butterworth Heinemann, 2002, pp 175–212.

Mitochondrial Disorders Due to Mutations in the Nuclear Genome

Michio Hirano

Disorders of mitochondria are clinically and genetically diverse because these mammalian organelles are under the control of two genomes, mitochondrial DNA (mtDNA) and nuclear DNA (nDNA). Defects of either genome can cause dysfunction of the mitochondrial respiratory chain, the common terminal pathway involved in oxidative phosphorylation, the aerobic production of energy in the form of ATP. Chapter 15 describes primary mtDNA mutations,[1] whereas this chapter focuses on the growing number of autosomal disorders of the mitochondrial respiratory chain.

When considering mitochondrial encephalomyopathies, it is important to keep in mind that mtDNA encodes only 13 structural polypeptide subunits of respiratory chain enzyme complexes, 22 transfer RNAs (tRNAs), and 2 ribosomal RNAs (rRNAs).[2] By contrast, the nuclear genome encodes hundreds of mitochondrial proteins that are vital for all functions of the organelles. Consequently, mutations of nDNA can affect the respiratory chain directly or indirectly, potentially impairing a wide variety of mitochondrial functions, such as mitochondrial motility, protein importation, maintenance of the membrane milieu, and intergenomic communication (Table 16–1).

Because of its relatively small size (16,569 base pairs), mutations in mtDNA have been identified rapidly. Over 115 pathogenic point mutations and numerous rearrangements of mtDNA are known, while the identification of nDNA mutations has lagged behind.[1]

CLINICAL PICTURE

Disorders of the mitochondrial respiratory chain present with diverse clinical phenotypes. Some patients have iso-lated myopathies, encephalopathies, or other single-organ disorders; however, most develop multisystem disorders. Despite the plethora of manifestations, some clinical features are common among individuals with mitochondrial disorders and can serve as clues to the diagnosis. For example, patients often complain of exercise intolerance owing to premature fatigue. Other typical clinical features of these patients include short stature, ptosis with progressive external ophthalmoparesis (PEO), sensorineural hearing loss, pigmentary retinopathy, optic atrophy, seizures, basal ganglia lesions, and diabetes mellitus. Clinical syndromes associated with defects of nDNA tend to be more stereotyped than disorders caused by mtDNA mutations, which are subject to the vagaries of heteroplasmy and tissue distribution.[1] The autosomal mitochondrial diseases are outlined in Table 16–2, and selected presentations are discussed below.

Leigh syndrome is the most common mitochondrial disorder in infants and children, but is rare in adults.[3] Infants may present symptoms at birth or may develop normally for months; however, onset is typically before age six months. The initial manifestations include hypotonia, psychomotor delay, and respiratory insufficiency followed by impaired vision, hearing loss, seizures, ataxia, limb weakness, pyramidal tract signs, and intellectual deterioration. Magnetic resonance imaging (MRI) of the brain reveals characteristic symmetric lesions of the basal ganglia and midline brainstem structures. The disorder can be inherited in an autosomal recessive, X linked, or maternal pattern.

Myopathy, often associated with cardiomyopathy, is another common presentation of mitochondrial disor-

TABLE 16–1. Nosological Classification of Mitochondrial Respiratory Chain Disorders due to Nuclear DNA Mutations

Biochemical defect	Clinical phenotype	Defective gene product (if known)
1. *Mutations in genes encoding structural subunits of respiratory chain enzymes*		
Complex I deficiency	Encephalomyopathy or Leigh syndrome	NDUFS2, NDUFS4, NDUFS8, NDUFV1, NDUFS1, NDUFS7
Complex II deficiency	Leigh syndrome	Flavoprotein subunit of SDH
Complex II deficiency	Hereditary paraganglioma or pheochromocytoma	SDHB, SDHC, SDHD
2. *Mutations in genes encoding assembly factors for respiratory chain enzymes*		
Complex III deficiency	Encephalopathy, tubulopathy, and hepatopathy	BCS1L
Complex IV deficiency	Leigh syndrome	SURF1
	Infantile cardioencephalopathy	SCO2
	Infantile encephalopathy	SCO1, COX10
3. *Defects of intergenomic communication*		
Autosomal recessive PEO with multiple Δ-mtDNA	MNGIE	Thymidine phosphorylase
	arPEO	POLG
	ARCO	Unknown
Autosomal dominant PEO with multiple Δ-mtDNA	adPEO	ANT1, Twinkle, POLG
MtDNA depletion	Infantile myopathy	TK2
	Infantile encephalopathy and hepatopathy	dGK
	Infantile myopathy or hepatopathy	Unknown
	Navaho neurohepatopathy	Unknown
4. *Defects of the mitochondrial membrane*		
Coenzyme Q10 deficiency	Myoglobinuria, encephalopathy, RRFs	Unknown
	Cerebellar ataxia	Unknown
Impaired processing of mitochondrial phospholipids	Barth syndrome	Tafazzin
5. *Defects of mitochondrial importation*		
Impaired importation of proteins	X-linked deafness-dystonia	Tim 8/9
6. *Defects of mitochondrial division*		
Impaired mitochondrial motility	Autosomal dominant optic atrophy 1	OPA1
7. *Defects of mitochondrial metal metabolism*		
Iron storage defect	Friedreich ataxia	Frataxin
Iron export defect	X-linked sideroblastic anemia	ABC7
8. *Other*	Hereditary spastic paraplegia	Paraplegin

ders. It is important for clinicians to recognize infantile myopathies with cytochrome *c* oxidase (COX) deficiency, because patients with *benign infantile myopathy* (BIM) can recover fully with proper medical care.[4] Both BIM and *fatal infantile myopathy* (FIM) with COX deficiency present with congenital generalized muscle weakness, respiratory muscle insufficiency, and lactic acidosis.

However, infants with FIM die within the first year of life despite aggressive medical interventions.[4]

Autosomal dominant and recessive progressive external ophthalmoplegia (adPEO or arPEO) are mendelian disorders with multiple deletions of mtDNA (multiple Δ-mtDNA).[5,6] Patients with adPEO gradually develop

TABLE 16–2. Clinical Features of Mitochondrial Diseases due to Nuclear DNA Mutations

Leigh syndrome

Onset typically in infancy or childhood, but can occur in adulthood

Infantile-onset

    Typically before age 6 months in a previously normal infant

    Developmental arrest or regression, hypotonia, feeding difficulty, respiratory abnormalities, vision loss, oculomotor palsies, and nystagmus

    Brain MRI reveals symmetric lesions of the basal ganglia and midline brainstem.

Childhood-onset

    Similar to infantile-onset patients, but PEO, dystonia, or ataxia may be prominent.

Infantile myoclonic epilepsy and leukodystrophy due to complex I deficiency (NDUFV1 mutations)

    Myoclonic epilepsy

    Hypotonia

    Developmental delay

    Leukodystrophy

Infantile cardioencephalomyopathy due to complex I deficiency (NDUFS2 mutations)

    Hypertrophic cardiomyopathy

    Encephalopathy (ataxia, pyramidal signs, basal ganglia, and white matter lesions)

    Myopathy

    Optic atrophy

Infantile cardioencephalopathy due to SCO_2 mutations

    Progressive hypertrophic cardiomyopathy

    Encephalopathy with seizures and variable atrophy, migrational defects, neuronal defects, and gliosis

    Respiratory insufficiency

    Hypotonia

Fatal infantile myopathy (FIM) with cytochrome *c* oxidase deficiency

    Diffuse weakness, hypotonia, and respiratory insufficiency due to myopathy

    Sometimes de Toni-Debré-Fanconi syndrome

Benign infantile myopathy (BIM) with cytochrome *c* oxidase deficiency

    Diffuse weakness, hypotonia, and respiratory insufficiency due to myopathy

    Spontaneous improvement by age 2–3 years

Autosomal dominant progressive external ophthalmoplegia (adPEO)

    Ptosis and PEO generally beginning in young adulthood

    Ragged-red and cytochrome *c* oxidase (COX) deficient fibers in skeletal muscle

    Multiple Δ-mtDNA

    Other features: proximal limb weakness, respiratory insufficiency, depression, peripheral neuropathy, sensorineural hearing loss, cataracts, endocrinopathies.

Mitochondrial neurogastrointestinal encephalomyopathy (MNGIE)

    Ptosis and PEO

    Gastrointestinal dysmotility

    Demyelinating peripheral neuropathy

    Cachexia

    Leukoencephalopathy on MRI scan

(Continued)

Table 16–2. *(continued)*

Autosomal recessive cardiomyopathy ophthalmoplegia (ARCO)

    Ptosis and PEO

    Proximal muscle weakness

    Hypertrophic cardiomyopathy

Infantile mtDNA depletion syndromes

Myopathic form

    Feeding difficulty, failure to thrive, hypotonia, weakness, and occasionally PEO

    Elevated serum creatine kinase (2–30 times the upper limit of normal)

    Myopathy with COX-deficient fibers and sometimes RRF

Hepatopathy

    Liver failure manifesting as persistent vomiting, failure to thrive, hypotonia, and hypoglycemia

Navajo neurohepatopathy (NNH); 4 of the following 6 criteria or 3 plus a positive family history of NNH

    Sensory neuropathy

    Motor neuropathy

    Corneal anesthesia, ulcers, or scars

    Liver disease

    Documented metabolic or immunologic derangement

    Central nervous system demyelination

Coenzyme Q10 deficiency

Myopathic form

    Myoglobinuria

    Encephalopathy (seizures or mental retardation)

    RRF in muscle biopsy

Cerebellar form

    Cerebellar ataxia with prominent cerebellar atrophy in brain MRI scans

Barth syndrome

    X-linked

    Dilated cardiomyopathy

    Neutropenia (due to impaired leukocyte maturation)

    Myopathy with abnormal mitochondria

Mohr-Tranebjaerg syndrome (X-linked deafness-dystonia syndrome)

    X-linked

    Sensorineural hearing loss

    Dystonia

    Other features: spasticity, dysphagia, intellectual decline, paranoia, cortical blindness

Autosomal dominant optic atrophy 1 (Kjer type optic atrophy)

    Childhood-onset of insidious optic atrophy manifesting as loss of visual acuity, color vision loss, temporal optic disc pallor, and centrocecal scotoma)

X-linked sideroblastic anemia with ataxia syndrome (XLSA/A)

    Hypochromic microcytic anemia

    Ring sideroblasts in bone marrow

    Ataxia

    Corticospinal tract signs

ptosis and ophthalmoparesis during early adulthood and may manifest other symptoms including proximal limb weakness, respiratory insufficiency, severe depression, peripheral neuropathy, sensorineural hearing loss, cataracts, and endocrine dysfunction.[6] By contrast, arPEO disorders begin in childhood or adolescence and manifest as multisystem disorders such as mitochondrial neurogastrointestinal encephalomyopathy (MNGIE) or autosomal recessive cardiomyopathy ophthalmoplegia (ARCO).[5] MNGIE is characterized by ptosis, PEO, peripheral neuropathy, and severe gastrointestinal dysmotility leading to cachexia.[7] Brain MRIs reveal striking diffuse leukoencephalopathy, and muscle biopsies show COX-deficient and ragged-red fibers (RRFs). ARCO was identified in two large families from the eastern Arabian peninsula with childhood-onset PEO, proximal muscle weakness, and severe hypertrophic cardiomyopathy.[8]

Coenzyme Q10 deficiency has a spectrum of presentations beginning in childhood and ranges from a predominantly myopathic form to a mainly cerebellar form. The myopathic form is characterized by the triad of recurrent myoglobinuria, encephalopathy (mental retardation or seizures), and mitochondrial myopathy with excessive lipid storage in muscle biopsies.[9] By contrast, some patients have had severe cerebellar ataxia with pyramidal signs, seizures, and normal muscle biopsies.[10] Diagnosis of coenzyme Q10 deficiency is particularly important because the condition is treatable.

Hereditary paragangliomas and pheochromocytoma, tumors of neural crest origin, have emerged as enigmatic consequences of mutations in subunits B, C, and D of succinate dehydrogenase.[11]

DIAGNOSTIC EVALUATION

A thorough clinical examination is required to evaluate patients with mitochondrial diseases that are often multisystemic. Ophthalmological signs such as mild ptosis, ophthalmoparesis, retinopathy, optic atrophy, and visual field defects are often present. Neurological evaluation is vital in most mitochondrial patients because of the high frequency of nervous system and muscle involvement.

The laboratory evaluation of patients suspected to have a mitochondrial disease should begin with routine blood tests including complete blood count, serum electrolytes, liver function tests, blood urea nitrogen, creatinine, lactate, and pyruvate. These tests may reveal evidence of kidney, liver, or parathyroid dysfunction. For patients whose clinical manifestations conform to one of the well-defined mitochondrial diseases, direct genetic testing can be performed using leukocyte DNA.

In patients with defects of the respiratory chain, serum lactate at rest is frequently elevated and out of proportion to pyruvate (e.g., lactate to pyruvate ratio of $\geq 20{:}1$);

however, many patients with well-documented mitochondrial diseases have normal baseline lactate levels. In such patients, moderate exercise can provoke an exaggerated rise of lactate. Measurement of oxidative metabolism during exercise provides more sensitive physiological tests for mitochondrial diseases. These tests include ^{31}P-magnetic resonance spectroscopy, near-infrared spectroscopy, cycle ergometry, and aerobic forearm exercise. Few facilities, however, routinely perform these tests.[12]

Muscle biopsies are useful in evaluating patients suspected of having a respiratory chain defect. Mitochondrial abnormalities can be detected in muscle by histologic, biochemical, or molecular genetic tests as described in the next section.

PATHOLOGY

Muscle Biopsy

In patients with mitochondrial disorders, skeletal muscle has been the most thoroughly studied tissue. Routine histological studies may reveal features of myopathy or neurogenic atrophy. Increased glycogen may be detected by periodic acid-Schiff (PAS) stain, while excess lipid can be identified by an oil red-O stain; both compounds may accumulate due to the downstream block in energy metabolism. The modified Gomori trichrome stain may reveal irregular bright red areas within the blue-green background (RRFs). These muscle fibers show marked proliferation of mitochondria in the subsarcolemmal regions. RRFs are generally associated with primary mtDNA mutations that affect mitochondrial protein synthesis, for example point mutations in tRNA genes or large-scale Δ-mtDNA that eliminate at least one tRNA gene. Both types of mutations lead to a paucity of mitochondrial tRNAs, and hence impaired protein synthesis. While none of the known primary nDNA mutations directly affects mitochondrial protein synthesis, defects of intergenomic communication lead to secondary depletion and multiple deletions of mtDNA, thereby producing RRF.

The histochemical stain for succinate dehydrogenase (SDH), which functions as complex II (succinate-CoQ reductase) of the mitochondrial respiratory chain, provides a more sensitive indicator of mitochondrial proliferation. Histochemical stain for COX (complex IV) often provides vital morphological information. In patients with a pathogenic nDNA mutation in a COX subunit or in a COX assembly factor, histochemistry will show a generalized reduction or absence of COX stain in skeletal muscle. By contrast, in patients with primary or secondary mtDNA mutations, COX histochemistry typically shows a mosaic pattern of fibers with normal and decreased staining.

Brain Pathology

Leigh syndrome or subacute necrotizing encephalomyopathy is defined by the characteristic neuropathology consisting of focal symmetric lesions affecting the brainstem tegmentum, basal ganglia, thalamus, cerebellum, optic nerves, and spinal cord.[3] Microscopically, these lesions show necrosis, vascular proliferation, demyelination, and astrocytosis. RRF are not seen in Leigh syndrome.

In infants with cardioencephalopathy due to SCO2 mutations, the neuropathological changes have been heterogeneous, with variable brain atrophy, migrational abnormalities, neuronal defects, gliosis, and, in one case, early capillary proliferation reminiscent of Leigh syndrome.[13]

Other Organs

Hypertrophic cardiomyopathy is a prominent clinical feature of SCO2 deficiency and Friedreich ataxia, but can also be seen in patients with Leigh syndrome.[3,13] Histological studies of the heart from patients with SCO2 defects have demonstrated vacuolization, proliferation of mitochondria, and myofibrillar disarray.[13]

Hepatopathy is a feature of mtDNA depletion syndromes, Leigh syndrome, and complex III (ubiquinol-cytochrome *c* reductase) deficiency due to mutations affecting the assembly factor BCS1L.[14,15] Hepatopathy can progress to cirrhosis.

BIOCHEMICAL FINDINGS

Measurement of mitochondrial respiratory enzymes in affected tissues is crucial to identify the specific biochemical defect(s) in mitochondrial patients. For example, Leigh syndrome can be due to defects of diverse mitochondrial enzymes, including pyruvate dehydrogenase complex and biotinidase, in addition to various components of the respiratory chain. Identification of an isolated enzyme deficiency pinpoints the biochemical problem and will focus molecular genetic analyses to identify the causative mutation.

In patients with primary or secondary mtDNA mutations affecting tRNA genes, variable defects of respiratory chain enzyme complexes I, III, and IV may be detected. By contrast, activity of succinate dehydrogenase (SDH) is normal or elevated because all subunits of this enzyme complex are encoded by nDNA.

In patients with deficiency of coenzyme Q10, activities of complexes I+III and complexes II+III will show defects. To confirm lack of coenzyme Q10, direct measurement of this compound can be performed by a straightforward high-performance liquid chromatography (HPLC) assay.[9,10]

For MNGIE patients, biochemical detection of elevated plasma thymidine or decreased thymidine phosphorylase activity in buffy coat provides more rapid and cost-effective screening tests than sequencing of the thymidine phosphorylase gene.[7]

IMMUNOCHEMICAL FINDINGS

Immunohistochemical and immunoblot assays have been successfully applied to research studies of mitochondrial disorders but have been of limited diagnostic use.

MOLECULAR GENETICS

In 1995, the identification of the first nDNA mutations causing SDH deficiency in two sisters with Leigh syndrome was the harbinger of a rapid expansion of nDNA defects associated with mitochondrial disorders.[16] In fact, Leigh syndrome illustrates recent advances in molecular genetics. While the biochemical diversity of Leigh syndrome has been well-documented over the last 3 decades, molecular genetic studies have revealed even greater genotypic heterogeneity. For instance, complex I deficiency, a common cause of Leigh and Leigh-like syndromes, has been associated with pathogenic mutations in 4 of the 36 nDNA-encoded subunits of this enzyme complex.[17] In addition, mutations in the complex I NDUFS2 subunit have been associated with cardiomyopathy and Leigh-like encephalopathy, while defects of the NDUFV1 subunit have been found in patients with leukoencephalopathy and myoclonic epilepsy.[17] Interestingly, defects of complex I or II have been associated with mutations in structural subunits of the enzymes, while defects of complexes III and IV have been associated with mutations in proteins (BCS1L, SURF1, SCO2, SCO1, and COX10) required for assembly of the enzymes, but not yet in structural components of these complexes.[13,15,18]

Linkage analysis and candidate gene screening, as well as in vitro studies using microcell-mediated chromosomal transfer experiments, have led to the identification of mutations in several nDNA genes that affect the mitochondrial respiratory chain through unanticipated pathogenic mechanisms. For example, loss-of-function mutations in the gene encoding the cytosolic protein thymidine phosphorylase led to the novel concept that nucleotide pool imbalances can affect mtDNA quantity and integrity (Fig. 16–1).[19] Subsequently, mutations in genes encoding mitochondrial deoxyguanosine kinase (dGK) and thymidine kinase (TK2) were found to cause mtDNA depletion, thus reinforcing the concept that defects of intergenomic communication are frequently caused by nucleotide pool imbalances (see Fig. 16–1).[14,20] In addition, mutations in the mitochondrial adenine nucleotide translocator 1, Twinkle, and polymerase gamma (POLG) have been identified as causes of adPEO.[21]

Identification of mutations in other autosomal genes is leading to new concepts of mitochondrial diseases. Identification of *DDP1* gene mutations in X-linked deafness-dystonia (Mohr-Tranebjaerg syndrome) is the first defect in a mitochondrial importation factor.[22] Similarly, mutations in the *OPA1* gene in autosomal dominant optic atrophy 1 (Kjer type optic atrophy) indicate

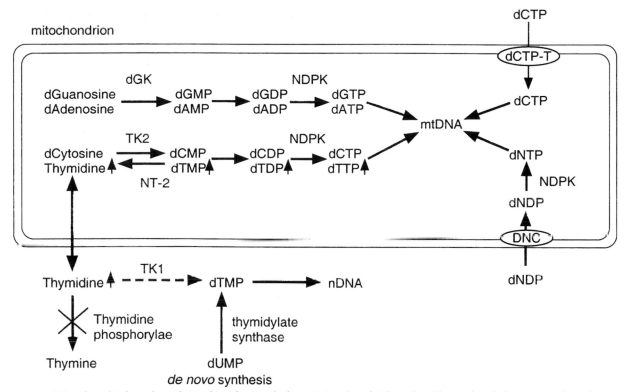

FIGURE 16–1. Mitochondrial nucleoside/nucleotide metabolism. Mitochondrial nucleotide pool imbalances are thought to produce depletion and multiple deletions of mitochondrial DNA (mtDNA). In MNGIE, thymidine phosphorylase deficiency leads to increased levels of plasma thymidine which, in turn, are thought to lead to abnormally high levels of dTTP in mitochondria. dCTP-T, deoxycytidine triphosphate transporter; dGK, deoxyguanosine kinase; DNC, mitochondrial deoxynucleotide carrier; NDP-K, nucleoside diphosphate kinase; NT-2, mitochondrial 5′-deoxy-ribonucleotidase; TK1, thymidine kinase 1; TK2, thymidine kinase 2; TP, thymidine phosphorylase.

that defects of mitochondrial division or biogenesis can cause diseases. Mutations in two genes have underscored the importance of mitochondrial metal metabolism; defects of the *ABC7* gene in X-linked sideroblastic anemia cause defects of iron export while mutations of frataxin in Friedreich ataxia are thought to affect mitochondrial iron storage.[23]

ANIMAL MODELS

Knockout mice have begun to shed light onto the pathomechanisms of mitochondrial diseases, although none of these animals have defects that are directly analogous to any known pathogenic mutations in human disorders. For example, ANT1-knockout mice have revealed features of human respiratory chain diseases including impaired oxidative-phosphorylation, lactic acidosis, exercise intolerance, and proliferation of muscle mitochondria.[24] Mitochondrial transcription factor A (Tfam) knockout mice have shown mtDNA depletion and respiratory chain defects.[25] Tissue-specific Tfam-knockout mice have produced focal mtDNA depletion and are important models of human diseases.[25]

THERAPY

While much progress has been achieved in understanding the molecular basis of human mitochondrial diseases due to nDNA mutations, therapy for these conditions remains unsatisfactory. Palliative therapies are important to treat various clinical manifestations, including antiepileptic drugs for seizures, insulin for diabetes mellitus, and cochlear implants for severe sensorineural hearing loss. Nutritional supplements have been recommended to maintain adequate levels of cofactors and metabolites. In patients with primary deficiency of coenzyme Q10, supplements of this molecule can produce significant clinical improvements.[9,10] MNGIE is another disorder that may be amenable to therapy because reducing toxic levels of thymidine may improve the hypothesized mitochondrial nucleotide pool imbalance.[7]

CONCLUSION

The number and spectrum of nDNA defects in human mitochondrial diseases are expanding rapidly. In fact, with the completion of the human genome project, the rate at which new nDNA mutations are identified is likely to accelerate. This expansion of information will deepen our understanding of these genetic diseases and will also provide new insights into the biological functions of mitochondria. Already, human disease mutations have fostered explorations of how mitochondrial respiratory chain enzyme complexes are assembled; how mitochondria process metals such as copper and iron; and how mitochondrial nucleotides are processed. Animal models will be important tools to study disease pathomechanisms and to test much-needed therapies to treat these devastating disorders.

Acknowledgments

MH is supported by NIH grants AR47989 and HD37529, and by a grant from the Muscular Dystrophy Association.

REFERENCES

1. DiMauro S: Disorders due to mutations in the mitochondrial genome. In Rosenberg RN, Prusiner SB, DiMauro S, et al (eds): The Molecular and Genetic Basis of Neurological and Psychiatric Disease. Boston, Butterworth-Heinemann, 2003, in press.

2. Anderson S, Bankier AT, Barrel BG, et al: Sequence and organization of the human mitochondrial genome. Nature 1981;290:457–465.

3. Leigh D: Subacute necrotizing encephalomyelopathy in an infant. J Neurol Neurosurg Psychiatry 1951;14:216–221.

4. DiMauro S, Lombes A, Nakase H, et al: Cytochrome c oxidase deficiency. Pediatr Res 1990;28:536–541.

5. Hirano M, Marti R, Ferreiro-Barros C, et al: Defects of intergenomic communication: Autosomal disorders that cause multiple deletions and depletion of mitochondrial DNA. Semin Cell Dev Biol 2001;12: 417–427.

6. Suomalainen A, Kaukonen J: Diseases caused by nuclear genes affecting mtDNA stability. Am J Med Genet 2001;106:53–61.

7. Nishino I, Spinazzola A, Papadimitriou A, et al: MNGIE: An autosomal recessive disorder due to thymidine phosphorylase mutations. Ann Neurol 2000; 47:792–800.

8. Bohlega S, Tanji K, Santorelli F, et al: Multiple mitochondrial DNA deletions associated with autosomal recessive ophthalmoplegia and severe cardiomyopathy. Neurology 1996;46:1329–1334.

9. Sobreira C, Hirano M, Shanske S, et al: Mitochondrial encephalomyopathy with coenzyme Q10 deficiency. Neurology 1997;48:1238–1243.

10. Musumeci O, Naini A, Slonim AE, et al: Familial cerebellar ataxia with muscle coenzyme Q10 deficiency. Neurology 2001;56:849–855.

11. Baysal BE, Rubinstein WS, Taschner PE: Phenotypic dichotomy in mitochondrial complex II genetic disorders. J Mol Med 2001;79:495–503.

12. Taivassalo T, Abbott A, Wyrick P, Haller RG: Venous oxygen levels during aerobic forearm exercise: An index of impaired oxidative metabolism in mitochondrial myopathy. Ann Neurol 2002;51:38–44.

13. Papadopoulou LC, Sue CM, Davidson MM, et al: Fatal infantile cardioencephalomyopathy with cytochrome c oxidase (COX) deficiency and mutations in SCO2, a human COX assembly gene. Nat Genet 1999;23:333–337.

14. Mandel H, Szargel R, Labay V, et al: The deoxyguanosine kinase gene is mutated in individuals with depleted hepatocerebral mitochondrial DNA. Nat Genet 2001;29:337–341.

15. de Lonlay P, Valnot I, Barrientos A, et al: A mutant mitochondrial respiratory chain assembly protein causes complex III deficiency in patients with tubulopathy, encephalopathy and liver failure. Nat Genet 2001;29:57–60.

16. Bourgeron T, Rustin P, Chretien D, et al: Mutation of a nuclear succinate dehydrogenase gene results in mitochondrial respiratory chain deficiency. Nat Genet 1995;11:144–149.

17. Triepels RH, Van Den Heuvel LP, Trijbels JM, Smeitink JA: Respiratory chain complex I deficiency. Am J Med Genet 2001;106:37–45.

18. Robinson BH: Human cytochrome oxidase deficiency. Pediatr Res 2000;48:581–585.

19. Nishino I, Spinazzola A, Hirano M: Thymidine phosphorylase gene mutations in MNGIE, a human mitochondrial disorder. Science 1999;283:689–692.

20. Saada A, Shaag A, Mandel H, et al: Mutant mitochondrial thymidine kinase in mitochondrial DNA depletion myopathy. Nat Genet 2001;29:342–344.

21. Hirano M, DiMauro S: ANT1, Twinkle, POLG, and TP: New genes open our eyes to ophthalmoplegia. Neurology 2001;57:2163–2165.

22. Koehler CM, Leuenberger D, Merchant S, et al: Human deafness dystonia syndrome is a mitochondrial disease. Proc Natl Acad Sci U S A 1999;96:2141–2146.

23. Patel PI, Isaya G: Friedreich ataxia: From GAA triplet-repeat expansion to frataxin deficiency. Am J Hum Genet 2001;69:15–24.

24. Graham BH, Waymire KG, Cottrell B, et al: A mouse model for mitochondrial myopathy and cardiomyopathy resulting from a deficiency in the heart/muscle isoform of the adenine nucleotide translocator. Nat Genet 1997;16:226–234.

25. Larsson NG, Rustin P: Animal models for respiratory chain disease. Trends Mol Med 2001;7:578–581.

Mitochondria in Neurodegenerative Disorders

Giovanni Manfredi

M. Flint Beal

Neurodegenerative diseases are heterogeneous and characterized by selective loss of specific populations of neurons. Genetic defects have been identified in some of these disorders, including Huntington's disease, Friedreich's ataxia, some hereditary forms of amyotrophic lateral sclerosis, Parkinson's disease, spastic paraplegia, and Alzheimer's disease. However, both etiologies and pathogenic mechanisms of many of these conditions remain unknown, and a role for mitochondrial dysfunction has been postulated in most of them (see reference 1 for a review).

Mitochondrial oxidative phosphorylation (OXPHOS) is the primary source of high-energy compounds in the cell. Dysfunction of mitochondrial metabolism causes decreased ATP production, but also impaired intracellular calcium buffering and increased generation of reactive oxygen species (ROS). All these factors play important roles in neuronal degeneration. Mitochondria are also involved in apoptosis. Although a decrease in mitochondrial membrane potential has been observed in the early phases of apoptosis, it is still not clear whether decreased membrane potential owing to OXPHOS defects is sufficient to activate apoptotic pathways.

Mitochondria are under the control of two genomes. Human mitochondria contain multiple copies of a 16-kb, double-stranded, circular DNA molecule (mtDNA), which is maternally inherited. The mtDNA encodes 13 polypeptides, all of which are components of the respiratory chain, and a set of rRNAs and tRNAs necessary for intraorganellar protein synthesis. Although nuclear DNA encodes most mitochondrial constituents, mtDNA defects can cause numerous diseases, many of which are associated with neuronal degeneration.

Here, we summarize evidence of mitochondrial involvement in the pathogenesis of paradigmatic examples of neurodegeneration. We will first analyze diseases in which genetic defects of mitochondrial or nuclear genes encoding mitochondrial proteins cause OXPHOS defects that are primarily responsible for the diseases. We will then attempt to summarize evidence in favor of and against the concept that mitochondrial dysfunction is involved in the pathogenesis of disorders whose genetic causes are still unknown or that are due to mutations in nonmitochondrial proteins.

MtDNA MUTATIONS

For a more detailed discussion of this group of disorders, see Chapter 15. Disorders owing to mtDNA abnormalities are typically characterized by heterogeneous clinical phenotypes. The majority of these disorders are multisystemic, affecting different tissues and organs to different degrees, depending on the vulnerability of each tissue to OXPHOS impairment and on the mutation load. Among a large number of mtDNA mutations that are loosely associated with specific syndromes, some tend to cause rather selective neuronal degeneration. This situation applies, for example, to mutations in the mtDNA genes coding for ATPase 6 and for complex I subunits.

Leber Optic Atrophy/Dystonia

MtDNA mutations in genes encoding complex I subunits (ND genes) have been specifically associated with Leber hereditary optic neuropathy (LHON), a subacute degeneration of the optic nerve that affects especially young males, with a 8:1 male-to-female ratio, causing severe bilateral visual failure. Some of the ND mutations cause marked decrease of complex I activity in cultured cells and in platelets of affected patients. One such mutation (G14459A) is associated with an "LHON-plus" syndrome, characterized pathologically by basal ganglia degeneration and clinically by dystonia with maternally inherited levodopa-responsive parkinsonism.

NARP/Leigh Syndrome

Mutations in the mtDNA ATPase 6 gene have been associated with a syndrome characterized by neuropathy, ataxia, and retinitis pigmentosa (NARP). When the proportion of mutant mtDNA is very high (>95%), onset is earlier and the clinical picture is more severe, manifesting as subacute necrotizing encephalopathy with clinical and pathologic features of Leigh syndrome. Studies in cultured cells from affected individuals have documented defective mitochondrial ATP synthesis of variable degree, depending on the mutation, the proportion of mutant mtDNA, and the type of cells.

NUCLEAR GENE MUTATIONS AFFECTING MITOCHONDRIAL PROTEINS OF THE RESPIRATORY CHAIN

For a more detailed discussion of this group of disorders, see Chapter 16.

Leigh Syndrome

Leigh syndrome (LS, MIM 256000) is a severe neurodegenerative condition pathologically characterized by subacute symmetrical necrotic lesions in the subcortical regions of the central nervous system including basal ganglia, thalamus, brainstem, and spinal cord. Demyelination, vascular proliferation, and gliosis are typical pathologic features. Onset is usually in early infancy or childhood, but may sometimes be in adult life. Symptoms include psychomotor regression, ataxia, dystonia, and abnormal breathing. Death generally occurs within 2 years of onset.

LS is the consequence of impaired mitochondrial energy metabolism, which can be due to a variety of molecular defects. As mentioned earlier, high levels of mutations in the mtDNA ATPase 6 gene are responsible for maternally inherited LS (MILS). Inheritance of LS can also be X-linked or autosomal recessive. A study of the genetic causes of LS in a large group of patients showed that approximately 19% of cases were due to mtDNA mutations, and 10% to X-linked pyruvate dehydrogenase complex (PDHC) defects. The remaining 71% were due to a variety of autosomal recessive mutations in nuclear genes encoding respiratory chain subunits or proteins involved in respiratory chain assembly. In most patients with PDHC deficiency and LS, the enzymatic defect resides in the catalytic E1α subunit of the complex.

Complex I deficiency is another important cause of LS, and mutations in the nuclear encoded 23-kD NDUFS8 subunit, 18-kD AQDQ NDUFS7 subunit, and NDUFV1 subunit, have been found in patients with LS. A less common molecular defect was identified in two siblings with LS born to consanguineous parents, who harbored a mutation in the gene coding for the flavoprotein of complex II (succinate dehydrogenase).

Cytochrome c oxidase (COX) deficiency is one of the most common causes of autosomal recessive LS. Using microcell mediated chromosome transfer techniques and linkage analysis, one molecular defect was assigned to a gene named SURF1 on chromosome 9q34. SURF1 is translocated to mitochondria, where its presequence is cleaved. Mature SURF1 is localized to the inner mitochondrial membrane, where it presumably participates in the assembly of COX. In a different form of LS and COX deficiency, clinically characterized by encephalopathy and severe cardiomyopathy, the gene defect is in another COX assembly gene named SCO2.[2,3] SCO proteins appear to be copper binding proteins required for the insertion of copper in COX subunit I and II. Mutations in two additional COX-assembly genes, SCO1 and COX10, have been associated with LS-like syndromes.

Friedreich's Ataxia

Friedreich's ataxia (FRDA) is the most common of the hereditary ataxias. It is clinically defined by autosomal recessive inheritance, onset before age 25 years, progressive limb and gait ataxia, absent tendon reflexes, axonal sensory neuropathy, and pyramidal signs. The FRDA gene, which encodes a protein labeled frataxin, has been mapped to chromosome 9q13. Frataxin expression is particularly abundant in the cerebellum and in the spinal cord. Homozygous GAA expansions in intron 1 or heterozygous point mutations compounded with heterozygous expansions cause decreased frataxin expression. Frataxin localizes to mitochondria, where the precursor protein is cleaved by mitochondrial peptidases to the mature form. In affected human tissues, iron concentration is increased and the activities of several mitochondrial enzymes (such as respiratory chain complexes I, II-III, and the matrix enzyme aconitase) are decreased. Mitochondrial enzyme deficiency and late-stage iron accumulation were also found in a frataxin knockout mouse model.[4] It is thought that loss of frataxin causes impaired mitochondrial iron storage and metabolism resulting in increased free iron.[5] The ensuing free radical generation by Fenton reaction leads to oxidative damage and inactivation of mitochondrial enzymes. For reasons that are not clear, antioxidant defenses (i.e., superoxide dismutase) are disabled in cultured cells from FRDA patients, making them more prone to oxidative damage.[6] The role of oxidative damage in the pathogenesis of FRDA is bolstered by the efficacy of the antioxidant idebenone in reducing myocardial hypertrophy and lowering markers of oxidative stress.[7]

Hereditary Spastic Paraplegia

Hereditary spastic paraplegia is a progressive disorder causing paraparesis in childhood or in early adulthood. Upper motor neuron dysfunction prevails, but additional symptoms, such as ataxia and retinitis, are common. Autosomal dominant, X linked, and autosomal recessive modes of inheritance have been described (Table 17–1). In families with a recessive form of the disease mapped to chromosome 16q24.3, the disease gene *(SPG7)*, encoding a protein called paraplegin, has been identified and cloned.[8] Although the underlying pathogenic mechanism is still unclear, homozygous deletions or frameshift mutations of the paraplegin gene cause OXPHOS dysfunction with COX deficiency and mitochondrial proliferation (i.e., ragged-red fibers) in muscle.[8] Paraplegin has a high degree of homology with yeast ATP-dependent zinc metalloproteases and may have chaperone-like activity in mitochondria.

Mohr-Tranebjaerg Syndrome

Mohr-Tranebjaerg syndrome, or deafness-dystonia syndrome, is an X-linked recessive disorder characterized by progressive sensorineural deafness, dystonia, cortical blindness, and psychiatric illness. It results from deletions or truncations of deafness/dystonia protein *(DDP1)*, homologous to yeast *Tim8*, a member of the inner mitochondrial membrane transport machinery *(Tim)* located in the mitochondrial intermembrane space. In fibroblasts from patients with mutant *DDP1*, the formation of the *Tim* machinery is defective, presumably resulting in a failure to import other mitochondrial proteins synthesized in the cytosol.[9]

TABLE 17–1. Genetic Types of Hereditary Spastic Paraplegia (HSP)

Inheritance	Chromosome	Locus	Protein (Function)	HSP Type
AD	2p22	SPG4	Spastin (microtubule-binding protein)	Uncomplicated
	2q24–34	SPG13	Hsp60 (mitochondrial chaperonin)	Uncomplicated
	8q23–q24	SPG8		Uncomplicated
	10q23.3–q24.2	SPG9		Complicated[1]
	11q12–q14	SPG17		Complicated[2]
	12q13	SPG10		Uncomplicated
	14q11–q21	SPG3A	Atlastin (GTPase similar to dynamins)	Uncomplicated
	15q11.1	SPG6		Uncomplicated
	19q13	SPG12		Uncomplicated
	9q33–q34	SPG19		Uncomplicated
AR	3q27–28	SPG14		Complicated[3]
	8q	SPG5		Uncomplicated
	15q	SPG11		Uncomplicated/complicated[4]
	16q	SPG7	Paraplegin (mitochondrial protein)	Uncomplicated/complicated[5]
	14q	SPG15		Complicated[6]
XR	Xq28	SPG1	L1CAM	Complicated[7]
	Xq28	SPG2	PLP	Complicated[8]
	Xq11.2	SPG16		Uncomplicated/complicated[9]

[1]Cataracts, gastroesophageal reflux, motor neuronopathy.
[2]Atrophy of hand muscles.
[3]Mental retardation, motor neuropathy.
[4]Mental retardation, arm weakness, dysarthria, nystagmus.
[5]Mitochondrial myopathy, dysarthria, dysphagia, optic atrophy, axonal neuropathy.
[6]Macular pigmentation, distal atrophy, dysarthria, mental retardation or dementia.
[7]Mental retardation, aphasia, hydrocephalus.
[8]White matter abnormality by MRI.
[9]Motor aphasia, decreased vision, mental retardation, bowel and bladder dysfunction.
Abbreviations: AD, autosomal dominant; AR, autosomal recessive; XR, X-linked recessive; SPG, spastic gait; Hsp, heat-shock protein; L1CAM, L1 cell adhesion molecule; PLP, proteolipid protein. *Uncomplicated* HSP is limited to lower limb spasticity and weakness; *complicated* HSP includes additional neurologic problems.[1–9]
From Fink JK: Ann Neurol 2002;51:669–672.

Other defects in the mitochondrial protein import machinery have been reported in humans, such as a deficit of *HSP60* (a mitochondrial chaperonin) in patients with severe multisystem disorder and multiple mitochondrial enzyme defects.

Wilson Disease

Wilson disease is an autosomal recessive condition characterized by movement disorders such as dystonia and parkinsonism, psychiatric symptoms, and liver failure, with onset in childhood or adolescence. A defect in copper homeostasis results in copper accumulation in liver, basal ganglia, and kidney. The disease-associated gene encodes a copper-transport P type ATPase, called WND. The WND protein exists in 2 isoforms, a 159-kDa form, which localizes to the trans-Golgi network, and a 140-kDa molecule, which localizes to mitochondria. Although the precise functions of the protein are not known, the mitochondrial localization of the 140-kDa WND suggests that this isoform may play a role in mitochondrial copper-dependent enzymes, such as cytochrome *c* oxidase. Mitochondria in affected tissues have characteristic morphologic abnormalities, which are also observed in the mitochondria of Long-Evans cinnamon rats, a spontaneous animal model of the disease. Increased levels of deleted species of mtDNA have been identified by PCR amplification in liver from patients with Wilson disease. Moreover, mitochondrial enzyme defects, especially complex I and aconitase deficiencies, have been demonstrated in liver mitochondria from patients with Wilson disease.[10] These findings suggest that oxidative damage mediated by mitochondrial copper accumulation may play a role in the pathogenesis of the disease.

MITOCHONDRIAL DYSFUNCTION IN DISORDERS ASSOCIATED WITH MUTATIONS OF NONMITOCHONDRIAL PROTEINS AND IN NEURODEGENERATIVE DISORDERS OF UNKNOWN CAUSES

Huntington's Disease

Huntington's disease (HD) is a chronic autosomal dominant disease with full penetrance by midadult life. The illness is characterized by choreoathetotic movements and by progressive emotional and cognitive disturbances. Selective degeneration of striatal neurons with marked atrophy of caudatum and putamen are the main pathologic features. By electron microscopy, nuclear inclusions have been observed in HD striatum and cortex. HD is caused by expansion of a CAG repeat in the *IT15* gene on chromosome 4, which encodes a protein of unknown function named huntingtin. A defect in energy metabolism has been proposed as one potential pathogenic

mechanism, based on evidence obtained both in vivo and in postmortem tissues. Lactate increase has been found by MRI spectroscopy in occipital cortex and basal ganglia of HD patients, who also had a reduced PCr/Pi ratio in muscle. In the striatum of experimental animals, the respiratory chain complex II inhibitor malonate produces pathologic lesions closely resembling those of HD. Defects of complexes II, III, and aconitase have been described in postmortem HD brains, particularly in the basal ganglia. Respiratory chain dysfunction and aconitase defects have been reported in some, but not all, transgenic mouse models of HD.[11,12]

Despite the increasing evidence of mitochondrial involvement in the pathogenesis of HD, the mechanisms through which mutant huntingtin causes mitochondrial dysfunction is not yet understood. Furthermore, it remains to be established whether mitochondrial dysfunction is an early event and primary cause of HD or whether it is secondary to neuronal damage mediated by other mechanisms, such as excitotoxicity.

Amyotrophic Lateral Sclerosis

Amyotrophic lateral sclerosis (ALS) is a neurodegenerative disease affecting the anterior horn cells of the spinal cord and cortical motor neurons. The disease generally starts in the fourth or fifth decade, progresses rapidly, and leads to paralysis and premature death. While the majority of cases are sporadic and due to unknown causes, about 5% to 10% are familial; of these, about 20% are associated with mutations in the superoxide dismutase 1 *(SOD1)* gene. As these mutations do not decrease significantly SOD1 activity, a toxic "gain of function" of the mutated protein has been postulated. Mouse models carrying these mutations develop severe motor neuron disease. One of the morphologic alterations in motor neurons of mutant *SOD1* mice is massive mitochondrial degeneration. In *G93A* mutant mice, symptoms are preceded by a transient explosive increase in the number of vacuoles derived from degenerating mitochondria in motor neurons. *G93A* mice also exhibit abnormal respiratory chain function. Accumulations of abnormal mitochondria were also observed in anterior horns of patients with sporadic ALS not related to SOD1 mutations. Because SOD1 concentrations comparable to the cytosolic ones have been found in the intermembrane space of mitochondria,[13,14] mutant SOD1 may directly cause damage to mitochondria. Transgenic mice expressing *G93A SOD1* show early activation of the mitochondrial-dependent apoptotic pathway with cytochrome *c* translocation to the cytosol and BAX translocation to mitochondria. Cytochrome *c* translocation appears to occur also in the spinal cord of sporadic ALS patients.[15] Moreover, mouse neuroblastoma cells expressing mutant SOD1 displayed impaired mitochondrial calcium buffering capacity, leading to increased cytoplasmic calcium, a potential stimulus for apoptotic cell death. Respiratory chain enzyme deficiency was also identified in spinal cord of sporadic ALS patients.[16] Another indication of mitochondrial dysfunction in ALS comes from the observation that supplementation with creatine, which takes part in the mitochondrial energy buffering and transfer system, improves motor performance and extends survival in *SOD1* mutant mice.

Taken together, these findings suggest that impairment of mitochondrial energy metabolism may play a role in the pathogenesis of both sporadic and familial ALS.

Progressive Supranuclear Palsy

Progressive supranuclear palsy (PSP) is a neurologic disorder with rapid progression that is characterized by cognitive impairment, extrapyramidal symptoms, and vertical gaze palsy of supranuclear origin. The pathologic hallmark of the disease is the presence of neurofibrillary filaments in the subcortical regions of the brain, with diffuse neuronal degeneration and gliosis. Genetic studies have established a significant association between an extended *tau* haplotype (H1) and PSP. The neurofilaments that accumulate in PSP contain hyperphosphorylated *tau*. There is evidence suggesting that mitochondrial energy metabolism may be affected in PSP. First, OXPHOS defects have been reported in muscle from patients. Second, postmortem PSP brains showed reduced activity of α-ketoglutarate dehydrogenase, a key enzyme of the Krebs cycle, vis-a-vis normal respiratory chain activities.[17,18] Third, malondialdehyde, a marker of lipid peroxidation, was also increased in PSP brains. It is conceivable that in PSP a combination of mitochondrial dysfunction and oxidative stress may generate a vicious cycle leading to further oxidative damage and neuronal degeneration.

Alzheimer's Disease

Alzheimer's disease (AD) is the most common form of dementia in the elderly. Approximately 5% of AD cases are inherited with autosomal dominant transmission. These cases are primarily due to mutations in the amyloid precursor protein *(APP)* or in presenilin genes. However, most patients with AD are sporadic cases without known genetic defects. The neuropathology of AD is characterized by neuronal loss and by the presence of amyloid plaques and neurofibrillary tangles. Aggregated β-amyloid peptide (Aβ 40–42 amino acid) is considered the principal culprit in the pathogenesis of AD. However, the mechanism through which Aβ 40–42 causes neurodegeneration is the subject of great controversy. Some investigators have even proposed that Aβ 40–42 accumulation might in fact represent a downstream phenomenon, maybe even a protective response to oxidative damage originating from mitochondrial dysfunction.[19] However, it has been shown that β-amyloid inhibits respiration when added to isolated mitochondria.[20] Moreover, cultured astrocytes from brain of patients with Down syndrome, which overexpress amyloid precursor protein, showed increased intracellular levels of Aβ 40–42 associated with impaired mitochondrial membrane potential.[21]

Reduced COX activity has been found in AD brains, and defects of COX have been identified in AD hippocampus by immunostaining for specific subunits of the complex.[22] Reduced immunoreactivity for COX subunits, more marked than for the mtDNA-encoded ones, was also found in AD Purkinje cells. COX deficiency has been described in platelets from AD. The enzyme defect was also found in cybrid cells (cytoplasmic hybrids) containing mtDNA from AD platelets and the nuclear DNA from a human osteosarcoma cell line, suggesting the presence of pathogenic mtDNA mutations. However, the mtDNA mutations initially identified in some patients were later shown to affect mtDNA nuclear pseudogenes. A number of studies have reported mtDNA changes in AD, but none of these has provided unequivocal evidence that mtDNA mutations play a role in the pathogenesis of AD (reviewed in reference 22). An increased burden of mitochondrial mtDNA mutations associated with decreased COX activity was found in postmortem brain of AD subjects compared to younger controls. However, there was no difference between AD and non-AD elderly subjects, suggesting that mtDNA mutations and mitochondrial dysfunction may develop in aging brain independently from AD.[23]

Parkinson's Disease

Parkinson's disease (PD) is a neurodegenerative disorder clinically characterized by bradykinesia, rigidity, and tremor. Pathologically, the hallmark of PD is loss of dopaminergic neurons in the substantia nigra. The causes of PD are unknown in the majority of cases. Rare familial forms have been associated with mutations in the α-synuclein gene, the parkin gene, and the gene for ubiquitin hydrolase, although the mechanism by which these mutations cause neuronal degeneration is not known.

Numerous findings have suggested mitochondrial involvement in the pathogenesis of PD. First, it was shown that the toxic effect of 1-methyl-4-phenyl-1,2,3,6-tetrahydropyridine (MPTP), which produces parkinsonism in humans and laboratory animals, is mediated by inhibition of respiratory chain complex I. Second, complex I deficiency and oxidative damage were demonstrated in the substantia nigra of PD patients, together with reduced immunoreactivity for complex I subunits. Because complex I is the principal source of free radicals in the cell, a dysfunctional complex I in the substantia nigra could be responsible for the increased lipid peroxidation and DNA damage found in PD brains. Cybrids containing mtDNA derived from PD platelets showed reduced complex I activity, suggesting that inherited and/or somatic mtDNA mutations may be responsible for the biochemical phenotype in PD. However, this latter finding was not confirmed in an independent series of cybrids from PD platelets.[24] In rare cases, mtDNA mutations appear to be the primary cause of PD, as maternally inherited forms of PD or parkinsonism with complex I deficiency have been reported.[25]

CONCLUSION

Impairment of mitochondrial energy metabolism appears to be involved in the pathogenesis of numerous neurodegenerative disorders. Some diseases, such as LS, LHON, and NARP, are caused by mutations in mtDNA or in nuclear genes that encode proteins involved in respiratory chain assembly and homeostasis. Others are caused by genetic defects of proteins with unknown functions but with clear mitochondrial localization, such as frataxin and paraplegin, which cause mitochondrial dysfunction with impaired respiratory chain activities. The evidence in favor of a mitochondrial role in the pathogenesis of PD,

HD, ALS, PSP, and AD is both circumstantial and somewhat controversial. Although there are many indications that mitochondria are defective, the mechanisms responsible for mitochondrial dysfunction are not clear. Nevertheless, mitochondrial dysfunction can still be relevant to the development of the disease. For example, an interaction between mitochondrial dysfunction and oxidative damage could trigger a vicious cycle, leading to neuronal degeneration and death. Figure 17–1 shows the complex interactions among mitochondrial and nuclear DNA mutations, the respiratory chain, energy metabolism, reactive oxygen species, and mitochondrial membrane potential in degenerating neurons. All of these factors are potential components of a detrimental cascade of events that may eventually result in neuronal degeneration and death. A better understanding of the role of mitochondria in neurodegenerative diseases may lead to the development of more effective therapeutic strategies that may include administration of free radical scavengers, antiapoptotic drugs that act at the mitochondrial level, or energy-buffering compounds such as creatine.

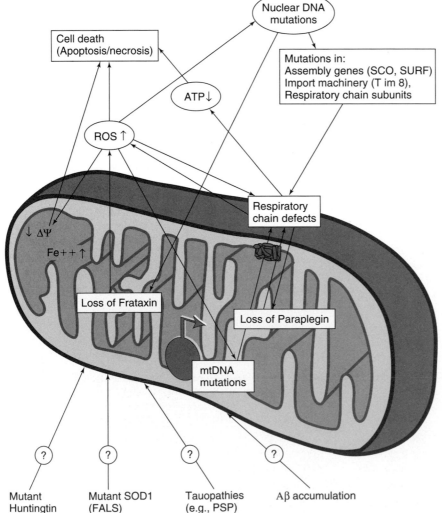

FIGURE 17–1. Schematic diagram of the complex interactions that may lead to mitochondrial dysfunction and neuronal cell death in the pathogenesis of neurodegenerative diseases. Some disorders are due to mutations in mitochondrial proteins such as paraplegin, frataxin, Tim 8, and respiratory chain subunits. In other disorders, nonmitochondrial proteins such as huntingtin, A-β, and hyperphosphorylated tau are thought to cause mitochondrial dysfunction through unknown mechanisms.

REFERENCES

1. Manfredi G, Beal MF: The role of mitochondria in the pathogenesis of neurodegenerative diseases. Brain Pathol 2000;10:462–472.

2. Papadopoulou LC, Sue CM, Davidson MM, et al: Fatal infantile cardioencephalomyopathy with COX deficiency and mutations in SCO2, a COX assembly gene. Nat Genet 1999;23:333–337.

3. Jaksch M: Mutations in SCO2 are associated with a distinct form of hypertrophic cardiomyopathy and cytochrome c oxidase deficiency. Hum Mol Genet 2000;9:795–801.

4. Puccio H: Mouse models for Friedreich ataxia exhibit cardiomyopathy, sensory nerve defect and Fe-S enzyme deficiency followed by intramitochondrial iron deposits. Nat Genet 2001;27:181–186.

5. Cavadini P, O'Neill HA, Benada O, Isaya G: Assembly and iron-binding properties of human frataxin, the protein deficient in Friedreich ataxia. Hum Mol Genet 2002;11:217–227.

6. Chantrel-Groussard K: Disabled early recruitment of antioxidant defenses in Friedreich's ataxia. Hum Mol Genet 2001;10:2061–2067.

7. Schulz JB, Dehmer T, Schols L, et al: Oxidative stress in patients with Friedreich ataxia. Neurology 2000;55:1719–1721.

8. Casari G, De Fusco M, Ciarmatori S, et al: Spastic paraplegia and OXPHOS impairment caused by mutations in paraplegin, a nuclear-encoded mitochondrial metalloprotease. Cell 1998;93:973–983.

9. Roesch K, Curran SP, Tranebjaerg L, Koehler CM: Human deafness dystonia syndrome is caused by a defect in assembly of the DDP1/TIMM8a–TIMM13 complex. Hum Mol Genet 2002;11:477–486.

10. Gu M, Cooper JM, Butler P, et al: Oxidative phosphorylation defects in liver of patients with Wilson's disease. Lancet 2000;356:469–474.

11. Tabrizi SJ, Workman J, Hart PE, et al: Mitochondrial dysfunction and free radical damage in the Huntington R6/2 transgenic mouse. Ann Neurol 2000;47:80–86.

12. Guidetti P, Charles V, Chen EY, et al: Early degenerative changes in transgenic mice expressing mutant huntingtin involve dendritic abnormalities but no impairment of mitochondrial energy production. Exp Neurol 2001;169:340–350.

13. Okado-Matsumoto A, Fridovich I: Subcellular distribution of superoxide dismutases (SOD) in rat liver: Cu,Zn SOD in mitochondria. J Biol Chem 2001;276:38388–38393.

14. Higgins CM, Jung C, Ding H, Xu Z: Mutant Cu, Zn superoxide dismutase that causes motorneuron degeneration is present in mitochondria in the CNS. J Neurosci 2002;22:RC215.

15. Guegan C, Vila M, Rosoklija G, et al: Recruitment of the mitochondrial-dependent apoptotic pathway in amyotrophic lateral sclerosis. J Neurosci 2001;21:6569–6576.

16. Wiedemann FR, Manfredi G, Mawrin C, et al: Mitochondrial DNA and respiratory chain function in spinal cords of ALS patients. J Neurochem 2002;80:616–625.

17. Albers DS, Augood SJ, Park LC, et al: Frontal lobe dysfunction in progressive supranuclear palsy: Evidence for oxidative stress and mitochondrial impairment. J Neurochem 2000;74:878–881.

18. Park LC, Albers DS, Xu H, et al: Mitochondrial impairment in the cerebellum of the patients with progressive supranuclear palsy. J Neurosci Res 2001;66:1028–1034.

19. Smith MA, Drew KL, Nunomura A, et al: Amyloid-beta, tau alterations and mitochondrial dysfunction in Alzheimer disease: The chickens or the eggs? Neurochem Int 2002;40:527–531.

20. Casley CS, Canevari L, Land JM, et al: Beta-amyloid inhibits integrated mitochondrial respiration and key enzyme activities. J Neurochem 2002;80:91–100.

21. Busciglio J, Pelsman A, Wong C, et al: Altered metabolism of the amyloid beta precursor protein is associated with mitochondrial dysfunction in Down's syndrome. Neuron 2002;33:677–688.

22. Bonilla E, Tanji K, Hirano M, et al: Mitochondrial involvement in Alzheimer's disease. Biochim Biophys Acta 1999;1410:171–182.

23. Lin MT, Simon DK, Ahn CH, et al: High aggregate burden of somatic mtDNA point mutations in aging and Alzheimer's disease brain. Hum Mol Genet 2002;11:133–145.

24. Aomi Y, Chen CS, Nakada K, et al: Cytoplasmic transfer of platelet mtDNA from elderly patients with Parkinson's disease to mtDNA-less HeLa cells restores complete mitochondrial respiratory function. Biochem Biophys Res Commun 2001;280:265–273.

25. Simon DK, Pulst SM, Sutton JP, et al: Familial multisystem degeneration with parkinsonism associated with the 11778 mitochondrial DNA mutation. Neurology 1999;53:1787–1793.

CHAPTER

18

Peroxisomal Disorders

Hugo W. Moser

A subcellular organelle, originally referred to as the microbody, was first described in the 1950s and characterized by de Duve and associates who later named it the peroxisome because of its role in the formation and degradation of hydrogen peroxide and because it also demonstrated a variety of other metabolic functions.[1] Its importance in mammalian metabolism was not recognized until it was shown later that several previously identified and named human disorders, such as Zellweger syndrome,[2] X-linked adrenoleukodystrophy (X-ALD),[3] and Refsum disease[4] were examples of peroxisomal malfunction. The human peroxisomal disorders are now divided into two major categories, the disorders of peroxisome biogenesis, in which the organelle fails to be formed normally, and those disorders in which a single peroxisomal enzyme is deficient. At present, 12 separate genetic defects have been identified for each of the two categories, but it is likely that the number will increase. This chapter provides a systematic description of the disorders of peroxisome biogenesis, X-ALD, and Refsum disease, and summarizes the other disorders that involve a single peroxisomal enzyme.

DISORDERS OF PEROXISOME BIOGENESIS

Key steps toward the understanding of the disorders of peroxisome biogenesis (PBD) were the demonstration that patients with Zellweger syndrome (ZS) lacked peroxisomes[5] and had a deficiency of plasmalogens, a class of lipids that had previously been shown to be synthesized in the peroxisome.[6] In 1988, Brul and colleagues[7] reported a series of cell fusion studies that showed that PBD could be subdivided into 12 complementation groups.[8] Progress in the understanding of PBD has been

aided by homology probing. Genetic studies in yeast have identified numerous genes required for peroxisome biogenesis, referred to as peroxins *(PEX)*. Computer-based searches of mammalian sequence databases identified many of their homologues.[9] Application of these studies to cell lines from patients belonging to specific complementation groups led to the demonstration that each of these groups was associated with defects of specific genes required for peroxisome import.[10]

Clinical Features

The disorders that are now known to belong to the PBD category were named and described clinically before it was recognized that they all are related to defective formation of this organelle. The historical names, Zellweger syndrome (ZS), neonatal adrenoleukodystrophy (NALD), infantile Refsum disease (IRD) and rhizomelic chondrodysplasia punctata (RCDP) have been retained. Studies of the complementation groups and the gene defects associated with each have shown that they can be grouped into two categories. The first is now referred to as the Zellweger spectrum. It includes the ZS, NALD, and IRD, which differ in respect to clinical severity. They often co-occur within a single complementation group. RCDP is the only representative of the second category. As noted subsequently, the clinical manifestations may also be mimicked by disorders that involve defects of single peroxisomal enzymes rather than defective import mechanisms.

The Zellweger Spectrum

Table 18–1 lists the main clinical features of patients with ZS, NALD, IRD; ZS is the most severe, IRD the least

TABLE 18–1. Major Clinical Features of Disorders of Peroxisome Assembly and Their Occurrence in Various Peroxisomal Disorders

Feature	ZS	NALD	IRD	Oxidase deficiency	Bifunctional enzyme deficiency	RCDP	DHAP synthase deficiency	DHAP Alkyl transferase deficiency
Average age at death or last follow-up (year)	0.76	2.2	6.4	4.0	0.75	1.0	0.5	?
Facial dysmorphism	++	+	+	0	73%	++	++	++
Cataract	80%	45%	7%	0	0	72%	+	+
Retinopathy	71%	82%	100%	2+	+	0	0	0
Impaired hearing	100%	100%	93%	2+	?	71%	33%	100%
Psychomotor delay	4+	3–4+	3+	2+	4+	4+	4+	?
Hypotonia	99%	82%	52%	+	4+	±	±	?
Neonatal seizures	80%	82%	20%	50%	93%	±	?	?
Large liver	100%	79%	83%	0	+	0	?	0
Renal cysts	93%	0	0	0	0	0	0	0
Rhizomelia	3%	0	0	0	0	93%	+	+
Chondrodysplasia punctata	69%	0	0	0	0	100%	+	+
Neuronal migration defect	67%	20%	±	?	88%	±	?	?
Coronal vertebral cleft	0	0	0	0	0	+	+	+
Demyelination	22%	50%	0	60%	75%	0	0	0

Percentages indicate the percentage of patients in whom the abnormality is present; 0, abnormality is absent; ± to 4+, degree to which an abnormality is present.

DHAP, dihydroacetone phosphate; IRD, infantile Refsum Disease; NALD, neonatal adrenoleukodystrophy; RCDP, rhizomelic chondrodysplasia punctata; ZS, Zellweger syndrome.

severe, and NALD is intermediate. It should be noted, however, that the range of phenotypic expression represents a continuum that is only imperfectly captured by these three designations. Figure 18–1 shows the facial appearance of patients with ZS. Infants with the ZS phenotype rarely live more than a few months due to the severe hypotonia, feeding difficulty, seizures, liver involvement, and apnea.[11] Some apparently classic ZS patients live longer.[9] Dysmorphic features are less striking in NALD than in ZS. The clinical course of NALD ranges from that of a severely involved infant who made no psychomotor gains and died at 4 months to patients who are stable but disabled in their midteens. IRD patients have moderate dysmorphic features. All have had sensorimotor hearing loss and pigmentary degeneration of the retina.

Rhizomelic Chondrodysplasia Punctata

The RCDP phenotype differs significantly from that of ZS. Patients with classic RCDP have rhizomelia with striking shortening of their proximal limbs. The facies are abnormal: flattened with frontal bossing, flat nasal bridge, and small nares (Fig. 18–2). Bilateral cataracts are present in 75% and 25% develop ichthyosis after birth.

Psychomotor retardation is profound. Endochondrial bone formation is profoundly disturbed. There is stippling of epiphyses especially at the knees, elbows, hips, and shoulders. Vertebral bodies have coronal clefts that are visualized on lateral roentgenograms of the spine. The majority of RCDP patients die in the first year or two of life, but several have survived longer, some into their teens.

Diagnosis

The diagnosis of PBD is suspected on the basis of clinical symptoms. The presence or absence of a peroxisomal disorder in affected persons can be determined on the basis of biochemical tests in plasma and red cells (Table 18–2). Definitive designation that the disorder is in the PBD category may require studies of cultured skin fibroblasts, because the clinical and biochemical abnormalities in peroxisomal single enzyme defects, particularly D-bifunctional enzyme deficiency, may mimic the Zellweger spectrum PBD disorders. Definition of the gene defect usually requires complementation analysis[8] and mutation analysis. Several reliable methods for prenatal diagnosis are available.[9] Heterozygote identification requires mutation analysis.

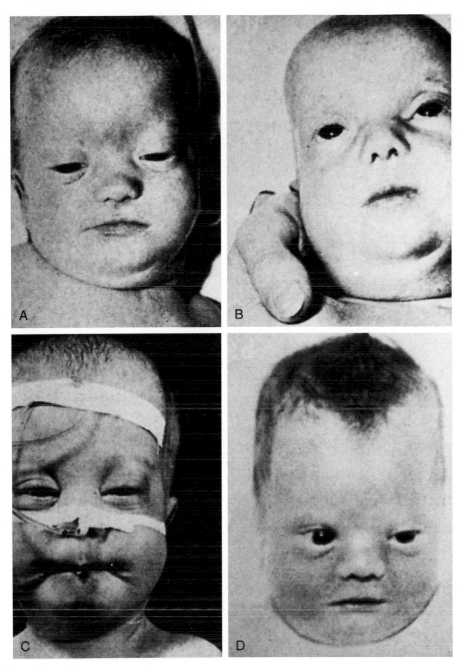

FIGURE 18–1. Newborn infants with the Zellweger syndrome. Note prominent forehead, hypertelorism, epicanthal folds, hypoplastic supraorbital ridge, and depressed bridge of nose. (From Lazarow M: Disorders of peroxisome biogenesis. In Scriver CR, Beaudet AL, Sly WS, Valle D [eds]: The Metabolic and Molecular Bases of Inherited Disease. New York, McGraw Hill, 1994, p 2297.)

Pathology

With subcellular localization of catalase as the criterion, peroxisomes are reduced or absent in all PBD patients who present as ZS, NALD, or IRD, that is, the Zellweger clinical continuum referred to previously. This abnormality can be demonstrated either by immunocytochemical methods[12] or by sedimentation methods. With these sedimentation methods, when peroxisomes are deficient, the catalase is found in the soluble fraction.[8] The degree of reduction of peroxisomes correlates roughly with clinical severity. When peroxisomal proteins are used as markers, most PBD patients can be shown to have membranous structures,

referred to as peroxisome ghosts, that contain peroxisome membrane proteins, but lack all or most peroxisomal matrix proteins.[13] Peroxisomes in patients with RCDP do not have demonstrable structural abnormalities.

Pathological changes are found in many organs. The liver is enlarged and fibrotic in most patients. Renal cysts are present in nearly all patients with the ZS phenotype but not in the milder PBD phenotypes. Calcific stippling of the patella and synchondrosis of the acetabulum occurs in 50% of ZS patients. The adrenal glands show striated cells in the reticularis fasciculata inner zone that contain lamellar inclusions similar to those in X-linked adrenoleukodystrophy. One of the most striking abnormalities is a

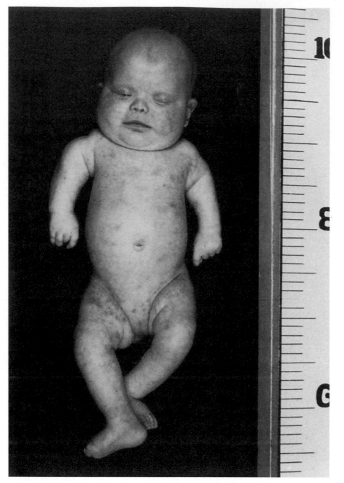

FIGURE 18–2. A newborn female with rhizomelic chondrodysplasia punctata (RCDP). Note severe shortening of proximal limbs, depressed bridge of nose, hypertelorism, and widespread erythematous and scaling skin lesions. (From Lazarow M: Disorders of peroxisome biogenesis. In Scriver CR, Beaudet AL, Sly WS, Valle D [eds]: The Metabolic and Molecular Bases of Inherited Disease. New York, McGraw Hill, 1994, p 2309.)

defect in neuronal migration.[14] This leads to characteristic and unique cytoarchitectonic abnormalities that involve the cerebral hemispheres, the cerebellum, and the inferior olivary complex. In the cerebral hemispheres, neurons that are normally destined for outer cortical layers are distributed within the inner cortical layers and in the underlying white matter. This migration failure causes the cerebral convolutions to be abnormally small (microgyria) or thick (pachygyria). The migration defect involves mainly the perisylvian and medially adjacent frontoparietal convexity. The pathogenesis of the migration defect is being investigated in the animal models of ZS.

Clinical Genetics

The PBD are inherited in an autosomal recessive manner and in the aggregate occur in approximately 1 in 50,000 live births.

Molecular Genetics

Table 18–3 lists the 12 complementation groups that have been identified so far, as well as the molecular defects associated with each. The defect associated with CG 8 has not yet been defined. Each of the defects involves one of the *PEX* genes, the genes that are required for peroxisome import. The studies of these cell lines with defined molecular defects have contributed to the understanding of the cell biology of the peroxisome.[9] PEX5 is the receptor for peroxisome targeting signal (PTS1). PTS1 targets proteins to the peroxisome, and is employed by most peroxisomal matrix proteins. The PTS1 signal is the S-K-L sequence at the carboxy terminus of the protein.[15] A structural model of the PEX5-PTS1 interaction has been proposed.[16] PEX5 is a predominantly cytoplasmic protein that shuttles between the cytoplasm and the peroxisome. Only four PEX5-deficient patients have been described. Two had the ZS phenotype, and two others the NALD. The ZS patients had a more severe import defect that involved proteins with the PTS-2 signal (discussed later) as well as those with the PTS-1 signal. In the more mildly involved NALD patients the import defect was confined to those carrying the PTS-1 signal.

PEX7 is the receptor for peroxisome targeting sequence-2 (PTS2).[17] The PTS-2 targeting sequence is located near the N-terminal and is contained in peroxisomal enzymes that play a role in ether phospholipid (plasmalogen) synthesis and in the alpha-oxidation of branched-chain fatty acids. *PEX7* deficiency has been demonstrated in all patients with the classic RCDP phenotype, referred to as RCDP type 1. The L292X mutation, which abolishes import of PTS2–containing proteins completely, is present in approximately two thirds of patients with RCDP type 1. Other mutations, which do not abolish import completely are associated with somewhat milder phenotypes that resemble Refsum disease.

PEX1 deficiency is the most common PBD. It accounts for about two thirds of cases; PEX 1 interacts closely with PEX6; and both function at late steps in the matrix protein import pathways. The high frequency appears to be caused by presence of two mutated PEX1 alleles in the general population: one that carries the G843D missense mutation and another that carries the frameshift mutation 2097insT. In vitro studies have shown that about 15% of import is maintained in cells with the G843D mutation, whereas, as expected, the frameshift mutation abolishes it completely. These differences are reflected in the phenotype.[18] Patients homozygous for the G843D mutation have the milder NALD phenotypes. One patient was able to function as a physical therapy assistant in young adulthood.[8] Patients homozygous for the 2097insT have the ZS phenotype, and persons who are compounds for the two mutations show phenotypes of intermediate severity.

PEX 2, 6, 10, 12, and 13 deficiencies all cause defects in the import of matrix enzymes. PEX 6 accounts

TABLE 18–2. Diagnostic Assays for Peroxisomal Disorders

	ZS-NALD-IRD	RCDP	X-ALD	Refsum Disease	D-Bifunctional Deficiency	Acyl-CoA Deficiency	Racemase Deficiency
Plasma							
VLCFA	Increased	Normal	Increased	Normal	Increased	Increased	Normal
THCA	Increased	Normal	Normal	Normal	Increased	Normal	Increased
Pristanic	Increased	Normal	Normal	Normal	Increased	Normal	Increased
Phytanic	Increased	Increased	Normal	Increased	Increased	Normal	Normal
Pristanic/ phytanic ratio	Normal	Decreased	Normal	Decreased	Increased	Normal	Increased
RBC							
Plasmalogen	Decreased 1–4+	Decreased 4+	Normal	Normal	Normal	Normal	Normal
Fibroblasts							
Catalase	Cytosol	Perox	Perox	Perox	Perox	Perox	Perox
Plasmalogen synthesis	Decreased 1–4+	Decreased 4	Normal	Normal	Normal	Normal	Normal
VLCFA	Increased	Normal	Increased	Normal	Increased	Increased	Normal

RCDP, rhizomelic chondrodyplasia punctata; VLCFA, very long chain fatty acids; X-ALD, X-linked adrenoleukodystrophy; ZS-NALD, Zellweger syndrome-neonatal adrenoleukodystrophy-infantile Refsum disease.

for 9% of PBD; the others are rare. The phenotypes in each of these disorders ranges from the severe ZS to the milder NALD and IRD. As in PEX 1 deficiency, the severity of the phenotype can often be correlated with the degree to which specific mutations impair import in vitro.

PEX 3, 9, and 16 deficiencies, although rare, are of special interest. Unlike the other PBD they do not contain "peroxisome ghosts," that is, structures that contain peroxisomal membrane proteins but lack matrix proteins. This observation, combined with other data,[9] has led to the conclusion that these three PEX proteins are required for the formation of membrane proteins. All have the severe ZS phenotype, presumably due to the complete lack of peroxisome function.

Animal Models

Two murine models with targeted disruption of PEX genes have been described: PEX 5[19] and PEX 2.[20] The affected animals showed intrauterine growth retardation and severe hypotonia and died a few days after birth. Both models show a defect in neuronal migration that resembles that seen in ZS patients, and thus provide the opportunity for determining the mechanism of this syndrome.

Treatment

The potential of postnatal treatment is limited by the multiple malformations that originate in fetal life. Based on the hypothesis that some of the biochemical defects secondary to peroxisomal malfunction may lead to additional progressive damage has led to therapeutic interventions aimed at correcting one or more of these biochemical abnormalities. These include the oral administration of ether lipids,[21] cholic and deoxycholic acid,[22] and a diet restricted in very long-chain fatty acids and phytanic acid (Moser HW, personal communication). Clinical documentation in each of these studies was limited. Martinez has reported that oral administration of docosahexaenoic acid (DHA) has improved clinical status, visual evoked responses, and brain MRI,[23] but evaluation of this therapy has been hampered by the great and unpredictable variability in natural history. Often overlooked, symptomatic therapy has been of benefit to children with ZS, NALD, IRD, and RCDP.

Future Directions

Continued study of import-deficient cell lines provides exciting opportunities for the understanding of the biologic role of the peroxisome and the disease mechanisms of each of the gene defects. Studies of the animal models will permit elucidation of the defects in neuronal migration. Until now, studies of peroxisomal disorders have focused strongly on gene defects that impair formation of the organelle. An exciting future benefit is that the increased understanding of peroxisome biology gained through study of these rare disorders will contribute to knowledge and therapy of common disorders, such as diabetes, obesity, vascular diseases, and cancer.

TABLE 18–3. Summary of Peroxisomal Biogenesis Disorders Complementation Groups, Number of Patients in Each Group and Their Phenotypes, Their Proportion of the PBD Patients, the Associated Gene Defects, Gene Map Position, and Peroxin Characteristics and Presumed Role in Peroxisome Biogenesis

CG	Phenotypes	%	Gene	Location	Peroxin size, distribution	Motifs	Function
1	75 ZS, 49 NALD, 26 IRD	57	PEX1	7q21-22	143 kDa, n.d.	AAA ATPase	Matrix protein import
2	1 ZS, 2 NALD, 1 IRD	1	PEX5	12p13	67 kDa, cytosolic/peroxisomal	TPR domain	Matrix protein import, PTS1 receptor
3	6 ZS, 2 NALD, 2 IRD	4	PEX12	—	41 kDa, integral PMP	Zinc RING	Matrix protein import, after docking
4	11 ZS, 11 NALD	9	PEX6	6p21.1	104 kDa, n.d.	AAA ATPase	Matrix protein import
7	4 ZS, 1 NALD	2	PEX10	1p36	37 kDa, integral PMP	Zinc RING	Matrix protein import, after docking
8	4 ZS, 5 NALD, 2 IRD	4	?	[Au]	?	?	Matrix protein import
9	1 ZS	<1	PEX16	—	39 kDa, integral PMP	None known	Peroxisome membrane biogenesis
10	5 ZS, 2 IRD	3	PEX2	8q21.1	35 kDa, integral PMP	Zinc RING	Matrix protein import, after docking
11	44 RCDP	17	PEX7	6q21-22.2	36 kDa, cytosolic/peroxisomal	WD-4C	Matrix protein import, PTS2 receptor
12	2 ZS	1	PEX3	6q23-24	42 kDa, integral PMP	None known	Peroxisome membrane biogenesis
13	1 ZS, 1 NALD	1	PEX13	2p14-16	44 kDa, integral PMP	SH3 domain	Matrix protein import, receptor docking
14	1 ZS	<1	PEX19	1q22	33 kDa, cytosolic/peroxisomal	Farnesylation	Membrane biogenesis, PMP receptor

CG - complementation group; IRD, infantile Refsum disease; NALD, neonatal adrenoleukodystrophy; n.d., no data; PBD, peroxisomal biogenesis disorders; RCDP, rhizomelic chondrodysplasia punctata; ZS, Zellweger syndrome.

From Gould SJ, Raymond GV, Valle D: The peroxisome biogenesis disorders. In Scriver CR, Beaudet AL, Sly WS, Valle D (eds): The Metabolic and Molecular Bases of Inherited Diseases. New York, McGraw Hill, 2001, p 3185.

Summary

Since the 1990s, remarkable advances have been achieved in the classification, diagnosis, and understanding of the disorders of peroxisome biogenesis (PBD). These advances have resulted from the mutual interaction between clinical studies and cell biology. The technique of complementation analysis led to delineation of 12 complementation groups, and the molecular defects in 11 of the 12 groups were defined in a period of a few years, and has also increased greatly the understanding of the biology of the organelle. Noninvasive diagnostic techniques permit accurate diagnosis post- and prenatally, but therapy is still very limited.

PEROXISOMAL DISORDERS DUE TO DEFECTS IN SINGLE PEROXISOMAL ENZYMES

Table 18–4 lists the peroxisomal disorders associated with defects in single peroxisomal enzymes. X-linked adrenoleukodystrophy (X-ALD) and Refsum disease will be described in detail, followed by brief comments about the other disorders.

X-LINKED ADRENOLEUKODYSTROPHY

MIM 300100

Although first reported in 1910, the first complete description of what is now referred to as X-linked adrenoleukodystrophy (Addison-Schilder disease) was provided by Siemerling and Creutzfeldt in 1923.[3] They reported a patient with an inflammatory myelopathy similar to the "encephalitis periaxialis diffusa" that had been described by Schilder but in whom the brain pathology was combined with adrenal atrophy. Adrenomyeloneuropathy (AMN), the adult form of the disease, was described in 1977. Lipid storage and the accumulation of saturated very long-chain fatty acids in the brain and adrenal gland were demonstrated in 1976[24] and were shown to be the result of the impaired capacity to degrade these substances,[25] a reaction that normally takes place in the peroxisome.[26] The defective gene, now referred to as *ABCD1*, was cloned in 1993.[27] It codes for a peroxisomal membrane protein, ALDP, that is a member of the ATP-binding cassette transporter superfamily of proteins.

Clinical Features

X-ALD displays a wide range of phenotypic expression (Table 18–5).[28–30] Three principal phenotypes occur in male patients: (1) *The cerebral forms.* In the aggregate these forms affect approximately 40% of male X-ALD patients. These are most common in childhood. The childhood cerebral form manifests most commonly between the ages of 4 and 8 years. The initial manifestations resemble those of attention deficit disorders, with later progression to dementia, more severe behavioral disturbances, impairment of vision, and hearing and motor deficits. It may progress to total disability within 2 to 3 years, and death ensues at varying intervals thereafter. The adolescent form resembles the childhood cerebral form but progresses more slowly. The adult cerebral form may present with focal neurologic deficits or with behavioral disturbances or dementia. All of the cerebral forms are associated with an inflammatory

TABLE 18–4. Single Peroxisomal Enzyme Defects

Disorder	Defective Protein	Reference No.
X-linked adrenoleukodystrophy	ALDP	27
CADDS	ALDP+	76
Acyl-CoA oxidase deficiency	Acyl-CoA oxidase	80
D-bifunctional protein deficiency	D-bifunctional	75
Racemase deficiency	Racemase	77
RCDP type 2	DHAPAT Acetyltransferase deficiency	78
RCDP type 3	Alkyl-DHAP synthase	79
Refsum disease	Phytanoyl-CoA hydroxylase deficiency	62
Mevalonate kinase deficiency	Mevalonate kinase	81
Glutaric aciduria type 3	Glytaryl-CoA oxidase	82
Acatalasemia	Catalase	83
Primary hyperoxaluria type 1	Alanine: glyoxylate Aminotransferase	84

RCDP, rhizomelic chrondrodysplasia punctata.

TABLE 18–5. Phenotypes in Males

Phenotype	Description	Estimated Relative Frequency
Childhood cerebral	Onset at 3–10 years of age. Progressive behavioral, cognitive and neurologic deficit, often leading to total disability within 3 years. Inflammatory brain demyelination	31%–35%
Adolescent	Like childhood cerebral. Onset age 11–21 years. Somewhat slower progression.	4%–7%
Adrenomyeloneuropathy (AMN)	Onset 28±9 years, progressive over decades. Involves spinal cord mainly, distal axonopathy inflammatory response mild or absent. Approximately 40% have or develop cerebral involvement with varying degrees of inflammatory response and more rapid progression.	40%–46%
Adult cerebral	Dementia, behavioral disturbances. Sometimes focal deficits, without preceding AMN. White matter inflammatory response present. Progression parallels that of childhood cerebral form.	2%–5%
Olivo-ponto-cerebellar	Mainly cerebellar and brain stem involvement in adolescence or adulthood.	1%–2%
"addison-only"	Primary adrenal insufficiency without apparent neurologic involvement. Onset common before 7.5 years. Most eventually develop AMN.	Varies with age. Up to 50% in childhood
Asymptomatic	Biochemical and gene abnormality without demonstrable adrenal or neurologic deficit. Detailed studies often show adrenal hypofunction or subtle signs of AMN.	Diminishes with age. Common <4 years. Very rare >40 years

myelinopathy. (2) *AMN*. Patients with AMN present most commonly in their twenties or thirties with a slowly progressive paraparesis with sphincter and sexual disturbances. These symptoms are often misdiagnosed as multiple sclerosis. Pathologically it is a noninflammatory axonopathy that affects mainly the dorsal columns and corticospinal tract in the spinal cord.[31] AMN is the most common X-ALD phenotype. It affects approximately 45% of male X-ALD patients. Approximately 30% of AMN patients also develop inflammatory cerebral involvement after or concurrent with the sensorimotor disturbances due to the myelinopathy, and when this occurs the disease may progress rapidly.[32] (3) *The "Addison only" phenotype.* Approximately 70% of patients with the cerebral forms and 50% to 70% of AMN patients also have primary adrenocortical insufficiency. In addition, 15% to 20% of patients (varies with age) have primary adrenocortical insufficiency without evidence of neurologic involvement. These patients cannot be distinguished clinically from patients with other forms of primary adrenal insufficiency. It is estimated that X-ALD is the cause of adrenal insufficiency in approximately 35% of boys with idiopathic Addison disease who are less than 7½ years old. Most X-ALD patients with the "Addison only" phenotype later also become neurologically involved. The various phenotypes often co-occur in the same family and phenotypic expression does not correlate with the nature of the molecular defect or the degree of elevation of very long-chain fatty acid (VLCFA) levels in plasma or cultured skin fibroblasts.

Women heterozygous for X-ALD remain asymptomatic in childhood and early adulthood, but up to 50% develop an AMN-like syndrome in middle age or later (Table 18–6). This syndrome is of later onset and milder than in the AMN patients, but occasionally patients require the use of a wheelchair.[29] Less than 1% of heterozygous women have cerebral involvement or adrenal insufficiency.

Diagnosis

The diagnosis of X-ALD is suspected on the basis of the clinical symptoms described earlier.

Confirmation of diagnosis is based most commonly on biochemical studies of plasma and, less frequently, on mutation analysis. Abnormalities in brain MRI may also provide the initial diagnostic clue.

The demonstration of increased levels of saturated very long-chain fatty acids in plasma[33] is the most frequently used diagnostic assay. Levels of hexacosanoic acid (C26:0) and the ratios of C26:0 and of tetracosanoic acid (C24:0) to docosahexaenoic acid (C22:0) are increased. This test is reliable for the diagnosis of affected males, irrespective of age. Levels are increased already on the day of birth. Plasma VLCFA levels are increased to a lesser degree in women who are heterozygous for X-ALD, but they are normal or borderline in 20% of obligate heterozygotes.[33] Mutation analysis[34] is the most reliable method for heterozygote identification. Prenatal diagnosis is achieved by demonstration of increased VLCFA levels in cultured chorion villus cells or amniocytes and by

TABLE 18–6. Phenotypes in Female X-ALD Carriers

Phenotype	Description	Estimated Relative Frequency
Asymptomatic	No evidence of adrenal or neurologic involvement	Diminishes with age. Most women <30 years neurologically uninvolved
Mild myelopathy	Increased deep tendon reflexes and distal sensory changes in lower extremities with absent or mild disability	Increases with age. Approximately 50% > 40 years
Moderate to severe myeloneuropathy	Symptoms and pathology resemble AMN, but are milder and of later onset.	Increases with age. Approximately 15% > 40 years
Cerebral involvement	Rarely seen in childhood and slightly more common in middle age and later	Approximately 2%
Clinically evident adrenal insufficiency	Rare at any age	Approximately 1%

mutation analysis.[35] MRI[36] and magnetic resonance spectroscopy (MRS)[37,38] show characteristic changes in patients with cerebral involvement but are normal in patients with AMN whose disease process is confined to the spinal cord. The most common MRI abnormality is symmetrical T-2 hyperintensity in the parieto-occipital region with contrast enhancement at the margin of the lesion. MRS shows decreased concentrations of *N*-acetyl aspartate and increased levels of choline.

Pathology

The pathology of the cerebral forms of X-ALD differs in important ways from that of AMN. An inflammatory demyelinating process with infiltration by T8 and T4 and B cells and increased cytokine and nitric oxide levels is a characteristic feature of the cerebral forms,[39] whereas AMN is a noninflammatory distal axonopathy that involves mainly the dorsal columns and the corticospinal tract.[31] The main biochemical abnormality is the abnormal accumulation of saturated VLCFA, most strikingly in the brain white matter and adrenocortical cells,[24] and to a lesser and varying extent in all other tissues. The VLCFA excess is present in a variety of lipid classes including cholesterol esters, sphingomyelin, glycerophospatides, and gangliosides.[28] The increase in VLCFA levels appears to be caused by the impaired capacity to degrade these substances,[25] a reaction that normally takes place in the peroxisome.[26] The peroxisomal beta-oxidation of VLCFA involves a series of four reactions. The first step is the formation of the Coenzyme A derivative and it is this reaction that is deficient in X-ALD.[40] This reaction is catalyzed by very long-chain acyl-CoA synthetase (VLCS). There are at least four different VLCS that differ in respect to substrate specificity and tissue distribution.[28,41] The pathogenesis of X-ALD is not well understood. VLCFA excess impairs membrane stability,[42] and it is proposed that this contributes to the axonopathy in AMN. The pathogenesis of the inflammatory response is not known. It may involve an immune-mediated inflammatory reaction to VLCFA excess. There may be additional as yet unidentified pathogenetic mechanisms that are unrelated to the VLCFA accumulation.

Clinical Genetics

The mode of inheritance is X-linked recessive. The minimum frequency in the United States is 1 in 21,000 males, and the combined frequency in men and women in the total population is 1 in 16,800.[43] X-ALD has been reported in all ethnic groups, and there is no evidence that there is significant variation in the frequency among them.

Molecular Genetics

The gene that is deficient in X-ALD is now referred to as *ABCD1*. It is located in Xq28. It occupies approximately 26 kb of genomic DNA. It is composed of 10 exons and encodes an mRNA of 4.3 kb and a predicted protein (ALDP) of 745 amino acids.[44] Surprisingly, the amino acid sequence is related to the superfamily of ATP-binding cassette (ABC) transporter proteins[45] and has no homology to VLCS. ALDP is a peroxisomal membrane protein. There exists another peroxisomal membrane protein, referred to as ALDR, which has 66% homology to ALDP and is encoded by the gene *ABCD2*, which is located on chromosome 12q11. Complementation studies have shown that expression of ABCD1 cDNA, and also of ABCD2 restores beta-oxidation of VLCFA in fibroblasts of X-ALD patients,[46,47] but the mechanism of this is not yet understood.[48] Mutations in the *ABCD1* gene have been identified in all X-ALD patients who have been studied in sufficient detail,[49] and are updated in the Web site www.x-ald.nl. More than 400 different mutations have been identified. Mutations are spread throughout the genome. Fifty-three percent are missense, 24% frameshift, 5% frame deletions or insertions, and 2.5% splicing defects. The majority of kindreds have private mutations; 68.5% were nonrecurrent. Immunofluorescence studies have shown that 67% of nonrecurrent mutations result in nondetectable ALDP. There is no correlation between the nature of the mutation and the phenotype.[49] The existence of a modifier gene has been proposed.[28]

Animal Models

Three laboratories have produced mouse models of X-ALD by targeted inactivation of ABCD1.[28,50] VLCFA levels in brain and adrenals are increased as in the human disease, but the animals appear to develop normally. The inflammatory brain disease observed in patients with the cerebral phenotypes has never been observed in the mouse model. It has been shown that the animals develop an AMN-like syndrome at the advanced age of 18 to 24 months.[51]

Therapy

Adrenal steroid replacement therapy is mandatory for all patients with impaired adrenocortical function. It can be life saving and improves general strength and well-being but does not affect neurologic status. There is no consistently effective therapy for the neurologic disability. Bone marrow transplantation has provided long-term stabilization and occasionally improvement in boys and adolescents with cerebral involvement that is still mild.[52,53] Key to success is the identification of patients with cerebral involvement that is still in the early stage. This is aided by monitoring of asymptomatic patients with MRI and MRS. Neuroimaging abnormalities precede clinical symptoms.[54] Semiannual or annual (depending on age) monitoring thus can help identify patients who are candidates for bone marrow transplantation (BMT). BMT carries a high risk; it is not recommended for patients who show no evidence of cerebral involvement, or for patients with AMN without cerebral involvement, or for those who already have advanced cerebral involvement. The promising results of BMT in patients with early cerebral involvement heightens the need to identify asymptomatic, or mildly symptomatic, patients by increasing awareness of the disease and by screening of at-risk family members.[43] Dietary therapy in which reduced fat intake is combined with the oral administration of a 4:1 mixture of glyceryl trioleate and glyceryl trierucate, also referred to as Lorenzo's oil, leads to rapid normalization of plasma VLCFA levels,[55] but its effect in patients who are already symptomatic has been disappointing.[56] An international study suggests that administration of Lorenzo's oil to boys who were younger than 6 years old, and were neurologically asymptomatic with normal MRI, reduces or delays the onset of subsequent neurologic involvement (Moser HW, unpublished observation). Other therapies that are undergoing clinical trials, and have been proposed on the basis of promising results in tissue culture or in the animal model (or both), are the oral administrations of 4 phenylbutyrate[47] and of lovastatin.[57] Gene therapy is under consideration for the future.

Future Directions

There is urgent need to obtain better understanding of the mechanism of action of ABCD1, both in respect to its effects on the metabolism of VLCFA and the exploration of possible actions that are not related to VLCFA.[58] Other priorities are the clarification of the mechanism of the inflammatory response. This would be aided by the development of an animal model that expresses the inflammatory response. Continued search for a modifier gene or other mechanisms that account for the great difference of phenotypic expression within the same family remains a high priority. The promising results obtained with bone marrow transplantation in the early stages of the disease process warrants the exploration of the feasibility of mass neonatal screening. Because X-ALD can be identified years before tissue damage occurs, it is also a prime candidate for gene and stem cell therapy.

Summary

X-ALD is the most common peroxisomal disorder, with a frequency that is equivalent to that of other more widely recognized metabolic disorders, such as phenylketonuria. X-ALD has a wide range of phenotypic expression. Reliable noninvasive diagnostic procedures are available. The gene defect has been identified. Therapy for the neurologic manifestations of the disease is a severe challenge, but results are encouraging for BMT in patients with cerebral involvement that is still mild.

REFSUM DISEASE

In 1946, the Norwegian neurologist, Sigvald Refsum, described a progressive familial disorder that he named heredopathia atactica polyneuritiformis[4] that has since been referred to as Refsum disease. In 1963, Klenk and Kahlke demonstrated that Refsum disease was associated with the accumulation of phytanic acid.[59] In 1966, Steinberg and coworkers demonstrated that the oxidation of phytanic acid involved an unusual initial alpha-oxidation and that this reaction was deficient in patients with Refsum disease.[60] They also showed that phytanic acid in man is of dietary origin exclusively and that dietary restriction of phytanic acid leads to clinical improvement.[61] The steps involved in the alpha oxidation of phytanic acid are complex and it was not until 1997 that Jansen and colleagues demonstrated that phytanoyl-coenzyme A hydroxylase is the enzyme that is deficient in Refsum disease.[62] The gene defect was defined only a short time later by two groups.[63] It has been shown that Refsum disease is genetically heterogeneous.[64] Classic Refsum disease is the disorder associated with phytanoyl-coenzyme A hydroxylase deficiency.

Clinical Features

The main clinical features in Refsum disease are retinitis pigmentosa, peripheral neuropathy, neurogenic hearing loss, anosmia, cardiac abnormalities, and ichthyosis.[65] Symptoms begin most commonly in the second decade. Pigmentary degeneration of the retina appears to be present in all patients and is an early manifestation. Night blindness may be present years before other clinical symptoms occur. Over the years concentric visual field constriction gradually develops until only tubular vision remains. A progressive polyneuropathy is another consistent manifestation but may not be recognized at the start of the illness. It is a mixed motor and sensory neuropathy that affects distal parts of the lower extremities most severely, with weakness, atrophy, and loss of deep tendon reflexes. Vibration and position sense are affected most severely, and peripheral nerves, mostly ulnar, peroneal, and great auricular, may be palpably enlarged and firm. Both the olfactory and the auditory nerves are affected. Anosmia along with pigmentary degeneration of the retina may be the earliest clinical manifestation. Loss of hearing is of the cochlear type and may be almost complete. Cardiomyopathy with cardiomegaly, heart failure, conduction disturbances, and electrocardiographic changes is common.[65] The involvement of the skin is highly variable. It ranges from slightly dry skin to florid ichthyosis, although some patients never develop it.

Diagnosis

Biochemical and genetic confirmation of the diagnosis is essential. Demonstration of abnormally high concentrations of phytanic acid in plasma is the key diagnostic assay. It is recommended that an assay procedure be used that measures levels of very long-chain fatty acid and of pristanic acid concurrently.[66] Plasma concentrations of phytanic acid are always increased except in early infancy. Normal concentration of phytanic acid in a patient who is one year or older thus rules out Refsum disease and related disorders, and permits distinction from the many other disorders that can cause retinitis pigmentosa or peripheral neuropathy. The concurrent measurements of VLCFA and pristanic acid permits distinction of Refsum disease from other disorders associated with increased levels of phytanic acid. In ZS, NALD, IRD, and bifunctional enzyme deficiency VLCFA levels are increased, whereas they are normal in Refsum disease. Pristanic acid levels are increased in racemase deficiency

and in bifunctional enzyme deficiency, whereas they are normal or decreased in classic Refsum disease. The phytanic and pristanic acid patterns in RCDP and in PEX 7 defects with milder manifestations resemble those in classic Refsum disease. Classic RCDP can be distinguished because its clinical presentation is totally different. Enzymatic assays or mutation analysis, or both, are required to distinguish classic Refsum disease from the milder forms of PEX 7 deficiency.[64]

Pathology
Biochemical Defect

The metabolism of phytanic acid is complex and has been clarified only recently.[64] An initial beta-oxidation is impossible because of the methyl group in the three position. The initial step is the formation of the coenzyme A derivative, followed by the formation of 2-hydroxyphytanoyl-CoA, catalyzed by phytanoyl-CoA hydroxylase (PHYH). PHYH is deficient in classic Refsum disease, owing to a variety of mutations (see Molecular Genetics later). It is located in the peroxisome and contains the PTS-2 targeting sequence.[67] PHYH activity is also deficient in RCDP (PEX 7 deficiency) and in ZS. The deficiency in RCDP results from the fact that PEX 7 is the receptor for proteins that contain the PTS-2 so that the enzyme is not targeted to the peroxisome and remains in the cytosolic compartment where it is unstable.

Pathogenesis

Steinberg and coworkers[61] demonstrated that phytanic acid in man is exclusively of dietary origin, a finding that forms the basis for current therapy. The impaired capacity to degrade it leads to striking abnormal accumulation of phytanic acid in many tissues. In some tissues, such as heart, phytanic acid may account for up to 50% of total fatty acids. The fact that lowering of phytanic acid levels by dietary restriction leads to clinical improvement suggests that the phytanic acid excess contributes to the pathogenesis. Several mechanisms have been proposed. These include the molecular distortion hypothesis, that is, that the increased cross-sectional area of methylated fatty acid when compared to that of straight chain fatty acids could cause membrane instability in myelin, and the hypothesis that phytanic acid may interfere with the formation of prenylated proteins. Of particular interest are studies that indicate that phytanic acid is a ligand for members of the nuclear receptor hormone receptor superfamily.[68]

Clinical Genetics

The pattern of inheritance is autosomal recessive. Refsum disease is rare. Approximately 150 cases had been reported up to 1996. Most cases seem to have come from Scandinavia, northern France, the British Islands, and

Ireland, a distribution that suggested the disease was spread by the Vikings. The disease has also been observed, however, in many other ethnic groups, and in many locations where any connection with the Vikings is unlikely.

Molecular Genetics

The *PHYH* gene spans 21,5 kb on chromosome 10p13 of the human genome and encodes an mRNA of about 1.6 kb. The 1014 nucleotides of the open-reading frame sequence are separated by eight introns. Nineteen different mutations have been identified in Refsum disease patients.[69] Interesting structure-function relationships have been described by Mukherji and colleagues.[70] The P29S does not abolish PHYH activity in vitro, but because it lies within the PTS2 targeting sequence, it may affect transport of the enzyme to the peroxisome. The R275W and the R275Q and R275A mutations affect the 2-oxoglutarate binding site, which impairs function because PHYH is an iron(II) 2-oxoglutarate-dependent oxygenase. Mukherji and coworkers[70] have noted that in the United Kingdom only about 45% of adult Refsum disease patients have defects in the function of PHYH. Other cases are associated with defects in PEX7. The A218V PEX7 mutation is associated with milder phenotypes that resemble adult Refsum disease. Indeed, one of the patients had been diagnosed as heredopathia atactica polyneuritiformis (Refsum disease) by Sigvald Refsum himself.[8]

Animal Model

No animal model of Refsum disease is available at this time.

Treatment

The prognosis of untreated patients with Refsum disease is poor. A survey in Norway found that 10 of 11 were blind and that one half had died before age 30 years.[71] Dietary therapy, based on restriction of phytanic acid intake, has revolutionized the prognosis. This therapy reduces the levels of phytanic acid in plasma from more than 100 mg/dL to less than 10. The dietary therapy improves the peripheral neuropathy and stabilizes the visual and auditory deficits, cardiomyopathy, and skin manifestations.[72] Because the diet does not appear to reverse deficits that are already present, except for the neuropathy, it is clear that the therapy should be begun early, hence the need for early diagnosis, including the screening of at-risk relatives. The phytanic acid content is highest in all kinds of dairy products. It may vary greatly in different geographic areas. Masters-Thomas and colleagues[73] provided a list of phytanic acid in foodstuffs and suggested a practical dietary regimen to maintain phytanic acid intake at less than 10 mg daily. Certain cautions in respect to dietary management are essential. The adipose tissues may contain an enormous amount of phytanic acid[9] (286 g in one patient). Release of phytanic acid may occur during periods of reduced food intake, including initiation of dietary therapy, dental or surgical procedures, or stress. It is essential, therefore, to maintain adequate caloric intake. Very high levels of phytanic acid (above 100 mg/dL) may precipitate toxic and life-threatening symptoms, such as cardiomyopathy or tetraparesis. Under these circumstances plasmapheresis has been successful as an emergency measure.[71]

Future Directions

Clarification of pathogenesis, with emphasis on the toxic role of phytanic acid, will be of great interest. This includes the creation of an animal model, additional studies on structure function relationships in mutant cell lines, and defining the role of phytanic acid as a ligand for members of the nucleic hormone receptor superfamily. Therapeutically, emphasis should be on presymptomatic diagnosis, because it is likely that dietary therapy could prevent all of the disease manifestations. Enzyme replacement or gene therapy, or both, may become available in the future.

Summary

Refsum disease can be viewed as a model of the successful interaction of clinical medicine and basic science. Sigvald Refsum delineated it as a clinical entity in 1946 in Norway. Phytanic acid, the storage substance, was identified in 1963 in Germany by Klenk and Kahlke. In 1966, Steinberg and associates in the United States made the crucial observation that phytanic acid in man is of dietary origin exclusively and this led to successful initiation of dietary therapy. Definition of the enzymatic defect was not achieved until 1997 by Jansen and Wanders in the Netherlands and this depended on understanding of the complex reactions of phytanic acid metabolism and peroxisome biology, which was based on research in the Netherlands, Australia, and the United States. The gene defect was then defined within the same year, concurrently by groups in the United States and the Netherlands. Current research focuses on better understanding of pathogenesis of the disease and on systems that will permit presymptomatic diagnosis, which would make it possible to apply therapies that may prevent the onset of clinical manifestations.

OTHER PEROXISOMAL SINGLE ENZYME DEFECTS WITH PHENOTYPES THAT RESEMBLE THE PEROXISOME BIOGENESIS DISORDERS

The phenotypes of peroxisomal acyl-CoA oxidase and D-bifunctional enzyme deficiencies resemble that of the PBD disorders with the ZS-NALD-IRD continuum.

Peroxisomal acyl-CoA oxidase deficiency, also referred to as pseudo-neonatal adrenoleukodystrophy, is a rare disorder, and its clinical manifestations are milder than those of bifunctional enzyme deficiency.[74] Bifunctional enzyme deficiency is more common. At the Kennedy Krieger Institute 15% of patients with the ZS-NALD-IRD phenotype were found to have bifunctional enzyme deficiency. The enzymatic and molecular basis of bifunctional enzyme deficiency has been clarified by Wanders and associates.[75] They demonstrated that the first patient reported to have this disorder, and who was thought to have a deficiency of L-bifunctional enzyme, actually had a deficiency of the D-bifunctional enzyme and that there is no documented case of human L-bifunctional enzyme deficiency. Furthermore, biochemical re-evaluation of the patient who was originally reported as an example of peroxisomal 3-oxoacyl-CoA thiolase 1 deficiency (pseudo-Zellweger syndrome) demonstrated that this patient also had D-bifunctional enzyme deficiency (Wanders R, personal communication). The phenotypic expression of D-bifunctional enzyme deficiency ranges from ZS to milder IRD-like phenotypes. The continuous deletion of the X-linked adrenoleukodystrophy gene and DXS1357E (CADDS) syndrome has been described.[76] Patients presented with a combination of cholestasis, hypotonia, and profound psychomotor retardation and the patients died during the first year. Their clinical presentation thus resembled that of a PBD. VLCFA levels were markedly increased and they lacked ALDP, but other peroxisomal functions were normal. Molecular analysis revealed that they had a contiguous deletion of ABCD1 and of DXS1357E. A point of great practical significance is that the mode of inheritance of CADDS is X-linked recessive, whereas that of the PBD is autosomal recessive. Patients with racemase deficiency[77] may present with a sensory motor neuropathy that bears some resemblance to Charcot-Marie-Tooth disease, Refsum disease, or a mild peroxisome biogenesis disorder. As shown in Table 18-2, the laboratory findings are characteristic. Dihydroxy-acetonephosphate (DHAP), acetyltransferase deficiency,[78] and alkyl-DHAP synthase[79] cannot be distinguished clinically from RCDP and this suggests that a deficit of ether lipids is sufficient to lead to this syndrome.

REFERENCES

1. De Duve C, Baudhuin P: Peroxisomes (microbodies and related particles). Physiol Rev 1966; 46:323–357.

2. Bowen PLCSN, Zellweger H, Lindenberg R: A familial syndrome of multiple congenital defects. Bull Johns Hopkins Hosp 1964;114:402–414.

3. Siemerling E, Creutzfeldt HG: Bronzekrankheit und Sklerosierende Encephalomyelitis. Arch Psychiatr Nervenkr 1923;68:217–244.

4. Refsum S: Hereditopathia atactica polyneuritiformis. Acta Psychiat Scan 1946;38:1–303.

5. Goldfischer S, Moore CL, Johnson AB, et al: Peroxisomal and mitochondrial defects in the cerebro-hepato-renal syndrome. Science 1973;182:62–64.

6. Heymans HS, Schutgens RB, Tan R, et al: Severe plasmalogen deficiency in tissues of infants without peroxisomes (Zellweger syndrome). Nature 1983; 306:69–70.

7. Brul S, Westerveld A, Strijland A, et al: Genetic heterogeneity in the cerebrohepatorenal (Zellweger) syndrome and other inherited disorders with a generalized impairment of peroxisomal functions. A study using complementation analysis. J Clin Invest 1988;81: 1710–1715.

8. Moser AB, Rasmussen M, Naidu S, et al: Phenotype of patients with peroxisomal disorders subdivided into sixteen complementation groups. J Pediatr 1995; 127:13–22.

9. Gould SJ, Raymond GV, Valle D: The peroxisome biogenesis disorders. In Scriver CR, Beaudet AL, Sly WS, Valle D (eds): The Metabolic and Molecular Bases of Inherited Diseases. New York, McGraw Hill, 2001, pp 3181–3217.

10. Distel B, Erdmann R, Gould SJ, et al: A unified nomenclature for peroxisome biogenesis factors. J Cell Biol 1996;135:1–3.

11. Wilson GN, Holmes RG, Custer J, et al: Zellweger syndrome: Diagnostic assays, syndrome delineation, and potential therapy. Am J Med Genet 1986;24:69–82.

12. Goldfischer S, Collins J, Rapin I, et al: Peroxisomal defects in neonatal-onset and X-linked adrenoleukodystrophies. Science 1985;227:67–70.

13. Santos MJ, Imanaka T, Shio H, et al: Peroxisomal membrane ghosts in Zellweger syndrome—aberrant organelle assembly. Science 1988; 239:1536–1538.

14. Evrard P, Caviness VS Jr, Prats-Vinas J, Lyon G: The mechanism of arrest of neuronal migration in the Zellweger malformation: An hypothesis based upon cytoarchitectonic analysis. Acta Neuropathol (Berl) 1978;41:109–117.

15. Gould SJ, Keller GA, Hosken N, et al: A conserved tripeptide sorts proteins to peroxisomes. J Cell Biol 1989;108:1657–1664.

16. Gatto GJJ, Geisbrecht BV, Gould SJ, Berg JM: A proposed model for the PEX5-peroxisomal targeting signal-1 recognition complex. Proteins 2000;38: 241–246.

17. Braverman N, Steel G, Obie C, et al: Human PEX7 encodes the peroxisomal PTS2 receptor and is responsible for rhizomelic chondrodysplasia punctata. Nat Genet 1997;15:369–376.

18. Reuber BE, Germain-Lee E, Collins CS, et al: Mutations in PEX1 are the most common cause of peroxisome biogenesis disorders. Nat Genet 1997;17: 445–448.

19. Baes M, Gressens P, Baumgart E, et al: A mouse model for Zellweger syndrome. Nat Genet 1997;17:49–57.

20. Faust PL, Hatten ME: Targeted deletion of the PEX2 peroxisome assembly gene in mice provides a model for Zellweger syndrome, a human neuronal migration disorder. J Cell Biol 1997;139:1293–1305.

21. Holmes RD, Wilson GN, Hajra A: Oral ether lipid therapy in patients with peroxisomal disorders. J Inher Metab Dis 1987;10:239.

22. Setchell KD, Bragetti P, Zimmer-Nechemias L, et al: Oral bile acid treatment and the patient with Zellweger syndrome. Hepatology 1992;15:198–207.

23. Martinez M, Vazquez E: MRI evidence that docosahexaenoic acid ethyl ester improves myelination in generalized peroxisomal disorders. Neurology 1998;51:26–32.

24. Igarashi M, Schaumburg HH, Powers J, et al: Fatty acid abnormality in adrenoleukodystrophy. J Neurochem 1976;26:851–860.

25. Singh I, Moser AE, Moser HW, Kishimoto Y: Adrenoleukodystrophy: Impaired oxidation of very long chain fatty acids in white blood cells, cultured skin fibroblasts, and amniocytes. Pediatr Res 1984; 18:286–290.

26. Singh I, Moser AE, Goldfischer S, Moser HW: Lignoceric acid is oxidized in the peroxisome: Implications for the Zellweger cerebro-hepato-renal syndrome and adrenoleukodystrophy. Proc Natl Acad Sci U S A 1984;81:4203–4207.

27. Mosser J, Douar AM, Sarde CO, et al: Putative X linked adrenoleukodystrophy gene shares unexpected homology with ABC transporters. Nature 1993; 361:726–730.

28. Moser HW, Smith KD, Watkins PA, et al: X-linked adrenoleukodystrophy. In Scriver CR, Beaudet AL, Sly WS, Valle D (eds): The Metabolic and Molecular Bases of Inherited Disease. New York, McGraw Hill, 2000, pp 3257–3301.

29. Moser HW: Adrenoleukodystrophy: Phenotype, genetics, pathogenesis and therapy. Brain 1997;120:1485–1508.

30. van Geel BM, Assies J, Wanders RJ, Barth PG: X linked adrenoleukodystrophy: Clinical presentation, diagnosis, and therapy. J Neurol Neurosurg Psychiatry 1997;63:4–14.

31. Powers JM, DeCiero DP, Ito M, et al: Adrenomyeloneuropathy: A neuropathologic review featuring its noninflammatory myelopathy. J Neuropathol Exp Neurol 2000;59:89–102.

32. van Geel BM, Bezman L, Loes DJ, et al: Evolution of phenotypes in adult male patients with X-linked adrenoleukodystrophy. Ann Neurol 2001; 49:186–194.

33. Moser AB, Kreiter N, Bezman L, et al: Plasma very long chain fatty acids in 3,000 peroxisome disease patients and 29,000 controls. Ann Neurol 1999; 45:100–110.

34. Boehm CD, Cutting GR, Lachtermacher MB, et al: Accurate DNA-based diagnostic and carrier testing for X-linked adrenoleukodystrophy. Mol Genet Metab 1999;66:128–136.

35. Moser AB, Moser HW: The prenatal diagnosis of X linked adrenoleukodystrophy. Prenat Diagn 1999;19:46–48.

36. Kumar AJ, Rosenbaum AE, Naidu S, et al: Adrenoleukodystrophy: Correlating MR imaging with CT. Radiology 1987;165:497–504.

37. Pouwels PJ, Kruse B, Korenke GC, et al: Quantitative proton magnetic resonance spectroscopy of childhood adrenoleukodystrophy. Neuropediatrics 1998;29:254–264.

38. Eichler FS, Barker PB, Cox C, et al: Proton MR spectroscopic imaging predicts lesion progression on MRI in X linked adrenoleukodystrophy. Neurology 2002;58:901–907.

39. Ito M, Blumberg BM, Mock DJ, et al: Potential environmental and host participants in the early white matter lesion of adreno-leukodystrophy: Morphologic evidence for CD8 cytotoxic T cells, cytolysis of oligodendrocytes, and CD1 mediated lipid antigen presentation. J Neuropathol Exp Neurol 2001;60:1004–1019.

40. Lazo O, Contreras M, Hashmi M, et al: Peroxisomal lignoceroyl-CoA ligase deficiency in childhood adrenoleukodystrophy and adrenomyeloneuropathy. Proc Natl Acad Sci U S A 1988;85: 7647–7651.

41. Steinberg SJ, Wang SJ, Kim DG, et al: Human very long-chain acyl-CoA synthetase: Cloning, topography, and relevance to branched-chain fatty acid metabolism. Biochem Biophys Res Commun 1999;257: 615–621.

42. Ho JK, Moser H, Kishimoto Y, Hamilton JA: Interactions of a very long chain fatty acid with model membranes and serum albumin. Implications for the pathogenesis of adrenoleukodystrophy. J Clin Invest 1995;96:1455–1463.

43. Bezman L, Moser AB, Raymond GV, et al: Adrenoleukodystrophy: Incidence, new mutation rate, and results of extended family screening. Ann Neurol 2001;49:512–517.

44. Sarde CO, Mosser J, Kioschis P, et al: Genomic organization of the adrenoleukodystrophy gene. Genomics 1994;22:13–20.

45. Higgins CF: ABC transporters: From microorganisms to man. Annu Rev Cell Biol 1992; 8:67–113.

46. Cartier N, Lopez J, Moullier P, et al: Retroviral mediated gene transfer corrects very-long-chain fatty acid metabolism in adrenoleukodystrophy fibroblasts. Proc Natl Acad Sci U S A 1995;92:1674–1678.

47. Kemp S, Wei HM, Lu JF, et al: Gene redundancy and pharmacological gene therapy: Implications for X-linked adrenoleukodystrophy. Nat Med 1998;4:1261–1268.

48. Steinberg SJ, Kemp S, Braiterman LT, Watkins PA: Role of very-long-chain acyl-coenzyme A synthetase in X-linked adrenoleukodystrophy. Ann Neurol 1999; 46:409–412.

49. Kemp S, Pujol A, Waterham HR, et al: ABCD1 mutations and the X-linked adrenoleukodystrophy mutation database: Role in diagnosis and clinical correlations. Hum Mutat 2001;18:499–515.

50. Lu JF, Lawler AM, Watkins PA, et al: A mouse model for X-linked adrenoleukodystrophy. Proc Natl Acad Sci U S A 1997;94:9366–9371.

51. Pujol A, Hindelang C, Callizot N, et al: Late onset neurological phenotype of the X-ALD gene inactivation in mice: A mouse model for adrenomyeloneuropathy. Hum Mol Genet 2002;11:499–505.

52. Aubourg P, Blanche S, Jambaque I, et al: Reversal of early neurologic and neuroradiologic manifestations of X-linked adrenoleukodystrophy by bone marrow transplantation. N Engl J Med 1990; 322:1860–1866.

53. Shapiro E, Krivit W, Lockman L, et al: Long-term effect of bone-marrow transplantation for childhood-onset cerebral X-linked adrenoleukodystrophy. Lancet 2000;56:713–718.

54. Moser HW, Loes DJ, Melhem ER, et al: X-Linked adrenoleukodystrophy: Overview and prognosis as a function of age and brain magnetic resonance imaging abnormality. A study involving 372 patients. Neuropediatrics 2000;31:227–239.

55. Rizzo WB, Leshner RT, Odone A, et al: Dietary erucic acid therapy for X-linked adrenoleukodystrophy. Neurology 1989;39:1415–1422.

56. van Geel BM, Assies J, Haverkort EB, et al: Progression of abnormalities in adrenomyeloneuropathy and neurologically asymptomatic X-linked adrenoleukodystrophy despite treatment with "Lorenzo's oil." J Neurol Neurosurg Psychiatry 1999;67:290–299.

57. Singh I, Khan M, Key L, Pai S: Lovastatin for X linked adrenoleukodystrophy. N Engl J Med 1998;339:702–703.

58. Aubourg P, Dubois-Dalcq M: X-linked adrenoleukodystrophy enigma: How does the ALD peroxisomal transporter mutation affect CNS glia? Glia 2000;29:186–190.

59. Klenk E, Kahlke W: Ueber das Vorkommen der 3,7,11,15 tetramethyldecansaure (phytansaure) in den cholesterinestern und anderen lipidfractionen der organe bei einem krankheitsfall unbekannter genese Verdacht auf Heredopathia atactica polyneuritiformis, Refsum's syndrome. Hoppe Seylers Z. Physiol Chem 1963;333:133.

60. Steinberg D, Herndon JH Jr, Uhlendorf BW, et al: Refsum's disease: Nature of the enzyme defect. Science 1967;156:1740–1742.

61. Steinberg D, Mize CE, Herndon JH Jr, et al: Phytanic acid in patients with Refsum's syndrome and response to dietary treatment. Arch Intern Med 1970; 125:75–87.

62. Jansen GA, Wanders RJ, Watkins PA, Mihalik SJ: Phytanoyl-coenzyme A hydroxylase deficiency—the enzyme defect in Refsum's disease. N Engl J Med 1997;337:133–134.

63. Jansen GA, Ofman R, Ferdinandusse S, et al: Refsum disease is caused by mutations in the phytanoyl-CoA hydroxylase gene. Nat Genet 1997;17:190–193.

64. Wierzbicki AS, Lloyd MD, Schofield CJ, et al: Refsum's disease: A peroxisomal disorder affecting phytanic acid alpha-oxidation. J Neurochem 2002;80: 727–735.

65. Wanders RJA, Jakobs C, Skjeldal OH: Refsum disease. In Scriver CR, Beaudet AL, Sly WS, Valle D (eds): The Metabolic and Molecular Bases of Inherited Disease. New York, McGraw-Hill, 2001, pp 3303–3321.

66. Vreken P, van Lint AE, Bootsma AH, et al: Rapid stable isotope dilution analysis of very-long-chain fatty acids, pristanic acid and phytanic acid using gas chromatography electron impact mass spectrometry. J Chromatogr B Biomed Sci Appl 1998; 713:281–287.

67. Jansen GA, Ofman R, Denis S, et al: Phytanoyl-CoA hydroxylase from rat liver. Protein purification and cDNA cloning with implications for the subcellular localization of phytanic acid alpha-oxidation. J Lipid Res 1999;40:2244–2254.

68. Wolfrum C, Ellinghaus P, Fobker M, et al: Phytanic acid is ligand and transcriptional activator of murine liver fatty acid binding protein. J Lipid Res 1999;40:708–714.

69. Jansen GA, Hogenhout EM, Ferdinandusse S, et al: Human phytanoyl-CoA hydroxylase: Resolution of the gene structure and the molecular basis of Refsum's disease. Hum Mol Genet 2000;9:1195–1200.

70. Mukherji M, Chien W, Kershaw NJ, et al: Structure function analysis of phytanoyl-CoA 2-hydroxylase mutations causing Refsum's disease. Hum Mol Genet 2001;10:1971–1982.

71. Wanders RJA, Barth PG, Heymans HSA: Single peroxisomal enzyme deficiencies. In Scriver CR, Beaudet AL, Sly WS, Valle D (eds): The Metabolic and Molecular Bases of Inherited Disease. New York, McGraw Hill, 2001, pp 3219–3256.

72. Gibberd FB, Billimoria JD, Page NG, Retsas S: Heredopathia atactica polyneuritiformis (Refsum's disease) treated by diet and plasma-exchange. Lancet 1979;1:575–578.

73. Masters-Thomas A, Bailes J, Billimoria JD, et al: Heredopathia atactica polyneuritiformis (Refsum's disease): 2. Estimation of phytanic acid in foods. J Hum Nutr 1980;34:251–254.

74. Watkins PA, McGuinness MC, Raymond GV, et al: Distinction between peroxisomal bifunctional enzyme and acyl-CoA oxidase deficiencies. Ann Neurol 1995;38:472.

75. van Grunsven EG, van Berkel E, Mooijer PA, et al: Peroxisomal bifunctional protein deficiency revisited: Resolution of its true enzymatic and molecular basis. Am J Hum Genet 1999;64:99–107.

76. Corzo D, Gibson W, Johnson K, et al: Contiguous deletion of the X-linked adrenoleukodystrophy gene (ABCD1) and DXS1357E: A novel neonatal phenotype similar to peroxisomal biogenesis disorders. Am J Hum Genet 2002;70:1520–1531.

77. Ferdinandusse S, Denis S, Clayton PT, et al: Mutations in the gene encoding peroxisomal alpha-methylacyl-CoA racemase cause adult-onset sensory motor neuropathy. Nat Genet 2000;24:188–191.

78. Wanders RJ, Schumacher H, Heikoop J, et al: Human dihydroxyacetonephosphate acyltransferase deficiency: A new peroxisomal disorder. J Inherit Metab Dis 1992;15:389–391.

79. Wanders RJ, Dekker C, Hovarth VA, et al: Human alkyldihydroxyacetonephosphate synthase deficiency: A new peroxisomal disorder. J Inherit Metab Dis 1994;17:315–318.

80. Poll-The BT, Roels F, Ogier H, et al: A new peroxisomal disorder with enlarged peroxisomes and a specific deficiency of acyl-CoA oxidase (pseudo-neonatal adrenoleukodystrophy). Am J Hum Genet 1988;42:422–434.

81. Hoffmann GF, Charpentier C, Mayatepek E, et al: Clinical and biochemical phenotype in 11 patients with mevalonic aciduria. Pediatrics 1993;91:915–921.

82. Bennett MJ, Pollitt RJ, Goodman SI, et al: Atypical riboflavin-responsive glutaric aciduria, and deficient peroxisomal glutaryl-CoA oxidase activity: A new peroxisomal disorder. J Inherit Metab Dis 1991;14:165–173.

83. Eaton JWMM: Actalasemia. In Scriver CR, Beaudet AL, Sly WS, Valle D (eds): The Metabolic and Molecular Bases of Inherited Disease. New York, McGraw Hill, 1994, pp 2371–2383.

84. Danpure CJ: Primary hyperoxaluria. In Scriver CR, Beaudet AL, Sly WS, Valle D (eds): The Metabolic and Molecular Bases of Inherited Disease. New York, McGraw Hill, 2001, pp 3323–3367.

CHAPTER

19

Gaucher Disease

Roscoe O. Brady

Raphael Schiffmann

Gaucher disease is the most prevalent hereditary metabolic storage disorder of humans. Patients have been classified into three phenotypes depending on whether the CNS is involved and the age of onset of clinical manifestations. The disorder is caused by insufficient activity of the sphingolipid hydrolase called *glucocerebrosidase,* resulting in accumulation of pathologic quantities of glucocerebroside throughout the body. Enzyme replacement therapy (ERT) provides spectacular benefit to patients with type 1 (non-neuronopathic) Gaucher disease, but it has not been convincingly beneficial regarding CNS involvement. Inhibition of glucocerebroside synthesis (substrate depletion) is being investigated for type 1 patients and for patients with chronic neuronopathic (type 3) Gaucher disease. Gene therapy has been undertaken in patients with type 1 Gaucher disease, but to date, no benefit has been demonstrated using this modality.

CLINICAL FEATURES AND DIAGNOSTIC EVALUATION

Patients with type 1 Gaucher disease, by far the most common phenotype, exhibit hepatosplenomegaly, anemia, thrombocytopenia, skeletal involvement, and to a lesser extent, pulmonary impairment. Signs of this form of Gaucher disease may become apparent as early as the first year, but initial manifestations can occur in childhood, middle years, or even late in life. The central nervous system (CNS) is not overtly affected, but rarely patients develop an atypical form of parkinsonism and dementia. Type 2 patients (with the rarest form of the disease) exhibit hepatosplenomegaly, developmental delay, bulbar signs, and strabismus early in infancy. They rarely live longer

than 4 years. Type 3 patients have varying systemic and neurologic manifestations that are usually apparent in childhood, early teen years, or adulthood. All neuronopathic patients have a predominantly horizontal supranuclear gaze palsy that can be the sole neurologic abnormality or can be associated with cognitive deficit. With ERT controlling the non-neurologic manifestations, most type 3 patients remain neurologically stable. Some patients deteriorate with a combination of seizures, myoclonus, and dementia. Brain stem deficit may progress with deteriorating eye movements to a complete gaze paralysis. Dysarthria, dysphagia, and respiratory abnormalities ensue, followed by death. Spasticity and hyperreflexia occur late, and we observed myoclonic dystonia in one patient. The progressive myoclonus seen in some patients is of the cortical type with a giant potential on the somatosensory-evoked potential (SEP). We found, however, that chronic neuronopathic patients without overt myoclonus have elevated cortical amplitude (P1-N2) on the SEP (Fig. 19–1). This amplitude inversely correlates with the patient's IQ, indicating that a deficit of cortical inhibition is a unifying feature of type 3 Gaucher disease.

The diagnosis of Gaucher disease is usually confirmed by assaying glucocerebrosidase activity in homogenates of leukocytes or cultured skin fibroblasts. The fluorogenic artificial substrate 4-methylumbelliferyl-β-D-glucoside is generally used for this assay. Most of the carriers of Gaucher disease can be identified with this test, but when the genotype is known, genotyping provides increased accuracy. Prenatal diagnosis is available through assays of glucocerebrosidase activity or genotyping using cultured amniocytes or chorionic villus biopsy specimens.

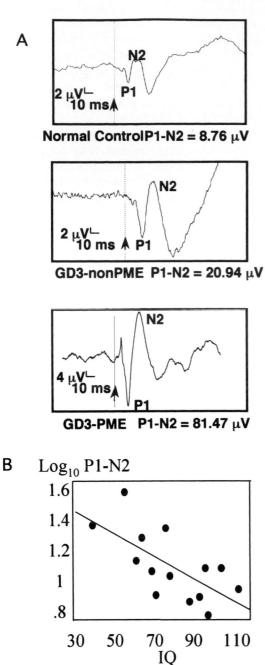

acoustic reflexes, poor medial olivocochlear suppression, and delayed or absent brain-stem–evoked potentials.

Systemic Pathology

The spleen contains enlarged histiocytes known as Gaucher cells that are engorged with lipid. The nucleus is displaced, and the cytoplasm has a crumpled tissue-paper appearance. The accumulating glucocerebroside occurs in a twisted tubular form under electron microscopy. The cells stain positively with the periodic acid-Schiff reagent for carbohydrate. Increased acid phosphatase activity is a prominent feature of Gaucher cells. They also show increased lysozyme activity and stain positively for iron. Kupffer cells are the principal storage elements in the liver. Gaucher cells are present to varying degrees in the bone marrow. In some patients, the entire bone marrow may become infiltrated with Gaucher cells, and extramedullary hematopoiesis becomes prominent. The cortices of the bones become demineralized, and there is extensive endosteal scalloping. Remodeling of the long bones is frequent and leads to flaring of the distal femoral metaphysis, which results in the so-called *Erlenmeyer flask* deformity. Fractures of the neck of the femur are common, and compression fractures of the vertebrae can produce progressive myelopathy. The lungs may contain Gaucher cells in alveolar capillaries and lymphatic vessels. Free Gaucher cells have been reported in the alveoli. These alterations occur most frequently in children who exhibit hypoxia, cyanosis, and clubbing. Gaucher cells are frequently found in lymph nodes, thymus, and pharyngeal tonsils, especially in type 2 and 3 phenotypes. There are Gaucher cells in Peyer's patches and other locations in the gastrointestinal tract. A significant percentage of children with Gaucher disease are delayed in growth and onset of menarche. Monoclonal and polyclonal gammopathies are not infrequent. Multiple myeloma, leukemia, Hodgkin's disease, cerebral astrocytoma, and bronchogenic carcinoma have been reported in association with Gaucher disease. Serum acid phosphatase, angiotensin-converting enzyme, lysozyme, and chitotrosidase are increased. Glucocerebroside is elevated in the blood, as much as 10-fold over normal.

FIGURE 19–1. *A,* Stretch-evoked somatosensory-evoked potentials (SEP) from *(top to bottom)* a 9-year-old healthy boy; a 4-year-old boy with type 3 Gaucher disease without progressive myoclonus epilepsy (GD3-nonPME); and a 33-year-old woman with type 3 Gaucher disease with PME (GD3-PME). Arrow on each panel indicates time of sensory stimulus (tap). *B,* Scatter plot showing linear regression of log10 P1-N2 SEP with IQ in all GD3-nonPME patients. Open circles represent individual patients. Regression equation: $Y = 1.65 - 0.007 \times X$; $r^2 = 0.455$; $p = 0.0082$.

Radiologic and Neurophysiologic Studies

MRI of the brain is often normal with cerebral atrophy seen in advanced cases of progressive myoclonic encephalopathy. Acoustic pathway studies show bilaterally raised

CNS Pathology

Closely packed Gaucher cells appear perivascularly in the Virchow-Robin spaces, even in type 1 brains. Perivascular gliosis is often observed. Neuronal storage material is very hard to find in neuronopathic Gaucher brains. Type 2 and 3 brains, and to a lesser extent type 1 brains, have in common selective regions of astrogliotic injury in the hippocampal CA4-2 region, cortical lamina 3 and 5, and calcarine layer 4b. In type 2 brains, typical lipid-laden macrophages (Gaucher cells) infiltrate these gliotic regions with evidence of extensive neuronophagia. Similar neuronophagocytic changes are seen patients with myoclonic epilepsy.

Biochemical Findings

Glucocerebroside is comprised of three components. The first is the long-chain amino alcohol sphingosine. The second is a long-chain fatty acid linked by an amide bond to the nitrogen atom on carbon atom 2 of sphingosine. The combination of sphingosine and fatty acid is called ceramide. In glucocerebroside, a single molecule of glucose is linked by a β-glycosidic bond to carbon 1 of the sphingosine moiety of ceramide. Glucocerebroside in systemic organs usually arises from the catabolism of larger sphingolipids such as globoside (ceramide-glucose-galactose-galactose-N-acetylgalactosamine) in red blood cells or ceramidelactoside (ceramide-glucose-galactose) from leukocytes. Glucocerebroside in neurons is thought to arise from the turnover of acidic glycolipids called gangliosides—for example, ceramide-glucose-galactose-(N-acetylneuraminic acid)-N-acetylgalactosamine, the so-called Tay-Sachs ganglioside. In neuronopathic Gaucher patients, a related compound called glucopsychosine (sphingosine-glucose) is also elevated in the brain. Glucopsychosine is particularly toxic to neurons. The enzyme glucocerebrosidase catalyzes the hydrolytic cleavage of the molecule of glucose from glucocerebroside and glucopsychosine.[1] Its activity is reduced from normal in all types of Gaucher disease,[2] and it is especially low in type 2 patients.[3] The hydrolysis of glucopsychosine catalyzed by glucocerebrosidase occurs at approximately 0.5% the rate of glucocerebroside. The hydrolysis of glucocerebroside by glucocerebrosidase requires the presence of an activator protein called saposin C. A very small number of patients who exhibit some resemblance to Gaucher disease have been described in which saposin C is not produced. Glucocerebrosidase activity is also stimulated by phosphatidyl serine.

Immunochemical Findings

We have undertaken an examination of the immunoreactivity of the lipid-laden cells in the Virchow-Robin space in patients with types 2 and 3 Gaucher disease. This investigation should resolve the origin of these cells.

Molecular-Genetic Data

The gene for glucocerebrosidase is located on human chromosome 1 at q21. More than 210 mutations in the glucocerebrosidase gene have been described. One of the most frequently encountered DNA base changes causes the substitution of serine for asparagine (Arg → Ser) at amino acid 370 of glucocerebrosidase. Patients with this mutation have considerable residual glucocerebrosidase activity. In fact, having this mutation on either allele typically prevents patients from having a neuronopathic form of Gaucher disease. Other common mutations are an Arg → His substitution at amino acid 496 and an Arg → Cys substitution at amino acid 463. Both are attended by mild phenotypes. A very common mutation is the Leu → Pro substitution at amino acid 444. This alteration is a frequent cause of neuronopathic Gaucher disease. Another frequent mutation is caused by an insertion of a molecule of guanine at nucleotide 84 in the glucocerebrosidase cDNA. This change results in a frameshift, and an allele with this mutation does not produce glucocerebrosidase protein. A severe phenotype is associated with this mutation. Another mutation that causes a severe phenotype is caused by a splice donor site mutation resulting in skipping of exon 2 in messenger RNA. Two additional mutations that result in a severe phenotypic effect are Val → Leu at amino acid 394 and Asp → His at amino acid 409.

Animal Models

Attempts have been made to produce glucocerebrosidase knockout mouse models of Gaucher disease. Mice with total ablation of glucocerebrosidase activity die in utero or within a few hours after birth. The cause of death was shown to be loss of water from the skin. This phenotype resembles neonatal Gaucher disease associated with hydrops fetalis. Neonates with this form of Gaucher disease die shortly after birth, and they have extremely low glucocerebrosidase activity. Attempts are underway to "knock-in" milder mutations in the murine glucocerebrosidase gene with the expectation that a less drastic phenotype with longer survival will be produced.

Therapy

Because macrophages in systemic organs arise from stem cells in the bone marrow, a number of Gaucher patients have received bone marrow transplantation. If the transplantation is successful, patients with type 1 Gaucher disease may be permanently cured. In chronic neuronopathic Gaucher disease, bone marrow transplantation cures the systemic disease but does not appreciably modify the CNS manifestations. Transplant rejection, graft-versus-host disease, and other untoward effects make this approach unattractive.

Enzyme Replacement Therapy

Intravenous administration of glucocerebrosidase purified from human placental tissue or produced recombinantly has been remarkably effective clinically. Virtually all of the systemic difficulties associated with this disorder respond satisfactorily. The effect of enzyme replacement therapt (ERT) on CNS manifestations has been less impressive,[4] although evidence for a decrease in the number of perivascular Gaucher cells has been found. This result was anticipated since the enzyme cannot cross the intact blood-brain barrier.

However, this therapy has dramatically altered the natural history of neuronopathic forms of Gaucher disease since patients no longer succumb to hematologic, hepatic, and pulmonary complications. Attempts have been made to deliver glucocerebrosidase to infants with type 2 Gaucher disease intrathecally, intracisternally, and intraventricularly. However, no benefit on the brain involvement could be documented. A number of attempts were made to temporarily alter the blood-brain barrier in experimental animals including primates. However, the penetration of enzymes into the brain under these circumstances has been so low that no clinical trials have been undertaken using this strategy.

Conclusion and Future Research Direction

The mechanism by which glucocerebrosidase deficiency causes neuronal dysfunction and death is not known. Glucocerebroside accumulation causes changes in calcium mobilization in a neuronal model of Gaucher disease, which results in neuronal dysfunction, hypersensitivity to neurotoxic agents (such as neurotoxic levels of glutamate), and altered patterns of phospholipid metabolism. Further study of the mechanism of disease will likely yield better therapeutic approaches, especially the use of small molecules that cross the blood-brain barrier.

Evidence has recently been obtained that intracerebral administration of human glucocerebrosidase using convection-enhanced delivery in experimental animals may be a feasible approach to ERT for patients with neuronopathic Gaucher disease.[5] The procedure was well-tolerated in rats. Glucocerebrosidase was taken up by neurons, the cells that are particularly susceptible to damage in patients with neuronopathic forms of Gaucher disease. Based on these results and additional safety trials to be undertaken in nonhuman primates, it is anticipated that phase 1 trials using this technique will be undertaken in patients with type 2 Gaucher disease and type 3A Gaucher disease with intractable myoclonic seizures. If the results indicate the feasibility of this approach, appropriate clinical efficacy trials can be expected.

Substrate Depletion

Treatment of patients with type 1 Gaucher disease by partial inhibition of enzymatic synthesis of glucocerebroside (using N-butyldeoxynojirimycin to inhibit transfer of glucose from UDP-glucose to ceramide) has recently been investigated. Some indication of clinical benefit has been reported.[6] We believe that its effect on CNS manifestations in patients with type 3 Gaucher disease merits investigation, and a phase 1/2 trial is under way.

Gene Therapy

Based on the findings in bone marrow transplantation trials, transduction of bone marrow stem and progenitor cells with retroviral vectors carrying the cDNA for human glucocerebrosidase were undertaken. A phase 1 gene therapy trial was carried out in two non–bone marrow–ablated patients with type 1 Gaucher disease.[7] In the first patient, there was no indication of expression of the transgene. Expression was demonstrated for a few months in the second recipient, but there was no discernible clinical effect. More efficient transduction methods need to be developed. Procedures for selecting transduced cells need to be developed, and enriched transduced cells should be administered to the patient. Consideration should be given to conditioning recipients so that engraftment will be more efficient. Experiments should be undertaken to increase the delivery of transduced cells to the bone marrow.

Gene therapy for patients with neuronopathic Gaucher disease must be carefully considered. Recent investigations of intracerebral injections with lentivirus and adeno-associated virus-based vectors into murine analogs of metachromatic leukodystrophy[8] and type VII mucopolysaccharidosis[9] indicate that the phenotypic abnormalities in these mice can be reversed. Transfer of gene products between central nervous system neurons using a recombinant lentivirus vector has recently been demonstrated.[10] These results bode well for eventual gene therapy for patients with neuronopathic Gaucher disease.

REFERENCES

1. Brady RO, Kanfer J, Shapiro D: The metabolism of glucocerebrosides. I. Purification and properties of a glucocerebroside-cleaving enzyme from spleen tissue. J Biol Chem 1965;240:39–42.

2. Brady RO, Kanfer JN, Shapiro D: The metabolism of glucocerebrosides. II. Evidence of an enzymatic deficiency in Gaucher's disease. Biochem Biophys Res Commun 1965;18:221–225.

3. Brady RO, Kanfer JN, Bradley RM, Shapiro D: Demonstration of a deficiency of glucocerebroside-cleaving enzyme in Gaucher's disease. J Clin Invest 1966;45:1112–1115.

4. Altarescu G, Hill S, Wiggs E, et al: The efficacy of enzyme replacement therapy in patients with chronic neuronopathic Gaucher's disease. J Pediatr 2001;138: 539–547.

5. Zirzow GC, Sanchez OA, Murray GJ, et al: Delivery, distribution and neuronal uptake of exogenous mannose-terminal glucocerebrosidase in the intact rat brain. Neurochemical Res 1999;24:301–305.

6. Cox T, Lachmann R, Hollak C, et al: Novel oral treatment of Gaucher's disease with N-butyldeoxynojirimycin (OGT 918) to decrease substrate biosynthesis. Lancet 2000;355:1481–1485.

7. Dunbar CE, Kohn DB, Schiffmann R, et al: Retroviral transfer of the glucocerebrosidase gene into CD34+ cells from patients with Gaucher disease: In vivo detection of transduced cells without myeloablation. Hum Gen Ther 1998;9: 2629–2640.

8. Consiglio A, Qattrini A, Martino S, et al: In vivo gene therapy for metachromatic leukodystrophy by lentiviral vectors: Correction of neuropathology and protection against learning impairments in affected mice. Nat Med 2001;7:310–316.

9. Frisella WA, O'Connor LH, Vogler CA, et al: Intracranial injection of recombinant adeno-associated virus improves cognitive function in a murine model of mucopolysaccharidosis Type VII. Mol Ther 2001;3: 351–358.

10. Lai A, Brady RO: Gene transfer into the central nervous system in vivo using a recombinant lentivirus vector. J Neurosci Res 2002;67:363–371.

The Niemann-Pick Diseases

Roscoe O. Brady

Raphael Schiffmann

Two distinct metabolic derangements are encompassed under the eponym Niemann-Pick disease (NPD). In the first group, excessive quantities of sphingomyelin accumulate in many organs and tissues. Patients with this abnormality are classified as having types A and B Niemann-Pick disease. Type A patients exhibit hepatosplenomegaly and profound central nervous system involvement. They rarely survive beyond the second year. Type B patients have hepatosplenomegaly and pathologic alterations of their lungs, but there are no signs of central nervous system involvement. Type B patients frequently live into their fourth decade. Both Types A and B Niemann-Pick disease are caused by a profound deficiency of the enzyme sphingomyelinase.[1] Patients in the second category are designated as having types C and D NPD. Patients may have mild hepatosplenomegaly, but the CNS is profoundly affected. Impaired intracellular trafficking of cholesterol causes both types C and D NPD.[2] Type D NPD is a genetic isolate originating from a common Nova Scotia ancestry. Therefore, in this chapter, both Types C and D NPD will be referred to as Type C NPD.

CLINICAL FEATURES AND DIAGNOSTIC EVALUATION

Type A NPD patients exhibit profound organomegaly within the first three months of life. A cherry-red spot is present in the macula in 50% of these infants. Developmental milestones are rarely attained, and psychomotor deterioration progresses rapidly. Patients become hypotonic and flaccid and rarely survive beyond the second year. Type B patients have no overt signs of CNS involvement, but hepatomegaly may be profound and accompanied by signs of liver failure. Serum lipids are often elevated. Type B patients usually exhibit moderate splenomegaly. The lungs are frequently involved, and pulmonary function is often compromised. There is often a reddish-brown halo surrounding the macula in the eyes of these patients. Because insufficient sphingomyelinase activity is the hallmark of Types A and B NPD, measurement of the activity of this enzyme in convenient cells such as circulating leukocytes or cultured skin fibroblasts is the standard confirmatory diagnostic procedure.[3]

Type C NPD is usually suspected in patients with vertical gaze impairment (Fig. 20–1), dysarthria, dementia, ataxia, dystonia, and mild hepatosplenomegaly. Some of these patients also have cataplexy and seizures. The diagnosis is usually confirmed by demonstrating an elevation of free cholesterol in cultured skin fibroblasts by staining with filipin and determination of the rate of cellular cholesterol esterification in these cells.[4]

RADIOLOGIC AND NEUROPHYSIOLOGIC STUDIES

Magnetic resonance imaging (MRI) of the brain in patients with types A and C NPD may be normal or reveal cerebral or cerebellar atrophy, sometimes with white matter hyperintensity on T2-weighted imaging. In patients with Type C NPD, magnetic resonance spectroscopic imaging reveals a reduction in the N-acetyl aspartate/creatine ratio indicating diffuse brain involvement consistent with the pathologic features of the disease. Brain stem auditory-evoked potentials are often delayed with absence of acoustic reflexes.

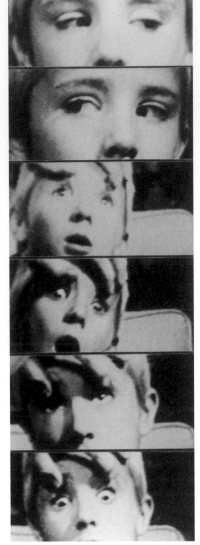

Left Gaze

Right Gaze

Saccadic
Up Gaze

Saccadic
Down Gaze

Pursuit
Up Gaze

Pursuit
Down Gaze

FIGURE 20–1. Vertical supranuclear gaze paresis in a patient with type C Niemann-Pick disease. (From Brady RO, Filling-Katz MR, Barton NW, et al: Niemann-Pick disease types C and D. Neurol Clin 1998;7:75.)

PATHOLOGY

Types A and B Niemann-Pick Disease

Large, lipid-laden cells are present in the liver, spleen, lymph nodes, adrenal cortex, and bone marrow. The cells have a mulberry appearance because of an accumulation of lipid droplets. They are autofluorescent and stain for phospholipids. Some cells are pigmented because of the presence of ceroid. The cells contain concentrically lamellated myelin-like figures. The brain of Niemann-Pick type A patients is usually atrophic. Ganglion cells are often swollen, and the cytoplasm is pale and vacuolated. Within these cells are membrane-bound inclusions. There is a loss of cells in the cerebral and cerebellar cortices along with gliosis in both gray and white matter. Some areas of the white matter show demyelination. Foam cells

are present in the leptomeninges, tela choroidea, endothelium, and perivascular spaces of cerebral blood vessels. The basal ganglia, brain stem, spinal cord, and autonomic ganglia may also show morphologic alterations. Little is known about structural changes in the brains of patients with type B Niemann-Pick disease.

Type C Niemann-Pick Disease

The spleen is infiltrated with foam cells that stain for cholesterol, phospholipid, and glycolipids. Kupffer cells and, to a lesser extent, hepatocytes in the liver are involved. In the infantile presentation, extensive hepatic vacuolization is seen along with cholestasis and giant cell formation. Foam cells are almost always present in the bone marrow. These cells have been termed sea-blue histiocytes. The cerebral cortex is atrophic, and ballooned neurons exhibit inclusions. The basal ganglia, thalamus, and brain stem are particularly involved. Cellular atrophy and lipid storage occurs in Purkinje cells and cells in the dentate nucleus of the cerebellum.

BIOCHEMICAL FINDINGS

The principal accumulating lipid in patients with types A and B Niemann-Pick disease is sphingomyelin (ceramide-phosphocholine). Sphingomyelin is a major component of the plasma membrane of all cells, and it is a principal phospholipid of the myelin sheath. In addition to sphingomyelin, elevated levels of bis(monoacylglycero) phosphate are prominent. Cholesterol, glucocerebroside, lactosylceramide, and gangliosides, particularly ganglioside GM_3, are elevated as well, but not so much as in type C Niemann-Pick disease. The cholesterol that accumulates in Type C NPD arises primarily from extracellular cholesterol associated with low-density lipoprotein. The enzymatic defect in Types A and B NPD is a lack of a sphingomyelinase isozyme called acid sphingomyelinase because its highest catalytic activity occurs at reduced pH. It catalyzes the hydrolytic cleavage of sphingomyelin-producing phosphocholine and ceramide (N-fatty acylsphingosine).

There are two protein abnormalities in Type C NPD. The most common (95%) is an alteration of a protein called NPC1, a glycoprotein with 13 transmembrane domains.[5] It has a high degree of homology with other proteins involved in intracellular cholesterol homeostasis. The second protein that is mutated in NPD Type C (NPC2) is a lysosomal protein called HEI whose function has not been identified.[6] It is frequently associated with severe clinical manifestations. NPC2 patients often die of respiratory failure due to extensive pulmonary involvement.

IMMUNOCHEMICAL FINDINGS

In Type C NPD, neurofibrillary tangles appear in neurons in the orbital gyrus, cingulate gyrus, entorhinal region, basal ganglia, thalamus, hypothalamus, inferior olivary nucleus, and spinal cord. The tangles stain with Alz 50, an antibody that reacts with phosphorylated tau proteins. Amyloid deposition has not been reported.

MECHANISM OF DISEASE

NPC1 and HE1 appear to be required for the vesicular shuttling of both lipids and fluid-phase constituents from multivesicular late endosomes to destinations such as the trans-Golgi network. However, the exact function and the mode of action of these proteins are unknown.

MOLECULAR GENETIC DATA

The gene that is mutated in Types A and B NPD is located on human chromosome 11 at p15.1 to p15.4. To date, less than 20 mutations have been identified in these patients.[7] Most of the mutations occur in exons 2 and 6. Similar to Tay-Sachs and Gaucher disease, there is a prevalence of Type A NPD among Ashkenazi Jews. Three common mutations have been described in this population. The first is a change of arginine to leucine (Arg → Leu) at amino acid 496. The second is Leu → Pro at amino acid 302, and the third is caused by a deletion resulting in a frameshift that causes a premature stop codon at amino acid 330. All patients with Type B NPD have considerable residual sphingomyelinase activity that is presumed to be sufficient to prevent CNS manifestations of the disorder.

The NPC1 gene is located on human chromosome 18. A variety of alterations have been described in Type C NPD patients including deletions, insertions, and missense mutations.[4] Several mutations in HE1 in NPC2 patients have recently been identified.[8]

ANIMAL MODELS

Canine and feline models of NPD Type A have been described, but no colonies are presently available. Knockout mice with some of the features of both types A and B NPD have been created by targeted disruption of the sphingomyelinase gene.[7] A spontaneously occurring murine analog of NPC1 provided much basic information concerning the nature of the metabolic abnormality in this condition.[9] In addition, feline and canine models of this disorder have been described.

THERAPY

Liver transplantation has been performed in several patients with Type B NPD.[10] Bone marrow transplantation caused some reduction of organomegaly and radiologic improvement of the lungs in Type B patients.[7] Similar investigations were performed in the knockout murine analog of this disorder as well as the spontaneous murine analog of Type C NPD.[11] Minimal benefit occurred with regard to CNS manifestations. Because the CNS is not involved in Type B NPD, enzyme replacement therapy is expected to be helpful in patients with this phenotype, but not in Type A NPD. This deduction is supported by studies with the sphingomyelinase knockout mouse.[12]

CONCLUSION

The heterogeneity of clinical phenotypes of NPD requires diagnostic sophistication. NPD is suspected in infants or children who present with hepatosplenomegaly and lipid-storing cells in the bone marrow. The CNS may (Type A NPD) or may not (Type B NPD) be involved. The diagnosis of these phenotypes is easily established by measuring sphingomyelinase activity in peripheral blood leukocytes or cultured skin fibroblasts. Type C NPD is suspected if a patient exhibits mild hepatosplenomegaly, "sea-blue" histiocytes in the bone marrow, and vertical gaze palsy (see Fig. 20–1) with or without other signs of CNS damage. The diagnosis of this condition can be confirmed by examining intracellular cholesterol esterification (vide supra). Future research directions involve elucidation of specific functions of the products of the NPC1 and the HE1 genes that are mutated in patients with Type C NPD and the development of specific therapies for patients with all forms of NPD.

REFERENCES

1. Brady RO, Kanfer JN, Mock MB, Fredrickson DS: The metabolism of sphingomyelin. II. Evidence of an enzymatic deficiency in Niemann-Pick disease. Proc Natl Acad Sci U S A 1966;55:366–369.

2. Pentchev PG, Comly ME, Kruth HS, et al: A defect in cholesterol esterification in Niemann-Pick disease (type C) patients. Proc Natl Acad Sci U S A 1985;82:8247–8251.

3. Gal AE, Brady RO, Hibbert SR, Pentchev PG: A practical chromogenic procedure for the detection of homozygotes and heterozygous carriers of Niemann-Pick disease. N Engl J Med 1975;293:632–636.

4. Patterson MC, Vanier MT, Suzuki K, et al: Niemann-Pick disease Type C: A lipid trafficking disorder. In Scriver CR, Beaudet AL, Sly WS, et al (eds): The Metabolic and Molecular Bases of Inherited Disease. New York, McGraw-Hill, 2001, pp 3611–3633.

5. Carstea ED, Morris JA, Coleman KG, et al: Niemann-Pick C1 disease gene: Homology to mediators of cholesterol homeostasis. Science 1997;277:228–232.

6. Naureckiene S, Sleat DE, Lackland H, et al: Identification of HE1 as the second gene of Niemann-Pick C disease. Science 2000;290:2298–2301.

7. Schuchman EH, Desnick RJ: Niemann-Pick disease Types A and B: Acid sphingomyelinase deficiency. In Scriver CR, Beaudet AL, Sly WS, et al (eds): The Metabolic and Molecular Bases of Inherited Disease. New York, McGraw-Hill, 2001, pp 3589–3610.

8. Millat G, Chikh K, Naureckiene S, et al: Niemann-Pick disease type C: Spectrum of HE1 mutations and genotype/phenotype correlations in the NPC2 group. Am J Hum Genet 2001;69:1013–1021.

9. Pentchev PG, Boothe A, Kruth H, et al: A genetic storage disorder in BALB/C mice with a metabolic block in the esterification of exogenous cholesterol. J Biol Chem 1984;259:5784–5791.

10. Smanik EJ, Tavill AS, Jacobs GH, et al: Orthotopic liver transplantation in two adults with Niemann-Pick's and Gaucher's disease—implications for the treatment of inherited metabolic disease. Hepatology 1993;17:42–49.

11. Boothe AD, Weintroub H, Pentchev PG, et al: A lysosomal storage disorder in the BALB/c mouse: Bone marrow transplantation. Vet Pathol 1984;21:432–441.

12. Miranda SR, He X, Simonaro CM, et al: Infusion of recombinant human acid sphingomyelinase into Niemann-Pick disease mice leads to visceral, but not neurological correction of the pathophysiology. FASEB J 2000;14:1988–1995.

CHAPTER 21

The G$_{M2}$-Gangliosidoses

Edwin H. Kolodny

Orit Neudorfer

In the 1880s, Tay[1] and Sachs[2] independently described a familial disorder characterized by progressive muscular weakness, mental deficiency, blindness, and death in infancy.[3] A half century later, Klenk[4] reported the storage of a lipid that he termed *ganglioside* because of its location within the ganglion cells of the nervous system. Okada and O'Brien[5] demonstrated the basis for this accumulation to be a deficiency of the lysosomal enzyme, β-N-acetyl-hexosaminidase A (Hex A). Thus, Tay-Sachs disease fulfilled the concept of an inborn lysosomal disease as defined by Hers.

Infantile, juvenile, and adult-onset forms of G$_{M2}$-gangliosidosis exist (Table 21–1). The infant with classic Tay-Sachs disease develops psychomotor retardation, blindness, seizures, and macrocephaly, with death occurring within a few years. Juvenile-onset cases have a more protracted course with blindness, increasing spasticity and rigidity, seizures and dementia, progressing to a vegetative state in 5 to 15 years. Others, with the late-onset variant, develop signs of cerebellar and anterior horn cell involvement, proximal muscle weakness and atrophy, dysmetria, ataxia, and tremor. Some also have psychiatric symptoms. Within neurons of all forms of G$_{M2}$-gangliosidosis can be found electron dense membranous cytoplasmic bodies.

Hex A consists of both α- and β-subunits.[6] Defects in the gene coding for the α-subunit are the most common cause of G$_{M2}$-gangliosidosis. Patients with the rare B$_1$ variant are able to degrade the artificial substrate 4-methylumbelliferone β-D-N-acetylglucosamine (4-MUG) but not its sulfated derivative, 4-MUGS. Mutations in the gene for the β-subunit result in deficiency of two hexosaminidases, Hex A and Hex B (the latter consisting entirely of β-subunits), and produce a condition known as Sandhoff disease. In addition to G$_{M2}$-ganglioside, tissues of patients with Sandhoff disease also store hexosamine-containing neutral glycolipids. Deficiency in the G$_{M2}$-activator protein results in the AB variant of G$_{M2}$-gangliosidosis.

G$_{M2}$-gangliosidosis is pan-ethnic, but until carrier screening and prenatal diagnosis became widely available, Tay-Sachs disease was most prevalent among Ashkenazi Jews. Three mutations in the α-chain gene account for nearly all the carriers in this population. In total, more than 100 α-chain mutations have been found, most associated with the classic infantile disease. Sandhoff disease is much rarer, with 30 known α-chain mutations of which a 16-kb deletion is the most common. Studies of the extremely rare AB variant revealed five mutations in the G$_{M2}$-activator protein gene, associated in each case with the classic infantile variant of the disease. No definitive treatment yet exists.

CLINICAL FEATURES

G$_{M2}$-gangliosidosis has been found in all age groups and follows an autosomal recessive pattern of inheritance. Generally, the later the onset, the slower the progression. Although in most instances genotype determines phenotype, differences in clinical expression may occur even among affected individuals within the same family.

Tay-Sachs Disease. The child may startle easily in the newborn period, appear listless and hypotonic, and fail to follow objects visually. Parents usually become concerned when the child is 3 to 6 months old, and loss of previously gained milestones is beginning to be noticed. The funduscopic examination shows a cherry-red macula,

TABLE 21–1. Clinical Variants of G_{M2}-Gangliosidoses

Variant	Ethnic Predilections	Enzyme Deficiency	Defective Protein	Gene Involved
Tay-Sachs disease	Ashkenazi Jewish French-Canadian	Hex A	α-subunit	HEXA
B$_1$ variant	Portuguese	Hex A (sulfated substrate only)	α-subunit	HEXA
Late-onset Tay-Sachs	Ashkenazi Jewish	Hex A	α-subunit	HEXA
Sandhoff disease		Hex A and B	β-subunit	HEXB
AB variant		GM2-ganglioside hydrolysis	G_{M2}-activator	GM2A

resulting from lipid deposition in the bipolar ganglion cells of the retina, causing a whitish halo that surrounds the fovea (Fig. 21–1). After age 1 year, the child becomes progressively more lethargic and immobile, and does not speak or reach for objects. There is an increase in muscle tone and deep tendon reflexes, and the plantar reflexes become extensor. Midway through the second year, spontaneous, symmetrical, small-amplitude myoclonic jerks may develop. Frank seizures occur with facial muscle twitching, tonic deviation of the eyes, and tonic-clonic movements of the extremities. Sound, light, or touch stimuli easily precipitate decerebrate posturing.

The electroencephalogram initially demonstrates high voltage slowing. With the development of seizures, multifocal spikes appear with progression to a more diffuse slow wave and then low voltage pattern. The computed tomography (CT) scan performed at age 11 to 14 months reveals low density signals in the basal ganglia and cerebral white matter and high signal intensity on T2 weighted magnetic resonance imaging (MRI). In a later phase, after age 2 years, the whole brain becomes atrophic with a diminution in white matter, mild to moderate ventricular dilation, and widening of the subarachnoid spaces.[7]

By age 2 years, the child is weaker, with poor gag and cough reflexes, and excessive drooling. Feeding is more difficult and there is severe constipation. The child is in a vegetative state, cortically blind, and requires constant nursing care. Autonomic disturbances are now frequent, with unexplained temperature elevations and spells of rubor, pallor, cyanosis, and irregular breathing. Progressive cachexia, dehydration, and aspiration pneumonia lead to death, usually by age 4 or 5 years.

B$_1$ Variant. The clinical presentation of this phenotype fits a juvenile-onset pattern but is more variable. In Portuguese B$_1$ variant patients, who are homozygous for the DN allele, gait or speech disturbances develop between ages 3 and 7 years.[8] All experience progressive mental deterioration with loss of speech and walking ability within a few years. Their life expectancy ranges from 11 to 22 years.

Other B$_1$ variant patients with earlier onset have also been described, with cherry-red spot, exaggerated startle response, and seizures or tremors.[9] These patients most likely represent compound heterozygotes with one B$_1$ allele and a second allele that codes for the classic form of G_{M2}-gangliosidosis. A form of the B$_1$ variant with survival into the third and fourth decades has also been described.

Late-Onset G_{M2}-Gangliosidosis. Most patients with this disorder are of Ashkenazi Jewish ancestry. They may be mistakenly classified as having Kugelberg-Welander disease, amyotrophic lateral sclerosis, spinal muscular atrophy, atypical motor neuron disease, spinocerebellar degeneration, or Friedreich ataxia.[10] The presentation is usually in childhood. Early development is normal, but the child is considered clumsy and unathletic. Many develop a dysarthric nasal speech that does not improve with speech therapy. Academic performance in grade school is usually satisfactory, although a few are labeled as *learning disabled*. They may also have difficulty relating to their peers.

During adolescence, proximal muscle weakness develops, there is difficulty climbing stairs, and fasciculations and muscle cramps occur. In the early 20s, walking becomes slightly broad-based and ataxic with high steppage. Weakness and ataxia lead to frequent falls. In about one half of patients psychiatric symptoms develop, including anxiety and depression. Episodes of frank psychosis can develop, with hallucinations, paranoid and suicidal ideation, looseness of associations, and withdrawal.[11] The optic fundi are normal, and vision is not impaired, but saccadic pursuit of the eyes is coarse. Swallowing difficulty may occur. The neck, forearm, and hand muscles are generally strong until late in the disease. There is a fine tremor of the outstretched arms, dysmetria, and ataxia. Atrophy of the shoulder and leg muscles is noticeable, and the patient cannot tandem walk. The knee jerk reflex is hyperactive, often with a crossed adductor response. Late in the illness, the plantar reflexes become extensor, and vibration sensation is diminished in the lower legs.

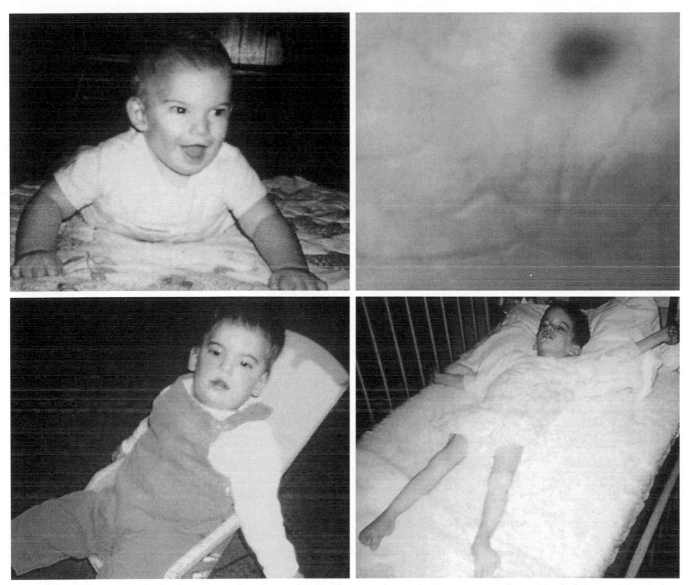

FIGURE 21–1. Classic Tay-Sachs disease. *A*, Age 3 months. *B*, Cherry-red macula (note surrounding white halo), age 15 months. *C*, Age 27 months. *D*, Age 41 months.

In patients age 50 years and older, swelling of the legs, with cool skin temperature and purplish discoloration, develops. A pattern of denervation atrophy is found on electromyography examination, but sensory nerve conduction is normal. Prominent cerebellar atrophy, particularly of the vermis, is seen by the early 20s in brain CT and MRI.[12] Patients may continue to ambulate independently, often with the help of walking aids, well into their fifth or sixth decade. Urinary urgency and frequency develop. Fertility is preserved in both men and women, and many have children. Most patients have a normal intellect or show only mild cognitive decline, but a few have been reported with progressive dementia.[13]

Progressive generalized dystonia may be encountered in the course of G$_{M2}$ gangliosidosis, usually associated with other extrapyramidal signs, decline in mental capacity, and muscle wasting.

Sandhoff Disease.   The late-infantile form is clinically similar to classic Tay-Sachs disease. Occasionally, the liver and spleen are slightly enlarged, and in a few patients, foam cells have been detected in the bone marrow. Juvenile Sandhoff disease begins after age 1 year, with clumsiness and unsteady gait. Seizures, tremors, and dystonic posturing may occur. There is no cherry-red spot in the macula. The late-onset form follows much the same clinical course as late-onset Tay-Sachs. Diarrhea and signs of autonomic dysfunction have also been described. A severe sensory loss can also occur in older patients, with painful neuropathy and dysesthesia.

AB Variant.   The few reported clinical cases of AB variant suggest close similarities to classic Tay-Sachs disease.[14]

DIAGNOSTIC EVALUATION

Serum and leukocyte assays employing the fluorogenic substrate 4-MUG detect most patients with G_{M2}-gangliosidosis. If the clinical picture is suggestive but the enzyme profile is normal, the sulfated 4-MUGS substrate should be used. Hydrolysis of 4-MUGS will be deficient in the B_1 variant. Diagnosis of the rare patient who has the AB variant may be suspected on the basis of a skin biopsy showing lamellated bodies in axons of the dermal nerves. In these instances, a G_{M2}-ganglioside loading test should be done.[15]

Carrier Screening and Prenatal Diagnosis. Since the introduction of Tay-Sachs carrier testing in 1970, the incidence of Tay-Sachs disease in the Jewish population has decreased by more than 90%. The Dor Yeshorim program, designed specifically for the Orthodox Jewish community, has gained acceptance within this community by preserving the anonymity of the tested individuals.

Population screening for carriers is customarily performed with the fluorogenic substrate 4-MUG. This means of testing does not identify carriers of the AB or B_1 variants or differentiate a disease-causing allele from a pseudodeficiency allele of *HEXA*. Therefore, the testing laboratory may elect to examine further those carriers identified by enzyme determinations for the pseudodeficiency mutation using DNA technologies. This approach is especially relevant to the non-Jewish population in whom more than one third of carriers identified by enzyme testing carry an allele for pseudodeficiency. In the case of carrier-carrier couples, knowledge of the specific mutations they carry is especially important, not only to rule out the possibility of a pseudodeficiency mutation, but also to provide for better specificity in the prenatal diagnosis of G_{M2}-gangliosidosis. By December 2000, more than 3200 pregnancies at risk have been monitored and the birth of more than 600 infants with Tay-Sachs disease has been prevented.[16]

In this era of genome-related discovery, although many new opportunities for genetic disease diagnosis are evident, some economic, social, ethical, and practical issues regarding screening arise. The Tay-Sachs screening program serves as a prototype for population-based screening.

PATHOLOGY

The brain of the Tay-Sachs child who survives beyond the third or fourth year shows cortical atrophy and loss of central white matter. In children younger than age 3 years, however, there is a 20% to 50% increase in brain weight greater than normal. Throughout the neuraxis, ballooned neurons are encountered with fine granular or vesicular cytoplasm that stains in frozen sections with periodic acid–Schiff (PAS) and Luxol fast blue. The nucleus is displaced, and the Nissl substance is reduced in amount. In the cerebellum, antler-like expansions occur at the bifurcation of Purkinje cell dendrites. Older patients show more neuronal loss with marked reduction in cerebellar Purkinje and granule cells. There is a loss of white matter accompanied by an intense gliosis with proliferation of protoplasmic astrocytes and microglia. Similar changes are also seen in the spinal cord, and the ganglion cells in the autonomic ganglia.

Golgi impregnation techniques and electron microscopic studies show the presence of torpedo-shaped swellings between the base of the perikaryon and the initial axonal segment. These *meganeurites* contain spine-like processes that are believed to form aberrant synapses that are possibly responsible for the neuronal hyperexcitability observed in late infantile G_{M2}-gangliosidosis. Within the nerve cells and their proximal axonal segment are numerous concentrically arranged electron dense lamellar structures known as membranous cytoplasmic bodies (MCBs). These have been detected in both myelinated and unmyelinated nerves of skin biopsy specimens, in astrocytes and in cultured skin fibroblasts.

The appearance of the brain in Sandhoff disease is similar to that in Tay-Sachs disease, with the exception of yellowing of the cerebral cortex and deeper structures. The MCBs are more pleomorphic, however, and zebra bodies are also encountered. Simultaneous damage of gray matter, in addition to white matter, is apparent in Sandhoff disease. There is widespread lipid storage within the viscera involving especially the kidneys and pancreas, without frank visceromegaly. Endocardial fibrosis is also found in Sandhoff disease. The inclusions in G_{M2}-activator deficiency are more pleomorphic and are prominent in glial cells as well as neurons.

BIOCHEMICAL AND MOLECULAR GENETICS

Storage Products. G_{M2}, the major accumulating material, is found almost exclusively in the central nervous system, where it is highly concentrated in neuronal plasma membranes. The hydrophobic ceramide portion of the molecule anchors it to the membrane, whereas the hydrophilic segment, an oligosaccharide, serves as a surface marker. Several other glycosphingolipids are found in lesser amounts in the G_{M2}-gangliosidoses. The structure of each of these compounds is shown in Table 21–2.

G_{A2}, the asialo derivative of G_{M2}, is also elevated in the G_{M2}-gangliosidoses, significantly more in Sandhoff disease and in G_{M2}-activator protein deficiency than in Tay-Sachs disease. The smaller accumulation in Tay-Sachs disease is due to an active Hex B, which in the presence of the G_{M2}-activator protein has a small but significant action toward G_{A2}. Generalized absence of hexosaminidase activity in patients with Sandhoff disease explains the presence of various N-acetylglucosaminyl oligosaccharides in their urine and visceral organs.

TABLE 21–2. Major Accumulating Glycolipids in G$_{M2}$ 1-1 Gangliosidoses

Compound	Structure
GM2	GalNAc($\beta1\to$ 4) [NeuAc($\alpha2\to$ 3)] Gal($\beta1\to$ 4)GLC($\beta1\to$ 1′)Cer
GA2	GalNAc($\beta1\to$ 4)Gal($\beta1\to$ 4)Glu($\beta1\to$ 1′)Cer
LysoGM2	GalNAc($\beta1\to$ 4)[NeuAc($\alpha2\to$ 3)]Gal($\beta1\to$ 4)Glu($\beta1\to$ 1′)Sph
LysoGA2	GalNAc($\beta1\to$ 4)Gal($\beta1\to$ 4)Glu($\beta1\to$ 1′)Sph
Globoside	GalNAc($\beta1\to$ 3)Gal($\alpha1\to$ 4)Gal($\beta1\to$ 4)Glu($\beta1\to$ 1′)Cer

Cer = ceramide; Gal = galactose; Glc = glucose; GalNAc = *N*-acetylgalactosamine; NeuNAc = *N*-acetyl-neuraminic acid; Sph = sphingosine.

Hexosaminidases A and B. Hex A is composed of one α-subunit and one β-subunit, whereas Hex B is composed of two slightly different β-subunits, β_a and β_b. Both the α-polypeptide and the β-polypeptide have active sites capable of hydrolyzing terminal β-linked *N*-acetyl-hexosamines, but neither is active in the monomeric form.[17] Dimerization to hexosaminidase A (αβ) or hexosaminidase B (ββ) is necessary for either subunit to function as a catalytically active enzyme. Both Hex A and Hex B are active toward neutral oligosaccharides, glycolipids, and glycoproteins, but only Hex A can hydrolyze negatively charged substrates such as G$_{M2}$-ganglioside (in concert with the G$_{M2}$-activator protein), β-linked glucosamine-6-sulfate containing glycosaminoglycans and 6-sulfated artificial substrates.

The gene for the α-subunit, known as *HEXA*, is 35-kb long and maps to chromosome 15q23–24. The β-subunit gene, *HEXB*, is 45-kb in length and maps to chromosome 5q11.2–13.3. Although they are encoded on separate chromosomes, the two genes have striking structural similarities. Both subunits are synthesized on the rough endoplasmic reticulum (ER) and transported into the lumen, where the *N*-terminal signal peptide is cleaved. At this point, they are *N*-glycosylated and disulfide bonds are formed. Subsequently, in the Golgi apparatus, the mannose-6-phosphate (M-6-P) recognition marker is attached. After dimerization and folding, the nascent protein containing the phosphomannosyl recognition marker binds to a receptor in the trans-Golgi from which it is transported in a protein-receptor complex by coated vesicles into the lysosome. Within the lysosome, the pro-Hex A and pro-Hex B molecules undergo further hydrolytic and glycolytic processing including removal of the M-6-P tag.

G$_{M2}$-Activator. This small 21–23-kd transport protein is a heat-stable glycosylated monomer of 162 amino acids that is probably processed and delivered to the lysosome in the same manner as Hex A and Hex B. It acts to overcome the steric hindrance by adjacent lipid molecules that interfere with access of Hex A to membrane-bound G$_{M2}$. *GM2A*, the gene encoding this protein, maps to chromo-

some 5q32–33, whereas a processed pseudogene has been localized to chromosome 3.

MUTATIONS

Up-to-date information about allelic variation at the *HEXA*, *HEXB*, and *GM2A* gene loci can be obtained at the G$_{M2}$-gangliosidoses database.[18]

HEXA Mutations. G$_{M2}$-gangliosidosis due to Hex A deficiency results from mutations in the α-subunit gene, *HEXA*. At least 100 alterations in its nucleotide sequence are now known, of which 85 are disease-causing mutations, mostly of the severe infantile type. Approximately 40% of mutations occur at CpG dinucleotides, which are considered mutational "hot spots." Disease expression correlates most closely with the biochemically less severe of the two alleles.

In French-Canadian patients of Quebec province, a 7.6-kb deletion in the 5′ end of the gene accounts for approximately 80% of the mutant Tay-Sachs alleles. The three mutations that are most prevalent in Ashkenazi Jews are a 4-bp insertion in exon 11, a G C transversion at the 5′ splice site of intron 12, and a point mutation at the 3′ end of exon 7 that causes serine to substitute for glycine at codon 269. A benign tryptophan for arginine substitution at codon 247, causing pseudodeficiency, is the most common alteration in the *HEXA* gene of non-Jewish enzyme-defined Tay-Sachs disease carriers, accounting for 32% to 42% of the total. The most common disease-causing mutation among non-Jews is a splice site mutation (G A) in the first nucleotide of intron 9 (+1 IVS-9). It results in a 17-bp insertion with activation of a cryptic donor site in the intron. It is seen in diverse populations but is especially frequent among subjects from the British Isles. This mutation and the C$_{739}$ T pseudodeficiency allele represent approximately one half of all the mutations present in non-Jews. The remainders are heterogeneous.

The Arg$_{178}$His mutation in exon 5 accounts for some cases of the B$_1$ variant form of G$_{M2}$-gangliosidosis with loss in the ability of Hex A to hydrolyze the sulfated synthetic substrate 4-MUGS and G_{M2}-ganglioside while retaining catalytic activity toward the unsulfated, electronically neutral substrate 4-MUG.

HEXB Mutations. Mutations in the *HEXB* gene cause deficiency of both Hex A and Hex B activity. Approximately 50% of patients with Sandhoff disease have a 16-kb deletion in one or both *HEXB* alleles that spans the promoter, exons 1–5, and part of intron 5. No transcription or translation occurs and the homozygote has the severe infantile form of Sandhoff disease. This mutation is found especially in French and French-Canadian patients.

GM2A Mutations. Of the five mutations recorded in the *GM2A* gene, three involve a single substitution and the other two are deletions.

ANIMAL MODELS

Naturally occurring G_{M2}-gangliosidosis has been detected in dogs, cats, Muntjac deer and Yorkshire swine. Mouse models of Tay-Sachs and Sandhoff diseases have also been created using murine *Hexa* and *Hexb*. The two genes are smaller than their human counterparts, but their cDNAs have 75% and 84% sequence homology to human *HEXA* and *HEXB*, respectively. Disruption in the *Hexa* gene results in biochemical and neuropathologic features of Tay-Sachs disease, but no clinical signs of disease. Disrupting the mouse Hexb gene in embryonic stem cells produces a dramatically different neurologic phenotype. The mice develop a fatal neurodegenerative disease, with spasticity, muscle weakness, rigidity, tremor, and ataxia. The difference in the clinical expression in these two models is due to the presence in the mouse of a sialidase that transforms G_{M2} to G_{A2} much more actively than in the human. The G_{A2} produced can then be further degraded by the Hex B activity of the Hex A-deficient Tay-Sachs mouse.

THERAPY

The only treatment currently available is symptomatic, and is aimed at maintaining function and quality of life for the affected child. To maintain adequate calorie-intake and positive fluid balance and prevent aspiration, a feeding tube may become necessary. Anticonvulsants used include diazepam, phenobarbital, or lamotrigine. Frequent turning, physical therapy, and chest therapy are helpful to minimize the tendency to contractures and infections. A bedside suction machine and positioning of the child can assist in preventing airway obstruction.

For the young adult with a later-onset form of G_{M2}-gangliosidosis, we recommend a regular regimen of physical exercise, speech therapy for patients who are dysarthric, and a mobility aid if there is a tendency to fall.

We protect the knees with pads and if the legs swell, elastic stockings are worn.

For behavioral or psychiatric symptoms, the major neuroleptic drugs should be avoided, as they are likely to worsen the basic disease and can lead to life-threatening complications, such as neuroleptic malignant syndrome.[19] An acute psychosis may be managed with a combination of lithium salts and lorazepam. Longer-term management of an affective disorder can be achieved with carbamazepine, valproic acid, lorazepam, or a combination of these medications, and depressive symptomatology can be managed with serotonin-reuptake inhibitors. Refractory cases may benefit from electro-convulsive therapy (ECT).

Several voluntary lay organizations provide parent and peer group support through telephone networks, educational programs, and regional and national conferences. These include the National Tay-Sachs and Allied Diseases Association and the Late-Onset Tay-Sachs Disease Foundation.

FUTURE THERAPIES

Potential strategies to remove the stored lipid include enzyme replacement therapy, bone marrow transplantation, neural stem cell therapy, gene therapy, and substrate deprivation. The blood-brain barrier (BBB) hinders transfer of enzyme to the CNS, whereas bone marrow transplantation (BMT) can theoretically transcend the BBB. However, trials of BMT have only slowed, but not halted, the progression of classic Tay-Sachs disease.[20]

Another potential source, neural stem cells, have shown efficacy in vitro but have not been tried in vivo.[21] Promising results have been obtained in a mouse model using gene therapy with transduced cells showing biochemical correction.[22] However, safety of this approach and targeting to the CNS are two of several aspects requiring further study.[23]

An alternative approach, substrate deprivation, has shown efficacy in the Sandhoff mouse.[24] It uses an iminosugar, *N*-butyldeoxynojirimycin, to inhibit the glucosyltransferase involved in the initial step in glycolipid synthesis. As a small molecule with CNS penetration that can be taken orally, its therapeutic potential rests with the ability of residual Hex A to remove the previously stored lipid.

CONCLUSIONS

Clinical variation in the G_{M2}-gangliosidoses can be correlated with the amount of residual enzyme activity present, which is, in turn, a function of the mutations that occur in each of three genes *HEXA*, *HEXB*, and *GM2A*. Predilection of classic Tay-Sachs disease for the Ashkenazi Jewish population has led to widespread carrier testing and prevention through prenatal diagnosis in couples found to be at risk for offspring with this autosomal recessive neurodegeneration. Medications used to treat adults with psychiatric manifestations must be carefully selected to avoid compromising the residual enzyme activity. The development of animal models now permits new therapeutic options to be explored, brightening prospects for future enzyme replacement and substrate synthesis inhibition.

REFERENCES

1. Tay W: Symmetrical changes in the region of the yellow spot in each eye of an infant. Trans Ophthalmol Soc UK 1981;1:55.

2. Sachs B: On arrested cerebral development with special reference to its cortical pathology. J Nerv Ment Dis 1987;14:541.

3. Evans PR: Tay-Sachs disease: A centenary. Arch Dis Child 1987;62:1056.

4. Klenk E: On gangliosides. Am J Dis Child 1959;711.

5. Okada S, O'Brien J: Tay-Sachs disease: Generalized absence of a beta-D-N-acetyl hexosaminidase element. Science 1969;165:698.

6. Desnick RJ, Kaback MM (eds): Tay-Sachs Disease. New York, Academic Press, 2001.

7. Yoshikawa H, Yamada K, Sakuragawa N: MRI in the early stage of Tay-Sachs disease. Neuroradiology 1992;34:394.

8. Maia MC, Alves D, Ribeiro MG, et al: Juvenile GM2-gangliosidoses variant B$_1$: Clinical and biochemical study in seven patients. Neuropediatrics 1990;21:18.

9. Gordon BA, Gordon KF, Hinton GG, et al: Tay-Sachs disease: B1 variant. Pediatr Neurol 1988;4:54.

10. Navon R, Argov Z, Frisch A: Hexosaminidase A deficiency in adults. Am J Hum Genet 1986;24:179.

11. MacQueen GM, Rosebush PI, Mazurek MF: Neuropsychiatric aspects of the adult variant of Tay-Sachs disease. J Neuropsychiatry Clin Neurosci 1998;10:10.

12. Streifler JY, Gornish M, Hadar H, et al: Brain imaging in late-onset G$_{M2}$ gangliosidosis. Neurology 1993;43:2055.

13. O'Neill B, Butler AB, Young E, et al: Adult-onset G$_{M2}$ gangliosidosis, seizures, dementia, and normal pressure hydrocephalus associated with glycolipid storage in the brain and arachnoid granulations. Neurology 1978;28:1117.

14. Hechtman P, Gordon BA, Ng Ying Kin NMK: Deficiency of the hexosaminidase A activator protein in a case of G$_{M2}$ gangliosidosis: Variant AB. Pediatr Res 1982;16:217.

15. Raghavan S, Krusell A, Lyerla TA, et al: G$_{M2}$-ganglioside metabolism in cultured human skin fibroblasts: Unambiguous diagnosis of G$_{M2}$-gangliosidosis. Biochim Biophys Acta 1985;834:238.

16. Kaback MM: Population-based genetic screening for reproductive counseling: The Tay-Sachs disease model. Eur J Pediatr 2000;159:S192.

17. Sonderfeld-Fresko S, Proia RL: Synthesis and assembly of a catalytically active lysosomal enzyme, β-hexosaminidase B, in a cell-free system. J Biol Chem 1988;263:13463.

18. Cordeiro P, Hechtman P, Kaplan F: The GM2 gangliosidoses databases: Allelic variation at the HEXA, HEXB, and GM2A gene loci. Genet Med 200;2:319.

19. Manor I, Hermesh H, Munitz H, Weizman A: Neuroleptic malignant syndrome with gangliosidosis type II. Biol Psychiatry 1997;41:1222.

20. Norflus F, Tifft CJ, McDonald MP, et al: Bone marrow transplantation prolongs life span and ameliorates neurologic manifestations in Sandhoff disease mice. J Clin Invest 1998;101:1881.

21. Flax JD, Aurora S, Yang C, et al: Engraftable human neural stem cells respond to developmental cues, replace neurons, and express foreign genes. Nat Biotechnol 1998;16:1033.

22. Teixeira CA, Sena-Esteves M, Lopes L, et al: Retrovirus-mediated transfer and expression of beta-hexosaminidase alpha-chain cDNA in human fibroblasts from G(M2)-gangliosidosis B1 variant. Hum Gene Ther 2001;12:1771.

23. Martino S, Emiliani C, Tancini B, et al: Absence of metabolic cross-correction in Tay-Sachs cells: Implications for gene therapy. J Biol Chem 2002;277:20177.

24. Jeyakumar M, Butters TD, Cortina-Borja M, et al: Delayed symptom onset and increased life expectancy in Sandhoff disease mice treated with N-butyldeoxynojirimycin. Proc Natl Acad Sci U S A 1999;96:6388.

CHAPTER 22

Metachromatic Leukodystrophy and Multiple Sulfatase Deficiency: Sulfatide Lipidosis

Edwin H. Kolodny, Orit Neudorfer

The sulfatide lipidoses are a group of inherited diseases affecting brain myelin metabolism. Onset may occur in childhood or adulthood, with mental regression, gait imbalance, and progressive spastic tetraparesis. Cerebroside sulfate accumulates as a result of a block in its catabolism owing to a deficiency of the lysosomal enzyme sulfatidase, or, in a few rare instances, a deficiency of cofactor saposin B (Sap-B), also required for substrate hydrolysis. There are two distinct clinical forms, metachromatic leukodystrophy (MLD) owing to arylsulfatase A deficiency, and multiple sulfatase deficiency in which at least seven different sulfatases are defective owing to an abnormality in their processing and functional maturation. The cloning of the genes for sulfatidase and Sap-B has led to the elucidation of mutations responsible for the various forms of MLD and a better understanding of the mechanisms that produce clinical heterogeneity in this class of genetic leukodystrophies.

CLINICAL FEATURES

MLD is an autosomal recessive disorder with an estimated frequency of 1:40,000. Table 22–1 lists six clinical variants. The majority of patients are equally divided between the late-infantile and juvenile forms of MLD. About 20% of patients have an onset in adolescence or later. Other variants are quite rare.

Late Infantile Metachromatic Leukodystrophy

Clinical signs usually appear between ages 15 months and 2 years, although a few children may show earlier developmental delay. Children with MLD begin to fall frequently. Then they lose the ability to walk and develop a flaccid weakness and peripheral neuropathy. Between ages 2 and 3 years, the child loses the ability to sit without support and exhibits truncal titubation. Speech is slow and less distinct, optic atrophy becomes apparent, and deep tendon reflexes are diminished and then lost. The arms remain hypotonic, but muscle tone increases in the legs. There is exquisite sensitivity to touch owing to spinal root and peripheral nerve involvement. Eventually the child becomes quadriplegic and spastic, with decerebrate, decorticate, or dystonic posturing. Loss of speech, seizures, hypertonic fits, bulbar palsy, and blindness characterize the late stage of this form of MLD. Death occurs 1 to 7 years after onset of symptoms.

Juvenile Metachromatic Leukodystrophy

Onset occurs between ages 4 and 12 years, with decline in school performance and disturbance in gait. The child becomes confused and unable to follow directions, speech becomes slurred, and postural abnormalities develop. Muscle tone increases, the ability to walk is lost, and flexion of the arms, scissoring of the legs, and equinovarus deformity of the feet occur (Fig. 22–1). Tremor, tonic spasms, and seizures may also occur. Eventually, the child becomes blind; however, hearing is retained, and even in a late stage of the illness, the child reacts appropriately to familiar voices. Peripheral neuropathy is common but not invariable. Recurrent seizures are common and may be observed at any stage of the disease, and in rare cases may even be the presenting symptom.[1] Seizures are usually of the complex partial type, whereas most patients with late-infantile form tend to have generalized seizures.[2] In the

TABLE 22–1. Classification of the Sulfatide Lipidoses

Type	Age at Onset (years)
Late infantile	1–2
Early juvenile	4–6
Late juvenile	6–12
Adult	>16
Multiple sulfatase deficiency	<1
Cerebroside sulfate sulfatase activator deficiency	<1–20s

early-onset juvenile form, which begins to manifest between ages 4 and 6 years, gait imbalance precedes the intellectual deterioration. In the later-onset variant, first noticed between ages 6 and 10 years, cognitive, behavioral, and social difficulties precede the gait disturbance. Most patients with juvenile MLD do not live into adulthood.

Adult Metachromatic Leukodystrophy

The widespread use of MRI and enzymatic assays in psychiatrically disturbed adolescents and adults has improved recognition of this variant.[3] Adult MLD begins insidiously in late adolescence or early adult life. School or work performance deteriorates, thinking becomes disorganized, memory is poor, and speech becomes cluttered and pressured. Bizarre behavior and paranoia may suggest schizophrenia-like psychosis. These patients may also present with depression or alcoholism. The patient seems bewildered, distracted, euphoric, or apathetic and is unable to care for himself or herself. The clinical picture may resemble psychosis[4] or dementia.[5]

The gait becomes wide-based and ataxic, muscle tone increases, and deep tendon reflexes are hyperactive. Incontinence can develop relatively early, and optic atrophy occurs; however, vision and the patient's contact with his or her surroundings are preserved until the end stage of the disease. Spastic tetraparesis, decorticate posturing, and pathologic reflexes are noted after 5 to 10 years, but survival for several decades is possible.

Multiple Sulfatase Deficiency

Development in a child with multiple sulfatase deficiency (MSD) is less advanced than that in a child with late-infantile MLD. Walking is delayed, and in the second

FIGURE 22–1. Metachromatic leukodystrophy, juvenile-onset variant. *A,* Age 3 years. *B,* Age 5½ years. Compare position of legs and feet of affected child *(right)* to normal sibling *(left)*. *C,* Age 6½ years. *D,* Age 8½ years (blind, aphonic, spastic quadriparesis, hearing retained).

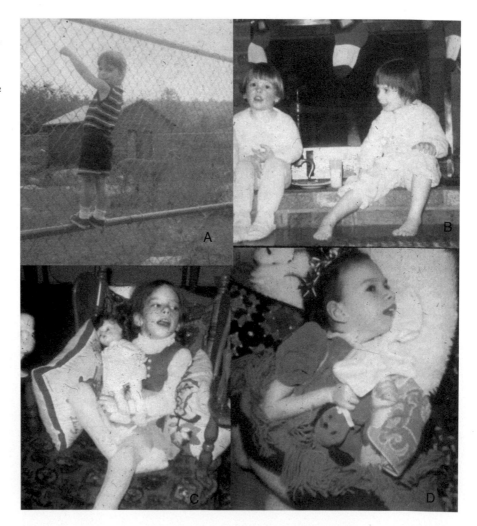

year, the child loses the ability to sit, stand, or speak. By the third year, staring spells, nystagmus, spasticity, and blindness occur. The facial features are coarsened, with a prominent forehead, midfacial hypoplasia, broad nose, upturned nares, and short neck. The liver is enlarged, and a characteristic ichthyotic rash, with dry and flaky skin, develops on the limbs, trunk, and scalp.[6] Skeletal abnormalities include rib flaring, rounding and beaking of the lumbar vertebrae, and deformities of the acetabulum. Feeding difficulty, frequent infections, and seizures are later complications. The MSD patient lives into the second decade bedridden and severely retarded.

Sulfatide Activator Protein Deficiency

Fewer than a dozen patients with this diagnosis have been described, with onset at various ages from birth to teenage years. The clinical course resembles the other MLD forms, according to the age of onset of symptoms.

LABORATORY AND IMAGING STUDIES

Cerebrospinal fluid protein level increases as the disease progresses in late-infantile and early-juvenile forms of MLD and may eventually exceed 100 mg/dL. Cerebrospinal fluid protein in later-onset juvenile and adult MLD may or may not be increased.

The electroencephalogram in patients with seizures discloses high-voltage slow waves and occasional irregular bursts of spikes, often with variable focal distribution. There is a good correlation between the severity of the EEG changes and the severity of the disease. Nerve conduction velocity (NCV) is reduced, most markedly in late-infantile MLD, initially noted to involve the afferent nerves; subsequently, motor conduction becomes more delayed than the sensory conduction. Both EEG and NCV abnormalities may be apparent in presymptomatic patients.[10] Brain stem auditory evoked response is also abnormal in late-infantile MLD, often before clinical symptoms appear, and may be abnormal in juvenile MLD but normal in adult MLD. Abnormalities of the visual and somatosensory evoked potentials have also been found in each form of MLD.

Neuroimaging studies can be especially helpful in the workup of patients with MLD. CT reveals abnormal low density in the cerebral white matter adjacent to the ventricles, progressive enlargement of the ventricles, and mild cerebral atrophy. An MRI T2-weighted image demonstrates confluent areas of high signal intensity in the periventricular white matter, suggesting more extensive involvement than that observed in CT scans. Early on, the arcuate fibers are preserved. There is preferential involvement of the subcortical white matter in the frontal regions, a fact that has been suggested[4] to explain the mental changes in MLD, especially in adolescent- and adult-onset cases. In late-infantile MLD, however, demyelination is more prominent in the occipital region.

T2-weighted images also reveal a bright signal in the corpus callosum, internal capsule, and corticospinal tract and a low-intensity signal for the basal ganglia and thalamus.[11] Radially oriented stripes of T2 prolongation, possibly representing areas of relative myelin sparing, are described as "tigroid" or "leopard skin." Although this pattern previously was considered to be pathognomonic of Pelizaeus-Merzbacher disease, it can also appear in MLD.[11]

Sulfatide deposits can also be found on the mucosal surface of the gallbladder and impair its function. Oral cholecystography, ultrasound, or radionuclide scanning of the gallbladder can demonstrate this defect. Polypoid filling defects can occur.

DIAGNOSTIC EVALUATION

Diagnosis of MLD is based on clinical symptoms and laboratory findings. Enzyme activity can be determined in peripheral blood leukocytes and cultured fibroblasts. The major problem in enzymatic diagnosis is the frequent occurrence of the pseudodeficiency (Pd) allele, which results in enzyme activity levels in the disease range without clinical disease. A useful diagnostic aid is the quantitative determination of urinary sulfatides. Sulfatide in the patient's urine is elevated by 10- to 100-fold. These sulfatides originate in the kidney, a major site for sulfatide storage in MLD. In contrast, urinary sulfatide levels in individuals with the Pd/Pd or Pd/MLD genotypes are normal or only slightly increased. Therefore, because of phenotypic heterogenicity, the overlap in biochemistry findings, and the PD allele, a combined approach is recommended for proper diagnosis, including determination of the enzyme activity, urine sulfatide levels, and screening for the mutations that lead to pseudodeficiency or disease. Attention to these requirements is necessary for carrier identification, and for prenatal diagnosis, the additional step of sulfatide loading of cultured amniocytes may be needed.[9]

PATHOLOGY

The principal findings in the central nervous system are a loss of myelin sheaths, reduced numbers of interfascicular oligodendroglia, and deposits of metachromatic granules. In areas of demyelination, the axis cylinders may be replaced by a reactive gliosis. Cavitation or spongy degeneration occurs in severely affected regions. There is sparing of nerve cells of the cerebral cortex, the subcortical U fibers, and the myelin sheaths in the central gray nuclei and optic radiation.

Metachromatic deposits are present in macrophages in perivascular spaces, in oligodendrocytes, and as free-lying bodies. They are spherical masses 15 mm to 20 mm in diameter that stain brown in frozen sections when exposed to a 1% solution of acidified cresyl violet. Under the electron microscope, these granules are arranged in characteristic shapes, primarily as prismatic and Tuffstone inclusions with a periodicity of 58 Å between lamellae.

The cerebellum is atrophic as a result of severe demyelination and accompanying gliosis, reduction in the number of Purkinje cells, and loss of axon terminals in the cerebellar granular and molecular layers. Demyelination also occurs in the brain stem and spinal cord. It is most pronounced in late-infantile MLD and less prominent in juvenile MLD. It does not occur in adult MLD.

Within the peripheral nervous system, MLD causes a reduction in the thickness of myelin sheaths and the loss of some myelinated fibers. Demyelination is segmental, with metachromatic granules present singly and in clusters between nerve fibers and in Schwann cells, endoneural macrophages, and Remak cells associated with unmyelinated nerve fibers. Metachromatic material is also deposited in the kidney, gallbladder, liver, pancreas, anterior pituitary, adrenal cortex, retina, sweat glands, testes, and rectal tissue.

BIOCHEMICAL FINDINGS

Lipid Alterations

The major accumulating lipid, sulfatide, is a sulfated glycosphingolipid consisting of equimolar amounts of sphingosine, fatty acid, galactose, and sulfate (Fig. 22–2). The sphingosine base consists primarily of C-18 sphingosine. The majority of the fatty acid is long-chain and contains the 2-hydroxy group. The sphingosine and fatty acid moieties are joined in an amide linkage forming the ceramide or lipid end of the molecule. The sulfate residue is attached to the galactose through an ester linkage at the C-3 position.

Sulfatide is the major sulfate-containing lipid in the nervous system. It accounts for 3.5% to 4% of the total lipids of myelin. In normal white matter, the galactocerebroside-to-sulfatide ratio is 3, but in late-infantile MLD this ratio is reduced to less than 1 owing to a 3- to 10-fold increase in sulfatide and a reduction in other myelin lipids. A marked increase in the concentration of lysosulfatide, the deacylated form of sulfatide, also occurs in MLD white matter, spinal cord, and kidney. Cytotoxicity of this compound is believed to contribute to the demyelination process in MLD.[12]

Arylsulfatase A and Saposin B

Degradation of sulfatide is catalyzed by the lysosomal enzyme arylsulfatase A (see Fig. 22–2). Arylsulfatase A (ASA) of normal human skin fibroblasts is synthesized as a precursor polypeptide of 62 kd that moves via mannose-6-phosphate receptor binding into a prelysosomal compartment, where it is cleaved to a 61.5-kd and 57-kd form before entering the lysosome. It contains three high-mannose N-linked oligosaccharide side-chains, the first and third of which are phosphorylated. It requires the heat-stable activator protein, Sap-B, to hydrolyze sulfatide in vivo. Sap-B is a 10-kd lysosomal glycoprotein of 80 amino acids containing one N-linked carbohydrate chain. It dimerizes and binds stoichiometrically with sulfatide to form a substrate complex on which the enzyme can act. Arylsulfatase A can hydrolyze several galactosyl-3-sulfates, including cerebroside sulfate, lactosyl sulfate, seminolipid, and lysosulfatide.

Classic Metachromatic Leukodystrophy

The tissues of patients with the classic forms of MLD are deficient in ASA activity. The amount of residual enzyme activity present directly correlates with the age of onset of the disease.

Multiple Sulfatase Deficiency

Patients with MSD also fail to degrade sulfatide. In this disease, however, a variety of sulfatases in addition to ASA are deficient (Table 22–2). This results in additional accumulation of mucopolysaccharides and steroid sulfates. The pathologic findings of MSD represent an overlap between a leukodystrophy and a mucopolysaccharidosis, and the pattern of enzyme deficiency in each patient is reflected in the relative contribution of each pathology to the whole clinicopathologic picture.[13]

Activator Protein Deficiency

Deficiency of the Sap-B activator protein can also cause MLD. In spite of ample ASA activity, cultured skin fibroblasts from patients with this form of MLD cannot degrade sulfatide in situ because of deficiency of the activator protein.

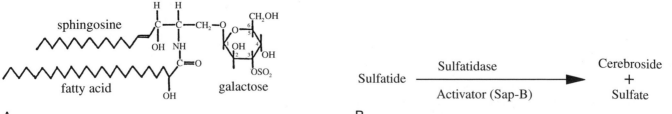

FIGURE 22–2. *A*, Chemical structure of cerebroside sulfate (sulfatide). *B*, Enzymatic hydrolysis of sulfatide.

TABLE 22–2. Human Arylsulfatases and Glycosaminoglycan Sulfatases

Enzyme	Natural Substrates	Deficiency States
Arylsulfatase A	Galactosyl sulfatide Lactosyl sulfatide Sulfogalactosylsphingosine Sulfogalactoglycerolipid Ascorbic acid-2-sulfate	Metachromatic leukodystrophy Multiple sulfatase deficiency
Arylsulfatase B (N-acetylgalactosamine- 4-sulfate sulfatase)	UDP-N-acetylgalactosamine-4-sulfate Dermatan sulfate Chondroitin-4-sulfate	Maroteaux-Lamy disease Multiple sulfatase deficiency
Arylsulfatase C	Dehydroepiandrosterone sulfate Pregnenolone sulfate Androstenediol-3-sulfate Estrone sulfate Cholesteryl sulfate	X-linked ichthyosis Multiple sulfatase deficiency
Iduronide-2-sulfate sulfatase	Dermatan sulfate Heparan sulfate	Hunter disease Multiple sulfatase deficiency
Heparan-N-sulfamidase	Heparan sulfate	Sanfilippo disease type A Multiple sulfatase deficiency
N-acetylgalactosamine-6-sulfate sulfatase	Keratan sulfate	Morquio disease type A Multiple sulfatase deficiency
N-acetylglucosamine-6-sulfate sulfatase	Chrondroitin-6-sulfate	Mucopolysaccharidosis VIII Multiple sulfatase deficiency

From Kolodny EH, Fluharty AL: Metachromatic leukodystrophy and multiple sulfatase deficiency: Sulfatide lipidosis. In Scriver CR, Beaudet AL, Sly WS, Valle D (eds): The Metabolic and Molecular Basis of Inherited Disease (7th ed). New York, McGraw-Hill, 1995, pp 2697.

Pseudodeficiency of Arylsulfatase A

Levels of ASA activity as low as 5% to 10% of control values without accumulation of sulfatide are frequently encountered in normal individuals and in some patients with neurologic or psychiatric symptoms.[3] Although these *pseudodeficient* individuals do not have MLD, as judged by normal levels of urine sulfatide and normal brain sulfatide concentration, some investigators have suggested that pseudodeficiency of ASA may predispose to other central nervous system diseases.[14] In a neuropsychological study of eight healthy family members of a child with MLD, each carrying a defective gene and five of whom also had a pseudodeficiency mutation, there was no tendency toward neuropsychological defects either in mutation carriers nor in those who also had a pseudodeficiency allele.[15]

MOLECULAR GENETICS

ARSA

The gene for ASA, *ARSA*, is located on human chromosome 22 distal to q13. It is 3.2 kb in length and contains 8 exons coding for 507 amino acids. Its amino acid sequence has substantial homology with another lysoso-

mal enzyme, arylsulfatase B (45%), and with steroid sulfatase, a nonlysosomal enzyme (35%).

Nearly 100 variations have been found in the human *ARSA* gene. The most common mutation in patients with late-infantile MLD is a G-to-A transition that eliminates the donor splice site at the start of intron 2.[16] This causes a loss of all enzyme activity, producing a severe early-onset form of the disease. In adults with MLD, the most frequent mutation is a C-to-T transition that results in substitution of a leucine for proline in amino acid 426 on exon 8.[16] Patients with this mutation have a small amount of residual enzyme activity and therefore exhibit a later-onset, more slowly progressive form of the disease. Compound heterozygosity for these two gene defects correlates with the juvenile (intermediate) form of MLD. Together, these two alleles account for approximately 50% of the mutations present in MLD patients from northern Europe. The remaining mutations are heterogeneous, most being confined to one family or only a few cases. In general, phenotypic characteristics of each mutation are inferred from their clinical expression in combination with other MLD mutations and from studies of site-directed mutagenesis. Variable onset of the disease in two siblings with the same genotype suggests that there may be other genetic or nongenetic factors, other than the genotype, that modifies the onset and course of the disease.[8]

Pseudodeficiency

The gene encoding ASA in individuals with pseudodeficiency usually contains two A-to-G transitions. One causes substitution of serine for asparagine at amino acid 350 and results in the loss of an N-glycosylation site. This change explains the reduced glycosylation and smaller size of ASA in fibroblasts of patients with pseudodeficiency. Loss of the N-glycosylation site, however, has no effect on the catalytic properties or stability of the enzyme. The other mutation changes the first polyadenylation signal downstream of the stop codon, causing a severe deficiency of the 2.1-kb mRNA species, the major mRNA for ASA expression. Loss of the N-glycosylation site may occur alone in about 3% of the population or together with the mutation in the polyadenylation site.[17] It is estimated that the combined effect of reduction in *ARSA* mRNA (due to the polyadenylation defect) and the lowering of ASA activity and aberrant targeting of the expressed N350S *ARSA* protein to the lysosome reduces the activity of the enzyme to 8% of normal in pseudodeficiency homozygotes. Estimates of the frequency of the Pd allele vary from 7% to 15% of the population.[17] Various laboratory procedures have been devised using the polymerase chain reaction to test for the presence of the Pd allele. Because of the high frequency of the Pd allele, it may coexist with a deleterious mutation causing MLD so the identification of the Pd allele does not necessarily rule out MLD. Therefore, molecular analysis of individuals with low levels of ASA activity needs to be supplemented with measurements of urine sulfatide excretion and sulfatide turnover in cultured cells.

Saposin B

Sap-B is one of four small, heat-stable glycoproteins (saposins) that stimulate the hydrolysis of sphingolipids. They are derived from proteolytic processing of a single 70-kd precursor protein, prosaposin. The gene for prosaposin has been mapped to chromosome 10. It is about 20 kb long and consists of approximately 13 exons, which encode a peptide of 524 amino acids. Sap-B is the second of the four prosaposins and is encoded by exons 5 to 7.

Seven mutations in Sap-B have been described, all associated with a clinical picture of infantile and juvenile forms of MLD.

ANIMAL MODEL

Because no naturally occurring animal model of metachromatic leukodystrophy is available, an ASA-deficient mouse was generated by means of targeted gene disruption, and is widely used in research. Clinically, young ASA-deficient mice show hyperactivity, and start developing neuromotor defects, with impaired coordination

and equilibrium, at the age of 6 to 12 months. Impaired learning and memory are apparent at age 12 months. Aged ASA-deficient mice show impaired performance, altered gait, ataxia, and tremor. In contrast to human MLD patients, their life span is normal.[19]

Mice with total SAP deficiency have also been generated. They show extensive neurovisceral storage, and do not survive beyond the age of 40 days. Neuronal storage is detected as early as postnatal day 1 and progressive neurologic symptoms are apparent by day 20. The pathologic ultrastructural features of the inclusions of accumulated lipid appeared unique and different from those seen in human cases of SAP deficiency and from other known sphingolipidoses.

THERAPY

Symptomatic treatment of leukodystrophy can help to maintain useful function and enable a child to participate meaningfully in activities at school and home. Supportive care for these patients includes maintenance of adequate nutrition, passive physical therapy, and drugs to reduce spasticity. For seizures, the use of nitrazepam or vigabatrin has been advocated. In addition to their antiepileptic action, they reduce muscle tone and should be considered as first choice antiepileptics in cases of MLD with marked spasticity.

Bone marrow transplantation (BMT) may be beneficial if the transplant is done before signs of nervous system involvement develop. Longitudinal neurologic, neuropsychologic, neurophysiologic, and neuroradiologic studies have demonstrated stabilization and even reversal of some signs in patients with the early and late juvenile forms of MLD.[20] Other reports describe further deterioration of the disease after transplantation, or a variable course resembling the natural history. A careful diagnostic evaluation is essential before deciding on transplantation to avoid the exposure of an individual with pseudodeficiency to the risk of an unnecessary procedure.

FUTURE THERAPY

The use of bone marrow transplantation to restore enzyme activity of the brain opens up the possibility that transduced autologous bone marrow cells may be used for gene correction in the CNS. Expression of enzyme activity after transduction of an adenovirus recombinant vector has been demonstrated in several cell types including oligodendrocytes and Schwann cells. In vivo trials with the ASA-deficient mouse using either transduced or stem cells or a recombinant lentiviral vector have also led to neuropathologic improvement.

CONCLUSION

The sulfatide lipidoses represent a family of autosomal recessive disorders characterized by partial or total inactivity of various sulfatases, causing demyelination in the central and peripheral nervous system. The clinical onset and severity show great variation, which correlates with the amount of residual activity of the enzyme. Diagnosis is based on clinical symptomatology, and the results of neuroimaging, enzyme activity testing, sulfatide urinary excretion, and mutation analysis. Overlap between normal and pathologic biochemical findings, and the presence of pseudodeficiency mutations complicate the diagnosis. There is no specific treatment for MLD or MSD. Bone marrow transplantation may be of benefit if performed early enough in the course of the disease. Stem cell and gene transfer experiments, using the mouse model developed for MLD, are in progress.

REFERENCES

1. Bostantjopoulou S, Katsarou Z, Michelakaki H, Kazis A: Seizures as a presenting feature of late onset metachromatic leukodystrophy. Acta Neurol Scand 2000;102:192.

2. Balslev T, Cortez MA, Blaser SI, Haslam RH: Recurrent seizures in metachromatic leukodystrophy. Pediatr Neurol 1997;17:150.

3. Hageman ATM, Gabreëls JM, de Jong GN, et al: Clinical symptoms of adult metachromatic leukodystrophy and arylsulfatase A pseudodeficiency. Arch Neurol 1995;52:408.

4. Hyde TM, Ziegler JC, Weinberger DR: Psychiatric disturbances in metachromatic leukodystrophy: Insights into the neurobiology of psychosis. Arch Neurol 1992;49:401.

5. Shapiro EG, Lockman LA, Knopman D, Krivit W: Characteristics of the dementia in late-onset metachromatic leukodystrophy. Neurology 1994;44:662.

6. Castano Suarez E, Segurado Rodriguez A, Guerra Tapia A, et al: Ichthyosis: The skin manifestation of multiple sulfatase deficiency. Pediatr Dermatol 1997;14:369.

7. Lu-ning W, Ke-wei H, Dong-gang W, Ze Yan L: Adult metachromatic leukodystrophy without deficiency of arylsulphatase. Chin Med J 1990;103:846.

8. Arbour LT, Silver K, Hechtman P, et al: Variable onset of metachromatic leukodystrophy in a Vietnamese family. Pediatr Neurol 2000;23:173.

9. Tylki-Szymanska AT, Czartoryska B, Lugowska A: Practical suggestions in diagnosing metachromatic leukodystrophy in probands and in testing family members. Eur Neurol 1998;40:67.

10. Philippart M, Nuwer MR, Packwood J: Presymptomatic adult-onset metachromatic leukodystrophy (MLD): Electrophysiological and clinical correlations. Neurology 1990;40:128.

11. Kim TS, Kim IO, Kim WS, et al: MR of childhood metachromatic leukodystrophy. AJNR Am J Neuroradiol 1997;18:733.

12. Toda K-I, Kobayashi T, Goto I, et al: Lysosulfatide (sulfogalactosylsphingosine) accumulation in tissues from patients with metachromatic leukodystrophy. J Neurochem 1990;55:1585.

13. Macaulay RJ, Lowry NJ, Casey RE: Pathologic findings of multiple sulfatase deficiency reflect the pattern of enzyme deficiencies. Pediatr Neurol 1998;19:372.

14. Hohenschutz C, Eich P, Friedl W, et al: Pseudodeficiency of arylsulfatase A: A common genetic polymorphism with possible disease implications. Hum Genet 1989;82:45.

15. Weber Byars AM, McKellop JM, Gyato K, et al: Metachromatic leukodystrophy and nonverbal learning disability: Neuropsychological and neuroradiological findings in heterozygous carriers. Neuropsychol Dev Cogn Sect C Child Neuropsychol 2001;7:54.

16. Polten A, Fluharty AL, Fluharty CB, et al: Molecular basis of different forms of metachromatic leukodystrophy. N Engl J Med 1991;324:18.

17. Nelson PV, Carey WF, Morris CP: Population frequency of the arylsulphatase A pseudo-deficiency allele. Hum Genet 1991;87:87.

18. Lullmann-Rauch R, Matzner U, Franken S, et al: Lysosomal sulfoglycolipid storage in the kidneys of mice deficient for arylsulfatase A (ASA) and of double-knockout mice deficient for ASA and galactosylceramide synthase. Histochem Cell Biol 2001;116:161.

19. Gieselmann V, Matzner U, Hess B, et al: Metachromatic leukodystrophy: Molecular genetics and an animal model. J Inherit Metab Dis 1998;21:564.

20. Krivit W, Aubourg P, Shapiro E, Peters C: Bone marrow transplantation for globoid cell leukodystrophy, adrenoleukodystrophy, metachromatic leukodystrophy, and Hurler syndrome. Curr Opin Hematol 1999;6:377.

21. Matzner U, Harzer K, Learish RD, et al: Long-term expression and transfer of arylsulfatase A into brain of arylsulfatase A-deficient mice transplanted with bone marrow expressing the arylsulfatase A cDNA from a retroviral vector. Gene Ther 2000;7:1250.

22. Matzner U, Hartmann D, Lullmann-Rauch R, et al: Bone marrow stem cell-based gene transfer in a mouse model for metachromatic leukodystrophy: Effects on visceral and nervous system disease manifestations. Gene Ther 2002;9:53.

23. Matzner U, Schestag F, Hartmann D, et al: Bone marrow stem cell gene therapy of arylsulfatase A-deficient mice, using an arylsulfatase A mutant that is hypersecreted from retrovirally transduced donor-type cells. Hum Gene Ther 2001;12:1021.

24. Consiglio A, Quattrini A, Martino S, et al: In vivo gene therapy of metachromatic leukodystrophy by lentiviral vectors: Correction of neuropathology and protection against learning impairments in affected mice. Nat Med 2001;7:310.

Krabbe Disease: Globoid Cell Leukodystrophy

David A. Wenger

Krabbe disease, or globoid cell leukodystrophy (GLD), is an autosomal recessive disorder affecting central and peripheral nervous system white matter. The initial descriptions of infants with *diffuse brain-sclerosis* or *diffuse gliosis* clearly describe patients we now recognize as having Krabbe disease.[1] In 1916, Krabbe[1] described five patients who had onset of symptoms at about 5 months of age. Symptoms included rigidity of musculature, violent tonic spasms, nystagmus, periodic elevations in temperature, progressive paresis, and early death. He noted the destruction of white matter in the cerebellum and degeneration of spinal nerve tracts with replacement by dense fibrillar glia. In 1924, Collier and Greenfield[2] used the term *globoid* to describe these abnormal scavenger cells, which are characteristic for this disorder. Excellent clinical and genetic studies on 32 Swedish patients by Hagberg et al[3] provide the basis for the clinical delineation of the infantile form of this disorder.

Early research suggested that these cells might contain a cerebroside similar to that stored in Gaucher disease. Chemical analysis and production of globoid cells by intracerebral injection of galactosylceramide into brains of experimental animals confirmed this.[4] In 1970 Malone[5] and Suzuki and Suzuki[6] reported that tissue samples from patients with Krabbe disease could not degrade galactosylceramide. The pathway for the formation of galactosylceramide from sulfatide and its degradation to ceramide and galactose is shown in Figure 23–1. The measurement of GALC activity in leukocytes, fibroblasts, and fetal-derived cells results in the accurate identification of patients prenatally and postnatally. Although modifications have been made in this basic method, it remains essentially unchanged today. Treatment is limited to HSCT in presymptomatic individuals and newborns.

The purification of GALC from human or animal tissues was very difficult due to its low abundance, extreme hydrophobicity, and tendency to aggregate into a high molecular weight complex. In 1993 GALC was first purified from human urine and brain.[7] This provided amino acid sequence information that was used to clone the human cDNA[8] and eventually the gene.[9] Many disease-causing mutations have been identified in human patients and the animal models.[10, 11]

Several animal models of globoid cell leukodystrophy are available.[12,13] They are useful to examine the chemical pathogenesis of this enzyme deficiency and to explore methods for effective therapy. In addition to bone marrow transplant, the mouse model has been used for some gene therapy trials as well as neural stem cell transplant. In general, these procedures have not been particularly successful. Although it has been over 30 years since the enzymatic defect was described, much more needs to be done before effective therapy for a majority of the patients is a reality.

CLINICAL PICTURE AND DIAGNOSTIC EVALUATION

Hagberg et al[3] described three stages in the progression of the most common infantile form of the disease. Stage I is characterized by general irritability, stiffness of limbs, arrest of mental and motor development, and episodes of temperature elevation without infection. During the stage II phase, patients are opisthotonic and have myoclonic-like jerks of the arms and legs, hypertonic fits, continued bouts of fever, and regression of any achieved abilities. By stage III, patients are severely decerebrate with no voluntary movements. They are hypotonic and cachectic, and they die of respiratory infections or

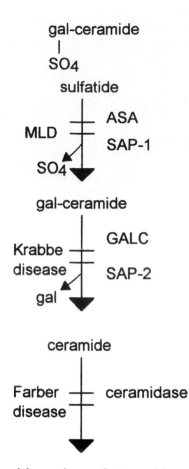

FIGURE 23–1. Pathway for the complete lysosomal degradation of sulfatide showing the required enzymes and sphingolipid activator proteins (saposins). Disorders resulting from defects in this pathway, including metachromatic leukodystrophy (MLD), Krabbe disease, and Farber disease, are noted.

cerebral hyperpyrexia. In Hagberg's study, the average age of onset was 4 months, and the average age at death was 13 months. We have diagnosed more than 400 patients with Krabbe disease since 1973, and 85% to 90% of them present before 6 months of age. Most die before 15 months of age. An increasing number of late infantile, juvenile, and adult cases are diagnosed in this laboratory, and this may partially reflect the liberal screening policy permitting all samples to be tested for GALC activity. The reader is referred to a number of papers that describe the clinical and molecular findings in late-onset patients.[14–18] Presenting symptoms in these patients can include vision problems, cerebellar ataxia, spastic hemiparesis, burning paresthesia, peripheral neuropathy, and dementia. While some individuals remain stable for long periods of time, others show a steady decline in intellect and develop seizures, severe dysarthria, and blindness leading to a vegetative state and death.

Initial studies in undiagnosed patients usually involve a battery of enzymatic studies in leukocytes or, in some cases, in cultured skin fibroblasts. Pathologic examination of white matter should show decreased levels of myelin followed by axonal degeneration and fibrous astrocytic proliferation. Pathologic changes are found in both the central and peripheral nervous systems. Hypomyelination of peripheral nerves has been reported in adult Krabbe disease. Few pathologic studies have been done on older patients (see "Pathology of Late-Onset GLD").

The definitive diagnosis rests on the finding of very low GALC activity (0% to 5% of our normal mean). Other laboratory studies are helpful in pointing to the diagnosis of a leukodystrophy. These include an elevated cerebrospinal fluid protein (75 to 500 mg/dl), decreased nerve conduction velocities, magnetic resonance images showing decreased myelination in the brainstem and cerebellum, and computed tomography showing lucencies in the white matter followed by diffuse cerebral atrophy in gray and white matter later in the disease. While these studies can indicate a diagnosis of a leukodystrophy, enzymatic testing is required to make a definitive diagnosis.

There are wide "normal" and carrier ranges for GALC activity due to the presence of polymorphisms in the GALC gene. Some healthy individuals have quite low GALC activity. This makes carrier testing in individuals other than immediate family members impossible. Of course, carrier testing in family members is relatively simple when the disease-causing mutation(s) is known. We no longer perform mutation analysis in newly diagnosed patients; however, we continue to test for the common 30 kb deletion first reported by this laboratory. This mutation makes up about 40% to 50% of the mutant alleles in patients with Krabbe disease.

Prenatal diagnosis of Krabbe disease has been available since 1971. Initial testing was done using cultured amniotic fluid cells. Since that time, hundreds of pregnancies from at-risk couples have been monitored using cultured amniotic fluid cells and chorionic villi samples. This laboratory alone has monitored nearly 500 pregnancies for Krabbe disease. Measurement of GALC activity is reliable, but if the mutations in the proband are known, the pregnancy can be monitored by DNA analysis. This adds neither speed nor reliability to the testing.

PATHOLOGY

Central Nervous System

In general the white matter is firm, reduced in volume, and whitish-gray in appearance with dilated ventricles. The gray matter appears relatively normal except for a moderate reduction of the cortical thickness. The major histopathologic changes are extensive demyelination, gliosis, and presence of unique macrophages (globoid cells) in the white matter. The fornix, hippocampus, mamillothalamic tract, and nerve fiber bundles in the basal centrum semiovale and the cerebellar white matter are significantly involved. In the spinal cord, the pyramidal tracts are more severely affected than the dorsal columns. In the areas of demyelination, the oligodendroglial cell population is severely diminished and globoid cells are often clustered around blood vessels. Both mononuclear and multinucleated globoid cells are similar ultrastructurally, except for the number of nuclei. They have prominent pseudopods, moderately electron-dense granular cytoplasm containing prominent rough endoplasmic reticulum, many free ribosomes, abundant fine filaments of approximately 9 to 10 nm, and scattered or clustered abnormal cytoplasmic inclusions. The inclusions have moderately electron-dense straight or curved hollow tubular profiles in longitudinal sections and appear irregularly crystalloid in cross sections. Scattered globoid cells with typical inclusions were found in the spinal cord in fetuses of 20 to 23 weeks' gestation.

Peripheral Nervous System

The peripheral nerves tend to be firm and abnormally thick and white on gross inspection. Major pathologic features are marked endoneurial fibrosis, proliferation of fibroblasts, demyelination, and infiltration or perivascular aggregation of histiocytes/macrophages containing PAS positive materials. Thinly myelinated fibers suggestive of remyelination may be present. Axonal degeneration of varying degrees has been reported. Ultrastructurally, inclusions similar to those in globoid cells in the brain are found in the cytoplasm of histiocytes/macrophages, as well as in the Schwann cells.

Pathology of Late-Onset GLD

Despite increasing clinical reports on late-onset cases in recent years, only limited information on their neuropathology has been reported. In late infantile and juvenile cases, neuropathologic changes are similar to those in typical infantile patients. Two identical twin females developed symptoms at about age 18 years. Both received allogeneic bone marrow transplants and both died of severe graft-versus-host disease within 2 months. Neuropathologic changes included degeneration of the fronto-parietal white matter and corticospinal tract. The fronto-parietal lesion consisted of multiple necrotic foci with calcified deposits and active degeneration of the surrounding white matter with globoid cell infiltration. Globoid cell infiltration was noted in the optic radiations. In a 73-year-old woman, the oldest reported case of GLD, sural nerve biopsy revealed a mild loss of myelinated fibers with disproportionately thin myelin sheaths, and Schwann cells contained needle-like inclusions.[14]

BIOCHEMICAL FINDINGS

All patients with Krabbe disease have a deficiency of GALC activity. This enzyme has specificity toward galactosylceramide, psychosine (galactosylsphingosine), monogalactosyldiglyceride, and lactosylceramide under specific assay conditions. The metabolism of the first two substrates is important to understanding the pathology of this disorder. It has been shown that globoid cells are composed of high concentrations of galactosylceramide and can be produced experimentally by injecting this lipid into the brain.[4] However, the pathogenic lipid may be psychosine, which has been demonstrated to inhibit key enzymes such as protein kinase C and induce apoptotic death in oligodendrocytes and Schwann cells. While it is a minor compound in a normal brain, psychosine is stored in relatively large amounts in brain white matter and peripheral nerves of humans and animal models with GALC deficiency. GALC is the only enzyme capable of hydrolyzing psychosine. It is synthesized during active myelination by the enzymatic transfer of galactose to sphingosine catalyzed by ceramide-galactosyltransferase. In people with sufficient GALC activity it is degraded, but in tissues of patients with Krabbe disease it accumulates.

We initially purified GALC from pooled human urine.[7] The most active fractions consist of three bands with estimated molecular weights between 50 and 53 kDa plus a 30-kDa band. From the cDNA sequence we know that it is produced as an 80-kDa precursor, and this must be proteolytically cut into two subunits to produce the active enzyme.

The role of a so-called sphingolipid activator protein (SAP) on stimulating GALC activity has also been investigated. In 1982, we showed that SAP-2 or saposin C could stimulate GALC activity in the presence of acidic lipids, including sulfatide and phosphatidylserine.[19] The gene coding for saposin C has been cloned, and it has been shown to encode four saposins, which are cleaved from one precursor species by proteolytic hydrolysis. Recently Matsuda et al[20] have produced a mouse model with a point mutation in the saposin A region. These mice have pathologic features resembling late-onset, chronic Krabbe disease. No human counterpart is known at this time. The role that activator proteins play in stimulating in vivo GALC activity and producing the observed clinical variability, especially in late-onset patients, remains to be determined.

MOLECULAR GENETICS

The gene for human GALC has been mapped to human chromosome 14 by linkage analysis and to the region 14q31 by in situ hybridization using a probe from the cDNA sequence. The cDNA is about 3.8 kb long, including 47 bp 5′ to the initiation start site, 2007 bp of open reading frame (the code for 669 amino acids), and 1741 bp of 3′ untranslated sequence.[8] The first 78 nucleotides of the open reading frame code for the 26 amino acid leader peptide. The remaining 643 amino acids plus glycosylation of 5 or 6 of the potential sites would constitute the 80 kDa precursor species. The 80 kDa precursor is processed into the 50 to 53 and 30 kDa mature forms by the action of proteases probably localized in lysosomes. The human GALC gene is nearly 58 kb long and contains 17 exons and 16 introns.[9] Other than the first and last exons, the other exons are relatively small ranging from 39 to 181 bp. The introns range in size from 247 bp for intron 2 to about 12 kb for intron 10.

With the available sequence information from the GALC cDNA and gene, mutation analysis on patients with all types of GLD is possible. Over 70 mutations have been identified, and a great majority have been reported in several recent reviews.[10,11] This laboratory does not do mutation analysis on new patients due to the time involved, and it adds little to the management of the patient or to the accuracy of prenatal diagnosis in future pregnancies. Knowing a patient's mutation(s) would improve carrier testing in immediate family members, however it does not help with carrier assessment in individuals who marry into such a family. We test all new patients for the most common mutation found in 40% to 50% of the disease-causing alleles for Krabbe disease. While this mutation probably originated in Sweden, it has spread throughout Europe and is also found in India and Mexico. It is a large deletion involving nearly 30 kb of the gene starting within intron 10 and proceeding past the 3' end of the gene. This eliminates all of the coding informa-tion for the 30 kDa subunit plus about 15% of the coding information for the 50 kDa subunit. Of the many mutations identified in this laboratory and reported by others, some have only been found in one family. However, some mutations do occur in a relatively higher frequency in the general population or are limited to one ethnic group. Table 23-1 shows the more common mutations identified in patients with Krabbe disease. Some only occur within small, defined populations such as in the Druze community of Northern Israel and in two villages of Moslem Arabs located near Jerusalem. Others have only been reported in the Japanese population. Many patients with a late onset form of Krabbe disease have one copy of the G809A (G270A) mutation. This missense mutation must result in the production of a small amount of active enzyme that delays the onset of the disease. This has never been proven because it is difficult to accurately measure very low levels of this enzyme in available tissue samples. This laboratory has identified six families who have this mutation on one allele and the 30-kb deletion on the other. The age of onset and clinical course of affected individuals are significantly different between and within families. Other genetic and/or environmental factors must be involved in the expression of the disease. Many patients are compound heterozygotes having different mutations in the two copies of the GALC gene. This makes genotype-phenotype correlations difficult. It is clear from mutation analysis that both 30- and 50-kD subunits must be functional to have an active enzyme. Many disease-causing mutations occur with additional

TABLE 23–1. Most Common Mutations Found in Patients with GLD*

Designation	Nucleotide Change	Effect	Polymorphic Background†	Comments
635del+ins	del 25 nts + ins 3 nts	del 5 aa + ins 2 aa	?	Infantile Japanese and Koreans
G809A	GGC>GAC	G270D	1637C	Results in a later-onset form of GLD when hom or het
502T/del	30 kb deletion	short mRNA	502T	About 40%–50% of mutant alleles
1424delA	ATAAGG>ATAGG	FS, PS	1637C	T1873C on same allele
C1538T	ACG>ATG	T513M	694A	Infantile
G1544A	CGC>CAC	R515H	?	Infantile Japanese
G1582A	GAT>AAT	D528N	1637C	Infantile Israeli Arab
A1652C	TAC>TCC	Y551S	1637C	Infantile
T1748G	ATT>AGT	I583S		Infantile Israeli Druze
T1853C	TTA>TCA	L618S	1637C	Adult Japanese

*All of these mutations have been found homozygous in patients from unrelated parents and/or heterozygous in other unrelated patients.
†The polymorphism examined includes C502T (R168C), G694A (D224N), and T1637C (1546T), with the most common nucleotide given first.
Abbreviations: hom, homozygous; het, heterozygous; FS, frame shift; PS, premature stop; del, deletion; ins, insertion; aa, amino acid.

polymorphic changes in the same copy of the GALC gene.[10,11] The possible role polymorphisms have in producing a clinical phenotype when three or more are inherited in one individual has been discussed elsewhere.[10]

ANIMAL MODELS

There are well-characterized animal models of GLD available for study. Several published reviews describe their clinical and pathologic features, molecular defects, and potential use as models to attempt therapeutic trials.[12,13] In addition to these naturally occurring models, a new transgenic mouse has been developed.[21] As has been demonstrated in human Krabbe disease, animal models have increased psychosine in nervous tissues, and mice have a large increase in galactosylceramide in kidney. Treatment of affected mice with bone marrow transplant has resulted in a prolonged life span.[24,25] There were significant elevations in GALC activity in lung, liver, heart, kidney, spleen, brain, and peripheral nervous system.[23] This rise in enzymatic activity was accompanied by a slower increase in the levels of psychosine in the brain. Histologically, there was disappearance of characteristic globoid cells and infiltration of donor-derived macrophages, which resulted in some remyelination in the central nervous system. Unfortunately, the major symptoms in the untreated twitcher mouse are related to severe demyelination in the peripheral nervous system. Although there was evidence for an increase in GALC activity in the peripheral nervous system, psychosine continued to increase, and the levels in the 100-day-old treated mice equaled those found in the 40-day-old untreated mice. Although the life span was more than doubled by the treatment, all affected mice died with severe neurologic disease. A number of mice received intracerebral injections of neural stem cells and viral vectors containing GALC cDNA with minimal positive results (unpublished observations).

Cairn and Westhighland white terriers with GLD have been known for many years, and a breeding colony has been established at the University of Pennsylvania School of Veterinary Medicine. This larger animal model has some advantages over the mouse model that could bridge the gap toward human trials once effective therapies are developed. We have used magnetization transfer imaging to evaluate these dogs.[24] As with the mice, bone marrow transplant slows the progression of the disease. A colony of rhesus monkeys that carry a mutation causing GLD is available at the Tulane Primate Research Center. Affected fetuses can be identified in utero using CVS early in pregnancy and treatment can be instituted. Although only a limited number of affected monkeys will be available, they can be utilized as a final step before human trials to investigate safety and effectiveness of new therapies.

THERAPY

At this time, more than 20 patients with Krabbe disease have undergone HSCT, and the outcomes have been generally positive.[25] While the long-term prognosis is unknown, there is clear evidence that transplant of presymptomatic infantile patients with HSC dramatically slows the clinical course of the disease, and transplanted individuals do not follow the clinical course and early death of untreated siblings. Transplant of mildly affected late-onset patients should be considered after careful neurologic examination and search for an acceptable donor.

Two juvenile-onset patients have done considerably well following bone marrow transplantation. An 18-year-old female with onset of symptoms at age 5 years received a bone marrow transplant from her homozygous normal brother. Ten years following the transplant, she is stably engrafted, maintaining normal leukocyte GALC activity. Her elevated cerebrospinal fluid protein concentration has decreased to normal, her school performance is normal, and she no longer experiences tremors or ataxia. There is an improvement in all of her neuropsychologic test results. An 8-year-old male was determined to be affected with GLD by enzyme studies using leukocytes. He is one of three affected siblings. He received a bone marrow transplant from his unaffected sister. Five years following the transplant, he is in excellent health and has a donor level of GALC activity. There has been a drop in cerebrospinal fluid protein from 125 to normal, a rise in his IQ, and an improvement in his MRI. Although it is too early to reach a conclusion regarding the role of HSCT in Krabbe disease, it should be seriously considered in presymptomatic infantile cases and in juvenile and late-onset cases if a suitable donor is available. In-utero bone marrow transplant has been tried with little success.

CONCLUSION

At this time, Krabbe disease remains readily diagnosable prenatally and postnatally by measuring GALC activity in available tissue samples. The cloning of the GALC gene and identification of mutations has led to improved carrier assessment in some families. No clear genotype-phenotype correlation can be assigned to novel mutations identified in newly diagnosed patients. In fact, there is considerable clinical variability in late-onset patients with the identical genotype. No completely satisfactory treatment is available, however HSCT in presymptomatic infantile patients and very mildly affected late-onset patients shows clear beneficial effects. Its use will require early diagnosis of affected individuals.

Very recent developments in the isolation and characterization of neural and embryonic stem cells and the production of hybrid viral vectors that can infect neural cells with genes of interest open the way to studies on GLD animal models. Potentially, stem cells can be transduced to produce high levels of GALC activity. Once injected, they could spread throughout the brain and supply either GALC activity to actively myelinating oligodendrocytes or repopulate large areas of the brain with oligodendrocytes that have sufficient GALC activity. Cultured oligodendrocytes from twitcher mice can be made to have a normal phenotype when GALC activity is supplied via viral transduction or uptake from neighboring cells.[26] While any treatment protocol should include a method for decreasing the level of psychosine in myelinating oligodendrocytes, a role for anti-apoptotic cytokines and growth factors may need to be considered in future protocols. Clearly, the rapid progression of the disease and the need to supply GALC activity globally throughout the CNS and PNS present significant challenges for the treatment of this disease.

Acknowledgments

The author thanks the many coworkers who have helped with the research on this disorder and the families with Krabbe disease who provided samples and support for our research. This research was supported in part by a grant from the National Institutes of Health (DK 38795).

REFERENCES

1. Krabbe K: A new familial, infantile form of diffuse brain sclerosis. Brain 1916;39:74–114.

2. Collier J, Greenfield J: The encephalitis periaxialis of Schilder: A clinical and pathological study, with an account of two cases, one of which was diagnosed during life. Brain 1924;47:489–519.

3. Hagberg B, Kollberg H, Sourander P, Akesson HO: Infantile globoid cell leukodystrophy (Krabbe's disease): A clinical and genetic study of 32 Swedish cases 1953–1967. Neuropaediatrie 1970;1:74–88.

4. Austin J, Lehfeldt D, Maxwell W: Experimental "globoid bodies" in white matter and chemical analysis in Krabbe's disease. J Neuropathol Exp Neurol 1961; 20:284–285.

5. Malone M: Deficiency in degradative enzyme system in globoid leukodystrophy. Trans Am Soc Neurochem 1970;1:56.

6. Suzuki K, Suzuki Y: Globoid cell leukodystrophy (Krabbe's disease): Deficiency of galactocerebroside β-galactosidase. Proc Natl Acad Sci U S A 1970;66: 302–309.

7. Chen YQ, Wenger DA: Galactocerebrosidase from human urine: Purification and partial characterization. Biochim Biophys Acta 1993;1170:53–61.

8. Chen YQ, Rafi MA, de Gala G, Wenger DA: Cloning and expression of cDNA encoding human galactocerebrosidase, the enzyme deficient in globoid cell leukodystrophy. Hum Mol Genet 1993;2:1841–1845.

9. Luzi P, Rafi MA, Wenger DA: Structure and organization of the human galactocerebrosidase (GALC) gene. Genomics 1995;26:407–409.

10. Wenger DA, Rafi MA, Luzi P, et al: Krabbe disease: Genetic aspects and progress toward therapy. Mol Genet Metab 2000;70:1–9.

11. Wenger DA, Suzuki K, Suzuki Y, Suzuki K: Galactosylceramide lipidosis: Globoid cell leukodystrophy (Krabbe disease). In Scriver CR, Beaudet AL, Sly WS, Valle D (eds): The Metabolic and Molecular Bases of Inherited Disease (8th ed). New York, McGraw-Hill, 2001, pp 3669–3694.

12. Suzuki K, Suzuki K: Genetic galactosylceramidase deficiency (globoid cell leukodystrophy, Krabbe disease) in different mammalian species. Neurochem Pathol 1985;3:53–68.

13. Wenger DA: Murine, canine and non-human primate models of Krabbe disease. Mol Med Today 2000;6:449–451.

14. Kolodny EH, Raghavan S, Krivit W: Late-onset Krabbe disease (globoid cell leukodystrophy): Clinical and biochemical features in 15 patients. Dev Neurosci 1991;13:232–239.

15. Luzi P, Rafi MA, Wenger DA: Multiple mutations in the GALC gene in a patient with adult-onset Krabbe disease. Ann Neurol 1996;40:116–119.

16. De Gasperi R, Gama Sosa MA, Sartorato EL, et al: Molecular heterogeneity of late-onset forms of globoid-cell leukodystrophy. Am J Hum Genet 1996; 59:1233–1242.

17. Furuya H, Kukita Y, Nagano S, et al: Adult onset globoid cell leukodystrophy (Krabbe disease): Analysis of galactosylceramidase cDNA from four Japanese patients. Hum Genet 1997;100:450–456.

18. De Stefano N, Dotti MT, Mortilla M, et al: Evidence of diffuse brain pathology and unspecific genetic characterization in a patient with a typical form of adult-onset Krabbe disease. J Neurol 2000;247: 226–228.

19. Wenger PA, Sattler M, Roth S: A protein activator of galactosylceramide β-galactosidase. Biochim Biophys Acta 1982;712:639–649.

20. Matsuda J, Vanier MT, Saito Y, et al: A mutation in the saposin A domain of the sphingolipid activator protein (prosaposin) gene results in a late-onset, chronic form of globoid cell leukodystrophy in the mouse. Hum Mol Genet 2001;10:1191–1199.

21. Luzi P, Rafi MA, Zaka M, et al: Generation of a mouse with low galactocerebrosidase activity by gene targeting: A new model of globoid cell leukodystrophy (Krabbe disease). Molec Genet Metab 2001;73:221–223.

22. Yeager AM, Brennan S, Tiffany C, et al: Prolonged survival and remyelination after hematopoietic cell transplantation in the twitcher mouse. Science 1984;225:1053–1054.

23. Ichioka T, Kishimoto Y, Brennan S, et al: Hematopoietic cell transplantation in murine globoid cell leukodystrophy (the twitcher mouse): Effects on levels of galactosylceramidase, psychosine, and galactocerebrosides. Proc Natl Acad Sci U S A 1987;84: 4259–4263.

24. McGowan JC, Haskins H, Wenger DA, Vite CL: Investigating demyelination in the brain in a canine model of globoid cell leukodystrophy (Krabbe disease) using magnetization transfer contrast: Preliminary results. J Comput Assist Tomogr 2000;24:316–321.

25. Krivit W, Shapiro EG, Peters C, et al: Hematopoietic stem-cell transplantation in globoid cell leukodystrophy. N Engl J Med 1998;338:1119–1126.

26. Luddi A, Volterrani M, Strazza M, et al: Retrovirus-mediated gene transfer and galactocerebrosidase uptake into twitcher glial cells results in appropriate localization and phenotype correction. Neurobiol Dis 2001;8:600–610.

The Mucopolysaccharidoses and the Mucolipidoses

Reuben Matalon

Kimberlee Michals Matalon

The mucopolysaccharidoses are a group of inherited disorders caused by specific enzyme deficiencies in the degradation of the glycosaminoglycans (mucopolysaccharides). Enzyme deficiencies result in the accumulation of glycosaminoglycans in lysosomes of various tissues and in the excessive excretion of partially degraded glycosaminoglycans in urine. Clinical manifestations of the mucopolysaccharidoses depend on the specific enzyme deficiency, the end organ affected, and the accumulation of glycosaminoglycans in the affected organs. In diseases in which the brain is not involved, there is no mental retardation. On the other hand, if the brain is affected and other somatic manifestations are minimal, the coarse features that are characteristic of the mucopolysaccharidoses are not as prominent. Specific degradative lysosomal enzyme deficiencies have been identified for all the mucopolysaccharidoses. The glycosaminoglycans that are stored and excreted in the urine of the various mucopolysaccharidoses are dermatan sulfate, heparan sulfate, keratan sulfate, and chondroitin 4/6 sulfates.[1-4]

The mucolipidoses have emerged as a separate group of inherited disorders that originally were considered to be part of the mucopolysaccharidoses. The storage material within tissues or cultured skin fibroblasts includes lipids and glycosaminoglycans.[5,6] These disorders are not characterized by mucopolysacchariduria.

HISTORY

Hunter in 1917[7] described two brothers that fit the clinical features of the X-linked recessive form of the mucopolysaccharidoses. Hurler in 1919[8] described two unrelated boys with clinical findings that conformed to the syndrome now associated with her name. Initially, all the mucopolysaccharidoses were referred to as Hurler syndrome. In 1936, Ellis et al[9] suggested the term *gargoylism* because of the coarse facial features of children with these diseases. In 1952, Brante identified storage of mucopolysaccharide in liver of patients with Hurler syndrome.[10] He then coined the term *mucopolysaccharidosis*. Further characterization of the mucopolysaccharides (glycosaminoglycans) in tissues and urine was instrumental for the delineation of the mucopolysaccharidoses.[1-4, 11]

The idea that the mucopolysaccharidoses are caused by defects of lysosomal hydrolases was proposed in 1964.[12] The liver from a patient with Hurler syndrome was studied, and distended lysosomes were found, suggesting storage within these organelles. Subsequent studies using cultured skin fibroblasts confirmed that fibroblasts from patients with mucopolysaccharidoses contained large amounts of glycosaminoglycans.[13,14] Studies showed that the accumulation of glycosaminoglycans in fibroblasts was indicative of faulty degradation and that mixing cells from various mucopolysaccharidoses led to cross-correction of the accumulation of glycosaminoglycans, which suggests that each mucopolysaccharide disorder is distinct from the other.[15, 16] Matalon et al[17] discovered the enzyme α-L-iduronidase in human and other mammalian tissues and that deficiency of this enzyme resulted in Hurler syndrome.[18] The discovery of this lysosomal defect led to the subsequent elucidation of the enzyme deficiencies in other mucopolysaccharidoses. Reviews dealing with the biochemistry of the glycosaminoglycans and mucopolysaccharidoses are available.[1-4]

MANIFESTATIONS OF THE MUCOPOLYSACCHARIDOSES

Hurler Syndrome

Hurler syndrome has been the prototype of the entire mucopolysaccharidoses. With the discovery of mucopolysacchariduria, however, delineation of the various mucopolysaccharidoses according to the urinary glycosaminoglycans emerged.[11] Further classification occurred following the enzyme deficiencies assigned for the various mucopolysaccharidoses (Table 24–1). For each enzyme deficiency, there is a spectrum of clinical manifestations. In α-L-iduronidase deficiency, the most severe form is Hurler syndrome (Fig. 24–1). The deficiency of α-L-iduronidase leads to the accumulation of dermatan sulfate and heparan sulfate and to the urinary excretion of these glycosaminoglycans.[19–21] In patients with Hurler syndrome, there is a wide occurrence of vacuolated cells containing engorged lysosomes with glycosaminoglycans.

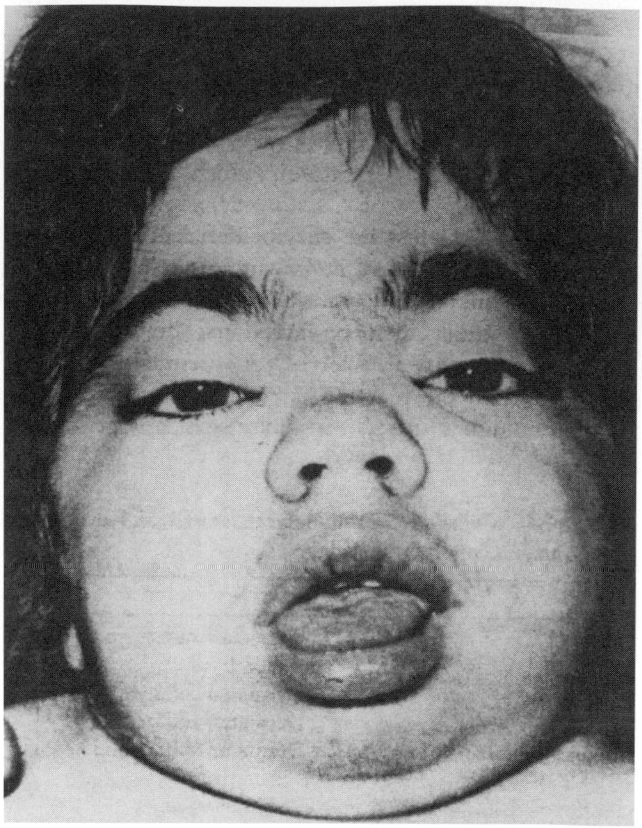

Clinical Findings

The infant with Hurler syndrome appears normal at birth, but after age 6 months, coarse facial appearance can be noted (Fig. 24–2). Hepatosplenomegaly can be detected, and umbilical and inguinal hernias may appear. Chronic rhinorrhea may suggest frequent colds. Recurrent upper-airway infection, otitis media, and hypertrophy of tonsils and adenoids may persist beyond early childhood. Hearing impairment may be secondary to such events. When these children attempt to sit, very mild kyphosis can be noticed. The kyphosis will progress as the child grows older to the gibbus that is typical of Hurler syndrome. Vision is impaired because of clouding of the corneas. Clouding of the cornea can be detected in the first year of life. Children with Hurler syndrome may sit, walk, and

FIGURE 24–1. Typical facial appearance of a child with Hurler syndrome showing coarse facial features, broad nasal bridge, frontal bossing, clouding of corneas, and large tongue.

develop early language skills, but soon these skills are lost. Severe mental retardation becomes apparent, and these children become bedridden (Fig. 24–3).

Before age 1 year, it is difficult to differentiate among the α-L-iduronidase deficiency syndromes clinically or enzymatically. This is important because of experimental

TABLE 24–1. Enzyme Deficiencies of the Mucopolysaccharidoses

Disease	Enzyme Deficiency	Inheritance
Hurler	α-L-iduronidase	Autosomal recessive
Hurler-Scheie	α-L-iduronidase	Autosomal recessive
Scheie	α-L-iduronidase	Autosomal recessive
Hunter (A and B)	Iduronosulfate sulfatase	X-linked recessive
Sanfilippo A	Sulfamidase	Autosomal recessive
Sanfilippo B	α-N-acetylglucosaminidase	Autosomal recessive
Sanfilippo C	Acetyl-CoA:α-glucosaminide N-acetyltransferase	Autosomal recessive
Sanfilippo D	N-acetylglucosamine-6-sulfate sulfatase	Autosomal recessive
Morquio A	N-acetylgalactosamine-6-sulfate sulfatase	Autosomal recessive
Morquio B	ß-galactosidase	Autosomal recessive
Maroteaux-Lamy	N-acetylgalactosamine-4-sulfate sulfatase	Autosomal recessive
ß-Sly	ß-glucuronidase	Autosomal recessive

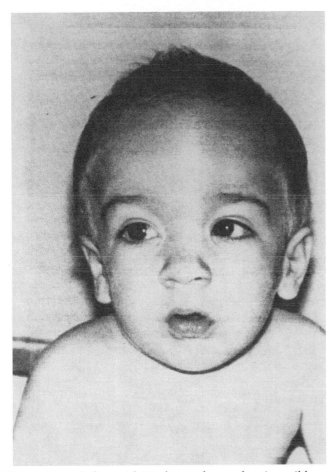

FIGURE 24–2. Infant with Hurler syndrome showing mild coarse features, presence of metopic sutures, mild corneal clouding, and chronic rhinorrhea.

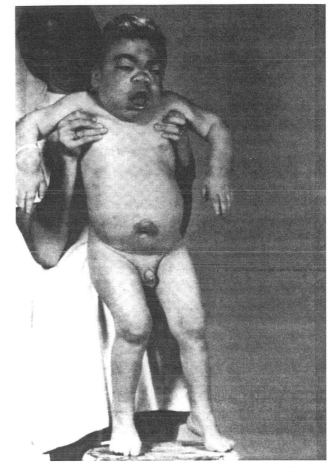

FIGURE 24–3. Severely retarded child with Hurler syndrome, with contracted joints, hepatosplenomegaly, umbilical hernia, and typical facial features.

therapy and because the milder forms of α-L-iduronidase defects may not require such therapeutic modalities (see section on therapy, discussed later). There have been several approaches to resolve this problem, including using enzyme kinetics and monoclonal antibodies for quantitation of α-L-iduronidase.[22] We have used two separate methods to differentiate these variants. The first approach is the analysis of urine for glycosaminoglycans. In Hurler syndrome, there is increased excretion of dermatan and heparan sulfate. In the mild forms (Hurler-Scheie and Scheie syndromes), there is excretion of only dermatan sulfate.[20] The second approach is the use of desulfated heparin as a natural substrate for α-L-iduronidase.[21] In Hurler syndrome, iduronic acid is not hydrolyzed from this substrate, whereas in Hurler-Scheie and Scheie syndromes, iduronic acid is hydrolyzed from desulfated heparin. Mutation analysis of the α-L-iduronidase gene may also be informative in some patients.

Hurler-Scheie Syndrome

Patients with Hurler-Scheie syndrome have severe joint involvement, short stature, small thorax, hepatosplenomegaly, coarse facial features, and corneal cloud-

ing but normal or near-normal mentality (Fig. 24–4). The small thorax and the cardiac involvement in this disease, usually mitral valve insufficiency, may be important to recognize because they are the major complicating events that lead to increased mortality.

Scheie Syndrome

Patients with Scheie syndrome usually attain normal height, and their hepatosplenomegaly may be very mild. Stiffness of joints may not be recognized early in life because these children are not retarded and they do not have coarse features. The dysostosis multiplex is very mild. Carpal tunnel syndrome or other joint stiffness may bring these patients to the physician. More commonly, ocular involvement such as corneal clouding and retinal degeneration may lead to the suspicion of mucopolysaccharide disorder. Usually the diagnosis is not made before age 10 years and frequently beyond age 20 years.

Roentgenographic Findings

The mucopolysaccharidoses have specific skeletal changes referred to as *dysostosis multiplex*. These changes may

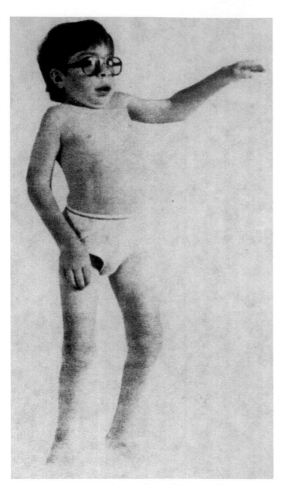

FIGURE 24–4. Patient with Hurler-Scheie syndrome who is mentally alert with short stature and contracted joints.

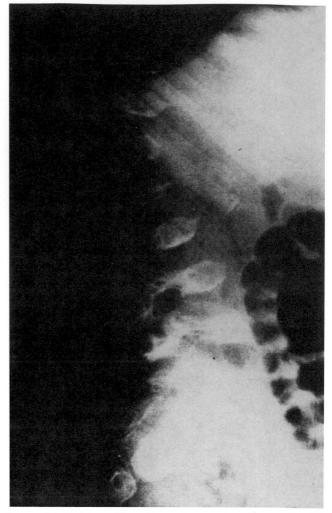

FIGURE 24–5. X-ray film of lateral spine showing ovoid and beaked vertebrae in a child with mucopolysaccharidosis.

vary in severity depending on the individual mucopolysaccharide disorder. Dysostosis multiplex can also be seen in diseases other than the mucopolysaccharidoses, especially glycoprotein storage diseases such as mannosidosis, aspartylglucosaminuria, and GM_1 gangliosidosis. The skull is usually dolichocephalic, and the calvarium is thickened with hyperostosis of the cranium. The sella turcica is large and/or boot-shaped. The clavicles are thickened, especially in the middle third. The vertebral bodies are ovoid with beaklike projections on their anterior lower margins. Thoracic vertebra (T-12) tends to be hypoplastic, which may result in a gibbus formation (Fig. 24–5). The ribs tend to widen distally, which gives them the shape of a spatula. The iliac bones are flared with shallow acetabula. The hips are deformed, and the head of the femur has changes that resemble aseptic necrosis. The hands show tapering of the terminal phalanges and tapering of the proximal ends of the metacarpals. The fifth metacarpal is usually the first to be affected. The long bones show areas of cortical thinning and irregular widening associated with expansion of the medullary cavity. The radius curves toward the ulna at the distal end, forming a V-shaped deformity (Fig. 24–6). The humerus is angulated, and the glenoid fossa is shallow.

All of the mucopolysaccharidoses have varying degrees of dysostosis multiplex.[3] Sanfilippo syndrome has the least severe radiologic changes.

Biochemical and Molecular Studies

α-L-iduronidase is required for the hydrolysis of α-L-iduronic acid from the terminal ends of dermatan and heparan sulfates. The gene for α-L-iduronidase has been localized to the short arm of chromosome 4 (4p16.3) in close proximity to the Huntington gene.[23–26] Mutation analysis indicates that a common allele leading to Hurler syndrome is substitution of the amino acid tryptophan to a stop codon ($Trp_{402} \rightarrow Ter$).[27] Another stop codon involving substitution of glutamine ($Gln_{70} \rightarrow Ter$) and substitution of proline to arginine ($Pro_{533} \rightarrow Arg$) results in a severe phenotype.[28] The $Trp_{402} \rightarrow Ter$ and $Gln_{70} \rightarrow Ter$ mutations account for 72% of alleles of children with Hurler syndrome in Europe.[29] Many other mutations have been described in individual patients and other ethnic groups.[29–31]

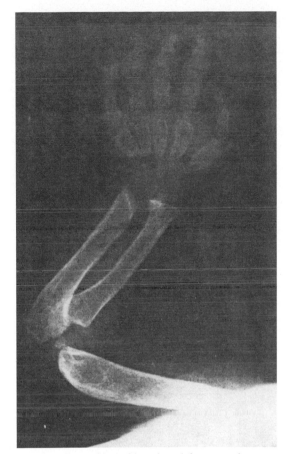

FIGURE 24–6. X-ray film of hand and forearm showing tapering of the proximal ends of the metacarpals, cortical thinning, and curving of the radius and ulna.

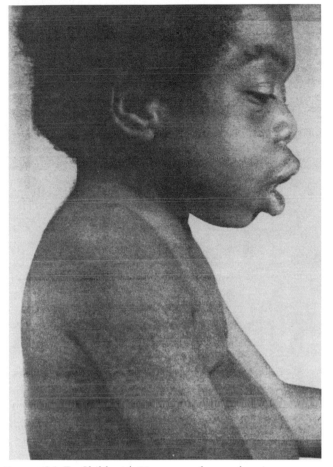

FIGURE 24–7. Child with Hunter syndrome showing coarse features, depressed nasal bridge, and characteristic rash on the arms and shoulders, frequently seen in Hunter syndrome.

The milder forms of iduronidase deficiency are associated with mutations that give some residual activity of iduronidase. The mutation that leads to the substitution of arginine to glutamine ($Arg_{89} \rightarrow Gln$) results in an intermediate phenotype.[32–33] The intronic mutation involving nucleotide in position 678 (g→a) results in Scheie syndrome.[32]

Canine models with α-L-iduronidase deficiency have been used to explore the efficacy of bone marrow transplant and enzyme therapy.[34–35] The cDNA for the canine α-L-iduronidase has been cloned.[36–37] The canine model for Hurler syndrome can be explored for gene therapy.

Hunter Syndrome (MPS II)

Hunter syndrome is the only X-linked recessive disease among the mucopolysaccharidoses. Phenotypically there are two forms of Hunter syndrome. One form is with mental retardation (Fig. 24–7), and the other is with no retardation. This disease may also represent a spectrum of severity. The facial features in both forms are similar, with slightly less coarseness in the mild form. In general, patients with Hunter syndrome look similar to patients with Hurler syndrome with a few

exceptions. The corneas are not involved in Hunter syndrome. This can be used as an important distinguishing feature, whereas hearing deteriorates rapidly with Hunter syndrome. In Hunter syndrome, the radiographic finding of dysostosis multiplex is found. The gibbus is not found until the second decade of life, and it is usually very mild. Patients with Hunter syndrome have skin rash over the arms, shoulders, and thighs. The rash is macular and may change in character (see Fig. 24–7). Patients with Hunter syndrome excrete dermatan and heparan sulfate similar to Hurler syndrome patients. The diagnosis of Hunter syndrome is confirmed by iduronosulfatase deficiency.[38–39]

As they grow older, patients with the mild variant of this disease develop severe hearing problems, carpal tunnel syndrome, and progressive upper-airway obstruction. Death may occur from upper-airway obstruction and heart failure. There are patients with Hunter syndrome who survived beyond the fifth or sixth decade of life.[1] In the α-L-iduronidase deficiency syndromes there is a difference in the urinary glycosaminoglycans between mild and severe forms. In Hunter patients there is no difference.

Biochemical and Molecular Studies

α-L-iduronic acid is sulfated on the C2 position. Iduronosulfatase is required to hydrolyze this ester sulfate as shown in Table 24–1.[38] The gene for iduronosulfatase has been localized to the Xq28 region close to the fragile X site.[40] The gene contains 9 exons and 8 introns.[41] Southern blot analysis of genomic DNA from Hunter patients suggests that a significant number of these patients have gross deletions in the iduronosulfatase gene.[42–45] Patients with complete deletion, partial deletion, or gross rearrangements of the gene all had severe phenotype.[46] Other mutations such as nonsense mutations, small deletions leading to frame shift or premature chain termination, splice mutations, and a point mutation eliminating a recognition site have been reported.[46–47] Several missense mutations have been described: $Ala_{68} \rightarrow Glu$, $Ser_{426} \rightarrow Ter$, $Ile_{485} \rightarrow Arg$, $Gln_{293} \rightarrow His$, and $Asp_{4/8} \rightarrow Gly$.[47] The gross deletion in some patients with Hunter syndrome further suggests that some of the pathology in these severely affected patients may be contributed by the deletion of other neighboring genes.[44] Isolation of the fragile X gene, distal to the iduronosulfatase gene, should make it possible to study whether there is interaction between the two genes.[48]

There have been reports of Hunter syndrome in females. In one such karyotypically normal girl, unbalanced inactivation of the wild type allele in the maternal chromosome has been suggested.[49] In another case, an X:autosome translocation was reported to span the iduronosulfatase locus.[40] The cDNA can be used to study female Hunter patients and has been used to improve carrier detection for females at risk.[50–51]

Sanfilippo Syndromes (MPS III)

There are four types of Sanfilippo syndrome. All have mild dysostosis multiplex and mild coarse facial features (Fig. 24–8). Children with Sanfilippo syndrome have hepatosplenomegaly, which is not as pronounced as in Hurler syndrome. As children with this disease grow older, the liver and spleen may resume normal size and hepatosplenomegaly will be missed. Hyperactivity, speech delay, and frank mental retardation are symptoms of this syndrome. By the end of the first decade of life, these children undergo rapid neurologic deterioration and become bedridden and die in their middle teens. Few Sanfilippo patients live beyond the second decade of life.

The mucopolysacchariduria is rather characteristic by increased levels of heparan sulfate only. There is no dermatan sulfate associated with the disease. The specific enzyme assay must be performed to determine which Sanfilippo syndrome the patient has.

Sanfilippo A is the most common of the Sanfilippo syndromes. The enzyme deficiency is sulfamidase, which can

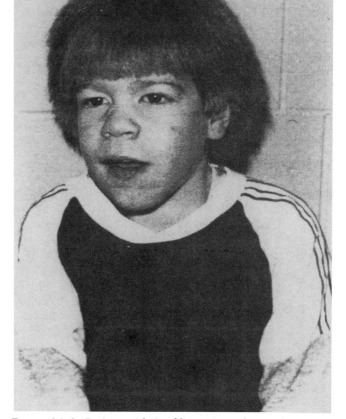

FIGURE 24–8. Patient with Sanfilippo A syndrome showing mild coarseness of facial features.

be assayed on white blood cells or cultured skin fibroblasts (see Table 24–1).[52–53]

Sanfilippo B syndrome is the second in frequency after Sanfilippo A. Clinically the presentation is similar. The enzyme deficiency in this syndrome is α-N-acetylhexosaminidase.[53]

Sanfilippo C is probably the mildest of the Sanfilippo syndromes in terms of mental retardation, dysostosis multiplex, and coarse features. Nevertheless, children show symptoms of hyperactivity and mental retardation as they grow older. Joint stiffness is not a prominent feature of Sanfilippo C. Heparan sulfaturia is a feature of this disease, and the enzyme deficiency is acetylCoA: α-glucosamide N-acetyltransferase.[55] This enzyme can be assayed on peripheral white blood cells and cultured skin fibroblasts.

Sanfilippo D is the rarest of the Sanfilippo syndromes. Phenotypically it is usually mild, and the physical findings are typical of the Sanfilippo syndromes. A case of Sanfilippo D was reported in which the patient did not have features of MPS III and presented only with speech delay.[56] The enzyme deficiency of N-acetylglucosamine-6-sulfate sulfatase can be assayed on white blood cells and cultured skin fibroblasts.[57] Sanfilippo D patients excrete not only heparan sulfate but also N-acetylglucosamine-6-sulfate. This is caused by the action of hexosaminidase A, which also cleaves sulfated glucosamine.

Biochemical and Molecular Studies

Sulfamidase is the enzyme that is specific for sulfate linked to the amino groups of glucosamine. The gene for sulfamidase has been cloned and localized to the long arm of chromosome 17 (17q25.3).[58] The most common mutation among those of European ancestry is $ARG_{245} \rightarrow HIS$.[59] Other mutations have been detected among other ethnic groups.[60–62] The common mutation $Arg_{245} \rightarrow His$ has been described in the Cayman Islands, indicating a founding father effect in a genetic isolate.[63]

α-N-Acetylglucosaminidase is required for the hydrolysis of N-acetylglucosamine residues from heparan sulfate. Deficiency of this enzyme leads to Sanfilippo B syndrome. The gene has been isolated and localized to chromosome 17q21.[64–65] Some mutations have been identified with no predominant mutation.[66–68] Heparan sulfate, which accumulates in the four types of Sanfilippo and in Hunter and Hurler syndromes, is unique among the glycosaminoglycans in two respects: N-acetylglucosamine is a-linked in heparan sulfate, and instead of N-acetylglucosamine there are N-sulfated groups on the glucosamine. Following the action of sulfamidase, the glucosamine moiety has to be cleaved. The free glucosamine to be hydrolyzed has to be acetylated by the specific enzyme acetyl-CoA: α-glucosaminide N-acetyltransferase. This is a lysosomal enzyme that catalyzes the acetylation of the free glucosamine on the polysaccharide terminus. The gene for this enzyme has not been cloned.

N-Acetylglucosamine-6-sulfatase hydrolyzes the sulfate on position 6 of the glucosamine of heparan sulfate. This enzyme is deficient in Sanfilippo D. The gene for N-acetylglucosamine-6-sulfatase has been cloned and localized to the long arm of chromosome 12 (12q14).[69,70]

Morquio Syndrome (MPS IV)

Morquio[71] and Brailsford[72] described this syndrome with severe skeletal dysplasia and keratan sulfaturia. The skeletal dysplasia can be severe, but also mild forms of Morquio syndrome have been observed. Morquio syndrome usually lacks mental involvement, and is associated with joint laxity, shortness of stature, and pectus carinatum. Skeletal abnormalities include shortened vertebrae (platyspondyly universalis), genu valgum, pes planus, and large joints (Fig. 24–9). The neck is short, and the odontoid process of the cervical

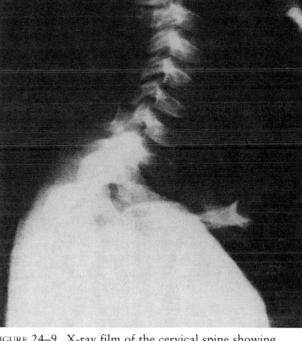

FIGURE 24–9. X-ray film of the cervical spine showing flattened ovoid shaped vertebrae typical of Morquio syndrome.

spine is underdeveloped. This may lead to atlantoaxial subluxation. Corneal clouding is present in 50% of cases. There is usually midfacial hypoplasia and protrusion of the mandible, which makes these children seem like they have a permanent grin. Hepatomegaly may be present, but it is not as prominent as in the other mucopolysaccharidoses. Cardiac involvement includes aortic regurgitation. Tooth enamel is severely affected and is usually very thin. Patients with Morquio syndrome usually survive until middle age. Because of the pectus carinatum and kyphoscoliosis, however, cor pulmonale may develop.

There is a wide range of variability in the phenotypic expression of this disease, and it is often difficult to distinguish Morquio syndrome from other skeletal dysplasias. Keratan sulfaturia, however, is specific for Morquio syndrome.

There are two types of Morquio syndrome: type A caused by deficiency of N-acetylgalactosamine-6-sulfate sulfatase[73] and type B caused by deficiency of β-galactosidase.[74] Type B usually lacks enamel hypoplasia. The enzyme deficiency in both conditions can be assayed in white blood cells and cultured skin fibroblasts.

Biochemical and Molecular Studies

Galactosamine-6-sulfate sulfatase, the enzyme that hydrolyzes sulfate from galactose-6-sulfate and N-acetyl-galactosamine-6-sulfate, is the enzyme deficient in Morquio type A. The gene for N-acetylgalactosamine-6-sulfatase has been cloned and has been localized to the long arm of chromosome 16 (16q24.3).[75–79] There have been more than 100 mutations reported in Morquio type A patients.[80–91]

β-galactosidase is also required for the sequential degradation of keratan sulfate. Deficiency of this enzyme leads to Morquio type B. The gene has been cloned and assigned to the short arm of chromosome 3 (3p21.33).[92–93] Several point mutations have been reported in the β-galactosidase gene: $Try_{273} \rightarrow Leu$, $Arg_{201} \rightarrow Cys$, $Ile_{51} \rightarrow Thr$, and $Arg_{482} \rightarrow His$.[94–96] ß-galactosidase deficiency can also be caused by a protective protein. Such a disease causes deficiency of sialidase and ß-galactosidase (mucolipidosis I).[75]

Maroteaux-Lamy Syndrome (MPS VI)

Maroteaux-Lamy syndrome resembles Hurler syndrome but lacks the mental retardation (Fig. 24–10). Patients have coarse facial features, corneal clouding, hepatosplenomegaly, and dysostosis multiplex.[97] Urinary mucopolysaccharides show increased excretion of dermatan sulfate, which is caused by the deficiency of N-acetylgalactosamine-4-sulfate sulfatase (arylsulfatase B) (see Table 24–1).[98–99] Maroteaux-Lamy syndrome also has a spectrum of severity, and in the severe form, children die from constricted chest and upper-airway obstruction.

Biochemical and Molecular Studies

N-acetylgalactosamine-4-sulfatase (arylsulfatase B) is a 38 to 41 kDa monomer enzyme isolated from liver.[100] The gene encoding for arylsulfatase B has been isolated

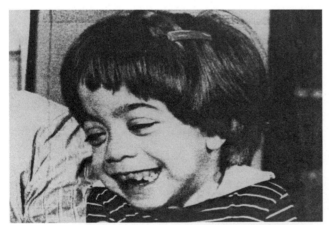

FIGURE 24–10. Patient with Maroteaux-Lamy syndrome with frontal bossing, large head, and mild coarse features.

and localized to chromosome 5 (5q13-5q14).[101–103] A feline model of MPS VI has been described and characterized biochemically and pathologically.[104] Mutations have been identified that cause severe, moderate, and mild forms of Maroteaux-Lamy, so genotype and phenotype can be correlated.[105–109]

ß-Glucuronidase Deficiency (MPS VII): Sly Disease

β-Glucuronidase deficiency (Sly disease) has a spectrum of clinical manifestations with mild and severe forms.[110] Sometimes these patients cannot be distinguished from patients with Hurler syndrome. The coarse facial features are usually milder, and the gibbus is not pronounced. The mucopolysacchariduria consisted mostly of chondroitin-4/6-sulfate.[111] The enzyme deficiency β-glucuronidase can be documented using white blood cells and cultured skin fibroblasts.

Biochemical and Molecular Studies

Glucuronic acid, found in heparan sulfate, dermatan sulfate, and chondroitin 4/6 sulfate, is hydrolyzed by β-glucuronidase. The gene for β-glucuronidase has been cloned both from human and mouse.[112–118] The exon-intron boundaries between the mouse and human genes are identical. The gene for human β-glucuronidase has been localized to the long arm of chromosome 7 (7q 21.11).[119–120]

Canine and mouse models with β-glucuronidase deficiency have been reported.[121–123] A feline colony with the disease has been reported.[124]

A variety of mutations have been identified to cause β-glucuronidase deficiency.[125–128] Two mutations ($Ala_{354} \rightarrow Val$ and $Arg_{611} \rightarrow Trp$) have been identified to result in hydrops fetalis.[129]

Multiple Sulfatase

Multiple sulfatase deficiency has been described where the protective moiety for the hydrolytic enzyme is required and may be deficient in patients with multiple sulfatase. Such patients will store and excrete in their urine various glycosaminoglycans.[130] We have described combined heparan and keratan sulfaturia with glucosamine-6-sulfatase deficiency, which is different than the enzyme deficiency in Sanfilippo D syndrome.[131,132] This unusual mucopolysacchariduria may be a result of a multiple sulfatase defect.

The basic defect for multiple sulfatase is not known. It has been postulated that either a co-translational or post-translational process results in deficient activity of various sulfatases.[133]

Although multiple sulfatase is not a mucopolysaccharide disease, such patients do accumulate and excrete glycosaminoglycans in addition to other sulfatides. These patients have coarse facial appearance and dysostosis multiplex similar to the mucopolysaccharidoses.

THERAPY FOR THE MUCOPOLYSACCHARIDOSES

Symptomatic treatment is needed to relieve hydrocephalus, cardiac disease, corneal clouding, and upper-airway obstruction. Medication for hyperactivity can be helpful. Experimental treatment by bone marrow transplant was reported by Hobbs et al in 1981.[134] According to these studies, coarse facial appearance, corneal clouding, hepatosplenomegaly, and mucopolysacchariduria improved. Mental function also seemed to improve. Subsequently, bone marrow transplant studies were performed in this country on a larger scale and support the earlier findings of Hobbs.[135] It seems that the best results can be obtained when bone marrow therapy is done early in life before the patient's IQ deteriorates. Bone marrow therapy has not been successful in Sanfilippo, Hunter, or Morquio syndromes. Enzyme replacement therapy has been tried on a mild form of iduronidase deficiency, mostly Hurler-Scheie. Treatment has been effective in reducing mucopolysacchariduria and hepatosplenomegaly. The skeletal tissues have not been affected by this treatment. Clinical trials are now underway.[136]

Experiments with gene therapy have not yet reached human clinical trials.[137] Animal studies have been used for this type of therapy and for early stem cell treatment.

MUCOLIPIDOSES

The mucolipidoses are a group of diseases that were once phenotypically confused with the mucopolysaccharidoses. The term mucolipidoses was coined because of combined storage of lipids and mucopolysaccharides in tissues and cells of these patients. There are four mucolipidoses that are considered here.

Sialidosis (Mucolipidosis I)

Sialidosis type I, which is due to neuraminidase deficiency as a specific entity that fit mucolipidosis I, was described by Kelly and Graetz in 1977.[138] These patients have myoclonic seizures and cherry-red spot.[139–140] The age of onset is variable, but visual difficulties, myoclonic seizures, and gait disturbances usually appear in the second decade of life. Eye involvement is usually progressive. Neuraminidase deficiency can be detected in cultured skin fibroblasts. The enzyme is unstable after freeze thawing. Caution should be exercised in assaying this enzyme. There are severe forms of neuraminidase deficiency that have been referred to as pseudo-Hurler syndrome. There is sometimes a distinction of type I and type II, with type I being the more severe form.

Biochemical and Molecular Studies

Neuraminidase and β-galactosidase exist in a protein complex in association with a protective protein.[141] Deficiency of the protective protein/cathepsin A (PPCA) leads to the secondary deficiency of ß-galactosidase and neuraminidase. This is referred to as galactosialidosis or severe form of mucolipidosis I.[142] The protective protein has the enzymatic activity of cathepsin A.[143]

The gene for neuraminidase has been cloned, and mutations have been identified.[144–145]

Galactosialidoses

Another form of neuraminidase deficiency, sialidosis type II, is associated with ß-galactosidase deficiency in addition to sialidase deficiency.[142, 146] Three forms of galactosialidosis have been described. There is a severe form called early infantile galactosialidosis and a mild form called late infantile galactosialidosis. The mildest form is the adult type. The onset of symptoms in most patients is early in life, and babies may be born with hydrops fetalis. These children are coarse and have dysostosis multiplex. Periosteal cloaking and hepatosplenomegaly may be present at birth. Foam cells and vacuolated lymphocytes are found in aspirated bone marrow. The storage material is oligosaccharide with N-acetylneuraminic acid at the nonreducing end. These compounds are excreted in excessive amounts in urine and can be detected using thin-layer chromatography or high-performance liquid chromatography.

Biochemical and Molecular Studies

Galactosidase and neuraminidase make a complex with a protective protein cathepsin A for activity. In sialidosis type II, the deficiency is in the protective protein. The gene for the protective protein was cloned by Galjart et al.[143] Mutations have been identified.[147]

I-Cell Disease (Mucolipidosis II)

In 1967, when cell culture for the study of the mucopolysaccharidoses became available, cultured fibroblasts from patients with I-cell disease were thought to exhibit inclusions typical for Hurler fibroblasts.[147–149] Later it was realized that those fibroblasts represented a different disease. Therefore, the letter *I* was used to indicate *inclusions,* and *I-cell* has become an accepted name for this disease.[150] Studies on the storage material in I-cell disease, thought to be a variant of Hurler syndrome, showed the storage of lipids and mucopolysaccharides in these cells.[6] Subsequent studies showed deficiency of multiple lysosomal enzymes in cultured fibroblasts, whereas the level of these enzymes was high in the culture medium.[151] Serum and urine of patients with I-cell disease also show high levels of lysosomal enzymes. These findings led to an important observation on the recognition site and targeting of lysosomal enzymes. Hickman and Neufeld[152] suggested that in I-cell disease the lysosomal enzymes are synthesized normally but lack a recognition marker that targets these enzymes to lysosomes; therefore they are excreted. Subsequent studies showed that mannose-6-phosphate was the recognition marker that targets lysosomal enzymes to the lysosome.[153] The mannose-6-phosphate is added to lysosomal enzymes by UDP-N-acetylglucosamine: N-acetylglucosaminyl-1-phosphotransferase.[154,155] There are two mucolipidoses associated with this enzyme deficiency: I-cell disease mucolipidosis II, which is the most severe, and mucolipidosis III, which is milder.[156, 157]

Coarse features and severe mental retardation characterize I-cell disease (Fig. 24–11). Radiologic findings are those of dysostosis multiplex, very similar to those found in Hurler syndrome. Usually coarse facial appearance, umbilical hernias, large liver and spleen, kyphoscoliosis, and lumbar gibbus are typical of I-cell disease. These clinical features are seen earlier than in Hurler syndrome. The thorax is usually small, joint movement is restricted, the tongue is large, and there is gingival hyperplasia. Corneal haziness is common. Cardiac involvement includes cardiomegaly and aortic insufficiency.

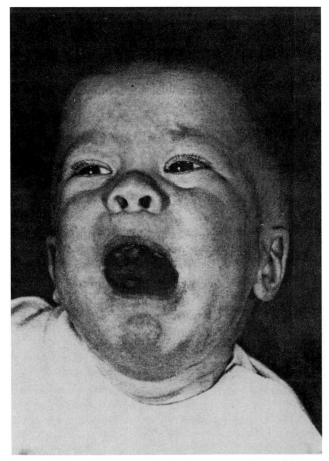

FIGURE 24–11. Patient with I-cell disease who has mild coarse features and gingival hyperplasia.

Usually these children die of cardiopulmonary insufficiency in the first decade of life.

A diagnosis is suggested by the lack of mucopolysacchariduria. Assaying lysosomal enzymes in plasma shows increased activity of lysosomal enzymes. Determining the N-acetylglucosaminyl-1-phosphotransferase should confirm the diagnosis.

Mucolipidosis III

Mucolipidosis III (pseudo-Hurler polydystrophy) is a milder form of mucolipidosis II with a late clinical onset, between 2 and 4 years.[156] Patients with this disease may live to adulthood, and some may not be retarded. Linear growth is severely affected, and they may experience joint stiffness, claw hand deformities, and aortic regurgitation. Coarseness of the face is minimal. Corneal clouding may be associated in some of the patients. Radiologic examination of the skeletal system shows moderate dysostosis multiplex. The enzyme deficiency in mucolipidosis III is a phosphotransferase similar to the one in I-cell disease. The biosynthetic pathway of mannose-6-phosphate, which is essential for lysosomal enzymes, showed that the defect in I-cell disease and mucolipidosis III is identical with the exception that in mucolipidosis III there is more residual activity of this enzyme. In general, there is a spectrum of deficiency level of this enzyme activity. In addition to this primary defect, fibroblasts from patients with mucolipidosis III similar to fibroblasts from I-cell disease show deficiency of a large number of lysosomal enzymes, whereas the culture media contain higher activity of these enzymes. Diagnosis can be made by increased activity of lysosomal enzymes in plasma or urine as well as by the direct assay of the N-acetylphosphotransferase.[156]

Mucolipidosis IV

Mucolipidosis IV is a disease in which the storage material in the fibroblasts is similar to what is observed in I-cell disease.[158] The basic defect has been identified as Mucolipin 1 (MCOLN1).[159] It is localized on the short arm of chromosome 19 (19p13.2-13.3).[160] Mucolipin is a membrane protein, and it is expressed in all tissues. Mutation analysis identified two founder mutations among Ashkenazi Jews.[161] Random blood samples indicated that 1:100 were carriers for this mutation.[162]

Children with mucolipidosis IV clinically share some phenotypic resemblance to other patients with storage diseases. Mucolipidosis IV patients were described with corneal clouding, psychomotor retardation, lack of facial dysmorphism, and no hepatosplenomegaly. Conjunctival biopsy specimens showed storage material within lysosomes, with lamellar configuration similar to those seen in Tay-Sachs disease.[163,164] The majority of these patients were of Ashkenazi Jewish extraction. All patients had striking findings in the conjunctival biopsy, but no dysostosis multiplex or mucopolysacchariduria was observed.

Suggestions of specific neuraminidase deficiency leading to this disease have not been adequately confirmed, and diagnosis relies primarily on the use of conjunctival biopsy.[165–167]

REFERENCES

1. Neufeld EF, Muenzer J: The mucopolysaccharidoses. In Scriver CR, Beaudet AL, Sly WS, Valle D (eds): The Metabolic and Molecular Bases of Inherited Disease (8th ed). New York, McGraw-Hill, 2001, pp 3421–3452.

2. Matalon R, Kaul R, Michals K: The mucopolysaccharidoses and the mucolipidosis. In Duckett S (ed): Pediatric Neuropathology. Baltimore, Williams & Wilkins, 1995, pp 525–544.

3. Matalon R: Mucopolysaccharidoses. In Gershwin ME, Robbins DL (eds): Musculoskeletal Diseases of Children. New York, Grune & Stratton, 1983, pp 381–445.

4. Kjellen L, Lindahl V: The proteoglycans structures and functions. In Richardson CC, Abelson JN, Meister A, Walsh CT (eds): Annual Reviews of Biochemistry. Palo Alto, Annual Reviews, 1991, 443–475.

5. Hof L, Matalon R, Dorfman A: Gangliosides in human skin fibroblasts and their enrichment in the "Hurler variant" and Krabbe's disease. Hoppe-Seylers Z Physiol Chem 1971;352:1329–1337.

6. Matalon R, Cifonelli HA, Zellweger H, Dorfman A: Lipid abnormalities in a variant of the Hurler syndrome. Proc Natl Acad Sci U S A 1968;59: 1097–1102.

7. Hunter C: A rare disease in two brothers. Proc R Soc Med 1917;10:104–116.

8. Hurler G: Uber Einen Type multipler Abortungen, Vorwiegent am Skelet System. Z Kinderheilkd 1919;24:220–234.

9. Ellis RWB, Sheldon W, Capon NB: Gargoylism (chondroosteo-dystrophy, corneal opacities, hepatosplenomegaly, and mental deficiency). Q J Med 1936;5:119–139.

10. Brante G: Gargoylism: A mucopolysaccharidosis. Scand J Clin Lab Invest 1952;4:43–46.

11. Dorfman A, Lorincz AE: Occurrence of acid mucopolysaccharides in the Hurler syndrome. Proc Natl Acad Sci U S A 1957;43:443–446.

12. Van Hoof F, Hers HG: The ultrastructure of hepatic cells in Hurler's disease (gargoylism). CR Hebd Seances Acad Sci (D) 1964;259:1281–1283.

13. Matalon R, Dorfman A: Biosynthesis of acid mucopolysaccharides in tissue culture. Proc Natl Acad Sci U S A 1966;56:1310–1316.

14. Danes BS, Bearn AG: Hurler's syndrome: Demonstration of an inherited disorder of connective tissue in cell culture. Science 1965;149:987–989.

15. Fratantoni JC, Hall CW, Neufeld EF: The defect in Hurler and Hunter's syndromes II: Deficiency of specific factors involved in mucopolysaccharide degradation. Proc Natl Acad Sci U S A 1969;64: 360–366.

16. Fratantoni JC, Hall CW, Neufeld EF: Hurler and Hunter syndromes: Mutual correction of the defect in cultured fibroblasts. Science 1968;162:570–572.

17. Matalon R, Cifonelli JC, Dorfman A: L-iduronidase in cultured human fibroblasts and liver. Biochem Biophys Res Commun 1971;42:340–345.

18. Matalon R, Dorfman A: Hurler's syndrome: Alpha-L-iduronidase deficiency. Biochem Biophys Res Commun 1972;47:959–964.

19. Bach GX, Friedman AX, Weissmann B, Neufeld EF: The defect in the Hurler and Scheie syndromes: Deficiency of alpha-L-iduronidase. Proc Natl Acad Sci U S A 1972;69:2048–2051.

20. Matalon R, Deanching M: The enzymic basis for the phenotypic variation of Hurler and Scheie syndromes. Pediatr Res 1977;11:513.

21. Matalon R, Deanching M, Omura K: Hurler, Scheie and Hurler-Scheie "compound" residual activity of alpha-L-iduronidase toward natural substrates suggesting allelic mutations. J Inher Metab Dis 1983;6: 133–134.

22. Clements PR, Brooks DA, McCourt AG, Hopwood JJ: Immunopurification and characterization of human α-L-iduronidase with the use of monoclonal antibodies. Biochem J 1989;259:199–208.

23. Scott HS, Anson DS, Osborn AM, et al: Human α-L-iduronidase: cDNA isolation and expression. Proc Natl Acad Sci U S A 1991;88:9695–9699.

24. Scott HS, Guo XII, Hopwood JJ, Morris CP: Structure and sequence of human α-L-iduronidase gene. Genomics 1992;13:1311–1313.

25. Scott HS, Ashton IJ, Eyre HJ, et al: Chromosomal localization of the human α-L-iduronidase gene (IDUA) to 4P16.3. Am J Hum Genet 1990;47:802–807.

26. MacDonald ME, Scott HS, Whaley WL, et al: Huntington-disease-linked locus D4Siii exposed as the α-L-iduronidase gene. Somat Cell Mol Genet 1991;17: 421–125.

27. Scott HS, Litjens T, Hopwood JJ, Morris CP: A common mutation for mucopolysaccharidosis type I associated with a severe Hurler syndrome phenotype. Hum Mutat 1992;1:103–108.

28. Scott HS, Litjens T, Nelson PV, et al: Alpha-L-iduronidase mutations (Q70X and P533R) associate with a severe Hurler phenotype. Hum Mutat 1992;1: 333–339.

29. Bunge S, Kleijer WJ, Steglich C, et al: Mucopolysaccharidosis type I: Identification of 8 novel mutations and determination of the frequency of the two common α-L-iduronidase mutations (W402X and Q/0X) among European patients. Hum Mol Genet 1994;3: 861–866.

30. Clarke LA, Nelson PV, Warrington CL, et al: Mutation Analysis of 19 North American mucopolysac-

charidosis type I patients: Identification of two additional frequent mutations. Hum Mutat 1994;3:275–282.

31. Tieu PT, Menon K, Neufeld EF: A mutant stop codon (TAG) in the IDUA gene is used as an acceptor splice site in a patient with Hurler syndrome (MPS IH). Hum Mutat 1994;3:333–336.

32. Scott HS, Litjens T, Nelson PV, et al: Identification of mutations in the alpha-L-iduronidase gene (IDUA) that cause Hurler and Scheie syndromes. Am J Hum Genet 1993;53:973–986.

33. Yamagishi A, Tamatsu S, Fukuda S, et al: Mucopolysaccharidosis type I: Identification of common mutations that cause Hurler and Scheie syndromes in Japanese population. Hum Mutat 1996;7:23–29.

34. Shull RM, Kakkis ED, McEntee MF, et al: Enzyme replacement in a canine model of Hurler syndrome. Proc Natl Acad Sci U S A 1994;91:12937–12941.

35. Schull RM, Bveider MA, Constantopoulos GC: Long term neurological effects of bone marrow transplantation in a canine lysosomal storage disease. Ped Res 1988;24:347–352.

36. Stoltzfus LJ, Uhrhammer N, Sosa-Pineda B, et al: Mucopolysaccharidosis I: Cloning and characterization of cDNA encoding canine α-L-iduronidase. Am J Hum Genet 1990;47:A167.

37. Menon KP, Tieu PT, Neufeld EF: Architecture of the canine IDUA gene and mutation underlying canine mucopolysaccharidosis I. Genomics 1992;14:763–768.

38. Sjoberg I, Fransson LA, Matalon R, Dorfman A: Hunter's syndrome: A deficiency of L-iduronosulfate sulfatase. Biochem Biophys Res Commun 1973;54: 1125–1132.

39. Bach G, Eisenberg F Jr, Cantz M, Neufeld EF. The defect in the Hunter syndrome: Deficiency of sulfoiduronate sulfatase. Proc Natl Acad Sci U S A 1973; 70:2134–2138.

40. Wilson PJ, Suthers GK, Callen DF, et al: Frequent deletions at xq28 indicate genetic heterogeneity in Hunter syndrome. Hum Genet 1991;86:505–508.

41. Flomen RH, Green EP, Green PM, et al: Determination of the organization of coding sequences within the iduronate sulphate sulphatase (IDS) gene. Hum Mol Genet 1993;2:5–10.

42. Wilson PJ, Morris CP, Anson DS, et al: Hunter syndrome: Isolation of an iduronate-2-sulfatase cDNA clone and analysis of patient DNA. Proc Natl Acad Sci U S A 1990;87:8531–8535.

43. Palmieri G, Capra V, Romano G, et al: The iduronate sulfatase gene: Isolation of a 1.2-Mb YAC contig spanning the entire gene and identification of heterogeneous deletions in patients with Hunter syndrome. Genomics 1992;12:52–57.

44. Wraith JE, Cooper A, Thornley M, et al: The clinical phenotype of two patients with a complete deletion of the iduronate-L-sulfatase gene (mucopolysaccharidosis II–Hunter syndrome). Hum Genet 1991;87: 205–206.

45. Wehnert M, Hopwood JJ, Schroder W, Herrmann FH: Structural gene aberrations in mucopolysaccharidosis II (Hunter). Hum Genet 1992;89:430–432.

46. Hopwood JJ, Bunge S, Morris CP, et al: Molecular basis of mucopolysaccharidosis type II: Mutations in the iduronate-2-sulphatase gene. Hum Mutat 1993;2:435–442.

47. Schroder W, Wulff K, Wehnert M, et al: Mutations of the iduronate-2-sulfatase (IDS) gene in patients with Hunter syndrome (mucopolysaccharidosis II). Hum Mutat 1994;4:128–131.

48. Giampietro PF, Haas BR, Matalon R, et al: Fragile X syndrome in two siblings with major congenital malformations. Am J Hum Genet 1994;55:449.

49. Clarke JT, Greer WL, Strasberg PM, et al: Hunter disease (Mucopolysaccharidosis type II) associated with unbalanced inactivation of the X-chromosomes in a karyotypically normal girl. Am J Hum Genet 1991;49:289–297.

50. Schroder W, Petruschka L, Wehnert M, et al: Carrier detection of Hunter syndrome (MPSII) by biochemical and DNA techniques in families at risk. J Med Genet 1993;30:210–213.

51. Gal A, Beck M, Sewell AC, et al: Gene diagnosis and carrier detection in Hunter syndrome by iduronate-2-sulphatase cDNA probe. J Inherit Metab Dis 1992;15:342–346.

52. Matalon R, Dorfman A: The Sanfilippo A syndrome: A sulfamidase deficiency. Pediatr Res 1973;7:156.

53. Matalon R, Dorfman A: Sanfilippo A syndrome: Sulfamidase deficiency in cultured skin fibroblasts and liver. J Clin Invest 1974;54:907–912.

54. O'Brien JS: Sanfilippo syndrome: Profound deficiency of alpha-acetylglycosaminidase activity in organs and skin fibroblasts from type B patients. Proc Natl Acad Sci U S A 1972;69:1720–1722.

55. Kresse H, vonFigura K, Klein U: A new biochemical subtype of the Sanfilippo syndrome: Characterization of the storage material in cultured fibroblasts of Sanfilippo C patients. Eur J Biochem 1978;92:333–339.

56. Ozand PT, Thompson JN, Gascon GG, et al: Sanfilippo Type D with acquired language disorder but without features of mucopolysaccharidosis. J Child Neuro 1994;9:408–411.

57. Kresse H, Paschke E, vonFigura K, et al: Sanfilippo disease type D: Deficiency of N-acetylglucosamine-6-sulfate sulfatase required for heparan sulfate degradation. Proc Natl Acad Sci U S A 1980; 77: 6822–6826.

58. Scott HS, Blanch L, Guo XH, et al: Cloning of the sulphamidase gene and identification of mutations in Sanfilippo A syndrome. Nat Genet 1995;11:465–467.

59. Weber B, Guo XH, Wraith JE, et al: Novel mutations in Sanfilippo A syndrome: Implications for enzyme function. Hum Mol Genet 1997;6:1573–1579.

60. Bunge S, Ince H, Steglich C, et al: Identification of 16 sulfamidase gene mutations including the common R74C in patients with mucopolysaccharidosis type IIIa (Sanfilippo A). Hum Mutat 1997;10:479–485.

61. Di Natale P, Balzano N, Esposito S, et al: Identification of molecular defects in Italian Sanfilippo A patients including 13 novel mutations. Hum Mutat 1998;11:313–320.

62. Montfort M, Vilageliu L, Garcia-Giralt N, et al: Mutation 109delC is highly prevalent in Spanish Sanfilippo syndrome type A patients. Hum Mutat 1998;12:274–279.

63. Rady P, Vu AT, Surendran S, et al: Founder mutation, R245H, of Sanfilippo syndrome A in the Cayman Islands. Genet Test 2002;6:in press.

64. Weber B, Blanch L, Clements PR, et al: Cloning and expression of the gene in Sanfilippo B syndrome (mucopolysaccharidosis III B). Hum Mol Genet 1996;5:771–777.

65. Zhao HG, Li HH, Bach G, et al: The molecular basis of Sanfilippo syndrome type B. Proc Natl Acad Sci U S A 1996;93:6101–6105.

66. Whitley CB: The mucopolysaccharidoses. In Beighton P (ed): McKusick's Heritable Disorders of Connective Tissue (5th ed). St Louis, CV Mosby, 1993, pp 367–499.

67. Schmidtchen A, Greenberg D, Zhao HG, et al: NAGLU mutations underlying Sanfilippo syndrome type B. Am J Hum Genet 1998;62:64–69.

68. Zhao HG, Aronovich EL, Whitley CB: Genotype-phenotype correspondence in Sanfilippo syndrome type B. Am J Hum Genet 1998;62:53–63.

69. Robertson DA, Freeman C, Nelson PV, et al: Human glucosamine-6-sulfatase cDNA reveals homology with steroid sulfatase. Biochem Biophys Res Commun 1988;157:218–224.

70. Robertson DA, Freeman C, Nelson PV, et al: Human glucosamine-6-sulfatase cDNA reveals homology with steroid sulfatase. Biochem Biophys Res Commun 1988;157:218–224.

71. Morquio L: Surune forme de dystrophie osseuse familiale. Bull Soc Pediatr (Paris) 1929;27:145–152.

72. Brailsford JF: Chondro-osteodystrophy: Roentgenographic and clinical features of child with dislocation of vertebrae. Am J Surg 1929;7:404–410.

73. Matalon R, Arbogast B, Justice P, et al: Morquio's syndrome: Deficiency of a chondroitin sulfate N-acetylhexosamine sulfate sulfatase. Biochem Biophys Res Commun 1974;61:759–765.

74. Arbisser AI, Donnell HA, Scott CI Jr, et al: Morquio-like syndrome with beta galactosidase deficiency and normal hexosamine sulfatase activity: Mucopolysaccharidosis IV B. Am J Med Genet 1977;1:195–205.

75. Masuno M, Tomatsu S, Nakashima Y, Hori T: Assignment of the human N-acetylgalactosamine-6-sulfate sulfatase (GALNS) gene to chromosome 16q24. Genomics 1993;16:777–778.

76. Baker E, Guo XH, Orsborn AM, et al: The Morquio A syndrome (Mucopolysaccharidosis IVA) gene maps to 16q24.3. Am J Hum Genet 1993;52: 96–98.

77. Tomatsu SS, Fukuda M, Masue K, et al: Morquio disease: Isolation, characterization and expression of full-length cDNA for human N-acetylgalactosamine-6-sulfate sulfatase. Biochem Biophys Res Commun 1991;181:677–681.

78. Morris CP, Guo XH, Apostolou S, et al: Morquio A syndrome: Cloning, sequence, and structure of the human N-acetylgalactosamine-6-sulfatase (GALNS) gene. Genomics 1994;22:652–654.

79. Nakashima Y, Tomatsu S, Hori T, et al: Mucopolysaccharidosis IV A: Molecular cloning of the human N-acetylgalactosamine-6-sulfate gene (GALNS) and analysis of the 5′-flanking region. Genomics 1994;20:99–104.

80. Tomatsu S, Fukuda S, Uchiyama A, et al: Molecular analysis by Southern blot for the N-acetyl-galactosamine-6-sulphate sulphatase gene causing mucopolysaccharidosis IVA in the Japanese population. J Inher Metab Dis 1994;17:601–605.

81. Ogawa T, Tomatsu S, Fukuda S, et al: Mucopolysaccharidosis IVA: Screening and identification of mutations of the N-acetylgalactosamine-6-sulfate sulfatase gene. Hum Mol Genet 1995;4:341–349.

82. Tomatsu S, Fukuda S, Cooper A, et al: Two new mutations, Q473X and N487S, in a Caucasian patient with mucopolysaccharidosis IVA (Morquio disease). Hum Mutat 1995;6:195–196.

83. Tomatsu S, Fukuda S, Cooper A, et al: Mucopolysaccharidosis type IVA: Identification of six novel mutations among non-Japanese patients. Hum Mol Genet 1995;4:741–743.

84. Fukuda S, Tomatsu S, Cooper A, et al: Mucopolysaccharidosis IVA (Morquio A): Three novel small deletions in the N-acetylgalactosamine-6-sulfate sulfatase gene. Hum Mutat 1996;8:187–190.

85. Tomatsu S, Fukuda S, Cooper A, et al: Mucopolysaccharidosis IVA: Identification of a common missense mutation I113F in the N-acetylgalactosamine-6-sulfate sulfate sulfatase gene. Am J Hum Genet 1995;57: 556–563.

86. Bunge S, Kleijer WJ, Tylki-Szymanska A, et al: Identification of 31 novel mutations in the N-acetylgalactosamine-6-sulfatase gene reveals excessive allelic heterogeneity among patients with Morquio A syndrome. Hum Mutat 1997;10:223–232.

87. Fukuda S, Tomatsu S, Masuno M, et al: Mucopolysaccharidosis IVA: Submicroscopic deletion of 16q24.3 and a novel R386C mutation of N-acetylgalactosamine-6-sulfate sulfatase gene in a classical Morquio disease. Hum Mutat 1996;7:123–134.

88. Yamada N, Fukuda S, Tomatsu S, et al: Molecular heterogeneity in mucopolysaccharidosis IVA in Australia and Northern Ireland: Nine novel mutations including T312S, a common allele that confers a mild phenotype. Hum Mutat 1998;11:202–208.

89. Fukuda S, Tomatsu S, Masue M, et al: Mucopolysaccharidosis type IV A: N-acetyl-galactosamine-6-sulfate sulfatase exonic point mutations in classical Morquio and mild cases. J Clin Invest 1992;90:1049–1053.

90. Tomatsu S, Fukuda S, Ogawa T, et al: A novel splice site mutation in intron 1 of the GALNS gene in a Japanese patient with mucopolysaccharidosis I VA. Hum Mol Genet 1994;3:1427–1428.

91. Tomatsu S, Fukuda S, Cooper A, et al: Mucopolysaccharidosis IVA: Structural gene alterations identified by Southern blot analysis and identification of racial differences. Hum Genet 1995;95:376–381.

92. Oshiwa A, Tsuji A, Nagao Y, et al: Cloning, sequencing and expression of cDNA for human beta-galactosidase. Biochem Biophys Res Commun 1988;157:238–244.

93. Morreau H, Galjart NJ, Gillemans N, et al: Alternative splicing of beta-galactosidase mRNA generates the classic lysosomal enzyme and a beta-galactosidase-related protein. J Biol Chem 1989;264:20655–20663.

94. Oshima A, Yoshida K, Shimmoto M, et al: Human β-galactosidase gene mutations in Morquio B disease. Am J Hum Genet 1991;49:1091–1093.

95. Oshima A, Yoshida K, Itoh K, et al: Intracellular processing and maturation of mutant gene products in hereditary beta-galactosidase deficiency (beta-galactosidosis). Hum Genet 1994;93:109–114.

96. Yoshida K, Oshima A, Shimmoto M, et al: β-Galactosidase gene mutations in GM$_1$-gangliosidase: A common mutation among Japanese adult/chronic cases. Am J Hum Genet 1991;49:435–442.

97. Maroteaux P, Lamy M: La pseudo-polydystrophy de Hurler. Presse Med 1966;74:2889–2892.

98. Matalon R, Arbogast B, Dorfman A: Deficiency of chondroitin sulfate N-acetylgalactosamine-4-sulfate sulfatase in Maroteaux-Lamy syndrome. Biochem Biophys Res Commun 1974;61:1450–1457.

99. Stumpf DA, Austin JH, Crocker AC, LaFrance M: Mucopolysaccharidosis type VI (Maroteaux-Lamy syndrome): Arylsulfatase B deficiency in tissue. Am J Dis Child 1973;126:747–756.

100. Shapira E, Nadler HL: Purification and some properties of soluble human liver arylsulfatase. Arch Biochem Biophys 1975;170:179–187.

101. Schuchman EH, Jackson CE, Desnick RJ: Human arylsulfatase B: MOPAC cloning, nucleotide sequence of a full length cDNA, and regions of amino acid identity with arylsulfatases A and C. Genomics 1990;6:149–158.

102. Peters C, Schmidt B, Rommerskirch W, et al: Phylogenetic conservation of arylsulfatases: cDNA cloning and expression of human arylsulfatase B. J Biol Chem 1990;265:3374–3381.

103. Litgens T, Baker EG, Beckmann KR, et al: Chromosomal localization of ARSB, the gene for human N-acetylgalactosamine-4-sulfatase. Hum Genet 1989;82:67–68.

104. Jackson CE, Yuhki N, Desnick RJ, et al: Feline arylsulfatase B (ARSB): Isolation and expression of the cDNA, comparison with human ARSB, and gene localization to feline chromosome A1. Genomics 1992;14:403–411.

105. Jin WD, Jackson CE, Desnick RJ, Schuchman EH: Mucopolysaccharidosis type VI: Identification of three mutations in the arylsulfatase B gene of patients with the severe and mild phenotypes provides molecular evidence for genetic heterogeneity. Am J Hum Genet 1992;50:795–800.

106. Litgens T, Morris CP, Robertson EF, et al: An N-acetylgalactosamine-4-sulfatase mutation (ΔG_{238}) results in a severe Maroteaux-Lamy phenotype. Hum Mutat 1992;1:397–402.

107. Isbrandt D, Arlt G, Brooks DA, et al: Mucopolysaccharidosis VI (Maroteaux-Lamy syndrome): Six unique arylsulfatase B gene alleles causing variable disease phenotypes. Am J Hum Genet 1994;54:454–463.

108. Wicker G, Prill V, Brooks D, et al: Mucopolysaccharidosis VI (Maroteaux-Lamy syndrome): An intermediate clinical phenotype caused by substitution of valine for glycine at position 137 of arylsulfatase B. J Biol Chem 1991;266:27386–27391.

109. Voskoboeva E, Isbrandt D, vonFigura K, et al: Four novel mutant alleles of the arylsulfatase B gene in two patients with intermediate form of mucopolysaccharidosis VI (Maroteaux-Lamy syndrome). Hum Genet 1994;93:259–264.

110. Sly WS, Quinton BA, McAllister WH, Rimoin DL. Beta-glucuronidase deficiency: Report of clinical radiologic and biochemical features of a new mucopolysaccharidosis. J Pediatr 1973;82:249–257.

111. Matalon R, Macias RV, Diekamp U, et al: Beta-glucuronidase deficiency: A mucopolysaccharidosis with chondroitin sulfaturia. Ped Res 1985;19(4):316.

112. Nishimura Y, Rosenfeld MG, Kriebich G, et al: Nucleotide sequence of rat preputial gland beta-glucuronidase cDNA and in vitro insertion of its encoded polypeptide into microsomal membrane. Proc Natl Acad Sci U S A 1986;83:7292–7296.

113. Oshima A, Kyle JW, Miller RD, et al: Cloning, sequencing and expression of cDNA for human beta-glucuronidase. Proc Natl Acad Sci U S A 1986;84:685–689.

114. Gallaghar PM, D'Amore MA, Lund SD, Ganshow RE: The complete nucleotide sequence of murine beta-glucuronidase mRNA and its deduced polypeptide. Genomics 1988;2:215–219.

115. Powell PP, Kyle JW, Miller RD, et al: Rat liver beta-glucuronidase: cDNA cloning, sequence comparisons and expression of a chimeric protein in COS cells. Biochem J 1988;250:547–555.

116. Miller RD, Hoffmann JW, Powell PP, et al: Cloning and characterization of beta-glucuronidase gene. Genomics 1990;7:280–283.

117. Funkenstein B, Leary SL, Stein JC, Catterall JF: Genomic organization and sequence of the GUS-S alpha allele of the murine beta-glucuronidase gene. Mol Cell Biol 1988;8:1160–1168.

118. Bevilacqua A, Erickson RP: Use of antisense RNA to help identify a genomic clone for 5' region of mouse beta-glucuronidase. Biochem Biophys Res Commun 1989;160:937–941.

119. Chitayat D, McGillivary BC, Wood S, et al: Interstitial 7q deletion (46,xx,del(7) (Pter-q21.1: : q22→ qter) and the location of genes for beta-glucuronidase and cystic fibrosis. Am J Med Genet 1988;31:655–661.

120. Allanson JE, Gemmill RN, Hecht BK, et al: Deletion mapping of beta-glucuronidase gene. Am J Med Genet 1988;29:517–522.

121. Haskins ME, Aguirre GD, Jezyk PE, et al: Mucopolysaccharidosis type VII (Sly syndrome): Beta-glucuronidase deficient mucopolysaccharidosis in the dog. Am J Pathol 1991;138:1553–1555.

122. Birkenmeier EH, Davisson MT, Neamer WG, et al: Murine mucopolysaccharidosis type VII: Characterization of a mouse with beta-glucuronidase deficiency. J Clin Invest 1989;83:1258–1266.

123. Schuchman EH, Toroyan TK, Haskins ME, Desnick RJ. Characterization of the defective ß-glucuronidase activity in canine mucopolysaccharidosis type VII. Enzyme 1989;42:174–180.

124. Gitzelmann R, Bosshard NU, Superti-Furga A, et al: Feline mucopolysaccharidosis VII due to β-glucuronidase deficiency. Vet Pathol. 1994;31:435–443.

125. Tomatsu S, Sukegawa K, Ikedo Y, et al: Molecular basis of mucopolysaccharidosis type VII: Replacement of ala 619 in beta-glucuronidase with val. Gene 1990;89:283–287.

126. Tomatsu S, Fukuda S, Sukegawa K, et al: Mucopolysaccharides type VII: Characterization of mutations and molecular heterogeneity. Am J Hum Gene 1991;48:89–96.

127. Shipley JM, Klinkenberg M, Wu BM, et al: Mutational analysis of a patient with mucopolysaccharidosis type VII, and identification of pseudogenes. Am J Hum Genet 1993;52:517–526.

128. Yamada S, Tomatsu S, Sly WS, et al: Four novel mutations in mucopolysaccharidosis type VII including a unique base substitution in exon 10 of β-glucuronidase gene that creates a novel 5'-splice site. Hum Mol Genet 1995;4:651–655.

129. Wu BM, Sly WS: Mutational studies in a patient with the hydrops fetalis form of mucopolysaccharidosis type VII. Hum Mutat 1993;2:446–457.

130. Kolodny EH, Fluharty AL: Metachromatic leukodystrophy and multiple sulfatase deficiency: Sulfatide liposis. In Scriver CR, Beaudet AL, Sly WS, Valle D (eds): The Metabolic and Molecular Bases of Inherited Disease (7th ed). New York, McGraw-Hill, 1995, pp 2693–2739.

131. Matalon R, Horwitz A, Wappner R, et al: Keratan and heparan sulfaturia: A new mucopolysaccharidosis with N-acetylglucosamine-6-sulfatase deficiency. Pediatr Res 1978;12:453.

132. Matalon R, Wappner R, Deanching M, et al: Keratan and heparan sulfaturia: Mucopolysaccharidosis with an enzyme defect not previously identified. J Inherited Metab Dis 1982;5:57–58.

133. Rommerskirch W, vonFigura K: Multiple sulfatase deficiency: Catalytically inactive sulfatases are expressed from retrovirally introduced sulfatase cDNAs. Proc Natl Acad Sci U S A 1992;89:2561–2565.

134. Hobbs JR, Hugh-Jones K, Barrett JA, et al: Reversal of clinical features of Hurler's disease and biochemical improvement after treatment by bone-marrow transplantation. Lancet 1981;2:709–712.

135. Krivit W, Shapiro EG: Bone marrow transplantation from storage diseases. In Desnick RJ (ed): Treatment of Genetic Diseases. New York, Churchill-Livingstone, 1991, pp 203–221.

136. Kakkis ED, Muenzer J, Tiller GE, et al: Enzyme-replacement therapy in mucopolysaccharidosis I. N Engl J Med 2001;18:182–188.

137. Desnick RJ, Schuchman EH: Human gene therapy: Strategies and prospects for inborn errors of metabolism. In Desnick RJ (ed): Treatment of Genetic Diseases. New York, Churchill-Livingstone, 1991, pp 239–259.

138. Kelly TE, Graetz G: Isolated acid neuraminidase deficiency: A distinct lysosomal storage disease. Am J Med Genet 1977;1:31–46.

139. Spranger JW, Gehler J, Cantz M: Mucolipidosis I: A sialidosis. Am J Med Genet 1977;1:21–29.

140. Durand P, Gatti R, Cavalieri S, et al: Sialidosis (mucolipidosis I). Helv Paediat Acta 1977;32: 391–400.

141. Hoogeveen AT, Verheijen FW, Galjaard H: The relation between human lysosomal beta-galactosidase and its protective protein. J Biol Chem 1983;258: 12143–12146.

142. Andria G, Del Giudice E, Reuser AJJ: Atypical expression of beta-galactosidase deficiency in a child with Hurler-Like features but without neurological abnormalities. Clin Genet 1978;14:16–23.

143. Galjart NJ, Gillemans N, Harris A, et al: Expression of cDNA encoding the human "protective protein" associated with lysosomal beta-galactosidase and neuraminidase: Homology to yeast protease. Cell 1988;54:755–764.

144. Bonten E, van der Spoel AV, Fornerod M, et al: Characterization of human lysosomal neuraminidase defines the molecular basis of the metabolic storage disorder sialidosis. Genes Dev 1996;10:3156–3159.

145. Pshezhetsky AV, Richard C, Michaud L, et al: Cloning, expression and chromosomal mapping of

human lysosomal sialidase and characterization of mutations in sialidosis. Nat Genet 1997;15:316–320.

146. Wenger DA, Tarby TJ, Wharton C: Macular cherry-red spots and myoclonus with dementia: Coexistent neuraminidase and beta-galactosidase deficiencies. Biochem Biophys Res Commun 1978;82: 589–595.

147. Zhou XY, van der Spoel A, Rottier R, et al: Molecular and biochemical analysis of protective protein/cathepsin A mutations: Correlation with clinical severity in galactosialidosis. Hum Mol Genet 1996;5:1977–1987.

148. DeMars R, Leroy JG: The remarkable cells cultured from a human with Hurler's syndrome: An approach to visual selection for in vitro genetic studies. In Vitro 1967;2:107.

149. Leroy JG, DeMars RI: Mutant enzymatic and cytological phenotypes in cultured human fibroblasts. Science 1967;157:804–806.

150. Leroy JG, Spranger JW, Feingold M, et al: I-cell disease: A clinical picture. J Pediatr 1971;79:360–365.

151. Wiesmann UN, Lightbody J, Vassella F, Herschkowitz NN: Multiple lysosomal enzyme deficiency due to leakage? N Engl J Med 1971;284:109–110.

152. Hickman S, Neufeld EF: Hypothesis for I-cell disease: Defective hydrolases that do not enter lysosomes. Biochem Biophys Res Commun 1972;49:992–999.

153. Sly WS, Fischer HD: The phosphomannosyl recognition systems for intracellular and intercellular transport of lysosomal enzymes. J Cell Biochem 1982;18:67–85.

154. Hasilik A, Waheed A, vonFigura K: Enzymatic phosphorylation of lysosomal enzymes in the presence of UDP-N-acetylglucosamine. Absence of the activity in I-cell fibroblasts. Biochem Biophys Res Commun 1981;98:761–767.

155. Reitman ML, Varki A, Kornfeld S: Fibroblasts from patients with I-cell disease and pseudo-Hurler polydystrophy are deficient in uridine-5-diphosphate-N-acetylglucosamine-glycoprotein N-acetylglucosaminyl-phosphotransferase activity. J Clin Invest 1981;67: 1574–1579.

156. Varki AP, Reitman ML, Kornfeld S: Identification of a variant of mucolipidosis III (pseudo Hurler Polydystrophy): A catalytically active N-acetyl-glucosaminylphosphotransferase that fails to phosphorylate lysosomal enzymes. Proc Natl Acad Sci U S A 1981; 78:7773–7777.

157. Kornfeld S, Sly WS: I-Cell disease and pseudo-Hurler polydystrophy: Disorders of lysosomal enzyme phosphorylation and localization. In Scriver CR, Beaudet AL, Sly WS, Valle D (eds): The Metabolic and Molecular Bases of Inherited Disease (7th ed). New York, McGraw-Hill, 1995, pp 2495–2508.

158. Amir N, Zlotogora J, Bach G: Mucolipidosis type IV: Clinical spectrum and natural history. Pediatrics 1987;79:953–959.

159. Bargal R, Avidan N, Ben Asher E, et al: Identification of the gene causing mucolipidosis type IV. Nat Genet 2000;26:118–123.

160. Sun M, Goldin E, Stahl S, et al: Mucolipidosis type IV is caused by mutations in a gene encoding a novel transient receptor potential channel. Hum Mol Genet 2000;9:2471–2478.

161. Bach G: Mucolipidosis type IV. Mol Genet Metab 2001;73:197–203.

162. Edelmann L, Dong J, Desnick RJ, et al: Mucolipidosis type IV in the American Ashkenazi Jewish population. Am J Hum Genet 2002;70:4.

163. Newell FW, Matalon R, Mayer S: A new mucolipidosis with psychomotor retardation, corneal clouding, and retinal degeneration. Am J Ophthal 1975; 80:440–449.

164. Merin S, Livni N, Berman ER, Yatziv S: Mucolipidosis IV: Ocular, systemic, and ultrastructural findings. Invest Ophthal 1975;14:437–448.

165. Bach G, Ziegler M, Schaap T, Kohn G: Mucolipidosis type IV: Ganglioside sialidase deficiency. Biochem Biophys Res Commun 1979;90:1341–1347.

166. Ben-Yoseph Y, Momoi T, Hahn LC, Nadler HL: Catalytically defective ganglioside neuraminidase in mucolipidosis IV. Clin Genet 1982;21:374–381.

167. Kiedel KG, Zwaan J, Kenyon KR, et al: Ocular abnormalities in mucolipidosis IV. Am J Ophthal 1985;99:125–136.

CHAPTER

25

Disorders of Glycoprotein Degradation: Sialidosis, Fucosidosis, Alpha-Mannosidosis, Beta-Mannosidosis, and Aspartylglycosaminuria

William G. Johnson

Disorders of glycoprotein degradation were originally recognized as having some clinical resemblance to Hurler syndrome but lacking mucopolysacchariduria. Spranger and Wiedemann in 1970 included these patients in the category of mucolipidosis, a somewhat heterogeneous category of disorders with storage of acid mucopolysaccharides, sphingolipids, or glycolipids in visceral and mesenchymal cells and with storage of abnormal amounts of sphingolipids or glycolipids in neural tissue. The mucolipidoses originally included GM1 gangliosidosis, fucosidosis, α-mannosidosis, juvenile sulfatidosis—Austin type (now known as mucosulfatidosis), mucolipidosis I (lipomucopolysaccharidosis, now known as sialidosis type II), mucolipidosis II (I-cell disease), and mucolipidosis III (pseudopolydystrophy). Disorders of glycoprotein degradation have also been included in the category of oligosaccharidoses because they have excessive urinary excretion of oligosaccharides or glycopeptides. This is the basis of useful diagnostic screening tests. Urinary oligosaccharides can be measured by high-performance liquid chromatography, by the simpler and less expensive thin-layer chromatography, or by other methods. Using these methods, abnormal urinary oligosaccharides are found in all disorders discussed in this chapter. In addition, the patterns of oligosaccharides differ from disorder to disorder. The diagnosis is confirmed by assay of the appropriate lysosomal hydrolase enzyme in leukocytes, cultured skin fibroblasts, and, in some cases, serum. Because oligosacchariduria may occasionally be absent, however, enzymatic testing should be carried out when these disorders are suspected. All of these disorders are inherited in the autosomal recessive pattern. There is no specific therapy, but bone marrow transplant has been carried out for a number of lysosomal disorders including fucosidosis, mannosidosis, and aspartylglucosaminuria and is reported to prolong survival for some patients. In 2001, Arvio et al. reported on the status of five patients with aspartylglycosaminuria who received successful bone marrow transplants and advised against this procedure for patients after infancy.

BIOSYNTHESIS AND BIODEGRADATION OF GLYCOPROTEINS

Glycoproteins consist of oligosaccharide chains attached to a protein core. The proteins are synthesized on polysomes in rough endoplasmic reticulum. Oligosaccharide chains are added as the polypeptides pass through smooth endoplasmic reticulum to the Golgi apparatus. Two types of oligosaccharide chains are made there: the N-glycosidic type (Figs. 25–1 and 25–2), which consists of substrates for the enzymes deficient in the diseases discussed in this chapter, and the O-glycosidic type, consisting mostly of those not involved in these diseases. The O-glycosidic linkage connects an N-acetylgalactosaminide moiety at the reducing end of the oligosaccharide chain through an O-glycosidic linkage to a serine or threonine residue of the polypeptide chain. These oligosaccharides are synthesized by sequential transfer of single sugar moieties from sugar-nucleotide intermediates to the end of a growing oligosaccharide chain. The

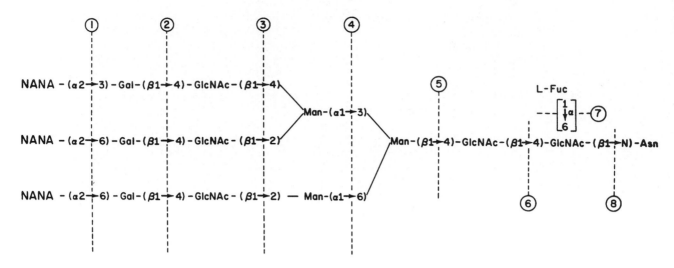

FIGURE 25–1. Structure of a complex-type triantennary oligosaccharide chain of an asparagine-linked glycoprotein consisting of asparagine, neutral sugars, hexosamine, and sialic acid. The mannose-6-phosphate recognition marker is formed by transfer of GlcNAc-1-P to the 6 hydroxyl groups of the α-linked mannose residues and the subsequent removal of the phosphate-linked GlcNAc residues. The numbers in circles indicate points of cleavage of lysosomal acid hydrolase enzymes that catabolize the oligosaccharide chain. Asn, asparagine; Gal, galactose; GlcNAc, N-acetylglucosamine; L-Fuc, L-fucose; Man, mannose; NANA, N-acetylneuraminic acid; 1 = glycoprotein sialidase; 2 = β-galactosidase; 3 = hexosaminidases A and B; 4 = α-mannosidase; 5 = β-mannosidase; 6 = endo-β-N-acetylglucosaminidase; 7 = α-L-fucosidase; 8 = aspartylglucosaminidase.

N-glycosidic linkage connects an N-acetylgalactosaminide moiety at the reducing end of the oligosaccharide chain through an N-glycosidic linkage to an asparagine residue of the polypeptide chain. These oligosaccharides are synthesized through the dolichol pathway.[1] A complex oligosaccharide intermediate attached to a lipid moiety, dolichol phosphate, is transferred to an N-glycosidic linkage with an asparagine residue of the polypeptide chain. Complex trimming and elongation to give the final N-glycosidic oligosaccharide then remodel this oligosaccharide chain. Two basic types of N-glycosidic oligosaccharide are important as sub-

strates for the diseases in this chapter: the complex-type oligosaccharides (see Fig. 25–1) and the high-mannose–type oligosaccharides (see Fig. 25–2). The high-mannose–type oligosaccharide chain is an intermediate in the synthesis of the complex-type oligosaccharide chain.[1]

Various lysosomal enzymes degrade N-glycosidic asparagine-linked glycoproteins sequentially (see Figs. 25–1 and 25–2 and Table 25–1). The polypeptide is catabolized by a variety of lysosomal peptidases. Sialic acid residues and α-L-fucoside residues occur only as terminal moieties and are removed by α-L-N-acetylneu-

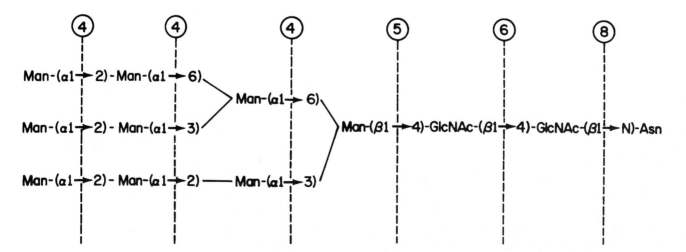

FIGURE 25–2. Structure of a high-mannose–type triantennary oligosaccharide chain of an asparagine-linked glycoprotein. This structure is an intermediate in the synthesis of the complex-type oligosaccharide chain (see Fig. 25–1). The components and enzyme cleavage points are numbered as in Figure 25–1.

TABLE 25–1. Genetic Features of Glycoprotein Degradation Disorders

Disease	Deficient Enzyme	Gene Symbol	Gene Locus (Human Chromosome and Band Number)
Sialidosis	α–L-N-Acetylneuraminidase	NEU, NEU1	Chromosome 6 (6p21.3)
Fucosidosis	α–L-Fucosidase	FUCA1	Chromosome 1 (1p34)
α–Mannosidosis	α–Mannosidase	MANB, MAN2B1	Chromosome 19 (19cen–q12)
β–Mannosidosis	β–Mannosidase	MANB1	Chromosome 4 (4q22-q25)
Aspartylglucosaminuria	Aspartylglucosaminidase	AGA	Chromosome 4 (4q23–q27)

raminidase, often called sialidase (see Fig. 25–1, reaction 1), and β-L-fucosidase (see Fig. 25–1, reaction 7). Acting next in sequence are β-galactosidase (see Fig. 25–1, reaction 2), hexosaminidases A and B (see Fig. 25–1, reaction 3), α-mannosidase (see Figs. 25–1 and 25–2, reaction 4), and β-mannosidase (see Figs. 25–1 and 25–2, reaction 5). All of these enzymes are exoglycosidases, that is, they remove a single sugar only when it is the terminal residue at the nonreducing end of the oligosaccharide chain. Endo-β-N-acetylglucosaminidase (see Figs. 25–1 and 25–2, reaction 6) cleaves the chitobiose linkage between two internal β-N-acetylglucosaminide residues. This enzyme, an endoglycosidase, can cleave in the middle of the oligosaccharide chain, thus removing the bulk of the oligosaccharide from the protein core. This can be an early step in glycoprotein catabolism. Finally, lysosomal aspartylglucosaminidase (see Figs. 25–1 and 25–2, reaction 8) cleaves the N-glycosidic bond linking β-N-acetylglucosamine to the asparagine residue of the peptide.

Besides peptide-linked oligosaccharides, the oligosaccharide portions of some glycolipids are substrates for α-L-fucosidase. Consequently, lipids along with oligosaccharides and glycopeptides are stored in fucosidosis.

SIALIDOSIS

History

This discussion focuses on the true sialidoses. These are genetic disorders in which damage to the gene for glycoprotein sialidase, an α-L-N-acetylneuraminidase, results in decreased activity of the enzyme. Patients with this enzyme deficiency were first described under the diagnosis of lipomucopolysaccharidosis and later placed in the category mucolipidosis I before the enzyme deficiency was found.

The true sialidoses, or isolated sialidoses, in which glycoprotein sialidase alone is deficient, have been divided into two groups[2,3]: the nondysmorphic group (sialidosis type I, also known as cherry-red spot–myoclonus syndrome) and the dysmorphic group (sialidosis type II, which includes mucolipidosis I).

Clinical Picture

Sialidosis Type I: Cherry-Red Spot–Myoclonus Syndrome

Onset of this striking disorder characteristically is between ages 8 and 15 years with myoclonus or decreasing visual acuity. There appears to be a predilection for Italian patients,[2] although patients of various backgrounds, including Japanese, German, Czech, and Saudi Arabian, have been described.

Action myoclonus develops, beginning in the limbs, and becomes increasingly debilitating. Patients may become unable to walk or stand and become bedridden. Cherry-red spots are found on funduscopy. Corneas are clear, but punctate lens opacities or lamellar cataracts may be seen. Grand mal seizures may occur. Hyperactive tendon reflexes may be found. Burning pain in the limbs, which is worse in hot weather, is reminiscent of that occurring in Fabry disease. Intelligence is usually normal but is occasionally impaired. Cerebellar ataxia may be present. Renal impairment is not a feature of this disorder, but severe renal involvement has occurred in two siblings with otherwise typical cherry-red spot–myoclonus syndrome. Coarse facial features, organ enlargement, and skeletal dysplasia are not features of this disorder. The cherry-red spot may disappear in the course of the disease. Consequently, absence of cherry-red spot is not grounds for excluding this diagnosis. Although there is no treatment for the underlying disorder, 5-hydroxytryptophan has been reported to cause dramatic or mild improvement of the action myoclonus.

Sialidosis Type II

Patients with deficiency of glycoprotein sialidase, without deficiency of β-galactosidase, and with clinical features of somatic dysmorphism (facial dysmorphism, skeletal dysmorphism, and organ enlargement) fall into the category of type II sialidosis.[2] There are various clinical phenotypes with onset at birth, in childhood, or later.

Congenital Sialidosis. This is the most severe form of sialidosis known and, in fact, the most severe phenotype of lysosomal disease. Affected neonates are born prematurely and have the clinical appearance of hydrops fetalis. They may be stillborn or may survive 1 to 3 months and perhaps longer. At birth, they are plethoric, hypotonic, and depressed, with generalized skin edema, ascites, hepatosplenomegaly, puffy face and eyelids, and a prominent telangiectatic skin rash. Seizures may occur, and neurologic development is arrested. The disorder is uncommon but not rare.

Because Rh-incompatibility is largely being prevented, it is no longer the most common cause of hydrops fetalis. Although there are many causes of the hydrops fetalis phenotype, metabolic disorders should be considered when such patients are seen. Gaucher disease type II, galactosialidosis, GM1-gangliosidosis, mucopolysaccharidosis types IVA and VII, Niemann-Pick type C, Farber disease, mucolipidosis II (I-cell disease), and infantile free sialic storage disease have all been found to produce this phenotype.

There is some resemblance to patients reported as having congenital lipidosis or congenital lipidosis of Norman and Wood in whom the biochemical defect was never defined.

Severe Infantile Sialidosis. Patients described as having severe infantile sialidosis show many similarities to patients with congenital sialidosis, but they survive into the second year. These patients have congenital ascites, progressive organomegaly, slowed neurologic development, and progressive renal disease in the second year. This phenotype lacks features present in congenital sialidosis including premature birth, anasarca, skin telangiectasis, vascular abnormalities, optic atrophy, and seizures. Sialidase levels were markedly decreased, and sialic acid content increased in fibroblast sonicates. It is not clear whether severe infantile sialidosis and congenital sialidosis are different manifestations of the same phenotype or different phenotypes. The same problem is seen if severe infantile sialidosis is compared with nephrosialidosis.

Nephrosialidosis. Nephrosialidosis was defined in studies that focused on the renal component of this disorder. These cases appear to have a milder phenotype than congenital sialidosis or severe infantile sialidosis. Infants come to medical attention at ages 4 to 6 months because of hernias, hepatosplenomegaly, facial dysmorphism, and psychomotor retardation. Late in the course, the patient develops severe progressive renal disease with proteinuria and cherry-red spot and fine corneal opacities. On autopsy at age 4½ years, one patient had storage in renal glomeruli and sympathetic ganglia. This was thought to distinguish nephrosialidosis from other sialidoses. The same findings, however, are seen in patients described as having severe infantile sialidosis or congenital sialidosis.

Mucolipidosis I (Lipomucopolysaccharidosis). The term *mucolipidosis I* is used for the forms of sialidosis

that may be noted in infancy but are more slowly progressive and are usually diagnosed in the juvenile period. This disorder was originally defined clinically, and some suspected cases turned out to be α-mannosidosis. The disorder was also termed GAL+ disease in the earlier literature because the lysosomal enzyme β-galactosidase was elevated. The term *mucolipidosis I,* however, now appropriately applies only to patients with the characteristic phenotype and sialidase deficiency without β-galactosidase deficiency.

These patients develop normally for the first 6 months, but motor development slows and mental delay is seen. Somatic abnormalities appear in the second or third year but are milder than those in Hurler syndrome. These include short trunk, sometimes with spinal deformity; relatively long limbs; mild coarsening of facial features; mild restriction of joint mobility; and inconsistent enlargement of liver and spleen. Impaired hearing, corneal opacity, and macular cherry-red spots are usually seen, and growth disturbance is common. Neurologic findings include slowly progressive gait ataxia, tremor, cerebellar signs, myoclonic jerks, hypotonia, muscle wasting, peripheral neuropathy, and seizures.

Laboratory Findings

Diagnosis is by the presence of abnormal sialo-oligosaccharides in the urine and demonstration of deficiency in glycoprotein sialidase activity in cultured skin fibroblasts, tissue, leukocytes, amniotic fluid cells, or chorionic villus samples. Patients do not have mucopolysacchariduria, and the amount of urinary uronic acid excretion is comparable to that of controls. Rectal biopsy is a useful confirmatory test because the stored material is visible on ultrastructure of rectal ganglion cells.

Roentgenographic Picture

Roentgenographic changes in mucolipidosis I are characteristically mild to moderate dysostosis multiplex. Kyphoscoliosis and hypoplastic odontoid have been described.

Pathologic Findings

On pathologic examination of cherry-red spot–myoclonus syndrome, the brain stem and spinal cord contain swollen, periodic acid-Schiff (PAS)-positive neurons. PAS-positive material was also seen in the nervous system in swollen dendrites of Purkinje cells, in Bergmann glia, in capillary endothelium, and in macrophages. PAS-positive material was also seen outside the nervous system. Electron microscopy showed atypical membranous cytoplasmic bodies.

Autopsy of a case of congenital sialidosis showed zebra bodies in the neurons of the spinal cord only. Neurons in the cerebral cortex and cerebellar cortex and autonomic ganglion cells showed only membrane-bound vacuoles but no membranous cytoplasmic bodies. Vacuolated cells were also found in the periphery: hepatocytes, endothelial cells, and Kupffer cells in the liver and glomerular and tubular epithelial cells in the kidney.

Vacuolated lymphocytes were plentiful on the peripheral smear, and vacuolated histiocytes were seen in the bone marrow. Foam cells were seen in large numbers in multiple tissues and in the placenta. Fibroblasts contained numerous vacuoles and whorled membranous structures on electron microscopy, although they appeared normal by high microscopy.

Ultrastructural study of cultured skin fibroblasts in sialidosis showed vacuolar inclusions of low electron density similar to those in α-mannosidosis and the mucopolysaccharidoses. A few myelin-like figures were seen. An unusual type of large round membrane-bound inclusion with many concentrically arranged tubules in a fine reticulogranular matrix was also seen.

The findings in nephrosialidosis by light and electron microscopy have been reported.

Stored Substances in the Sialidoses

Sialic acid content is increased in tissue. In one study of autopsy tissue, water-soluble-bound sialic acid was increased between 10-fold and 17-fold in visceral organs but only about 2-fold in brain. Lipid-bound sialic acid was increased up to eightfold in visceral organs but was not elevated in brain. The increase in viscera resulted from elevated amounts of GD4 and probable GM4 and LM1. This pattern of accumulation supported the idea that ganglioside accumulation in the sialidoses was a secondary phenomenon, perhaps induced by inhibition of a ganglioside sialidase by substances stored because of the primary sialidase deficiency. Gangliosides such as GM3 and GD1a, which contain only $\alpha(2\rightarrow3)$-linked sialic acid moieties, are apparently not substrates for glycoprotein sialidase but are cleaved by a different enzyme.

Substrates for glycoprotein sialidase include sialyloligosaccharides containing terminal $\alpha(2\rightarrow6)$-linked or $\alpha(2\rightarrow3)$-linked sialic acid residues. Sialyloligosaccharides containing these linkages have been found in urine and cultured fibroblasts. Urinary glycopeptides have also been found.

Enzyme Deficiency in the Sialidoses

Lysosomal sialidase activity (see Fig. 25–1, reaction 1), or α-L-N-acetylneuraminidase activity, is markedly deficient in both type I and type II sialidoses. Because sialic acid is N-acetylneuraminic acid, sialidase is properly equated with α-N-acetylneuraminidase, although the terms *sialidase* and *neuraminidase* are often used interchangeably. The sialidase deficient in the sialidoses appears to cleave both

$\alpha(2\rightarrow6)$-linked and $\alpha(2\rightarrow3)$-linked sialyloligosaccharides. Because 80% of the accumulating sialyloligosaccharides have the $\alpha(2\rightarrow6)$-linkage, it has been suggested that the mutant enzyme retains greater residual activity for $\alpha(2\rightarrow3)$-linkages. Carrier detection and prenatal diagnosis are possible in this disorder.

The Alpha-L-N-Acetylneuraminidase Gene

There are three distinct genetic classes of disorders in which glycoprotein sialidase activity is deficient. In the first group, discussed in this chapter, glycoprotein sialidase alone is deficient. These disorders, the sialidoses proper, or isolated sialidase deficiencies, result from mutations of *NEU*, the structural gene for glycoprotein sialidase that has been localized to chromosome 6 (6p21.3). In the second group, both glycoprotein sialidase activity and β-galactosidase (GM1 ganglioside β-galactosidase) activity are secondarily deficient owing to primary deficiency of a protective protein, which is required for activity of both enzymes and which is coded by a gene on chromosome 20 (see Fig. 25–1, reaction 2). This protective protein has cathepsin A–like activity, which is distinct from its protective function and appears to be present in the lysosome bound to β-galactosidase and sialidase in a multienzymic complex.[4] There is evidence that the protective protein is identical to a multifunctional protein with esterase/deamidase/carboxypeptidase activities. Another name for this protein is PPCA (protective protein/cathepsin A). This group of disorders is referred to as galactosialidosis. In the third type, sialidase and multiple lysosomal enzymes are decreased owing to deficient post-translational modification. This is the case in mucolipidosis types II and III.

Now that the glycoprotein sialidase gene has been cloned, specific mutations of the gene are being reported. Most reported mutations are missense mutations. Frameshift mutations, a nonsense mutation, and a splice donor site mutation have also been reported. In 2001, Lukong et al reported mutations that interfered with binding of sialidase to its multienzyme complex.[5] In 2000, Bonten et al classified mutations into three groups according to whether the resulting enzyme protein was catalytically active or inactive and whether it was localized in the lysosome.[6]

FUCOSIDOSIS

History

The first case of fucosidosis was described in 1966 by Durand et al, who later documented the presence of fucose-rich storage material in multiple organs. In 1968, Van Hoof and Hers found the cause of the disorder and documented absence of α-L-fucosidase activity.

Clinical Picture

Patients with fucosidosis differ greatly in the kind of clinical involvement and the severity of their illness. Some patients (type I) present with severe, progressive neurologic disorder. Others with milder disease (type II) resemble the Hurler phenotype. Some patients have survived into the second, third, or fourth decade. Usually, however, they become symptomatic in childhood. Some authors refer to these adult cases as type II, whereas others recognize a type III. Types I and II may appear in the same family.

In severely affected infants (type I), symptoms develop in the first year of life with psychomotor retardation and hypotonia. Patients then develop hypertonia, and, later in the course, spasticity, tremor, and mental deterioration leading to loss of contact with their environment. Dystonia has been reported. Patients have thick skin and excessive sweating and may lose gallbladder function. They have only mild facial coarsening, radiographic bone changes, and organ enlargement. Cardiac enlargement may occur. Some patients die at age 4 or 5 years. Others (with type II) have onset of symptoms in the second year of life with more markedly coarsened facial features and greater resemblance to Hurler syndrome. These patients also deteriorate mentally and die around age 5 years. Other patients with infantile or juvenile onset have a milder course, with coarsened facial features, skeletal changes, and dwarfing; skin changes resembling the angiokeratoma of Fabry disease; and survival into the third decade. Angiokeratoma is characteristic of patients with longer survival. Besides Fabry disease and fucosidosis, angiokeratoma corporis diffusum has also been reported in sialidosis, α-mannosidosis, β-mannosidosis, aspartylglucosaminuria, galactosialidosis, and other disorders. Recurrent respiratory infections may occur.

In a review of 77 patients, Willems et al[7] did not find evidence for a rapidly progressive type I and slowly progressive type II fucosidosis, but found a wide continuous clinical spectrum. They tabulated the percentage of cases with various clinical signs and symptoms: progressive mental deterioration (95%), motor deterioration (87%), coarse facies (79%), growth retardation (78%), recurrent infections (78%), dysostosis multiplex (58%), angiokeratoma corporis diffusum (52%), visceromegaly (44%), and seizures (38%).

Laboratory Findings

All of these phenotypes have marked deficiency of the lysosomal enzyme α-L-fucosidase. Diagnosis requires a high index of suspicion because of the diverse clinical pictures. Abnormal urinary oligosaccharides are present in characteristic pattern.

Diagnosis is by finding abnormal oligosaccharides in urine and demonstration of severely decreased α-L-fucosidase in serum, leukocytes, and cultured skin fibro-

blasts. Residual fucosidase in occasional unusual patients may be 60% of control values but with heat-labile enzyme. Therefore, it is important to analyze urine for oligosaccharides because otherwise these patients may be missed. On the other hand, false-positive diagnosis of fucosidosis was made in a patient with pseudohypoparathyroidism because serum and fibroblast α-fucosidase activity was about 10% of control values.

It is important to realize that 6% to 11% of the normal population have a polymorphism in which serum α-L-fucosidase but not leukocyte α-L-fucosidase is markedly decreased to less than 10% of the mean value in controls. Therefore, serum and plasma by themselves are not suitable for enzymatic diagnosis of fucosidosis.

Roentgenographic Picture

Roentgenographic changes are those of a mild dysostosis multiplex but are most marked in the pelvis, hips, and spine. These are not in themselves diagnostic but should point the way to more specific studies. Imaging abnormalities have been reported in thalamus, globus pallidus, internal capsule, and supratentorial white matter.[8]

Pathologic Findings

Rectal biopsy specimens have been found to contain three kinds of inclusions in vascular endothelial cells: clear vacuoles, dark vacuoles, and mixed vacuoles. Clear vacuoles and dark vacuoles appeared to contain fucosyloligosaccharides, and the presence of these two types together has been considered pathognomonic of fucosidosis. Lectin histochemistry on paraffin-embedded tissue sections can distinguish between α-mannosidosis, β-mannosidosis, fucosidosis, and sialidosis. Fucosidosis tissue stained with UEA-I, whereas the others did not.

Stored Substances in Alpha-L-Fucosidosis

Fucose residues form part of the structure of oligosaccharides, glycoproteins, glycolipids, and keratan sulfate. α-L-Fucoside residues occur in both N-glycosidic and O-glycosidic types of glycoproteins. Like α-L-N-acetylneuraminic acid residues, α-L-fucoside residues are usually located at the terminal nonreducing position in an oligosaccharide chain.

In fucosidosis, oligosaccharides, glycopeptides, glycolipids, and keratan sulfate may be stored. In brain, the main stored material is oligosaccharide, chiefly the decasaccharide Fuc-$\alpha(1{\rightarrow}2)$-Gal-$\beta(1{\rightarrow}4)$-GlcNAc-$\beta(1{\rightarrow}2)$-Man-[Fuc-$\beta(1{\rightarrow}2)$-Gal-$\beta(1{\rightarrow}4)$-GlcNAc-$\beta(1{\rightarrow}2)$-Man-]$\alpha(1{\rightarrow}3/6)$-Man-$\beta(1{\rightarrow}4)$-GlcNAc, and the disaccharide Fuc-$\alpha(1{\rightarrow}6)$-GlcNAc. Oligosaccharides are stored in other viscera also. In liver, the glycolipid Fuc-$\alpha(1{\rightarrow}2)$-Gal-$\beta(1{\rightarrow}3)$-GlcNAc-$\beta(1{\rightarrow}4)$-Gal-$\beta(1{\rightarrow}4)$-Glc-ceramide is stored and has H-antigen specificity. Because α-L-fucoside residues are important components of blood group antigens, the red cells and body fluids of patients with fucosidosis contain increased amounts of blood group–specific compounds as well as abnormal blood group phenotypes. In the urine, a large number of fucose-containing oligosaccharides and glycopeptides of the N-glycosidic type have been recovered.

Enzyme Deficiency in Fucosidosis

In patients with fucosidosis, the lysosomal enzyme, α-L-fucosidase, is deficient in serum, leukocytes, and cultured skin fibroblasts. The normal enzyme is a tetramer consisting of 50-kd subunits, which are processed from a 53-kd precursor. The enzyme is subject to post-translational processing, and abnormalities of processing have been found in patients with fucosidosis. Eleven patients with severe fucosidase deficiency usually synthesized no precursor, but two synthesized a precursor that was not processed and one synthesized small amounts of cross-reacting material.

Approximately 6% to 7% of healthy unaffected individuals have markedly low α-L-fucosidase in serum, but leukocyte and tissue values are within normal limits and they do not have fucosidosis. This trait for low serum fucosidase levels is inherited in mendelian fashion and is governed by a gene locus on chromosome 6.

The Alpha-L-Fucosidase Gene

The α-L-fucosidase gene (structural gene *FUCA1*) has been mapped to human chromosome 1 (1p34-p36). The gene has been cloned and sequenced.[9] Two restriction fragment length polymorphisms have allowed demonstration of genetic linkage between fucosidosis and its structural gene. Willems et al reviewed 22 mutations detected in fucosidosis.[10] These mutations included missense mutation, large and small deletions, an insertion, a deletion, a splice site mutation, and stop codon mutations. It was not clear how these mutations resulted in the different fucosidosis phenotypes, because all appeared to result in nearly total enzyme activity loss. The gene coding for the quantitative polymorphism of serum α-L-fucosidase occurring in normal individuals has been mapped to chromosome 6. An α-L-fucosidase pseudogene, *FUCA1P*, has been mapped to chromosome 2.

Fucosidosis in Other Species

Fucosidosis has been found in dogs. Bone marrow transplant in canine fucosidosis was not reported to have any beneficial clinical effect and was later reported to show improvement in neurologic signs and tissue storage. Cloned human cDNA encoding for human α-L-fucosidase has been successfully inserted into canine hematopoietic cells using retroviral vectors, and this model may become useful for assessing the effectiveness of gene therapy. α-L-Fucosidase has been studied in a number of mammalian species.

ALPHA-MANNOSIDOSIS

History

Alpha-mannosidosis (α-mannosidosis) was first described in 1967 by Ockerman. The initial patient was tall for his age with large hands and feet, slight hepatosplenomegaly, and mild psychomotor retardation. The patient developed slowed growth, lumbar kyphosis, somewhat coarse features, enlarged tongue, and small cloudy lenticular opacities (although corneas were clear). Subsequently, the patient developed mental and motor deterioration, hypotonia and hyperreflexia, and Babinski signs. He died in his fifth year during an attack of suspected increased intracranial pressure. This patient and others had deficiency of α-mannosidase, and the disorder was called mannosidosis. Subsequently, patients have been found with deficiencies of β-mannosidase, a disorder referred to as β-mannosidosis. Although the term *mannosidosis* still refers to patients with α-mannosidase deficiency, it is clearer to call this disorder α-mannosidosis.

Clinical Picture

The clinical picture of α-mannosidosis is quite varied. More than 70 cases have been reported. These patients may have severe disease, as with the index case just described, or a milder disorder. Patients with a severe form have hepatomegaly, splenomegaly, severe infections, and early death. Severely affected patients have been confused with mucolipidosis I patients.

Other patients have had slower progression of the disorder with greater dysmorphism, corneal opacities, and longer survival. Others have presented primarily with marked mental defect, striking gingival hyperplasia, and survival into the third decade or longer. Facial dysmorphism, skeletal involvement, and organ enlargement have been slight in these patients. This more common mild form shows no clinical abnormalities or nonspecific abnormalities in the first year of life (psychomotor delay, speech delay, or frequent infections), and only later do sensorineural hearing loss, gait and limb ataxia, mild then moderate or severe mental defect, coarse facial features, and dysostosis multiplex develop. Patients develop short stature and may survive into adulthood, at least until age 41, without hepatomegaly. The cognitive and language impairments do not correlate well with the amount of residual α-mannosidase activity measured with an artificial substrate. Pancytopenia with antiplatelet and antineutrophil antibodies may occur. Destructive synovitis may occur with damage at the ankle, knee, or spine. Multiple suture synostosis, macrocephaly, and papilledema with increased intracranial pressure have been reported. Immunodeficiency affecting both cellular and humoral immunity often occurs and may account for the frequent infections.[11]

Laboratory Findings

Diagnosis requires a high index of suspicion, findings of abnormal urinary oligosaccharides, and demonstration of decreased α-mannosidase in leukocytes and cultured skin fibroblasts. Diagnosis has also been made using transformed lymphoblasts.

Roentgenographic Picture

The most notable roentgenographic finding is dense thickening of the calvaria; dysostosis multiplex tends to be mild and in some cases decreases in prominence with the age of the patient. The roentgenographic elements of dysostosis multiplex in α-mannosidosis include flattened vertebral bodies, oar-shaped ribs, hypoplastic ilia, and abnormalities of the small bones of the hands. Poor pneumatization of the sphenoid may be seen. Tight foramen magnum and cervical syrinx have been reported.[12] Results of computed tomography scans may be normal or may show an increase of subarachnoid spaces and hypodensity of the white matter.

Pathologic Findings

The pathology of α-mannosidosis is characterized by the appearance in multiple cell types of enlarged membrane-bound vacuoles that may contain storage material of reticulofibrillar appearance or appear almost empty. These vacuoles appear to be enlarged lysosomes and are not specific for α-mannosidosis. Ultrastructural study of cultured skin fibroblasts in α-mannosidosis showed vacuolar inclusions containing fine reticulogranular material with low electron density similar to those in sialidosis and the mucopolysaccharidoses.

Skeletal muscle is not involved symptomatically in α-mannosidosis; however, muscle biopsy may show ultrastructural abnormalities. A 32-year-old patient had numerous membrane-bound inclusions in biopsied skeletal muscle as well as interstitial fibroblasts and some endothelial cells. The inclusions were small (0.5 to 5.0 μm) and membrane-bound, and they contained dark granules as well as electron-lucent spaces. They were not believed to cause the patient's mild muscle weakness. In another patient, with generalized muscle weakness and spastic paraplegia, muscle pathology may have contributed to the weakness.

Lectin histochemistry on paraffin-embedded tissue sections can distinguish between α-mannosidosis, β-mannosidosis, fucosidosis, and sialidosis. α-Mannosidosis tissue showed staining with concanavalin A (Con A), wheat germ agglutinin (WGA), and succinyl-wheat germ agglutinin (S-WGA). Fucosidosis tissue stained with UEA-I. Sialidosis tissue stained with WGA but not S-WGA. β-Mannosidosis did not stain with Con A, WGA, S-WGA, UEA-I, or PNA.

Stored Substances in Alpha-Mannosidosis

In the initial report, mannose-rich storage material was reported in tissues; however, most subsequent studies have examined compounds in the urine. The compounds found have been oligosaccharides, both linear and branching, containing one or more terminal α-mannoside residues at the nonreducing end of the molecule. The most abundant and characteristic oligosaccharide found has been the trisaccharide Man-α(1→3)-Man-β(1→4)-GlcNAc. This trisaccharide may result from partial catabolism of a complex-type oligosaccharide chain (see Fig. 25–1). After release of the oligosaccharide from the protein core by endo-β-N-acetylglucosaminidase (see Fig. 25–1, reaction 6), stepwise cleavage by exoglycosidases would result in the trisaccharide. This would require removal of an α(1→6)-mannoside; presumably patients with α-mannosidosis have an enzyme that can catabolize this linkage. More than a dozen other oligosaccharides have been isolated from patients' urine, up to decasaccharides in size. Most of these may result from partial catabolism of a complex (see Fig. 25–1) or high-mannose–type (see Fig. 25–2) oligosaccharide chain. Some may result from partial catabolism of the dolichol-linked oligosaccharide precursor.[1]

Enzyme Deficiency in Alpha-Mannosidosis

Patients with α-mannosidosis have deficiency of lysosomal acid α-mannosidase (see Figs. 25–1 and 25–2, reaction 4). A variety of α-mannosidases is known, and their genetic origins, relationships, and natural substrate specificities are not well understood. α-Mannosidase activity with acid pH-optimum is found in lysosomes. α-Mannosidase activity with neutral or intermediate pH-optimum is found in cytoplasm and the Golgi apparatus. Tissue α-mannosidase activity has been separated into three forms: A, B, and C. α-Mannosidases A and B are lysosomal forms with a pH-optimum of 4.4; α-mannosidase C is a cytoplasmic form with a pH-optimum of 6.0. An intermediate form of α-mannosidase with pH-optimum 5.5 has also been reported. The neutral cytoplasmic form, α-mannosidase C, is coded for by a gene on chromosome 15, localized to 15q11-q13, and designated MANA. The acidic, lysosomal forms, α-mannosidases A and B (which are deficient in α-mannosidosis), are coded for by a gene on chromosome 19, localized to 19p13.2-q12, and designated MANB. The relationship between α-mannosidases A and B is not clear. Both, however, have been reported deficient in α-mannosidosis, and both have been converted to a common, apparently identical, form.

When assayed with artificial substrate 4-methyl-umbelliferyl-α-D-mannopyranoside, leukocytes and fibroblasts show marked deficiency of acid α-mannosidase because lysosomal acid α-mannosidases are the largest fraction of the α-mannosidases in these cells.

Serum, by contrast, contains a small fraction of acid (lysosomal α-mannosidases) and is not useful for diagnosis of α-mannosidosis.

The Alpha-Mannosidase Gene

The α-mannosidosis gene, *MANB*, has been cloned.[13] Berg et al reviewed the spectrum of mutations found in α-mannosidosis patients from 39 families.[14] One missense mutation, the R750W substitution, accounted for 21% of the disease alleles. Other disease alleles included splicing mutants, nonsense mutations, deletions, insertions, and other missense mutations. There seemed to be no correlation between mutation type and phenotype. Gotoda et al. reviewed the spectrum of mutations in Japanese patients with α-mannosidosis.[15]

Alpha-Mannosidosis in Other Species

Besides the human disease, α-mannosidosis occurs in cats. Ingestion of swainsonine, an inhibitor of α-mannosidase, causes an α-mannosidosis-like disorder in cattle, sheep, and horses. Bone marrow transplant in cats with α-mannosidosis has been reported to arrest progression of neurologic signs and prevent neuronal storage; functional acid α-mannosidase activity was demonstrated within neurons and other cells.

BETA-MANNOSIDOSIS

History

β-Mannosidosis, deficiency of β-mannosidase, is unusual because the disease was described first in goats.[16] Five years later, the disease was recognized by two groups in humans.[17,18]

Clinical Picture

In humans, the disorder presents with mental retardation, angiokeratoma, and tortuousness of conjunctival vessels.[17] Just over a dozen cases have been reported. Hearing loss has been reported in some patients,[18] but not others.[17] Peripheral neuropathy with thenar and hypothenar atrophy has been reported.[19] One patient from consanguineous parents had hypotonia and feeding difficulties in the first few months of life; it is not clear whether the abnormalities of swallowing and esophageal motility and achalasia at age 2 years, which required surgery, were part of her β-mannosidosis. Intrafamilial heterogeneity has been noted. As in Fabry disease, the angiokeratomas are distributed on the buttocks and lower limbs and in males may be seen on the shaft of the penis and scrotum. In 1996, Rodriguez-Serna et al reported on a 22-year-old woman who had had angiokeratomas since age 12 years as her only manifestation. She had β-mannosidase deficiency in serum, leukocytes, and cul-

tured skin fibroblasts, and her parents had intermediate levels consistent with autosomal recessive inheritance. One patient[18] had dysmorphic features, dysostosis multiplex, and sulfamidase deficiency (the enzyme deficient in Sanfilippo syndrome type A), in addition to β-mannosidase deficiency, and may have had two diseases. The other patients did not show dysmorphic features. Seizures or peripheral neuropathy may be prominent.

Laboratory Findings

Diagnosis is by demonstration of the characteristic oligosacchariduria and by demonstration of the enzyme deficiency in plasma, leukocytes, and fibroblasts. Heterozygotes can be detected, and the disease could presumably be detected during prenatal diagnosis in humans as has been done in goats. Ethanolaminuria has been noted in association with β-mannosidosis.

Lectin histochemistry on paraffin-embedded tissue sections can distinguish between α-mannosidosis, β-mannosidosis, fucosidosis, and sialidosis. α-Mannosidosis tissue showed staining with Con A, WGA, and S-WGA. β-Mannosidosis did not stain with Con A, WGA, S-WGA, UEA-I, or PNA.

Stored Substances in Beta-Mannosidosis

Oligosaccharides accumulate in cells and in urine in β-mannosidosis. The major oligosaccharide in the human disease is mannosyl-β(1→4)-N-acetylglucosamine, which has been found in leukocytes. Sialyl-α(2→6)-mannosyl-β(1→4)-N-acetylglucosamine has also been found. In goats, a trisaccharide accumulates. Oligosacchariduria is present[17,18] and is easily detected by thin-layer chromatography. The disaccharide mannosyl-β(1→4)-N-acetylglucosamine, however, requires a special solvent system to distinguish it from lactose.

Enzyme Deficiency in Beta-Mannosidosis

In β-mannosidosis, the deficient enzyme is lysosomal acid β-mannosidase (see Figs. 25–1 and 25–2, reaction 5). β-Mannosidase in humans is measurable in plasma, where it varies with age (but not with sex, as in goats); leukocytes; fibroblasts; and urine. β-Mannosidase is deficient in all of these in β-mannosidosis. Of interest, β-mannosidase activity in human fibroblasts is 10 times as high as in goat fibroblasts.

The Beta-Mannosidase Gene

Human β-mannosidase has been mapped to 4q22-q25 and cloned. Homozygosity for a splice acceptor site mutation was found in one family of Czech Gypsy origin.[20]

Beta-Mannosidosis in Other Species

β-Mannosidosis was identified in goats[16] before the defect was found in humans. The disease in goats differs from that in humans. In goats, there is ataxia, pendular nystagmus, inability to stand, dysmorphism, and marked intention tremor. The disorder is present at birth. A major element of the neuropathology is a myelin defect, perhaps caused by an oligodendrocyte defect. In addition, there were axonal lesions with axonal spheroids. In the peripheral nervous system, there were vacuolated Schwann cells and axonal spheroids. Characteristic lysosomal storage vacuoles were seen in all tissues in most cell types. The caprine gene has been cloned and a single base deletion identified that causes a frame shift with premature termination of the protein.

Subsequently, the disorder has been diagnosed in Salers cattle. Neuropathology in Salers calves showed hydrocephalus and myelin deficiency in the cerebral hemispheres, cerebellum, and brain stem. On microscopic examination, cytoplasmic vacuolation, myelin deficiency, and axonal spheroids were found. In general, the neuropathologic features in the calves resembled those in goats. In goats, the extent of demyelination did not correlate with the concentration of stored oligosaccharides or the degree of deficiency. The degree of oligosaccharide storage, however, did correlate with the regional β-mannosidase activity levels in control goats. The thyroid gland seems to be the site of severe involvement in goats with β-mannosidosis. Affected neonatal animals have decreased thyroid hormone levels. It has been hypothesized that this hypothyroidism plays a role in the pathogenesis of hypomyelination in affected animals.

ASPARTYLGLYCOSAMINURIA

History

Aspartylglycosaminuria was first reported in 1968 in England. Although cases from other countries have been reported, most come from Finland, especially Eastern Finland. In Eastern Finland, aspartylglycosaminuria is the third most common genetic cause of mental retardation after trisomy 21 and fragile X syndrome.[21,22] Carrier screening and prenatal diagnosis appear to be effective and are being evaluated in a university-based clinic in Eastern Finland.[23]

Clinical Picture

Other than rapid infantile growth, often the first clinical sign of aspartylglycosaminuria, patients present as clinically normal until age 1 to 5 years, when progressive somatic and mental changes develop. Progressive coarsening of facial features is noted with depressed nasal bridge, anteverted nostrils, broad nose, broad face, and rosy cheeks. Skeletal changes include thickening of the skull, cranial asymmetry, short neck, joint hypermobility, thinned cortex of the long bones, short stature, and thoracic or lumbar scoliosis. Development is slowed. Diarrhea, frequent respiratory infections, and cutaneous manifestations may be seen. Intellectual deterioration occurs leading to severe mental defect in the adult. Episodic hyperactivity, psychotic behavior, speech defects, and seizures may occur. Some patients have subcapsular, crystal-like lens opacities. Macroglossia, cardiac murmur, or hernia may occur. Angiokeratoma corporis diffusum and pubertal macro-orchidism have been observed. Inheritance is autosomal recessive.

Laboratory Findings

Diagnosis is by the characteristic clinical and genetic features, findings of aspartylglycosamine in urine, and demonstration of deficiency of aspartylglucosaminidase (N-aspartyl-β-glucosaminidase). Aspartylglycosamine is easily detected with thin-layer chromatography of urine for oligosaccharides, with liquid chromatography, with the amino acid analyzer, or from urine specimens recovered from absorbent filter paper. Aspartylglycosaminuria has been demonstrated in amniotic fluid and fetal urine. Aspartylglucosaminidase deficiency can be demonstrated most satisfactorily in cultured skin fibroblasts, although the deficiency is also found in plasma, seminal fluid, and tissue. Elevated serum dolichol levels have been found in aspartylglycosaminuria, as in other neurologic disorders.

Roentgenographic Picture

Chief roentgenographic findings include thickening of the calvaria, osteochondrosis of the vertebrae leading to wedge-shaped vertebral bodies with narrowing of the intervertebral spaces, and generalized osteoporosis. Cranial asymmetry may be noted. The cortex of the long bones is thin. Kyphosis or scoliosis may be noted.

Pathologic Findings

A wide variety of tissues and cell types show lysosomal storage. The chief ultrastructural finding is enlarged lysosomal vacuoles, which contain fibrillar or granular material. Vacuolated lymphocytes are also seen.

Stored Substances in Aspartylglycosaminuria

Patients excrete in their urine large amounts of aspartylglycosamine [(2-acetamido-1-β'-L-aspartamido)-1,2-dideoxyglucose] and more complex compounds containing this moiety. Aspartylglycosamine is also the chief storage material in tissues.

Enzyme Deficiency in Aspartylglycosaminuria

The disease results from deficiency of the lysosomal enzyme aspartylglucosaminidase (N-aspartyl-β-glucosaminidase), an amidase that cleaves aspartylglycosamine. This bond constitutes the linkage region between the protein portion and saccharide portion of one class of glycoproteins and of keratan sulfate. The enzyme aspartylglucosaminidase has been purified from urine, where it was found to consist of two heavy chains and two light chains. Purified from leukocytes, the enzyme was composed of two nonidentical polypeptides, which gave rise to the tetrameric enzyme protein. Both polypeptides appear to be products of the same structural gene. A 34.6-kd propeptide is cleaved into a 19.5-kd α-subunit and a 15-kd β-subunit. The enzyme subunits are glycosylated to form the final tetrameric protein.

The Aspartylglucosaminidase Gene

The aspartylglucosaminidase gene has been localized to the long arm of human chromosome 4 (4q23-q27). The gene has been cloned and sequenced. Mutations responsible for aspartylglycosaminuria have been identified. Nearly all Finnish patients have the C163S mutation, but other mutations have been found in patients born outside Finland.[24] In 2001, Saarela et al. reviewed the consequences of known mutations of the aspartylglucosaminidase gene.[25] They found that some mutations affected the active site, destroying enzyme activity and affecting precursor maturation, but others affected the dimer interface of the protein, thus preventing dimerization.

Two mouse knockout models for aspartylglycosaminuria have been constructed that develop neurologic degeneration, ataxia, progressive motor disease, impaired bladder function, and early death. These may be useful for the development of effective therapy.

REFERENCES

1. Kornfeld S, Li E, Tabas I: Synthesis of complex-type oligosaccharides II: Characterization of the processing intermediates in the synthesis of the complex oligosaccharide units of the vesicular stomatitis virus G1 protein. J Biol Chem 1978;253:7771.

2. Lowden JA, O'Brien JS: Sialidosis: A review of human neuraminidase deficiency. Am J Hum Genet 1979;31:1.

3. O'Brien JS, Warner TG: Sialidosis: Delineation of subtypes by neuraminidase assay. Clin Genet 1980;17:35.

4. Galjart NJ, Morreau H, Willemsen R, et al: Human lysosomal protective protein has cathepsin A-like activity distinct from its protective function. J Biol Chem 1991;266:14754.

5. Lukong KE, Landry K, Elsliger MA, et al: Mutations in sialidosis impair sialidase binding to the lysosomal multienzyme complex. J Biol Chem 2001;276:17286.

6. Bonten EJ, Arts WF, Beck M, et al: Novel mutations in lysosomal neuraminidase identify functional domains and determine clinical severity in sialidosis. Hum Mol Genet 2000;9:2715.

7. Willems PJ, Gatti R, Darby JK, et al: Fucosidosis revisited: A review of 77 patients. Am J Med Genet 1991;38:111.

8. Terespolsky D, Clarke JT, Blaser SI, et al: Evolution of the neuroimaging changes in fucosidosis type II. J Inherit Metab Dis 1996;19:775.

9. Fukushima H, de Wet JR, O'Brien JS: Molecular cloning of a cDNA for human alpha-L-fucosidase. Proc Natl Acad Sci U S A 1985;82:1262.

10. Willems PJ, Seo HC, Coucke P, et al: Spectrum of mutations in fucosidosis. Eur J Hum Genet 1999;7:60.

11. Malm D, Halvorsen DS, Tranebjaerg L, et al: Immunodeficiency in alpha-mannosidosis: A matched case-control study on immunoglobulins, complement factors, receptor density, phagocytosis and intracellular killing in leucocytes. Eur J Pediatr 2000;159:699.

12. Patlas M, Shapira MY, Nagler A, et al: MRI of mannosidosis. Neuroradiology 2001;43:941.

13. Nebes V, Schmidt MC: Human lysosomal alpha-mannosidase: Isolation and nucleotide sequence of the full-length cDNA. Biochem Biophys Res Commun 1994;200:239.

14. Berg T, Riise HM, Hansen GM, et al: Spectrum of mutations in alpha-mannosidosis. Am J Hum Genet 1999;64:77–88.

15. Gotoda Y, Wakamatsu N, Kawai H, et al: Missense and nonsense mutations in the lysosomal alpha-mannosidase gene (MANB) in severe and mild forms of alpha-mannosidosis. Am J Hum Genet 1998;63:1015.

16. Jones MZ, Dawson G: Caprine beta-mannosidosis. J Biol Chem 1981;256:5185.

17. Cooper A, Sardharwalla IB, Roberts MM: Human beta-mannosidase deficiency. N Engl J Med 1986;315:1231.

18. Wenger DA, Sujansky E, Fennessey PV, et al: Human beta-mannosidase deficiency. N Engl J Med 1986;315:1201.

19. Levade T, Graber D, Flurin V, et al: Human beta-mannosidase deficiency associated with peripheral neuropathy. Ann Neurol 1994;35:116.

20. Alkhayat AH, Kraemer SA, Leipprandt JR, et al: Human beta-mannosidase cDNA characterization and first identification of a mutation associated with human beta-mannosidosis. Hum Mol Genet 1998;7:75.

21. Matilainen R, Airaksinen E, Mononen T, et al: A population-based study on the causes of mild and severe mental retardation. Acta Paediatr 1995;84:261.

22. Mononen T, Mononen I, Matilainen R, et al: High prevalence of aspartylglycosaminuria among

school-age children in eastern Finland. Hum Genet 1991;87:266.

23. Kallinen J, Marin K, Heinonen S, et al: Wide scope prenatal diagnosis at Kuopio University Hospital 1997–1998: Integration of gene tests and fetal karyotyping. BJOG 2001;108:505.

24. Fisher KJ, Aronson NN, Jr: Characterization of the mutation responsible for aspartylglucosaminuria in three Finnish patients: Amino acid substitution Cys[163]Ser abolishes the activity of lysosomal glycosylasparaginase and its conversion into subunits. J Biol Chem 1991;266:12105.

25. Saarela J, Laine M, Oinonen C, et al: Molecular pathogenesis of a disease: Structural consequences of aspartylglucosaminuria mutations. Hum Mol Genet 2001;10:983.

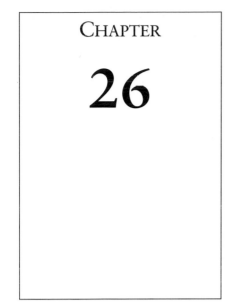

CHAPTER

26

Beta-Galactosidase Deficiency: GM1 Gangliosidosis, Morquio B Disease, and Galactosialidosis

Kunihiko Suzuki

Genetic deficiency of lysosomal acid β-galactosidase (EC 3.2.1.23) in humans causes GM1 gangliosidosis, a neurologic disorder, and Morquio B disease, which is primarily a skeletal-connective tissue disorder.[1] Clinical manifestations of GM1 gangliosidosis are highly variable. The classic infantile form is a severe, rapidly progressive neurologic and systemic disorder, and patients rarely survive for more than a few years. Patients with clinically, pathologically, and biochemically less severe juvenile and adult forms, however, have later onset, slower progression, and in many adult patients, little mental involvement. Although it has been clear for many years that the underlying cause of these various clinical phenotypes is genetic deficiency of acid β-galactosidase activity, numerous attempts at their enzymologic delineation have failed. Availability of cDNA clones coding for the human acid β-galactosidase made it feasible to examine the underlying abnormalities on the gene level in different clinical phenotypes of GM1 gangliosidosis. The line between GM1 gangliosidosis and Morquio B disease is increasingly blurred because certain mutations have been found to cause intermediate phenotypes with both neurodegenerative and skeletal manifestations. Both GM1 gangliosidosis and Morquio B disease can be diagnosed definitively by assay of acid β-galactosidase activity with artificial chromogenic or fluorogenic substrates, provided appropriate precautions are taken to exclude galactosialidosis. Diagnosis based on specific mutations is possible. It is highly specific and unambiguous, particularly in heterozygote diagnosis. It is, however, often too specific and can never entirely replace enzymatic diagnosis, which tests for the functional abnormality of the enzyme whatever the underlying mutation might be.

Galactosialidosis was initially thought to be a variant of genetic β-galactosidase deficiency. It was later recognized that these patients are deficient in activities of both β-galactosidase and α-neuraminidase.[2] It has since been established that galactosialidosis is genetically distinct from β-galactosidase deficiencies and that the underlying cause is genetic defects in the protective protein, the product of another unrelated gene. The gene coding for the *protective protein* has also been cloned. The gene product has since been identified as a lysosomal protease, cathepsin A.

Naturally occurring animal models of genetic β-galactosidase and protective protein deficiencies are known among larger animals. Cloning and characterization of full-length cDNA and the gene coding for mouse β-galactosidase and protective protein opened the way to generate authentic genetic murine models by the homologous recombination and transgenic technologies. Two lines of GM1 gangliosidosis mouse models and a galactosialidosis mouse line have been successfully produced.

GM1 GANGLIOSIDOSIS AND MORQUIO B DISEASE

GM1 gangliosidosis and Morquio B disease are traditionally classified as entirely different diseases. Their basic relationship is not obvious because their typical clinical phenotypes are so different. Conceptually, however, these two diseases merely represent the extremes of phenotypic variations of the same disorder caused by genetic deficiency of acid β-galactosidase activity. The term *β-galactosidosis* has been suggested as an inclusive nomenclature of both GM1 gangliosidosis and Morquio B disease.[1]

GM1 GANGLIOSIDOSIS

Clinical Picture and Diagnostic Evaluation

Until the mid-1960s, the only known *ganglioside storage disease* was the classic Tay-Sachs disease (a GM2 gangliosidosis). Existence of another entirely different category of gangliosidosis, GM1 gangliosidosis, was firmly established by 1965.[3–5] Advances in the technology of ganglioside analysis were the key for this development because, in retrospect, the disease had been described earlier without definitive chemical evidence. GM1 gangliosidosis is transmitted as a mendelian autosomal recessive disorder. Although the most important clinical manifestations are for the most part neurologic, the disease involves systemic organs, such as the liver and spleen, and the skeletal structure. It is pragmatically convenient to divide the phenotype into *infantile, juvenile*, and *adult* forms according to the time of onset and the rate of progression.

Patients with the infantile form of GM1 gangliosidosis generally experience clinical onset by 6 months, although facial and bony abnormalities are often recognized at birth. In early stages, patients appear dull and hypotonic with retarded psychomotor development. Regression soon becomes evident, leading to later manifestations, such as spasticity and seizures. Eventually patients become deaf and blind, totally unresponsive to external stimuli. Macular cherry spots are common but not consistent. The entire clinical course rarely exceeds 2 to 3 years, and inevitable death occurs most commonly as a result of concurrent infections. Neurologic manifestations are primarily those of gray matter. White matter and peripheral nerve involvement is relatively minor. Infantile patients show, in addition to the previously mentioned neurologic manifestations, clinical features that are similar to those in mucopolysaccharidoses, including facial deformity, macroglossia, radiologic bone abnormalities, and visceromegaly.

The late infantile or juvenile form of the disease manifests itself later, usually after age 1 year, with milder neurologic signs and slower progression. Systemic involvement, prominent in infantile patients, is less and may be absent. Patients with this phenotype often survive beyond 10 years. A typical case of this form was described early by Derry et al.[6]

The adult or chronic form is very variable clinically. The clinical onset can be any time between a few to 30 years or older. Perhaps the first clearly delineated patients were described in 1977 by Suzuki et al.[7] This phenotype appears to be relatively common in Japan, but cases are known in other ethnic groups. Slowly progressive dysarthria, gait difficulties, dystonic movements, and other extrapyramidal signs are most prominent. Patients are often slightly or moderately impaired intellectually. Signs prominent in the younger forms, such as macular cherry-red spots, facial abnormalities, and visceromegaly, are not associated with the adult form. Bony abnormalities

are recorded, however, sometimes causing symptoms owing to spinal compression. Clinical diagnosis of adult GM1 gangliosidosis is difficult, and patients with the above-mentioned clinical picture should be screened for the possibility with appropriate enzymatic assays.

Pathology

Pathology of the infantile and juvenile forms is qualitatively similar, with the infantile form being generally more severe. The gray matter is affected, whereas the white matter and the peripheral nerves are relatively spared. Essentially all neurons throughout the body are enlarged and contain faintly granular material, which actually consists of discrete abnormal lamellar bodies (membranous cytoplasmic bodies) under the electron microscope. The pathology of cortical neurons is for all practical purposes indistinguishable from that of classic Tay-Sachs disease (GM2 gangliosidosis). Many reactive astrocytes also contain abnormal cytoplasmic bodies. White matter often shows mild myelin loss with sudanophilia, presumably secondary to neuronal loss. Many reticuloendothelial organs, such as lung, liver, spleen, lymph nodes, and bone marrow, contain swollen foamy histiocytes with intracellular vacuoles containing strongly PAS-positive materials. This systemic pathology is present even in juvenile patients, who show relatively few clinical signs of systemic organ involvement. Ultrastructure of the systemic organs more closely resembles that of mucopolysaccharidoses and is different from neuropathology. Clear vacuoles in these cells, however, contain interwoven bundles of tubular structures.

The characteristic finding in the neuropathology of adult GM1 gangliosidosis is its selective distribution of lesions within the central nervous system. Unlike in the younger phenotypes, cortical neurons tend to be relatively spared, and those in the basal ganglia are primarily affected. Even within the same region, severely swollen neurons can be found next to others that appear relatively normal or pyknotic. The ultrastructural features of affected neurons, however, are qualitatively similar to those in the younger forms. This selective involvement of the basal ganglia can explain, at least on the phenomenologic level, the predominant extrapyramidal manifestations in the adult disease. Again, systemic organs can show pathology similar to the younger forms even when there is no clinical evidence of their involvement.

Biochemistry and Enzymology

GM1 gangliosidosis was originally recognized as a distinct disease by a massive accumulation of GM1 ganglioside in the brain. The total concentration of ganglioside in the brain at the terminal stage in the infantile disease can be three to five times normal. GM1 ganglioside, normally present at 22 to 25 molar percent of total ganglioside, is present at 90 to 95 molar percent in patients' gray matter.[8] Thus the increase in GM1 ganglioside in the gray matter is actually up to 20 times normal. There is also an abnormal increase in GM1 ganglioside in systemic organs, although the absolute amounts remain small. GM1 gangliosidosis was named early as *generalized gangliosidosis* because of the abnormal accumulation of GM1 ganglioside in systemic organs. This terminology, however, is a misnomer. Similar degrees of abnormal accumulation of the affected ganglioside, GM2, also occur in systemic organs of patients with Tay-Sachs disease without clinical signs of visceromegaly. There is very limited information available for analytical biochemistry of the adult GM1 gangliosidosis because of the long survival of patients. In one well-characterized patient, abnormal accumulation of GM1 ganglioside paralleled with the distribution of pathologic lesions in that the basal ganglia clearly contained a much larger quantity of GM1 ganglioside than cerebral cortex.[9]

The main storage materials in the systemic organs are heterogeneous galactose-rich fragments of varying molecular weights derived from glycoproteins, keratan sulfate, and other carbohydrate-containing materials. The most insoluble of these was first described as *keratan sulfate–like* based on its behavior in preparative procedures, electrophoretic properties, and the sugar composition.[10] When all of these materials are combined, the amount in patients' tissues can be more than 20 times normal. Many compounds of similar molecular weight also appear in excess in patients' urine. Several extensive characterizations have been done on these materials, which appear to be for the most part derived from glycoproteins. These materials should, *a priori*, have a terminal β-galactose moiety at the nonreducing end because their accumulation is a consequence of the genetic defect in acid β-galactosidase.

The underlying cause of GM1 gangliosidosis is a genetic deficiency of the lysosomal acid β-galactosidase.[5,11,12] The defect can be readily demonstrated either with conventional chromogenic or fluorogenic artificial substrate or with the natural substrate, GM1 ganglioside. Among several glycolipids that have the terminal β-galactosidase residue, GM1 ganglioside, asialo-GM1 ganglioside, and lactosylceramide are natural substrates for the enzyme. There is no prominent abnormal accumulation of lactosylceramide in GM1 gangliosidosis, however, because the other lysosomal β-galactosidase, galactosylceramidase, also hydrolyzes lactosylceramide. Genetic deficiency of galactosylceramidase is the cause of globoid cell leukodystrophy (Krabbe disease), and this enzyme is normal in GM1 gangliosidosis.

MORQUIO B DISEASE

Clinical Picture and Diagnostic Evaluation

Morquio B disease was originally classified as a form of mucopolysaccharidosis because of its clinical and pathologic similarity to other forms of Morquio disease. Unlike GM1 gangliosidosis, Morquio B disease is a primary skele-

tal disease without neurologic manifestations except those caused by bone deformity. Progressive skeletal dysplasia starts during the first several years of life, often most prominent in vertebral and pelvic bones. Many patients are of short stature. Severe spinal deformities are common. Odontoid hypoplasia is always present and is the cause of potentially serious complications due to cervical cord compression. Mild corneal opacity, mild organomegaly, and cardiac lesions are frequent manifestations besides bony abnormalities. As in all forms of GM1 gangliosidosis, patients with Morquio B disease also excrete excess amounts of galactose-containing materials into urine.

Pathology

Because Morquio B disease was recognized relatively recently as a genetic disorder distinct from other forms of mucopolysaccharidosis IV, information on pathology pertaining specifically to this disease is limited.

Biochemistry and Enzymology

As in other clinical forms of Morquio disease, patients with Morquio B disease excrete keratan sulfate into urine, in addition to galactose-rich fragments of glycoproteins. The first two steps of keratan sulfate degradation are desulfation by N-acetylgalactosamine 6-sulfatase (galactose-6-sulfatase) and then cleavage of the β-galactosidic bond by β-galactosidase. A genetic block at the first step causes the classic type A disease, whereas that of the second step causes type B disease. Deficient activities of β-galactosidase can be demonstrated using conventional chromogenic or fluorogenic substrates. The fundamental enzymatic defect underlying Morquio B disease involves the same enzyme that is defective in GM1 gangliosidosis. Therefore, it is likely that the mutations underlying the respective disorders differentially affect the specificity of the enzyme toward various natural substrates, resulting in dramatically different clinical pictures. Paschke and Kresse[13] have presented findings consistent with this prediction. Their finding was that the capacity of the β-galactosidase from Morquio B patients to hydrolyze GM1 ganglioside could be activated by the natural activator protein, saposin B, up to 20% of the normal activity, whereas it could not be activated to hydrolyze the β-galactose residue from keratan sulfate.

Molecular Genetics of β-Galactosidase Deficiency

In the past several years, knowledge of GM1 gangliosidosis and Morquio B disease entered the molecular biology phase. This occurred when cDNA coding for the normal human acid β-galactosidase was cloned and characterized.[14] The genomic organization of the human β-galactosidase gene has also been characterized.[15] The human β-galactosidase gene is located on chromosome 3.

TABLE 26–1. Identified Mutations in Acid β-Galactosidase That Cause GM1 Gangliosidosis or Morquio B Disease

Mutation	Phenotype	Mutation	Phenotype
GM1 Gangliosidosis		$Asp^{332}\rightarrow Asn$	infantile
20-bp insertion from intron 2, caused by a base insertion in the 5' donor site	adult	$Arg^{351}\rightarrow Ter$	infantile
		$Ser^{434}\rightarrow Leu$	infantile
		$Arg^{457}\rightarrow Ter$	infantile
23-bp duplication in exon 3	infantile	$Arg^{457}\rightarrow Gln$	adult
duplication of exons 11 and 12 in mRNA	infantile	$Asp^{491}\rightarrow Asn$	infantile
		$Gly^{494}\rightarrow Cys$	infantile
9-base in-frame insertion in exon 6 (GluAsnPhe)	adult	$Trp^{509}\rightarrow Cys$	infantile? Found in a heteroallelic patient with Morquio B disease
9-base insertion due to a base change at the acceptor site of intron 6	juvenile	$Lys^{578}\rightarrow Arg$	infantile
1-base insertion at nucleotide #896	infantile	$Arg^{590}\rightarrow His$	juvenile or adult
		$Thr^{610}\rightarrow Ala$	juvenile
1-base insertion at nucleotide #1627	infantile	$Glu^{632}\rightarrow Gly$	juvenile or adult
		$Lys^{655}\rightarrow Arg$	juvenile
$Arg^{49}\rightarrow Cys$	infantile		
$Arg^{59}\rightarrow His$	infantile	**Morquio B Disease**	
$Ile^{51}\rightarrow Thr$	adult	32-bp insertion from intron 2, caused by a mutation at the 3' acceptor site	juvenile Morquio B
$Thr^{82}\rightarrow Met$	very mild adult?		
$Arg^{121}\rightarrow Ser$	infantile		
$Gly^{123}\rightarrow Arg$	infantile	$Tyr^{83}\rightarrow His$	juvenile Morquio B
$Arg^{148}\rightarrow Ser$	infantile	$Arg^{208}\rightarrow His$	GM1/Morquio B intermediate
$Arg^{201}\rightarrow Cys$	juvenile	$Pro^{263}\rightarrow Ser$	GM1/Morquio B intermediate
$Arg^{201}\rightarrow His$	adult	$Trp^{273}\rightarrow Leu$	adult Morquio B (one gene dose sufficient for the Morquio B phenotype)
$Arg^{208}\rightarrow Cys$	infantile		
$Val^{216}\rightarrow Ala$	infantile		
$Val^{240}\rightarrow Met$	infantile	$Asn^{318}\rightarrow His$	GM1/Morquio B intermediate
$Asn^{266}\rightarrow Ser$	adult	$Arg^{482}\rightarrow His$	infantile/Morquio intermediate
$Tyr^{316}\rightarrow Cys$	infantile	$Arg^{482}\rightarrow Cys$	Morquio

The boundary between the phenotypes of GM1 gangliosidosis and Morquio B disease is often ill-defined, particularly in older patients. Original sources that recorded these mutations are available in references 1 and 25.

Reports on disease-causing mutations have been rapidly increasing in the past several years (Table 26–1). Initially, nine mutations responsible for GM1 gangliosidosis were found, by coincidence, among Japanese patients. Within this population and within the relatively limited number of patients examined, one mutation each could be characterized as the cause of the juvenile and adult forms of the disease. It was noteworthy that $Ile^{51}\rightarrow Thr$ was found in 27 of 32 mutant alleles among 16 Japanese adult patients. Some residual activity of the juvenile mutant enzyme and even higher residual activity in the adult mutant enzyme in an ASVGM1-4 cell expression system are consistent with the hypothesis that each mutation causes less severe, more slowly progressive clin-

ical phenotypes. In contrast to the older forms, mutations responsible for the infantile form of GM1 gangliosidosis are highly heterogeneous. The initial series of mutation analyses among Japanese patients was followed by studies with Caucasian patients. As expected, most disease-causing mutations found among the Caucasian population were different from those among Japanese patients. The mutation, $Thr^{82}\rightarrow Met$, was found among three adult patients from two unrelated families of Scandinavian extraction.

A single mutation was found by Oshima et al[14] in three patients with Morquio B disease, although two were siblings. The mutation is an unusual double substitution of two adjacent nucleotides (TGG to CTG). The enzyme protein generated from this mutant gene gave 8% of the normal activity in the ASVGM1-4 cells. This finding is consistent with the relatively mild clinical features compared with severe GM1 gangliosidosis. However, it would be of great interest to test its catalytic activity toward different natural substrates as to whether the enzyme retains its activity toward GM1 ganglioside but is inactive toward desulfated keratan sulfate or equivalent oligosaccharide substrates. Such a finding would not only support the hypothesis regarding the enzymology of β-galactosidase mutations, but also would provide, taken together with the precise knowledge of the primary structure of the mutant enzyme, the essential information concerning the functional domains of β-galactosidase. Additional mutations underlying the typical Morquio B phenotype and also a clinical phenotype of combined neurologic manifestations and Morquio-like skeletal abnormalities have been described (see Table 26–1).

As in other genetic disorders, the traditional classification of genetic β-galactosidase deficiency based on the clinical phenotype now faces fundamental as well as pragmatic complications. The fundamental question is how to define a *disease* or its *variant*. There are already so many mutations known to cause inactivation of catalytic activity of the gene product. Except for consanguineous cases, compound heterozygosity would be the norm rather than the exception. The number of possible combinations would be enormous. Thus it becomes impossible to define a disease on the basis of the genotype for any given patient. Nevertheless, for pragmatic purposes, one hopes that the traditional clinical classification can be useful. Prediction, however, is not very reassuring. In compound heterozygous individuals, two abnormal alleles contribute to the phenotypic expression. If one makes a reasonable assumption that clinical phenotypes depend on the residual activity of the mutant enzyme protein in vivo, a mutant enzyme with higher residual activity tends to override that with less residual activity. Thus it is likely that patients who have at least one allele with the adult mutation are all of the adult phenotype, regardless of the nature of the other allele. In contrast, one juvenile mutant allele will define the juvenile phenotype only if the other allele carries either a juvenile or an infantile mutation. If the other allele carries an adult mutation, the patient will be of the adult phenotype. Then patients with the infantile phenotype must carry two infantile mutations. This analysis holds only if there are *adult, juvenile*, and *infantile* mutations with discontinuous ranges of residual activities. Probability dictates that it is far more likely that the degree of residual activities of all individual mutations will be continuous between the *normal* activity to zero activity. Any degree of discontinuity among individual mutations will further be smoothed out by the additive nature of the contributions by the two mutant alleles in autosomal recessive disorders, such as GM1 gangliosidosis. In the case of β-galactosidase, the diverse natural substrates and possible differential effect of any

mutation on different substrates further complicate the eventual phenomena. The range of the final outcome of the *residual activity* contributed by the two mutant genes in any given patient defies any hope for discrete clinical phenotypes and consequently any orderly clinical classification. The traditional line between the primarily neurologic GM1 gangliosidosis and the exclusively skeletal Morquio B disease is increasingly blurred. The term *β-galactosidosis* encompasses all clinical phenotypes, from purely neurologic to purely skeletal. In fact, the argument advanced here finds parallels in all genetic disorders, particularly in those of the autosomal recessive inheritance.

GALACTOSIALIDOSIS

Although included here, galactosialidosis is a genetic disorder entirely distinct from GM1 gangliosidosis/Morquio B disease.[2] The acid β-galactosidase gene is not affected in this disorder. Because patients show deficiencies of both β-galactosidase and sialidase (α-neuraminidase), they were often diagnosed erroneously as having either a variant of GM1 gangliosidosis or sialidosis. For example, an early somatic cell hybridization study showed that fibroblasts from a group of patients then classified as a GM1 gangliosidosis variant gave genetic complementation when fused with cells from patients with other phenotypes of GM1 gangliosidosis, indicating that a different gene is involved in these patients. Wenger was first to point out a combined deficiency of β-galactosidase and sialidase in many of these *variant* patients.[16] Controversy followed as to which of the two enzymatic deficiencies is the primary cause of this disease. Then it was shown that β-galactosidase in fibroblasts from galactosialidosis patients had an abnormally short half-life because of rapid proteolytic degradation in vivo. This led to the definitive delineation of this disorder as a genetic *protective protein* deficiency.[17] Knowledge about the nature of this protective protein is evolving, and it is now known as a lysosomal cathepsin A–like carboxypeptidase. Endothelin has been implicated as an endogenous natural substrate.[18]

Clinical Picture and Diagnostic Evaluation

The mode of inheritance of galactosialidosis is autosomal recessive. The clinical phenotype is heterogeneous, ranging from an early-onset, severe, and rapidly progressive infantile form to a late-onset, slowly progressive adult form. Patients with the infantile form may closely resemble those with infantile GM1 gangliosidosis, with severe central nervous system involvement, macular cherry-red spots, visceromegaly, renal insufficiency, coarse facies, and skeletal abnormalities. The late infantile form is essentially a later onset, milder phenotype of the infantile disease. The juvenile/adult form of the disease appears to have a much higher incidence in Japan. The main clinical manifestations are slowly progressive central nervous system symptoms, including motor disturbance and mental retardation, skeletal abnormalities, dysmorphism, macular cherry-red spots, and angiokeratoma. Patients survive well into adulthood. Galactosialidosis patients of all clinical types excrete excess amounts of a complex mixture of glycopeptide fragments that are rich in sialic acid.

Pathology

Relatively little is known about the pathology of patients with verified galactosialidosis. The neuropathology of a 13-year old Japanese patient was recently described in some detail. Severe neuronal loss was seen in the basal ganglia, lateral geniculate body, and nucleus gracilis, as well as loss of Purkinje cells and retinal ganglion cells. On the other hand, remaining neurons in the cerebral cortex, motor neurons, spinal cord, and trigeminal and spinal ganglia were distended, containing complex membranous cytoplasmic bodies, lipofuscin-like materials, and cytoplasmic vacuoles.

Biochemistry and Enzymology

Very little is known about the analytic biochemistry of tissue constituents of patients with galactosialidosis. Storage materials in cultured fibroblasts and fetal placenta and those excreted into urine, however, have been characterized in detail. They are predominantly sialylated glycopeptides, similar to those found in sialidosis patients.

The enzymatic characteristic of galactosialidosis is the simultaneous deficiency of both β-galactosidase and α-neuraminidase.[17] It was noted earlier that when β-galactosidase was purified, its molecular weight appeared to be approximately 54 K but that another protein component of approximately 32 K always copurified with the 54 K component. d'Azzo et al[17] found that, in galactosialidosis, the 32 K component was lacking. On the basis of this finding and the earlier finding that the half-life of β-galactosidase in galactosialidosis patients was abnormally short but that it could be prolonged by addition of protease inhibitors, it was proposed that the function of the 32 K protein is to protect ß-galactosidase and neuraminidase from proteolytic digestion within the lysosome by forming a complex with them and that genetic abnormality in this *protective protein* is the underlying cause of galactosialidosis.

Molecular Genetics of Protective Protein [Cathepsin A] Deficiency

The human gene coding for the *protective protein* is present on chromosome 20. Galjart et al[19] cloned human and murine cDNA coding for the *protective protein* of the respective species. Unexpectedly, the primary structure was homologous with carboxypeptidase. Consistent with this observation, simultaneous deficiency of carboxypepti-

dase has been described in galactosialidosis. The exact mechanism by which the *protective protein* stabilizes β-galactosidase and neuraminidase is still not well understood because of this apparent contradiction: the *protective protein*, which is supposed to protect the two enzymes from proteolytic degradation, is itself a peptidase.

Several specific mutations responsible for human galactosialidosis are known. The common mutation in the late onset form of the disease prevalent in Japan results in missplicing of the transcript. A substitution of a G at the third base from the 5′ donor site of intron 7 to A appears to cause skipping of exon 7 during processing of the transcript. All nine Japanese patients with the late-onset form had this mutation. A generally clear genotype/phenotype correlation was observed among 19 Japanese patients. No patients with infantile, severe form of the disease had this mutation, all late-onset, mild adult patients were homoallelic, and most patients with an intermediate phenotype were compound heterozygotes with one allele carrying this mutation. More recently, five additional disease-causing mutations have been recorded. Four of them, Gln^{49}→Arg, Trp^{65}→Arg, Ser^{90}→Lys (a double base substitution), and Tyr^{395}→Cys were found among Japanese patients, while Tyr^{249}→Asn was found in a French German patient. Particularly Tyr^{395}→Cys appeared common among infantile/childhood Japanese patients.

ANIMAL MODELS

Over the years, genetic β-galactosidase deficiency has been described in domestic and farm animals. The species include dogs, cats, and cattle. Similar animal models for galactosialidosis have also been reported in sheep. However, this model appears to have GM1 gangliosidosis with low α-neuraminidase activity because the cells from sick sheep genetically complemented the human galactosialidosis cells. On the other hand, a disease described in Schipperke dog may well be a model for human galactosialidosis. Because the human diseases are rare and because ethical considerations limit experiments on human patients, these animal models provide unique opportunities to study biology and possible treatment of these devastating genetic diseases. The feline and canine models have, in fact, been used for such experimental purposes. No naturally occurring model, however, is known among small laboratory animals, which would give further advantage for certain types of studies. The cloning and complete characterization of the murine β-galactosidase cDNA and gene, however, opened the way for experimental production of a murine strain with genetic acid β-galactosidase deficiency by the homologous recombination and transgenic technologies. Such acid β-galactosidase "knockout" mouse lines have been generated in two laboratories independently.[20,21] Similarly, a mouse galactosialidosis model has also been generated.[22] These mouse models are being utilized actively in studies of the pathogenetic mechanism and of therapeutic trials of these disorders.

STATUS AND FUTURE POSSIBILITY OF THERAPY

Pragmatically effective therapy is not yet available for human patients. Many laboratories actively investigate the gene therapy approach, but it remains experimental.[23] In the mouse model of galactosialidosis, lesions in systemic organs could be corrected almost completely using erythroid cells that were made to overexpress the protective protein by ex vivo transfection of normal gene.[22] However, despite the almost complete "cure" of the systemic pathology, brain lesions were not corrected. A conceptually novel approach is activation of mutant enzyme with the use of galactonojirimycin derivatives, which inhibit glycolipid synthesis.[24,25] Future prospect for effective therapy must include the following consideration: If the effectiveness of a treatment can only be demonstrated by well-controlled experiments and perhaps with sophisticated statistical analysis, it is biologically significant but probably not sufficiently effective for clinical therapy. Clinically meaningful therapy requires a different order of magnitude in its effectiveness. From this perspective, pragmatically effective treatment still seems many years off.

REFERENCES

1. Suzuki Y, Oshima A, Nanba E: β-Galactosidase deficiency (β-galactosidosis): GM1 gangliosidosis and Morquio B disease. In Scriver CR, Beaudet AL, Sly WS, et al (eds): The Metabolic and Molecular Basis of Inherited Disease (8th ed). New York, McGraw-Hill, 2001, pp 3775–3809.

2. d'Azzo A, Andria G, Strisciuglio P, Galjaard H: Galactosialidosis. In Scriver CR, Beaudet AL, Sly WS, et al (eds): The Metabolic and Molecular Basis of Inherited Disease (8th ed). New York, McGraw-Hill, 2001, pp 3811–3826.

3. Jatzkewitz H, Sandhoff K: On a biochemically special form of infantile amaurotic idiocy. Biochim Biophys Acta 1963;70:354–356.

4. Gonatas NK, Gonatas J: Ultrastructural and biochemical observations on a case of systemic late infantile lipidosis and its relationship to Tay-Sachs disease and gargoylism. J Neuropathol Exp Neurol 1965;24: 318–340.

5. Okada S, O'Brien JS: Generalized gangliosidosis: Beta galactosidase deficiency. Science 1968;160: 1002–1004.

6. Derry DM, Fawcett JS, Andermann F, Wolfe LS: Late infantile systemic lipidosis. Major monosialogangliosidosis: Delineation of two types. Neurology 1968; 18:340–348.

7. Suzuki Y, Nakamura N, Fukuoka K, et al: β-Galactosidase deficiency in juvenile and adult patients: Report of six Japanese cases and review of literature. Hum Genet 1977;36:219–229.

8. Suzuki K, Suzuki K, Kamoshita S: Chemical pathology of GM1-gangliosidosis (generalized gangliosidosis). J Neuropathol Exp Neurol 1969;28:25–73.

9. Kobayashi T, Suzuki K: Chronic GM1-gangliosidosis presenting as dystonia. II. Biochemistry. Ann Neurol 1981;9:476–483.

10. Suzuki K: Cerebral GM1-gangliosidosis: Chemical pathology of visceral organs. Science 1968; 159:1471–1472.

11. Sacrez R, Juif JG, Gigonnet JM, Gruner JE: La maladie de Landing, ou idiotie amaurotique infantile précose avec gangliosidose généralisée de type GM1. Pédiatrie 1967;22:143–162.

12. Seringe P, Plainfosse B, Lautmann F, et al: Gangliosidose généralisée, du type Norman Landing, à GM1. Etude à propos d'un diagnostiqué du vivant du malade. Ann Pédiat 1968;44:165–184.

13. Paschke E, Kresse E: Morquio disease, type B: Activation of GM1-beta-galactosidase by GM1-activator protein. Biochem Biophys Res Commun 1982;109:568–575.

14. Oshima A, Tsuji A, Nagano Y, et al: Cloning, sequencing and expression of cDNA for human beta-galactosidase. Biochem Biophys Res Commun 1988;157: 238–244.

15. Morreau H, Bonten E, Zhou X-Y, d'Azzo A: Organization of the gene encoding human lysosomal β-galactosidase. DNA Cell Biol 1991;10:495–504.

16. Wenger DA, Tarby TJ, Wharton C: Macular cherry-red spots and myoclonus with dementia: Coexistent neuraminidase and beta-galactosidase deficiencies. Biochem Biophys Res Commun 1978;82: 589–595.

17. d'Azzo A, Hoogeveen A, Reuser AJJ, et al: Molecular defect in combined beta-galactosidase and neuraminidase deficiency in man. Proc Nat Acad Sci U S A 1982;79:4535–4539.

18. Itoh K, Kase R, Shimmoto M, et al: Protective protein as an endogenous endothelin degradative enzyme in human tissues. J Biol Chem 1995;270:515–518.

19. Galjart NJ, Gillemans N, Meijer D, d'Azzo A: Mouse "protective protein": cDNA cloning, sequence comparison and expression. J Biol Chem 1990;265: 4678–4684.

20. Matsuda J, Suzuki O, Oshima A, et al: β-galactosidase-deficient mouse as an animal model for GM1-gangliosidosis. Glycoconj J 1997;14:729–736.

21. Hahn CN, Martin MD, Schröder M, et al: Generalized CNS disease and massive GM1-ganglioside accumulation in mice defective in lysosomal acid β-galactosidase. Hum Mol Genet 1997;6:205–211.

22. Zhou XY, Morreau H, Rottier R, et al: Mouse model for the lysosomal disorder galactosialidosis and

correction of the phenotype with overexpressing erythroid precursor cells. Genes Dev 1995;9:2623–2634.

23. Sena-Esteves M, Camp SM, Alroy J, et al: Correction of acid ß-galactosidase deficiency in GM1 gangliosidosis human fibroblasts by retrovirus vector-mediated gene transfer: Higher efficiency of release and cross-correction by the murine enzyme. Hum Gene Ther 2000;11:715–727.

24. Tominaga L, Ogawa Y, Taniguchi M, et al: Galactonojirimycin derivatives restore mutant human β-galactosidase activities expressed in fibroblasts from enzyme-deficient knockout mouse. Brain Dev 2001; 23:284–287.

25. Callahan JW: Molecular basis of GM1 gangliosidosis and Morquio disease, type B: Structure-function studies of lysosomal β-galactosidase and the non-lysosomal β-galactosidase–like protein. Biochim Biophys Acta Mol Basis Dis 1999;1455:85–103.

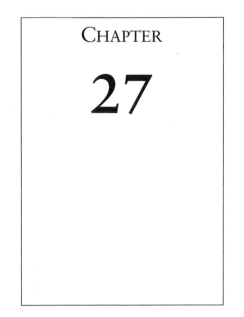

CHAPTER 27

Farber Disease: Acid Ceramidase Deficiency, Farber Lipogranulomatosis

Hugo W. Moser

In 1957 Sidney Farber[1] reported three patients, two of whom were siblings, in whom granulomatous inflammatory lesions in the skin, joints, and larynx were associated with neuronal storage of a complex glycosphingolipid. He found this disorder of special interest because it appeared to be a bridge between true metabolic disorders such as Tay-Sachs or Niemann-Pick Disease, and the inflammatory histiocytoses. Farber named this disorder lipogranulomatosis. In 1967 Prensky et al[2] demonstrated that this disorder was associated with the abnormal accumulation of ceramide, and in 1972 Sugita et al[3] demonstrated the deficiency of lysosomal acid ceramidase. In 1996 Koch et al[4] purified and cloned acid ceramidase. In 1999 Li et al[5] characterized the gene that codes for acid ceramidase and demonstrated pathogenic mutations in patients with Farber lipogranulomatosis.

Clinical Picture

Table 27–1 summarizes the clinical manifestations in 75 Farber disease (FD) patients who have been reported in the literature or are known to the author. Diagnosis was confirmed by acid ceramidase assay or by morphologic and/or biochemical studies of biopsy or autopsy tissue. They have been provisionally subdivided into seven subtypes.[6]

Type 1. Classic FD is the most common phenotype. The clinical presentation is so characteristic that diagnosis can almost be made at a glance.[1,7] Characteristic features are painful swelling of joints (particularly the interphalangeal, metacarpal, ankle, wrist, knee, and elbow); palpable subcutaneous nodules in relation to affected joints and over pressure points (Fig. 27–1) and also in the conjunctiva external

ear and nostrils; hoarse cry that may progress to aphonia; feeding and respiratory difficulties; poor weight gain; and intermittent fever. Symptoms usually appear between ages 2 weeks and 4 months. Disturbances in swallowing, vomiting, and repeated episodes of pulmonary consolidations associated with fever occur frequently, and pulmonary disease is the usual cause of death. Other organs are also involved and include hepatosplenomegaly, generalized lymphadenopathy, and cardiac murmurs secondary to valvular involvement. Diminished deep tendon reflexes, hypotonia, and muscular atrophy are due to involvement of anterior horn cells and peripheral neuropathy. Initial psychomotor development may be normal, but seizures and progressive cognitive decline may occur later. Diffuse, grayish opacification of the retina about the foveola, with a cherry-red center, is present in approximately one third of the patients (although there is no disturbance of visual function, and it is subtler than the cherry-red spot in Tay-Sachs disease).[8]

Types 2 and 3. Intermediate and mild phenotypes. Twenty-five of the 78 patients belonged to this category. The arthropathy and subcutaneous nodules in these patients may be as severe as in the classic phenotype, but the lungs, visceral organs, and nervous system are less involved. Eleven of the patients survived to age 16 years or older. In 14 patients, neurologic function was normal at time of last follow-up at ages ranging from 4 to 16 years.

Type 4. Neonatal phenotype. Six patients in this category are known. They are extremely ill during the neonatal period with severe hepatosplenomegaly. The most severe patient presented as hydrops fetalis and died on the third day.[9]

299

TABLE 27–1. Farber Disease Clinical Findings

	1, Classic	2, Intermediate	3, Mild	4, Neonatal	5, Neurologic Progressive	6, Combined with Sandhoff	7, Prosaposin Deficiency
Number of Cases	35	14	11	6	7	1	1
Mean age (years)							
Onset	0.3	0.66	1.6	0	1.66	0.13	0
Death	1.45	6.25	15.8	0.16	3.6	1.1	0.3
Last follow-up	1.1	5.6	13.0		3.9		
Nodules	100%	100%	100%	1/3	7/7	1/1	0/1
Joint involvement	100%	100%	100%	2/3	7/7	1/1	0/1
Hoarseness	100%	100%	100%	0/3	6/6	1/1	0/1
Large liver	14/20	3/7	3/7	100%	1/5	1/1	1/1
Large spleen	7/15	3/7	3/7	100%	1/5	1/1	1/1
Lung infiltrates	16/19	1/8	2/11		0/4	0/1	
Macular cherry-red spot	4/15	0/6	0/9		3/4	0/1	0/1
Lower motor neuron involvement	11/13	2/5	2/4		1/1		
Central nervous system impaired	15/22	3/10	5/9		7/7	1/1	1/1

Type 5. Neurologic progressive. Progressive neurologic deterioration and seizures were the most prominent manifestations. Joint manifestations and subcutaneous nodules were relatively mild in the seven patients in this category. Neurologic manifestations included loss of speech, ataxia and progressive paraparesis, and macular cherry-red spots.

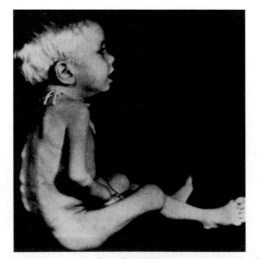

FIGURE 27-1. Type 3 Farber disease patient at 23 months. Note joint swelling and contractures and subcutaneous nodules over spinous processes. Tracheostomy was performed as a lifesaving procedure at age 15 months. (From Zetterstrom R: Disseminated lipogranulomatosis: Farber disease. Acta Paediatr 1958;47:501.)

Type 6. Combined Farber disease and Sandhoff disease. One patient with this combination had been reported, but subsequent genetic studies indicated that this represented a coincidental combination of two distinct disease entities.[10]

Type 7. Prosaposin deficiency. A homoallelic A-to-T transversion in the initiation codon of the precursor protein of the sphingolipid activator prosaposin has been reported in a single patient and his 20-week-old fetal sibling.[11] Ceramide and sulfatide levels were increased, and activities of acid ceramidase, glucoceramidase, and galactoceramidase were diminished. Clinical manifestations resembled those of Gaucher disease type II. There was no arthropathy, and subcutaneous nodules were not present.

Diagnosis

Clinical diagnosis of classic type 1 FD can be easily made because the triad of subcutaneous nodules, arthropathy, and laryngeal involvement appears to be unique for FD. In our experience, acid ceramidase activity has been diminished in all patients with this clinical presentation. Diagnostic challenges arise when one or more of these features is missing or mild. Joint and/or skin manifestations that resemble FD may occur in juvenile rheumatoid arthritis, multicentric histiocytosis, and fibromatosis hyalina multiplex juvenilis. Acid ceramidase activity is normal in these disorders. Patients with the neonatal forms of FD do not show the classic clinical triad, and diagnosis depends upon demonstration of reduced acid ceramidase activity. Other patients in whom the clinical manifestations were dominated by hepatosplenomegaly or by psychomotor deterioration and in whom joint and skin abnormalities were mild have been misdiagnosed as histiocytosis or Tay-Sachs disease.

Deficiency of Acid Ceramidase

In vitro acid ceramidase activity in FD patients is usually less than 6 percent of control values. The test can be applied to white blood cells,[12] cultured skin fibroblasts,[13] amniocytes,[14] and also to plasma[12] and postmortem tissues.[3] N-lauroylsphingosine is the preferred substrate.[12]

Accumulation of Ceramide in Plasma and Urine

Increased levels of ceramide are demonstrable in subcutaneous nodules. Ceramide levels were also increased in the urine of one patient,[15] but this increase was not demonstrable in the urine of four other patients.[6]

Studies of Ceramide Turnover

Impaired degradation of ceramides in FD can also be demonstrated by loading studies with labeled precursors, such as [14C] acid-labeled cerebroside sulfate. Abnormal retention of this substrate in the ceramide fraction has been demonstrated in FD cultured skin fibroblasts,[16,17] but results in FD lymphocytes do not differ from normal, presumably owing to the presence of an alternative degradative pathway in these cells.[17] Use of LDL-associated [3H] sphingomyelin demonstrates impaired degradation of lysosomal ceramides in both FD cultured skin fibroblasts and transformed lymphocytes, and the degree of impairment correlates to some extent with the clinical disease severity.[18] Long-term studies with [14C] serine, a substrate for a committed step in the de novo synthesis of ceramide and complex sphingolipids,[19] can also demonstrate impaired synthesis of ceramide in FD and has added valuable information about the dynamics of ceramide metabolism in this disorder.

Morphologic Studies

Biopsies of subcutaneous nodules demonstrate granulomas and the presence of lipid cytoplasmic inclusions that are PAS-positive and are extracted by lipid solvents. Under the electron microscope, they have a characteristic curvilinear tubular structure, and are referred to as Farber bodies or Banana bodies (Fig. 27–2).[20]

Identification of Heterozygotes

All of the obligate heterozygotes tested so far had reduced acid ceramidase activity in cultured skin fibroblasts or white blood cells.[6,13] Mutation analysis is used in families in which the molecular defect has been defined.

Prenatal Diagnosis

Prenatal diagnosis has been achieved by measurement of acid ceramidase activity in cultured amniocytes[14] or loading studies in either cultured amniocytes or chorion villus samples.[10]

PATHOLOGY

Histopathology

Studies with the light microscope show granulomatous infiltrations in the subcutaneous tissues and joints. The earliest lesions appear to be the accumulation of macrophages or histiocytes. Foam cells are prominent. These lesions have also been found in the larynx, lungs, heart valves, lymph nodes, intestine, liver, spleen, gall bladder, tongue, and thymus.[6] The nervous system is also involved in most cases. The main abnormality is the accumulation of storage material in neuronal cytoplasm. The accumulation is most prominent in the anterior horn cells in the spinal cord, but large cells (nerve cells of the brain stem nuclei, basal ganglia, and cerebellum; retinal ganglion cells; autonomic ganglia; Schwann cells; and, to a lesser extent, cortical neurons) are also involved. The storage material is PAS-positive and is extracted with lipid solvents.[7] Ultrastructural studies show characteristic curvilinear inclusions (see Fig. 27–2).[20]

Chemical Pathology

Abnormally high ceramide levels, as high as 60-fold normal, have been found in all FD patients in whom the levels

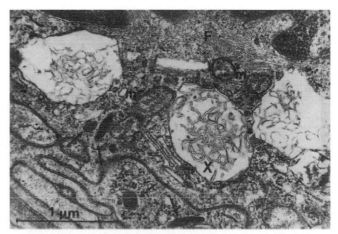

FIGURE 27–2. Farber disease. Thin section of an endothelial cell with filaments (F), Wiebel-Palade bodies *(arrows)*, mitochondria (m), and three vacuoles, one of which (X) contains "Farber bodies." Reduced from ×45,000. (From Schmoeckel C, Hohlfed M: A specific ultrastructural marker for disseminated lipogranulomatosis [Farber]. Arch Dermatol Res 1979;266:187–196.)

of this lipid have been analyzed. In the subcutaneous nodule, they may make up 20% of total lipids. They are also increased in the kidney. For other tissues, the extent of ceramide excess appears to vary with the severity of the disease. Severely affected patients showed high ceramide levels in the liver, lungs, and brain,[7] whereas mildly affected patients had normal ceramide levels in these tissues.[21] Unlike those of normal subjects, the ceramides of patients with FD may contain significant proportions of 2-hydroxy fatty acids.[7] Levels of gangliosides may also be increased.[7]

Enzyme Deficiency

Acid ceramidase (EC 3.5.1.23), the enzyme that is deficient in FD,[3] catalyzes the reaction

$$Ceramide + H_2O \rightarrow Sphingosine + FA$$

The enzyme has been purified.[22] It is a heterodimeric glycoprotein with a molecular weight of approximately 50 kDa. It is comprised of two subunits. The alpha subunit has an approximate molecular weight of 13 kDa. The beta unit (molecular weight approximately 40 kDa) contains 5 or 6 N-linked oligosaccharide units, whereas the alpha unit is not glycosylated. Both subunits arise from a single chain precursor of approximately 55 kDa. Proteolytic processing of the precursor takes place in either the late endosomal and/or lysosomal compartments, and preliminary studies indicate that targeting of the enzyme is dependent on the mannose-6-phosphate pathway. Degradation of membrane-bound ceramide by acid ceramidase requires the presence of sphingolipid activator proteins[23] with SAP-C-and SAP-D being most active. As noted, FD type 7 is due to a genetic defect in the synthesis of the prosaposin precursor. Negatively charged lipids, particularly Bis (monoacylglycerol) phosphate (BMP) are also required. It is proposed that the degradation of ceramide by acid ceramidase takes place on lysosomal vesicles that contain the substrate, acid ceramidase, SAP-C, SAP-D, and BMP. Several neutral and alkaline ceramidases have been identified. The activities of these enzymes are not deficient in FD.[6]

Pathogenesis

The ceramide that accumulates in FD is located in the lysosome. Turnover studies show that it results from the impaired capacity to hydrolyze the ceramide generated during the degradation of complex sphingolipids. The rate of ceramide synthesis is the same as in normal cells, and newly synthesized ceramides in FD fibroblasts are directed to the synthesis of complex sphingolipids as they are in normal cells.[19] The distribution of lesions in FD and the variability of the expression of the disease can only be partially explained. Neuronal storage is not unexpected because ceramide metabolism in brain is known to be active. The striking involvement of subcutaneous tissues may be accounted for by the observation that ceramide has an important role in normal skin. Ceramide forms an essential part of the skin barrier that preserves water impermeability in normal skin.[24] Ceramide accumulation appears to be the cause of the granuloma formation. Granulomatous lesions that resemble those in FD were produced by the subcutaneous injection of ceramide in rats.[7] It is of interest that bone marrow transplant leads to regression of the subcutaneous nodules, possibly by removing this stimulus of granuloma formation.[25] Ceramide appears to play a critical, but not fully understood, role in many aspects of cell biology,[26] such as apoptosis, response to stress, and expression of cytokines. This led to inquiry about whether the ceramide that accumulates in FD could affect these critical processes. This does not seem to be the case, however. Apoptosis was not demonstrable in FD fibroblasts in spite of the increased ceramide level.[27] This appears to be a consequence of compartmentalization of the ceramide. Biomodulatory actions appear to be exerted by those ceramides located in the inner leaflets of the plasma membrane and at the cell surface in caveolae.[28] The ceramide that accumulates in FD appears to be confined to the lysosome[29] and thus does not exert these biomodulatory effects.

CLINICAL GENETICS

The mode of inheritance of FD is autosomal recessive. Except for the Jewish population, all ethnic groups appear to be affected. The prevalence of FD is unknown. The fact that we have been able to document only 78 cases and that consanguinity was present in 11 of 50 families suggests that it is rare.

MOLECULAR GENETICS

The human acid ceramidase gene spans about 30 kb and contains a total of 14 exons. It has been mapped to chromosomal region 8p21.3/22.[5] The full-length cDNA contains an 1185-bp open reading frame that encodes 395 amino acids, an 1110-bp 3′-untranslated sequence, and an 18-bp poly (A) tail. Twelve different pathogenic mutations have been described so far (Table 27–2) as well as 2 polymorphisms (M72V and V931) that have no effect on enzymatic activity.

ANIMAL MODEL

At this time there is no animal model of acid ceramidase deficiency. Targeted disruption of the mouse sphingolipid activator protein[30] leads to a complex phenotype including severe leukodystrophy, and axonal abnormalities and storage of multiple sphingolipids.

TABLE 27–2. Pathogenic Mutations of the Acid Ceramidase (AC) Gene in Farber Disease Patients

Mutations in AC cDNA	Predicted Amino Acid Substitution	Reference
66→C	Q22H	32
67C→G	H23B	32
107A→G	Y36C	33
423A→T	E138V	5
del1383-457	del128-152	33
665C→A	T222K	4
760A→G	R254G	5
958A→G	N320D	33
991G→A	D331	33
del1042-1048	del1348-366	33
1085T→G	P362R	5
1204insT	X402L	32

THERAPY

Therapy is symptomatic. Bone marrow transplant has led to regression of subcutaneous nodules and arthropathy but did not alter neurologic deterioration. It should be considered in patients without neurologic involvement, such as the one reported by Samuelsson.[21] Gene therapy may become possible in the future. Introduction of cDNA of human acid ceramidase into FD disease fibroblasts with a retroviral vector restored enzyme activity completely and normalized ceramide levels and lysosomal turnover.[31]

FUTURE DIRECTIONS

Future directions include the development of an animal model of acid ceramidase deficiency, purification of the enzyme in sufficient quantity to test the possibility of enzyme replacement therapy, and other therapeutic approaches such as stem cell therapy.

CONCLUSION

Farber disease (MIM 22800) is a genetically determined disorder of lipid metabolism associated with the deficiency of lysosomal acid ceramidase and accumulation of ceramide in the lysosome. The disorder presents most commonly during the first few months of life with a unique triad of symptoms: painful and progressively deformed joints, subcutaneous nodules, and progressive laryngeal involvement leading to hoarseness and respiratory impairment. The involved tissues show granulomas and lipid-laden macrophages with characteristic inclusions. Progressive involvement of lungs, heart valves, liver, spleen, peripheral nerves, and brain follow and often lead to death during the first few years of life. Other phenotypes occur, including neonatal, adolescent, and adult forms in which the nervous system may be spared, and a form in which progressive neurologic deterioration is the main feature. Acid ceramidase (EC 3.5.1.23) has been purified and cloned. The full-length DNA contains an 1185 bp open reading frame. Twelve different mutations have been identified in FD patients. The ceramide that accumulates is confined to the lysosome and does not appear to contribute to the multiple biomodulatory roles attributed to ceramides in other compartments. Laboratory diagnosis is achieved by demonstration of reduced acid ceramidase activity in white blood cells, cultured skin fibroblasts, and amniocytes. Prenatal diagnosis is possible. The disease is rare. Data on 78 patients in a variety of ethnic groups have been assembled. The mode of inheritance is autosomal recessive. Rarely, ceramide accumulation may also be caused by a deficiency of a sphingolipid activator protein (prosaposin). There is no effective therapy. Bone marrow transplant can lead to regression of joint manifestations and subcutaneous nodules and relieves the hoarseness, but it does not alter progressive neurologic deterioration. It should be considered for patients without neurologic involvement.[32,33]

REFERENCES

1. Farber S, Cohen J, Uzman LL: Lipogranulomatosis: A new lipoglyco-protein storage disease. Mt Sinai J Med 1957;24:816–837.

2. Prensky AL, Ferreira G, Carr S, Moser HW: Ceramide and ganglioside accumulation in Farber's lipogranulomatosis. Proc Soc Exp Biol Med 1967;126:725–728.

3. Sugita M, Dulaney JT, Moser HW: Ceramidase deficiency in Farber's disease (lipogranulomatosis). Science 1972;178:1100–1102.

4. Koch J, Gartner S, Li CM, et al: Molecular cloning and characterization of a full-length complementary DNA encoding human acid ceramidase: Identification of the first molecular lesion causing Farber disease. J Biol Chem 1996;271:33110–33115.

5. Li CM, Park JH, He X, et al: The human acid ceramidase gene (ASAH): Structure, chromosomal location, mutation analysis, and expression. Genomics 1999;62:223–231.

6. Moser HW, Linke T, Fensom AH, et al: Acid ceramidase deficiency: Farber lipogranulomatosis. In Scriver CR, Beaudet AL, Sly WS, et al (eds): The Metabolic and Molecular Basis of Inherited Disease, 8th ed. New York, McGraw-Hill, 2001, pp 3573–3588.

7. Moser HW, Prensky AL, Wolfe HJ, Rosman NP: Farber's lipogranulomatosis: Report of a case and demonstration of an excess of free ceramide and ganglioside. Am J Med 1969;47:869–890.

8. Cogan DG, Kuwabara T, Moser H, Hazard GW: Retinopathy in a case of Farber's lipogranulomatosis. Arch Ophthalmol 1966;75:752–757.

9. Kattner E, Schafer A, Harzer K: Hydrops fetalis: Manifestation in lysosomal storage diseases including Farber disease. Eur J Pediatr 1997;156:292–295.

10. Levade T, Enders H, Schliephacke M, Harzer K: A family with combined Farber and Sandhoff, isolated Sandhoff and isolated fetal Farber disease: Postnatal exclusion and prenatal diagnosis of Farber disease using lipid loading tests on intact cultured cells. Eur J Pediatr 1995;154:643–648.

11. Bradova V, Smid F, Ulrich-Bott B, et al: Prosaposin deficiency—further characterization of the sphingolipid activator protein-deficient sibs: Multiple glycolipid elevations (including lactosylceramidosis), partial enzyme deficiencies and ultrastructure of the skin in this generalized sphingolipid storage disease. Hum Genet 1993;92:143–152.

12. Ben-Yoseph Y, Gagne R, Parvathy MR, et al: Leukocyte and plasma N-laurylsphingosine deacylase (ceramidase) in Farber disease. Clin Genet 1989;36:38–42.

13. Dulaney JT, Milunsky A, Sidbury JB, et al: Diagnosis of lipogranulomatosis (Farber disease) by use of cultured fibroblasts. J Pediatr 1976;89:59–61.

14. Fensom AH, Benson PF, Neville BR, et al: Prenatal diagnosis of Farber's disease. Lancet 1979;2:990–992.

15. Sugita M, Iwamori M, Evans J, et al: High performance liquid chromatography of ceramides: Application to analysis in human tissues and demonstration of ceramide excess in Farber's disease. J Lipid Res 1974;15:223–226.

16. Kudoh T, Wenger DA: Diagnosis of metachromatic leukodystrophy, Krabbe disease, and Farber disease after uptake of fatty acid-labeled cerebroside sulfate into cultured skin fibroblasts. J Clin Invest 1982;70:89–97.

17. Levade T, Tempesta MC, Moser HW, et al: Sulfatide and sphingomyelin loading of living cells as tools for the study of ceramide turnover by lysosomal ceramidase: Implications for the diagnosis of Farber disease. Biochem Mol Med 1995;54:117–125.

18. Levade T, Moser HW, Fensom AH, et al: Neurodegenerative course in ceramidase deficiency (Farber disease) correlates with the residual lysosomal ceramide turnover in cultured living patient cells. J Neurol Sci 1995;134:108–114.

19. van Echten-Deckert G, Klein A, Linke T, et al: Turnover of endogenous ceramide in cultured normal and Farber fibroblasts. J Lipid Res 1997;38: 2569–2579.

20. Schmoeckel C, Hohlfed M: A specific ultrastructural marker for disseminated lipogranulomatosis (Farber). Arch Dermatol Res 1979;266:187–196.

21. Samuelsson K, Zetterstrom R: Ceramides in a patient with lipogranulomatosis (Farber's disease) with chronic course. Scand J Clin Lab Invest 1971;27:393–405.

22. Bernardo K, Hurwitz R, Zenk T, et al: Purification, characterization, and biosynthesis of human acid ceramidase. J Biol Chem 1995;270:11098–11102.

23. Kishimoto Y, Hiraiwa M, O'Brien JS: Saposins: Structure, function, distribution, and molecular genetics. J Lipid Res 1992;33:1255–1267.

24. Doering T, Holleran WM, Potratz A, et al: Sphingolipid activator proteins are required for epidermal permeability barrier formation. J Biol Chem 1999;274:11038–11045.

25. Yeager AM, Uhas KA, Coles CD, et al: Bone marrow transplantation for infantile ceramidase deficiency (Farber disease). Bone Marrow Transplant 2000;26:357–363.

26. Perry DK, Hannun YA: The role of ceramide in cell signaling. Biochim Biophys Acta 1998;1436: 233–243.

27. Tohyama J, Oya Y, Ezoe T, et al: Ceramide accumulation is associated with increased apoptotic cell death in cultured fibroblasts of sphingolipid activator protein-deficient mouse but not in fibroblasts of patients with Farber disease. J Inherit Metab Dis 1999;22:649–662.

28. Liu P, Anderson RG: Compartmentalized production of ceramide at the cell surface. J Biol Chem 1995;270:27179–27185.

29. Chatelut M, Leruth M, Harzer K, et al: Natural ceramide is unable to escape the lysosome, in contrast to a fluorescent analogue. FEBS Lett 1998;426:102–106.

30. Oya Y, Nakayasu H, Fujita N, et al: Pathological study of mice with total deficiency of sphingolipid activator proteins (SAP knockout mice). Acta Neuropathol (Berl) 1998;96:29–40.

31. Medin JA, Takenaka T, Carpentier S, et al: Retrovirus-mediated correction of the metabolic defect in cultured Farber disease cells. Hum Gene Ther 1999;10: 1321–1329.

32. Zhang Z, Mandal AK, Mital A, et al: Human acid ceramidase gene: Novel mutations in Farber disease. Mol Genet Metab 2000;70:301–309.

33. Bär J, Linke T, Ferlinz K, et al: Molecular analysis of acid ceramidase deficiency in patients with Farber disease. Hum Mutat 2001;17:199–209.

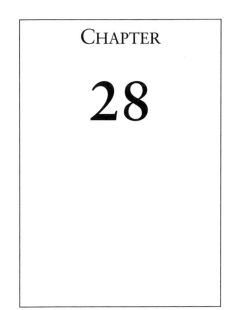

CHAPTER

28

Wolman Disease

Rita Alam

Frank M. Yatsu

Lysosomal acid lipase/cholesteryl-ester hydrolase (LAL; EC 3.1.1.13) is a 43 kDa protein whose gene has been cloned and sequenced and is required for the intracellular hydrolysis of cholesteryl-esters and triglyceride, and thus is important in cholesterol regulation and its role for cell growth and membrane functions.[1–6] Two autosomal recessive genetic disorders exist for this gene/lysosomal enzyme, one of which results in a marked reduction in activity, causing Wolman disease (WD), and the other a milder decrease, resulting in cholesteryl ester storage disease (CESD). In WD, the onset is in infancy, and the signs are failure to thrive, persistent vomiting, hepatosplenomegaly, steatorrhea, and other gastrointestinal signs. These infants die in the first year of life and are found to have massive collections of cholesteryl esters and triglycerides in their livers, leading to cirrhosis. In CESD, residual LAL activity exists, resulting in milder symptoms and signs, occurring clinically in adults, primarily with hepatomegaly and premature atherosclerosis with hyperlipoproteinemia. Because the pathology in both WD and CESD is primarily in the periphery, particularly the liver, and notably absent in the brain, it has been considered a prototypic disease for which gene transfer or gene therapy might be beneficial.

Although CESD has a milder clinical picture, it has been established that both CESD and WD have mutation in LAL gene. Elucidation of cDNA sequence[7] and the respective gene structure,[8–10] which is composed of 10 exons located within a 38.8 kb region on human chromosome 10,[11] has allowed identification of mutation responsible for WD and CESD (Fig. 28–1). Human LAL purified from various sources shows different molecular sizes. Fibroblasts, for instance, express two molecular forms of 41 and 49 kDa,[12] and LAL purified from human liver show two molecular forms of 41 and 56 kDa.[7]

Comparison of the protein sequences of LAL with those of known lipases reveals significant amino acid homologies with human gastric lipase, rat lingual lipase, and bovine pregastric esterase, establishing the enzymes as members of a gene family of highly conserved acid lipases.[13,14] Structure-function studies of LAL have focused on delineating the roles of serine residues in the two Gly-X-Ser-X-Gly consensus sequences of LAL, demonstrating that S153 is important for hydrolysis of triolein and cholesteryl esters, whereas S99 does not affect the enzymatic activity of LAL.[15,16] This has been substantiated by the three-dimensional model building of LAL based on the crystal structure of human gastric lipase.[17] Depending on the specific mutation, HLAL deficiency can manifest either as the milder clinical picture of CESD or as the severe phenotype of WD. Both diseases are extremely rare. It has been pointed out by Wolman[18] that the true incidence of growth disorders cannot be determined with certainty because CESD is sometimes very difficult to diagnose, as illustrated by clinically asymptomatic and purely accidentally diagnosed disease. A number of LAL mutations have been identified in WD patients. Various missense mutations, such as L179P, G321W, and nonsense mutations T22X, Q277X, Y303X, have been found in the LAL gene.[8,19–22] Insertion mutations, such as 635insT, 351insA,[8] and deletion mutations, such as Δ159–166, Δ435–436,[8,23] and Δexon8 have also been encountered in pedigrees with WD.[24] In the rat model of WD, a deletion of 4.5 kb and 60-bp substitution resulted in a premature stop codon at amino acid position 368 and a consecutively truncated LAL protein.[25] Zschenker et al, reported a case with single-base deletion leading to a premature stop codon at amino acid position 106, a homozygote for a signal peptide mutation and a missense mutation at amino acid

```
                                                           39
       gcggagtctccgaggcacttcccggtggctggctgctctgattggCTGAA...Exon 1...TCCAGgtgagagtgccggcgccggcgtgccaggtgcgggtgcggcgtggaagctggtgc

EX2F                          40                 151                                                       EX2R
gtgggagcattaagttaccagaatcattt.(39).tattatacagAATGA...Exon 2...ATGTGgtaagtttctcaaagttatgtacttttaaaatgcatctatttccccgatcca

E3F                   152              269                                                    E3bR
gtttcagattctgtccacccaatttccat.(6)..tttctctacagAGTGA...Exon 3...CAAAGgtatgggaaggctcttaaaagtaaaaaccagaattcttctgggttttgtg

     EXN3F                     270             468                                                      EXN3R
     gaagcttggtgctactgcctcctaaacaatgaatgtttttcagGTCCC...Exon 4...TTCAGgtatatatgaa.(20).tttccttagtactcttaaagcagacaacaggcttccag

EXN4F                        469             578                                                EXN4R
catactcagtatgtgtgtgctctattttta.(25).tggattacagTTATG...Exon 5...TATAGgtatgtatg.(15).gttgatataaattcttcattacagagtttgtactttc

EXN5F2                      579             715                                               EXN5R
ggaaatcccagatgatggaattcctgtt.(10).tgttctcacagGTTTT...Exon 6...TTAAGgtacttggaccccctcccatccctctcctctccccgcagatttcctcctgaga

EXN6F                      716             862                                                EXN6R
tatgcaccagagtgaaatgctgagatg.(14).tttattttgtagGACTT...Exon 7...ATATGgtatgcatgtt.(37).atgatatgggagaggtgggaatgacctcatcagaact

EX7aF                       863             934                                               EX7AR
tcaatgccaccttaatgctgtttttcat.(16).tttattttgcagTCTAG...Exon 8...GCCAGgtaggcattcca.(27).caacatcagaaaggnctgggcatgcaaaaccctttcc

EXN7BF                      935             1006                                              EXN7BR2
gttggatttccgaggttgtggctagctc.(56).tcttctttttagGCTGT...Exon 9...ACCAGgtaaagtttt.(28).aactcattaagaaagccagcctggcctatcaggattctg

       EXN8F                  1007             Ter                                           EXN8R
       aacaacgaggcttctctggttcctttcattgtagAGTTA...Exon 10...AAATATCAGTGAAAGCTGGACTTGAGCTGTGTGTACCACCAAGTCA....
```

FIGURE 28–1. Exon/intron junctions are shown for the human lysosomal acid lipase/cholesteryl ester hydrolase with partial intron sequences in lower case letters and exon sequences in upper case letters. Numbers above sequences refer to nucleotide positions on the gene locus given by Anderson and Sando.[7] The numbers in parentheses represent deleted nucleotides to show sequences and positions of primers used in PCR amplification; the primers are underlined. Ter refers to the translation termination site. (Reproduced with permission from Anderson RA, Byrum RS, Coates PM, Sando GN: Mutations at the lysosomal acid cholesteryl ester hydrolase gene locus in Wolman disease. Proc Natl Acad Sci 1994;91:2718–2722.)

position 60. Single and double mutants, G60V and S106X, G-5R/G60V, when expressed in Spodoptera frugiperda cells, show single peptide mutant retains lipase activity in cell extracts and drastic reduction of enzyme activity in culture supernatant, indicating that mutation may affect secretion of active enzymes from cells.[26]

Although the current understanding of a genotype/phenotype correlation in WD and CESD is not complete, nonsense mutations of LAL have produced conflicting data with respect to genotype–phenotype correlations. In certain families of WD, homozygosity for mutations in the LAL gene is *unique* and associated with almost a complete absence of enzymatic activity. Although it has been suggested that a residual lipase activity remains in CESD individuals, resulting in a more benign clinical course than WD,[22,23,25] other investigators have presented data on LAL mutants not supporting of this concept.[27–29] Additional mechanism besides a deficiency of LAL may play a role in the production of two phenotypes, WD and CESD.

WOLMAN DISEASE: THERAPEUTIC INTERVENTIONS

Treatment strategies to minimize the effects of lysosomal acid lipase (LAL) deficiency have been limited to either reducing cholesterol synthesis, in the expectation of decreasing the amount of esterified cholesterol formed, or reconstituting the LAL gene deficiency by liver or bone marrow transplantation or by viral vector use such as adenovirus or adeno-associated virus (AAV). This section will emphasize primarily the last techniques and its applicability in vivo to humans.

Although use of drugs to reduce cholesterol synthesis has the logic of decreasing substrate-derived compounds, such as cholesterol synthesis rate-limiting drugs, namely, HMG CoA reductase inhibitors, they have been only minimally beneficial. Thus far, use of liver and bone marrow transplantation to replenish LAL deficiency has not been successful, but successes in other gene deficiency states suggest that these techniques have not been exhausted for either WD or CESD.[18,30]

Direct transfer of the LAL gene using an adenoviral vector has been investigated by Tietge et al,[31] in vitro using fibroblast cells from a patient with WD, as well as in vivo in normal CS7BL/6 mice. These studies demonstrated, as detailed subsequently, that increased levels of LAL can be achieved in the WD fibroblasts, as well as COS cells, but also in the liver of the C57BL/7 mice. In these treated WD fibroblasts, reduced cholesteryl esters and triglycerides are inversely reduced to increased amounts of LAL introduced. The last also correlates with increased amounts of LAL protein synthesized, quantitated by Western blotting, and electron microscopic morphology becomes normalized. Because a mouse model resembling CESD has been developed by targeted disruption of the LAL gene and because a naturally occurring rat model similar to WD exists,[32,33] it is anticipated that successes noted earlier with gene transfer will be achieved in these two human disease models.

Construction of Recombinant Adenoviruses. In the investigation on human LAL by Tietge et al,[31] LAL cDNA was excised from pBluescriptllKS-hLAL with *HindIll* and subcloned into the *HindIll* site of pAdCMV link, containing adenoviral 0–1 mU, CMV immediate-early promoter and enhancer, SV4O polyadenylation signal, and adenoviral 9–16 mU. This plasmid, designated pAdCMVhLAL, was cotransfected into cells with adenoviral DNA that contains a temperature-sensitive mutation (ts 125) in the E2A gene, making the recombinant adenovirus unable to replicate at 39°C. After incubation, plaques were screened by PCR, and positive cells for hLAL cDNA were repurified. Aliquots of purified adenoviruses were stored in 10% glycerol-phosphate-buffered saline (PBS) at -80°C until used.

Wolman Disease Fibroblast Cell Culture and Adenoviral Infection. Fibroblasts from a patient with WD (GM 11851) and a normal individual (GM 03468A) were cultured in a standard fashion, plated, and infected with various multiplicities of infections (MOIs) with either AdhILAL or Adnull with analyses at various time points after two hours of incubation at 37°C.

Human Adenovirus LAL Expression in Normal C57BL/6 Mice. In the studies by Tietge et al,[31] 8-week-old C57BL/6 mice were injected with 1×10^{11} particles of either AdhLAL or Adnull in the tail veins; after 5 days, the mice were sacrificed, the livers were harvested, and their LAL activities were analyzed. The basal and control (Adnull) levels of LAL were 0.04 ± 0.02 nmol/mg/hr and increased significantly to 0.54 ± 0.07 nmol/mg/hr, a 13.5-fold increase. These in vivo results in normal animals suggest that the same results can be achieved in humans, including those with genetic LAL deficiency.

SUMMARY

Success in normalizing LAL levels and their enzymatic activities in vitro using WD fibroblasts with an adenoviral vector, plus a statistically significant ($P < 0.001$) 13.5-fold increase hepatic LAL in normal C57BL/6 mice suggests that experimental WD and CESD will respond to gene transfer, perhaps using the more favored adeno-associated virus. Although the short duration of gene expression, toxicity, and issues related to insertional mutagenesis are concerns with gene transfer, the future appears promising for beneficial therapeutic interventions in these human genetic conditions.

REFERENCES

1. Yatsu FM, Alam R: Wolman Disease. In Rosenberg RN, Prusiner SB, DiMauro, S, Barchi, RL (eds): The Molecular and Genetic Basis of Neurological Disease, 2nd ed. Boston, Butterworth Heinemann, 1977, pp 371–378.

2. Assman G, Seedorf U: Acid lipase deficiency: Wolman disease and cholesteryl ester storage disease. In Scriver CR, Beaudet AL, Sly WS, Valle D (eds): The Metabolic and Molecular Basis of Inherited Disease. New York, McGraw-Hill, 1995, pp 2563–2587.

3. Goldstein JL, Dana SE, Faust JR, et al: Role of lysosomal acid lipase in the metabolism of plasma low density lipoprotein. Observations in cultured fibroblasts from a patient with cholesteryl ester storage. J Biol Chem 1975;250:8487 8495.

4. Brown MS, Goldstein JL: Receptor-mediated control of cholesterol metabolism. Science 1976;191: 150–154.

5. Coates PM, Langert T, Cortner JA: Genetic variation of human mononuclear leukocyte lysosomal acid lipase activity. Relationship to atherosclerosis. Atherosclerosis 1986;62:11–20.

6. Yatsu F, Hagemenas F, Manaugh L, Galumbos T: Cholesteryl ester hydrolase activity in human symptomatic atherosclerosis. Lipids 1980;15:1019–1022.

7. Anderson RA, Sando GN: Cloning and expression of cDNA encoding human lysosomal acid lipase/cholesteryl ester hydrolase. J Biol Chem 1991;266: 2479–2484.

8. Anderson RA, Byrum RS, Coates PM, Sando GN: Mutations at the lysosomal acid cholesteryl ester hydrolase gene locus in Wolman disease. Proc Natl Acad Sci 1994;91:2718–2722.

9. Aslanidis C, Klima H, Lackner KJ, Schmitz G: Genomic organization of the human lysosomal acid lipase gene (LIPA). Genomics 1994;20:329–331.

10. Lohse P, Lohse P, Chahrokh-Zadeh S, Seidel D: The acid lipase gene family: Three enzymes, one highly conserved gene structure. J Lipid Res 1997;38:880–891.

11. Anderson RA, Rao N, Byrum RS, et al: In situ localization of the genetic locus encoding the lysosomal acid lipase/cholesteryl esterase (LIPA) deficient in Wolman disease to chromosome 10q23.2-q23.3. Genomics 1993;5:245–247.

12. Sando GN, Rosenbaum LM: Human lysosomal acid lipase/cholesteryl ester hydrolase: Purification and properties of the form secreted by fibroblasts in microcarrier culture. J Biol Chem 1985;260:15186–15193.

13. Ameis D, Merkel M, Eckerskorn C, Greten H: Purification, characterization and molecular cloning of human hepatic lysosomal acid lipase. Eur J Biochem 1994;219:905–914.

14. Lohse P, Lohse P, Chahrokh-Zadeh S, Seidel D: The acid lipase gene family: Three enzymes, one highly conserved gene structure. J Lipid Res 1997;38: 880–891.

15. Sheriff S, Du H, Grabowski GA: Characterization of lysosomal acid lipase by site-directed mutagenesis and heterologous expression. J Biol Chem 1995;270: 27766–27772.

16. Lohse P, Chahrokh-Zadeh S, Lohse P, Seidel D: Human lysosomal acid lipase/cholesteryl ester hydrolase and human gastric lipase: Identification of the catalytically active serine, aspartic acid, and histidine residues. J Lipid Res 1997;38:892–903.

17. Roussel A, Canaan S, Egloff MP, et al: Crystal structure of human gastric lipase and model of lysosomal acid lipase, two lipolytic enzymes of medical interest. J Biol Chem 1999;274: 16995–17002.

18. Wolman M: Wolman disease and its treatment. Clin Pediatr (Phila) 1995;34:207–212.

19. Lohse P, Maas S, Lohse P, et al: Molecular defects underlying Wolman disease appear to be more heterogeneous than those resulting in cholesteryl ester storage disease. J Lipid Res 1999;40:221–228.

20. Fujiwama J, Sakuraba H, Kuriyama M, et al: A new mutation (LIPA Tyr22X) of lysosomal acid lipase gene in a Japanese patient with Wolman disease. Hum Mutat 1996;8:377–380.

21. Ries S, Aslanidis C, Fehringer P, et al: A new mutation in the gene for lysosomal acid lipase leads to Wolman disease in an African kindred. J Lipid Res 1996;37:1761–1765.

22. Pagani F, Pariyarath R, Garcia R, et al: New lysosomal acid lipase gene mutants explain the phenotype of Wolman disease and cholesteryl ester storage disease. J Lipid Res 1998;39:1382–1388.

23. Seedorf U, Wiebusch H, Muntoni S, et al: Wolman disease due to homozygosity for a novel truncated variant of lysosomal acid lipase (351insA) associated with complete in situ acid lipase deficiency. Circulation 1996;35:0196.

24. Aslanidis C, Ries S, Fehringer P, et al: Genetic and biochemical evidence that CESD and Wolman disease are distinguished by residual lysosomal lipase activity. Genomics 1996;33:85–93.

25. Nakagawa H, Matsubara S, Kuriyama M, et al: Cloning of rat lysosomal acid lipase cDNA and identification of the mutation in the rat model of Wolman's disease. J Lipid Res 1995;36:2212–2218.

26. Zschenker O, Jung N, Rethmeier J, et el: Characterization of lysosomal acid lipase mutations in the signal peptide and mature polypeptide region causing Wolman disease. J Lipid Res 2001;42:1033–1040.

27. Du H, Sheriff S, Bezerra J, et al: Molecular and enzymatic analyses of lysosomal acid lipase in cholesteryl ester storage disease. Mol Genet Metab 1998;64: 126–134.

28. Mayatepek E, Seedorf U, Wiebusch H, et al: Fatal genetic defect causing Wolman disease. J Inherit Metab Dis 1999;22: 93–94.

29. Redonnet-Vernhet I, Chatelut M, Salvayre R, Levade T: A novel lysosomal acid lipase gene mutation in a patient with cholesteryl ester storage disease. Hum Mutat 1998;11:335–336.

30. Kale AS, Ferry GD, Hawkins EP: End-stage renal disease in a patient with cholesteryl ester storage disease following successful liver transplantation and cyclosporine immunosuppression. J Pediatr Gastroenterol 1995;20:95–97.

31. Tietge UWE, Sun G, Czarnecki S, et al: Phenotypic correction of lipid storage and growth arrest in Wolman Disease fibroblasts by gene transfer of lysomal acid lipid. Hum Gene Ther 2001;12: 279–289.

32. Kuriyama M, Yoshida H, Suzuki M, et al: Lysosomal acid lipase deficiency in rats: Lipid analyses and lipase activities in liver and spleen. J Lipid Res 1990;31:1605–1612.

33. Yoshida H, Kuriyama M: Genetic lipid storage disease with lysosomal acid lipase deficiency in rats. Lab Anim Sci 1990;40:486–489.

Lysosomal Membrane Disorders—LAMP-2 Deficiency

Ichizo Nishino

In normal skeletal muscle, lysosomes have morphologically unremarkable structures. By electron microscopy, they are very hard to find and appear to be totally devoid of internal structure compared with other organelles such as mitochondria. Nevertheless, lysosomes have important physiologic roles in the skeletal muscle since a number of muscle diseases are accompanied by structurally abnormal lysosomes. Among these disorders, two have been genetically defined, acid maltase deficiency and Danon disease. In this chapter, I will focus on Danon disease, which is due to a primary deficiency of lysosome-associated membrane protein (LAMP-2), a major lysosomal membrane protein, and is the only known human muscle disorder caused by a lysosomal membrane protein defect.

DANON DISEASE

In 1981, Danon and colleagues reported two unrelated 16-year-old boys with similar phenotypes.[1] Both patients presented with a clinical triad of hypertrophic cardiomyopathy, myopathy, and mental retardation. In addition to the clinical manifestations, the disorder was characterized by a vacuolar myopathy with increased muscle glycogen resembling glycogen storage disease type II; however, acid maltase activity was normal. Accordingly, the disease was called "lysosomal glycogen storage disease with normal acid maltase." However, the disease is not a glycogen storage disease because glycogen is not always increased and because the defective molecule, LAMP-2, is a structural protein rather than a glycolytic enzyme.[2] Therefore, "Danon disease" has been redefined as X-linked vacuolar cardiomyopathy and myopathy due to LAMP-2 deficiency.[2]

Clinical Features

The disease is clinically characterized by hypertrophic cardiomyopathy, myopathy, and mental retardation.[2,3] All probands have been male, but females have had milder, later-onset cardiomyopathy; therefore, the disease was thought to be transmitted in the X-linked dominant mode of inheritance before the underlying defect was identified. In fact, the causative gene for Danon disease, *lamp-2*, is present on chromosome Xq24.[4]

Both male and female patients have been born through normal pregnancies and deliveries. Ages at onset in a study of 20 male and 18 female patients varied from 10 months to 19 years in males and from 12 to 53 years in females.[3] The actual onset could be earlier, but goes undetected because of the subacute insidious nature and slow progression of the disease. For example, two male patients were identified when isolated increases in serum creatine kinase (CK) were noted, and two others because they had abnormal electrocardiograms (ECGs) preceding any cardiac symptoms. Only one male patient developed dyspnea in the infantile period. Most commonly, onset is in childhood. Delayed milestones with mild mental retardation have been observed in 15% of male patients.

All patients develop cardiomyopathy, which is the most severe and life-threatening manifestation. In male patients, cardiac symptoms, such as exertional dyspnea, begin during their teenage years. Hypertrophic cardiomyopathy and cardiac arrhythmia are common features. In a study of 38 patients with genetically-confirmed Danon disease, ages at death were 19 + 6 (mean ± standard deviation [SD]) years for males and 40 ± 7 years for females, obviously reflecting the milder phenotype in female patients.[3]

Skeletal myopathy is usually mild and is present in most male patients (90%), but is seen in only a minority of female patients (33%).[3] All patients have been able to walk throughout their lives despite the myopathy. Weakness and atrophy affect shoulder-girdle and neck muscles predominantly, but distal muscles can also be involved. Interestingly, all male patients show serum creatine kinase levels 5- to 10-fold above upper limits of normal even in the preclinical state. Therefore, Danon disease should be considered in a differential diagnosis in boys with cardiomyopathies and high serum CKs. Other muscle enzymes including serum AST, ALT, and LDH are also increased. In contrast, serum CK is elevated in only 63% of female patients; therefore, serum CK levels can be normal in females. Electrophysiologically, myopathic units have been seen in all male patients studied. In addition, myotonic discharges were recorded in 3 of 10 male patients.[3]

Although both original patients reported by Danon and colleagues had mental retardation, this manifestation is mild and is absent in 30% of male patients. In our study, there has been only one female patient with mental retardation (1/18, 6%).[3] Brain MRI is usually normal. In two autopsy cases, we found vacuolar changes in the cytoplasm of red nucleus; however, this abnormality does not directly account for the mental retardation.[5]

Hepatomegaly has been noted in 36% of male patients and splenomegaly has been seen in one male patient. In *LAMP-2* knockout mice, a wider variety of organs is affected, including liver, kidney, pancreas, small intestine, thymus, and spleen, in addition to heart and skeletal muscle.[6] Similarly, autopsy study showed vacuolar changes in a wide variety of tissues including all kinds of muscles, that is, cardiac, skeletal and smooth muscles, and liver.[5] Therefore, potentially other organs can be involved in this disease.

Muscle Pathology

Currently, muscle biopsy is crucial to make the diagnosis. As discussed below, the genetic test is now available and can be performed instead of a muscle biopsy; however, considering the rarity of the disease and absence of a mutation hotspot, it is not cost-effective to screen patients for a mutation in *lamp-2* without a biopsy demonstrating vacuolar myopathy.

In muscle biopsies of Danon disease patients, variation of fiber size is mild to moderate and necrotic fibers are usually not seen. Muscle samples show many scattered intracytoplasmic vacuoles, which, on hematoxylin and eosin staining, often look like solid basophilic granules. These vacuoles are so tiny that they can easily be overlooked (Fig. 29–1). Interestingly, the vacuolar membranes have activity for acetylcholinesterase and thus they are highlighted in the histochemical stainings for acetylcholinesterase (see Fig. 29–1) and nonspecific esterase.[3,7,8] Acetylcholinesterase is present in specialized

sarcolemma at the neuromuscular junctions called junctional folds. Therefore, the presence of acetylcholinesterase activity indicates that the vacuolar membrane has features of sarcolemma. This characteristic has been confirmed by immunohistochemical study for other sarcolemma-specific proteins.[3,7,8] The sarcolemmal proteins that we found associated with the vacuolar membrane include dystrophin, α-, β-, γ-, and δ-sarcoglycans, α- and β-dystroglycans, dystrobrevin, utrophin, dysferlin, perlecan, caveolin-3, collagen IV, and fibronectin (paper in preparation) (see Fig. 29–1). Therefore, the vacuolar membrane appears to have an extensive set of sarcolemmal proteins.

By electron microscopy, the intracytoplasmic vacuoles typically contain myelin figures, electron-dense

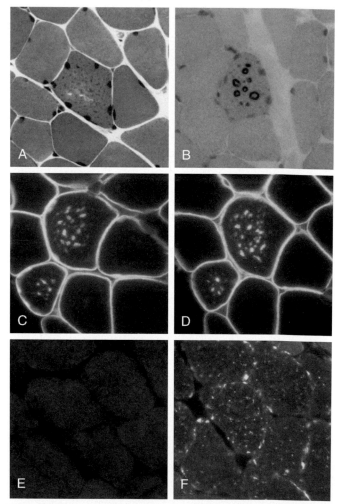

FIGURE 29–1. Muscle pathology of Danon disease. With hematoxylin and eosin staining, tiny autophagic vacuoles often look like solid basophilic granules rather than vacuoles, and can be overlooked easily (A). Immunohistochemical analyses for dystrophin (B) and merosin (C) show that the vacuolar membrane has features of sarcolemma. Interestingly, the vacuolar membrane has acetylcholinesterase activity (D). Immunostaining for LAMP-2 clearly demonstrates the complete absence of the LAMP-2 protein (E) in contrast to control (F).

bodies, and various cytoplasmic debris; therefore, they are autophagic vacuoles.[3,7,8] Interestingly, basal lamina is sometimes seen along the inner surface of autophagic vacuoles; this observation provides further evidence that the vacuolar membrane has features of sarcolemma. Occasionally, sarcolemma and vacuolar membranes appear to be connected, suggesting that the unusual vacuolar membrane may arise from indentations of the sarcolemma.[8]

The unusual combination of autophagic vacuoles with sarcolemmal features is a pathologic hallmark of Danon disease, but has been seen in other autophagic vacuolar myopathies, including X-linked myopathy with excessive autophagy (XMEA)[9] and infantile autophagic vacuolar myopathy.[10] Although genetically distinct from Danon disease, these disorders have pathologic similarities indicating a common pathomechanism. Therefore, autophagic vacuolar myopathies should be categorized as a distinct group of disorders.

By immunohistochemical and Western blot analyses, LAMP-2 protein is absent in the skeletal muscles regardless of the specific LAMP-2 gene mutation (see Fig. 29–1).[2,3] Western blot analysis of the cardiac muscle in one patient also showed a complete absence of LAMP-2 protein.[2] In contrast, other lysosomal membrane proteins, such as lysosomal integral membrane protein-I, are associated with the autophagic vacuoles in Danon disease.[2,3]

LAMP-2

LAMP-2 is a type 1 membrane protein with a large luminal domain connected to a transmembrane region and a short cytoplasmic tail. The luminal domain can be divided into two internally homologous domains separated by a hinge region rich in proline, serine, or threonine. Each of the two homologous regions contains four cysteines that are linked in pairs by disulfide bonding between neighboring residues creating two loops in each domain. The luminal domain is heavily glycosylated; most of the potential N-linked glycosylation sites are utilized, yielding a molecular mass of 90 to 120 kDa for the approximately 40-kDa core protein. LAMP-2 is abundantly expressed and is thought to coat the inner surface of the lysosomal membrane together with its autosomal paralogue, LAMP-1. Therefore, the topographical distribution of LAMPs, together with the fact that LAMP-2 is one of the most heavily glycosylated proteins, indicates that LAMPs probably protect lysosomal membrane and thus cytoplasm from proteolytic enzymes within the lysosomes.[11]

The cytoplasmic tail of LAMP-2 is short, consisting of only 11 amino acids, but has a well-conserved tyrosine residue which is thought to provide a crucial signal for trafficking of LAMP-2 molecules to lysosomes. Moreover, the cytoplasmic tail of LAMP-2 is thought to function as a receptor for the uptake of certain proteins

into lysosome for degradation in association with the 73 kDa heat shock cognate protein.[12]

The expression of LAMP-2 is increased in a variety of situations, whereas LAMP-1 seems rather constitutively expressed; therefore, the expression of LAMP-2 is likely to be specifically regulated.[13] Interestingly, a small fraction (2% to 3%) of LAMP-2 is present in the plasma membrane[11] and its expression in the cell surface is increased in certain situations, including malignancy[14] and scleroderma.[15] Although the functional significance of LAMP-2 expression at the cell surface is not yet known, this phenomenon may be related to the development of the unusual autophagic vacuoles with sarcolemmal features.

LAMP-2 Gene Mutation

The LAMP-2 gene is located on Xq24, whereas the gene for LAMP-1 is on 13q34.[4] The *lamp-2* open reading frame consists of 1233 nucleotides and encodes 410 amino acids. Exons 1 through 8 and part of exon 9 encode a luminal domain, whereas the remainder of exon 9 encodes both a transmembrane domain and a cytoplasmic domain. Human exon 9 exists in two forms, 9a and 9b, that are alternatively spliced and produce two isoforms, LAMP-2a and LAMP-2b, respectively. LAMP-2a is expressed rather ubiquitously whereas LAMP-2b is expressed specifically in heart and skeletal muscles.[16]

To date, we have identified 11 different LAMP-2 gene mutations in 13 pedigrees,[2,3] including the original family in the report by Danon et al (Table 29–1).[1] Genetically-confirmed Danon disease patients have been ethnically diverse, suggesting that this disorder can be seen in any ethnic group. All but one of the mutations have been stop-codon or out-of-frame mutations that are predicted to truncate the protein, resulting in loss of the transmembrane and cytoplasmic domains. Therefore, the mutated products cannot function as a lysosomal membrane protein. The total absence of the LAMP-2 protein in Danon disease muscles suggests that the abnormal proteins are unstable and are immediately degraded.

An exon-skipping mutation is predicted to cause an in-frame deletion of one of the four loop structures and several potential glycosylation sites in the luminal domain, resulting in severe structural changes.[2] The patient with this particular mutation also had complete absence of the LAMP-2 protein in the skeletal muscle, suggesting that this mutation is as harmful as other null-type mutations.

In a patient harboring a mutation in exon 9b, Western blot analysis revealed a trace amount of the LAMP-2 protein.[2] This signal most likely represents LAMP-2a because the mutation in exon 9b should affect only the LAMP-2b isoform. This particular patient is alive at age 34 years; therefore, this mutation apparently causes an exceptionally mild phenotype.[3] Usually, Danon disease is clinically uniform in male patients. No other

TABLE 29–1. LAMP-2 Gene Mutations

Gene mutation	Site	Effect of mutation	Ethnic background
G14del	E1	frameshift	Greek
G138A	E2	nonsense	Spanish
T440A	E4	nonsense	Japanese
GT554/555TA*	E4	nonsense	Italian
g5c	I6	E6 skipping (in-frame)	Japanese
g1a	I5	6-bp insertion creating stop codon	Japanese, Afro-American[†], Anglo-Saxon
10-bp deletion	I5/E6 junction	10 bp deletion at the 5′ end of E6 resulting in frameshift of the codon	Japanese
883insT	E7	framshift	Japanese
C813G	E8	nonsense	African-American
T974AA	E8	frameshift	Italian
2-bp del	E9b	frameshift	Japanese

*Two nucleotides, GT, at nt 554 and 555 are mutated to TA.
[†]One of the patients in the original case report by Danon et al.

apparent genotype-phenotype correlation has been seen.[3] The mutation in this patient not only supports the idea that LAMP-2b is the major isoform in cardiac and skeletal muscles, but also suggests that a deficiency of LAMP-2b by itself is sufficient to cause the disease, albeit a milder form.

LAMP-2 Knockout Mouse

LAMP-2 deficient mice produced by a German group provide confirmatory evidence that LAMP-2 deficiency causes Danon disease.[6] About 50% of LAMP-2 deficient mice die between postnatal day 20 and 40 irrespective of sex and genetic background. Surviving mice are smaller and have cardiac hypertrophy, but the life span is normal. LAMP-2 deficient mice have autophagic vacuoles in various tissues including heart and skeletal muscles (analogous to the patients), liver, pancreas, spleen, and kidney. Mice that die early often have stenoses or segmental hemorrhagic infarcts of the small intestine and pancreatic lesions. In addition, apoptotic cell loss is pathologically increased in thymus and the demarcation of white and red pulp is absent. Together with the fact that the LAMP-2 gene mutations segregate with Danon disease, the findings in LAMP-2 knockout mice clearly demonstrate that Danon disease is primary LAMP-2 deficiency. Furthermore, the abnormalities in a wider variety of organs in LAMP-2 deficient mice suggest that more variable organs could potentially be involved in Danon disease and the patient might develop other symptoms, in addition to classical triads of manifestations.

Curiously, in contrast to LAMP-2 knockout mice, LAMP-1 deficient mice show normal lysosomal mor-

phology and function and do not develop any symptoms.[17] This is probably due to the compensatory upregulation of LAMP-2 in LAMP-1 knockout mice, whereas the LAMP-1 is not upregulated in LAMP-2 knockout mice.[6] This result indicates that expression patterns of these highly homologous proteins are regulated differently and further suggests that they may have different functional roles in the body.

Other Autophagic Vacuolar Myopathies

In 1988, Kalimo et al reported a type of autophagic vacuolar myopathy in a Finnish family.[9] The disease is transmitted in an X-linked recessive manner. Clinically, the disease is characterized by slowly progressive muscle weakness and atrophy that spares cardiac and respiratory muscles. Muscle biopsy shows many tiny vacuoles and the vacuolar membranes have features of plasma membrane as in Danon disease, that is, sarcolemmal proteins, such as dystrophin, are present in the vacuolar membrane. Autophagic vacuoles are seen in the cytoplasm. The muscle pathology resembles that of Danon disease; therefore, the two diseases are likely to share similar molecular pathomechanisms.

The characteristic pathologic findings in XMEA are depositions of complement C5b-9 over the surface of muscle fibers and multilayered basal lamina along the sarcolemma,[18] which are not seen in Danon disease.[3] Furthermore the presence of LAMP-2 in XMEA muscle clearly demonstrates that XMEA is distinct from Danon disease.[2] In addition, the XMEA locus has been mapped to Xq28, whereas the gene encoding LAMP-2 is present on Xq24.[19,20]

There have been two well-documented reports of infants with autophagic vacuolar myopathy described as having the infantile form of "lysosomal glycogen storage disease with normal acid maltase."[21,22] Both patients presented with muscle weakness and hypotonia at birth and died early in their lives. Muscle biopsies showed extensive vacuolar changes with increased glycogen, but acid maltase activity was normal in both patients; hence, the diagnosis seemed to be clear. Nevertheless, the infantile disease is distinct from Danon disease because LAMP-2 protein is not deficient in the skeletal muscle and sequences of the LAMP-2 gene are normal. Interestingly, as in XMEA muscle, complement C5b-9 stained muscle sarcolemma in one infantile patient. On electron microscopy, many vacuoles containing membrane-bound glycogen particles, free glycogen particles, and cytoplasmic degradation products scattered in the cytoplasm. In addition, duplication of basal lamina into two layers was observed along portions of the sarcolemma. Multilayered basal lamina was also seen in some fibers. Material exocytosed from vacuoles accumulated under and between the multiple layers of basal lamina. The deposition of complement C5b-9 over the surface of muscle fibers and the multiplication of basal lamina suggest that the pathologic features of infantile autophagic vacuolar myopathy are more similar to those of XMEA than of Danon disease.[10]

Although details of pathologic features are different in Danon disease, XMEA, and infantile autophagic vacuolar myopathy, they are most likely to be able to categorized into a distinct group of myopathies because they commonly show unusual autophagic vacuoles with sarcolemmal features. Unlike other types of lysosomal myopathies characterized by the presence of rimmed vacuoles, such as distal myopathy with rimmed vacuoles and inclusion body myopathy, which are probably secondary lysosomal myopathies, it seems rational to hypothesize that the defects reside primarily in lysosomes in autophagic vacuolar myopathies as has been demonstrated in Danon disease.

The identification of causative genes for XMEA and infantile autophagic vacuolar myopathy should provide information about a common pathway for the production of these peculiar autophagic vacuoles. Most likely there will be other diseases in this group of myopathy and we expect that the list will expand rapidly.

REFERENCES

1. Danon MJ, Oh SJ, DiMauro S, et al: Lysosomal glycogen storage disease with normal acid maltase. Neurology 1981;31:51–57.

2. Nishino I, Fu J, Tanji K, et al: Primary LAMP-2 deficiency causes X-linked vacuolar cardiomyopathy and myopathy (Danon disease). Nature 2000;406:906–910.

3. Sugie K, Yamamoto A, Murayama K, et al: Clinicopathological features of genetically-confirmed Danon disease. Neurology 2002;58:1773–1778.

4. Mattei M-G, Maaterson J, Chen JW, et al: Two human lysosomal membrane glycoproteins, h-lamp-1 and h-lamp-2, are encoded by genes localized to chromosome 13q34 and chromosome Xq24-25, respectively. J Biol Chem 1990;265:7458–7551.

5. Nishino I, Yamamoto A, Tokonami F, et al: Two autopsy cases of Danon disease(Abstr). Neuromuscul Disord 2001;11:668–669.

6. Tanaka Y, Guhde G, Suter A, et al: Accumulation of autophagic vacuoles and cardiomyopathy in LAMP-2-deficient mice. Nature 2000;406: 902–906.

7. Muntoni F, Catani G, Mateddu A, et al: Familial cardiomyopathy, mental retardation and myopathy associated with desmin-type intermediate filaments. Neuromusc Disord 1994;4:233–241.

8. Murakami N, Goto YI, Itoh M, et al: Sarcolemmal indentation in cardiomyopathy with mental retardation and vacuolar myopathy. Neuromuscul Disord 1995;5:149–155.

9. Kalimo H, Savontaus ML, Lang H, et al: X-linked myopathy with excessive autophagy: A new hereditary muscle disease. Ann Neurol 1988;23: 258–265.

10. Yamamoto A, Morisawa Y, Verloes A, et al: Infantile autophagic vacuolar myopathy is distinct from Danon disease. Neurology 2001;57:903–905.

11. Fukuda M: Biogenesis of the lysosomal membrane. Subcell Biochem 1994;22:199–230.

12. Cuervo AM, Dice JF: A receptor for the selective uptake and degradation of proteins by lysosomes. Science 1996;273:501–503.

13. Sawada R, Jardine KA, Fukuda M: The genes of major lysosomal membrane glycoproteins, lamp-1 and lamp-2. The 5'-flanking sequence of lamp-2 gene and comparison of exon organization in two genes. J Biol Chem 1993;268.9014–9022.

14. Kannan K, Divers SG, Lurie AA, et al: Cell surface expression of lysosome-associated membrane protein-2 (lamp2) and CD63 as markers of in vivo platelet activation in maligancy. Eur J Haematol 1995;55: 145–151.

15. Holcombe RF, Baethge BA, Stewart RM, et al: Cell surface expression of lysosome-associated membrane proteins (LAMPs) in scleroderma: Relationship of lamp-2 to disease duration, anti-Scl70 antibodies, serum interleukin-8, and soluble interleukin-2 receptor levels. Clin Immunol Immunopathol 1993;67:31–39.

16. Konecki DS, Foctisch K, Zimmer KP, et al: An alternatively spliced form of the human lysosome-associated membrane protein-2 gene is expressed in a tissue-specific manner. Biochem Biophys Res Commun 1995;215:757–767.

17. Andrejewski N, Punnonen EL, Guhde G, et al: Normal lysosomal morphology and function in LAMP-1-deficient mice. J Biol Chem 1999;274:12692–12701.

18. Villanova M, Louboutin JP, Chateau D, et al: X-linked vacuolated myopathy: Complement membrane

attack complex on surface membrane of injured muscle fibers. Ann Neurol 1995;37:637–645.

19. Villard L, des Portes V, Levy N, et al: Linkage of X-linked myopathy with excessive autophagy (XMEA) to Xq28. Eur J Hum Genet 2000;8:125–129.

20. Auranen M, Villanova M, Muntoni F, et al: X-linked vacuolar myopathies: Two separate loci and refined genetic mapping. Ann Neurol 2000;47:666–669.

21. Verloes A, Massin M, Lombet J, et al: Nosology of lysosomal glycogen storage diseases without in vitro acid maltase deficiency. Delineation of a neonatal form. Am J Med Genet 1997;72:135–142.

22. Morisawa Y, Fujieda M, Murakami N, et al: Lysosomal glycogen storage disease with normal acid maltase with early fatal outcome. J Neurol Sci 1998;160:175–179.

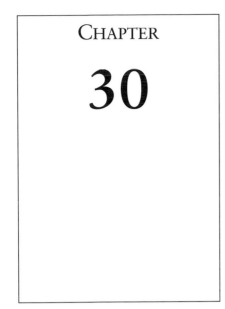

CHAPTER
30

Fabry Disease: α-Galactosidase A Deficiency

Robert J. Desnick

Fabry disease is an X-linked recessive disorder resulting from the deficient activity of the lysosomal hydrolase α-galactosidase A (Fig. 30–1).[1] The enzymatic defect leads to the progressive accumulation of neutral glycosphingolipids with terminal α-galactosyl moieties, particularly globotriaosylceramide (GL-3), in the plasma and in the lysosomes of tissues throughout the body. In classically affected males, who have no detectable α-Gal A activity, GL-3 accumulation in the vascular endothelium causes the major disease manifestations. Clinical onset in childhood or adolescence is characterized by severe acroparesthesias, angiokeratoma, hypohidrosis, and corneal/lenticular opacities. With advancing age, the progressive lysosomal GL-3 accumulation, particularly in the microvasculature, leads to renal failure, vascular disease of the heart and brain, and premature demise, typically in the fourth or fifth decade of life. Atypical variants, who have residual α-Gal A activity and no vascular endothelial involvement, are asymptomatic or have mild manifestations usually limited to the heart (i.e., the "cardiac variants"). Diagnosis of affected males with the classical or variant phenotype by enzyme assay is reliable, whereas the identification of carrier females may require identification of the specific mutation in the α-Gal A gene, in which over 200 mutations have been identified. Dilantin, tegretol or gabapentin can provide prophylaxis for the painful acroparesthesias. Specific treatment by enzyme replacement therapy with recombinant human α-Gal A has been shown to be safe and effective in clinical trials.[2–5]

CLINICAL FEATURES AND DIAGNOSTIC EVALUATION

Fabry disease is inherited as an X-linked recessive trait.[1] The α-Gal A gene is fully penetrant; however, different mutations result in variable clinical expressivity in affected males. The disease is rare, and it is estimated that the incidence is about one in 40,000 to 60,000 males. Of more than 400 cases described in the literature, most are white; however, black, Latin, American Indian, Arab, and Asian cases have been observed.

Classic Phenotype

Clinical onset in classically affected males with severely deficient, if any, α-Gal A activity, usually occurs during childhood or adolescence (Table 30–1). Early manifestations include periodic crises of severe pain in the extremities (acroparesthesias), angiokeratoma, hypohidrosis, and characteristic corneal and lenticular opacities. With advancing age, progressive vascular glycosphingolipid deposition causes ischemia and infarction leading to cardiac, cerebral, and renal vascular disease with death typically occurring in the fourth or fifth decade of life. Affected individuals who have blood group antigen B or AB may have a more severe clinical course because the blood group B substances also accumulate owing to deficient α-Gal A activity. The clinical and pathologic features of the disease have been comprehensively reviewed,[1] but are briefly described later. Death most often results from uremia or vascular disease of the heart or brain. The mean age of death for affected males who did not receive hemodialysis or renal transplantation was 41 years.[6]

Acroparesthesias. The single most debilitating symptom of this disease is the pain. Typically, affected males experience episodic crises of excruciating burning pain in the fingers and toes in childhood, which may become

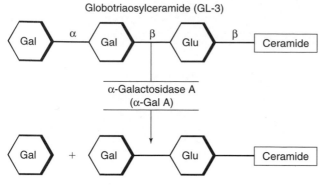

FIGURE 30–1. The metabolic defect in Fabry disease. The deficient activity of α-galactosidase A results in the accumulation of globotriaosylceramide (GL-3) and other glycoconjugates with terminal α-galactosyl moieties.

TABLE 30–1. Fabry Disease: Major Manifestations in Classical and Cardiac Variant Patients

Manifestation	Classical Type	Cardiac Variant
Age at onset	4–8 yr	>40 yr
Average age of death	41 yr	>60 yr
Angiokeratoma	++	–
Acroparesthesias	++	–
Hypohidrosis/anhidrosis	++	–
Corneal/lenticular opacity	+	–
Heart	Ischemia/MI	LVH/Cardio-myopathy
Brain	TIA[†]/Strokes	–
Kidney	Renal Failure	Mild Proteinuria
Residual α-Gal A activity	<1%	<10%

LVH, left ventricular hypertrophy; MI, myocardial infarction; TIA, transient ischemic attack; +, present; –, absent.

more frequent and severe in adolescence. These painful acroparesthesias may last several days to weeks and are associated with low-grade fevers and elevations of the erythrocyte sedimentation rate. During the second and third decades of life, these recurrent painful episodes may occur less frequently, usually associated with a fever. In a few patients, however, they may become progressively more frequent and severe, radiate to proximal extremities, and occasionally persist for 1 to 2 weeks. Affected individuals may be incapacitated for prolonged periods of time with pain that is so severe that suicide has been attempted. It has been suggested that the etiology of the acroparesthesias may be due to spasms of the ischemic microvasculature, impaired autonomic function,[7] and peripheral nervous system involvement.[8]

Angiokeratoma. The cutaneous vascular lesions (angiokeratoma) are telangiectases, which usually appear as clusters of individual punctate, dark-red to blue angiectases in the superficial layers of the skin. The lesions may be flat or slightly raised and do not blanch with pressure. There may be a slight hyperkeratosis over these lesions. They usually appear during childhood and progressively increase in size and number with age. Characteristically, these lesions are most dense between the umbilicus and the knees and have a tendency toward bilateral symmetry. These lesions frequently are found on the oral mucosa and conjunctiva as well as on other mucosal areas. Variants without the characteristic skin lesions have been described.[9] Hypohidrosis is common, and atrophic or sparse sweat and sebaceous glands have been reported.

Ophthalmologic Features. Ocular manifestations include aneurysmal dilatation and tortuosity of conjunctival and retinal vessels as well as characteristic corneal and lenticular changes.[10] The conjunctival and retinal vascular lesions are common and part of the diffuse sys-

temic vascular involvement. The keratopathy is characterized by diffuse haziness or whorled streaks extending from a central vortex in the corneal epithelium. The corneal lesions resemble the changes seen in patients taking chloroquine or amiodarone and must be observed by slit-lamp microscopy; they occur in all classically affected males and in about 70% to 80% of carrier females from classically affected families, but are usually absent in the cardiac variants (discussed later). The lenticular changes include a granular anterior capsular or subcapsular deposit seen in about 30% of affected males and a unique linear opacity, termed the *Fabry cataract*, in affected males and some carrier females. The cataracts are best observed by retroillumination and appear as whitish, spotlike deposits of fine, granular material near the posterior capsule. These lesions do not impair vision.

Renal, Cardiac, and Cerebral Vascular Involvement. With increasing age, the major morbid signs result from the progressive involvement of the vascular system. Early in the course of the disease, casts, red cells, and lipid inclusions with characteristic birefringent *Maltese crosses* appear in the urinary sediment. Proteinuria, isosthenuria, gradual deterioration of renal function, and development of azotemia occur in the second to fourth decade of life. Cardiovascular findings may include hypertension, left ventricular hypertrophy, anginal chest pain, myocardial ischemia or infarction, and congestive heart failure. Mitral insufficiency is the most common valvular lesion. Abnormal electrocardiographic and echocardiographic findings are common. Cerebrovascular manifestations result primarily from multifocal small vessel involvement.

Other Features. Nausea, vomiting, diarrhea, and abdominal or flank pain are common gastrointestinal symptoms. Other less frequent features include massive lymphedema of the legs and dyspnea. Musculoskeletal system findings have included a permanent deformity of the distal interphalangeal joints of the fingers and avascular necrosis of the head of the femur and talus. Mild normochromic, normocytic anemia, presumably as a result of decreased red cell survival, has been observed. Many affected males appear to have growth retardation or delayed puberty.

Cardiac Variant

Affected males with a variant phenotype have been described who were essentially asymptomatic at ages when classical hemizygotes would be severely affected or would have expired from the disease.[11–13] Many of these variants were identified serendipitously during evaluation of unrelated medical problems. In contrast to patients with the classical phenotype who have no detectable α-Gal A activity, these variants have residual activity compatible with their milder phenotypes. These patients presented with late-onset cardiac disease, including cardiomegaly, typically involving the left ventricular wall and interventricular septum, and electrocardiographic abnormalities consistent with a cardiomyopathy. Others had hypertrophic cardiomyopathy or myocardial infarctions, or both. They were essentially asymptomatic during most of their lives and did not experience the early classical manifestations, including acroparesthesias, angiokeratoma, corneal and lenticular opacities, and hypohidrosis. Most were diagnosed after the onset of cardiac manifestations and most were found to have mild proteinuria, but their renal function was generally normal for their age.

Carrier Females

The clinical course and prognosis of affected males and affected carrier females from families with the classical phenotype differ significantly.[1] Most carrier females experience little difficulty in adult life at ages when affected males already have severe renal or cardiac involvement, or both. Although most molecularly documented carriers are asymptomatic throughout a normal life span, with increasing age some manifest minor symptoms of the disease. Approximately 50% of carriers have a few, isolated skin lesions, at least 30% have acroparesthesias, and about 70% to 80% have the whorl-like corneal dystrophy. Renal findings in carriers include hyposthenuria; the occurrence of erythrocytes, leukocytes, and granular and hyaline casts in the urinary sediment; proteinuria; and other signs of renal impairment. Some carriers develop cardiac involvement with advanced age. A few carriers have been described with disease as severe as that observed in classically affected males due to random X-chromosomal inactivation. To date, limited information is available on the clinical manifestations of carrier females in families with the cardiac variant phenotype.

Diagnostic Evaluation

All suspect cases should be confirmed enzymatically by the demonstration of deficient α-Gal A activity in plasma or isolated leukocytes.[14] Prenatal detection can be accomplished by the demonstration of deficient α-Gal A activity in chorionic villi obtained in the first trimester or in cultured amniocytes obtained by amniocentesis in the second trimester of pregnancy. Carrier females may have intermediate levels of α-Gal A enzymatic activity,[14] but can be more accurately diagnosed by demonstration of the family's α-Gal A mutation (see later).

Classically affected hemizygotes with Fabry disease have no detectable α-Gal A activity. The physical and kinetic properties of the residual α-Gal A activities (1% to 10% of normal) in atypical variants who are asymptomatic or have mild manifestations have been described.[1–9] Studies of α-Gal A biosynthesis in fibroblasts from unrelated classical and atypical Fabry hemizygotes demonstrated several types of enzyme defects, consistent with the occurrence of different mutations that affect α-Gal A synthesis, maturation, and stability.[15]

PATHOLOGY

The glycosphingolipid substrates progressively accumulate in most cells of classically affected males. The major manifestations result from deposition in the lysosomes of the endothelial cells of blood vessels throughout the body. Presumably, the small vessel involvement leads to the cerebrovascular complications and the minor electroencephalogram and electromyelogram abnormalities in these patients. In addition, vascular ischemia and lipid deposition in the perineurium may cause the peripheral nerve conduction abnormalities of slowed conduction velocities and distal latency. In classically affected males and carrier females, glycosphingolipid deposition in nervous tissue appears to be limited to perineural sheath cells of peripheral nerves, neurons of the peripheral and central autonomic nervous system, and certain primary neurons of somatic afferent pathways. Glycosphingolipid deposition has been observed in Schwann cells by some, but not by other investigators. Qualitative and quantitative studies of peripheral sensory neurons in sural nerves and spinal ganglia have shown preferential loss of small myelinated and unmyelinated fibers as well as small cell bodies of spinal ganglia.

Brain stem centers in which lipid deposition has been observed include the nuclei gracilis and cuneatus, dorsal autonomic vagal nuclei, salivary nuclei, nucleus ambiguus, thalamus, reticular substance, mesencephalic nucleus of the fifth nerve, and substantia nigra. Hemisphere involvement has been noted in the amygdaloid, hypothalamic, and hippocampal nuclei. Studies have revealed abnormal lipid deposits in the fifth and sixth cortical layers of the inferior temporal gyrus, the Edinger-Westphal nucleus, the parasympathetic cell column, and the midline nucleus. Lipid storage in neuronal cells of the anterior and posterior lobes of the pituitary also has been described. Immunocytochemical studies using a sensitive anti-globotriaosylceramide monoclonal antibody revealed a highly selective pattern of neuronal involvement. Deposition was observed in selected neurons in the spinal cord and ganglia, brain stem, amygdala, hypothalamus, and entorhinal cortex; however, adjacent areas were spared, including the nucleus basalis, striatum, globus pallidus, and thalamus.

The involvement of peripheral and central autonomic nerve cells may be responsible for the paresthesias, pain, hypohidrosis, such gastrointestinal symptoms as nausea and diarrhea, and a variety of vague neurologic signs and symptoms. Marked degeneration of the secretory cells and myoepithelial cells of sweat glands has been observed by electron microscopy, suggesting that the hypohidrosis was due to local lipid deposition rather than autonomic nervous system involvement. The episodic fevers may be related to lesions of the hypothalamus. The observation of a selective decrease in the number of unmyelinated and small myelinated fibers in peripheral nerves has led to the suggestion that the selective damage to these fibers may account for the pain production and hypohidrosis in this disorder. Studies of autonomic function revealed sympathetic and parasympathetic dysfunction, particularly in distal cutaneous responses. The exclusive glycolipid deposition in dorsal root ganglia observed at autopsy of one affected male leads to the suggestion that the pain resulted from sensory root ganglia involvement.[16] Histochemical evidence of glycosphingolipid accumulation in neurons and nerve fibers of intestinal nerve plexuses and smooth muscle[16] may account for the uncoordinated intestinal smooth-muscle activity which may lead to complaints of chronic diarrhea or constipation. Glycosphingolipid deposition in the myenteric and submucosal plexuses and a marked decrease in argyrophilic neurons were observed in an involved segment of bowel from an affected male who had jejunal diverticulosis and perforation. Detailed reviews of the neurologic findings are available.[1,16,17]

BIOCHEMISTRY

The deficient activity of the lysosomal enzyme, α-Gal A, results in the accumulation of glycosphingolipids and glycoconjugates with terminal α-galactosyl moieties in most visceral tissues and body fluids. The predominant glycosphingolipid accumulated is GL-3, galactosyl-(α1 4)-galactosyl-(β1 4)-glycosyl-(β1 1')-ceramide [Gal (α1 4) Gal (β1 4) Glc (β1 1') Cer]. A second neutral glycosphingolipid, galabiosylceramide [Gal (α1 4) Gal (β1 1') Cer], also accumulates in Fabry hemizygotes to abnormally high concentrations. Galabiosylceramide deposition

appears to be tissue-specific, because this substrate has been detected only in the pancreas, right heart, lung, kidney, and urinary sediment. In addition, the blood group B-specific substances, which have terminal α-galactosyl moieties, [Gal (α1 3) Gal (2 1α Fuc) (β1 3) GlcNAc (β1 3) Gal (β1 4) Glc (β1 1') Cer] and the blood group B1 glycosphingolipid [Gal (α1 3) Gal (2 1α Fuc) (β1 4) GlcNAc (β1 3) Gal (β1 4) Glc (β1 1') Cer] accumulate in patients who have the blood group B antigens. Thus, Fabry hemizygotes and carriers who have blood group B and AB accumulate four major glycosphingolipid substrates and appear to have a more rapid disease course.

Human α-Gal A is a homodimeric glycoprotein with native and subunit molecular masses of ~101 and ~46 kDa. The enzyme has a pH optimum of 4.6 and hydrolyzes the α-linked galactosyl moieties from glycolipids and glycopeptides. Isoelectric focusing studies of the enzyme from various sources reveal multiple forms with pI values ranging from 4.2 to 5.1, owing to glycoforms with varying sialylation and phosphorylation. Biosynthetic studies indicated that the α-Gal A subunit in cultured fibroblasts is normally synthesized as a precursor glycopeptide of ~50 kDa.[15] After cleavage of the signal peptide and carbohydrate modifications in the Golgi apparatus and lysosomes, the mature enzyme subunits of ~46 kDa form the active, homodimeric enzyme, which contains complex, hybrid, and high-mannose type oligosaccharide moieties. A comprehensive review of glycosphingolipid metabolism, the biochemistry of α-Gal A, and the metabolic defect in Fabry disease is available.[1]

MOLECULAR GENETIC DATA

α-Gal A Gene and Transcript

Human α-Gal A is encoded by a single housekeeping gene, localized to Xq22.1.[1] The 12 kb α-Gal A gene has been completely sequenced and characterized.[18,19] The gene contains 7 exons ranging from 92 to 291 bp and 6 introns ranging from 0.2 to 3.8 kb. The full-length 1437 bp α-Gal A cDNA encodes a precursor peptide of 429 amino acids, including a 31-residue signal peptide. The mature 398 amino acid subunit contains four N-glycosylation consensus sequences.[18,19]

Characterization of the Molecular Lesions Causing Fabry Disease

Over 200 α-Gal A mutations have been reported (Human Gene Mutation Database http://archive.uwcm.ac.uk/ uwcm/mg/hgmd0.html) including large and small gene rearrangements, splicing defects, and missense or nonsense mutations.[20] All of the asymptomatic or mildly affected cardiac variants had missense mutations or splicing lesions that expressed residual α-Gal A activity. Most of the reported mutations have been private (i.e., confined to a single Fabry pedigree). Several mutations have been found in unrelated families of different ethnic or geographic backgrounds. These include N215S, R227Q, R227X, and R342Q mutations. The N215S was found in several unrelated cardiac variants who were asymptomatic or had mild disease manifestations. R227Q and R227X, which occurred at a CpG nucleotide, were the most common mutations causing the classical phenotype. Efforts to establish genotype/phenotype correlations have been limited because most Fabry patients had private mutations, and attempts to predict the phenotype require more extensive clinical information from unrelated patients with the same genotype.

TREATMENT

Medical Management

The single most debilitating and morbid aspect of Fabry disease is the excruciating pain. Prophylactic administration of low maintenance dosages of diphenylhydantoin, carbamazepine, or gabapentin has been found to provide relief from the periodic crises of excruciating pain and constant discomfort in hemizygotes and carriers.[21] Diphenylhydantoin and carbamazepine may be used in combination if either alone has not significantly reduced the pain. Otherwise, care of patients with regard to cardiac, pulmonary, and cerebrovascular manifestations remains nonspecific and symptomatic.

Dialysis and Renal Transplantation

Because renal insufficiency is the most frequent late complication in patients with this disease, chronic hemodialysis and renal transplantation have become life-saving procedures. Successful transplantation will correct renal function. The α-Gal A in the allograft will catabolize the turnover of endogenous renal glycosphingolipid substrates. Renal transplantation also provides an in situ source of the normal enzyme. Renal transplantation, however, should be undertaken only in patients with clinically significant renal failure. Transplantation of kidneys from Fabry carriers, which already may contain significant substrate deposition, should be avoided.

Enzyme Replacement Therapy

Based on extensive preclinical evaluations in α-Gal A–deficient mice,[22] enzyme replacement therapy with recombinant human α-Gal A has been evaluated in clinical trials.[2-5] Although the two enzymes used in these trials were produced by different companies, a study comparing their specific activity, biochemical compositions, and cell uptake found that the proteins were essentially the same with comparable glycosylation and specific activities.[23]

Phase 1 and 1/2 Clinical Trials. A Phase 1 trial involving 10 classically affected males demonstrated that a single dose of recombinant human α-Gal A could reduce the accumulated GL-3 in the liver and urinary sediment.[2] A Phase 1/2 open-label, dose-escalation trial involving 15 classically affected males evaluated the safety and effectiveness of five doses of α-Gal A (Fabrazyme, Genzyme Corp.) in dose regimens of 0.3, 1.0, or 3.0 mg/kg every 14 days or 1.0 or 3.0 mg/kg every 48 h.[3] Intravenously administered α-Gal A was cleared from the circulation in a dose-dependent manner, via both saturable and nonsaturable pathways. The enzyme was well tolerated and rapid and marked reductions in plasma and tissue GL-3 were observed biochemically, histologically, and ultrastructurally. Mean GL-3 content decreased 84% in liver ($n = 13$) and was markedly reduced in kidney in 4 of 5 patients who had pre- and post-treatment biopsies. GL-3 deposits also were reduced in the vascular endothelium of the kidney, heart, skin, and liver by light and electron microscopic evaluation. In addition, patients reported decreased pain, increased ability to perspire, and improved quality of life.

Phase 2 and 3 Clinical Trials. A single center, double-blind, placebo-controlled, Phase 2 trial of α-Gal A replacement involved 26 male patients with neuropathic pain who received 0.2 mg/kg every 2 weeks for 22 weeks (12 doses).[3] The primary efficacy endpoint was pain at its worst and pain medication was withdrawn before evaluations. The mean (SE) Brief Pain Inventory neuropathic pain severity score declined from 6.2 to 4.3 in patients treated with α-Gal A ($n = 14$) versus no significant change in the placebo group ($n = 12$) ($P = .02$). Mean creatinine clearance increased by 2.1 mL/min for patients receiving α-Gal A versus a decrease of 16.1 mL/min for the patients receiving the placebo ($P = .02$). One patient in the placebo group advanced to renal failure. Plasma GL-3 levels decreased approximately 50% in patients treated with α-Gal A.

A Phase 3 multinational, multicenter, randomized placebo-controlled, double-blind study evaluated the safety and effectiveness of enzyme replacement in 58 patients who received 1 mg/kg of α-Gal A (Fabrazyme, Genzyme Corp.) or placebo every 2 weeks for 20 weeks (11 doses).[4] The primary efficacy endpoint was the percentage of patients whose renal capillary endothelial GL-3 deposits cleared to normal or near normal. Also evaluated were the histologic clearance of microvascular endothelial GL-3 deposits in the heart and skin and changes in pain (Short Form McGill Pain Questionnaire) and in quality of life (Short Form-36 Health Status Survey). In this study, 20 of 29 α-Gal A–treated patients (69%) cleared the accumulated GL-3 from the renal capillary endothelium versus 0 of 29 placebo-treated patients ($P < 0.001$). Compared with the placebo group, α-Gal A treated patients also had markedly decreased microvascular endothelial GL-3 in the skin ($P < 0.001$) and heart ($P < 0.001$). Patients receiving α-Gal A cleared the accumulated GL-3 in plasma to nondetectable levels. Pain and quality-of-life assessments improved in both treatment groups in comparison to baseline, indistinguishable from a placebo effect. Note that patients in this study were not selected for pain nor were pain medications discontinued during treatment.

All 58 patients who completed the Phase 3 trial received α-Gal A in an extension study. After 6 months of the open-label therapy, all 22 former placebo and 20 of 21 α-Gal A–treated patients (42 of 43; 98%) who had biopsies achieved or maintained normal or near normal renal capillary endothelial histology. Similar results were observed for skin capillary endothelium; 96% of both former placebo patients (22 of 23) and of α-Gal A patients (23 of 24) who had biopsies achieved normal or near normal histology. In the capillary endothelium of the heart, histology scores improved with duration of treatment. Among patients who had heart biopsies, 10 of the 15 (67%) former placebo patients (6 months of treatment) and 14 of 17 (82%) of the α-Gal A patients (12 months of treatment) attained normal or near normal histology. In addition, histologic examination of other renal, cardiac, and skin cell types revealed complete or partial clearance of accumulated GL-3. For example, in the kidney, GL-3 clearance to normal or near normal levels was observed in renal, glomerular and nonglomerular capillary endothelial cells, mesangial cells, and interstitial cells after 6 to 12 months of treatment.

Treatment with α-Gal A was well tolerated; the adverse event incidence and profiles were similar for both treatment groups in the Phase 3 trial, except for mild to moderate infusion reactions to α-Gal A, which were managed conservatively. Although IgG seroconversion occurred in 51 of 58 α-Gal A–treated patients, GL-3 clearance was not impaired, and titers decreased with continued treatment.

In summary, enzyme replacement with α-Gal A has been shown to safely reverse the pathogenesis of the major clinical manifestations, to decrease pain, and to stabilize renal function in patients with Fabry disease. All patients who participated in clinical trials are continuing in open-label extension trials. The European Agency for Evaluation of Medical Products has approved the treatment, and the U.S. Food and Drug Administration is currently reviewing it.

Acknowledgments

The author thanks Kenneth H. Astrin for his assistance with this manuscript. This work was supported, in part, by grants from the National Institutes of Health including a research grant (R37 DK 34045 Merit Award), a grant (5 MO1 RR00071) for the Mount Sinai General Clinical Research Center Program from the National Center for Research Resources, a grant (5 P30 HD28822) for the Mount Sinai Child Health Research Center, and a research grant from the Genzyme Corporation.

REFERENCES

1. Desnick RJ, Ioannou YA, Eng CM: α-Galactosidase A deficiency: Fabry disease. In Scriver CR, Beaudet AL, Sly WS, et al (eds): The Metabolic and Molecular Bases of Inherited Disease, 8th ed. New York, McGraw-Hill, 2001, pp 3733–3774.
2. Schiffmann R, Kopp JB, Austin H, et al: Infusion of α-galactosidase A reduces tissue globotriaosylceramide storage in patients with Fabry disease. Proc Natl Acad Sci U S A 2000;97:365–370.
3. Eng CM, Banikazemi M, Gordon R, et al: A phase 1/2 clinical trial of enzyme replacement in Fabry disease: Pharmacokinetic, substrate clearance, and safety studies. Am J Hum Genet 2001;68:711–722.
4. Eng CM, Guffon N, Wilcox WR, et al: Safety and efficacy of recombinant human α-galactosidase A replacement therapy in Fabry's disease. N Engl J Med 2001;345:9–16.
5. Schiffmann R, Kopp JB, Austin HA, 3rd, et al: Enzyme replacement therapy in Fabry disease: A randomized controlled trial. JAMA 2001;285:2743–2749.
6. Colombi A, Kostyal A, Bracher R, et al: Angiokeratoma corporis diffusum—Fabry's disease. Helv Med Acta 1967;34:67–83.
7. Cable WJ, Kolodny EH, Adams RD: Fabry disease: Impaired autonomic function. Neurology 1982;32:498–502.
8. Ohnishi A, Dyck P: Loss of small peripheral sensory neurons in Fabry disease. Histologic and morphometric evaluation of cutaneous nerves, spinal ganglia, and posterior columns. Arch Neurol 1974;31:120.
9. Clarke JT, Knaack J, Crawhall JC, Wolfe LS: Ceramide trihexosidosis (Fabry's disease) without skin lesions. N Engl J Med 1971;284:233–235.
10. Sher NA, Letson RD, Desnick RJ: The ocular manifestations in Fabry's disease. Arch Ophthalmol 1979;97:671–676.
11. von Scheidt W, Eng CM, Fitzmaurice TF, et al: An atypical variant of Fabry's disease with manifestations confined to the myocardium. N Engl J Med 1991;324:395–399.
12. Elleder M, Bradova V, Smid F, et al: Cardiocyte storage and hypertrophy as a sole manifestation of Fabry's disease. Report on a case simulating hypertrophic non-obstructive cardiomyopathy. Virchows Arch A Pathol Anat Histopathol 1990;417:449–455.
13. Nakao S, Takenaka T, Maeda M, et al: An atypical variant of Fabry's disease in men with left ventricular hypertrophy. N Engl J Med 1995;333:288–293.
14. Desnick RJ, Allen KY, Desnick SJ, et al: Fabry's disease: Enzymatic diagnosis of hemizygotes and heterozygotes. α-Galactosidase activities in plasma, serum, urine, and leukocytes. J Lab Clin Med 1973;81:157–171.
15. Lemansky P, Bishop DF, Desnick RJ, et al: Synthesis and processing of α-galactosidase A in human

fibroblasts. Evidence for different mutations in Fabry disease. J Biol Chem 1987;262:2062–2065.

16. Sung JH: Autonomic neurons affected by lipid storage in the spinal cord in Fabry's disease: Distribution of autonomic neurons in the sacral cord. J Neuropathol Exp Neurol 1979;38:87–98.

17. Morgan SH, Rudge P, Smith SJ, et al: The neurological complications of Anderson-Fabry disease (α- galactosidase A deficiency)—Investigation of symptomatic and presymptomatic patients. Q J Med 1990;75: 491–507.

18. Kornreich R, Desnick RJ, Bishop DF: Nucleotide sequence of the human α-galactosidase A gene. Nucl Acids Res 1989;17:3301–3302.

19. Bishop DF, Kornreich R, Desnick RJ: Structural organization of the human α-galactosidase A gene: Further evidence for the absence of a 3′ untranslated region. Proc Natl Acad Sci U S A 1988;85:3903–3907.

20. Ashley GA, Shabbeer J, Yasuda M, et al: Fabry disease: Twenty novel α-galactosidase A mutations causing the classical phenotype. J Hum Genet 2001;46: 192–196.

21. Lockman LA, Hunninghake DB, Krivit W, Desnick RJ: Relief of pain of Fabry's disease by diphenylhydantoin. Neurology 1973;23:871–875.

22. Ioannou YA, Zeidner KM, Gordon RE, Desnick RJ: Fabry disease: Preclinical studies demonstrate the effectiveness of α-galactosidase A replacement in enzyme-deficient mice. Am J Hum Genet 2001;68:14–25.

23. Edmunds T, Lee K, Barngrover D: Biochemical comparison of Fabrazyme™ and Replagal™. Genet Med 2002;4:184.

Schindler Disease: Deficient α-*N*-Acetylgalactosaminidase Activity

Robert J. Desnick

Detlev Schindler

Schindler disease is a recently recognized autosomal recessive disorder resulting from the deficient activity of α-*N*-acetylgalactosaminidase, the lysosomal glycohydrolase previously known as α-galactosidase B.[1] The enzymatic defect leads to the cellular accumulation and increased urinary excretion of glycoconjugates, mostly glycopeptides and oligosaccharides containing α-*N*-acetylgalactosaminyl residues. The disease is clinically heterogeneous with three major subtypes. The clinical, biochemical, and molecular defects in patients with type I, II, or III Schindler disease have been characterized based on the findings in three related German cases with the infantile-onset type I disease,[2,3] two unrelated adult Japanese women[4,5] and two adult Spanish siblings[6] with type II disease, and five children of Dutch,[7] Moroccan,[8] and French/Italian/Albanian descent with type III disease.[9] Patients with type I disease have early-onset neuroaxonal dystrophy with the characteristic neuropathology, while type II patients have angiokeratoma corporis diffusum, mild intellectual impairment, and sensory nerve involvement with neuroaxonal degeneration of peripheral nerves. Patients with type III disease have an intermediate and variable phenotype with manifestations ranging from seizures and moderate psychomotor retardation in infancy to a milder autistic presentation. All three subtypes have very low levels of α-*N*-acetylgalactosaminidase activity, have essentially the same patterns of glycoconjugate accumulation in the urine, and are inherited as autosomal recessive traits. Here, the clinical, pathologic, biochemical, and molecular findings in the severe infantile and milder later-onset forms of this neuroaxonal dystrophy are described.

CLINICAL FEATURES AND DIAGNOSTIC EVALUATION

Type I Disease

α-*N*-acetylgalactosaminidase deficiency was first recognized in two German brothers, the offspring of fourth cousins of German descent.[1] The clinical course of these patients was characterized by three stages: (1) apparently normal development in the first 9 to 12 months of life; (2) a period of developmental delay followed by rapid regression starting in the second year of life; and (3) increasing neurologic impairment, resulting by age 3 to 4 years in profound psychomotor retardation, spasticity, seizures, blindness, and decorticate posturing (Fig. 31–1).

Clinical onset of disease in the older brother was signaled by poor gait coordination, clumsiness, episodes of falling, and startle reactions at 12 months. In the younger brother, grand mal seizures began at 8 months and occurred five times during the next 6 months. Peak development was achieved at about 15 months in both sibs. Thereafter, each experienced a retrogressive course, with the final loss of all mental and motor skills acquired previously. Along with the progressive psychomotor deterioration, both siblings developed strabismus, nystagmus, visual impairment, spasticity, and frequent myoclonic movements. By age 3 to 4 years, both brothers had profound psychomotor retardation, were immobile and incontinent, and had little or no contact with the environment. Since then, they have survived in a vegetative state, dependent on

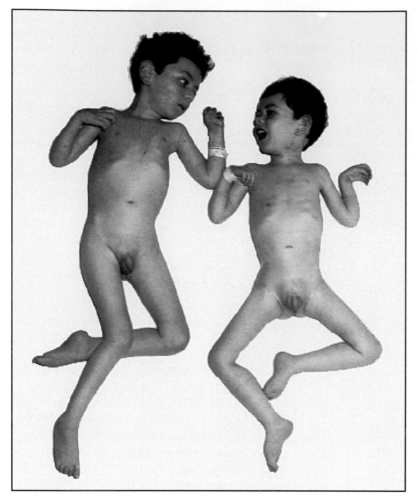

FIGURE 31–1. The affected German siblings with type I disease at 5 years 3 months *(left)* and at 4 years *(right)* of age. (From Desnick RJ, Schindler D: α-N-Acetylgalactosaminidase deficiency: Schindler disease. In Scriver CR, Beaudet AL, Sly WS, Valle D [eds]: The Metabolic and Molecular Bases of Inherited Disease, 8th ed. New York, McGraw-Hill, 2001, pp 3483–3505.)

liquid nutrition, intermittent tube feeding, and regular nasopharyngeal suctioning. They remain alive in their teens because of the diligent nursing efforts of their parents.

At ages 16 and 17 years, neither sib has voluntary movement (except for frequent myoclonic jerks and occasional seizures) or response to optical or acoustic stimuli. They are relatively hypotonic distally and hypertonic proximally. They have bilateral pyramidal tract involvement with symmetric hyperreflexia and clonus. Bilateral optic atrophy is evident. Their developmental skills are at the newborn level, and they do not have ocular, cutaneous, skeletal, or other visceral signs of a storage disease.

A third patient with type I disease, a maternal third and paternal fourth infant cousin of the original sibs, was diagnosed posthumously.[3] This patient experienced several severe grand mal seizures from age 7 months, most occurring with febrile episodes during respiratory tract infections. Developmental progress also was halted from 15 months of age. He died unexpectedly at 18 months from apnea during prolonged convulsions. An autopsy was not performed. However, fibroblasts were preserved, and the diagnosis of α-N-acetylgalactosaminidase deficiency was made.

Pertinent Laboratory and Imaging Findings

Routine laboratory studies including complete blood counts and blood and cerebrospinal fluid chemistries were within normal limits.[10] Skeletal radiography showed systemic, diffuse, and severe osteopenia, and bilateral subluxation of the hips. The EEG indicated diffuse brain dysfunction and disclosed irritative features such as multifocal isolated spikes and spike-wave complexes. Quantitative EEG and brain mapping showed marked slowing with substantially increased β and δ activity, in particular over the central and parieto-occipital regions. The brain stem auditory, somatosensory, and visual-evoked potentials had low amplitude, delayed responses, or both. These findings were consistent with cortical blindness and deafness, although some residual informational processing was retained. Electroretinography showed increased voltages under all conditions, in a manner consistent with the exclusion of the peripheral visual pathway from the disease process. Nerve conduction velocities were low normal. CT and MRI studies showed marked atrophy of the cervical spinal cord, the brainstem, and the cerebellum. The optic tracts and cranial nerves were hypotrophic. Brain atrophy was generalized and also extended to supratentorial regions including the cerebral white matter and cortical structures. These findings were consistent with an overall reduced cerebral glucose metabolism compared to normal values for age, seen on PET studies using 2-[^{18}F] fluoro-2-deoxy-D-glucose.[11] In addition, the extent of regional glucose hypometabolism was directly correlated with the degree of brain atrophy seen on MRI.

Type II Disease

Type II α-N-acetylgalactosaminidase deficiency is an adult-onset disorder characterized by angiokeratoma corporis diffusum, mild intellectual impairment, sensory nerve involvement, and lymphedema. To date, four affected adults in three unrelated consanguineous families have been identified.[4–6] Angiokeratoma corporis diffusum was first noted at about 30 years of age in the unrelated Japanese patients.[4,5] The eruption spread slowly over their bodies, essentially in an appearance and distribution similar to that of affected males with Fabry disease. There was no family history of individuals with similar dermatologic findings. Both patients were products of first-cousin marriages.

Dermatologically, these patients had densely peppered, tiny, deep red to purple maculopapules ranging in diameter from less than 1 mm to 3 mm. The lesions were distributed over the entire body, including the face and fingers, but they were more dense on the axillae, breasts, lower abdomen, groin, buttocks, and upper thighs. Telangiectasia was present on the lips, and on the oral pharyngeal mucosa. Dilated blood vessels also were present on the ocular conjunctiva and were observed with a corkscrew-like tortuousness in the fundi. There were no retinal hemorrhages, macular changes, or corneal opacities. Cardiac examination and electrocardiographic findings were normal at rest and with exercise. There was no organomegaly, lymphadenopathy, or skeletal abnormality. On neurologic examination, the first Japanese patient had a dull affect and was mentally slow.

The second Japanese patient experienced tinnitus and hearing loss that started before age 20 years, and recurrent attacks of vertigo from age 25 years.[5] She was diagnosed as having Menière's syndrome and underwent surgery for vestibular dysfunction twice, without success. She appeared to be of normal intelligence.

In 1994, two consanguineous adult sibs of Spanish descent with type II disease were reported.[6] At diagnosis, the male proband was 42 years old, and his sister was 38 years old. The affected male had a slightly coarse facies with thick lips and enlarged nasal tip. Both sibs developed angiokeratoma corporis diffusum in adulthood, with the lesions in the male distributed between umbilicus and the upper thighs and those in the female isolated on the abdomen, breasts, and gingival mucosa. Both sibs had tortuous conjunctival vessels, and the male also had tortuous retinal vessels. In the male, massive lymphedema of the lower extremities developed at age 10 to 14 years,

whereas the female had a milder involvement. The male had diffuse haziness in the corneal epithelial layer, which differed from the typical whorllike opacities seen in Fabry disease, and he had moderate cardiomegaly. His neurologic status was unremarkable.

Pertinent Laboratory Findings

Routine hematologies and serum and urinary chemistries were normal. Various endocrine studies, a chest radiograph, and a skeletal survey also were normal. Psychometric evaluations showed a low intelligence quotient in the first Japanese type II patient using the Wechsler adult intelligence scale.[4] Verbal IQ and performance IQ also were below normal. The electroencephalogram was unremarkable. Magnetic resonance imaging of the brain showed a few small lacunar infarctions; no gross atrophy of the parenchyma was observed. Nerve conduction studies of the right peroneal nerve showed normal conduction amplitude and velocity in the motor fibers. There was, however, a marked decrease in amplitude (0.5 µV; normal measurement, 1.2 µV to 9 µV) with normal velocity in the sensory fibers. Similar results were obtained from the right median nerve. Results of electromyograms of the muscles innervated by these nerves were normal. The second Japanese patient also had markedly decreased conduction amplitude with normal velocity, whereas the amplitude and velocity in motor nerves were normal.[5] These results were indicative of peripheral neuroaxonal degeneration.

In the Spanish sibs, motor and sensory conduction velocities of the median nerve and motor conduction of the peroneal nerve were within normal ranges. Psychomotor examination of the male showed an IQ of 84 with normal verbal and low performance IQ values.[6]

Type III Disease

Five children with type III α-N-acetylgalactosaminidase deficiency from three unrelated families have been described with an intermediate phenotype, designated type III disease.[7–9] In a Dutch family, twins were affected.[7] The female was essentially well until she experienced severe asymmetric convulsions at age 11 months. She had a high fever that precipitated uncontrollable grand mal seizures, and attacks of apnea and bradycardia that required admission to an intensive care unit. Although the fever and convulsions responded to medication, a few days after detubation she developed pneumonia, a high fever, sepsis, and multiple organ failure from which she slowly recovered. Psychomotor retardation was noted later. She walked by herself and spoke only single words at age 21 months. On examination at age 2 years, mild psychomotor retardation was evident and strabismus was observed. After age 2.4 years, she had four convulsions, mostly associated with fever, despite treatment with antiepileptic drugs. She did not have dysmorphic features, organomegaly, cutaneous lesions, or vacuolated lymphocytes. A CT scan of the brain appeared normal at age 2 years. The diagnosis was made by the characteristic urinary oligosaccharide patterns and by the demonstration of α-N-acetylgalactosaminidase deficiency in fibroblasts and leukocytes.

Her twin brother also was mildly affected. At age 9 months, his developmental performance was reported to be within normal limits, but probably less advanced than that of his twin sister. At age 4 years, he had some developmental delay, particularly in language skills, but neurologic tests had not been performed. Of interest, the mother was an effectively treated epileptic, and epilepsy also occurred in the father's family.

A third patient with type III disease was recently recognized in France.[9] The proband was the only child of unrelated parents of French, Italian, and Albanian descent. Pregnancy, labor, and delivery were uneventful. The boy's early development was reportedly normal; however, he sat alone at age 9 months and walked independently at age 18 months. His parents sought medical advice at age 2 years because he did not speak or interact with others. On physical examination, at age 6 years, he had no dysmorphic features, organomegaly, skeletal or cutaneous abnormalities, or abnormal neurologic findings. Weight, height, and head circumference were at -0.5 SD for age. He was characterized as having a restless attitude, diminished attention span, emotional instability and irritability, and fits of anger with stereotyped and ritualistic behavior. His intellectual development was impaired and he only had rudimentary syntax. These behavioral findings led to the diagnosis of autism. Brain MRI and spine x-rays were unremarkable. At age 8 years, he did not exhibit seizures or neurologic regression. Psychometric evaluation was difficult because of his behavior; however, his global IQ was markedly decreased (48), the verbal IQ was 58, and the performance IQ was 46. Routine laboratory studies, including complete blood cell counts, blood glucose, serum electrolytes and protein, and liver enzymes were all within normal limits. Vacuolated lymphocytes were not found in blood smears. Serum and urinary amino acid profiles were normal, as were the urinary organic acids.

Two sibs of Moroccan descent with type III disease also have recently been reported.[8] The proband was the 3-year-old son of consanguineous parents. He was evaluated for abnormal eye movements at 4 weeks. Urinary oligosaccharide screening that showed an abnormal pattern. He had neuromotor developmental delay. At 3 years of age, he was unable to walk without support, but had normal hand coordination and speech development. A brain MRI showed diffuse white matter abnormalities and secondary symmetrical demyelinization, while an ophthalmologic examination showed bilateral cataracts. The proband's 7-year-old brother, identified by urinary oligosaccharide screening and deficient α-N-acetylgalactosaminidase activity, had no clinical or neurologic symptoms.[8]

DIAGNOSTIC EVALUATION

Children with developmental delay and retrogression in the first or second year of life and clinical manifestations compatible with an infantile neuroaxonal dystrophy should be examined for type I disease. Patients with manifestations ranging from seizures and moderate psychomotor retardation in infancy to a milder autistic presentation with speech and language delay, and marked behavioral difficulties in early childhood may be investigated for type III disease. In adolescents and adults with mild intellectual impairment and angiokeratoma, type II disease should be considered. Initial screening for all subtypes can be performed by analysis of the urinary oligosaccharide and glycopeptide profiles.[12] Definitive diagnosis of all forms is made by demonstration of deficient α-N-acetylgalactosaminidase activity in plasma, isolated leukocytes, or cultured lymphoblasts or fibroblasts using the chromogenic substrate, p-nitrophenol-α-N-acetylgalactosaminide, or better, the fluorogenic substrate, 4-methylumbelliferyl-α-N-acetylgalactosaminide.[1] Prenatal diagnosis can be accomplished by determining the enzymatic activity in chorionic villi obtained at 10 menstrual weeks or in cultured amniocytes obtained by amniocentesis at 15 to 16 menstrual weeks.

PATHOLOGY

Light microscopic examination of blood, bone marrow, liver, skeletal muscle, skin, peripheral nerve, conjunctiva, and jejunal and rectal wall from the type I patients appeared normal. Electron microscopy of blood leukocytes, secretory cells of eccrine sweat glands, myelinated axons of cutaneous nerves, and cultured fibroblasts from both type I and II patients showed the presence of inclusions with lamellar, fibrillar, vesicular, and granular material in single membrane-bound organelles.[1]

Ultrastructural studies of rectal mucosa from the type I patients showed abnormal tubulovesicular material free in the cytoplasm in only a few preterminal and terminal (intraganglionic) axons in the myenteric plexus.[1,21] Examination of a frontal lobe biopsy revealed the characteristic neuropathology of infantile neuroaxonal dystrophy.[21] There were numerous large, dense axonal swellings, or spheroids, throughout the neocortex, with no apparent laminar distribution; few such formations were observed in axons in the white matter. On light microscopy, the deposits were sharply demarcated, rounded, or polygonal structures that contained prominent angular or curving clefts with a darker, amorphous background. Ultrastructurally, these abnormal formations appeared exclusively within the preterminal and terminal axons and were not observed in the neuronal perikarya, dendrites, axons in white matter, small axon terminals in the cortical neuropil, astrocytes, oligodendrocytes, microglia, endothelial cells, or arachnoid cells. The accumulations were morphologically heterogeneous, comprising dense, labyrinthine membranous tubulovesicular formations, lamelliform membranous arrays, and prominent acicular electron-lucent clefts, all admixed with a few mitochondria, lysosomes, and occasional microtubules. These aggregates were free in the electron-dense axoplasmic matrix and limited by a plasmalemma facing an epithelial interspace. Based on the neocortical findings, the rectal biopsies from the sibs were re-examined, and spheroids were unequivocally identified in the myenteric plexus and ganglionic neurophil.

In Giemsa-stained peripheral blood smears from the probands with type II disease, small cytoplasmic vacuoles were observed in granulocytes, monocytes, and lymphocytes. These vacuoles did not stain positive with periodic acid-Schiff, alcian blue, or toluidine blue. Histopathologic examination of the skin lesions showed localized hyperkeratosis and dilated thin-walled blood vessels.[13,14] Dilated lymphatic vessels were observed in the mid dermis as well as the upper dermis. Ultrastructural examination of both involved and uninvolved skin of type II patients revealed numerous cytoplasmic vacuoles in several cell types, including endothelial cells in blood and lymphatic vessels, pericytes, fibroblasts, fat cells, Schwann cells, axons, arrector smooth-muscle cells, and eccrine sweat gland cells. They were most prominent in vascular endothelial cells and the secretory portion of sweat gland cells. These membrane-lined vacuoles were electron-lucent or contained filamentous material. Electron-dense multilayered structures were observed only in vacuoles of the sweat gland cells. Vascular endothelial cells of the kidney had similar lysosomal vacuolization as those in skin, but the epithelial cells appeared normal. Similar, but smaller, vacuoles also were observed in peripheral leukocytes.

To date, the pathologic studies of type III disease have been limited to peripheral blood cells. In the Dutch sibs, histologic and electron microscopic examination of

lymphocytes, granulocytes, and monocytes were normal and no vacuolization was observed.[3] Similar findings were noted in the French type III patient.

BIOCHEMISTRY

The deficient activity of lysosomal α-N-acetylgalactosaminidase is the specific enzymatic defect in types I, II, and III disease.[1] Heterozygotes for both subtypes have approximately half-normal levels of activity. The enzymatic defect results in the accumulation of glycoconjugates with terminal or internal α-N-acetylgalactosaminyl moieties, including O-linked and N-linked glycopeptides and glycoproteins (e.g., mucins, blood group A substances), glycosphingolipids (e.g., A-type glycolipids), and proteoglycans (e.g., cartilage keratin sulfate II).[1] Structural analysis of the accumulated urinary compounds showed the presence of the glycopeptide, oligosaccharide, and glycosphingolipid structures (Tables 31–1 and 31–2).

MOLECULAR GENETICS

Types I, II, and III diseases are inherited as autosomal recessive traits and are very rare. The human α-N-acetyl galactosaminidase gene has been mapped to the chromosomal region 22q11. The full-length cDNA and complete genomic sequence encoding α-N-acetylgalactosaminidase have been isolated.[15,16] The 13,709-bp genomic sequence has nine exons ranging from 95 to 2028 bp and intronic sequences of 304 to 2684 bp. Analysis of 1.4 kb of 5′ flanking sequence showed three *Sp*1 and two CAAT-like promoter elements. The α-N-acetylgalactosaminidase gene is transcribed into two transcripts of 2.2 and 3.6 kb, the latter resulting from a second downstream polyadenylation signal in the 3′ untranslated region. Both transcripts have a 1236-bp open reading frame, which

Table 31–1. Accumulated urinary compounds in α-N-acetylgalactosaminidase deficiency

Glycopeptides:

1 GalNAcα1→O-Ser/Thr

2 NeuNAcα2→3Galβ1→3GalNAcα1→O-Ser/Thr

3 Galβ1→3(NeuNAcα2→6)GalNAcα1→O-Ser/Thr

4 NeuNAcα2→3Galβ1→3(NeuNAcα2→6)GalNAcα1→O-Ser/Thr[1]

5 NeuNAcα2→3Galβ1→3(Galβ1→4GlcNAcβ1→6)GalNAcα1→O-Ser/Thr

6 Galβ1→3(NeuNAcα2→3Galβ1→4GlcNAcβ1→6)GalNAcα1→O-Ser/Thr

7 NeuNAcα2→3Galβ1→3(NeuNAcα2→3Galβ1→4GlcNAcβ1→6)GalNAcα1→O-Ser/Thr

8 (NeuNAc)$_2$(Galβ1→4GlcNAc)$_2$Galβ1→3GalNAcα1→O-Ser/Thr

Oligosaccharide:

Blood group A Trisaccharide[2] GalNAcα1→3(Fucα1→?)Gal

Glycosphingolipid:

Blood group A-6-22 GalNAcα1→3(Fucα1→2)Galβ1→4GlcNAcβ1→3Galβ1→4Glcβ1→1′Cer

[1]Major accumulated component underlined.
[2]Only in patients with blood group A.

Table 31–2. Mutations in the α-N-acetylgalactosaminidase gene causing Schindler disease

Disease Type	Ancestry	cDNA Change	Genotype	Reference
I	German	973G>A	E325K/E325K	(3, 18)
II	Japanese A	985C>T	R329W/R329W	(21)
	Japanese B	986G>A	R329G/R329G	(5)
	Spanish	577G>T	E193X/E193X	(3)
III	Dutch	479C>G / 973G>A	S160/E325K	(3)
	Moroccan	973G>A	E325K/E325K	(8)
	French/Albanian/Italian	973G>A / 1099G>A	E325K/E367K	(1)

[1]Numbering according to reference 15, EMBL database accession no. M59199.

encodes 411 amino acids, including a 17-residue signal peptide. The mature 394 amino acid lysosomal polypeptide contains six putative N-glycosylation sites.

Mutations causing the three subtypes of α-N-acetylgalactosaminidase deficiency have been determined for each of the affected probands.[3,8,17,18] Causative mutations include homozygosity for E325K (type I disease); homozygosity for R329W, R329Q, or E193X (type II disease); and heterozygosity for S160C and E367K or homozygosity for E325K (type III disease). The crystal structure of chicken α-N-acetylgalactosaminidase has been solved at 1.9 Å.[19] Based on the homology of the human and chicken proteins, the mutations causing α-N-acetylgalactosaminidase deficiency were modeled. Notably, none of the mutations were localized to the enzyme's active site. Thus, the disease-causing mutations presumably impaired the stability of the enzyme, consistent with the biosynthetic studies of the mutant proteins.[1]

ANIMAL MODEL

There is no identified natural animal model for α-N-acetylgalactosaminidase deficiency. However, knockout mice with α-N-acetylgalactosaminidase deficiency have been generated by targeted gene disruption.[20] The homozygous mice with no detectable α-N-acetylgalactosaminidase activity appeared normal, were fertile and bred, lived a normal life span, and appeared to have no clinically evident neurologic or other disease. In contrast, there was remarkable cellular pathomorphology. Two main lesions were identified: (1) widespread lysosomal storage of abnormal material in the central nervous system and in other organs and (2) focal axonal swellings or spheroids in the central nervous system.[1]

Lysosomal storage was histologically and ultrastructurally observed in numerous cell types throughout the central and peripheral nervous system and in many other organs. Neuronal storage varied from minimal to profound. Perivascular macrophages, either within the neuroparenchyma or in the subarachnoid space, consistently contained the most storage material. Ultrastructurally, the enlarged lysosomes contained flocculent, particulate material, concentric lamellar figures, and multivesicular and dense formations.

The second pathologic finding was neuroaxonal dystrophy. Axonal spheroids were found more frequently in the spinal cord, where they were observed throughout its entire length in a distribution limited to the dorsal gray and white matter, than in the brain. The spheroid content varied from homogeneous to complex. The murine knockout model appears to mimic the characteristic pathologies of the human disease subtypes. However, in absence of autopsied human material, comparisons remain preliminary. Notably, the spheroids in the spinal cord of the knockout mice had remarkable ultrastructural similarity to the cortical spheroids in type I human disease and to those observed in the central nervous system of infantile neuroaxonal dystrophy (Seitelberger disease). Although the definitive distribution of spheroids in type I disease has not been determined, in Seitelberger disease, spheroids are found in large numbers in the spinal cord and medulla and less so in the cerebrum.

THERAPY

There is no treatment for this disease. Supportive care should be implemented to optimize patient comfort.

FUTURE RESEARCH DIRECTIONS

The neuropathology in the murine knockout model, which is similar to the neuroaxonal dystrophy in type I α-N-acetylgalactosaminidase deficient patients, should permit investigation of the role of α-N-acetylgalactosaminidase in neuroaxonal transport. Moreover, studies in the knockout mouse should facilitate future evaluation of various neuron-targeted therapeutic strategies, including gene therapy.

Acknowledgments

This work was supported in part by grants from the National Institutes of Health, including a Merit Award research grant (5 R37 DK34045), a grant for the Mount Sinai General Clinical Research Center from the National Center for Research Resources (5 Mo1 RR00071), and a program project grant for the Mount Sinai Child Health Research Center (5 P01 HD28822).

REFERENCES

1. Desnick RJ, Schindler D: α-N-Acetylgalactosaminidase deficiency: Schindler disease. In Scriver CR, Beaudet AL, Sly WS, Valle D (eds): The Metabolic and Molecular Bases of Inherited Disease, 8th ed. New York, McGraw-Hill, 2001, pp 3483–3505.

2. van Diggelen O, Schindler D, Kleijer W, et al: Lysosomal α-N-acetylgalactosaminidase deficiency: A new inherited metabolic disease. Lancet 1987;2:804.

3. Keulemans JLM, Reuser AJJ, Froos MA, et al: Human α-N-acetylgalactosaminidase (α-NAGA) deficiency: New mutations and the paradox between genotype and phenotype. J Med Genet 1996;33:458–465.

4. Kanzaki T, Yokota M, Mizuno N, et al: Novel lysosomal glycoaminoacid storage disease with angiokeratoma corporis diffusum. Lancet 1989;1:875–877.

5. Kodama K, Kobayashi H, Abe R, et al: A new case of α-N-acetylgalactosaminidase deficiency with angiokeratoma corporis diffusum, with Menierc's syndrome and without mental retardation. Br J Dermatol 2001;144:363–368.

6. Chabas A, Coll MJ, Aparicio M, Rodriguez Diaz E: Mild phenotypic expression of α-N-acetylgalactosaminidase deficiency in two adult siblings. J Inherit Metab Dis 1994;17:724–731.

7. de Jong J, van den Berg C, Wijburg H, et al: α-N-Acetylgalactosaminidase deficiency with mild clinical manifestations and difficult biochemical diagnosis. J Pediatr 1994;125:385–391.

8. Bakker HD, de Sonnaville ML, Vreken P, et al: Human α-N-acetylgalactosaminidase (α-NAGA) deficiency: No association with neuroaxonal dystrophy? Eur J Hum Genet 2001;9:91–96.

9. Blanchon YC, Gay C, Gilbert G, Lauras B: A case of N-acetylgalactosaminidase deficiency (Schindler disease) associated with autism. J Autism Dev Disord 2002;32:145–146.

10. Schindler D, Bishop DF, Wolfe DE, et al: Neuroaxonal dystrophy due to lysosomal α-N-acetyl-galactosaminidase deficiency. N Engl J Med 1989;320: 1735–1740.

11. Rudolf J, Grond M, Schindler D, et al: Cerebral glucose metabolism in type I α-N-acetylgalactosaminidase deficiency: An infantile neuroaxonal dystrophy. J Child Neurol 1999;14:543–547.

12. Schindler D, Kanzaki T, Desnick RJ: A method for the rapid detection of urinary glycopeptides in α-N-acetylgalactosaminidase deficiency and other lysosomal storage diseases. Clin Chim Acta 1990;190:81–91.

13. Kanzaki T, Wang AM, Desnick RJ: Lysosomal α-N-acetylgalactosaminidase deficiency, the enzymatic defect in angiokeratoma corporis diffusum with glycopeptiduria. J Clin Invest 1991;88:707–711.

14. Kanzaki T, Yokota M, Irie F, et al: Angiokeratoma corporis diffusum with glycopeptiduria due to deficient lysosomal α-N-acetylgalactosaminidase activity. Arch Dermatol 1993;129:460–465.

15. Wang A, Bishop D, Desnick R: Human α-N-acetylgalactosaminidase: Molecular cloning, nucleotide sequence, and expression of a full-length cDNA. J Biol Chem 1990;265:21859–21866.

16. Wang AM, Desnick RJ: Structural organization and complete sequence of the human α-N-acetylgalactosaminidase gene: Homology with the α galactosidase A gene proves evidence for evolution from a common ancestral gene. Genomics 1991;10:133–142.

17. Wang AM, Kanzaki T, Desnick RJ: The molecular lesion in the α-N-acetylgalactosaminidase gene that causes angiokeratoma corporis diffusum with glycopeptiduria. J Clin Invest 1994;94:839–845.

18. Wang A, Schindler D, Desnick R: Schindler disease: The molecular lesion in the α-N-acetylgalactosaminidase gene that causes an infantile neuroaxonal dystrophy. J Clin Invest 1990;86:1752–1756.

19. Garman SC, Hannick L, Zhu A, Garboczi DN: The 1.9 Å structure of α-N-acetylgalactosaminidase: Molecular basis of glycosidase deficiency diseases. Structure (Camb) 2002;10:425–434.

20. Wang AM, Stewart CL, Desnick RJ: Schindler disease: Generation of a murine model by targeted disruption of the α-N-acetylgalactosaminidase gene. Pediatr Res 1994;35:155A.

21. Wolfe D, Schindler D, Desnick R: Neuroaxonal dystrophy in infantile α-N-acetylgalactosaminidase deficiency. J Neurol Sci 1995;132:44–56.

Alzheimer's Disease

Dennis J. Selkoe

The remarkably successful aging of the population that occurred during the twentieth century has made Alzheimer's disease (AD) one of the most common disorders of late life. An insidious loss of memory, cognition, reasoning, and behavioral stability leads inexorably to global dementia and premature death of the patient. At autopsy, one finds myriad amyloid plaques and neurofibrillary tangles in limbic and association cortices. These lesions have served as the starting point for an intensive biochemical and molecular biologic attack on the disorder. In particular, progress in unraveling the genotype-to-phenotype relationships of inherited forms of AD has provided growing support for the hypothesis that cerebral accumulation of the amyloid β (Aβ) protein is an early, invariant, and necessary step in the development of the disease.

At least seven kinds of evidence support a central role for excessive accumulation of Aβ in the initiation and progression of the disease: (1) Immunocytochemical studies on the brains of subjects with Down syndrome, Alzheimer's disease, or normal aging all suggest that amorphous, nonfibrillar deposits of Aβ—referred to as diffuse or preamyloid plaques—are the earliest detectable AD-type lesion and precede the development of other neuropathologic features of the disease. (2) Missense mutations immediately surrounding the Aβ region of the amyloid β precursor protein *(APP)* gene are a specific cause of AD, and each of these mutations has been shown to lead to excess production of amyloidogenic Aβ peptides, particularly $A\beta_{1-42}$. (3) Altered levels of $A\beta_{1-42}$ peptide in the serum and/or cerebrospinal fluid (CSF) can precede the onset of AD symptoms by many years or decades, as observed, for example, in individuals harboring mutations in the presenilin *(PS)* 1 or 2 genes.[1] (4) Cortical levels of $A\beta_{1-42}$ determined by enzyme-linked immunosorbent assay (ELISA) correlate tightly with both the presence and the degree of cognitive impairment[2] (5) Aggregated Aβ peptides have been shown reproducibly to exert cytotoxicity on neurons and smooth muscle cells and to activate astrocytes and microglia, in both in vitro and in vivo studies. (6) Transgenic overexpression of AD-causing mutations in *APP* and/or *PS1* has provided mouse models that, while not perfect, reproduce much of the characteristic neuritic and glial cytopathology of AD, supporting the concept that Aβ accumulation can initiate neuritic dystrophy, gliosis, synaptic loss, and perhaps even neurofibrillary tangle formation.[3] (7) Treatments that lower cerebral Aβ levels in vivo, for example, an Aβ vaccine, lead to less neuropathology and improved learning behavior in APP transgenic mice.[4,5]

This chapter reviews these and other recent molecular advances in the context of the complex clinicopathologic phenotype of the Alzheimer syndrome. The influence of the known genetic factors underlying familial forms of AD on the development of Aβ deposition and subsequent neuronal dysfunction is discussed. A model of the disease process that links Aβ accumulation to many other features of the AD phenotype is presented, and emerging points of therapeutic intervention are considered.

CLINICAL FEATURES AND DIAGNOSIS

Alzheimer Syndrome

Most AD patients present with subtle deficits in recent memory, particularly retention of the minor details of everyday life—what they did yesterday, whom they telephoned this morning, what was said to them 5 minutes ago. It is the family, not the patient, who usually becomes concerned about these intermittent lapses in short-term memory. Time and again, patients either deny the memory problem or reluctantly admit to minor symptoms but dismiss them as common to older people. They usually seem to be unconcerned about the lapses their relatives point out, or they hide any concerns they may have quite effectively. The patient who comes to the office earnestly worried that he or she is developing specific symptoms of AD usually turns out not to have the disorder. Most patients show surprising equanimity about their symptoms, making up a variety of excuses for why it should not be surprising that they cannot remember this or that. This characteristic lack of interest in one's own mental errors may be explained by the patient's gradual loss of insight and judgment—the inability to sense one's situation in life—that so often accompanies the classical memory deficits of AD.

A salient feature of the clinical presentation is its remarkable insidious onset. Neither patient nor family can pinpoint when it all began. Once they become convinced that there is something wrong, the family searches retrospectively for the first clue. Often, past events of major or minor import, perhaps a medical illness, accident, or emotional upset, will be viewed by the spouse or children as the starting point. But when one considers the biology of the process, one recognizes that the biochemical and pathologic phenotype has been building very slowly over a long time, almost certainly for many years. Accordingly, the first symptoms are so subtle and occur so infrequently that they blend with everyday behavior.

As patients progress over the first few years, they usually develop increasing forgetfulness, disorientation, confusion about mathematical and geographical concepts, decreased abstraction, and word-finding difficulty and other language problems. As these deficits accrue, many patients also develop intermittent behavioral symptoms—agitation, restlessness (e.g., pacing), insomnia, paranoia, angry outbursts, and sometimes frank delusions and hallucinations. But the sensorium remains clear, and alertness is preserved through most of the illness. Motor function usually remains normal until extrapyramidal signs (rigidity, bradykinesia) and slowed gait develops after several years of cognitive decline. In later years, global dementia is accompanied by motor impairment, incontinence of bladder and bowel, and an increasingly mute, immobile state. Death often comes after one to two decades of progressive symptomatology, with minor respiratory difficulty, aspiration, or pneumonia serving as common terminal events.

Much has been written in the popular press about the difficulty that doctors have in diagnosing AD. It seems that because AD can only be diagnosed definitively at postmortem examination, an assumption has developed that it is almost impossible to come to a diagnosis during life. This is no more true for AD than for many commonly diagnosed systemic diseases in which the symptoms, signs, and laboratory tests point clearly to a particular diagnosis but definitive proof requires tissue examination. Experienced clinicians can distinguish AD from most other dementias with a rather high degree of accuracy. Indeed, autopsy series from clinics specializing in dementia indicate that the accuracy of a clinical diagnosis of AD can exceed 95%. In the general medical community, this rate is likely to be somewhat lower, perhaps 70% to 80%.

Until recently, the diagnostic work-up for AD was largely a matter of obtaining negative blood tests and a normal brain imaging study that helped rule out other causes of dementia. Now, positive evidence for the presence of AD has emerged from imaging studies such as SPECT and functional MRI, and from the measurement of elevated tau and decreased $A\beta_{42}$ levels in the CSF. Psychometric tests can solidify the clinical diagnosis and quantify deterioration over time. Psychiatric consultation can help determine whether behavioral symptoms are due to dementia and suggest how they should be treated pharmacologically. It is likely that quantitative imaging of the neuropathology itself—particularly the cerebral $A\beta$ deposits—will become possible in the future. For now, prolonged follow-up usually clarifies diagnostic dilemmas and reveals the rather stereotyped clinical pattern of AD.

PATHOLOGY

Neuropathology of AD Provides the Basis for Molecular Advances

In contrast to numerous other hereditary neurologic and psychiatric disorders in which the identification of causative genes by linkage analysis and positional cloning provided the first insights into disease mechanism, genetic advances in AD have derived in considerable part from the detailed characterization of the neuropathologic phenotype. The morphologic signature provided by the presence of amyloid plaques and neurofibrillary tangles has given rise to countless biochemical, molecular biologic, and cell biologic studies that have cumulatively helped to explain the pathogenesis of AD. Based on Alzheimer's original description of the disease as well as formal consensus about its pathodiagnostic criteria, all cases of AD have amyloid-bearing neuritic plaques in densities substantially greater than those found in nondemented subjects of similar age. These plaques are complex, multicellular lesions, the temporal development of which appears to be very gradual, as judged by studies of young adults with Down syndrome. The mature neuritic plaque generally contains a central extracellular deposit of $A\beta$ that is largely in filamentous form (i.e., amyloid fibrils of 6 nm to 10 nm) and is intimately associated with dilated, ultrastructurally abnormal dendrites and axons (dystrophic neurites). In addition, the neuritic plaques are usually associated with activated microglia located within the amyloid deposit and reactive fibrillary astrocytes immediately surrounding the lesion.

The other hallmark lesion of AD, the neurofibrillary tangle, usually occurs abundantly in entorhinal cortex; hippocampus; amygdala; association cortices of the frontal, temporal, and parietal lobes; and certain subcortical nuclei that project to these regions. Tangles are non-membrane-bound masses of abnormal paired helical filaments (PHF) and straight filaments found in the perinuclear cytoplasm of selected neurons. Smaller bundles of highly similar or identical PHF are present in many of the dystrophic neurites of the neuritic plaque. In addition to sensitively detecting tangles and plaque-associated neurites, silver stains also highlight widely scattered dystrophic neurites that contain PHF and are found throughout much of the cortical neuropil in most cases of AD, particularly those with high tangle densities. The occurrence of this diffuse neuritic abnormality in affected brain regions indicates that neuritic dystrophy is by no means confined to the immediate periplaque region.

The subunit protein of the PHF is the microtubule-associated protein, tau. Biochemical studies reveal that the tau found in the tangles and also in many of the dystrophic neurites within and outside of the plaques constitutes hyperphosphorylated, largely insoluble forms of this normally highly soluble cytosolic protein. The insoluble tau aggregates in the tangles are often conjugated with ubiquitin, a feature they share with other intraneuronal proteinaceous inclusions in etiologically diverse disorders such as Parkinson's disease and diffuse Lewy body disease. If this ubiquitination represents an attempt to rid the cytoplasm of the tau aggregates by way of the proteasome, it appears to be largely unsuccessful. Tangles also occur in a dozen or more relatively uncommon neurodegenerative diseases in which one usually finds no Aβ deposits and neuritic plaques. One particularly important example is frontotemporal dementia with parkinsonism linked to chromosome 17 *(FTDP-17)*, which is reviewed in Chapter 33.

In addition to the presence of abundant neuritic plaques, neurofibrillary tangles, and dystrophic neurites in almost all AD cases, shrinkage and loss of limbic and cortical neurons and, in particular, loss of their synaptic endings are a prominent feature of the pathology. Cortical synaptic loss shows a particularly strong quantitative correlation with the degree of dementia that a patient experienced during life. Robust reactive astrocytosis and microgliosis are observed immediately surrounding and between amyloid-bearing neuritic plaques. Granulovacuolar degeneration in the cytoplasm of selected pyramidal neurons, primarily in the hippocampus, is found in many AD brains.

The purification and partial sequencing of Aβ by Glenner and Wong[6] and the subsequent development of antibodies to Aβ led to the recognition that diffuse Aβ deposits lacking neuritic and glial alterations are more abundant than amyloid-bearing neuritic plaques in AD brain tissue. Moreover, substantial numbers of diffuse plaques occur in brain areas not obviously implicated in the classical symptomatology of AD, such as the cerebellum, striatum, and thalamus. The presence of abundant diffuse plaques in these cytopathologically and clinically

"unaffected" areas of brain, as well as their very early appearance in the course of the AD pathology of Down syndrome, provides strong evidence that Aβ accumulation and deposition can precede neuritic and glial alteration rather than follow it.

Because some aged, nondemented humans show moderate or even high densities of cortical Aβ deposits at postmortem examination, the relevance of Aβ deposition to the pathogenesis of the clinical disease has been questioned. However, these age-related deposits are almost entirely diffuse plaques lacking detectable neuritic and glial pathology. Indeed, if significant numbers of amyloid-bearing neuritic plaques were present, a pathologic diagnosis of AD would usually ensue. Thus, the presence of some, or occasionally many, diffuse Aβ deposits in humans lacking measurable cognitive impairment does not rule against a critical role for Aβ accumulation in the disease but rather suggests that associated neuritic and glial cytopathology must develop for clinical symptoms to appear. The very occurrence of diffuse Aβ deposits in otherwise normal brain tissue of healthy older humans clearly supports the concept that Aβ production and initial deposition do not require pre-existing cellular abnormalities. Biochemical quantification of cortical Aβ in normal aged and minimally cognitively impaired individuals has revealed that cerebral Aβ concentrations are substantially elevated before the first symptoms of dementia become apparent.[7]

In addition to abundant Aβ deposits of varying morphologies, almost all AD brains have at least modest and often substantial amounts of fibrillar Aβ deposits in the basement membranes of cerebral capillaries and cerebral and meningeal arterioles and small arteries (i.e., amyloid angiopathy). Because the amount of vascular amyloid deposition often correlates poorly with the generally high levels of amyloid plaques in AD, the relationship of the processes that lead to these two types of β-amyloid deposits remains unsettled. The Aβ species that appears to be initially deposited in diffuse plaques and that remains the major constituent of most mature (neuritic) plaques ends at Aβ residue 42, whereas the principal Aβ peptide in vascular amyloid ends at residue 40, with some $Aβ_{42}$ species also present (discussed later). AD brains often show typical amyloid plaques that are intimately associated with capillaries as well as cylindrical Aβ tissue deposits immediately surrounding amyloid-bearing cortical vessels (dysphoric angiopathy). The reasons for this microvascular predilection of some Aβ deposits are only poorly understood.

BIOCHEMICAL FINDINGS

Biochemistry of Amyloid Deposits Leads to the Characterization of APP

Biochemical analyses of isolated amyloid plaques indicate that they contain Aβ peptides ending at $alanine_{42}$ as their major constituent but show substantial N-and C-terminal heterogeneity, including species that begin at native or modified residues between aspartate$_1$ and glutamate$_{11}$ and that end at Val$_{40}$, Ala$_{42}$, or other nearby residues. Among the modified N-terminal species are peptides that begin at residue 3 with the conversion of glutamate to pyroglutamate or at residue 1 with the conversion of L-aspartate to D-aspartate or L-isoaspartate, each of which provides a blocked N-terminus. The pathogenic significance of this N-terminal heterogeneity in AD is unclear, and it is likely that at least some of the modifications occur after years of storage of Aβ_{1-42} and Aβ_{1-40} in plaques. Highly specific ELISAs performed on total cortical extracts demonstrate that the major species that accumulates in AD cortex ends at residue 42 but that brains having robust amyloid angiopathy also contain abundant Aβ peptides ending at residue 40.

Immunocytochemistry with antibodies that are specific for particular N- or C-termini of Aβ largely confirms the findings obtained by compositional analysis and indicates that Aβ peptides ending at Ala$_{42}$ are the initially deposited species in plaques.[8] Vascular amyloid generally reacts with antibodies specific for Val$_{40}$, although it is likely that the Aβ_{42} peptide is the initially deposited species in vessels, as it is in brain parenchyma. The heterogeneity found at both ends of Aβ purified from cerebral amyloid deposits correlates in part with the variety of soluble Aβ peptides that are normally secreted by cells (discussed later).

The provision of the protein sequences for vascular and plaque Aβ led to the cloning of their large precursor protein, APP. Aβ was shown to be a proteolytic fragment comprising the last 28 residues of the APP ectodomain just prior to the membrane plus the first 12–14 residues of the transmembrane region (Fig. 32–1). APP is a single membrane-spanning, receptor-like glycoprotein that is inserted in part at the plasma membrane but occurs to a much greater extent in internal vesicular membranes, including the Golgi apparatus and endosomes. As expected from this distribution, APP has a signal peptide for translocation into the endoplasmic reticulum (ER), after which it is processed through the secretory pathway, undergoing first N- and then O-linked glycosylation. In addition to post-translational events, APP undergoes alternative splicing of several exons in its ectodomain, including a motif homologous to the Kunitz family of serine protease inhibitors that suggests one function of the ectodomain, namely as a secreted protease inhibitor.

Cellular Trafficking of APP: Nonamyloidogenic and Amyloidogenic Pathways

Intensive studies of the cellular trafficking and proteolytic processing of APP have revealed the alternative metabolic fates that this molecule can undergo. APP is expressed in virtually all neuronal and non-neuronal cells, although the expression of alternate transcripts shows some cell and tissue differences. Transcripts containing the Kunitz protease inhibitor (KPI) insert in the midregion of the ectodomain (APP$_{751}$ and APP$_{770}$) are the most abundantly expressed isoforms in all non-neuronal tissues and in glial, endothelial, and smooth muscle cells in the brain. The transcript lacking the KPI insert (APP$_{695}$) is the major species expressed in neurons, with substantially lower amounts of APP$_{751/770}$ also expressed in these cells. The trafficking and processing of APP vary only modestly as a function of cell type; the findings about to be described are generalized from studies conducted primarily in non-neuronal cells.

Newly synthesized APP molecules are translocated into the ER, with the N-terminal ectodomain projecting into the lumen of the vesicle and the C-terminus located in the cytoplasm. Following addition of N- and O-linked sugars in the Golgi, a subset of APP molecules is trafficked via secretory vesicles to the cell surface. The percentage of total cellular APP that exists at the cell surface at any one point is relatively small in most cell types. Those precursors that arrive at the cell surface can undergo one of two fates: α-secretase cleavage 12 residues N-terminal to the beginning of the transmembrane domain to release the large soluble ectodomain (APP$_s$) or re-internalization of the holoprotein and trafficking through the endosomal/lysosomal system (reviewed in reference 9). The likelihood that some APP molecules are internalized from the cell surface was initially raised by the observation that APP contains a consensus sequence (Arg-Pro-Thr-Tyr) for clathrin-mediated endocytosis near the end of its cytoplasmic domain, and this route has been confirmed in several cell types, including primary neurons. Following endocytosis, some APP molecules recycle rapidly to the cell surface. Because no natural ligand that binds the APP ectodomain at the surface has yet been identified, it is unclear what signal triggers the internalization and recycling of the molecule. However, the finding that chimeric APP molecules containing a heterologous transactivating domain in the cytoplasmic tail can drive the transcription of reporter genes in the nucleus strongly suggests that APP functions as a signaling receptor.[10] In accord, the free cytoplasmic domain generated by γ-secretase reaches the nucleus.[11]

Current data suggest that surface-derived APP present in recycling endosomes may serve as the major precursor of Aβ. A portion of the endocytosed APP C-terminal fragments (C83 and C99) are trafficked on to late endosomes and lysosomes, but there is no evidence that the fragments reaching these later compartments actually give rise to Aβ and p3; they may be directed to lysosomes for complete catabolism. It appears that nonamyloidogenic (α-secretase) and amyloidogenic (β-secretase) processing of APP can occur in part in the secretory pathway as well. For example, the generation of α-APP$_s$ by α-secretase has been demonstrated intracellularly during the exocytic trafficking of APP, presumably in the trans-Golgi network (TGN) or in secretory vesicles

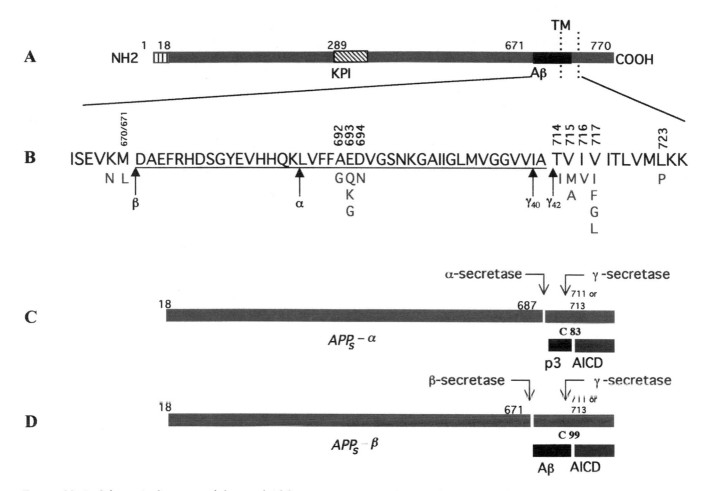

FIGURE 32–1. Schematic diagrams of the amyloid β precursor protein (APP) and its principal metabolic derivatives. *A*, Diagram showing the largest of the known APP alternate splice forms comprising 770 amino acids. Regions of interest are indicated at their correct relative positions. A 17-residue signal peptide occurs at the N-terminus *(vertical lines)*. Two alternatively spliced exons of 56 and 19 amino acids are inserted at residue 289; the first contains a serine protease inhibitor domain of the Kunitz type (KPI). A single transmembrane domain (TM) at amino acids 700–723 is shown *(vertical dotted lines)*. The amyloid β (Aβ) protein fragment includes 28 residues just outside the membrane plus the first 12–14 residues of the transmembrane domain. *B*, Expanded sequence within APP that contains the Aβ and transmembrane regions. The $A\beta_{1-42}$ peptide *(underlined residues)* is shown. Currently known missense mutations identified in certain patients with AD and/or hereditary cerebral hemorrhage with amyloidosis *(letters below the wild-type sequence)* are also shown. Three-digit numbers shown above the sequence represent the codon number (βAPP_{770} isoform). *C*, Site of cleavage after residue 687 *(arrows)* by α-secretase that enables secretion of the large soluble ectodomain of APP (APP$_S$-α) into the medium, and retention of the 83-residue C-terminal fragment (C83) in the membrane. C83 can undergo cleavage by the protease called γ-secretase at residue 711 or 713 to release the p3 peptides. *D*, Alternative proteolytic cleavage after residue 671 by β-secretase that results in the secretion of the slightly truncated APP$_S$-β molecule and the retention of a 99-residue C-terminal fragment (C99). C99 can also undergo cleavage by γ-secretase at either residue 711 or 713 to release the Aβ peptides. Cleavage of both C83 and C99 by γ-secretase releases the APP intracellular domain (AICD) into the cytoplasm.

budding from it. Moreover, at least the Swedish mutant form of APP, which is a particularly attractive substrate for β-secretase, appears to undergo some cleavage by this enzyme on the way to the cell surface, while the wild-type substrate may do less.

Although Aβ was originally identified as the subunit of amyloid fibrils in AD, it is now known that this fragment is constitutively secreted by APP-expressing cells during normal metabolism throughout life and is present in extracellular fluids such as CSF and plasma

(reviewed in reference 9). Therefore, the terms *nonamyloidogenic processing* (α-secretase) and *amyloidogenic processing* (β-secretase) do not imply normal and abnormal processing, respectively. Various influences on the cell, both normal events such as activation of certain signal transduction cascades and pathologic events such as mutations in APP, seem to shift the relative processing of APP between these two alternate cleavage events. For example, activation of cell-surface receptors for several different first messenger systems, including acetylcholine, bradykinin, vasopressin, and other neurotransmitters or modulators that act via the phospholipase C/protein kinase C-dependent pathway, can enhance the fraction of APP holoproteins undergoing α-secretory cleavage and thereby presumably reduce Aβ production. Electrical stimulation of brain slices has also been shown to increase α-APP$_s$ release in vitro. Such information suggests that a variety of pharmacologic manipulations may be able to shift APP metabolism away from Aβ production and toward α-secretase processing. Of course, these would also increase production of α-APP$_s$, which appears to have several discrete functions.

The distribution and trafficking of APP shows special features in polarized cells. APP is brought down the axon from the cell body via fast axonal transport. In cultured neurons, the molecule is primarily distributed on the axonal surface in cells that have established mature axonal and somatodendritic compartments. Despite this preferential axonal location, surface APP appears to be sparsely present on axonal growth cones. Surface APP at axonal terminals can be endocytosed and retrogradely transported up the axon. Moreover, some of these molecules are fully transcytosed into the somatodendritic compartment of the neuron. Although the polarized trafficking of APP has been demonstrated in neurons, it has not been possible to specify whether Aβ release occurs at axonal, somatic, and/or dendritic sites. Resolution of this issue would help address whether axonal terminals could be the immediate local source of the extracellular Aβ deposits that lead to neuritic plaques.

MOLECULAR GENETIC DATA

Genetics

It has been known for at least several decades that clinically typical AD can cluster in families and sometimes be inherited in an autosomal dominant fashion. Estimates of the fraction of all AD cases determined by genetic factors have varied widely from as low as 5% to 10% to as high as 50% or more. Some investigators believe that in the fullness of time, a large majority of AD cases will be shown to have underlying genetic determinants, many of which may appear as polymorphic alleles that predispose to the disease but do not invariably cause it. Determining how frequently genetic factors underlie the disease is difficult in a late-onset disorder such as AD, particularly one that was not specifically diagnosed and studied prior to the last two decades. Moreover, the recognition that polymorphic alleles of ApoE can predispose humans to develop AD in their 60s and 70s suggests that other polymorphic genes could predispose to the disorder but may be difficult to detect in genetic epidemiologic studies because they do not always produce the disease and thus will not show high penetrance.

Despite the uncertainty about the extent to which AD is accounted for by genetic factors, phenotypic analy-

ses of familial and nonfamilial ("sporadic") cases make clear that these two forms are highly similar or indistinguishable phenotypically, except for the generally earlier age of onset of the known autosomal dominant forms. The histologic phenotype of early-onset familial cases is usually impossible to distinguish from that of common late-onset patients. Similarly, the clinical manifestations of dominantly inherited AD are often quite similar or indistinguishable from those of the sporadic cases, although some families show distinctive clinical signs (e.g., myoclonus, seizures, early and prominent extrapyramidal signs). This phenotypic similarity strongly suggests that information about the mechanism of dominant forms caused by mutations in the APP and presenilin genes is directly relevant to the pathogenesis of the common, presumably nonfamilial forms.

Missense Mutations in APP

The first specific genetic cause of AD to be identified was the occurrence of missense mutations in APP.[12] Families harboring APP missense mutations that cause AD generally have the onset of symptoms before age 65 years, often in their 50s. Such mutations have only been confirmed in some two dozen or so families worldwide. Nevertheless, the location of the mutations (see Fig. 32–1) and the subsequent delineation of their genotype-phenotype relationships have provided critical insights into the pathogenesis of AD. The mutations are strategically located either immediately prior to the β-secretase cleavage site, shortly following the α-secretase site, or just C-terminal to the γ-secretase cleavage site. No other mutations in the 770-residue APP protein that causes AD have been discovered. This strongly suggests that these substitutions lead to AD by altering the proteolytic processing at the secretase sites or, in the case of the intra-Aβ mutations, enhancing the aggregation properties of the resultant Aβ peptides. This hypothesis has been confirmed by detailed analysis of each mutation, initially in transfected cells and/or primary cells from patients and later in transgenic mouse models (reviewed in reference 13).

Alterations in the APP gene predispose to the development of AD in another way. The overexpression of structurally normal APP owing to elevated gene dosage in trisomy 21 (Down syndrome) leads to the premature occurrence of classical AD neuropathology (neuritic plaques and neurofibrillary tangles) during the middle adult years. A lifelong increase in APP expression owing to duplication of either the entire chromosome 21 (or in the case of translocation Down syndrome, of a portion of 21q containing the APP gene), results in overproduction of Aβ$_{40}$ and Aβ$_{42}$ peptides dating from birth. This is assumed to be responsible for the remarkably early appearance of many Aβ$_{42}$ diffuse plaques, which can occur as early as age 12 years. Down syndrome subjects display diffuse plaques composed principally of Aβ$_{42}$ in their teens and 20s, with accrual of Aβ$_{40}$ peptides onto these plaques and the appearance of associated microgliosis, astrocytosis, and surrounding neuritic dystrophy usually beginning in the late 20s or 30s. This sequence supports the importance of $A\beta_{42}$ accumulation as a seminal event in the development of AD-type pathology. The appearance of neurofibrillary tangles is also delayed until the late 20s, 30s, or at a later age in Down syndrome patients. The gradual accrual of AD-type brain lesions in these individuals, who are retarded from birth for other reasons, appears to be associated in many cases with progressive loss of cognitive and behavioral function after their 30s.

Because the entire chromosome 21 is duplicated in the vast majority of Down syndrome subjects, it has been difficult to attribute the AD phenotype that they develop directly to APP gene dosage. However, this issue has been essentially resolved by the evaluation of a patient with translocation Down syndrome, in which the obligate Down syndrome region in the distal portion of chromosome 21 was duplicated, but the break point was telomeric to the APP gene. The subject bearing this translocation had typical phenotypic features of Down syndrome but did not develop evidence of behavioral deterioration during middle age. At autopsy, no significant $A\beta$ deposition or other Alzheimer-type neuropathology was observed.[14] The clinicopathologic findings in this unusual case provide further support for the primacy of $A\beta$ deposition in the development of AD neuropathology.

Missense Mutations in the Presenilins

The realization that autosomal dominant AD is genetically heterogeneous led to intensive searches for loci in the genome besides APP that could explain the many families that did not link to chromosome 21. Establishment of a linkage of some families to chromosome 14 led to further linkage analyses and positional cloning that ultimately identified a novel gene on chromosome 14q now known as presenilin 1 (PS1).[15] Missense mutations appear to be causative of AD in certain families with clinical onset in their 40s and 50s, and sometimes as early as their 20s. A homologous gene (PS2) was discovered on chromosome 1, in which mutations explain the early-onset families referred to as the Volga German kindred and in an Italian AD family. Further genetic surveys have identified as many as 80 missense mutations in PS1 and at least six in PS2 as molecular causes of early-onset AD in several hundred families worldwide (reviewed in reference 15). PS1 missense mutations cause the earliest and most aggressive form of AD, commonly leading to onset of symptoms before age 45 years and demise of the patient during his or her 60s. These mutations have been instructive for understanding both the role of presenilins (PS) in AD and the normal functions of these interesting polytopic membrane proteins.

Apolipoprotein ε4: A Major Risk Factor for Late-Onset Alzheimer's Disease

Whereas the autosomal dominant mutations in APP, PS1, or PS2 are relatively infrequent causes of AD, the discovery that the ε4 allele of apolipoprotein E (ApoE) predisposes to AD provided a major genetic risk factor for the disorder in the typical late-onset period. Studies initiated by searching for proteins in human CSF that bound $A\beta$ peptides led to the identification of ApoE and its gene localized to chromosome 19q, in a region previously linked to AD in some late-onset families.[16] Further genetic analyses indicated that the ε4 allele of ApoE is overrepresented in subjects with AD compared with the general population, and that inheritance of one or two ε4 alleles heightens the likelihood of developing AD and makes its mean age of onset earlier than in subjects harboring ε2 and/or ε3 alleles. Thus, ApoE4 protein helps precipitate the disorder primarily in subjects in their 60s and 70s. There is also evidence that inheritance of the ε2 allele confers protection against the development of AD. Although inheritance of a single ε4 allele may increase the likelihood of patients developing AD in their 60s and 70s from twofold to fivefold, and two ε4 alleles may increase the risk fivefold to eightfold, it should be emphasized that ApoE4 is a risk factor for, not an invariant cause of, AD. Some humans homozygous for the E4 isoform still show no Alzheimer symptoms in their ninth decade of life and beyond. Conversely, many humans develop AD without harboring ε4 alleles.

The discovery of tau mutations clarifies the roles of $A\beta$ and tau in AD.

All of the genetic alterations discussed that are associated with AD have been shown to promote the accumulation of $A\beta$ in the brain. The finding of missense and splicing mutations in the tau gene on chromosome 17 in patients with frontotemporal dementia with parkinsonism (FTDP-17) helped settle the long-standing debate over whether plaques or tangles have temporal primacy in AD. Mutant tau in FTDP-17 produces profound neurofibrillary tangle formation and neuronal cell loss, resulting in a severe dementia and the ultimate demise of the host. But no $A\beta$ accumulation is detected in these patients, unless they survive long enough to develop some diffuse plaques associated with aging. Therefore, primary $A\beta$ buildup in autosomal dominant AD precedes secondary alterations of wild-type tau, whereas primary defects in tau in FTDP-17 do not lead to $A\beta$ buildup.

Genotype-Phenotype Conversions in Familial Alzheimer's Disease

Experiments to decipher genotype-phenotype relationships of AD genes have been conducted in cell culture, in transgenic mice and, most importantly, in patients who actually harbor the relevant genetic alterations. For all four genes unequivocally confirmed to date (APP, ApoE,

PS1, and *PS2*), inherited alterations in the gene products have been credibly linked to increases in the production and/or cerebral deposition of Aβ peptides. Such studies have provided the strongest support for the hypothesis that cerebral accumulation of Aβ is an early, invariant, and necessary event in the genesis of AD.

APP Mutations Increase the Production of $A\beta_{42}$ Peptides

The missense mutations in APP currently linked to familial AD (see Fig. 32–1) have been found to increase Aβ production by somewhat different mechanisms. A double mutation in the two amino acids immediately preceding the β-secretase cleavage site (often referred to as the "Swedish" APP mutation, based on the ethnic origin of the relevant family) induces increased cleavage by β-secretase to generate more $A\beta_{40}$ and $A\beta_{42}$. Mutations occurring just C-terminal to the γ-secretase cleavage sites appear in slightly different ways to enhance the relative production of Aβ species ending at residue 42. Among the mutations located near the middle of the Aβ sequence, it is possible that some may serve to decrease the efficiency of α-secretase and thus allow relative increases in cleavages by β-secretase. However, there is more evidence that these internal mutations enhance or alter the aggregation propensity of the peptide and thus lead to cytopathology. Among the mutations associated with prominent microvascular deposition, the *E22Q* ("Dutch") peptide has been shown to aggregate on the surfaces of smooth muscle and endothelial cells and thus confer local toxicity that could lead to the hyaline necrosis and vessel rupture seen in families with hereditary cerebral hemorrhage with amyloidosis of the Dutch type (HCHWA-D).[17] It should be noted that all patients with APP mutations are heterozygotes. In accord, microvascular Aβ deposits have been shown to contain mixtures of peptides derived from the mutant and wild-type alleles.

Presenilin Mutations Increase $A\beta_{42}$ Production

Perhaps the most intriguing genotype-phenotype relationships in AD involve the presenilin mutations. When *PS1* and *PS2* were first cloned, the mechanism by which mutations produced the AD phenotype was an open matter and not necessarily expected to involve enhanced Aβ production. However, direct assays of $A\beta_{40}$ and $A\beta_{42}$ in the plasma and cultured skin fibroblast media of humans harboring these mutations soon revealed a selective ~twofold elevation of $A\beta_{42}$ levels.[1] Extensive modeling of these mutations in cultured cells and transgenic mice has confirmed this finding.[9,13] A particularly important observation has been the finding that crossing mice transgenic for human *APP* with mice expressing a *PS1* missense mutation leads to a substantially accelerated AD-like phenotype in the offspring, with $A\beta_{42}$ plaques

(first diffuse and then mature) occurring as early as age 3 to 4 months.[18] Quantitative immunohistochemistry of brain amyloid deposits in patients with PS mutations has directly demonstrated a 1.5-fold to 3-fold increase in the relative abundance of plaques containing $A\beta_{42}$ peptides, as compared to levels observed in sporadic AD.[19] The molecular mechanism by which missense mutations in PS selectively increase the γ-secretase cleavage of C99 (and also C83) to yield relatively more peptides ending at $A\beta_{42}$ will be discussed later, after current knowledge of the biology of presenilin is reviewed.

Inheritance of ApoE4 Alleles Increases Brain Aβ Levels

Even before ApoE4 was recognized as a genetic risk factor for late-onset disease, immunohistochemistry had demonstrated the presence of ApoE protein in a high percentage of Aβ deposits in AD brain tissue. Once the genetic connection between AD and ApoE4 inheritance was made, immunohistochemistry on brains of patients lacking or expressing ApoE4 showed that inheritance of this allele was associated with a significantly higher Aβ plaque burden than was observed in patients lacking ApoE4. Importantly, studies in nonagenarians who died without showing clinical symptoms of AD demonstrated that the ApoE4 genotype was again linked to enhanced amounts of diffuse $A\beta_{42}$ plaques in the brain, suggesting that the Aβ-elevating effects associated with ApoE4 inheritance could be observed presymptomatically and in hosts who would not necessarily develop clinical AD.

The mechanism by which ApoE4 protein leads to increased Aβ deposition has been difficult to pinpoint. No evidence has emerged that ApoE4 specifically elevates Aβ production. Rather, ApoE4 seems to enhance the steady-state levels of Aβ peptides, presumably by decreasing its clearance from the brain tissue in some way. In vitro studies quantifying the degree of Aβ fibrillogenesis using synthetic peptides suggest that the presence of ApoE4 increases the number of fibrils, compared to levels obtained in the presence of ApoE.[20] Therefore, ApoE4 may serve either as a less effective inhibitor of Aβ fibrillogenesis or as a more potent stimulator. An alternative mechanism for the AD-promoting effect of ApoE4 inheritance emerges from evidence in transgenic mice expressing either the ε4 or ε3 human protein. Mice expressing ε4 appear to have decreased neuritic outgrowth of cultured neurons and decreased maintenance of established neurites. These studies suggest that ApoE4 protein is less supportive of normal neuronal form and function than are ApoE3 or ε2 proteins. However, such a neuronal vulnerability in ApoE4 gene carriers may not be the actual mechanism of the ApoE4 effect on the AD phenotype, given the fact that ApoE4, in a gene dose-dependent fashion, enhances deposition of Aβ into cerebral and meningeal vessels to produce amyloid angiopathy, even in the absence of AD-type neuropathology.[21] The fact that

ApoE4 alleles have enhanced Aβ deposition in parenchymal plaque deposits as well as microvessels outside of the brain parenchyma (and in the absence of AD) potentially separates the ApoE4 effect in promoting the AD cerebral phenotype (i.e., neuritic plaques) from any deleterious effects ApoE4 may have on neuronal/neuritic function in general. Thus, the most parsimonious explanation for ApoE4 effects vis-à-vis AD is that this isoform enhances the deposition or decreases the clearance of Aβ peptides in both the cerebral cortex and its microvasculature.

Such a mechanism is supported by studies in which mice transgenic for mutant human APP are crossed with mice in which the endogenous mouse ApoE gene is deleted. The resultant offspring show substantially decreased Aβ burden compared to that seen in the parental APP line, and the Aβ deposits that develop are overwhelmingly diffuse (nonfibrillar). Moreover, mice lacking endogenous ApoE that transgenically express human APP and either human ApoE3 or ε4 initially show even less Aβ deposits than mice expressing no ApoE at all. But as the mice develop deposits with age, the presence of the ε4 isoform leads to far more fibrillar (neuritic) plaques than does the ε3 isoform.[22]

Cell Biology of PS: A Major Molecular Switch in Signaling

How do missense mutations in *PS1* and *PS2* enhance the amyloidogenic processing of APP? The first clue came from deleting the *PS1* gene in mice, which results in markedly altered skeletal and brain development in utero and perinatal mortality. Embryonic neurons cultured from $PS1^{-/-}$ mice showed a striking 60% to 70% decrease in total Aβ production, both of $Aβ_{40}$ and $Aβ_{42}$.[23] In addition, a small fraction of APP molecules was found to coimmunoprecipitate with *PS1,* suggesting that the two formed transient complexes.[9] Separate work using designed peptidomimetic inhibitors of γ-secretase suggested that this unknown enzyme had the properties of an aspartyl protease. Putting these and other observations together, we hypothesized that presenilin might actually be γ-secretase.[24] Close inspection of the sequence of presenilin revealed two conserved aspartate residues in adjacent transmembrane regions (TM 6 and 7) of all PS family members (Fig. 32–2). Mutation of either aspartate in *PS1* decreased cellular Aβ production by ~60%, akin to the effect of ablating the entire *PS1* gene.[24] Moreover, mutation of either TM aspartate prevented the endoproteolysis of *PS1*. The co-expression of *PS1* and PS2 in which each had one of its TM aspartates mutated decreased cellular Aβ production to zero.

These results suggest that the two aspartates constitute the active site of γ-secretase, an unprecedented intramembranous aspartyl protease activated by an autoproteolytic cleavage to create the biologically active heterodimeric form. This interpretation is provocative, given the lack of precedent for a polytopic aspartyl protease with

its active site in the membrane. But the findings are reminiscent of the observation that the metalloprotease responsible for cleaving the sterol regulatory-element–binding protein implicated in cholesterol homeostasis had its active site in the membrane. Strong support for the model has come from the subsequent finding that γ-secretase inhibitors designed to mimic the transition state of a substrate with an aspartyl protease bound directly to PS heterodimers and no other cellular proteins.[25] Moreover, the region immediately around one of the two TM aspartates has homology to part of the active site of a known bacterial aspartyl protease.[26] Definitive confirmation of *PS1* and *PS2* as γ-secretases will require full purification of the protease complex and identification of its protein cofactors, allowing reconstitution of Aβ-generating activity.

The multiple lines of evidence that PS constitutes the active site of γ-secretase are in agreement with the "amyloid hypothesis" (Aβ hypothesis) of AD causation.[9] All of the genetic mutations known to cause autosomal dominant forms of AD to date are found either in the substrate (APP) or the protease (PS) of the γ-secretase reaction. AD-causing missense mutations in PS might subtly alter the conformation of one or more of the PS TM domains to decrease the interaction of the two TM aspartates with the $Aβ_{40-41}$ peptide bond in the APP TM domain and/or increase their interaction with the $Aβ_{42-43}$ peptide bond. The result would be a relative increase in the production of the highly self-aggregating $Aβ_{1-42}$ species throughout life.

As the work just reviewed was proceeding, it became apparent that PS had another, biologically more important substrate than APP: the Notch family of cell-surface receptors (reviewed in reference 27). Shortly after the human presenilins were cloned, the homologous gene in *Caenorhabditis elegans (sel-12)* was shown to be a facilitator of signaling by *lin-12,* the worm homologue of Notch. Notch is a major regulator of cell fate determination in all metazoans. The binding of protein ligands such as Delta or Jagged to the Notch ectodomain leads to signaling of the Notch cytoplasmic domain by regulating the transcription of target genes in the nucleus. But how the cytoplasmic domain of Notch reached the nucleus was initially a matter of lively debate. Mounting evidence has suggested that it does so as the result of two sequential proteolytic cleavages: first by ADAM 17 (TNFα-converting enzyme) just 12 amino acids outside the TM domain (highly similar to the α-secretase cleavage of APP) and then by a γ-secretase–like scission within the Notch TM domain that releases the Notch intracellular domain (NICD) (see Fig. 32–2). Loss of function mutations in the *Drosophila melanogaster* presenilin gene produce a phenotype closely resembling that of deleting Notch function, and the generation of the NICD fragment is abrogated.[28] Furthermore, γ-secretase inhibitors lower the proteolytic formation of NICD in a fashion indistinguishable from their effects on Aβ.[27] Deletion of both *PS1* and *PS2* in mammalian embryonic stem cells abolishes

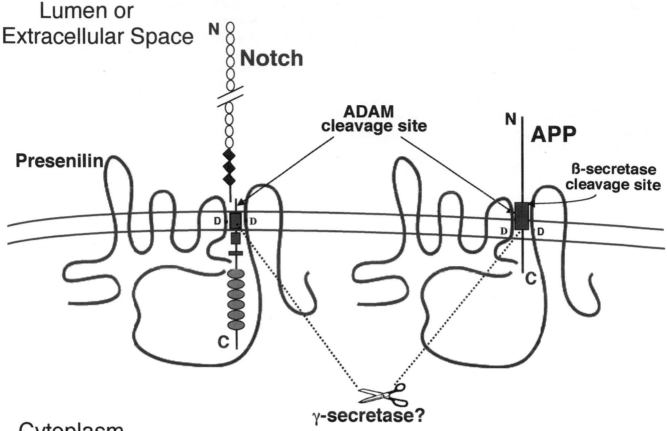

FIGURE 32–2. Model of the role of presenilin (PS) in Notch and APP processing based on current information. The diagram shows the predicted eight TM domain topology of PS, which occurs principally as a cleaved heterodimer. Some Notch and APP molecules form complexes with PS, together with other protein cofactors. Two aspartate residues (D) in TM6 and TM7 of PS are required for the cleavages of Notch and APP within their TM domains, and these are predicted to align with the respective sites of intramembrane cleavage in the two substrates. It is likely that PS directly affects these cleavages, but it remains possible that a still unidentified aspartyl protease (γ-secretase) present in the complexes does so. Ectodomain shedding effected by certain ADAM proteases precedes the PS-mediated proteolysis of both Notch and APP. In the case of APP, a small subset of holoproteins undergoes alternative ectodomain shedding by β-secretase. Several motifs are depicted in Notch: EGF-like repeats *(yellow ovals)*, LNG repeats *(red diamonds)*, a single TM *(orange rectangle)*, the RAM23 domain *(blue square)*, a nuclear localization sequence *(red rectangle)*, and six cdc10/ankyrin repeats *(green ovals)*. Following the putative intramembranous cleavage mediated by PS, the Notch intracellular domain is released to the nucleus to activate transcription of target genes. APP contains the Aβ region *(blue rectangle)*, which is released into the lumen after sequential cleavages of APP by β-secretase and γ-secretase/PS. The APP intracellular domain is released to the nucleus as well.

both NICD and Aβ production. The parallels continue with the discovery that the APP intracellular domain (AICD) participates in multiprotein complexes capable of driving gene transcription in the nucleus.[10,11] Thus, the normal function of APP, like Notch, is probably as a signaling receptor, and its ligand(s) and the genes whose transcription it regulates are under investigation.

Accumulating evidence from numerous laboratories now supports the concept that the presenilins are key molecular switches that allow the release of cytoplasmic signaling domains from various single-TM polypeptides. Thus, work that began with a focus on the pathobiology

of AD has uncovered a common proteolytic mechanism that is required in what may be a large number of different signaling pathways. On this basis, one can postulate that AD arose in the human population because a highly conserved proteolytic machine crucial for developmental decisions in all multicellular organisms has as one of its substrates a protein whose membrane-derived fragment (Aβ) can slowly aggregate and accumulate in the brain during postreproductive life. This accumulation occurs in virtually all old humans to some degree, and mutations in the substrate or the protease markedly accelerate the process, with devastating clinical consequences.

THERAPY

Therapeutic Approaches Emerge from Understanding the Molecular Cascade of Alzheimer's Disease

The identification of at least four genes that predispose to AD and the existence of several additional undefined loci led to the clear conclusion that AD is a syndrome that can be initiated by distinct molecular alterations that trigger a common pathologic cascade. Such a model predicts that the earliest molecular events in AD differ among the distinct genetic forms of the disease but that these converge to result in a common pathogenic mechanism: a critical imbalance between Aβ production and Aβ clearance in cerebral tissue. This imbalance, the degree of which may well be regulated by numerous gene products, results in the gradual cerebral accumulation of $A\beta_{42}$ peptides, a fraction of which undergoes conformational alteration into a β-pleated sheet-rich form and aggregates over time into soluble oligomers and, later, insoluble filamentous polymers (amyloid fibrils). The gradual accrual of Aβ oligomers and their apparent triggering of microgliosis and astrocytosis, and the secretion of inflammatory mediators (e.g., complement factors, cytokines, acute phase proteins) may lead first to subtle and later more profound synaptic pathology that ultimately produces the symptoms of progressive neuronal dysfunction. The pathogenic cascade includes the dissociation of tau from microtubules and its aggregation into PHF within innumerable neurites and neuronal cell bodies. In vivo evidence that Aβ accumulation can drive tau alteration and tangle formation has arisen from the crossing of mutant human tau transgenic mice to mutant human Aβ transgenic mice.[3] The consequences of the neuronal dysfunction and loss induced by the putative synaptotoxic and inflammatory effects of Aβ oligomers ultimately include the multiple neurotransmitter deficiencies of the disease. The precise temporal sequence of the complex molecular and cellular alterations that occur in the disease and their relative importance in producing progressive neuronal dysfunction and hence dementia remain incompletely understood but will be addressed in part by further characterization of APP, presenilin, and/or tau transgenic mice and other models.

The Aβ hypothesis of AD has the greatest amount of supporting experimental data among various hypotheses that have been proposed to explain the etiology and mechanism of the disorder. The model of Alzheimer's disease reviewed here points to new therapeutic strategies aimed at one or more critical steps in its molecular progression: (1) One could partially inhibit the proteolytic activities (β- and γ-secretases) that liberate Aβ from its precursor. (2) One could decrease the production and release of Aβ by a variety of means other than protease inhibition, for example, by pharmacologically diverting some APP molecules from the amyloidogenic (β-secretase) to the non-amyloidogenic (α-secretase) processing

pathway. (3) One could attempt to inhibit the oligomerization of Aβ monomers that precedes fibrillogenesis, but one would probably need to block the monomer-to-dimer conversion, as blockage thereafter could risk increasing the levels of potentially synaptotoxic dimers.[29] (4) One could try to clear Aβ peptides (both monomers and oligomers) from the cortex. This may be the mechanism of Aβ vaccines and related immunologic approaches. (5) One could interfere with the activities of microglia and astrocytes that contribute to the development of a chronic inflammatory process around Aβ deposits. (6) One could attempt to block the molecules on the surface of neurons or their intracellular effectors that mediate the neurotoxic effects of Aβ oligomers and proteins intimately associated with them, although these molecules have not been clearly identified as yet.

None of these pharmacologic objectives will be easy to reach. But the confluence of data emerging from many laboratories suggests that these six steps are rational therapeutic targets that offer the best hope of slowing or arresting the progression of Alzheimer's disease early during its course.

REFERENCES

1. Scheuner D, Eckman C, Jensen M, et al: Secreted amyloid β-protein similar to that in the senile plaques of Alzheimer's disease is increased *in vivo* by the presenilin 1 and 2 and APP mutations linked to familial Alzheimer's disease. Nat Med 1996;2:864–870.
2. Näslund J, Haroutunian V, Mohs R, et al: Correlation between elevated levels of amyloid beta-peptide in the brain and cognitive decline. JAMA 2000;283:1571–1577.
3. Lewis J, Dickson DW, Lin WL, et al: Enhanced neurofibrillary degeneration in transgenic mice expressing mutant tau and APP. Science 2001;293:1487–1491.
4. Janus C, Pearson J, McLaurin J, et al: A beta peptide immunization reduces behavioural impairment and plaques in a model of Alzheimer's disease. Nature 2000;408:979–982.
5. Morgan D, Diamond DM, Gottschall PE, et al: A beta peptide vaccination prevents memory loss in an animal model of Alzheimer's disease. Nature 2000;408:982–985.
6. Glenner GG, Wong CW: Alzheimer's disease: Initial report of the purification and characterization of a novel cerebrovascular amyloid protein. Biochem Biophys Res Commun 1984;120:885–890.
7. Näslund J, Haroutunian V, Mohs R, et al: Correlation between elevated levels of amyloid beta-peptide in the brain and cognitive decline. JAMA 2000;283:1571–1577.
8. Iwatsubo T, Mann DM, Odaka A, et al: Amyloid β protein (Aβ) deposition: Aβ42(43) precedes Aβ40 in Down syndrome. Ann Neurol 1995;37:294–299.

9. Selkoe DJ: Alzheimer's disease: Genes, proteins and therapies. Physiol Rev 2001;81:742–761.

10. Cao X, Sudhof TC: A transcriptionally active complex of APP with Fe65 and histone acetyltransferase Tip60. Science 2001;293:115–120.

11. Kimberly WT, Zheng JB, Guenette SY, et al: The intracellular domain of the beta-amyloid precursor protein is stabilized by Fe65 and translocates to the nucleus in a notch-like manner. J Biol Chem 2001;276: 40288–40292.

12. Hardy J: The Alzheimer family of diseases: Many etiologies, one pathogenesis? Proc Natl Acad Sci U S A 1997;94:2095–2097.

13. Price DL, Wong PC, Markowska AL, et al: The value of transgenic models for the study of neurodegenerative diseases. Ann N Y Acad Sci 2000;920:179–191.

14. Prasher VP, Farrer MJ, Kessling AM, et al: Molecular mapping of Alzheimer-type dementia in Down's syndrome. Ann Neurol 1998;43:380–383.

15. St. George-Hyslop PH: Molecular genetics of Alzheimer's disease. Biol Psychiatry 2000;47:183–199.

16. Corder EH, Saunders AM, Strittmatter WJ, et al: Gene dose of apolipoprotein E type 4 allele and the risk of Alzheimer's disease in late onset families. Science 1993;261:921–923.

17. Van Nostrand WE, Melchor JP: Disruption of pathologic amyloid beta-protein fibril assembly on the surface of cultured human cerebrovascular smooth muscle cells. Amyloid 2001;8:20–27.

18. Holcomb L, Gordon MN, McGowan E, et al: Accelerated Alzheimer-type phenotype in transgenic mice carrying both mutant amyloid precursor protein and presenilin 1 transgenes. Nat Med 1998;4:97–100.

19. Lemere CA, Lopera F, Kosik KS, et al: The E280A presenilin 1 Alzheimer mutation produces increased Ab42 deposition and severe cerebellar pathology. Nat Med 1996;2:1146–1150.

20. Ma J, Yee A, Brewer HB Jr, et al: The amyloid-associated proteins a1-antichymotrypsin and apolipoprotein E promote the assembly of the Alzheimer b-protein into filaments. Nature 1994;372:92–94.

21. Greenberg SM, Rebeck GW, Vonsattel JPG, et al: Apolipoprotein E e4 and cerebral hemorrhage associated with amyloid angiopathy. Ann Neurol 1995;38: 254–259.

22. Holtzman DM, Bales KR, Tenkova T, et al: Apolipoprotein E isoform-dependent amyloid deposition and neuritic degeneration in a mouse model of Alzheimer's disease. Proc Natl Acad Sci U S A 2000;97:2892–2897.

23. De Strooper B, Saftig P, Craessaerts K, et al: Deficiency of presenilin-1 inhibits the normal cleavage of amyloid precursor protein. Nature 1998;391:387–390.

24. Wolfe MS, Xia W, Ostaszewski BL, et al: Two transmembrane aspartates in presenilin-1 required for presenilin endoproteolysis and γ-secretase activity. Nature 1999;398:513–517.

25. Esler WP, Wolfe MS: A portrait of Alzheimer secretases—new features and familiar faces. Science 2001;293:1449–1454.

26. Steiner H, Kostka M, Romig H, et al: Glycine 384 is required for presenilin-1 function and is conserved in bacterial polytopic aspartyl proteases. Nat Cell Biol 2000;2:848–851.

27. Haass C, De Strooper B: The presenilins in Alzheimer's disease—proteolysis holds the key. Science 1999;286:916–919.

28. Struhl G, Greenwald I: Presenilin is required for activity and nuclear access of notch in drosophila. Nature 1999;398:522–525.

29. Walsh D, Klyubin I, Fadeeva J, et al: Naturally secreted oligomers of the Alzheimer amyloid β-protein potently inhibit hippocampal long-term potentiation in vivo. Nature 2002;416:535–539.

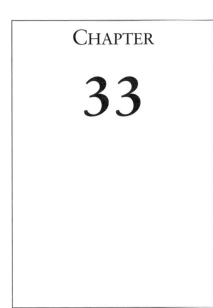

Frontotemporal Dementias

John Q. Trojanowski

Virginia M.-Y. Lee

Frontotemporal dementia (FTD) refers to a heterogeneous group of sporadic and familial neurodegenerative disorders in which clinical manifestations are linked to pathologic processes that specifically and primarily target the frontal and anterior temporal lobes, leading to relentlessly progressive and selective brain degeneration. Clinically, FTDs are most commonly recognized as distinct neurodegenerative syndromes characterized by profound neurobehavioral deficits including abnormal social conduct, loss of executive functions, and personality changes, but subsequently more generalized cognitive impairments develop. While the clinical manifestations of FTDs reflect the selective damage to brain regions that are affected by a neurodegenerative disease process, a number of other diverse disorders including Alzheimer's disease (AD), multisystem atrophies, Huntington's disease, and prion disorders also may present with behavioral symptoms that closely resemble those seen in classic FTDs. Since prominent tau abnormalities are now recognized as the defining neuropathology of nearly all well-studied FTDs, most of these unique dementing disorders are classified neuropathologically as tauopathies. Although these neurodegenerative diseases are heterogeneous, they are grouped together because they result from accumulations of insoluble hyperphosphorylated tau proteins in neurons, glial cells, or both neurons and glia that are readily demonstrated to be the most prominent lesions in the postmortem brains of affected patients. Additionally, some hereditary and sporadic disorders that present with the clinical features of FTDs also are called tauopathies because they show a loss or marked reduction in the levels of brain tau proteins relative to normal age-matched controls. Further, some FTD-like neurodegenerative disorders with prominent tau pathologies share some of the neuropathologic features that are characteristic of tauopathies, but they are not classified as such because they also show evidence of other diagnostic brain lesions. For example, AD, dementia pugilistica, and Down syndrome are characterized by prominent tau pathologics in addition to abundant extracellular amyloid deposits of aggregated Aβ peptides or fibrils.

After studies were reported showing linkage of chromosome 17q21–22 to disease in several families with hereditary FTDs, additional families with a remarkable variety of clinical and pathologic phenotypes also were reported to show linkage to this region of chromosome 17 that harbors the *tau* gene locus. Since some of these familial disorders also showed evidence of parkinsonism, they all have been collectively referred to as FTD with parkinsonism linked to chromosome 17 (FTDP-17). Significantly, the major neuropathologic features of FTDP-17 are neurofibrillary lesions made of hyperphosphorylated tau proteins with little or no Aβ amyloid pathology or other diagnostic brain abnormalities. For this reason, it was logical to scrutinize the *tau* gene for evidence of mutations pathogenic for FTDP-17 syndromes. The suspicion that FTDP-17 syndromes may be caused by autosomal dominant *tau* gene mutations was substantiated by a series of remarkable discoveries beginning in 1998 showing that more than 20 mutations in the gene encoding the tau protein were pathogenic for these disorders. Thus, these findings provided unequivocal proof that tau abnormalities were sufficient to cause neurodegenerative diseases. Since 1998, FTDs, FTDP-17 syndromes, and the pathologic significance of tau abnormalities for mechanisms of brain degeneration have become an increasingly intense focus of basic and clinical research as well as the topic of a number of comprehensive reviews.[1-14] Accordingly, this review is not intended to present an encyclopedic summary of this voluminous literature, but rather it is designed to provide an updated overview of the rapidly evolving concept of FTDs as a distinct class of neurodegenerative disorders.

EMERGENCE OF THE CONCEPT OF FTDS

FTDs are commonly mistaken for AD or other progressive dementing disorders of the elderly, but FTDs are clearly recognized now to be a heterogeneous group of sporadic and familial neuropsychiatric diseases. The initial emergence of the concept of FTDs began nearly 100 years ago with reports by Dr. A. Pick, who described cases of dementia with severe circumscribed atrophy of frontotemporal regions. As sharper definitions of the clinical and pathologic features of these dementing disorders were formulated, those characterized by the presence of argyrophilic intraneuronal inclusions (known as Pick bodies) and ballooned neurons in the postmortem brain were initially referred to as Pick's disease (PiD). This was because such lesions distinguished these cases from other types of dementias such as AD. However, it became increasingly clear that many patients with PiD-like clinical features did not show neuropathologic evidence of frontotemporal lobar atrophy, typical Pick bodies, or ballooned neurons. This resulted in a plethora of alternative terms for these non-PiD and non-AD dementias. For example, the more common diagnostic terms used by different investigators over the past several decades have included FTD, frontal lobe degeneration, frontotemporal lobar degeneration, dementia lacking distinctive histopathology, progressive aphasia, semantic dementia, corticobasal degeneration (CBD), progressive supranuclear palsy (PSP), and FTD with motor neuron disease, depending on the prominence of various clinical and neuropathologic features of a given patient.[15-23] Not surprisingly, this nomenclature and the classification of FTDs have been fraught with controversy due in large part to substantial gaps in understanding of the cellular and molecular neuropathologic correlates of the clinical manifestations of FTDs. For example, not all investigators have included CBD and PSP among the FTDs. However, basic and clinical research on FTDs in the 1990s began to clarify the underlying neuropathology of different FTD variants, and this is leading to new insights into possible mechanisms of brain degeneration in FTDs. Further, similar to variants of sporadic and familial AD, it now is very clear that the clinical manifestations of different FTD variants do not enable prediction of the neuropathologic or genetic basis of the dementia in a given patient. For these reasons, an international panel of FTD investigators recently reviewed clinical and basic research advances on FTD. They recommended that the clinically diverse variants of FTD be referred to collectively as FTD to emphasize the shared clinical features that enable FTDs to be distinguished during life from other dementias, but without making assumptions about their neuropathologic correlates or underlying disease processes.[9]

CLINICAL MANIFESTATIONS OF FTDS

FTDs affect men and women in equal numbers with clinical onset of disease typically between ages 35 and 75. (For more details on the clinical aspects of FTDs, see references 9 and 15 through 23.) Remarkably, 20% to 40% of patients report a family history of an FTD-like disorder. The clinical onset of FTD is manifested by a change in social or personal behavior such as inappropriate impulsiveness or social deviancy (e.g., theft, self-destructive acts, bizarre sexual behavior, altered dietary habits, neglect of personal hygiene) without evidence of AD-like memory impairments until later in the disease process. However, FTD patients often lack insight into the consequences of their activities, and this may lead them to come to the attention of the criminal justice system before that of health care providers. Alternatively, FTDs can present with prominent language impairments (e.g., reading or word-finding difficulties) that progress to aphasia or mutism as well as the emergence of the behavioral abnormalities mentioned above and memory impairments. A small minority of FTD patients also may develop motor impairments that mimic those seen in motor neuron diseases such as amyotrophic lateral sclerosis, and parkinsonism is a feature of some FTDP-17 syndromes as well as sporadic variants of FTDs such as PSP and CBD. Imaging studies of FTD patients commonly reveal bilateral or asymmetric frontal and anterior temporal lobe atrophy early in the disease, but brain atrophy becomes more generalized with the progression of FTD to eventually resemble that seen in AD and related neurodegenerative dementias. Although no laboratory tests provide definitive confirmation for the diagnosis of sporadic FTD in living patients, the hereditary form of FTD known as FTDP-17 can be diagnosed in affected members of a kindred during life by detecting one of the *tau* gene mutations that are pathogenic for FTDP-17.

These diagnostic limitations notwithstanding, the Work Group on Frontotemporal Dementia and Pick's Disease[9] suggested the following criteria for establishing a diagnosis of FTD in patients:

1. The appearance of behavioral/cognitive deficits exemplified by either early and progressive personality/behavioral changes or early and progressive language impairments.
2. The deficits in 1 lead to a decline in prior social/occupational functions.
3. The onset of impairments in 1 and 2 is gradual but progressive.
4. The deficits in 1 and 2 are not caused by other neuropsychiatric disorders, substance-induced conditions, or delirium.

NEUROPATHOLOGY, BIOCHEMISTRY, AND GENETICS OF FTDS

Growing evidence has led to the realization that many sporadic and familial neurodegenerative diseases are characterized by distinct hallmark brain lesions formed by filamentous deposits of abnormal brain proteins, and a group of heterogeneous disorders characterized neuropathologically by prominent intracellular accumulations of abnormal tau filaments may share common disease mechanisms. (For reviews, see references 1 through 8, 11, and 14.) Despite diverse phenotypic manifestations, these disorders are known as tauopathies (Table 33–1), and the absence of other disease-specific brain abnormalities provided circumstantial evidence implicating tau abnormalities in the onset and progression of brain degeneration in these diseases. Following controversy about the underlying brain pathology in FTDP-17, in 1998 multiple *tau* gene mutations were discovered in members of several FTDP-17 kindreds. This discovery provided unequivocal evidence that tau abnormalities alone can cause neurodegenerative disease.[1-14] This opened up new avenues for investigating the role of tau abnormalities in mechanisms of brain dysfunction and degeneration in FTDs as well as in AD and related disorders.

Overview of the Biology of Normal Tau

Tau isoforms are low-molecular-weight microtubule (MT)–associated proteins that are expressed predominantly in axons of central nervous system (CNS) neurons, and they also are found in axons of peripheral nervous system (PNS) neurons. However, they are barely detectable in CNS astrocytes and oligodendrocytes. (For detailed reviews of the normal biology and pathobiology of tau, see references 1 through 4, 6 through 8, and 11 through 14). Human tau is encoded by a single gene with 16 exons on chromosome 17q21, and the CNS tau isoforms are generated by alternative mRNA splicing of 11 exons. In the adult human brain, alternative splicing of exons 2 (E2), 3 (E3), and 10 (E10) generates six tau isoforms ranging from 352 to 441 amino acids in length. These isoforms differ by the presence of either three (3R-tau) or four (4R-tau) carboxy-terminal tandem MT binding repeat sequences of 31 or 32 amino acids encoded by E9, E10, E11, and E12. Further, 3R-tau and 4R-tau isoforms differ due to alternative splicing of E2 and E3 to produce tau isoforms without (0N) or with either 29 (1N) or 58 (2N) amino acid inserts of unknown function. The ratio of 3R-tau to 4R-tau isoforms is approximately 1 in adult human brains, but the 1N, 0N, and 2N tau isoforms comprise about 54%, 37% and 9% of total tau, respectively. However, tau is developmentally regulated such that only the shortest tau isoform (3R0N) is expressed in fetal brain followed by the expression of all six isoforms in the postnatal and adult human brain. Finally, the inclusion of E4a in the amino-terminal half of tau results in the expression of the largest tau isoform in the PNS.

Several functions of tau have been documented (reviewed in references 1, 3, 4, 8, 11, and 14), including the ability of tau to bind to and stabilize MTs and promote MT polymerization through MT-binding domains in the carboxy-terminal half of tau. These domains are composed of highly conserved 18-amino-acid–long binding elements separated by less conserved 13- to 14-amino-acid–long interrepeat sequences, but the binding of tau to MTs is a complex process mediated by several sites distributed throughout the MT binding repeats, interrepeat sequences, and by amino acids flanking the MT binding repeats. The 4R-tau isoforms are more efficient at promoting MT assembly and have a greater MT-binding affinity than 3R-tau isoforms. However, the interrepeat sequence between the first and second MT-binding domains has more than two times the binding affinity of any of the MT-binding repeats, and this region is unique to 4R-tau, which may account for the higher MT-binding affinity of 4R-tau versus 3R-tau isoforms.

Tau phosphorylation is developmentally regulated. Fetal tau is more highly phosphorylated in the embryonic compared to the adult CNS, while the degree of phosphorylation of the six adult tau isoforms decreases with age

TABLE 33–1. Neurodegenerative Diseases with Prominent tau Pathology

Alzheimer's disease

Amyotrophic lateral sclerosis/parkinsonism-dementia complex*

Argyrophilic grain dementia*

Corticobasal degeneration*

Dementia pugilistica*

Diffuse neurofibrillary tangles with calcification*

Down syndrome

Frontotemporal dementia with parkinsonism linked to chromosome 17*

Multiple system atrophy

Myotonic dystrophy

Neurodegeneration with brain iron accumulation type 1 (formerly Hallevorden-Spatz disease)

Niemann-Pick disease, type C

Pick's disease*

Post-encephalitic parkinsonism

Prion diseases

Progressive subcortical gliosis*

Progressive supranuclear palsy*

Subacute sclerosing panencephalitis

Tangle only dementia*

*Diseases in which tau pathologies are the most predominant neurodegenerative brain lesions.

(reviewed in references 1, 3, 4, 8, 11, and 14). The tau phosphorylation sites are clustered in regions flanking the MT-binding repeats. There are 79 potential serine (Ser) and threonine (Thr) phosphate acceptor residues present in the longest tau isoform. Phosphorylation at approximately 30 of these sites has been reported in normal tau, the increasing phosphorylation of which negatively regulates MT binding. Although the relative importance of individual sites for regulating the binding of tau to MTs is unclear, phosphorylation of Ser-262 has been reported to play a dominant role in reducing the binding of tau to MTs. A similar role has been ascribed to phosphorylation of Ser-396, while other studies suggest that neither of these sites dominantly regulate binding of tau to MTs. However, both sites are phosphorylated in fetal tau, and they are hyperphosphorylated in all six adult human brain tau isoforms that form paired helical filaments (PHFs) in AD neurofibrillary tangles (NFTs). Further, it has been suggested that a sequence of residues amino-terminal to the MT-binding domains ($_{224}$KKVAVVR$_{230}$) promotes MT binding in combination with the repeat regions, and it is likely that phosphorylation at multiple phosphate acceptor sites regulates the binding of tau to MTs.

Although the kinases and protein phosphatases that regulate tau phosphorylation (and a large number of Ser/Thr protein kinases have been suggested to play a role in regulating tau functions in vivo), this aspect of tau biology remains controversial (reviewed in references 1, 3, 4, 8, 11, and 14). The major candidate tau kinases include mitogen-activated protein kinase, glycogen synthase kinase 3 (gsk3), cyclin-dependent kinase 2 (cdk2), cyclin-dependent kinase 5 (cdk5), cAMP-dependent protein kinase, Ca^{2+}/calmodulin-dependent protein kinase II, MT-affinity regulating kinase, and stress-activated protein kinases. However, the relative contributions of individual kinases to tau phosphorylation in vivo remain to be elucidated.

Protein phosphatases also have been the focus of research on tau since they counterbalance the effects of tau kinases. Studies have implicated protein phosphatase 1 (PP1), 2A (PP2A), 2B (PP2B), and 2C (PP2C) in regulating tau phosphorylation, although their role in vivo is unclear (reviewed in references 1, 3, 4, 8, 11, and 14). Both PP2A and PP2B are present in human brain tissue, and they dephosphorylate tau in a site-specific manner. For example, both enzymes dephosphorylate Ser396, but PP2A also dephosphorylates tau at additional sites, and PP2A shows major activity in brain on tau phosphorylated by a number of kinases. PP1 and PP2A bind to tau, possibly mediating an association with MTs, and PP2A also binds directly to MTs. As with tau kinases, the specific role of individual phosphatases in the in vivo regulation of tau phosphorylation remains to be determined.

Pathologic Tau in FTDs

In contrast to tauopathies, wherein filamentous neuronal and/or glial tau inclusions are the key defining neuropatho-

logic features in affected brain regions, tau-rich NFTs and neuropil threads co-occur with deposits of Aβ fibrils in the extracellular space as diffuse and senile plaques as well as in blood vessel walls of AD brains (reviewed in references 1 through 5, 7, and 8). However, until relatively recently, the majority of studies of tau pathology focused on AD, and most of the early discoveries about the molecular mechanisms leading to the formation of tau inclusions came from research on AD. Indeed, the neurofibrillary tau lesions in AD brains were first shown to be stained with antitau antibodies in the mid-1980s, whereas earlier electron microscopical (EM) studies had revealed that the major structural components of NFTs were paired helical filaments (PHFs) and to a lesser extent straight filaments (SFs). Subsequent EM studies demonstrated that PHFs contain two strands of fibrils twisted around one another with a periodicity of 80 nm and a width between 8 nm and 20 nm, while SFs do not demonstrate a similar helical periodicity. However, after the appearance of a number of conflicting reports on the composition of these filaments in the early 1980s, the building block subunits of both PHFs and SFs were shown to be abnormally phosphorylated tau proteins. For example, biochemical analysis of PHFs purified from AD brains revealed three major bands of approximately 68-, 64- and 60-kDa, in addition to a minor 72-kDa band, but after enzymatic dephosphorylation, six protein bands corresponding to the six adult human brain tau isoforms were evident. Indeed, the relative abundance of each of the six tau isoforms in AD PHFs (PHFtau) was indistinguishable from the six soluble tau isoforms in the normal adult human brain. Moreover, nearly all the phosphorylated residues in PHFtau also were found in tau isolated from biopsies of normal human brain, but relative to normal soluble adult brain tau isoforms, PHFtau was more extensively phosphorylated (i.e., hyperphosphorylated) at these sites.

Numerous kinases and protein phosphatases were implicated in the aberrant phosphorylation tau in the AD brain (reviewed in references 1, 3, 4, 8, 11, and 14). However, cdk5 abnormally activated by p25, a truncated form of p35, may play a mechanistic role in the conversion of normal tau into PHFtau in AD. While the precise role of tau phosphorylation in AD brain degeneration remains uncertain, it is possible that hyperphosphorylation of tau disengages tau from MTs, thereby increasing the pool of unbound tau that then may aggregate into insoluble filamentous inclusions. There is no consensus on this hypothetical scenario at this time, but it may be beneficial to increase the ability of pathologic tau to interact with MTs. The organic osmolytes trimethylamine N-oxide (TMAO), betaine, or related compounds may have therapeutic potential in AD and related tauopathies because they appear to increase tau-mediated MT assembly and restore the ability of phosphorylated tau to promote this assembly. Nonetheless, while tau hyperphosphorylation is likely an early step in the generation of

PHFtau from normal soluble tau, it is unclear if it directly mediates tau fibrillization in vivo. Indeed, a number of early studies of tau fibrillization showed that PHF-like filaments can be assembled in vitro from bacterially expressed nonphosphorylated 3R-tau fragments, although PHFs from AD brain consist of full-length tau. In subsequent studies, sulfated glycosaminoglycans (GAGs) were shown to stimulate phosphorylation of tau by a number of protein kinases and induce fibrillization of full-length tau, while a short amino acid sequence (VQIVYK) in the third MT-binding repeat was suggested to be essential for heparin-induced filament assembly. Further, tau fibrillization may occur in a nucleation-dependent manner. Moreover, RNA and arachidonic acid also were shown to induce fibrillization of full-length recombinant tau, and the detection of GAGs and RNA colocalized with PHFtau in NFTs suggests that these in vitro findings may be relevant to tau fibrillization in the AD brain.

Despite controversies about the role of tau pathology in AD, indirect evidence of a causative role for tau protein abnormalities in brain degeneration comes from studies of pure tauopathies wherein there is abundant filamentous tau pathology and brain degeneration in the absence of extracellular amyloid deposits or other brain lesions (see Table 33–1). This is exemplified by sporadic tauopathies such as PSP and CBD (for which specific tau haplotypes appear to be genetic risk factors), and PiD (reviewed in references 1, 3, 4, 8, 11, and 14). Moreover, as a result of a large number of studies of tau pathologies in AD as well as sporadic and familial tauopathies, several important similarities and differences between the pathobiology of AD and other sporadic and hereditary neurodegenerative tauopathies emerged: (1) The sarkosyl-insoluble brain tau in many tauopathies, including those caused by pathogenic *tau* gene mutations, is recognized by the same tau epitope specific antibodies that bind PHFtau isolated from AD brains; (2) A triplet of AD PHFtau-like bands with an Mr of 68, 64, and 60 kDa is seen in several tauopathies (e.g., some FTDP-17 kindreds), but only the 64 and 60 kDa PHFtau-like bands or only the 68 and 64 kDa PHFtau-like bands are seen in some sporadic (PiD versus PSP and CBD, respectively) and hereditary tauopathies; (3) While there is little or no white matter tau pathology in AD, tau inclusions and dystrophic neurites as well as accumulations of insoluble tau are common and sometimes abundant in several sporadic and hereditary tauopathy variants; (4) Filamentous tau inclusions are the defining neuropathologic hallmarks of all tauopathies except for a novel group of possibly related disorders wherein tau levels are absent or reduced, presumably leading to losses of tau function similar to mutation-induced functional impairments in tau in some FTDP-17 kindreds; and (5) Sporadic tauopathies and familial variants thereof (e.g., FTDP-17 syndromes) are caused by different tau pathologies.

However, the most compelling evidence implicating tau abnormalities in human neurodegenerative diseases came from studies of FTDP-17 syndromes that are autosomal dominant neurodegenerative diseases with diverse, but overlapping, clinical and neuropathologic features including prominent filamentous tau inclusions in neurons and/or glial cells. For example, in 1998, several groups identified pathogenic mutations in the *tau* gene that segregated with FTDP-17, and within four years more than 20 distinct pathogenic mutations in the *tau* gene had been identified in a large number of new FTDP-17 families. As reviewed elsewhere,[1,3,4,8,11,14] these include missense mutations in coding regions of the *tau* gene involving E9 (e.g., K257T, I260V, G272V), E10 (e.g., N279K, P301L, P301S, S305N), E12 (e.g., V337M, E342V), and E13 (e.g., G389R, R406W); silent mutations in E10 (e.g., L284L, N296N, S305S); and a deletion mutation (ΔK280). Substitutions in several different positions in the intron following E10 have been identified (at positions +3, +12, +13, +14, and +16). Other pathogenic *tau* gene mutations continue to be reported in meetings, and more mutations are likely to be discovered as research on the *tau* gene and FTDP-17 syndromes continues. Further studies of FTDP-17 brains from several laboratories add increasing support to the hypothesis that FTDP-17 mutations lead to tau dysfunction and neurodegenerative disease by one or more distinct mechanisms, including losses of tau functions and/or gains of toxic properties. Experimental confirmation of this notion is emerging from studies of a number of transgenic mice and other model systems of tauopathies (reviewed in references 1, 3, 4, 8, 11, and 14).

Recommended Neuropathologic Classification of FTDs

The neuropathologic classification of FTDs recommended by the Work Group on Frontotemporal Dementia and Pick's Disease has been informed by the advances in tau pathobiology summarized in this chapter.[9,12] The FTD experts in this work group incorporated genetic and biochemical findings into the neuropathologic classification of FTDs for the first time. They noted that the neurodegenerative abnormalities detected by histochemical, immunohistochemical, biochemical, molecular biologic, and other methods in the postmortem brains of patients with well-documented clinical evidence of FTD probably will enable the establishment of a neuropathologic diagnosis of the underlying disease in most FTD patients. Thus, the systematic examination of postmortem brains of FTD patients that was recommended by the work group will facilitate the detection of neurodegenerative and other lesions, an estimation of the regional distribution and abundance of these abnormalities, and the formulation of one or more neuropathologic diagnoses to account for FTD. However, they also acknowledged that this may not be possible in all cases owing to extensive gaps in current understanding of FTDs and the mechanisms leading to the onset and progression of these disorders.

Briefly, the distribution and severity of brain atrophy seen on macroscopic examination of the postmortem brain should be documented, but it is not specific for a particular neurodegenerative disorder. For this reason, microscopic examination is necessary and should be performed on a variety of brain regions using contemporary histochemical and immunohistochemical methods to detect brain lesions diagnostic of other well-recognized disorders such as AD, synucleinopathies caused by accumulations of Lewy bodies (LBs), and Lewy neurites.[9,12] Thus, in addition to traditional histochemical staining procedures, sensitive methods for detecting tau pathology by immunohistochemistry with tau specific antibodies are essential for the neuropathologic evaluation of FTD brains. Further, since some of the inclusions found in FTDs are negative for tau yet positive for ubiquitin, immunohistochemical studies with ubiquitin specific antibodies also are important in the routine evaluation of FTDs. In addition, immunohistochemistry performed with anti-alpha-synuclein and other antibodies also is helpful for detecting LBs, Lewy neurites, and additional pathologies that support or exclude specific neuropathologic diagnoses. For example, ballooned or achromatic neurons that are found in several of the disorders associated with FTD are best appreciated with immunostaining for neurofilament or alpha-β-crystallin. Thus, the increasing application of immunohistochemical methods is likely to continue to foster a more modern and reliable neuropathologic classification of FTDs and other neurodegenerative disorders characterized by filamentous protein aggregates or inclusions.

A number of other specialized techniques can be performed on postmortem brain samples. These techniques show promise in helping to establish a neuropathologic diagnosis in patients with FTDs.[9,12] For example, EM analysis of the nature of the filaments that accumulate within neurons and glia may provide additional information of diagnostic relevance to FTDs. However, EM studies usually are not required for diagnosis of FTDs. On the other hand, biochemical analyses of tau protein abnormalities appear increasingly useful in the rational classification of FTDs. This is because fractionation of tau proteins from brain separates disorders into those with and without measurable amounts of insoluble tau. Further characterization of this abnormal insoluble tau differentiates FTD cases and other disorders into those with a predominance of tau with 3 MT-binding repeats (3R tau), 4 MT-binding repeats (4R tau), or a combination of 3R tau and 4R tau. Notably, recent studies suggest that some FTDs show a selective loss or marked reduction of all tau proteins in the soluble fractions of postmortem brains in the setting of normal levels of tau mRNA, and that the profile of tau proteins in other FTDs can be heterogeneous, especially in gray versus white matter.[24–26] While these studies need to be extended and confirmed, they point out the utility of biochemical analyses of soluble and insoluble tau in diagnostic neuropathologic studies of postmortem brains from patients with FTDs and other neurodegenerative diseases.

However, the correlation of neuropathologic findings with FTD in a patient does not prove a cause-and-effect relationship, since more than one brain abnormality may contribute to the manifestations of dementia and there is evidence that alpha-synuclein, tau, and Aβ pathology may co-occur in some neurodegenerative diseases including AD and other tauopathies. (See references 8, 27 through 29, and other citations therein.) Thus, it must be recognized that neuropathologic findings alone cannot establish unequivocally that the patient had FTD in the absence of documented clinical information. This notwithstanding, the classification of FTD recommended by the Work Group on Frontotemporal Dementia and Pick's Disease[9,12] requires exclusion of other CNS diseases that may account for the clinical syndrome, and demonstration of a plausible correlation between the neuropathologic findings and clinical evidence of FTD (Table 33–2).

CONCLUSION

Despite earlier uncertainties about the role of tau pathology in AD, the discovery of multiple mutations in the *tau* gene that lead to the abnormal aggregation of tau and the onset/progression of FTDP-17 demonstrates that tau dysfunction is sufficient to produce neurodegenerative disease. The mutations lead to specific cellular alterations, including altered expression, function, and biochemistry of tau. The finding that specific *tau* gene mutations lead to diverse FTDP-17 phenotypes raises the possibility that the clinical and pathologic expression of hereditary and related sporadic tauopathies may be influenced by *tau* gene polymorphisms, other genetic factors, and epigenetic events. However, the precise mechanisms whereby tau assembles into filaments and causes neurodegeneration in the human brain remain to be elucidated, but further investigation into the mechanisms of tau dysfunction, as well as the identification of potential disease-modifying factors, will provide additional insight into novel strategies for the treatment and prevention of FTDs and related disorders. Moreover, development of additional animal models of tauopathies that more closely recapitulate human diseases will facilitate this undertaking. This is likely to have implications for other neurodegenerative disorders because the aggregation of tau in FTDs and related diseases is an example of abnormal protein-protein interactions resulting in the intracellular accumulation of filamentous proteins common in many fatal CNS diseases characterized by relentlessly progressive brain degeneration. (For more detailed reviews, see references 1 through 8 and 29.) Thus, the fibrillization

TABLE 33–2. Neuropathologic Classification of FTDs[*]

When the neuropathology is tau-positive inclusions, neuron loss, gliosis, and insoluble 3R tau predominates, the most likely diagnoses are:

  Pick's disease

  FTDP-17 (with documentation of a pathogenic *tau* gene mutation)

  Other

When the neuropathology is tau-positive inclusions, neuron loss, gliosis, and insoluble 4R tau predominates, the most likely diagnoses are:

  Corticobasal degeneration

  Progressive supranuclear palsy

  FTDP-17 (with documentation of a pathogenic *tau* gene mutation)

  Other

When the neuropathology is tau-positive inclusions, neuron loss, gliosis, and insoluble 3R tau and 4R tau occur, the most likely diagnoses are:

  Neurofibrillary tangle dementia

  FTDP-17 (with documentation of a pathogenic *tau* gene mutation)

  Other

When the neuropathology is frontotemporal neuronal loss and gliosis without tau- or ubiquitin-positive inclusions and without insoluble tau, the most likely diagnoses are:

  FTLD (also known as DLDH)

  Other

When the neuropathology is frontotemporal neuronal loss and gliosis with ubiquitin-positive, tau-negative inclusions and without insoluble tau (with or without MND), the most likely diagnoses are:

  FTLD with MND

  FTLD with MND-type inclusions, but without MND

  Other

---

[*]As described in the text, this table summarizes the recently revised neuropathologic classification of FTDs. This classification incorporates a number of advances in understanding the pathobiology of these disorders, including data from genetic and biochemical studies of FTDs For further details, see McKhann GM, Albert MS, Grossman M, et al. Clinical and pathological diagnosis of front temporal dementia: Report of Work Group on Frontotemporal Dementia and Pick's Disease. Arch Neurol 2001; 581: 1803–1809 and Trojanwski, JQ, Dickson DW; Update on the neuropathological diagnosis of frontotemporal dementias. J Neuropath Exper Neurol 2001, 60: 1123–1126.

and aggregation of proteins in the brain is a common theme in a diverse group of neurodegenerative disorders. Insight into the pathogenesis of any of these disorders may have implications for understanding the mecha-

nisms that underlie all of these diseases as well as for the discovery of better treatment strategies.

Indeed, there may be multiple pathways that lead to pathologic protein misfolding with the subsequent formation of toxic amyloid deposits, and a much larger array of proteins than previously anticipated may be vulnerable to fibrillize and cause disease as a result of a variety of noxious or stressful cellular perturbations.[29] Thus, more intense research efforts are needed to elucidate these processes to develop more effective therapies for protein-misfolding diseases (including FTDs) and other neurodegenerative brain amyloidoses (such as AD, synucleinopathies, and prionopathies). For example, compounds have been identified that prevent the conversion of normal proteins into abnormal conformers or variants with conformations that predispose the pathologic proteins to form potentially toxic filamentous aggregates.[30–32] It is also plausible to speculate that some of these agents may have therapeutic efficacy in more than one neurodegenerative brain amyloidosis. Thus, as further research yields more substantial insights into abnormal protein-protein interactions and protein misfolding, these insights can be exploited for the discovery of new and better therapies for FTDs and for other neurodegenerative disorders caused by abnormal filamentous aggregates.

Acknowledgments

Virginia M-Y Lee is the John H. Ware Third Chair of Alzheimer's disease research at the University of Pennsylvania. Work done in the laboratories of the authors is supported by grants from the National Institute of Aging of the National Institutes of Health and the Alzheimer's Association. We also thank our many collaborators and the past and current members of the Center for Neurodegenerative Disease Research (CNDR) for contributions to the research from CNDR summarized in this chapter. Finally, the support of the families of our patients has made this research possible. For additional information on the neurodegenerative diseases reviewed, please visit the CNDR web site at http://www.med.upenn.edu/cndr.

REFERENCES

1. Buee L, Bussiere T, Buee-Scherre V, et al: Tau protein isoforms, phosphorylation and role in neurodegenerative disorders. Brain Res Rev 2000;33:95–130.

2. Dickson DW: Neuropathology of Alzheimer's disease and other dementias. Clin Geriatr Med 2001;17:209–228.

3. Forman MS, Lee VM-Y, Trojanowski JQ: New insights into genetic and molecular mechanisms of brain degeneration in tauopathies. J Chem Neuroanat 2000;20:225–244.

4. Goedert M, Spillantini MG: Tau gene mutations and neurodegeneration. Biochem Soc Symp 2001;67:59–71.

5. Hardy J, Gwinn-Hardy K: Genetic classification of primary neurodegenerative disease. Science 1998;282: 1075–1079.

6. Higuchi M, Trojanowski JQ, Lee VM-Y: Tau protein and tauopathies. In Davis KL, Charney D, Coyle J, Nemeroff CN (eds): Neuro-psychopharmacology: Fifth Generation of Progress. Philadelphia, Lippincott Williams & Wilkins, 2002, pp 1339–1354.

7. Hutton M: Missense and splice site mutations in tau associated with FTDP-17: Multiple pathogenic mechanisms. Neurol 2001;56(11 Suppl 4): 21–25.

8. Lee VM-Y, Goedert M, Trojanowski JQ: Neurodegenerative tauopathies. Annu Rev Neurosci 2001; 24:1121–1159.

9. McKhann GM, Albert MS, Grossman M, et al: Clinical and pathological diagnosis of frontotemporal dementia: Report of Work Group on Frontotemporal Dementia and Pick's Disease. Arch Neurol 2001;58: 1803–1809.

10. Morris HR, Khan MN, Janssen JC, et al: The genetic and pathological classification of familial frontotemporal dementia. Arch Neurol 2001;58: 1813–1816.

11. Spillantini MG, Goedert M: Tau gene mutations and tau pathology in frontotemporal dementia and parkinsonism linked to chromosome 17. Adv Exp Med Biol 2001;487:21–37.

12. Trojanowski JQ, Dickson DW: Update on the neuropathological diagnosis of frontotemporal dementias. J Neuropath Exper Neurol 2001;60: 1123–1126.

13. Wilhelmsen KC, Clark LN, Miller BL, Geschwind DH: Tau mutations in frontotemporal dementia. Dement Geriatr Cogn Disord 1999;10 (Suppl 1): 88–92.

14. Yoshiyama Y, Lee VM-Y, Trojanowski JQ: Frontotemporal dementias and tauopathy. Curr Neurol Neurosci Rep 2001;1:413–421.

15. Brun A, England B, Gustafson L, et al: Clinical and neuropathological criteria for frontotemporal dementia: The Lund and Manchester Groups. J Neurol Neurosurg Psychiatry 1994;57:416–418.

16. Gustafson L: Frontal lobe degeneration of non-Alzheimer type II: Clinical picture and differential diagnosis. Arch Gerontol Geriat 1987;6:209–223.

17. Gustafson L: Clinical picture of frontal lobe degeneration of non-Alzheimer type. Dementia 1993;4: 143–148.

18. Hauw JJ, Duyckaerts C, Seilhean D, et al: The neuropathologic diagnostic criteria of frontal lobe dementia revisited—A study of ten consecutive cases. J Neural Transm Suppl 1996;47:47–59.

19. Knopman DS: Overview of dementia lacking distinctive histology: Pathological designation of a progressive dementia. Dementia 1993;4:132–136.

20. Lowe J: Establishing a pathological diagnosis in degenerative dementias. Brain Pathol 1998;8: 403–406.

21. Mann DM, South P, Snowden JS, Neary D: Dementia of frontal lobe type: Neuropathology and immunohistochemistry. J Neurol Neurosurg Psychiatry 1993;56:605–614.

22. Neary D, Snowden JS, Mann DM, et al: Frontal lobe dementia and motor neuron disease. J Neurol Neurosurg Psychiatry 1990;53:23–33.

23. Neary D, Snowden JS, Gustafson L, et al: Frontotemporal lobar degeneration: A consensus on clinical diagnostic criteria. Neurology 1998;51: 1546–1554.

24. Forman MS, Zhukareva V, Bergeron C, et al: Signature tau neuropathology in gray and white matter of corticobasal degeneration. Am J Pathol 2002;160: 2045–2053.

25. Zhukareva V, Vogelsberg-Ragaglia V, Van Deerlin VMD, et al: Loss of brain tau defines novel sporadic and familial tauopathies with frontotemporal dementia. Ann Neurol 2001;49:165–175.

26. Zhukareva V, Mann D, Pickering-Brown S, et al: Sporadic Pick's disease: A tauopathy characterized by a spectrum of pathological tau isoforms in gray and white matter. Ann Neurol 2002;51:730–739.

27. Forman MS, Schmidt ML, Kasturi S, et al: Tau and alpha-synuclein pathology in amygdala of Parkinsonism-Dementia Complex patients of Guam. Am J Pathol 2002;160:1713–1725.

28. Judkins AR, Forman MS, Uryu K, et al: Co-occurrence of Parkinson's disease with progressive supranuclear palsy. Acta Neuropathol 2002;103: 525–530.

29. Trojanowski JQ: Tauists, Baptists, Syners, apostates and new data. Ann Neurol 2002;52:263–265.

30. Irizarry MC, Hyman BT: Alzheimer disease therapeutics. J Neuropathol Exp Neurol 2001;60: 923–928.

31. Mayeux R, Sano M: Treatment of Alzheimer's disease. N Engl J Med 1999;341:1670–1679.

32. Trojanowski JQ: Emerging Alzheimer's disease therapies: Focusing on the future. Neurobiol Aging 2002;23:985–990.

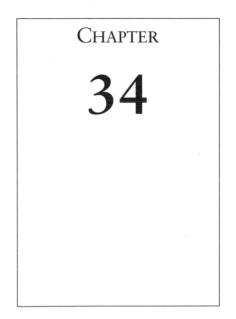

Genetics of Movement Disorders

Juliette M. Harris

Stanley Fahn

Movement disorders can be defined as neurological syndromes in which there is either an excess of movement or a paucity of voluntary and automatic movements, unrelated to weakness or spasticity. The former are commonly referred to as *hyperkinesias* (excessive movements), *dyskinesias* (unnatural movements), and *abnormal involuntary movements*. We commonly use the term dyskinesias, but all are interchangeable. The five major categories of dyskinesias, in alphabetical order, are: chorea, dystonia, myoclonus, tics, and tremor. The paucity of movement group can be referred to as *hypokinesia* (decreased amplitude of movement), but *bradykinesia* (slowness of movement) and *akinesia* (loss of movement) are alternative names. The parkinsonian syndromes are the most common cause of such paucity of movement; other hypokinetic disorders affect only a small group of patients. Basically, movement disorders can be conveniently divided into parkinsonism and all other types. The parkinsonian syndromes, in turn, are divided into primary parkinsonism (i.e., Parkinson disease [PD]) and a variety of Parkinson-plus states such as progressive nuclear palsy, multiple system atrophy, cortical-basal ganglionic degeneration, and other entities. The genetics of PD have evolved so that 10 different monogenetic disorders have now been elucidated. Whereas PD has been considered to be of unknown etiology, with the discovery of these genetic forms, it is better to describe it as primary parkinsonism rather than idiopathic parkinsonism. Genetic research is rapidly revealing the cause of many of the familial movement disorders and shedding light on mechanisms of disease process. In this chapter we review the genetic highlights of the parkinsonian syndromes and of the hyperkinetic conditions.

Parkinson Disease

Parkinsonism is characterized clinically by any combination of rest tremor, bradykinesia, rigidity, postural instability, flexed posture (Fig. 34–1), and freezing phenomena. It is conveniently divided into PD, secondary parkinsonism (insults to the brain), Parkinson-plus syndromes, and heredodegenerative disorders in which parkinsonism is not the primary clinical feature (e.g., Wilson disease, juvenile Huntington disease). PD is the most common form of parkinsonism encountered by neurologists and the second most common neurodegenerative disorder. It affects 1% to 2% of people older than 65 years.

The classical neuropathology of PD is loss of dopaminergic neurons and presence of eosinophilic intracytoplasmic inclusions (Lewy bodies) that contain ubiquitin and α-synuclein in the *substantia nigra pars compacta*. PD is differentiated from Parkinson-plus syndromes because the latter have pathology involving other areas of the basal ganglia and other parts of the brain, producing symptoms beyond those of pure parkinsonism.

The observation of families with autosomal dominant PD and of individuals with PD who were exposed to 1-methyl-4-phenyl-1,2,3,6-tetrahydropyridine (MPTP), now known to be a potent neurotoxin, suggested both genetic and environmental causes of PD. It is now accepted that the cause of PD for individuals with sporadic late-onset PD is probably a combination of both factors. Findings from a recent twin study segregating individuals into young- and old-onset groups suggest a genetic component in individuals with young-onset PD only. A community-based study identified a lifetime risk

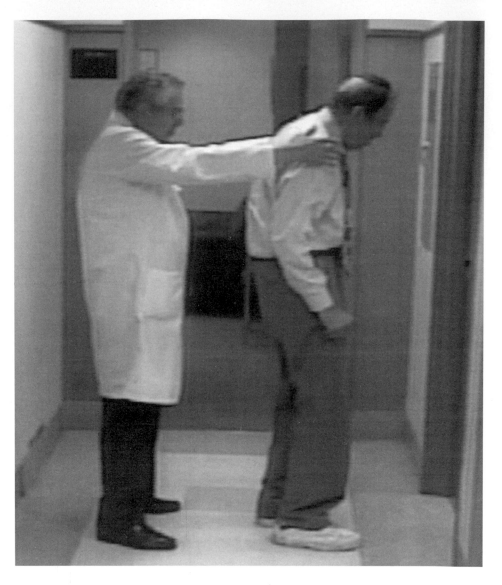

FIGURE 34–1. Flexed posture and pull test in a patient with Parkinson disease. The physician is performing a pull test to determine postural instability.

of PD in a parent or a sibling of an individual with PD as approximately 2% as opposed to a lifetime risk of PD of 1% in controls, suggesting multifactorial inheritance.

Four genes and six loci have been associated with familial PD. Understanding the rare forms of familial PD is a crucial first step in uncovering the biochemical pathways that lead to sporadic late-onset PD. Autosomal dominant, highly penetrant, Lewy body parkinsonism caused by a mutation in the α-synuclein gene on chromosome 4q21.3-q22 (SNCA, formerly called PARK1) was the first gene to be associated with PD (Table 34–1). Two mutations have so far been discovered in a small number of families of Italian and Greek (A53T) and German (A30P) ancestry. The clinical and pathological picture is similar to sporadic late-onset PD, but early onset, rapid progression, and dementia are also frequent features. Interestingly, aggregated, fibrillar α-synuclein proteins are a major component of Lewy bodies in sporadic late-onset PD. So far, one gene and three other loci have been linked to autosomal dominant PD, all of which are rare.

They are listed here in the order in which they were discovered: (1) A small group of European families with incomplete penetrance have been linked to 2p13 (PARK3) and have clinical and pathologic findings similar to sporadic late-onset PD, including age of onset; (2) A specific haplotype on chromosome 4p15 (PARK4) was found to segregate with familial Lewy body parkinsonism in a North American family called the "Iowa kindred." The haplotype was found to occur not only in family members with Lewy body parkinsonism but also in those with isolated postural tremor, consistent with essential tremor. The pattern of striatal dopamine depletion in this family was not consistent with sporadic late-onset PD; (3) A missense mutation in the *Ubiquitin Carboxy Terminal Hydrolase L1 (UCH-L1)* gene on 4p14-16.3 was identified in a Northern German family with autosomal dominant PD (formerly PARK5). Interestingly, UCH-L1 is involved in the ubiquitin-proteasomal degradation pathway, and is a component of Lewy bodies in the brains of individuals with sporadic

TABLE 34–1. A List of Monogenic Forms of Parkinson Disease

Disease name	Inheritance	Location	Protein	Protein function
SNCA (formerly PARK1)	AD	4q21.3-q22	α-synuclein	synaptic protein
PARK2 (Juvenile PD/Parkin)	AR	6q25.2-q27	Parkin	ubiquitin-protein ligase
PARK3	AD	2p13	N/I	–
PARK4	AD	4p15	N/I	–
UCHL1 (formerly PARK5)	AD	4p14	Ubiquitin Carboxy Terminal Hydrolase	ubiquitin hydrolase
PARK6	AR	1p35-36	N/I	.
PARK7	AR	1p36	DJ-1	transcription cofactor
PARK8	AD	12p11.2-q13.1	N/I	–
PARK9 (Kufor-Rakeb)	AR	1p36	N/I	–
PARK10	Susceptibility locus?	1p32	N/I	–

AD, autosomal dominant; AR, autosomal recessive; N/I, not identified.

late-onset PD. (4) A Japanese family with levodopa-responsive PD (mean age at onset, 51 years) with features similar to sporadic late-onset PD, and an absence of Lewy bodies has been linked to chromosome 12p11.2-q13.1 (PARK8).

A number of loci have been linked to families with autosomal recessive PD. Mutations in the *Parkin* gene on chromosome 6q25.2-q27 (PARK2) were initially identified in Japanese individuals with juvenile-onset PD. Parkin mutations have now been identified pan-ethnically and are thought to be the cause of approximately 50% of familial young-onset PD and 15% to 20% of sporadic young-onset PD (younger than 50 years). More than 70 mutations, including exon rearrangements, point mutations, and deletions have been identified, many of them recurrent in different populations. The identification of Parkin mutations is inversely correlated with age of onset, with the earliest age of onset having the greatest association. However, PARK2 does not appear to be restricted to young-onset PD, and Parkin mutations have been identified in individuals older than 50 years. Recent findings suggest that juvenile Parkin-related PD is associated with mutations in both Parkin alleles (homozygotes or compound heterozygotes), and that a single Parkin mutation may be responsible for later onset PD. This is a crucial finding in the search for the cause of sporadic late-onset PD and it is clear that of all the loci and genes discovered to date, Parkin is the most important. The frequency and penetrance of Parkin mutations have yet to be determined. PARK2, especially in juvenile cases, has been characterized by slow progression, sustained response to levodopa, levodopa-induced dyskinesias, dystonia, sleep-benefit, and hyperreflexia, but these findings have not been consistent. Some individuals with PARK2, especially with later onset, are clinically indistinguishable from sporadic

adult-onset PD. PARK2 is characterized pathologically by loss of neurons in pigmented nuclei, and interestingly, by absence of Lewy bodies, although a recent case report identified Lewy bodies in a compound heterozygous individual. Parkin interacts with the ubiquitin-conjugating enzyme UbcH7 and is a ubiquitin ligase, involved in the ubiquitin-proteasome pathway.[1]

A number of families of European ancestry with autosomal recessive early-onset PD have been linked to 1p35-36 (PARK6). PARK6 is characterized by early onset, slow progression, and sustained response to levodopa. Individuals with later onset have been observed, with clinical symptoms similar to sporadic late-onset PD. Mutations in the *DJ-1* gene (PARK7) on chromosome 1p36 have been found to cause autosomal recessive early-onset PD in Europeans, which is characterized by slow progression and a good response to levodopa. The DJ-1 protein appears to have a role as a transcription cofactor. The contribution that PARK7 mutations make to young-onset PD remains to be investigated. A Parkinson-plus syndrome with autosomal recessive inheritance called Kufor-Rakeb syndrome has been linked to chromosome 1p36, close to PARK6 and PARK7, and is characterized by juvenile-onset pallidopyramidal degeneration with spasticity, supranuclear upgaze paresis, and dementia, and has been designated PARK9, making this syndrome a Parkinson-plus disorder, rather than PD.

A late onset susceptibility locus on chromosome 1p32, close to PARK6, 7, and 9, was recently identified using a genome-wide scan involving multiple PD families in the Icelandic population (PARK10). Other genome scans involving sibling studies have yielded more than 10 other possible loci that are only suggestive of linkage.

Other candidate PD genes are those involved in the development and maintenance of dopaminergic neurons in the *substantia nigra*, such as *Nurr1*. A homozygous polymorphism in this gene has been found at a significantly higher frequency in individuals with PD than in controls. In addition, reduction in complex I mitochondrial activity has been observed in PD, and a mutation in the complex I ND4 subunit gene of mitochondrial DNA (mtDNA) is suggestive of a pathogenic role for ND4 in a subset of PD patients.

Although we are discovering the genes associated with familial and young-onset PD, the big challenge will be to identify the cause of sporadic late-onset PD and to understand how genetic factors interact with the environment to cause disease. So far, the implication from genetic studies is that abnormalities in protein degradation play a major role, leading to accumulation of toxic proteins.

Parkinson-Plus Syndromes

A number of the Parkinson-plus syndromes involve abnormal accumulation of aberrantly phosphorylated microtubule-associated protein tau in the central nervous system. These Parkinson-plus syndromes together with other diseases with characteristic abnormal tau accumulation are collectively described as "tauopathies."

Frontotemporal dementia and parkinsonism linked to chromosome 17 (FTDP-17) is an autosomal dominant tauopathy caused by mutations in the *tau* gene on chromosome 17 and characterized by parkinsonism with cognitive and behavioral changes. Familial FTDP-17 only accounts for a small proportion of all cases, and individuals with sporadic FTD are much more common.

Six major isoforms of tau protein are expressed in the adult brain and are generated by alternate splicing of exons 2, 3, and 10. Alternate splicing of exon 10 generates 2 major isoforms termed 10+ and 10–. Specifically, exon 10 encodes a microtubule-binding domain. Alternate splicing of exon 10 is an important step in the generation of the isoforms. Splice site mutations of the intron downstream of exon 10 appear to be a major cause of FTDP-17. More than 10 other missense mutations and dosage changes clustered in exons 9 to 13 have also been discovered. There is marked intrafamilial variation of disease phenotype among FTDP-17 family members with the same mutation, suggesting that other factors, genetic or environmental, contribute to the expression of the disease.

An extended haplotype that covers the human *tau* gene has recently been associated with the tauopathy *progressive supranuclear palsy* (PSP), a Parkinson-plus syndrome that is usually sporadic and is characterized by supranuclear vertical gaze palsy, postural instability, freezing, and falling. Having two copies of the common haplotype (H1) in the *tau* gene is associated with increased risk to develop PSP in Europeans. It is not known at the present time which specific region of the haplotype increases susceptibility to PSP. The same tau haplotype has also been associated with *corticobasal ganglionic degeneration* (CBGD).[2] The finding that the same

tau isoform accumulates in PSP and CBGD adds weight to the theory that a shared pathway contributes to the development of PSP and CBGD. Clinically, PSP and CBGD have many overlapping features, although cortical features, such as myoclonus, cortical sensory loss, apraxia, and alien limb strongly favor CBGD, as do unilateral rigidity and dystonia.

Multiple system atrophy (MSA) is a sporadic neurodegenerative Parkinson-plus syndrome characterized by any combination of cerebellar symptoms, parkinsonism, and pyramidal and autonomic dysfunctions. Different clinical forms are recognized, including olivopontocerebellar atrophy, Shy-Drager syndrome, and striatonigral degeneration. The presence of oligodendroglial inclusions containing α-synuclein is a pathologic feature characteristic of all clinical variants. Thus MSA, along with PD, is considered a synucleinopathy. The expression of *ZNF231*, a brain-specific gene on chromosome 3p21 encoding neuronal double zinc finger protein, is enhanced in brains of individuals with MSA, suggesting that genetic factors may play a role in the etiology. In addition, the distribution of polymorphisms in the *cytokine* gene, interleukin-1β, in MSA cases versus controls suggests that abnormal cytokine expression may be implicated in the pathogenesis of MSA.

Essential Tremor

Essential tremor (ET) is a progressive neurological condition characterized by a 4 to 12 Hz kinetic tremor of the hands, head, or vocal cords that can severely affect basic daily activities (Fig. 34–2). ET is the most common form of tremor, and in some age groups has been estimated to be approximately 20 times more prevalent than PD. In addition to action tremor, patients with ET often have postural tremor, and later in the disease some individuals develop tandem gait abnormalities. It is common for the tremor to lessen remarkably following alcohol consumption. There are familial and nonfamilial forms of ET, and a number of autosomal dominant families have been described. Sporadic and familial forms of ET are clinically indistinguishable.

The challenge to researchers has been to identify the etiology of idiopathic ET. A community-based case-control study found that first-degree relatives of ET patients are 5 times more likely to develop the disease than are members of the general population and 10 times more likely if the proband's tremor began at an early age. However, relative risk to second-degree relatives was found to be similar to the general population, and not half of the risk of their first-degree relatives, as would be predicted in a simple autosomal dominant model.[3] These results, together with twin studies, support a mutifactorial role for inheritance of ET, with both genetic and environmental components. Interestingly, a number of studies have suggested that the genetic component of ET is greater than that shown by epidemiological studies, but

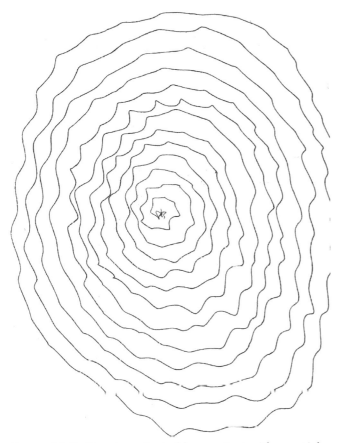

FIGURE 34–2. Drawing of spiral by a patient with essential tremor.

this may reflect biased experimental methods, such as lack of case-controls. The complex inheritance of ET has made it a challenge to identify susceptibility loci. Because ET is a relatively common condition, it has been postulated that some "ET families" may, in fact, consist of numerous sporadic individuals, coincidentally occurring in a single family, thus confusing analysis.

Researchers focusing on large Czech and Icelandic ET families have, however, discovered linkage to chromosome 2p22 and 3q13. These findings were not reproducible in Italian ET families. This may reflect etiologic variants, including genetic heterogeneity and population-based differences.

Dystonia

Dystonia refers to twisting movements that tend to be sustained at the peak of the movement, are frequently repetitive, and often progress to prolonged abnormal postures. In contrast to chorea, dystonic movements repeatedly involve the same group of muscles (i.e., they are patterned). Agonist and antagonist muscles contract simultaneously (co-contraction) to produce the sustained quality of dystonic movements. The speed of the movement varies widely from slow (athetotic dystonia) to shocklike (myoclonic dystonia). When the contractions

are very brief (e.g., less than a second), they are referred to as dystonic spasms. When they are sustained for several seconds, they are called dystonic movements. And when they last minutes to hours, they are known as dystonic postures. When present for weeks or longer, the postures can lead to permanent fixed contractures.

There are numerous types of dystonia that can present in different regions of the body. Dystonia can involve a single body part (focal dystonia), can be segmental or generalized, and can present early or late in life. Many focal dystonias have specific names based on the body part involved, such as blepharospasm, oromandibular dystonia, spasmodic dysphonia, spasmodic torticollis, and occupational cramps or writer's cramp. Etiologic classification distinguishes into primary dystonia (no degenerative pathology detected and no other neurological features except dystonia and sometimes kinetic tremor), secondary dystonia (brain injuries), dystonia-plus (no degeneration, but other neurological features are present, such as parkinsonism or myoclonus), and heredodegenerative disorders (hereditary and degenerative). Genetics has allowed classification of the different types of dystonia into 13 sub-types, designated DYT1 to 13, including both primary and heredodegenerative dystonias. It should be emphasized, though, that the vast majority of individuals with dystonia are sporadic, non-familial, and of adult onset.

Oppenheim dystonia, named after Hermann Oppenheim, who described dystonia in 1911, is an autosomal dominant disorder of young onset (almost always before age 26 years) starting in a limb. Rarely does it begin in the neck or cranial region. It is the most common form of early onset primary dystonia. Oppenheim dystonia is caused by a 3 base-pair GAG deletion in the *DYT1* gene on chromosome 9q34 (Table 34–2). *DYT1* encodes an ATP-binding protein called TorsinA. The GAG deletion removes a glutamic acid residue in a conserved region of the ATP binding domain. DYT1 is highly expressed in the dopamine neurons of the *substantia nigra pars compacta*, but many other regions of the brain also express this protein, including the cholinergic intrastriatal neurons. Intellect is normal. It is rare for DYT1 carriers to develop symptoms after their mid-20s and diagnostic guidelines for genetic testing reflect this finding, recommending DYT1 testing for individuals with onset of limb dystonia under age 26 years.[4] No other gene test for primary dystonias is currently available. Oppenheim dystonia has been found in all ethnic groups, worldwide, with the same GAG deletion. The risk in the Ashkenazi Jewish population is particularly high due to a founder effect: One out of 2000 are gene carriers. Ten percent and 50% of individuals of Ashkenazi Jewish and non-Jewish ancestry, respectively, have a DYT1 phenotype but no identifiable mutation, suggesting genetic heterogeneity. Only 30% of individuals who carry the DYT1 GAG deletion manifest dystonia, and symptoms can vary both between and within families and can manifest as focal limb dystonia, hand cramps

TABLE 34–2. A List of Hereditary Forms of Primary Dystonia (DYT1,6,7,13), Dystonia-plus Syndromes (DYT5,11,12), and One Degenerative Form of Dystonia (DYT3)

Name	Clinical features	Inheritance pattern	Location	Protein	Mutations identified
DYTI, Early onset-torsion dystonia	Limb onset, may generalize	AD, incomplete penetrance, increased in Ashkenazi Jews	9q34	TorsinA	3 bp deletion (GAG)
DYT3 (with parkinsonism) (Lubag)	Usually generalized	X-linked recessive, increased in the Philippines, mosaic gliosis in striatum	Xq13.1	N/I	–
GCH1 Dopa-responsive dystonia (formerly DYT5)	Childhood-onset dystonia, responsive to L-dopa	AD, incomplete penetrance; F>M	14q22.1-q22.2	GTP Cyclohydro-lase I	> 80
DYT6, adult-onset, mixed type	Cranial-cervical dystonia	AD, incomplete penetrance, in Mennonites of German ancestry	8p21-p22	N/I	–
DYT7, adult-onset focal dystonia	Focal dystonia-torticollis, adult onset	AD, incomplete penetrance, in Germans	18p	N/I	–
DYT11 (SGCE) myoclonus-dystonia	Myoclonus or dystonia or both	AD, imprinting effect	7q21	ε-sarcoglycan	>15
DYT12, Rapid-onset dystonia-parkinsonism	Rapid-onset dystonia-parkinsonism	AD, incomplete penetrance	19q13	N/I	–
DYT13	Cranial/cervical dystonia	AD, incomplete penetrance	1p36	N/I	–

AD, autosomal dominant; N/I, not identified.

(Fig. 34–3), or other manifestations. The variability of symptoms and incomplete penetrance of Oppenheim dystonia suggests a role for modifier genes and possibly environmental interactions. No consistent pathology has been found, but fluorodeoxyglucose (FDG) positron emission tomography (PET) scans reveal high lenticular and reduced thalamic regional metabolism.

Lubag or DYT3 is a rare neurodegenerative, adult-onset, highly penetrant X-linked recessive form of dystonia-parkinsonism characterized by generalized dystonia and levodopa-unresponsive parkinsonism. When onset is during adulthood, focal cranial dystonia (jaw/tongue) is common. DYT3 is located on Xq13.1 and is restricted almost exclusively to males whose ancestors originated from the Philippines, presumably due to a founder effect.

Dopa responsive dystonia (DRD) (Segawa syndrome) is an autosomal dominant disease with incomplete penetrance caused by mutations in the GTP cyclohydrolase 1 (GCH1) gene on chromosome 14q22.1-q22.2. DRD manifests as childhood-onset lower-limb dystonia/gait disorder, often with marked diurnal fluctuation. It may be accompanied by parkinsonian features such as hypomimia, bradykinesia, and loss of postural reflexes, and it demonstrates a dramatic and sustained resolution of symptoms with low doses of levodopa. GCH1 is an enzyme in the biosynthetic pathway of tetrahydrobiopterin, the cofactor for tyrosine hydroxylase, which in turn is the rate-limiting enzyme in the synthesis of dopamine.[5] Interestingly, DRD is more penetrant in females (87%) than in males (38%). More than 85 mutations in the GCH1 gene have been identified. This limits the utility of genetic testing, and current molecular techniques detect mutations in 60% of families with DRD. It is unknown whether this is due to genetic heterogeneity or whether the presence of dosage or noncoding mutations result in reduced detection rates. DRD can also present, albeit with different symptoms, as an infantile, autosomal recessive parkinsonism, caused by mutations in the tyrosine hydroxylase gene on chromosome 11p15.5. A leading differential diagnosis is Parkin-related PD (PARK2), which can present with parkinsonism or dystonia. The differential diagnosis is resolved by FDOPA PET scans, which show no deficit in DRD, but a loss of FDOPA uptake in PARK2.

Adult-onset idiopathic torsion dystonia of the mixed type (DYT6) causes autosomal dominant dystonia with incomplete penetrance in a few Mennonite families of German ancestry. It is characterized by focal or generalizable dystonia, with cranial, cervical, or limb involvement and has been linked to chromosome 8p21-p22.

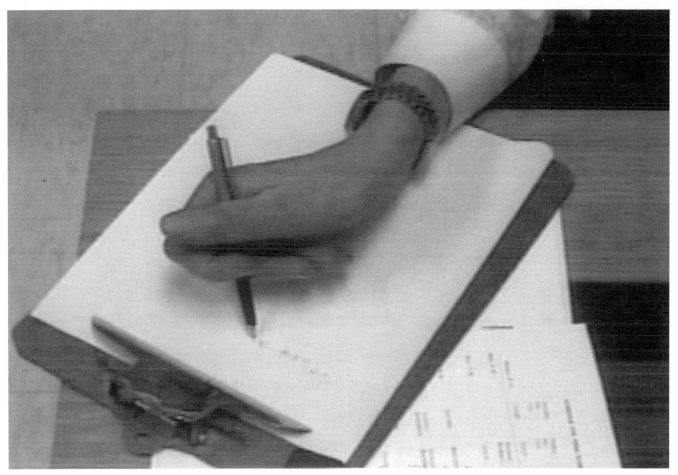

FIGURE 34–3. Oppenheim dystonia manifested as difficulty in writing (writer's cramp).

Adult-onset focal dystonia (DYT7) is the cause of autosomal dominant focal dystonia (cervical and laryngeal dystonia with or without postural tremor) with reduced penetrance in individuals of German ancestry and has been linked to chromosome 18p. However, linkage of German individuals with the proposed DYT7 phenotype to the 18p locus has not shown a consistent association. It should be noted that individuals with 18p-syndrome not only have dystonic features, but also a deletion that spans the putative DYT7 locus.

Myoclonus-dystonia (DYT11) is an autosomal dominant movement disorder characterized by sudden jerking movements and dystonia of variable expression and penetrance. It is caused by mutations in the epsilon sarcoglycan gene (SGCE) on chromosome 7q21, which encodes one member of the dystrophin glycoprotein complex. Myoclonus-dystonia can obviously be inherited maternally or paternally; however, a maternal imprinting effect leads to penetrance mainly when inherited through the paternal line. Psychiatric abnormalities such as obsessive-compulsive disorder are associated with the disease. Alcohol alleviates symptoms of the myoclonus component, leading some individuals to alcohol addiction. A mutation in the D2 dopamine receptor gene has also been

associated with myoclonus-dystonia in a large family; however, subsequent studies did not support a major role for the DR2 locus as a cause of DYT11.

Rapid-onset dystonia-parkinsonism is a rare autosomal dominant disease with incomplete penetrance. Onset is sudden and symptoms progress within weeks to a plateau state; it usually occurs in adolescence. This disease has been linked to chromosome 19q13 (DYT12). The discovery of the causal gene may provide important insights into the dopaminergic pathway responsible for both dystonia and PD. DYT13 was recently linked to 1p36 in an Italian family with cranial-cervical or upper limb onset dystonia and incomplete penetrance. The disease is characterized by juvenile or early-adult onset, a mild course, and occasional generalization.

Dystonia is manifested in a number of heredodegenerative diseases. Neurodegeneration with iron accumulation in the brain is a feature of Pantothenate Kinase Associated Neurodegeneration (PKAN), formerly called Hallervorden-Spatz disease, an autosomal recessive disease with childhood onset caused by mutations in the pantothenate kinase gene 2 (PANK2) on chromosome 20p12.3-p13.[6] Clinical features include dystonia, progressive extrapyramidal dysfunction, dementia, and eye findings. Histological findings reveal iron deposits in the basal ganglia visualized as brown discolorations. PANK2 is involved in coenzyme A production, which has a crucial role in fatty acid metabolism. Mutations in *PANK2* also cause hypoprebetalipoproteinemia, acanthocytosis, retinitis pigmentosa, and pallidal degeneration (HARP), a rare syndrome overlapping clinically with PKAN. A number of individuals with PKAN do not have mutations in *PANK2,* suggesting genetic heterogeneity. Recently, the *hGFRalpha-4* gene, encoding a member of the glial-derived neurotrophic factor family, was proposed as another candidate PKAN locus.

Neuroferritinopathy is an autosomal dominant disease of the basal ganglia caused by mutations in the gene encoding ferritin light polypeptide on chromosome 19q13.3, and is characterized by extrapyramidal features with symptoms of both Huntington disease and parkinsonism. Histological findings reveal abnormal deposition of ferritin and iron in the basal ganglia. Iron accumulation has been associated with a number of neurodegenerative diseases and occurs naturally with age.

Huntington Disease

Huntington disease (HD) is a neurodegenerative autosomal dominant disease caused by CAG triplet repeat expansions in exon 1 of the *IT15* gene on chromosome 4p16.3 coding for the huntingtin protein. Abnormal involuntary movements, cognitive decline, and psychiatric disturbance characterize HD. Mean age of onset is 35 to 44 years. The triplet repeat expansion results in a gain of function mutation causing substantial loss of spiny neurons in the striatum. The elucidation of the cause of HD in 1993 was one of the first genetic discoveries in movement disorders. HD research has since led the way as a model of the polyglutamine diseases. In addition, genetic testing protocols first developed for HD are now templates for other adult-onset diseases. We have therefore placed special emphasis on genetic testing, clinical features, and pathogenesis of HD.

Genetics and Genetic Testing

The HD triplet repeat expansion translates into an expanded polyglutamine tract close to the "N" terminus of the huntingtin protein. In normal individuals, the number of repeats in the *ITIS* gene is 26 or less. Triplet repeat lengths of 27 to 35 repeats do not cause HD, but may expand into the "HD" range during gametogenesis, placing children of carriers in this range at risk to develop HD. Thirty-six to 39 CAG repeats cause HD with variable penetrance—an individual with a repeat length in this range may or may not develop symptoms of HD, and may also be at risk for offspring with an expansion in the "HD" range. Finally, individuals with 40 or more repeats develop fully penetrant HD. Triplet repeat length between "normal" and "HD" is termed "intermediate range."[7]

There is a loosely inverse relationship between repeat length and age of onset. However, it is clear that factors other than repeat length also determine age of onset. No association between repeat length and clinical features or rate of progression has consistently been reported. Twenty-five percent of individuals with HD develop symptoms after age 50 years. Seven percent of individuals with HD have the juvenile form with onset before age 20 years and with large expansions (over 55, up to 121 repeats). Individuals with later-onset HD may have a more slowly progressing disease when compared to those with juvenile-onset HD. Eighty percent of individuals with juvenile HD inherit an expanded paternal allele. This phenomenon is called "anticipation" and produces ever-larger HD expansions from generation to generation, resulting in earlier ages of onset in successive generations. An unknown mechanism specific to spermatogenesis causes CAG repeat instability and expansion. The children of females with HD have smaller shifts in triplet repeat lengths, and these may take the form of contractions or expansions. Approximately 10% of patients with symptoms of HD do not have a family history. After discounting nonpaternity, early death of family members, and other causes of incomplete family history, it has been suggested that the remaining individuals may represent new expansions, possibly from a parent with a repeat length in the intermediate range.

Genetic testing for individuals with HD and other neurodegenerative genetic diseases is a lengthy and complex process that involves pre- and post-counseling sessions with a genetic counselor or geneticist, who is trained to address not only the complex details of inheritance, but also the psychosocial issues that frequently occur in either the individual coming to terms with having HD or in at-risk family members. Protocols designed by neurologists and geneticists addressing the genetic testing of at-risk, asymptomatic individuals recommend long-term counseling. Presymptomatic testing of minors is strongly discouraged owing to issues of informed consent and the lack of therapies to prevent onset of the disease. When ordering genetic tests for HD, it should be noted that very large CAG repeat lengths that cause juvenile HD may not be detected by conventional diagnostic PCR techniques and may only be detected by Southern blot analysis.

The prevalence of HD is approximately 5 to 10/100,000 in the United States but recent epidemiology studies have not been done. The prevalence is as high as 1/10,000 in the United Kingdom and as low as 1/1 million in African and Asian populations. This finding may be related to the observation that alleles with high-normal numbers of repeats are higher in Europeans than in Africans or Asians.

Clinical Symptoms of HD

The symptoms of HD can vary greatly, and although chorea, psychiatric, and cognitive changes are the hallmarks of HD, some patients do not develop dementia or chorea. The majority of patients present with movement disorders such as chorea (usually minor involuntary movements), clumsiness, dropping of objects (negative chorea), or impaired coordination of voluntary movements, but often report prior depression or difficulty planning or concentrating. Studies currently under way observe at-risk individuals to determine signs of HD before onset of abnormal movements.

Gait disturbance (prancing, stuttering, unsteady gait) (Fig. 34–4), dysarthria, dysphagia, bradykinesia, rigidity, or dystonia often appear further on in the course of the disease. Psychiatric and cognitive changes such as psychosis, agitation, apathy, impulsiveness, depression, mania, paranoia, delusions, sexual disorders, hallucinations, memory loss, and poor judgment may occur. HD is often fatal between 15 and 20 years after onset of symptoms.

Juvenile HD is characterized by progressive parkinsonism (bradykinesia and rigidity), dementia, ataxia, and seizures and can present as declining cognitive function, behavioral disturbance (such as violence or suicidal ideation), rigidity of limb or trunk, and seizures. Chorea can be absent. Juvenile HD is often associated with a family history of HD (usually paternal). The constellation of features that characterize juvenile HD differ from adult-onset HD and can lead to misdiagnosis. Juvenile HD is not only characterized by loss of neurons in the striatum but may also show cerebellar atrophy.

Symptoms of HD may overlap with those of other genetic disease such as dentatorubro-pallidoluysian atrophy (DRPLA), Wilson disease, neuroacanthocytosis, benign hereditary chorea, familial ataxia, HD-like 2 disease (described later), familial prion disease, and nongenetic causes of chorea-like illnesses (e.g., tardive dyskinesia, thyrotoxicosis, cerebral lupus, polycythemia).

Therapy for HD includes antidepressants, antipsychotic and anti-anxiety medication, and neuroleptics (but these may induce tardive dyskinesia). Supportive therapy, including occupational and physical therapy, has proven very effective in managing symptoms.

Pathogenesis of HD

It is still not clear how the polyglutamine expansion causes neurodegeneration. Mice, transgenic for human

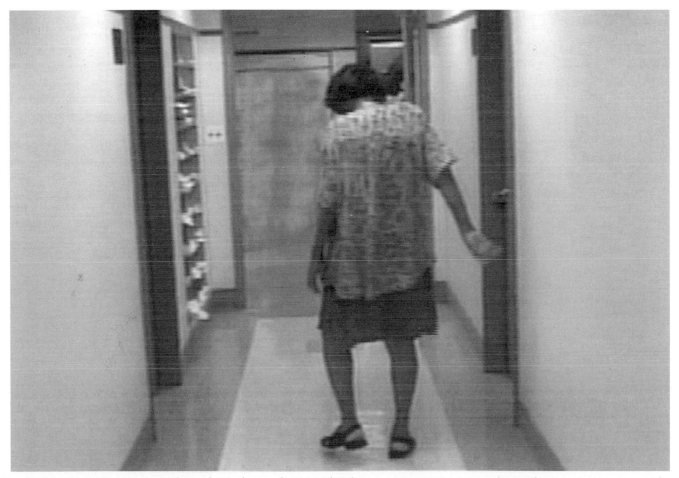

FIGURE 34–4. Stuttering, uncoordinated gait due to chorea and right arm posturing owing to chorea/dystonia in a patient with Huntington disease.

exon 1 containing the expansion, develop symptoms of HD, supporting a gain of function role. Observations on the normal role of huntingtin and its mutated version also give clues as to the pathogenesis of the disease. Normal and expanded huntingtin are both expressed in the brain and body. However, the brains of individuals with HD contain large intracellular aggregates or inclusions containing huntingtin and also ubiquitin. The length of huntingtin and its polyglutamine tract is directly proportional to the frequency of intracellular aggregates. The aggregates contain only part of the huntingtin protein that include the expanded polyglutamine tract, cleaved from the rest of the protein by caspases. The presence of the abnormal tract may induce apoptosis and it is hypothesized that normal huntingtin may have an anti-apoptotic role. Trials involving caspase inhibitors such as minocycline are under way to determine whether the inhibition of caspase will prevent cleavage of huntingtin and the formation of the aggregates that result in neuronal death.

Formation of the aggregates may, however, be a compensatory mechanism, sequestering the expanded huntingtin. This is supported by the observation that aggregates are often found in surviving neurons. Alternatively, the expanded polyglutamine tract may interact abnormally with a number of transcription factors containing short polyglutamine tracts, thereby altering gene expression. One such protein is the transcriptional coactivator cAMP responsive element-binding protein (CREB) binding protein (CBP), which is thought to bind the expanded polyglutamine tract, thus reducing the normal acetyl transferase activity of CBP, decreasing acetylation of histones, and leading to reduced gene transcription, possibly affecting cell survival.[8] One possibility is that trials involving histone deacetylator inhibitors could prevent HD-related degeneration.

It is also clear that there is a cellular energy dysfunction in HD. Mutant huntingtin binds to neuronal synaptic vesicles. This adversely affects glutamate levels in the striatum resulting in mitochondrial calcium abnormalities and high levels of free radicals. Trials using antioxidant therapy involving coenzyme Q10 and creatine are in process.

Polyglutamine tract expansions are now known to cause a number of neurodegenerative diseases. It is hoped that the expanding research in the field of HD may help shed light on how triplet repeat expansions cause disease.

Huntington Disease-like Phenotypes

An autosomal dominant HD-phenotype pedigree has been linked to chromosome 20p12 (HD-like 1). Affected individuals present with adult-onset psychiatric or behavioral disturbance and develop cognitive decline, personality change, motor disturbance with chorea, dysarthria, and ataxia together with atrophy of the basal ganglia. Some affected family members also develop epileptic seizures, which is atypical for adult-onset HD.

The discovery of an expansion in the coding region of the prion protein gene led to the diagnosis of familial prion disease. This important finding reveals that prion protein gene repeat-expansion mutations can provoke an autosomal-dominant, early-onset, slowly progressing, atypical prion disease with features overlapping those of HD. This finding has important implications for genetic testing.

Another disease with HD-like symptoms, termed "Huntington disease-like 2" (HDL2), has recently been described.[9] The causative mutation is a CTG expansion in exon 2A of *JPH3* (encoding junctophilin-3) on chromosome 16q24.3. *JPH3* is primarily expressed in the brain, and appears to be involved in the formation of junctional membrane structures. Exon 2A is variably spliced, and does not appear in the full-length JPH3 transcript. Three different versions of a truncated transcript containing only exon 1 and exon 2A have been identified, each with a different splice junction that alters the reading frame, so that the CTG repeat may encode polyalanine or polyleucine, or fall in 3'UTR. The normal repeat is 7 to 28 triplets in length, with expansions ranging in length from 41 to 57 triplets; the precise range of normal and abnormal repeat lengths will undoubtedly change as repeat length is determined in more individuals. Expansions in the shorter range may be associated with more prominent chorea and a slower rate of progression, while individuals with longer repeat lengths may initially present with more rigidity and dystonia, resembling juvenile HD. Findings on MRI and autopsy are indistinguishable from HD, with prominent striatal atrophy in a dorsal to ventral gradient. Surprisingly, and just as in HD, intranuclear inclusions have been detected in HDL2 brain tissue by an antibody thought to be specific for expanded tracts of polyglutamine residues; the implications of this finding remain unclear.

Available evidence suggests that HDL2 may be quite rare or nonexistent in populations of European descent, as most reported cases have been of African ethnicity, in addition to one Mexican pedigree and an isolated case from Morocco. Overall, the rate of HDL2 in the population with HD-like symptoms but without the HD mutation may be about 1% if the phenotype is broadly defined. The prevalence is likely to be much higher among individuals with a more classic HD phenotype, autosomal dominant inheritance, and African ethnicity (RL Margolis, personal communication).

An autosomal recessive neurodegenerative "Huntington disease-like 3" (HDL-3) disorder segregating in a consanguineous family from Saudi Arabia has been mapped to 4p15.3, in close proximity to the HD locus at 4p16.3. The disease manifests at approximately 3 to 4 years and is characterized by both pyramidal and extrapyramidal abnormalities, including chorea, dystonia, ataxia, gait instability, spasticity, seizures, mutism, and intellectual impairment. Brain magnetic resonance imaging (MRI) findings include progressive frontal cortical atrophy and bilateral caudate atrophy.

It is likely that other genetic causes of the HD phenotype will eventually be identified.

Dentatorubral-Pallidoluysian Atrophy

Dentatorubral-pallidoluysian atrophy (DRPLA) is a progressive neurodegenerative autosomal dominant disease, caused by an expansion of a CAG triplet repeat in exon 5 of the *DRPLA* gene on chromosome 12p13.31. It is characterized by ataxia, choreoathetosis, progressive dementia, and cognitive decline. The triplet-repeat expansion causes combined systemic degeneration of the dentatofugal and pallidofugal pathways visualized histologically by ubiquitinated neuronal intranuclear inclusions. The relative quantities of DRPLA mRNA and protein in individuals with DRPLA and without are the same, suggesting that the *DRPLA* expansion acts as a gain of function mutation possibly by interfering with CREB-dependent transcriptional activation resulting in neuronal toxicity.

Unaffected individuals have up to 35 CAG repeats in the *DRPLA* gene, but there is an undetermined group of patients who have between 36 and 48 repeats, and affected individuals have 49 or more. DRPLA demonstrates anticipation, especially when inherited through the paternal line.

Age of onset varies from 1 to 62 years, with an average of 30 years. CAG triple repeat length has been shown to be inversely proportional to age, with earlier age of onset usually accompanying greater expansions. Two main phenotypes have been described: progressive myoclonus epilepsy phenotype (62 to 79 repeats), age of onset 21 years and younger, usually caused by a paternal expansion. In addition to classical symptoms of DRPLA, individuals with young-onset DRPLA may exhibit myoclonus, epilepsy, and mental retardation.[10] The second phenotype is characterized by nonprogressive myoclonus epilepsy (54 to 67 repeats) and a later age at onset (older than 21); it is clinically similar to HD and other spinocerebellar ataxias, but the chorea component of the DRPLA phenotype can mask the presence of the ataxia. Individuals with very small expansions (49 to 55) can exhibit solely ataxia, also complicating the diagnostic process.

The prevalence of both DRPLA and HD in the Japanese population is estimated to be 0.2 to 0.7/100,000. Only a small number of families of European descent, however, have been described with DRPLA. A neurodegenerative disease in an African-American family described as having "Haw River Syndrome" was later found to be caused by a *DRPLA* expansion. Interestingly, the increased prevalence of DRPLA in the Japanese population corresponds to the increased frequency of triplet repeats in the high-normal range of the *DRPLA* gene in Japanese when compared to Europeans.

Neuroacanthocytosis

Neuroacanthocytosis (chorea acanthocytosis) is a rare neurodegenerative autosomal recessive disorder characterized by chorea, buccal dyskinesias, tics, cognitive decline, seizures, dementia, parkinsonism, absent tendon reflexes, and occasional myopathy. Epilepsy is the initial manifestation in half of individuals with this disease. The mean age of onset is 35 years, but both young- and late-onset cases have been described. Computerized tomography (CT) and MRI reveal atrophy of the caudate nuclei with dilatation of the anterior horns. Acanthocytes are present in up to 50% of red blood cells of affected individuals, although rarely they are absent, and in some patients, they are present only in the latter stages of the disease. Myopathy is usually accompanied by increased serum concentration of muscle creatine phosphokinase. Neuroacanthocytosis is caused by mutations in the *CHAC* gene on chromosome 9q21, which codes for the protein "chorein."[11] So far, 17 mutations have been described, dispersed throughout the gene, including missense, deletion, and frameshift mutations. Between 200 and 250 people with neuroacanthocytosis have been identified worldwide, 20% of whom are Japanese—suggesting a founder effect in this population.

Although neuroacanthocytosis is a rare disease, it is noticeable for its clinical overlap with McLeod syndrome and HD. In addition, it can mimic Tourette syndrome with vocal tics, obsessive-compulsive behavior, and impaired impulse control.

Genetic testing is not currently used to diagnose neuroacanthocytosis, and diagnosis rests on assays for acanthocytes in blood smears.

Benign Hereditary Chorea

Benign hereditary chorea is an autosomal dominant condition linked to chromosome 14q and characterized by non-progressive, benign, early-onset chorea with an absence of mental deterioration, dystonia, myoclonic jerks, or dysarthria. Onset of chorea usually begins by age 5 years, and stabilizes between age 10 and 20 years. For some, symptoms abate during adulthood. A greater penetrance in males than females has been reported, and there is both intra- and inter-familial variability. Haplotype analysis has found no suggestion of a common founder for families linked to 14q. Major cerebral changes have not been detected by MRI. A number of families with benign hereditary chorea do not show linkage to chromosome 14q. These families, in addition to symptoms of chorea, tend to have more heterogeneous symptoms (such as ataxia, dysarthria, or mental disturbance) and a wider range of age of onset.[12]

Wilson Disease

Wilson disease (WD) is an autosomal recessive neurodegenerative disease with hepatic, renal, neurologic, and psychiatric manifestations. It is caused by mutations in the *ATP7B* gene on chromosome 13q14-q21 leading to defective copper transport and accumulation of copper.

ATP7B is homologous to the cation-transporting P-type adenosinetriphosphatase (ATPase) gene family, including the gene responsible for Menkes syndrome.

Symptoms of WD are caused by defective biliary copper excretion from hepatocytes. In addition, copper fails to be incorporated into ceruloplasmin. These defects result in copper deposition at toxic levels in the brain, liver, and kidney. Diagnosis of WD is aided by the following findings: low serum ceruloplasmin concentration, and increased urinary and hepatic copper concentration. However, a normal serum ceruloplasmin concentration is found in at least 5% of patients with WD with neurologic symptoms and in up to 40% of patients with hepatic symptoms. Some heterozygotes may also have some of these findings, but are asymptomatic. In addition, Kayser-Fleischer (K-F) rings in the outer circumference of the cornea are caused by copper deposition in Descemet's membrane of the corneal endothelium and can be detected by slit-lamp examination. K-F rings are observed in approximately 50% of individuals with WD presenting with hepatic disease and in approximately 90% of those presenting with neurologic or psychiatric manifestations. However, K-F rings are not unique to WD. Assaying for both serum ceruloplasmin and K-F rings by slit-lamp examination may be necessary if one suspects or wants to rule out neurologic WD.

Age of onset of WD ranges from 6 to 50 years, and symptoms are variable. Liver disease is the first manifestation in 40% of individuals with WD and is usually the first manifestation in early-onset WD. Initial presentation of neurologic or psychiatric symptoms often occurs at a later age. Interestingly, mutations that eliminate gene function (null mutations) appear to correlate with young-onset WD and hence initial presentation with liver disease. Neurological findings can include incoordination, tremor of any type including wing-beating postural tremor, dystonia (Fig. 34–5), rigidity, chorea, and a risus sardonicus dystonic facial grin with open mouth. Presentation can also be unilateral. Psychiatric symptoms can include depression, cognitive decline, and compulsive behavior. The range of symptoms and variability of initial symptoms can lead to differential diagnoses as wide-ranging as PD, juvenile PD, HD, DRPLA, ataxia, or Niemann-Pick type C disease. Early diagnosis of symptomatic and presymptomatic individuals is crucial since copper chelation therapy has proven very effective, with reversible symptoms in the early stages of the disease.

The prevalence of WD is approximately 1/30,000 (with a 1/90 carrier frequency), but is higher in Asia and

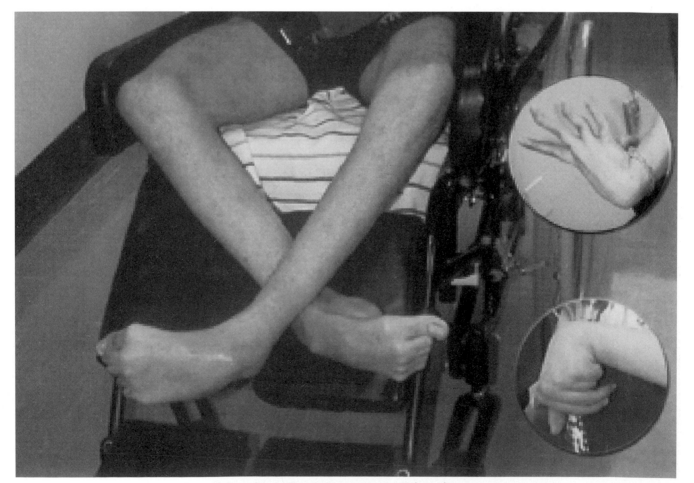

FIGURE 34–5. Dystonic postures in Wilson disease.

Europe. A single mutation (His 1069 Glu) is thought to account for more than 30% of European cases of WD. More than 200 other mutations have been described across the world, most of which are rare ("private mutations"). As a result, most patients are compound heterozygotes (they have a different mutation on each allele). The variety of mutations in this gene make genetic testing a difficult, unreliable, and expensive option. However, both European and Asian populations appear to have, to some degree, individual founders. As more becomes known about the genetics of WD, mutation panels targeted to specific populations may allow development of molecular diagnostic protocols for WD. At the present time, it is possible for an individual with WD to undergo linkage studies so that the disease status of other family members can be determined. This can be useful for prenatal diagnosis or to identify asymptomatic family members so that prophylactic copper chelation therapy can be administered to offset symptoms.

A naturally occurring rat model of WD, called the Long-Evans Cinnamon (LEC) rat, has played a large role in the elucidation of the underlying defect of WD. The rat homologue of the human *ATP7B* gene is abnormal in the LEC rat. Recently, the LEC rat has been used successfully to investigate gene therapy of WD using adenoviral gene transfer.

Myoclonus Epilepsy of Unverricht-Lundborg Type

There are several genetic causes of progressive myoclonus epilepsy, the most common being Myoclonus Epilepsy of Unverricht-Lundborg disease (EPM1). This autosomal recessive disease is caused by a dodecamer (12-mer) minisatellite repeat expansion (CCC CGC CCC GCG) located about 70 nucleotides upstream of the transcription start site nearest to the 5′ end of the *Cystatin B* gene on chromosome 21q22.3. Cystatin B codes for a cysteine protease inhibitor, which has a crucial role in the programming of cell apoptosis and is widely expressed in neurons but not glial cells. The expansion results in loss of expression of Cystatin B leading to uncontrolled cell apoptosis and neuronal cell death (without inclusion bodies). Onset is usually between age 6 and 15 years and is characterized by stimulus-sensitive myoclonus, tonic-clonic seizures, and typical electroencephalogram (EEG) findings. Neurodegenerative changes such as ataxia and dementia are common, and cognitive function typically declines 10 to 20 years after onset of symptoms.

Expansion of the dodecamer repeat in Cystatin B was also found to cause Baltic Mediterranean progressive myoclonus epilepsy, proving that these two diseases are in fact a single disease entity. Founder effects are thought to be responsible for the increased incidence of EPM1 that has been reported in both Finland (where the incidence is 1/20,000) and North Africa.

Normal alleles of the Cystatin B gene contain 2 or 3 copies of this dodecamer repeat whereas mutant alleles contain more than 30 repeats. Premutation repeats with 12 to 17 repeats show marked instability when transmitted to offspring. Evidence of the instability of the repeat is also provided by the observation that affected siblings can have widely differing repeat lengths. While the majority of EPM1 mutated alleles contain expansions of the dodecamer repeat (85% to 90%), the remaining are caused by smaller mutations, such as point mutations in the Cystatin B gene. The majority of laboratories that offer Cystatin B testing only analyze the dodecamer repeat expansion, reducing the sensitivity of the test. No correlation has been found between the size of the repeat and age of onset or severity.[10]

Neuronal Ceroid Lipofuscinoses

The neuronal ceroid lipofuscinoses (NCLs) are a group of neurodegenerative genetic lysosomal-storage diseases characterized by seizures, progressive deterioration of cognition (dementia and speech abnormalities) and motor function (involuntary movement, ataxia, and spasticity), blindness, and the accumulation of autofluorescent lipopigment material in neurons and other cell types, probably caused by an underlying defect in protein degradation. Characteristic inclusion bodies representing lysosomal storage material such as Saposins A and D and subunit c of mitochondrial ATPase are detectable on electron microscopy for some forms of the disease.

Collectively, this group of diseases account for the most common cause of childhood onset neurodegeneration with an incidence of approximately 1/25,000, but with wide geographical variation, most common in Northern Europe. The NCLs are named according to age of onset and symptom presentation. The discovery of the causative genes has helped to delineate this group of disorders. However, there is significant overlap in presentation between the NCLs. For example, individuals with mutations in the *CLN1* gene present mainly as infantile NCL, but can also present as late-infantile, juvenile, and adult NCL (Table 34–3). This is probably due to genotype-phenotype interactions.

Infantile NCL (INCL) is characterized by normal early development, onset of retinal blindness and seizures by age 2 years, myoclonic jerks, progressive mental deterioration, and death between age 8 and 11 years. INCL is caused by mutations in palmitoyl-protein thioesterase 1 (*PPT1*). Myoclonic epilepsy manifesting between age 2 to 4 years is usually the first sign of late INCL (LINCL). Loss of motor and mental milestones and vision, dementia; ataxia; extrapyramidal and pyramidal signs; and death between age 6 and 30 years are other characteristics of this disease. Finnish, Gypsy/Indian, and Turkish variants of LINCL are caused by mutations in *CLN5*, *CLN6*, and *CLN7*, respectively.

TABLE 34–3. Classification of the Neuronal Ceroid Lipofuscinoses

Name/s	Inheritance pattern	Gene/location	Protein	Mutations identified (n)
Infantile NCL/Santavuori-Haltia CLN1 mutations also cause classic late infantile, juvenile, and adult NCL	AR	CLN1/1p32	Palmitoyl-protein thioesterase	>38 3 common
Classic late infantile/Jansky-Bielschowsky. CLN2 mutations also cause juvenile NCL	AR	CLN2/11p15	Tripeptidyl-peptidase 1	>40 2 common
Juvenile/Batten Disease/Spielmeyer-Vogt-Sjögren. CLN3 mutations also cause adult NCL	AR	CLN3/16p12.1	Battenin (membrane protein)	>31 1 common
Adult NCL/Kuf's disease	AD/AR	CLN4/N/I	–	–
Late infantile Finnish variant	AR	CLN5/13q21.2-32	Membrane protein	>5, Northern Europe only
Late infantile/early juvenile Variant/Gypsy/Indian	AR	CLN6/15q21-23	Putative membrane protein	>6, increased in Southern Mediterranean
Turkish variant (may be allelic to CLN8)	AR	CLN7/8p23	–	–
Northern epilepsy (NE)/Progressive epilepsy with mental retardation	AR	CLN8/8p23 (see CLN7)	Putative membrane protein	1, in Finland

AD, autosomal dominant; AR, autosomal recessive; N/I, not identified.

Juvenile NCL (JNCL) usually begins with retinal visual failure between age 4 and 10 years. Other symptoms include epilepsy with generalized clonic-tonic seizures, complex-partial or myoclonic seizures, behavioral problems, extrapyramidal signs, and death in the late teens. Adult NCL (ANCL) occurs around age 30 years and is characterized by ataxia, dementia, athetosis and dyskinesias, pyramidal and extra-pyramidal signs, and progressive myoclonic epilepsy and death approximately 10 years from onset. ANCL is not characterized by vision loss, however. Northern Epilepsy (NE) results in onset of epilepsy between age 5 and 10 years and is characterized by progressive epilepsy with mental retardation, no vision loss, and a protracted course.[13]

Differential diagnoses include other progressive neurodegenerative diseases such as Tay-Sachs, Krabbe disease, Canavan disease, Rett syndrome, metachromatic leukodystrophy, Niemann-Pick A and B, and other lysosomal storage disorders. Treatment usually involves management of symptoms and control of seizures. Enzyme assay for CLN1 and CLN2 is available, as is clinical gene testing for CLN 1, 2, and 3, and research-based testing for CLN5 and 6. Animal models, both naturally occurring (with mutations in CLN6 and 8 homologues) and genetically manipulated (CLN2 and 3) are helping researchers to understand how mutations in NCL genes cause disease. It is hoped that the NCLs will be good candidates for enzyme replacement therapy since they are caused by loss of protein function.

Rett Syndrome

Rett syndrome is an X-linked dominant neurodegenerative disease characterized by normal presentation at birth with loss of acquired skills beginning between age 6 and 18 months, gradual deceleration of head growth and the development of all or some of the following features: ataxia, seizures, stereotyped hand movements, gait apraxia, tremors, and dystonia. Rett syndrome is usually embryonic lethal in males. It is caused by mutations in the methyl-CpG binding protein 2 (MECP2) gene on Xq28.

Molecular genetic testing for Rett syndrome leads to identification of a mutation in MECP2 in approximately 80% of cases. Nonsense, missense, and frameshift mutations have all been described. Mutations in MECP2 also cause atypical Rett syndrome (either a more severe phenotype with early onset and infantile spasms, or a more benign phenotype), as well as autism, behavioral disorders, and mental retardation with tremor/spasticity. Rarely, afflicted males have severe neonatal hypotonia or encephalopathy. A small number of males with classical Rett syndrome have been reported. Most cases are due to mosaicism, reducing the severity of the phenotype.

The prevalence of classic Rett syndrome is estimated to be 1/10,000 to 1/15,000 and nearly all cases are sporadic. However, multiple siblings with Rett syndrome have been described. This can be due to gonadal (germline) mosaicism. Alternatively, the mother may be a mutation carrier, but due to favorable (random) X inactivation, have mild or no symptoms. It is therefore advisable to offer the mother of a child with a known *MECP2* mutation genetic testing to determine carrier status. If negative, the family should appreciate that there is still a possible recurrence risk owing to gonadal mosaicism.

The function of MECP2 is to down-regulate transcription of other genes by binding to methylated CpG dinucleotides and recruiting histone deacetylases. Mutations in *MECP2* cause disease due to loss of normal gene function and hence over-expression of those genes. Missense mutations resulting in only partial loss of function have been reported to cause a less severe phenotype than nonsense/frameshift mutations that obliterate gene function. In addition, a number of males with mental retardation, cognitive delay, and movement disorders such as tremor and bradykinesia have MECP2 mutations that have not been described in females with classic Rett syndrome.

The clinical and developmental features of Rett syndrome suggest that dysfunction of subcortical regulator systems, brain stem, basal forebrain nuclei, and basal ganglia cause abnormal development of the cortex in late infancy. Immaturity of the respiratory regulator is thought to be a crucial step in the development of the disease. A number of diseases share features with Rett syndrome and must be considered in the differential diagnosis, such as infantile neuronal ceroid-lipofuscinosis and Angelman syndrome. A typical EEG pattern is associated with Rett syndrome, but is not unique to the disease. Current management of patients with Rett syndrome focuses on supportive and symptomatic therapy.

MECP2 mouse knockouts have been generated by gene targeting. The mice are born normal and develop symptoms of tremor, behavioral change, and deceleration of head growth from about age 6 weeks. They typically die between age 8 and 12 weeks.[14] Research has shown that mutations in MECP2, a widely expressed gene, appear to selectively affect neurons.

Paroxysmal Dyskinesias

The majority of hyperkinetic movement disorders have symptoms that are continuously present. There is a rare group of hyperkinetic movement disorders that are characterized by transient symptoms of varying frequency, severity, duration, and aggravating factors. Symptoms that manifest as dyskinesias of the choreoathetotic and dystonic type are called "paroxysmal" and those of the ataxic type are described as "episodic."

Episodic ataxia-1 (EA1) is a rare autosomal dominant condition characterized by episodes of ataxia and dysarthria, without vertigo, lasting seconds to minutes with symptoms of myokymia (rippling of muscles, diagnosable by electromyography) during and between episodes, with near normal neurological function in between attacks. It is triggered by exercise, startle, or

stress. It is caused by mutations in a voltage-gated (delayed rectifier) potassium channel gene *KCNA1* on chromosome 12p13. Individuals with EA1 may also have epilepsy.

Episodic ataxia 2 (EA2) is a rare autosomal dominant condition. EA2 often manifests with vertigo and is associated with episodic ataxia lasting hours with nystagmus between episodes. It is caused by mutations in the calcium channel, voltage-dependent, P/Q type, alpha 1A subunit gene (*CACNA1A*), which is highly expressed in the cerebellum and is located on chromosome 19p13. More than 50% of patients have vertigo, nausea, and vomiting during attacks and about half have migraine headaches. Like EA1, EA2 is triggered by exercise, startle, or stress. EA2 is responsive to acetozolamide treatment. Familial hemiplegic migraine is also caused by mutations in *CACNA1A* and SCA6, with a triplet repeat in the 3′ end of *CACNA1A*. Spinocerebellar ataxia can be distinguished from EA2 by progressive rather than episodic ataxia and a later age of onset, although there is an overlap of symptoms.

Paroxysmal kinesigenic dyskinesia (PKD) is a rare autosomal dominant disease characterized by recurrent, brief attacks of dystonia, chorea, ballistic, or athetoid involuntary movements induced by sudden voluntary movements. It has been mapped to chromosome 16p11.2-q12.1 (DYT10) in a number of Japanese PKD families.[5] Episodes often begin in late childhood and can last seconds to minutes and occur up to 100 times a day (Fig. 34–6). Some patients with PKD have a history of infantile afebrile convulsions with a favorable outcome. EEG, neuroimages, and pathology are normal in individuals with PKD. Individuals with PKD are very responsive to antiepileptics, such as carbamazepine. A PKD Afro-Caribbean family mapped to a second locus in the same region (16p11.2-q11.2). An Indian PKD family has been linked to 16q13-q22.1.

Benign familial infantile convulsions and paroxysmal choreoathetosis (ICCA) is a rare autosomal dominant condition linked to the pericentromeric region of chromosome 16p12-16cen, very close to the locus for PKD. ICCA is characterized by nonfebrile seizures that occur spontaneously or are induced by a variety of stimuli, with the first attack occurring between 3 and 12 months of age. Rolandic epilepsy, paroxysmal exercise-induced dystonia, and writer's cramp (RE-PED-WC) is an autosomal recessive condition linked to 16p12-11.2 overlapping with the ICCA chromosomal region. It is characterized by dystonia (mostly affecting the feet) induced by continuous exercise like walking or running. Clinical analogies and linkage findings suggest that the same gene could be responsible for RE-PED-WC and ICCA, with specific mutations accounting for each of these conditions.

The fact that PKD, with or without other findings, maps to a number of regions on chromosome 16p may be due to an ion gene family in this region caused by gene

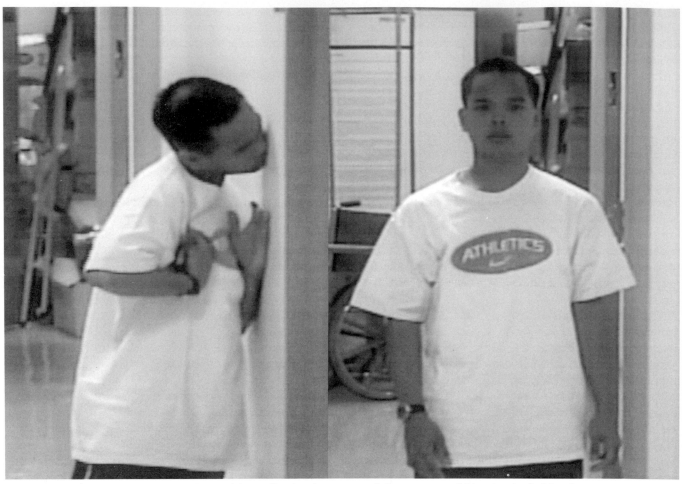

FIGURE 34–6. During and immediately after an attack in paroxysmal kinesigenic dyskinesia.

duplication. However, some PKD families do not show linkage to this region, suggesting further genetic heterogeneity. A large pedigree with paroxysmal choreoathetosis/spasticity has shown linkage to chromosome 1p (DYT9), close to a cluster of potassium channel genes.

Families with autosomal dominant paroxysmal nonkinesigenic dyskinesias (PNKD) (dystonic choreoathetosis, familial paroxysmal dyskinesia, or Mount-Reback syndrome) have been linked to chromosome 2q33-35 (DYT8), close to a cluster of ion channel genes. PNKD differs from PKD in that movements are characterized by attacks of involuntary movements such as dystonia, chorea, and athetosis that last up to several hours; are triggered by caffeine or alcohol consumption, stress, or hormonal changes; but do not follow sudden voluntary movement.[5]

Paroxysmal nocturnal dyskinesia is now known to be a form of nocturnal frontal lobe epilepsy with autosomal dominant (ADNFLE) and sporadic presentation. It is characterized by childhood-onset partial epilepsy causing frequent, violent, brief seizures at night. The seizures mainly consist of motor elements, which can be dystonic, tonic, or hyperkinetic. ADNFLE is caused by mutations in genes encoding the cholinergic receptor, nicotinic,

alpha polypeptide subunit 4 (CHRNA4) or beta polypeptide subunit 2 (CHRNB2) of the neuronal nicotinic acetylcholine receptor on chromosome 20q13.2 and 1q21 respectively. Other families have been linked to chromosome15q24.

Hereditary Hyperekplexia

Hereditary hyperekplexia, otherwise known as familial startle disease (STHE) or stiff baby syndrome, is caused by mutations in the alpha 1 subunit of the inhibitory glycine receptor gene (GLRA1) on chromosome 5q31.2. GLRA1 is a ligand-gated chloride channel composed of three ligand-binding alpha1-subunits and two structural beta-subunits that are clustered on the postsynaptic membrane of inhibitory glycinergic neurons. Dominant and rare recessive forms of the disease have been described. STHE can begin in the neonatal period. The exaggerated startle reflex (such as when performing the Moro reflex or tapping the infant on the nose, or in response to unexpected acoustic or tactile stimuli) can result in sustained myoclonus that produces continuous increased muscle tone. Occasionally, this startle reflex results in fatal apneic attacks. Muscle tone usually returns to normal during the first years of life, but the startle reflex continues to be manifested. Additional symptoms may include excessive hypnic jerks (including periodic limb movements in sleep) and exaggerated head retraction reflex. Onset can be later in childhood, with the excessive startle reflex causing the patient to become stiff and unable to maintain a standing position, leading to falls. Some individuals with STHE benefit from clonazepam.

More than five mutations have been discovered in the GLRA1 gene. A small number of individuals with "sporadic" STHE were found to be homozygotes (due to consanguinity). A compound heterozygote has also been reported. Mutations appear to be clustered in exons 7 and 8. The mouse mutant "spasmodic," which exhibits a phenotype similar to STHE, is caused by mutations in the mouse homologue of GLRA1.

The normal function of GLRA1 involves mediating neuronal inhibition in the brain stem and spinal cord resulting in the control of muscle tone. GLRA1 belongs to an ion channel family that also includes gamma-aminobutyric, serotonin, and nicotinic acetylcholine receptors. Like other members of the family, GLRA1 has both N- and C-terminal extracellular components on either side of four transmembrane regions.

A minor form of STHE has also been characterized with excessive startle response without the accompanying hypertonia. Mutations in GLRA1 have not been identified for the majority of individuals with the minor form, suggesting alternative genetic loci. In addition, a number of individuals with sporadic STHE do not have mutations in GLRA1. Further research will lead to elucidation of other genes involved in hyperekplexia.

Tourette Syndrome

Tourette syndrome (TS) is a neurologic condition characterized by motor and phonic tics and behavioral symptoms (such as loss of impulse control), which usually manifest in childhood. TS is usually familial and is often accompanied by attention-deficit hyperactivity disorder (ADHD), obsessive-compulsive disorder (OCD), and other behavioral problems. Current theories suggest that TS is a gender-influenced autosomal dominant disease with nearly complete penetrance in males and lower penetrance in females (56%). Twin studies showing high concordance for TS in monozygotic twins provide evidence for a genetic involvement in TS. It has also been proposed that TS is a semi-dominant, semi-recessive disease supported by evidence that parents with partial symptoms of TS are at increased risk to have children manifesting full-blown TS. Interestingly, it appears that individuals with TS undergo assortative mating, which may contribute to this phenomenon (affected individuals non-randomly choosing likewise affected partners).

Inter- and intra-familial variability of TS symptoms has been widely reported. OCD and ADHD are often seen in family members of individuals with TS, and can often appear alongside symptoms of TS. The spectrum of conditions, including other behavioral disorders, that may occur under the "umbrella" of TS can make diagnosis a confusing task. The lack of clear definition as to what constitutes TS may also contribute to the difficulties of locating susceptibility genes and may adversely affect linkage analyses. Numerous susceptibility loci have so far been tested for linkage to TS (including dopamine D1, D2, D3, D4, D5 receptors, dopamine beta hydroxylase, tyrosinase, and tyrosine hydroxylase), but none have consistently been associated with the disease and more than 95% of the genome has so far been excluded. However, it is still believed that there is one major locus. Interestingly, recent results show evidence for TS susceptibility loci on 2p11, 8q22, and 11q23 using French-Canadian and Afrikaner family studies.[15]

A candidate region on chromosome 7q31 is also being investigated due to the observation of an individual with a chromosomal rearrangement in this region and TS. It is hoped that examining the breakpoint may help locate genes causal to TS.

Movement Disorders, Genetics, Multidisciplinary Care, and the Future

The practice of neurology is entering a new era. With the advent of confirmatory genetic testing, we have the tools to diagnose neurogenetic disorders in a way that is unparalleled. But this gain in diagnostic power means that neurologists will need a multidisciplinary team, including genetic counselors and social workers, who can assist patients with the added burden of genetic disease. Genetic counseling for neurogenetic conditions includes not only discussions of mechanisms of inheritance, risk to relatives, and psychosocial counseling, but also encompasses issues such as confidentiality of genetic information and the unknown risk of discrimination by life and health insurance companies (for more details, see www.nsgc.org). In addition, asymptomatic individuals at 50% risk to inherit a neurogenetic disease can now choose to learn of their future disease status through genetic testing. The enormously difficult predicament that these individuals experience requires lengthy and complex pre- and post-test genetic counseling sessions to enable a fully informed decision.

Genetic discovery has greatly expanded our knowledge of movement disorders and will continue to change the way we approach understanding of disease, and hopefully in the future, treatment. The ethical, legal, and social implications of genetics, along with its diagnostic power, will change our medical practice in a way that is unparalleled in the history of medicine.

REFERENCES

1. Lansbury P, Brice A: Genetics of Parkinson's disease and biochemical studies of implicated gene products: Commentary. Curr Opin Cell Biol 2002;14:653.

2. Houlden H, Baker M, Morris HR, et al: Corticobasal degeneration and progressive supranuclear palsy share a common tau haplotype. Neurology 2001;56:1702–1706.

3. Louis ED, Ford B, Frucht S, et al: Risk of tremor and impairment from tremor in relatives of patients with essential tremor: A community-based family study. Ann Neurol 2001;49:761–769.

4. Bressman SB, Sabatti C, Raymond D, et al: The DYT1 phenotype and guidelines for diagnostic testing. Neurology 2000;9:1746–1752.

5. Nemeth AH: The genetics of primary dystonias and related disorders. Brain 2002;125:695–721.

6. Zhou B, Westaway SK, Levinson B, et al: A novel pantothenate kinase gene (PANK2) is defective in Hallervorden-Spatz syndrome. Nat Genet 2001;28: 345–349.

7. The American College of Medical Genetics/ American Society of Human Genetics Huntington Disease Genetic Testing Working Group (ACMG/ ASHG) statement: Laboratory guidelines for Huntington disease genetic testing. Am J Hum Genet 1998;62:1243–1247.

8. Nucifora FC Jr, Sasaki M, Peters MF, et al: Interference by huntingtin and atrophin-1 with cbp-mediated transcription leading to cellular toxicity. Science 2001;291:2423–2428.

9. Holmes SE, O'Hearn E, Rosenblatt A, et al: A repeat expansion in the gene encoding junctophilin-3 is associated with Huntington disease-like 2. Nat Genet 2001;29:377–8.

10. Delgado-Escueta AV, Ganesh S, Yamakawa K: Advances in the genetics of progressive myoclonus epilepsy. Am J Med Genet 2001;106:129–138.

11. Rampoldi L, Dobson-Stone C, Rubio JP, et al: A conserved sorting-associated protein is mutant in chorea-acanthocytosis. Nat Genet 2001;28:119–120.

12. Breedveld GJ, Percy AK, MacDonald ME, et al: Clinical and genetic heterogeneity in benign hereditary chorea. Neurology 2002;59:579–584.

13. Mitchison HM, Mole SE: Neurodegenerative disease: The neuronal ceroid lipofuscinoses (Batten disease). Curr Opin Neurol 2001;14:795–803.

14. Guy J, Hendrich B, Holmes M, et al: A mouse Mecp2-null mutation causes neurological symptoms that mimic Rett syndrome. Nat Genet 2001;27:322–6.

15. Simonic I, Nyholt DR, Gericke GS, et al: Further evidence for linkage of Gilles de la Tourette syndrome (GTS) susceptibility loci on chromosomes 2p11, 8q22 and 11q23–24 in South African Afrikaners. Am J Med Genet 2001;105:163–167.

RELEVANT WEB SITES

http://www.ncbi.nlm.nih.gov/Omim/
http://www.nsgc.org
http://www.geneclinics.org/
http://www.gene.ucl.ac.uk/nomenclature/

CHAPTER 35

The Inherited Ataxias

Roger N. Rosenberg

Henry L. Paulson

THE INHERITED ATAXIAS

Of the syndromes constituting the inherited ataxias, some show autosomal dominant or recessive inheritance, whereas others are caused by mitochondrial mutations and thus show maternal inheritance. Significant progress has been made in defining the molecular basis of these syndromes (Table 35–1), so that a genotype classification[1] now supersedes previous ones based on clinical features alone.[2]

The clinical manifestations and neuropathologic findings of cerebellar disease typically dominate the clinical picture, but depending on the type of ataxia, there may also be characteristic changes in the basal ganglia, brain stem, spinal cord, optic nerves, retina, and peripheral nerves. In large families with dominantly inherited disease, there are many gradations from purely cerebellar manifestations to mixed cerebellar and brain stem disorders, cerebellar and basal ganglia syndromes, and spinal cord or peripheral nerve disease. The clinical picture may be consistent within a family with dominantly inherited ataxia, but sometimes most affected family members show one characteristic syndrome whereas one or several members have a much different phenotype.[1]

Thus far, the genetically identified autosomal dominant spinocerebellar ataxias (known as the SCAs) and the most common recessively inherited ataxia, Friedreich ataxia (FA), have proved to be caused by dynamic expansions of simple sequence repeats in specific genes. All but one of these are trinucleotide repeat expansions. The greatest number of SCAs are caused by expanded CAG repeats that encode a glutamine repeat, or polyglutamine tract, in the disease protein. These polyglutamine ataxias include SCA1,[3,4] SCA2, SCA3 (also known as Machado-

Joseph disease),[5] SCA6, SCA7, and SCA17. The three other genetically identified SCAs are SCA8 (due to an untranslated CTG repeat), SCA12 (linked to an untranslated CAG repeat), and SCA10 (caused by an untranslated pentanucleotide repeat). The clinical phenotypes of the SCAs overlap, thus one cannot reliably diagnose a particular SCA on clinical grounds alone. A single familial phenotype can be caused by several different genotypes; conversely, a single genotype can manifest as several different familial phenotypes. This phenotypic complexity is explained by the dynamic nature of expanded repeats and the tendency for disease features to vary with the size of the expansion.

New knowledge of the genetic basis of ataxias has settled the formerly vexing issue of classification, and genetic testing has simplified the route to diagnosis in many cases. Here we review the clinical and molecular genetic features of inherited ataxias, discuss current views on mechanisms of pathogenesis, and describe potential therapeutic approaches to these currently untreatable diseases. A classification of the inherited ataxias based on genotype is emphasized.[1]

Autosomal Dominant Ataxias

Previously, descriptive neuropathologic terms such as *olivopontocerebellar atrophy* and *cerebellar cortical atrophy* were applied to the class of dominantly inherited ataxias now known as spinocerebellar ataxias (SCAs). The explosion of genetic data has shown that these descriptive syndromes encompass many different genetic disorders with overlapping clinical features. As presented in Table 35–1, the genetic classification of dominant

Table 35–1. Genotype Classification of the Spinocerebellar Ataxias

Name	Locus	Phenotype
SCA1 (autosomal dominant type 1)	6p22-p23 with CAG repeats (Exonic) Ataxin1	Ataxia with ophthalmoparesis, pyramidal and extrapyramidal findings
SCA2 (autosomal dominant type 2)	12q23-q24.1 with CAG repeats (Exonic) Ataxin2	Ataxia with slow saccades and minimal pyramidal and extrapyramidal findings
Machado-Joseph disease/SCA3 (autosomal dominant type 3)	14q24.3-q32 with CAG repeats (Exonic) MJD-Ataxin3	Ataxia with ophthalmoparesis and variable pyramidal, extrapyramidal, and amyotrophic signs
SCA4 (autosomal dominant type 4)	16q24-ter	Ataxia with normal eye movements, sensory axonal neuropathy, and pyramidal signs
SCA5 (autosomal dominant type 5)	Centromeric region of chromosome II	Ataxia and dysarthria
SCA6 (autosomal dominant type 6)	19p13.2 with CAG repeats in α_{1a}-voltage-dependent calcium channel gene (Exonic)	Ataxia and dysarthria, nystagmus, mild proprioceptive sensory loss
SCA7 (autosomal dominant type 7)	3p14.1-p21.1 with CAG repeats (Exonic) Ataxin7	Ophthalmoparesis; visual loss; ataxia; dysarthria, extensor plantar response; pigmentary retinal degeneration
SCA8 (autosomal dominant type 8)	13q21 with CTG repeats; non-coding	Gait ataxia, dysarthria, nystagmus; leg spasticity and reduced vibratory sensation
SCA10 (autosomal dominant type 10)	22q; ATTCT repeat; non-coding	Gait ataxia, dysarthria, nystagmus; partial complex and generalized motor seizures; polyneuropathy
SCA11 (autosomal dominant type 11)	15q14-q21.3 by linkage	Slowly progressive gait and extremity ataxia, dysarthria, vertical nystagmus, hyperreflexia
SCA12 (autosomal dominant type 12)	5q31-q33 by linkage; CAG repeat; protein phosphatase 2A	Tremor, decreased movement, increased reflexes, dystonia, ataxia, dysautonomia, dementia, dysarthria
SCA13 (autosomal dominant type 13)	19q13.3-q14.4	Mutation unknown in 1 family
SCA14 (autosomal dominant type 14)	19q-13.4	Mutation unknown in 1 family
SCA15 (autosomal dominant type 15)	Mutation unknown in 1 family; other known loci were excluded	Gait and extremity ataxia, dysarthria
SCA16 (autosomal dominant type 16)	8q22.1-q24.1	Mutation unknown in 1 family; pure cerebellar ataxia and head tremor; gait ataxia and dysarthria; horizontal gaze-evoked nystagmus
SCA17 (autosomal dominant type 17)	6q27; CAG expansion in the TATA-binding protein (TBP) gene	Gait ataxia, dementia; parkinsonism; dystonia; chorea; seizures; MRI shows cerebral & cerebellar atrophy
SCA18 (autosomal dominant type 18)	7q22-q32	Ataxia motor/sensory neuropathy
SCA19 (autosomal dominant type 19)	1p21-q21	Ataxia, tremor, cognitive impairment, myoclonus
SCA20 (assigned but not yet published)		
SCA21 (autosomal dominant type 21)	7p21.3-p15.1	Ataxia, extrapyramidal features of akinesia, rigidity, tremor, cognitive defect
SCA22 (assigned but not yet published)		
Dentatorubropallidoluysian atrophy (autosomal dominant)	12p12-ter with CAG repeats (Exonic) Atrophin	Ataxia, choreoathetosis, dystonia, seizures, myoclonus, dementia

(Continued)

TABLE 35–1. (*Continued*)

Name	Locus	Phenotype
Friedreich's ataxia (autosomal recessive)	9q13-q21.1 with intronic GAA repeats Frataxin	Ataxia, areflexia, extensor plantar responses, position sense deficits, cardiomyopathy, diabetes mellitus, scoliosis, foot deformities; defective iron transport from mitochondria
Friedreich's ataxia (autosomal recessive)	8q13.1-q13.3; α-TTP deficiency	Same as phenotype that maps to 9q but associated with vitamin E deficiency
Autosomal recessive spastic ataxia of Charlevoix-Saguenay (ARSACS)	Chromosome 13; SACS gene; loss of Sacsin peptide activity	Childhood onset of ataxia, spasticity, dysarthria, distal muscle wasting, foot deformity, retinal striations, mitral valve prolapse
Kearns-Sayre syndrome (sporadic)	mtDNA deletion and duplication mutations	Ptosis, ophthalmoplegia, pigmentary retinal degeneration, cardiomyopathy, diabetes mellitus, deafness, heart block, increased CSF protein, ataxia
Myoclonus epilepsy and ragged red fiber syndrome (MERRF) (maternal inheritance)	Mutation in mtDNA of the tRNA^{lys} at 8344: also mutation at 8356	Myoclonic epilepsy, ragged red fiber myopathy, ataxia
Mitochondrial encephalopathy, lactic acidosis, and stroke syndrome (MELAS) (maternal inheritance)	tRNA^{leu} mutation at 3243; also at 3271 and 3252	Headache, stroke, lactic acidosis, ataxia
Leigh's disease; subacute necrotizing encephalopathy (maternal inheritance or autosomal recessive)	mtDNA complex V defect (ATPase gene at 8993) or mitochondrial protein synthesis defect (both maternally inherited); or complex IV defect (autosomal recessive)	Obtundation, hypotonia, cranial nerve defects, respiratory failure, hyperintense or signals on T2-weighted magnetic resonance images in basal ganglia, cerebellum, or brainstem; ataxia
Episodic ataxia, type I (EA-1) (autosomal dominant)	12p; potassium channel gene KCNA1	Episodic ataxia for minutes: provoked by startle or exercise; with facial and hand myokymia; cerebellar signs are not progressive; responds to phenytoin
Episodic ataxia, type II (EA-2) (autosomal dominant)	19p-13(CACNA1A) (allelic with SCA6) (α_{1a}-voltage dependent calcium channel subunit)	Episodic ataxia for days: provoked by stress, fatigue; with down-gaze nystagmus; cerebellar atrophy results; progressive cerebellar signs; responds to acetazolamide
Ataxia telangiectasia (autosomal recessive)	11q22-q23; ATM gene for regulation of cell cycle. Mitogenic signal transduction, and meiotic recombination	Telangiectasia, ataxia, dysarthria, pulmonary infections, neoplasms of lymphatic system; IgA and IgG deficiencies; diabetes mellitus, breast cancer
Infantile-onset spinocerebellar ataxia of Nikali et al (autosomal recessive)	10q23.3-q24.1	Infantile ataxia, sensory neuropathy; athetosis, hearing deficit, ophthalmoplegia, optic atrophy; primary hypogonadism in females
Hypoceruloplasminemia with ataxia & dysarthria (autosomal recessive)	Ceruloplasmin gene; 3q23-q25 (trp 858 ter)	Gait ataxia and dysarthria; hyperreflexia; cerebellar atrophy by MRI; iron deposition in cerebellum, basal ganglia; thalamus and liver; onset in the 4th decade
Spinocerebellar ataxia with neuropathy (SCA1) (autosomal recessive)	Tyrosyl-DNA phosphodiesterase-1 (TDP-1) 14q31-q32	Onset in 2nd decade; gait ataxia; dysarthria; seizures; cerebellar vermis atrophy on MRI, dysmetria

ataxia currently includes SCA types 1 through 22, as well as dentatorubropallidoluysian atrophy (DRPLA), and episodic ataxia (EA) types 1 and 2 (EA-1 and EA-2).[1]

SCA1. SCA1 was the first genetic locus identified for a dominantly inherited ataxia. Although SCA1 is not as common as several other SCAs, studies of this disease continue to advance our understanding of the entire class of glutamine-repeat diseases to which it belongs.

Symptoms and Signs. The clinical syndrome of SCA1 is typically characterized by the development in adult or late middle life of progressive cerebellar ataxia of the trunk and limbs, impairment of equilibrium and gait, slowness of voluntary movements, scanning speech, nystagmoid jerks, and tremor of the head and trunk. Dysarthria and dysphagia usually develop in most patients during the course of the illness and oculomotor and facial palsies may also occur. Rarely, extrapyramidal symptoms may include rigidity, immobile facies, and parkinsonian tremor. We think Parkinsonism is rather rare in this disease, unlike SCA3/Machado-Joseph disease. The reflexes are usually normal, but knee and ankle jerks may be lost, and extensor plantar responses may occur. Dementia may occur but is usually mild. Impairment of sphincter function is common, with urinary and, sometimes, fecal incontinence. Cerebellar and brain stem atrophy are evident on MRI in affected individuals (Fig. 35–1).

Marked shrinkage of the ventral half of the pons, disappearance of the olivary eminence on the ventral surface of the medulla, and atrophy of the cerebellum are evident

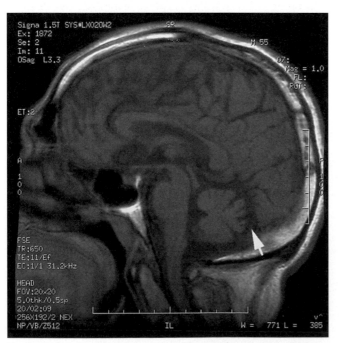

FIGURE 35–1. Sagittal MRI of the brain of a 60-year-old man with SCA1 showing cerebellar and brain stem atrophy.

on gross post-mortem inspection of the brain. Variable loss of Purkinje cells, reduction in the number of cells in the molecular and granular layer, demyelination of the middle cerebellar peduncle, and the cerebellar hemispheres, and severe loss of cells in the pontine nuclei and olives are found on histologic examination. Degenerative changes in the striatum, especially the putamen, and loss of the pigmented cells of the substantia nigra may be found in cases with extrapyramidal features. More widespread degeneration in the central nervous system (CNS), including involvement of the posterior columns and the spinocerebellar fibers, is often present, especially in the cases with autosomal dominant inheritance.

Genetics. SCA1 was the first genetically defined SCA. In 1993, Drs. Orr, Zoghbi, and colleagues determined that SCA1 is due to a CAG repeat expansion in the *SCA1* gene on chromosome 6 (6p22-p23).[6] The mutant allele has a CAG repeat of 39 or more repeats in length, whereas alleles from control subjects have 6 to 44 repeats. Disease causing expanded repeats are pure, uninterrupted CAG repeats, whereas normal alleles greater than 20 repeats in length are interrupted by one or more CAT repeat units that encode histidine instead of glutamine. There is a direct correlation between increasingly large repeat sizes and younger age of onset for SCA1, with juvenile onset cases having the highest repeat numbers. Anticipation is frequently present in subsequent generations owing to further expansion of disease repeats on transmission. The CAG repeat lies in the protein coding portion of the gene, in frame to encode a pure stretch of glutamine in the disease protein, hence the term *glutamine-repeat* or *polyglutamine* diseases. The SCA1 disease protein, ataxin-1, is a novel nuclear protein of unknown function. Ubiquinated, intranuclear inclusions containing the disease protein have been described in neurons of select brain regions, including the pons and dentate nucleus of the cerebellum.[4] Studies led by Drs. Zoghbi and Orr have shed light on many molecular features of SCA1 and other polyglutamine diseases. As discussed later, pathogenesis seems to be mediated by a novel toxic property of the disease protein that requires nuclear localization. Although the details of pathogenesis are still being defined, increasing evidence implicates protein misfolding in the pathogenesis of this and other polyglutamine diseases.

SCA2: Symptoms and Signs. A second clinical phenotype, SCA2, was initially described in a large Cuban population that may represent the largest homogeneous group of ataxic patients described. Since the discovery of its genetic defect, SCA2 has been found to be one of the more common forms of ataxia in the United States. The age of onset ranges from 2 to 65 years, and there is considerable clinical variability within various families. The most common features are ataxia, dysarthria, slow saccades, neuropathy, and relatively little corticospinal or extrapyramidal involvement. Dementia and facial myokymia are also relatively common.[1]

SCA2: Genetics. After the SCA2 locus was mapped to chromosome 12, three separate groups identified the disease gene. The mutation proved to be an expanded CAG repeat that encodes polyglutamine in the disease protein, ataxin-2. Normal alleles contain 15 to 32 repeats, whereas mutant alleles have 35 to 77 repeats. There is a zone of reduced penetrance (32 to 34 repeats) within which not all individuals will develop signs of disease in a normal life span. Occasionally, sporadic cases of SCA2 are identified with no family history. In such cases, an intermediate-sized allele from an asymptomatic parent presumably underwent further expansion when transmitted to the affected individual.[1]

SCA3/Machado-Joseph Disease. SCA3/MJD was first described among the Portuguese and their descendants in New England and California. Subsequently, SCA3/MJD has been found in families from Portugal, Australia, Brazil, Canada, China, England, France, India, Israel, Italy, Japan, Spain, Taiwan, and the United States. In many populations, it is the most common autosomal dominant ataxia.[1]

Symptoms and Signs. The phenotypic spectrum in SCA3/MJD is remarkably broad, ranging from early-onset dystonia to late-onset ataxia with neuropathy. This broad spectrum has led some to classify SCA3/MJD into three clinical types. In type 1 SCA3/MJD (amyotrophic lateral sclerosis-parkinsonism-dystonia type), neurologic deficits appear in the first two decades and involve weakness and spasticity of extremities, especially the legs, often with dystonia of the face, neck, trunk, and extremities. Patellar and ankle clonus are common, as are extensor plantar responses. The gait is more spastic than ataxic—slow and stiff, with a slightly broadened base and lurching from side to side. Pharyngeal weakness and spasticity cause difficulty with speech and swallowing. Ophthalmoparesis, ocular prominence, and facial and lingual fasciculations are common and early manifestations. In type 2 SCA3/MJD (ataxic type), which is the most common form of disease, signs and symptoms begin in the second to fourth decade. True cerebellar deficits predominate, including dysarthria, gait and extremity ataxia, along with corticospinal and extrapyramidal deficits of spasticity, rigidity, and dystonia. Ophthalmoparesis, upward vertical gaze deficits, and facial and lingual fasciculations are also commonly present. Type 3 SCA3/MJD (ataxic-amyotrophic type) occurs in the fifth to the seventh decade with a cerebellar disorder that includes dysarthria, gait, and extremity ataxia. Distal sensory loss involving pain, touch, vibration, and position senses and distal atrophy are prominent, indicating the presence of peripheral neuropathy. The deep tendon reflexes are depressed to absent, and no corticospinal or extrapyramidal findings occur. Neurologic deficits progress and lead to death from debilitation within 15 years of onset, especially in patients with types 1 and 2 disease. Usually, patients retain full intellectual function.

The major pathologic findings are variable loss of neurons and glial replacement in the corpus striatum and severe loss in the zona compacta portion of the substantia nigra. A moderate loss of neurons occurs in the dentate nucleus of the cerebellum, the red nucleus, and cranial nerve motor nuclei. Purkinje cell loss and granule cell loss are found in the cerebellar cortex. Relative sparing of the inferior olives distinguishes SCA3/MJD from several other dominantly inherited ataxias.[4a,4b]

Genetics. In 1994, Kawaguchi and colleagues identified the mutation in SCA3/MJD as a CAG repeat expansion in the *MJD1* gene on chromosome 14.[5] Soon afterward, the genetic defect in what had been thought to be a separate dominant ataxia, SCA3, was found to be the same mutation. Hence SCA3 and SCA3/MJD are genotypically the same disorder. The CAG repeat in normal control subjects is between 12 and 40 CAG repeats, and is expanded in disease to between 60 to 84 CAG repeats. The expanded CAG repeat encodes an expanded polyglutamine tract in the disease protein, ataxin-3, and earlier age of onset is associated with longer repeats. In diseased brain, aggregates of ataxin-3 have been observed in neuronal nuclei in the pons, midbrain, and other regions undergoing neuropathologic degeneration.[1,6,7]

SCA4. A single family with progressive ataxia, pyramidal tract deficits, and prominent sensory axonal neuropathy has been described in which the trait has autosomal dominant transmission and is mapped to chromosome 16q24-ter.[1]

SCA5. Another family is reported that has two major branches, both descended from the paternal grandparents of Abraham Lincoln, in which dominantly inherited, relatively pure cerebellar ataxia (SCA5) is mapped to chromosome 11.[1]

SCA6. Along with SCA2 and SCA3/MJD, SCA6 represents one of the more common dominantly inherited ataxias. It is a milder, later onset disease characterized by slowly progressive ataxia, dysarthria, nystagmus, and sensory loss. In some cases, SCA6 occurs sporadically with no family history of similar disease. SCA6 is caused by a relatively small CAG repeat expansion (21 to 30 triplets in patients; 3 to 17 triplets in normal subjects) in an α_{1a} voltage-dependent calcium channel subunit gene (CACNAIA4) on chromosome 19p13.2. Interestingly, other mutations in the same gene cause two additional neurologic disorders. Episodic ataxia type 2 (EA-2) is usually caused by nonsense mutations resulting in truncation of the channel protein. A few missense mutations in CACNAIA4 have also been reported in EA-2. More commonly, however, missense mutations in the CACNAIA4 gene result in a different disease, familial hemiplegic migraine. Some patients with familial hemiplegic migraine also develop progressive ataxia with cerebellar atrophy.[8]

SCA7. This autosomal dominant ataxia is distinguished from all other SCAs by the presence of retinal pigmentary degeneration. The visual abnormalities first appear as blue-yellow color blindness and proceed to frank visual loss with macular degeneration. In almost all other respects, SCA7 resembles several other SCAs in which ataxia is accompanied by various noncerebellar findings, including ophthalmoparesis and extensor plantar responses. The genetic defect is an expanded CAG repeat in the SCA7 gene, which maps to 3p14.1-p21.1. Repeats on normal alleles contain 4 to 19 CAG repeats, and disease alleles range from 37 to greater than 200 CAG repeats. The expanded repeat size in SCA7 is highly variable. Consistent with this, the severity of clinical findings varies from essentially asymptomatic to mild late-onset symptoms to severe, aggressive disease in childhood with rapid progression. Marked anticipation has been recorded, especially with paternal transmission. The disease protein, ataxin-7, forms aggregates in nuclei of affected neurons, as has also been described for SCA1 and MJD/SCA3.[9–11]

SCA8. This form of ataxia is caused by a CTG repeat expansion in an untranslated region of a gene on chromosome 13q21. There is marked maternal bias in transmission, perhaps reflecting contractions of the repeat during spermatogenesis. Normal CTG alleles are between 16 and 37 repeats and affected alleles are more than 80 repeats (usually between 107 and 127). The mutation is not fully penetrant as there are some individuals with very large expansions who do not develop disease. Symptoms include dysarthria and gait ataxia beginning about age 40 years with a range between 20 and 65 years. Other features include nystagmus, leg spasticity, and reduced vibratory sensation. Patients have slowly progressive disease but severely affected individuals are nonambulatory by the fourth to sixth decade. MRI shows cerebellar atrophy consistent with the clinical features.[12] The molecular mechanism of disease is not known but may involve a dominant "toxic" effect occurring at the RNA level, as occurs in myotonic dystrophy.

SCA10. This form of ataxia has been reported in families of Mexican origin. It occurs with gait ataxia, dysarthria, and nystagmus. Partial complex and generalized motor seizures occur in a segment of affected patients.[13] The genetic defect in SCA10 was discovered to be a new type of dynamic repeat expansion, an extremely large expansion of a pentanucleotide repeat (ATTCT) in an intron of the SCA10 gene. The mechanism of pathogenesis of this novel expansion is uncertain.

SCA11. Two British families have been described with a relatively benign, slowly progressive form of gait and limb ataxia that maps to chromosome 15q14-q21.3. This SCA represents a relatively "pure" cerebellar syndrome with mild pyramidal signs. The mean age at onset is roughly 25 with a normal life expectancy.[14]

SCA12. Two families have been described with this autosomal dominant ataxia. Patients develop a syndrome—between ages 8 and 55 years—of extremity tremor, hyperreflexia, decreased movement, ophthalmoparesis, focal dystonia, dysautonomia, gait ataxia, and dementia. Cerebellar and cerebral atrophy are present on MRI studies. The disease is linked to a CAG repeat expansion in the 5′ untranslated region of a gene at 5q32 that encodes a regulatory subunit for the protein phosphatase 2A. The repeat is 7 to 28 triplets in length in control subjects and greater than 65 repeats in patients. The mechanism of pathogenesis is uncertain.[15]

SCA13 and SCA14. These both map to chromosome 19q, and each represents a progressive autosomal dominant ataxia in a single family. The genetic basis for disease has not been found.[16]

SCA15. This is an autosomal dominant, progressive pure ataxia described in an Australian family in whom known loci have been excluded.[16]

SCA16. This is a slowly progressive dominant cerebellar ataxia occurring in a four-generation Japanese family between ages 20 and 66 years. One third of the patients had a head tremor. Dysarthria, horizontal gaze-evoked nystagmus, and impaired smooth movement of the eyes were also present in some patients. Linkage analysis suggested linkage to a locus on chromosome 8q22.1-q24.1.[17]

SCA17. Nakamura and colleagues described four Japanese pedigrees with an autosomal dominant cerebellar ataxia caused by an abnormal CAG expansion in the TATA-binding protein (TBP) gene (6q27), a general transcription initiation factor. The abnormal expansion of glutamine tracts in TBP has 47 to 55 CAG repeats, whereas the normal repeat number ranges from 29 to 42. A postmortem brain with 48 CAG repeats had neuronal intranuclear inclusion bodies that stained with anti-ubiquitin antibody, anti-TBP antibody, and with IC2 antibody that recognizes specifically expanded pathologic polyglutamine tracts. Age at onset ranged from 19 to 48 years. An inverse correlation was noted between age at onset and the number of CAG repeats in the TBP gene. Most patients presented in the third decade with gait ataxia and dementia progressing over decades to produce bradykinesia, dysmetria, dysdiadochokinesia, hyperreflexia and reduced motor movements. Parkinsonian features in some patients included bradykinesia, shuffling gait, postural reflex disturbance (retropulsion), tremor, and rigidity. Dystonia and chorea were noted in some patients. Seizures were present in some patients as well. Eye movements were normal. MRI findings included cerebral and cerebellar atrophy.[18]

SCA18: Sensory-Motor Ataxia with Neuropathy. This phenotype includes autosomal dominant spinocerebellar ataxia present in a five-generation American family of Irish ancestry with variable expressivity and severity of symptoms, including sensory loss, pyramidal tract signs, and muscle weakness. Onset was in the second decade of life and was slowly progressive. Gait ataxia, dysmetria, and nystagmus were present in all affected patients. Nerve conduction studies were consistent with a sensory axonal neuropathy. A muscle biopsy showed neurogenic atrophy, and brain MRI showed mild cerebellar atrophy. It links to ch 7q22-q32.[18a] It is a phenotype that comprises ataxia (SCA) and hereditary motor/sensory neuropathy (HMSN).

SCA19. This syndrome was described in a Dutch family as autosomal dominant with onset between ages 20 and 45 years. Gait ataxia, nystagmus, postural tremor, cognitive impairment, myoclonus, and sensory neuropathy are the typical clinical features. MRI shows marked atrophy of the cerebellar hemispheres with mild vermal and cerebral atrophy. It maps to ch 1p21-q21.

SCA20. This phenotype is assigned but not yet published.

SCA21. A four-generation French family is described with dominantly inherited gait and limb ataxia, akinesia, hyporeflexia, and mild cognitive impairment. The average age at onset was 17 years; age ranged from 6 to 30 years. Several patients had prominent extrapyramidal features. It links to 7p21.3-p15.1.[18b]

SCA22. This phenotype is assigned but not yet published.

Dentatorubropallidoluysian Atrophy (DRPLA). DRPLA is a disorder of variable clinical presentation that is characterized by progressive ataxia, choreoathetosis, dystonia, seizures, myoclonus, and dementia. DRPLA is due to a CAG triplet repeat expansion in the DRPLA gene, encoding atrophin on chromosome 12p12-ter. As in other CAG repeat diseases, larger expansions at the DRPLA locus cause more severe disease, manifesting earlier in life, and anticipation occurs particularly with paternal transmission. The number of repeats is greater than or equal to 49 in patients with DRPLA, and less than or equal to 26 in control individuals. It is most prevalent in Japan and rare in the United States. One well characterized family in North Carolina has a phenotypic variant known as the Haw River Syndrome, formerly thought to be a separate disease and now recognized to be caused by the DRPLA mutation.[1]

Episodic Ataxia Types 1 and 2. These rare, dominant disorders are caused by mutations in a voltage-gated potassium and calcium channel, respectively. In EA-1, which is due to mutations in the KCNA1 gene on 12p13, patients typically have brief episodes of ataxia lasting only minutes, in some cases precipitated by sudden change in posture, stress, or exercise. Myokymia is a common feature of EA-1. In EA-2, which is due to mutations in the CACNAIA4 gene on 19p13 (and thus is allelic with SCA6 and familial hemiplegic migraine), patients have episodes of ataxia that can last for hours or days, often precipitated by stress, exercise, or fatigue. Acetazolamide may be therapeutic for either episodic ataxia, but particularly for EA-2.[1,8]

Autosomal Recessive Ataxias

Friedreich Ataxia. This is the most common form of inherited ataxia, constituting about one-half of all hereditary ataxia. It is an autosomal recessive disorder, typically characterized by ataxia and lower limb areflexia beginning in late childhood. Since the discovery of the underlying genetic defect, however, it has become clear that FA also manifests as an "atypical" adult onset form that differs in many respects from the "classic" presentation.

Symptoms and Signs. Friedreich ataxia classically occurs before 25 years of age with progressive ataxic gait and titubation. The lower extremities are more severely involved than are the upper ones. Patients occasionally present with symptoms of dysarthria. Progressive scoliosis, foot deformity, nystagmus, or cardiopathy are rarely initial signs.[19]

In classic FA, the neurologic examination reveals nystagmus and square wave jerks, slowing of saccadic eye movements, truncal titubation, dysarthria, dysmetria, and gait and limb ataxia. Extensor plantar responses (with normal tone in trunk and extremities), absent deep tendon reflexes in the legs, and weakness (greater distally than proximally) are usually found. Loss of vibratory and proprioceptive sensation occurs. The median age of death is approximately 35 years.

Cardiac involvement occurs in 90% of patients with classic Friedreich ataxia. Cardiomegaly, symmetrical hypertrophy, murmurs, and conduction defects are reported. Moderate mental retardation or psychiatric syndromes are present in a small percentage of patients. An unusually high incidence of diabetes (20%) is found and is associated with insulin resistance, pancreatic beta-cell dysfunction, and type 1 diabetes. Musculoskeletal deformities are common and include pes cavus, pes equinovarus, and scoliosis. MRI of the spinal cord shows significant cord atrophy in affected patients (Fig. 35–2).

Onset before age 25 years was once a hallmark of FA. Now, however, genetic testing shows that "atypical" adult onset disease is not uncommon, accounting for perhaps as many as one-fourth of patients. Adult onset disease is less severe, progresses more slowly, and is less frequently accompanied by foot deformities, muscle wasting, areflexia, and cardiomyopathy. In any adult with unexplained progressive ataxia, FA should be among the first diseases considered in the differential diagnosis.[19,20]

The primary site of pathology is the spinal cord, dorsal root ganglion cells, and the peripheral nerves. Sclerosis and degeneration are seen predominantly in the spinocerebellar tracts, lateral corticospinal tracts, and posterior columns. Degeneration of the glossopharyngeal, vagus, hypoglossal, and deep cerebellar nuclei is described. Slight atrophy of the cerebellum and cerebral gyri may occur. The cerebral cortex is histologically normal except for loss of Betz cells in the precentral gyri.

Peripheral nerves are extensively involved, with a loss of large myelinated fibers. The density of small myelinated fibers is normal, but axonal size and myelin thickness are diminished.

Cardiac pathology consists of myocytic hypertrophy and fibrosis, focal vascular fibromuscular dysplasia with subintimal or medial deposition of periodic acid-Schiff (PAS)–positive material, myocytopathy with unusual pleomorphic nuclei, and focal degeneration of myelinated and unmyelinated nerves and cardiac ganglia.

Genetics. All cases of FA are due to mutations in the *FRDA* gene on chromosome 9q13-q21. In more than 95% of patients, the mutation is an expanded GAA triplet repeat occurring in the first intron of the *FRDA* gene and present on both alleles. In other words, most patients are homozygous for the expansion. A few patients, however, are compound heterozygotes, having an expansion in one allele and a point mutation or deletion in the second allele. Normal alleles have 7 to 34 GAA repeats and disease alleles have 120 to approximately 1700 GAA repeats. Patients with FA have very low levels of frataxin mRNA and protein, and thus the fundamental problem in this disease seems to be reduced frataxin expression. Frataxin is an essential, iron-binding mitochondrial protein involved in iron homeostasis. Studies of disease tissue have confirmed a deficiency in iron/sulfur cluster-containing mitochondrial enzymes, decreased mitochondrial ATP production, and accumulation of iron in heart. Thus, FA can be thought of as a mitochondrial disorder in which iron-mediated oxidative stress likely plays an important role in pathogenesis.[19,21]

Genetic Causes of Vitamin E Deficiency

Classic FA must be compared and contrasted with the similar ataxic presentation associated with vitamin E

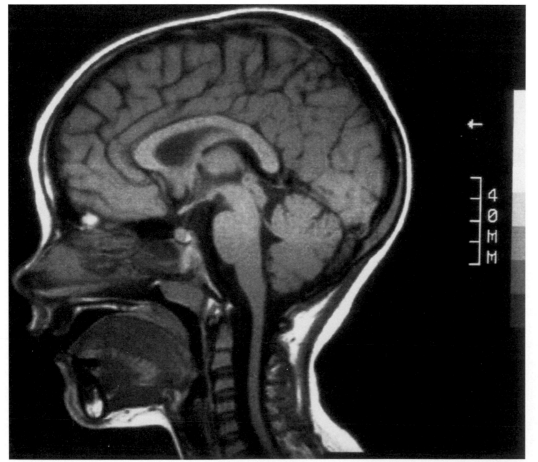

FIGURE 35–2. Sagittal MRI of the brain and spinal cord showing significant spinal cord atrophy in a 6-year-old girl with Friedreich ataxia.

deficiency. Two forms of recessively inherited ataxia associated with abnormalities in vitamin E (α-tocopherol) have been identified: *Ataxia with vitamin E deficiency* (AVED), and *abetalipoproteinemia* (Bassen-Kornzweig syndrome). The clinical features of AVED are indistinguishable from those of classic FA, but the presence of retinopathy helps to distinguish abetalipoproteinemia from FA. AVED is due to mutations in the gene for α-tocopherol transfer protein (α-TTP) on chromosome 8 (8q13). These patients have an impaired ability to incorporate vitamin E into the VLDL produced and secreted by the liver, resulting in a deficiency of vitamin E in peripheral tissues. Abetalipoproteinemia is caused by mutations in the gene coding for a subunit of the microsomal triglyceride transfer protein (MTP). Defects in MTP result in impaired formation and secretion of VLDL in the liver. This defect results in deficient delivery of vitamin E to tissues, including the nervous system, as VLDL is the transport molecule for vitamin E and other fat-soluble substitutes. Hence, either impaired incorporation of vitamin E into VLDL (AVED) or the absence of VLDL (abetalipoproteinemia) causes an ataxic syndrome similar to FA.[22,23] *Marinesco-Sjögren syndrome* is another rare disorder in which progressive cerebellar deficits can occur in association with other features (cataracts, mental retardation, multiple skeletal abnormalities, hypogonadotropic hypogonadism). The genetic basis is unknown, but a study raises the possibility that the underlying biochemical defect also leads to severe vitamin E deficiency.[24]

Ataxia Telangiectasia (AT).　Though much less common than Friedreich ataxia, this recessively inherited ataxia has received considerable attention because of its association with cancer.

Symptoms and Signs.　Patients usually present in the first decade of life with progressive telangiectatic lesions associated with cerebellar ataxia and nystagmus. The neurologic manifestations are similar to those seen in FA except that extrapyramidal features (including myoclonic jerks, dystonia, and athetosis) are more common and areflexia is less common. There is a high incidence of recurrent pulmonary infections and neoplasms of the lymphatic and reticuloendothelial system in patients with AT. Lymphomas, Hodgkin disease, and acute leukemias are the most common cancers. Chromosomal translocations occur frequently, particularly between chromosomes 7 and 14. Thymic hypoplasia with cellular and humoral immunodeficiencies (particularly IgA and IgG2), premature aging, and endocrine disorders, such as insulin-dependent diabetes mellitus, are also described. Elevated levels of alpha-fetoprotein and carcinoembryonic antigen are useful markers of disease. Fibroblasts can be screened for increased x-ray sensitivity and radioresistant DNA synthesis, two hallmarks of AT. The mean age of death is

approximately 20 years, usually from infection or cancer. There may also be an increased incidence of breast cancer in women who are ATM heterozygotes, though the data on this point are still controversial.

The most striking neuropathologic changes include loss of Purkinje, granule, and basket cells in the cerebellar cortex and of neurons in the deep cerebellar nuclei. The inferior olives of the medulla also may have neuronal loss. There is a loss of anterior horn neurons in the spinal cord and of dorsal root ganglion cells associated with posterior column spinal cord demyelination. A poorly developed or absent thymus gland is the most consistent defect of the lymphoid system.

Genetics.　More than 200 mutations have been found in the *ATM* gene (ataxia-telangiectasia, mutated) on chromosome 11, broadly distributed throughout the gene. Most mutations that cause AT are null mutations; rarer mutations that act in a dominant negative manner may be especially prone to predispose heterozygous carriers to cancer. The *ATM* gene encodes a large protein kinase (3056 amino acids) that is homologous to cell cycle checkpoint genes in other organisms. Evidence from cellular studies and knockout mice indicates that the ATM protein serves as a regulator of the cell cycle checkpoint in response to double strand breaks in DNA. By phosphorylating various cell cycle proteins, DNA repair proteins and kinases, ATM controls signaling pathways activated during genotoxic stress.[25,26]

Autosomal Recessive Spastic Ataxia.　Autosomal recessive spastic ataxia (ARSACS) has been reported in the Charlevoix-Saguenay region of Quebec. This childhood onset, progressive ataxia is also characterized by spasticity, dysarthria, distal muscle wasting, foot deformities, truncal ataxia, absence of somatosensory evoked potentials in the lower limb, retinal striations visible on funduscopic examination, and the frequent presence of mitral valve prolapse. ARSACS is caused by a mutation in the *SACS* gene on chromosome 13, resulting in loss of expression of the novel disease protein, sacsin.[27] A similar-appearing inherited spastic ataxia in a Tunisian family maps to the same region of chromosome 13, raising the possibility that these two ataxias may be caused by different mutations in the same gene.[28] Troyer syndrome, another spastic ataxia that resembles ARSACS, has been shown to be due to mutations in the *SPG20* gene encoding spastin.

Mitochondrial Ataxias.　Spinocerebellar syndromes have been identified with mutations in mitochondrial DNA (mtDNA). More than 30 pathogenic mtDNA point mutations and more than 60 different types of mtDNA deletions are known, and several of these mutations cause or are associated with ataxia.

Xeroderma Pigmentosum.　Xeroderma pigmentosum is a rare autosomal recessive neurocutaneous disorder caused by mutatons in enzymes necessary for nucleotide excision DNA repair. In addition to skin lesions, patients may show progressive mental deterioration, microcephaly, ataxia, spasticity, choreoathetosis, and hypogonadism. Nerve deafness, peripheral neuropathy (predominantly axonal), electroencephalographic abnormalities, and seizures are reported. Neuronal death is noted in pyramidal cells, cerebellar Purkinje cells, the deep nuclei of the cerebellum, the brain stem, the spinal cord, and peripheral nerves.

Cockayne Syndrome.   This is a rare autosomal recessive disorder first described by Cockayne in 1936. Like xeroderma pigmentosum, Cockayne syndrome is due to mutations in enzymes of nucleotide excision repair. Clinical features are mental retardation, optic atrophy, dwarfism, neural deafness, hypersensitivity of skin to sunlight, cataracts, and retinal pigmentary degeneration. Cerebellar, pyramidal, and extrapyramidal deficits and peripheral neuropathy may occur, with bird-headed facies and normal-pressure hydrocephalus. Skin fibroblasts show defective DNA repair when exposed to ultraviolet light.[29]

Spinocerebellar Ataxia and Axonal Neuropathy. Spinocerebellar ataxia with axonal neuropathy (SCAN1) has been described with autosomal recessive inheritance. It is caused by a homozygous mutation in tyrosol DNA phosphodiesterase 1 (TDP1) that results in the substitution of histidine 493 with an arginine residue. Loss-of-function mutations in TDP1 may cause SCAN1 either by interfering with DNA transcription or by inducing apoptosis in postmitotic neurons. Affected persons had gait ataxia, cerebellar vermis atrophy on MRI, axonal neuropathy, and normal intelligence. Onset of symptoms occurred in the second decade of life in a Saudi Arabian family. This phenotype maps to 14q31-q32.[29a]

Molecular Genetics

DNA repeat expansions are a common cause of hereditary ataxia.   The classification of hereditary ataxias was formerly confusing because of the highly variable pheno-

type. Even in the same family, age of onset and disease severity can vary widely. Further confounding attempts at classification was the fact that many late-onset ataxias show anticipation, the tendency for disease to manifest earlier in successive generations. These unusual clinical features are now explained by the particular type of genetic defect underlying most late-onset ataxias: dynamic expansions of DNA repeats within specific disease genes.

DNA repeat expansions as the cause of human disease were first noted in 1991.[30] Yet it is already clear that they represent a major cause of hereditary neurologic disorders.[31] At least 18 diseases—all neurologic—are known to be caused by dynamic repeat expansions (Fig. 35–3). Most often these are trinucleotide repeat expansions, but tetranucleotide, pentanucleotide, and dodecanucleotide repeats have also been reported.[32,33] The mechanism by which expanded repeats cause disease differs, depending on at least three key points: the sequence of the repeat, the nature of the gene, and the place in the gene where the expansion resides. Several repeat expansions fall outside the protein coding region of the gene and cause disease by reducing gene expression (fragile X syndromes and FA) or through an RNA-based effect (myotonic dystrophy types 1 and 2; possibly SCA8). However, the greatest number of repeat expansion diseases, including many SCAs, are caused by a CAG repeat that codes for expanded polyglutamine in the disease protein.[6,34] To date, this group includes six dominantly inherited spinocerebellar ataxias (SCA types 1, 2, 3, 6, 7, and 17) as well as DRPLA, Huntington disease (HD), and spinobulbar muscular atrophy (SBMA).

The discovery of dynamic repeat expansions has important ramifications for both the clinician and the patient. Particular inherited ataxias can now be diagnosed by simple, sensitive, and specific genetic tests that are commercially available. A positive test result carries profound implications for the patient and his or her family. Thus, genetic testing should be performed only after the patient has been counseled on the potential consequences of the results, both positive and negative. Because currently there are no proven therapies for any hereditary ataxia, the only clear benefit of testing for the

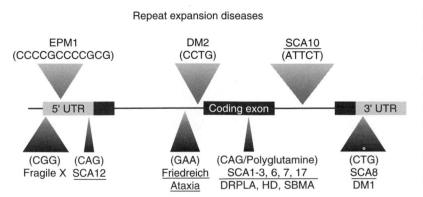

Repeat expansion diseases

FIGURE 35–3. Shown is a schematic of a gene indicating the diseases and repeat sequence and location within the gene. All but one CAG repeat (SCA12) are in the protein-coding region, encoding polyglutamine in the disease protein. All other repeats are untranslated and cause disease through several different mechanisms at the transcriptional or post-transcriptional level. Hereditary ataxias are underlined. (DM1, DM2 = myotonic dystrophies, types 1 and 2, EPM1 = progressive myoclonic epilepsy of Unverricht Lundborg.)

patient and his or her family is obtaining the knowledge that their disease is a particular genetic ataxia. Genetic testing is a highly personal decision that the patient must reach without undue pressure from the physician; in the absence of a definitive therapy, many patients forego testing. In families in whom the genetic cause has already been identified, presymptomatic testing of at-risk individuals should be undertaken only after appropriate genetic counseling.

General Features of Polyglutamine Neurodegenerative Disease

The polyglutamine diseases have generated excitement because of their similarity to more common neurodegenerative diseases, such as Alzheimer and Parkinson disease, in which abnormal protein folding or accumulation also seems to play an important role in pathogenesis. Several shared features (discussed subsequently) of polyglutamine diseases, discussed subsequently, provide insight into the underlying biology.

All are progressive neurodegenerative diseases. The inexorable progression of clinical signs probably reflects both an increasing physiological dysfunction of "sick" neurons and, later on, the frank loss of neurons through cell death. In each disease, selective neurotoxicity and regional brain vulnerability occur, despite the fact that the disease proteins are expressed widely in the brain and elsewhere in the body. Why are neurons especially vulnerable? Modifying factors must exist that make neurons more susceptible than other cell types, including their long-lived, postmitotic state, high metabolic demands, and the stress of recurrent ion fluxes during depolarization.

Longer repeats cause more severe disease. Each disease shows a strong inverse correlation between repeat length and age of onset: the longer the repeat, the earlier the disease. Repeat length accounts for roughly 70% of the variability in age of onset, differing slightly for each disease. Clearly, the toxicity of CAG/polyglutamine must increase with greater repeat lengths. Moreover, most polyglutamine diseases conform to a similar threshold length of approximately 35 repeats, beyond which repeats undergo a transition from normal to pathogenic. One notable exception is SCA6, in which repeats as short as 21 can cause disease. Taken together, these facts suggest that a glutamine repeat of approximately 35 or more is increasingly prone to undergo a toxic conformational change. Yet the probability that this conformational change and its deleterious consequences will occur must be influenced by the protein context in which expanded polyglutamine resides. In other words, even though different expanded polyglutamine tracts behave similarly, they are not identical. The relative "toxicity" depends significantly on the protein context, which differs for each protein. Indeed, despite the shared features among poly-

glutamine diseases, the various mutant proteins are entirely dissimilar and there is no evidence that they serve related cellular functions.

Most are pure dominant disorders. The polyglutamine diseases are autosomal dominant diseases, except SBMA, which, as an X-linked disorder involving the male hormone receptor, may be a special case. Data from patients and from transgenic models demonstrate that a single mutant allele is sufficient to cause disease. The very rare, homozygous patient will develop disease similar to that of heterozygotes except that onset may be earlier. This has been shown in a few SCA3/MJD and SCA6 patients. Yet there is renewed interest in the possibility that the dominant toxic effect also may result in a loss of the *normal* function of the disease gene.[35,36] This loss of normal function could occur if the mutant protein adopted a conformation that makes the protein nonfunctional or depletes the cell of *normal* protein by sequestering it in aggregates.

Clinical anticipation is common. Expanded CAG repeats are "dynamic" mutations that tend to change size when passed from one generation to the next, with further expansions occurring more commonly than contractions. This trend toward further expansion, coupled with the fact that longer repeats cause more severe disease, explains the phenomenon of anticipation. In most polyglutamine diseases, paternal transmission is more likely than maternal transmission to lead to further expansion. Thus, juvenile onset patients are more likely to have inherited the mutant allele from their father.

Phenotype can vary greatly. The highly variable size of expanded repeats explains the marked variability in phenotype. SCA3/MJD illustrates this point particularly well. This disease most commonly manifests as a progressive ataxia in young adults, but can also occur as dystonia in younger-onset patients (typically with longer repeats), or as parkinsonism or sensorimotor neuropathy in older patients (typically, the shortest expansions). With the very longest expansions, the various polyglutamine diseases lose some of their unique clinicopathologic features and instead become characterized by more widespread neurodegeneration with increasing extrapyramidal signs.

The molecular mechanism is toxic gain of function at the protein level. Most evidence supports a protein-based mechanism of disease, starting with the essential fact that all polyglutamine disease proteins are expressed in the correct brain regions to cause disease. Moreover, isolated stretches of expanded polyglutamine are cytotoxic, whereas untranslated expanded CAG RNA is not. Polyglutamine expansion thus seems to confer on the disease protein a novel, dominant, toxic property. Even though the expanded polyglutamine domain may itself be the primary toxic element, its particular protein context must influence where in the brain, and to what degree, its toxicity becomes manifested.

Protein misfolding is central to pathogenesis. Many lines of evidence suggest that expanded polyglutamine adopts a novel, abnormal conformation with deleterious consequences for the neuron. In the test tube, expanded polyglutamine self-associates into amyloid-like fibrils with a repeat threshold that precisely mirrors that of disease.[37] In cell culture and animals, expanded polyglutamine proteins (and fragments derived from the full protein) have been shown to form insoluble intracellular complexes.[38] In diseased brain, the mutant proteins accumulate in intraneuronal, ubiquitinated inclusions in select neurons.[38] These inclusions most often occur in the nucleus, but in some diseases (HD, SCA2, and SCA6) they have also been observed in the cytoplasm or in neurites. Further evidence supporting a role for protein misfolding in pathogenesis is the fact that specific heat shock proteins—molecular chaperones that help maintain protein homeostasis within the cell—can suppress polyglutamine aggregation and/or toxicity in vitro and in vivo.[39–44]

A second line of evidence indicating that perturbed protein homeostasis is a key event in pathogenesis comes from studies of proteasome-mediated protein degradation. Proteasomal degradation is the major route by which cytoplasmic proteins are degraded. When the proteasome is inhibited pharmacologically or genetically, polyglutamine aggregation increases and toxicity is exacerbated, further implicating the protein quality control machinery of the cell in pathogenesis.[39,40] Moreover, aggregates of polyglutamine protein sequester the proteasome, thereby inhibiting the cell's ability to clear abnormal proteins.[45] Thus, the proteasome represents a first-line cellular defense against misfolded polyglutamine protein that, as polyglutamine protein accumulates over time, becomes less effective at clearing the abnormal protein.

Nuclear dysfunction is implicated in polyglutamine diseases. The discovery of nuclear inclusions immediately focused attention on the nucleus as a major site of pathogenesis. Even though studies have since shown that nuclear inclusions are not necessary for toxicity,[41] nuclear localization of the disease protein is clearly required for some polyglutamine diseases. Current thinking is that the mutant proteins probably engage in aberrant protein interactions in the nucleus, even before inclusion formation. Aberrant protein interactions could perturb important nuclear events, such as gene transcription, RNA splicing, or nuclear transport. Polyglutamine disease proteins, for example, bind several important transcription factors and cofactors, and thus could alter gene expression. Considerable attention has focused on the ubiquitous coactivator, CREB-binding protein (CBP). Polyglutamine proteins sequester CBP in inclusions and inhibit CBP-dependent gene expression in cellular models; conversely, overexpression of CBP mitigates polyglutamine toxicity in cellular models.[46,47] In addition,

studies of transgenic animal models have begun to identify early changes in gene expression that may contribute to pathogenesis.[48,49] Whether such gene changes are critical to the disease process or are merely secondary phenomena, still needs to be determined.

Treatment and Future Research

Currently, the only known effective therapies for hereditary ataxia are acetazolamide for episodic ataxia and vitamin E replacement for inherited vitamin E deficiencies. There are no preventive or symptomatic therapies for the progressive spinocerebellar ataxias. The task of developing therapeutics for inherited ataxias is daunting. The rarity of most of these ataxias, the diverse array of genes involved, and the fact that ataxia can occur from damage to essentially any region of the neuraxis conspire to make the development of effective therapies a tremendous challenge. Despite these difficulties, triplet repeat diseases represent promising avenues for developing therapeutics, especially for Friedreich ataxia and the polyglutamine diseases.

In Friedreich ataxia, new insights into the molecular mechanism suggest that mitochondrial dysfunction and oxidative stress are central to pathogenesis. Consistent with this, preliminary clinical trials indicate that the free-radical scavenger, idebenone, may protect heart muscle from iron-induced injury and decrease myocardial hypertrophy. Larger trials must confirm this finding before it can be recommended for patients, but the results do raise the promise of antioxidant strategies in this disease.[50] Other therapeutic strategies in FA address the fundamental problem in FA: markedly reduced levels of frataxin. Gene replacement therapy is one such approach. A second approach is to adapt antisense strategies to block the formation of a sticky DNA or triplex structures that expand GAA repeat forms and that inhibit frataxin gene expression. The creation of a conditional knockout mouse for frataxin now makes it possible to test such therapeutics in vivo.[51]

In polyglutamine diseases, the fact that they share features raises hope that a therapy may prove effective for the entire class. Progress in this field has been pushed by the development of powerful animal models of disease in mice and flies. Screens in *Drosophila* have already identified genes and cellular pathways involved in pathogenesis, including several molecular chaperones.[41,42] Thus, compounds or genes that facilitate the elimination of abnormally folded polyglutamine protein may be useful therapeutically. A second major advance has been the development of cellular and invertebrate models of disease that will permit high throughput screening for compounds that suppress aggregation, toxicity, or both. Another strategy is to inhibit caspaces, cell death proteases that carry out the apoptotic cascade. This strategy has already shown some efficacy in transgenic HD mice,[52] and could prove to be effective in humans if, as some researchers suspect, there is chronic activation of caspases in the disease state. Low-level caspase activity has been proposed to cleave mutant polyglutamine proteins into toxic, aggregation-prone fragments, thereby accelerating disease progression. Finally, RNA interference (RNAi) strategies to reduce expression of the toxic disease gene are a promising new therapeutic direction.

In the absence of established therapies, the physician's task is to identify treatable acquired diseases that can resemble inherited ataxias. Malignancies may appear with chronic progressive ataxia either directly, with a mass effect in the posterior fossa, or indirectly by paraneoplastic degeneration. Inherited and acquired vitamin E deficiency states (e.g., malabsorption syndromes) must always be considered, and serum vitamin E levels measured. Vitamin E therapy is indicated for these rare patients. Hypothyroidism may also produce ataxia. Aminoacidopathies, leukodystrophies, urea-cycle abnormalities, and mitochondrial encephalomyopathies may produce ataxia, and some dietary or metabolic therapies are available. The further identification of gene defects in ataxia and continued investigations of the molecular mechanisms will, it is hoped, lead to specific pharmacologic therapies for the remarkably diverse array of genetic diseases.

REFERENCES

1. Rosenberg RN: Ataxic disorders. In Harrison's Textbook of Medicine, 15th ed. New York, McGraw-Hill, 2001, pp 2406–2412.

2. Harding AE: Clinical features and classification of inherited ataxias. Adv Neurol 1993;61:1.

3. Orr HTM, Chung MY, Banfi S, et al: Expansion of an unstable trinucleotide CAG repeat in spinocerebellar ataxia type 1. Nat Genet 1993;4:221.

4. Klement IA, Skinner PJ, Kaytor MD, et al: Ataxin-1 nuclear localization and aggregation: Role in polyglutamine disease in SCA1 transgenic mice. Cell 1998;95:41–53.

4a. Rosenberg RN, Nyhan WL, Bay C et al: Autosomal dominant striatonigral degeneration: A clinical, pathological, and biochemical study of new genetic disorder. Neurology 1976; 26: 703–714.

4b. Rosenberg RN, Nyhan WL, Coutinho P, and Bay C: Joseph's Disease: An Autosomal dominant neurological disease in the Portuguese of the United States and the Azores Islands. In Kark RAP, Rosenberg RN and Schut L, eds. Advances in Neurology, Vol. 21. New York, Raven Press, 1978, pp 33–57.

5. Kawaguchi Y, Okamoto T, Taniwaki M, et al: CAG expansions in a novel gene for Machado-Joseph disease at chromosome 14q32.1. Nat Genet 1994;8:221.

6. Zoghbi HY, Orr HT: Glutamine repeats and neurodegeneration. Ann Rev Neurosci 2000;23: 217–247.

7. Paulson HL, Perez MK, Trottier Y, et al: Intranuclear inclusions of expanded polyglutamine protein in spinocerebellar ataxia type 3. Neuron 1997; 19: 333–344.

8. Zhuchenko O, Bailey J, Bonnen P, et al: Autosomal dominant cerebellar ataxia (SCA6) associated with small polyglutamine expansions in the α_{1a}-voltage-dependent calcium channel. Nat Genet 1997; 15:62.

9. Holmberg M, Duyckaerts C, Dürr A, et al: Spinocerebellar ataxia type 7 (SCA7): A neurodegenerative disorder with neuronal intranuclear inclusions. Human Molec Genet 1998;7:913–918.

10. Kaytor MD, Duvick LA, Skinner PJ, et al: Nuclear localization of the spinocerebellar ataxia type 7 protein, ataxin 7. Human Molec Genet 1999;8: 1657–1664.

11. David G, Abbas N, Stevanin G, et al: Cloning of the SCA7 gene reveals a highly unstable CAG repeat expansion. Nat Genet 1997;17:65–70.

12. Koob M, Mosely M, Schut L, et al: An untranslated CTG expansion causes a novel form of spinocerebellar ataxia (SCA8). Nat Genet 1999;21:379–384.

13. Matsuura T, Yamagata T, Burgess DL, et al: Large expansion of the ATTCT pentanucleotide repeat in spinocerebellar ataxia type 10. Nat Genet 2000;26: 191–194.

14. Worth, PF, Guinti P, Gardner-Thorpe C, et al: Autosomal dominant cerebellar ataxia type III: Linkage in a large British family to a 7.6 cM region on chromosome 15q14-q21.3. Am J Hum Genet 1999;65:420–426.

15. Holmes SE, O'Hearn EE, McInnis MG, et al: Expansion of a novel CAG trinucleotide repeat in the 5' region of PPP2R2B is associated with SCA12. Nat Genet 1999;23:391–392.

16. Subramony SH, Filla A: Autosomal dominant spinocerebellar ataxias ad infinitum? Neurology 2001; 56:287–289.

17. Miyoshi Y, Yamada T, Tanimura M, et al: A novel autosomal dominant spinocerebellar ataxia (SCA16) linked to chromosome 8q22.1-24.1. Neurology 2001;57:96–100.

18. Nakamura K, Jeong S-Y, Uchihara T, et al: SCA 17, a novel autosomal dominant cerebellar ataxia caused by an expanded polyglutamine in TATA binding protein. Human Molec Genet 2001;10:1441–1448.

18a. Brkanac Z, Fern M, Matsushita M, et al: Autosomal dominant sensory motor neuropathy with ataxia (SMNA). Am J Med Genet 2002;114:450–457.

18b. Vuillaume I, Devos D, Schraen-Maschke S: A new locus for spinocerebellar ataxia (SCA21) maps to chromosome 7p21.3-p15.1. Ann Neurol 2002;52:666–670.

19. Durr A, Cossee M, Agid Y, et al: Clinical and genetic abnormalities in patients with Friedreich's ataxia. N Engl J Med 1996;335:1169–1175.

20. Pandolfo M, Montermini L: Molecular genetics of the hereditary ataxias. Adv Genet 1998;38:31–68.

21. Campuzano V, Montermini L, Molto MD, et al: Friedreich's ataxia: Autosomal recessive disease caused by an intronic GAA triplet repeat expansion. Science 1996;271:1423–1427.

22. Ouahchi K, Arita M, Kayden H, et al: Ataxia with isolated vitamin E deficiency is caused by mutations in the alpha-tocopherol transfer protein. Nat Genet 1995;9:141.

23. Sharp D, Blinderman L, Combs KA, et al: Cloning and gene defects in microsomal triglyceride

transfer protein associated with abetalipoproteinaemia. Nature 1993;365:65–69.

24. Aguglia U, Annesi G, Pasquinelli G, et al: Vitamin E deficiency due to chylomicron retention disease in Marinesco-Sjogren syndrome. Ann Neurol 2000; 47:260–264.

25. Shiloh Y: ATM and ATR: Networking cellular responses to DNA damage. Curr Opin Genet Dev 2001; 11:71–77.

26. Savitsky K, Bar-Shira A, Gilad S, et al: A single ataxia telangiectasia gene with a product similar to PI-3 kinase. Science 1995;268:1749–1753.

27. Engert JC, Berube P, Mercier J, et al: ARSACS, a spastic ataxia common in northeastern Quebec, is caused by mutations in a new gene encoding an 11.5-kb ORF. Nat Genet 2000;24:120—125.

28. Mrissa N, Belal S, Ben Hamida C, et al: Linkage to chromosome 13q11-12 of an autosomal recessive cerebellar ataxia in a Tunisian family. Neurology 2000; 54:1408–1414.

29. Nance MA, Berry S: Cockayne syndrome: Review of 140 cases. Am J Med Genet 1992;42:68–84.

29a. Takashina H, Boerkoel C, John J, et al: Mutation of TDP-1 encoding a topoisomerase 1-dependent DNA damage repair enzyme in spinocerebellar ataxia with axonal neuropathy. Nat Genet 2002;32:267–272.

30. La Spada AR, Berry SA: Androgen receptor gene mutations in X-linked spinal and bulbar muscular atrophy. Nature 1991;352:77–79.

31. Cummings CJ, Zoghbi HY: Fourteen and counting: Unraveling trinucleotide repeat diseases. Hum Mol Genet 2000;9:909–916.

32. Liquori CL, Ricker K, Moseley ML, et al: Myotonic dystrophy type 2 caused by a CCTG expansion in intron 1 of ZNF9. Science 2001;293:864–867.

33. LaFreniere RG, Rochefort DL, Chrestien N, et al: Unstable insertion in the 5′ flanking region of the cystatin B gene is the most common mutation in progressive myoclonus epilepsy type 1, EPM1. Nat Genet 1997; 15(3):298–302.

34. MacDonald ME: Molecular genetics: Unmasking polyglutamine triggers in neurodegenerative disease. Nat Rev Neurosci 2000;1:109–115.

35. Cattaneo E, Rigamonti D, Goffredo D, et al: Loss of normal huntingtin function: New developments in Huntington's disease research. Trends Neurosci 2001; 24(3):182–188.

36. Zuccato C, Ciammola A, Rigamonti D, et al: Loss of huntingtin-mediated BDNF gene transcription in Huntington's disease. Science 2001;293:493–498.

37. Scherzinger E, Lurz R, Turmaine M, et al: Huntingtin-encoded polyglutamine expansions form amyloid-like protein aggregates in vitro and in vivo. Cell 1997;90:549–558.

38. Paulson HL: Protein fate in neurodegenerative proteinopathies: Polyglutamine diseases join the (mis)fold. Am J Hum Genet 1999;64:339–345.

39. Cummings CJ, Mancini MA, Antalffy B, et al: Chaperone suppression of aggregation and altered subcellular proteosome localization imply protein misfolding in SCA1. Nat Genet 1998;19:148–154.

40. Cha Y, Koppenhafer S, Shoesmith S, et al: Evidence for proteasome involvement in polyglutamine disease: Localization to nuclear inclusions in SCA3/MJD and suppression of polyglutamine aggregation in vitro. Hum Mol Genet 1999;8:673–682.

41. Warrick JM, Chan HY, Gray-Board GL, et al: Suppression of polyglutamine-mediated neurodegeneration in Drosophila by the molecular chaperone Hsp70. Nat Genet 1999;23:425–428.

42. Fernandez-Funez P, Nino-Rosales ML, De Gouyon B, et al: Identification of genes that modify ataxin-1-induced neurodegeneration. Nature 2000; 408:101–106.

43. Satyal SH, Schmidt E, Kitagawa K, et al: Polyglutamine aggregates alter protein-folding homeostasis in Caenorhabditis elegans. Proc Natl Acad Sci U S A 2000;97:5750–5755.

44. Cummings CJ, Sun Y, Opal P, et al: Overexpression of inducible HSP70 chaperone suppresses neuropathology and improves motor function in SCA1 mice. Hum Mol Genet 2001;10(14):1511–1518.

45. Bence NF, Sampat RM, Kopito RR: Impairment of the ubiquitin-proteasome system by protein aggregation. Science 2001;292:1552–1555.

46. McCampbell A, Taylor JP, Taye AA, et al: CREB-binding protein sequestration by expanded polyglutamine. Hum Mol Genet 2000;9:2197–2202.

47. Nucifora FC Jr, Sasaki M, Peters MF, et al: Interference by huntingtin and atrophin-1 with CBP-mediated transcription leading to cellular toxicity. Science 2001;291:2423–2428.

48. Luthi-Carter R, Strand A, Peters NL, et al: Decreased expression of striatal signaling genes in a mouse model of Huntington's disease. Hum Mol Genet 2000;9:1259–1271.

49. Lin X, Antalffy B, Kang D, et al: Polyglutamine expansion down-regulates specific neuronal genes before pathologic changes in SCA1. Nat Neurosci 2000; 3:157–163.

50. Rustin P, von Kleist-Retzow J-C, Chantrel-Groussard K, et al: Effect of idebenone on cardiomyopathy in Friedreich's ataxia: A preliminary study. Lancet 1999;354:477–479.

51. Puccio H, Simon D, Cossee M, et al: Mouse models for Friedreich's ataxia exhibit cardiomyopathy, sensory nerve defect and Fe-S enzyme deficiency followed by intramitochondrial iron deposits. Nat Genet 2001;27:181–186.

52. Ona VO, Li M, Vonsattel JPG, et al: Inhibition of caspase-1 slows disease progression in a mouse model of Huntington's disease. Nature 1999;399:263–267.

CHAPTER

36

Canavan Disease

Reuben Matalon
Kimberlee Michals Matalon

Spongy degeneration of the brain, Canavan disease, is an autosomal recessive leukodystrophy prevalent among individuals of Ashkenazi Jewish extraction. Clinically, severe mental retardation, developmental delays, and early death characterize Canavan disease. Urinary excretion of excessive amounts of N-acetylaspartic acid and elevated levels in brain and body fluids are the diagnostic markers of Canavan disease. Deficiency of the enzyme aspartoacylase causes the increased level of N-acetylaspartic acid.[1-3] Cloning of the gene for aspartoacylase and identification of mutations allows for reliable diagnosis. Since only two mutations are found in 99% of Jews, carrier screening is available in this ethnic group. In other ethnic groups, the mutations are different from those found in Jewish individuals. Prenatal diagnosis can be done when mutations are identified. Levels of N-acetylaspartic acid can be used for prenatal diagnosis when mutations are not known.

HISTORY

Spongy degeneration of white matter of the brain was described more than 70 years ago by Canavan, Globus, and Strauss.[4,5] Van Bogaert and Bertrand in 1949 recognized Canavan disease as a new entity.[6] It became clear that Canavan disease has an autosomal recessive mode of inheritance with high prevalence among Ashkenazi Jews.[7-17]

Elevated N-acetylaspartic acid in the urine and the deficiency of aspartoacylase in cultured skin fibroblasts were described by Matalon et al. in 1988.[1,3] N-Acetylaspartic aciduria and the deficiency of aspartoacylase in Canavan disease have been confirmed by other groups.[18-25]

The incidence of Canavan disease is about 1:6,000 to 1:13,000 in Ashkenazi Jews and less frequent in other ethnic groups.

BASIC DEFECT

Aspartoacylase deficiency causes Canavan disease. This leads to accumulation of N-acetylaspartic acid in brain and body fluids. Tallan et al. discovered the compound N-acetylaspartic acid in 1956.[26] The synthesis of N-acetylaspartic acid is catalyzed by L-aspartate-N-acetyltransferase and has been found only in the central nervous system.[27-29] It is found in high concentration in the brain of most vertebrates. The concentration in the human brain is 6 to 7 μmol/g tissue, with the highest concentration in the cerebral cortex and the lowest in the medulla.[30-32]

The concentration of N-acetylaspartic acid is second only to glutamic acid in the free amino acid pool of the brain and is higher in concentration than gamma aminobutyric acid (GABA). In spite of its abundance in the brain, the function of N-acetylaspartic acid is not known, and it is often referred to as an inert compound.[27,33] Recent studies suggest that the acetate moiety is an essential component in a series of reactions required for the conversion of lignoceric acid to cerebronic acid, a component of myelin.[34-36] A review by Baslow suggests that NAA may serve as a molecular water pump.[37]

Aspartoacylase hydrolyzes N-acetylaspartic acid to acetate and aspartate. The enzyme was first characterized in pig kidney homogenate as aminoacylase II and was shown to be specific for the hydrolysis of N-acetylaspartic acid. Aminoacylase I was shown to hydrolyze the

N-acetyl derivatives of all the amino acids other than N-acetylaspartic acid.[38,39]

CLINICAL FEATURES

Adachi et al.[11] reported three clinical variants of Canavan disease: a congenital form in which the disease is apparent at birth or shortly thereafter; an infantile form, which is most common, in which symptoms manifest after the first 6 months of life; and a juvenile form, in which the disease manifests after the first 5 years of life. Since the discovery of the enzyme deficiency, milder forms of Canavan disease have not been observed.[40]

In general, babies with Canavan disease do not present clinical features of the disease early in life. Delayed development, however, may be noted at about age 3 months. An important feature of Canavan disease that should alert the physician is persistent hypotonia and head lag. Macrocephaly is another symptom, although head circumference in early infancy may not be remarkably increased and may remain in the upper limit of normal. The triad of hypotonia, head lag, and macrocephaly should suggest Canavan disease in the differential diagnosis. As the infant grows older, hypotonia gives in to spasticity, so these children are labeled as having cerebral palsy. Head control remains very poor. Seizures usually develop in the second year, and optic atrophy may become a feature of the disease. Patients with Canavan disease become irritable with sleep disturbance and often have fevers of unknown origin. As the disease progresses, problems with gastroesophageal reflux become prominent, leading to feeding difficulties and poor weight gain. Swallowing deteriorates, and some of these children require nasogastric feeding or permanent feeding gastrostomy. Most patients with Canavan disease die in the first decade of life. With improved medical care and nursing, however, more of these children are surviving into the second and even the third decade of life.[41]

DIAGNOSIS

Computed tomography (CT) or magnetic resonance imaging (MRI) scan of the brain reveals diffuse white matter degeneration in Canavan disease.[42–44] The involvement is primarily in the cerebral hemispheres, with less involvement in the cerebellum and brainstem. The MRI of a patient with Canavan disease at 9 months of age was thought to be nondiagnostic (Fig. 36-1A), whereas at age 2 years, MRI shows the progression of the disease with severe white matter degeneration (Fig. 36-1B). Nuclear magnetic resonance (NMR) spectroscopy of the Canavan brain as compared with the normal brain has revealed large accumulation of N-acetylaspartic acid in the Canavan brain.[42,45]

Excessive levels of N-acetylaspartic acid in the urine has become the most reliable test for Canavan disease since 1988.[40] The levels of N-acetylaspartic acid in normal urine, as determined by gas chromatography-mass spectroscopy, are less than 10 µmol/mmol creatinine, whereas in Canavan patients, they are in the range of 3000 ± 1800 µmol/mmol creatinine.[3] High levels of N-acetylaspartic acid in plasma, cerebrospinal fluid, and brain tissue can also be detected.[42]

The enzyme diagnosis requires cultured skin fibroblasts for the determination of aspartoacylase. However, urinary elevation of NAA should be the diagnostic test.

DIFFERENTIAL DIAGNOSIS

Macrocephaly associated with white matter disease can be found in Alexander's disease, benign megalencephaly with leukodystrophy, Krabbe disease, and vacuolating leukodystrophy. Canavan disease is not a rapidly progressive disease, and often such children are diagnosed with static encephalopathy. The child remains relatively stable with severe development delays and no obvious deterioration. These infants are often diagnosed as having cerebral palsy. This leads to a delay in diagnosis in a disease that can be prevented by counseling.

EPIDEMIOLOGY

Canavan disease is pan-ethnic; however, it is most prevalent among Jews of East European ancestry. Canavan disease is more common among non-Jewish individuals than is Tay-Sachs disease.

Screening of healthy Jewish individuals revealed that 1:37 to 1:58 is a carrier for Canavan disease.[46–48] The incidence for Canavan disease in this population is about 1:6000 to 1:13,000. The high incidence and the accuracy of carrier testing using mutation analysis make screening desirable in this population.[49]

Non-Jewish patients have mutations that are more diverse. Canavan disease has been reported among European, Middle-Eastern, Turkish, Gypsy, African-American, and Japanese populations.

MOLECULAR BASIS

The gene encoding for aspartoacylase has been isolated, and mutations in patients with Canavan disease have been identified.[50] The human aspartoacylase gene is 20 kb, and the cDNA is comprised of 6 exons. The gene has been mapped to chromosome 17 p-ter. The cDNA for aspartoacylase codes for 313 amino acid protein with a molecular mass of 36 kDa. The aspartoacylase gene is conserved among species. The coding sequence of the bovine and mouse cDNA shows 92% and 86% identity with the human cDNA, respectively.[51]

Two predominant mutations occur in Jewish patients. The first is a missense mutation on exon 6, 285Glu→Ala, in 86% of the alleles. The other is a nonsense mutation on exon 5, 231Try→X, (termination codon) in 13.6% of the alleles. More than 99% of all

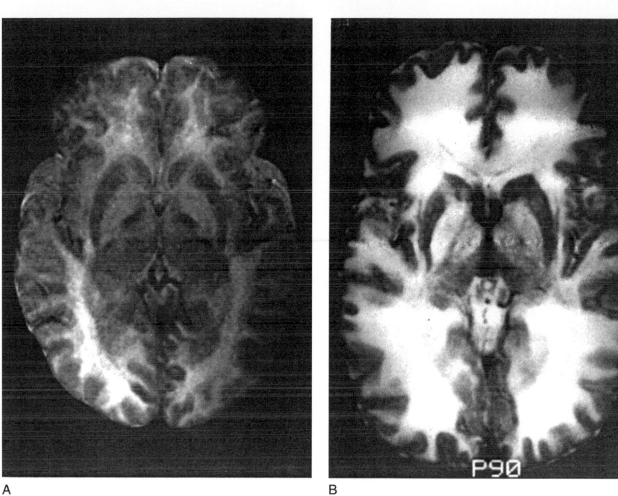

A   B

FIGURE 36-1. *A*, Axial T2-weighted MRI scan taken of a patient with Canavan disease at 9 months of age was initially interpreted as normal. Closer evaluation, however, reveals moderate expansion of medullary and subcortical white matter. *B*, Axial T2-weighted MRI scan taken of a patient with Canavan disease at age 2 years reveals extensive thickening of the white matter radiation.

Jewish patients with Canavan disease have these two mutations.[52]

A common mutation found in non-Jewish Canavan disease patients of European ancestry is Ala305→Glu on exon 6. Thus far, there have been more than 30 mutations among non-Jewish individuals identified.[52-57] Because of the diversity of the mutations, screening programs are not possible.

PRENATAL DIAGNOSIS

When the mutations are known, DNA diagnosis is feasible with amniocentesis or chorionic villus samples (CVS). This diagnosis can be readily made in patients of Jewish ancestry because of the two known Jewish mutations. Among non-Jewish individuals, attempts should be made to identify the mutation in the proband so that molecular prenatal diagnosis can be made.[58,59]

Elevation of NAA in amniotic fluid can be measured, but the elevation is less than the increase found in urine. Stable isotope dilution increases the accuracy for measuring NAA in amniotic fluid. This requires specialized laboratories with experience in doing this test.[60,61]

THERAPY

There is no treatment for Canavan disease. Experiments with gene therapy have been ongoing on a limited number of patients. The results are being evaluated.[62]

KNOCKOUT MOUSE FOR CANAVAN DISEASE AND FUTURE RESEARCH

A knockout mouse for Canavan disease has been engineered.[63] The mouse has a phenotype of neurodegenerative disease. The mouse has spongy degeneration of the brain, increased NAA in urine, and aspartoacylase deficiency. This mouse is used for experimentation with gene therapy and for understanding the pathogenesis of Canavan disease. A rat with aspartoacylase deficiency, tremor rat, was discovered in Japan. The rat has spongy degeneration of the brain and increased NAA.[64]

REFERENCES

1. Matalon R, Michals K, Sebasta D, et al: Aspartoacylase deficiency and N-acetylaspartic aciduria in patients with Canavan disease. Am J Med Genet 1988;29:463–471.

2. Matalon R, Kaul RK, Casanova J, et al: Aspartoacylase deficiency: The enzyme defect in Canavan disease. J Inherit Metab Dis 1989;12: 329–331.

3. Kaul R, Michals K, Casanova J, Matalon R: The role of N-acetylaspartic acid in brain metabolism and the pathogenesis in Canavan disease. Int Pediatrics 1991;6:40–43.

4. Canavan MM: Schilder's encephalitis periaxialis diffusa. Arch Neurol Psychiatr 1931;25:299–308.

5. Globus JH, Strauss I: Progressive degenerative subcortical encephalopathy: Schilder's disease. Arch Neurol Psychiatr 1928;20:1190–1228.

6. van Bogaert L, Bertrand I: Sur une idiotie familiale avec degerescence sponglieuse de neuraxe (note preliminaire). Acta Neurol Belg 1949;49:572–587.

7. Banker BQ, Robertson JJ, Victor M: Spongy degeneration of the central nervous system in infancy. Neurology 1964;14:981–1001.

8. Buchanan DS, Davis RL: Spongy degeneration of the nervous system: A report of 4 cases with a review of the literature. Neurology 1965;15:207–222.

9. Sacks O, Brown WJ, Aguilar MJ: Spongy degeneration of white matter: Canavan's sclerosis. Neurology 1965;15:165–171.

10. Gamberti P, Mellman WJ, Gonatas NK: Familial spongy degeneration of the central nervous system: van Bogaert–Bertrand disease. Acta Neuropathol 1969;12:103–115.

11. Adachi M, Schneck L, Cazara J, Volk BW: Spongy degeneration of the central nervous system: van Bogaert and Bertrand type; Canavan's disease. Hum Pathol 1973;4:331–346.

12. Ungar M, Goodman RM: Spongy degeneration of the brain in Israel: A retrospective study. Clin Genet 1983;23:23–29.

13. Menkes JH: Textbook of Child Neurology, 3rd ed. Philadelphia, Lea & Febiger, 1985.

14. van Bogaert L, Bertrand I: Spongy Degeneration of Brain in Infancy. Amsterdam, North Holland, 1967.

15. Banker BQ, Victor H: Spongy degeneration of infancy. In Goodman RM, Motulsky AG (eds): Genetic Disease among Ashkenazi Jews. New York, Raven Press, 1979, pp 201–217.

16. Hogan GR, Richardson EP Jr: Spongy degeneration of the nervous system (Canavan's disease): Report of a case in an Irish-American family. Pediatrics 1965;35:284–294.

17. Mahdi AH, Elidirssy ATH, Wright EA: Spongy degeneration of the central nervous system (van Bogaert-Bertrand disease): Report of a case in a Saudi family. J Child Neurol 1986;1:61–63.

18. Kvittingen EA, Guldal G, Borsting S, et al: N-Acetylaspartic aciduria in a child with a progressive cerebral atrophy. Clin Chim Acta 1986;158:217–227.

19. Hagenfeldt L, Bollgren I, Venizelos N: N-Acetylaspartic aciduria due to aspartoacylase deficiency: A new etiology of childhood leukodystrophy. J Inherit Metab Dis 1987;10:135–141.

20. Divry P, Viamey-Liaund C, Gay C, et al: N-Acetylaspartic aciduria: Report of three cases in children with a neurological syndrome associating macrocephaly and leukodystrophy. J Inherit Metab Dis 1988;11: 307–308.

21. Gason GG, Ozand PT, Mahdi A, et al: Infantile CNS spongy degeneration—14 cases: Clinical update. Neurology 1990;40:1876–1882.

22. Ozand PT, Gascon G, Dhalla M: Aspartoacylase deficiency and Canavan disease in Saudi Arabia. Am J Med Genet 1990;35:266–268.

23. Echeme B, Divry P, Viamey-Liaud C: Spongy degeneration of the neuraxis (Canavan-van Bogaert's disease) and N-acetylaspartic aciduria. Neuropediatrics 1989;20:179–181.

24. de Coo IFM, Bakkeren JAJM, Gabreels FJM: Canavan disease: Value of N-acetylaspartic aciduria? Neuropediatrics 1991;22:3.

25. Michelakakis H, Giouroukos S, Divry P, et al: Canavan disease: Findings in four new cases. J Inherit Metab Dis 1991;14:267–268.

26. Tallan HH, Moore S, Stein WH: N-Acetyl-L-aspartic acid in brain. J Biol Chem 1956;219:257–264.

27. Jacobson HB: Studies on the role of N-acetylaspartic acid on mammalian brain. J Gen Physiol 1957;43:323–333.

28. Hnizley H. The enzymatic synthesis of N-acetyl-L-aspartic acid by a water-insoluble preparation of a cat brain acetone powder. J Biol Chem 1967;242: 4619–4622.

29. Margolis RU, Barkulis SS, Geiger A: A comparison between 14C from glucose into N-acetyl-L-aspartic acid and aspartic acid in brain perfusion experiments. J Neurochem 1960;5:379–382.

30. Birken DL, Oldendorf WH: N-Acetyl-L-aspartic acid: A literature review of a compound prominent in `H-NMR spectroscopic studies of brain. Neurosci Behav Rev 1989;13: 23–31.

31. Miyake M, Kakimoto Y, Sorimachi M: A gas chromatographic method for the determination of N-acetyl-L-aspartic acid, N-acetylalpha-aspartylglutamic acid and beta-citryl-L-glutamic acid and their distributions in the brain and other organs of various species of animals. J Neurochem 1980;36:804–810.

32. Kaul RK, Casanova J, Johnson A, et al: Purification, characterization and localization of aspartoacylase from bovine brain. J Neurochem 1991;56: 129–135.

33. McIntosh JM, Cooper JR: Studies on the function of N-acetylaspartic acid in the brain. J Neurochem 1965;12:825–835.

34. Shigematsu H, Okamura N, Shimeno H, et al: Purification and characterization of the heat stable factors essential for conversion of lignoceric acid to cerebronic acid and glutamic acid: Identification of N-acetyl-L-aspartic acid. J Neurochem 1983;40: 814–820.

35. Miyake M, Kakimoto Y: Developmental changes of N-acetyl-L-aspartic acid, N-acetyl-alpha-aspartylglutamic acid and beta-citryl-L-glutamic acid in different brain regions and spinal cords of rat and guinea pig. J Neurochem 1981;37:1064–1067.

36. Chakraborty G, Mekala P, Yahya D, et al: Intraneuronal N-acetylaspartate supplies acetyl groups for myelin lipid synthesis: Evidence for myelin-associated aspartoacylase. J Neurochem 2001;78:736–745.

37. Baslow MH: Evidence supporting a role of N-acetyl-L-aspartate as a molecular water pump in myelinated neurons in the central nervous system. An analytical review. Neurochem Int 2002;40:295–300.

38. Birnbaum SM, Levintow L, Kingsley RB, Greenstein JP: Specificity of amino acid acylases. J Biol Chem 1952;194:455–462.

39. Birnbaum SM: Amino acid acylases I and II from hog kidney. Methods Enzymol 1955;2:115–119.

40. Matalon RM, Michals-Matalon K: Spongy degeneration of the brain (Canavan disease): Biochemical and molecular findings. Front Biosci 2000;5:307–311.

41. Matalon R, Michals-Matalon K: Biochemistry and molecular biology of Canavan disease. Neurochem Res 1999;24:507–513.

42. Matalon R, Michals K, Kaul R, Mafee M: Spongy degeneration of the brain: Canavan disease. Int Pediatrics 1990;5:121–124.

43. Brismar J, Brismar G, Gascon G, Ozand P: Canavan disease: CT and MR imaging of the brain. Am J Neuroradiol 1990;11:805–810.

44. Rushton AR, Shaywitz BA, Dumen CC, et al: Computerized tomography in the diagnosis of Canavan's disease. Ann Neurol 1981;10:57–60.

45. Grodd W, Kragelh-Mann I, Peterson D, et al: In vivo assessment of N-acetylaspartate in brain in spongy degeneration (Canavan's disease) by proton spectroscopy. Lancet 1990;336:437–438.

46. Matalon R, Kaul R, Michals K: Carrier rate of Canavan disease among Ashkenazi Jewish individuals. Am J Hum Genet 1994;55:A908.

47. Kronn D, Oddoux C, Phillips J, Ostrer H: Prevalence of Canavan disease heterozygotes in the New York metropolitan Ashkenazi Jewish population. Am J Hum Genet 1995;5:1250–1252.

48. Sugarman EA, Allitto BA: Carrier testing for seven diseases common in the Ashkenazi Jewish population: Implications for counseling and testing. Obstet Gynecol 2001;5.38–39.

49. ACOG committee opinion. Screening for Canavan disease. Committee on Genetics. American College of Obstetrician Gynecologists, Number 212, November 1998. Int J Gynaecol Obstet 1999;1: 91–92.

50. Kaul R, Gao GP, Balamurugan K, Matalon R: Human aspartoacylase cDNA and mis-sense mutation in Canavan disease. Nat Genet 1993;5:118–123.

51. Kaul R, Balamurugan K, Gao GP, Matalon R: Canavan disease: Genomic organization and localization of human ASPA to 17p13-ter and conservation of the ASPA gene during evolution. Genomics 1994;21: 364–370.

52. Kaul R, Gao GP, Aloya M, et al: Canavan disease: Mutations among Jewish and non-Jewish patients. Am J Hum Genet 1994;55:34–41.

53. Elpeleg ON, Shaag A: The spectrum of mutations of the aspartoacylase gene in Canavan disease in non-Jewish patients. J Inherit Metab Dis 1999;4: 531–534.

54. Kaul R, Gao GP, Matalon R, et al: Identification and expression of eight novel mutations among non-Jewish patients with Canavan disease. Am J Hum Genet 1996;59:95–102.

55. Shaag A, Anikster Y, Christensen E, et al: The molecular basis of Canavan (aspartoacylase deficiency) disease in European non-Jewish patients. Am J Hum Genet 1995;57:572–580.

56. Sistermans EA, de Coo RF, van Beerendonk HM, et al: Mutation detection in the aspartoacylase gene in 17 patients with Canavan disease: Four new mutations in the non-Jewish population. Eur J Hum Genet 2000;7:557–560.

57. Tahmaz FE, Sam S, Hoganson GE, Quan F: A partial deletion of the aspartoacylase gene is the cause of Canavan disease family from Mexico. J Med Genet 2001;9:38.

58. Matalon R, Kaul R, Gao GP, et al: Prenatal diagnosis for Canavan disease: The use of DNA markers. J Inherit Metab Dis 1995;18:215–217.

59. Matalon R, Michals-Matalon K. Prenatal diagnosis of Canavan disease. Prenat Diagn 1999;7:669–670.

60. Bennett MJ, Gibson KM, Sherwood WG, et al: Reliable prenatal diagnosis of Canavan disease (aspartoacylase deficiency): Comparison of enzymatic and metabolite analysis. J Inherit Metab Dis 1993;16: 831–836.

61. Kelley RI: Prenatal diagnosis of Canavan disease by measurement of N-acetyl-L-aspartate in amniotic fluid. J Inherit Metab Dis 1993;16:918–919.

62. Leone P, Janson CG, Bilaniuk L, et al: Aspartoacylase gene transfer to the mammalian central nervous system with therapeutic implications for Canavan disease. Ann Neurol 2000;1:27–38.

63. Matalon R, Rady PL, Platt KA, et al: Knock-out mouse for Canavan disease: A model for gene transfer to the central nervous system. J Gene Med 2000;3:165–175.

64. Kitada K, Akimitsu T, Shigematsi Y, et al: Accumulation of N-acetyl-L-aspartate in the brain of the tremor rat, a mutant exhibiting absence-like seizure and spongiform degeneration in the central nervous system. J Neurochem 2000;6:2512–2519.

CHAPTER

37

Neuro-Oncology: The Neurofibromatoses

Christina A. Gurnett

David H. Gutmann

Tumors of the nervous system typically occur in a sporadic fashion without a pre-existing familial predisposition. The uncommon tumors that arise in the context of a tumor predisposition syndrome can provide valuable insights into the critical genetic events important for tumorigenesis in the nervous system. Two such syndromes, neurofibromatosis type 1 (NF1) and neurofibromatosis type 2 (NF2), are autosomal dominant disorders characterized by an increased susceptibility to both benign and malignant tumors. The genes responsible for NF1 (neurofibromin) and NF2 (merlin/schwannomin) were identified by positional cloning and they encode proteins that function as negative growth regulators. This chapter will focus on the nervous system tumors in NF1 and NF2.

CLINICAL FEATURES AND DIAGNOSTIC EVALUATION

Neurofibromatosis Type 1

NF1 is a relatively common autosomal dominant disorder with an incidence of 1 in 3500 individuals worldwide.[1] NF1 was previously known as *peripheral neurofibromatosis* or *von Recklinghausen disease* in honor of Frederick von Recklinghausen, who first described the condition in 1882. Occasionally, NF1 has been incorrectly referred to as the "Elephant Man" disease, based on the affliction of Joseph Merrick, who instead suffered from a completely distinct clinical disorder, Proteus syndrome. Although many of the organ systems involved in this disorder arise from neural crest cells (i.e., Schwann cells, peripheral nerves, melanocytes, adrenal medulla, and select skull bones), the clinical manifes-

tations are not limited to these cell types. For this reason, it is not accurate to classify NF1 as a *neurocristopathy*. Because of its preponderance of "spots," NF1 has also been grouped with a collection of disorders, that include tuberous sclerosis complex and Cowden syndrome, termed the *phakomatoses*. Although these classification schemes may highlight some of the similarities between distinct medical conditions, they have often resulted in confusion and clinical misdiagnoses.

Most individuals with NF1 present in infancy or early childhood with pigmented cutaneous lesions such as café-au-lait macules, skinfold freckling, or Lisch nodules. The diagnostic criteria for NF1, originally formulated by the National Institutes of Health Consensus Panel, are shown in Table 37–1. In order for an individual to be given the diagnosis of NF1, two of these seven diagnostic criteria must be present. Other non-tumor phenotypes include cognitive deficits, renal and cerebral artery stenosis, and bony abnormalities, including sphenoid wing dysplasia, distinctive bony lesions, and scoliosis. Other characteristic features are short stature, with 13% of all patients being more than 2 standard deviations below the mean, and macrocephaly, with more than 24% being more than 2 standard deviations above the mean.

Café-au-lait macules occur in 99% of individuals with NF1 and are frequently the earliest manifestation of the disorder (Fig. 37–1A). Although it is not uncommon for one or two café-au-lait macules to be seen in unaffected individuals in the general population, patients with NF1 have many more café-au-lait macules. Café-au-lait macules are frequently noted at birth and tend to increase in number during the first two years of life. Typically, these macules have smooth, regular borders and demonstrate homogenous pigmentation.

Often times, café-au-lait macules fade in adults with NF1, making the diagnosis of NF1 difficult in an adult in whom the childhood history is lacking. Histopathologically, café-au-lait macules are associated with increased numbers of large melanosomes called *macromelanosomes*.

Like café-au-lait macules, freckling is also an early diagnostic sign and is seen in 80% of children by age 6. Freckling typically occurs in regions where there is frequent skin friction, such as the axilla, inguinal region, and beneath the chin. In women, freckling may be seen under the breasts. Lisch nodules are benign pigmented nodules of the iris that are not clinically significant except for diagnostic purposes. Lisch nodules do not interfere with vision. Although only about 30% of NF1 patients have Lisch nodules by age 6 years, nearly all NF1 patients have them by adulthood. Slit lamp examinations are usually required to accurately identify these lesions.

The most common tumor seen in individuals with NF1 is the benign neurofibroma, composed of Schwann cells, fibroblasts, and mast cells (Fig. 37–1*B*). These tumors may appear as defined cutaneous or subcutaneous lesions or as larger, more extensive tumors involving multiple nerves. The number of dermal neurofibromas typically increases as a function of age, with tumors first appearing around the time of puberty. Discrete neurofibromas are always benign tumors and harbor no risk of malignant transformation.

Neurofibromas may be a source of skin irritation when they occur in particular locations and may become a major cosmetic problem when abundant.

Plexiform neurofibromas likely represent congenital lesions, found in approximately 25% of patients with NF1. They may grow anywhere along the length of major peripheral nerves and may result in bony abnormalities or functional impairment. While often considered congenital lesions present in infancy, they may arise from deeper structures and remain clinically silent until later in life. Plexiform neurofibromas may be extensive and involve multiple tissues, including skin, fascia, muscle, bone, and internal organs. Their presence may stimulate underlying bone growth to result in leg length discrepancy or scoliosis. Orbital plexiform neurofibromas may be associated with sphenoid wing dysplasia, often resulting in intracranial extension and exophthalmos. Surgical removal of plexiform neurofibromas may be difficult because these tumors cross tissue planes and are nearly impossible to completely resect. In addition, plexiform neurofibromas often exhibit significant vascularity and may result in tremendous blood loss during surgery.

Unlike the discrete neurofibroma, plexiform neurofibromas may transform into aggressive malignant peripheral nerve sheath tumors (MPNSTs) in about 5% to 10% of patients. The two most predictive clinical signs suggestive of malignant transformation are pain and

TABLE 37–1. Diagnostic Criteria for Neurofibromatosis 1 and Neurofibromatosis 2

Neurofibromatosis Type 1

Two or more of the following features are required:

(1) Six or more café-au-lait spots with diameters greater than 0.5 mm before puberty or 1.5 cm after puberty

(2) Two or more neurofibromas or a single plexiform neurofibroma

(3) Freckling in the axillary or inguinal regions

(4) Optic pathway tumor

(5) Lisch nodules (hamartomas of the iris)

(6) A distinctive bony lesion: dysplasia of the sphenoid bone or dysplasia/thinning of long bone cortex

(7) A first-degree relative diagnosed with NF1

Neurofibromatosis Type 2

Definite NF2

   (1) Bilateral vestibular schwannomas (VS) or

   (2) Family history of NF2 plus either

      (A) unilateral VS at <30 years old, or

      (B) Any two of the following: meningioma, glioma, schwannoma, juvenile posterior subcapsular lenticular opacities/juvenile cortical cataract

Probable NF2

   (1) Unilateral VS at <30 years old, plus at least one of any of the following: meningioma, glioma, schwannoma, juvenile posterior subcapsular lenticular opacities/juvenile cortical cataract, or

   (2) Multiple meningiomas (two or more) plus unilateral VS at <30 years old, or

   (3) Any one of the following: glioma, schwannoma, juvenile posterior subcapsular lenticular opacities/juvenile cortical cataract

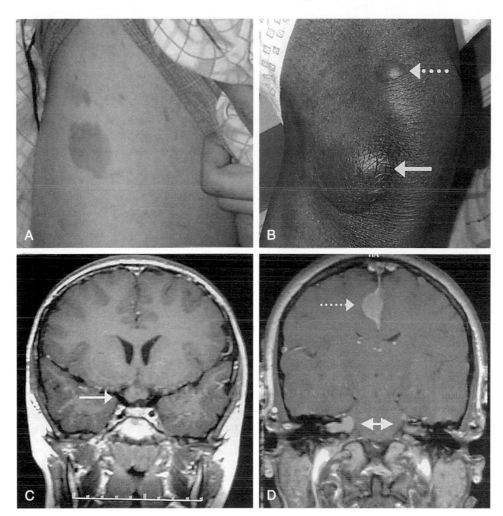

FIGURE 37–1. Clinical Features of NF1 and NF2. *A*, Café-au-lait macule in an individual with NF1. *B*, Dermal neurofibroma *(dotted arrow)* and plexiform neurofibroma *(solid arrow)* in an adult with NF1. *C*, Optic pathway glioma predominantly involving the right optic nerve on cranial MRI in a young child with NF1. *D*, Para-sagittal meningioma *(dotted arrow)* and bilateral vestibular schwannomas *(double-headed arrow)* on cranial MRI in a teenager with NF2.

neurologic deficit.[2] Unfortunately, reliable signs of malignant transformation are lacking. Individuals with clinical signs suspicious for malignancy require prompt and aggressive management. Studies have evaluated the role of 18-fluorodeoxyglucose positron emission tomography (PET) for distinguishing malignant from benign peripheral nerve sheath tumors.[3] Based on these preliminary observations, PET might become an adjunct diagnostic tool in the evaluation of an NF1 patient in whom MPNST is suspected. MPNSTs also have the propensity for distant metastasis to bone and lung. New onset of bone pain or fracture in an NF1 patient with an MPNST warrants a search for metastases. Unfortunately, MPNSTs are not typically sensitive to conventional chemotherapy and radiation. Local radiotherapy after wide surgical excision of an MPNST may delay the time to local recurrence, but does not improve the overall long-term survival.

The second most frequent tumor in NF1 is the optic pathway glioma, occurring in 15% of individuals with NF1 (Fig. 37–1C). These tumors are almost entirely restricted to childhood, with a mean age at presentation of 4.5 years. The optic pathway glioma in NF1 is almost always a low-grade (WHO grade I) pilocytic astrocytoma. These tumors may arise anywhere along the length

of the optic pathway from the retrobulbar optic nerve to the post-chiasmatic optic radiations. They may also extend into the hypothalamus to cause neuroendocrine dysfunction, such as precocious puberty. Many of these tumors are detected incidentally on brain magnetic resonance imaging (MRI), and only about one third of these are clinically symptomatic. Some NF1-associated optic pathway gliomas have been reported to regress without treatment. Clinical surveillance includes annual ophthalmologic evaluations in the first decade of life to identify visual impairment resulting from these tumors.[4] Routine brain imaging in asymptomatic individuals is not recommended, as the decision to treat is based on clinical symptoms. NF1-associated gliomas may also involve the brain stem. Compared with the brain stem gliomas seen in individuals without NF1, NF1-associated brain stem tumors are more likely to be located in the medulla, but are less likely to progress clinically or radiographically. Although sporadic brain stem gliomas carry a poor prognosis, NF1-associated brain stem tumors are more often low-grade lesions with lower morbidity and mortality.

Gliomas have sometimes been misdiagnosed in individuals with NF1 who have other intracranial signal abnormalities uniquely found in NF1 patients on brain

MRI. High signal intensity lesions on T2 weighted images, referred to as unidentified bright objects (UBOs), are seen in more than one half of NF1 children. These non-enhancing lesions are most often found in the brain stem, thalamus, cerebellum, and basal ganglia. Pathologically, these lesions may represent regions of vacuolar or spongiotic change. UBOs have no known potential for neoplastic degeneration, but may enlarge and be misdiagnosed as gliomas. Multiple studies have investigated a potential correlation between the number of these lesions and cognitive deficits, yet no consensus exists as to their clinical significance. Notably, most UBOs disappear by late adolescence or early adulthood in individuals with NF1.

NF1 patients are also at higher risk for specific bony and vascular abnormalities as well as rare tumors. Scoliosis occurs in 10% to 20% of patients with NF1. The scoliosis in children with NF1 may resemble the idiopathic form, or patients may present earlier when scoliosis is related to vertebral dysplasia or secondary to paravertebral neurofibromas. Scoliosis resulting from a paravertebral neurofibroma may manifest with a dramatic abrupt angle curvature, unusual for non–NF1-associated cases. Tibial pseudarthrosis and sphenoid wing dysplasia are osseous lesions that are quite specific to patients with NF1. These distinctive bony lesions typically are obvious in early infancy. Bowing of the long bones may be the result of cortical thinning or dysplastic bony changes and may lead to pathologic fracture in NF1. Repeated fracture and incomplete healing produces the appearance of a "false joint" or pseudarthrosis. Early recognition is essential to avoid limb amputation. Sphenoid wing dysplasia will usually manifest as an orbital deformity. Skull radiographs should readily identify this bony defect. Vascular abnormalities, including renal artery stenosis, which may cause hypertension, and moya-moya, a cerebral vessel abnormality that can result in stroke, are unusual complications of NF1, found in less than 1% of patients. NF1 patients are also at a higher risk for other malignancies, including pheochromocytoma and juvenile chronic myeloid leukemia.

One of the hallmark features of NF1 is phenotypic variability. There is typically as much difference in the spectrum of clinical features between individuals within a single family who all harbor an identical germline NF1 mutation as there is between individuals from different families. Parents with few clinical features of NF1 (e.g., café-au-lait macules, skinfold freckles) can have children with more clinically serious manifestations (e.g., MPNSTs, optic pathway gliomas). This variability suggests that factors other than the germline NF1 mutation determine the clinical expression of the disorder. Some studies have implicated injury as an inciting stimulus for tumor formation in NF1. For example, cutaneous neurofibromas sometimes grow at sites of previous wounds or skin grafts. Further work will be required to determine what effects these factors have on tumor formation and growth in NF1.

Rare individuals have been identified with segmental NF1, affecting only a single region of the body.[5] Some of these patients are genetically mosaic for mutations in the NF1 gene and therefore are known to harbor the mutation in only a subset of their cells. Mosaicism, resulting from a somatic mutation occurring at a later stage in fetal development, is more likely to affect fewer cells and yield a more restricted somatic distribution of clinical abnormalities. Given that mosaicism also potentially affects gonadal tissues, the probability of transmission of NF1 may be as high as 50%, as seen in typical cases of NF1, but generally is lower. Although the parent may have a mosaic or segmental pattern of NF1, affected offspring will have the generalized NF1 phenotype, because they would have inherited a germline NF1 mutation in all cells.

The diagnosis of NF1 can be made accurately and early based on clinical examination findings and history alone (see Table 37–1). Although only 26% of sporadic patients meet criteria by 1 year of age, almost all (97%) meet criteria for diagnosis by 8 years of age because many of the cutaneous signs develop during early childhood.[6] Although NF1 gene mutation analysis is available for diagnostic purposes, it is costly and time consuming, given the large size of the gene and lack of mutation clustering. For this reason, the diagnosis of NF1 remains a clinical one.

Neurofibromatosis Type 2

NF2 is much less common than NF1 and has an incidence of 1 in 30,000 to 42,000.[1] It is characterized by the early development of multiple schwannomas affecting cranial, spinal, and peripheral nerves. The hallmark of the disorder is the development of bilateral vestibular schwannomas (Fig. 37–1D). The diagnostic criteria for NF2 are shown in Table 37–1. In contrast to NF1, the large tumor burden often results in a diminished life expectancy. Nearly all individuals with NF2 will develop schwannomas and in about one half of affected patients, meningiomas, ependymomas and, less commonly, astrocytomas will be observed. In addition to nervous system tumors, common ocular findings include posterior subcapsular lenticular opacities (cataracts). Although NF2 is often referred to as a neurocutaneous disorder, the presence of cutaneous features is much less common than in NF1. Fusiform subcutaneous schwannomas may be palpated in patients with NF2, but are never present in the hundreds, as may occur with cutaneous neurofibromas in NF1.

The majority of adult patients with NF2 present with unilateral hearing loss, often associated with imbalance and tinnitus. Children, who have more serious disease, due to an early onset and more rapidly progressive clinical course, are more likely to present with tumors involving other cranial and peripheral nerves. In some families with NF2, the onset and severity are similar in all affected individuals, suggesting a relationship between the phenotype and the underlying genetic mutation (genotype-phenotype correlation).[7]

The most common tumor found in NF2 is the schwannoma, which is composed of neoplastic Schwann cells. Clinically, schwannomas from individuals with NF2 are not different from their sporadic counterparts, except that they are often multiple and typically occur at an earlier age. Despite the misnomer "acoustic neuroma," schwannomas most frequently affect the vestibular branch of the eighth cranial nerve, although other cranial nerves may be affected. Similarly, extramedullary spinal schwannomas may arise at any vertebral level. Vestibular schwannomas are so common in NF2 patients that they are required for a definite diagnosis of the disorder. Likewise, spinal schwannomas are identified in nearly 80% to 90% of individuals with NF2 using gadolinium-enhanced MRI.

Meningioma is the second most common tumor in NF2 and occurs both intracranially and within the spinal cord (see Fig. 37–1D). Most are supratentorial, occurring in the parasagittal region, cerebral convexities, or sphenoid ridge. Like schwannomas, meningiomas are also common sporadic tumors; however, only 1% of individuals with a single meningioma meet criteria for NF2. The recognition of multiple meningiomas in a child or young adult should prompt a search for other signs of NF2, because meningiomas are typically found in older adults in the general population.

The initial diagnostic workup for patients at risk for NF2 includes full cranial and spinal MRI to evaluate for schwannomas, meningiomas, and intramedullary tumors. Brain MRI, neurologic examinations, and audiologic assessments are recommended and should be dictated by clinical findings.[8] Brain stem auditory evoked responses may also be helpful in assessing eighth cranial nerve function. Brain MRI also serves as an effective screening examination for asymptomatic individuals, because a normal MRI scan at age 30 years makes a diagnosis of NF2 extremely unlikely.

Because of the difficulty involved in identifying NF2 gene mutations as a rapid screening test for NF2, clinical examination and history remain the standard for diagnosis. Mutation scanning, using single strand conformation polymorphism (SSCP) followed by direct sequencing, reveals about 65% of causative mutations. Linkage studies can also be performed on families with multiple affected individuals.

There are also rare patients with schwannomatosis, a disorder defined by multiple noncranial schwannomas in the absence of meningiomas, ependymomas, or astrocytomas. These patients tend to develop schwannomas later in life and, therefore, have a longer life expectancy. In contrast to patients with NF2, these individuals do not harbor germline mutations in the NF2 gene, but their schwannomas contain somatic mutations in both NF2 alleles. Schwannomatosis patients provide a unique opportunity to study the mechanisms by which somatic mutations arise in the NF2 gene and the genetic factors that contribute to tumorigenesis.

Another subset of patients with NF2 has disease-related tumors restricted to one region of the nervous system, such as localized meningiomas and unilateral vestibular schwannomas.[5] These patients have segmental or mosaic NF2, characterized by somatic mutations in the NF2 gene occurring later during fetal development, much as described earlier for segmental NF1. Mosaicism is much more common in NF2 than in NF1, accounting for up to 20% of patients with no previous family history.

PATHOLOGY

Although there have been studies that suggest differences in the histopathologic appearance of NF-associated and sporadic tumors, there are no conclusive data to support such claims. In general, the tumor types seen in NF1 and NF2 are relatively indistinguishable from those that arise in the general population.[9] Distinguishing features of NF-associated tumors include the number of tumors, the age at presentation, and the clinical context in which they arise.

Astrocytomas in children with NF1 are nearly always pilocytic astrocytomas. Pilocytic astrocytomas are the most common glioma in children. Pilocytic astrocytomas often occur in the cerebellum in children without NF1, but the most frequent sites in the context of NF1 are the optic nerve, optic chiasm, hypothalamus, and brain stem. Macroscopically, these tumors are soft, gray masses with frequent cyst formation. They demonstrate low cellularity and high vascularity associated with brightly eosinophilic corkscrew-shaped structures, termed *Rosenthal fibers*. These tumors are often highly fibrillated and stain positively for glial fibrillary acidic protein (GFAP).

Schwannomas are globoid masses composed of spindle-shaped neoplastic Schwann cells with alternating areas of compact elongated cells (Antoni A pattern) and less cellular, loosely textured areas (Antoni B pattern). They typically arise eccentric to the associated nerve and often appear encapsulated. In contrast, neurofibromas are composed of neoplastic and non-neoplastic Schwann cells, perineurial-like cells, and fibroblasts in a matrix of collagen fibers. Frequently, these tumors have entrapped mast cells. Patients with neurofibromas typically present with a cutaneous nodule, but subcutaneous or visceral tumors associated with a nerve may also occur. Unlike the schwannoma, nerve fibers course through the neurofibroma tumor mass. Plexiform neurofibromas form in association with multiple nerve fascicles and may represent embryological or early developmental neoplastic lesions. They may be associated with a rich vasculature and carry a lifetime risk of degeneration into malignant peripheral nerve sheath tumors (MPNSTs). MPNSTs are highly malignant and metastatic cancers that appear as globoid or fusiform pseudo-encapsulated masses with a firm consistency. They may exhibit areas of frank hemorrhage or necrosis. Histologically, these tumors contain tightly packed, hyperchromatic, spindle-shaped neoplastic Schwann cells that often express the S-100 protein.

Meningiomas arise from leptomeningeal arachnoidal cap cells as slow-growing tumors, sometimes associated with calcification. Most meningiomas are rubbery, well-demarcated masses demonstrating dural attachment. Although these tumors typically cause neurologic problems by compression of adjacent brain, meningiomas can be brain-invasive or invade through dura to involve the skull. Histopathologic analysis reveals several different tumor appearances including meningothelial, fibrous, and transitional subtypes. Meningothelial meningioma tumor cells form lobules surrounded by collagen and exhibit whorls and psammoma bodies. Fibrous (or fibroblastic) tumor cells form interlacing bundles with infrequent whorls and psammoma bodies. Lastly, transitional meningiomas have histologic features shared by both meningothelial and fibrous meningiomas.

MOLECULAR-GENETIC DATA

The NF1 gene on the long arm of chromosome 17 was identified by positional cloning and spans over 350 kb of genomic DNA.[10] The NF1 gene encodes an mRNA of 11 to 13 kb with at least 59 exons and a protein of 2818 amino acids. Neurofibromin, the 220-kDa NF1 gene product, is most abundant in neurons, oligodendrocytes, and Schwann cells, but is also expressed in astrocytes, leukocytes, and the adrenal medulla. Neurofibromin

expression is more widespread during embryonic development, suggesting a role as a negative growth regulator in developing tissues.

Sequence analysis has revealed homology between neurofibromin (exons 20a to 27a) and a family of molecules, termed GTPase activating proteins (GAPs), involved in the down-regulation of RAS activity (Fig. 37–2A). RAS is a low molecular weight GTPase protein involved in stimulating cell growth and promoting tumor formation. RAS exists in an active form when bound to GTP and an inactive form when guanosine diphosphate (GDP)-bound. GAP proteins, like neurofibromin, inhibit RAS by stimulating its intrinsic GTPase activity and accelerating the conversion of GTP-bound active RAS to the inactive GDP-bound form. Failure to inactivate RAS, as a result of loss of neurofibromin function due to NF1 gene inactivation, leads to increased cell proliferation and tumor formation.

Multiple alternatively spliced NF1 transcripts have been identified as a result of the alternative use of three exons (9a, 23a, and 48a). These three alternatively spliced exons are differentially expressed and may contribute to potentially unique functions of neurofibromin in specific tissues during development. Exon 48a is expressed only in muscle tissues, whereas exon 9a expression is restricted to forebrain neurons in a developmentally regulated manner. Exon 23a encodes an additional 21 amino acids within the GAP-related domain, such that neurofibromin containing exon 23a is less effective at RAS regulation than neurofibromin that lacks this alternatively spliced exon.

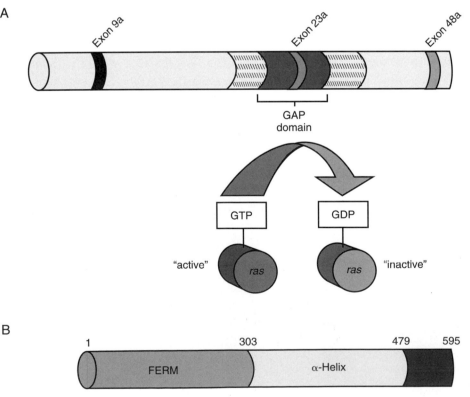

FIGURE 37–2. NF1 and NF2 gene products. A, The NF1 gene product, neurofibromin, contains three alternatively spliced exons (9a, 23a, and 48a). The central region of the protein contains a domain (GAP domain) with structural and functional similarity to GTPase activating proteins (GAPs) that accelerate the conversion of RAS from its active GTP-bound form to an inactive GDP-bound form. Active RAS provides a mitogenic signal for many cell types. B, The NF2 gene product, merlin, contains three regions of structural significance, including an amino terminal FERM domain (residues 1–302), a central alpha helical region (residues 303–478), and a unique carboxyl terminal domain (residues 479–595) lacking the conventional actin-binding sequences in other ERM proteins.

NF1 mutational analyses have not demonstrated a correlation between the mutation type or location and the phenotype of an affected individual. There is relatively little clustering of *NF1* gene mutations, with the exception of exon 10 and 37, where 30% of germline mutations have been identified.[11] Most mutations are unique to a single family. Aside from specific mutations within the GAP domain, most mutations are thought to result in a truncated or nonfunctional protein.

The *NF2* gene was identified by positional cloning in 1993 and is located on the long arm of chromosome 22.[10] The *NF2* gene encodes a 2.2 kb messenger RNA and a 595 amino acid protein named merlin (or schwannomin). Merlin is expressed in neurons, lens fibers, blood vessels, leptomeningeal cells, astrocytes, gonadal tissue, and Schwann cells, but similar to neurofibromin there is more widespread expression during embryonic development. Merlin is a member of the protein 4.1 family, whose members link the actin cytoskeleton to cell surface glycoproteins. Merlin consists of an amino terminal FERM domain followed by a predicted alpha helical region, both of which are conserved in the ERM (ezrin, radixin, and moesin) subclass of protein 4.1 molecules (Fig. 37–2B). However, merlin is the only ERM protein known to function as a tumor suppressor.

The carboxyl terminal of merlin lacks similarity to any other protein and, significantly, lacks the actin-binding domain found in ERM proteins. Weak actin binding does occur, however, through residues in the amino terminus of merlin. Merlin may also indirectly associate with actin through its interaction with the actin binding protein, βII-spectrin. The importance of the potential interaction of merlin with actin is supported by observations that actin cytoskeleton-related abnormalities are seen in *NF2*-deficient Schwann cells and that actin-dependent processes, such as cell attachment, spreading, and motility are affected by *NF2* gene overexpression in rat schwannoma cells.

Merlin exists in at least two states, open and closed, as a result of intramolecular associations between the carboxyl and amino termini. The alpha helical middle portion of the protein is believed to function as a hinge to facilitate these interactions. Cycling between the two states may be regulated by merlin phosphorylation.[12,13] Several lines of evidence suggest that merlin is able to mediate growth arrest in the closed, dephosphorylated conformation, where it can interact with specific proteins, such as CD44.

Similar to ERM proteins, merlin binds to cell surface glycoproteins through its conserved amino terminal (FERM) domain. Notably, merlin associates with CD44, a transmembrane receptor involved in cell-to-cell and cell-to-matrix signaling, to modulate cell growth.[12] In the growth-permissive state, merlin is phosphorylated, perhaps by Rac1,[13] and resides in an inactive, "open" conformation. Dephosphorylation of merlin permits merlin folding and activation, allowing merlin to bind to the cytoplasmic tail of CD44 and to abrogate the CD44-mediated growth signal. The mechanism by which merlin transduces its growth suppressor message is not known; however, studies have suggested that merlin interacts with a number of potential effector molecules that might propagate this signal. One of these molecules, hepatocyte growth factor (HGF)–regulated tyrosine kinase receptor substrate (HRS), is involved in HGF mitogenic signaling, which is important for Schwann cell proliferation. Further studies will be required to determine whether HRS is required for merlin growth suppression.

Like NF1, at least 50% of the mutations associated with NF2 represent new mutations. A significant percentage of patients (20%) without a family history have localized disease and are mosaic for an *NF2* gene mutation. Germ line mutations in NF2 patients are heterogeneous, involving frequent deletions, splice site mutations, nonsense mutations, and less commonly, missense mutations. An early onset and more severe clinical phenotype is often associated with mutations that result in early protein truncation (e.g., frameshift mutations). SSCP analysis, used to screen patients, can identify mutations in about two thirds of all patients with NF2.[7]

Both NF1 and NF2 are considered tumor suppressor disorders. The mechanism by which autosomal dominant tumor suppressor genes result in the formation of tumors is explained by the Knudson "two hit" hypothesis, whereby affected individuals start life with a germ line mutation in the *NF1* (or *NF2*) gene in all cells. Random somatic mutation in the one remaining functional *NF1* or *NF2* gene, the "second hit," is then required for loss of tumor suppressor expression and tumor formation. These second mutations are stochastic and may be affected by other genetic factors, resulting in differential expression of the disorder, even in individuals within the same family. Although the disorder is inherited as an autosomal dominant trait, tumor formation is autosomal recessive at the cellular level because both genes need to be inactivated to result in dysregulated cell growth.

Further support for the Knudson two-hit hypothesis has been provided by studies demonstrating loss of either neurofibromin or merlin expression in tumor specimens from patients with NF1 and NF2, respectively. Loss of *NF1* gene expression and, therefore, loss of neurofibromin protein has been demonstrated in malignant peripheral nerve sheath tumors, pheochromocytomas, myeloid leukemia cells, plexiform neurofibromas, cutaneous neurofibromas, and pilocytic astrocytomas in patients with NF1. In support of the role of neurofibromin as a negative regulator (inhibitor) of RAS, studies have also demonstrated increased levels of activated RAS in tumor cells from NF1 patients with malignant tumors.

Consistent with the lack of pathologic and clinical differences between sporadic and NF2-associated meningiomas and schwannomas, the molecular basis of these tumors is also remarkably similar. Loss of *NF2* expression has been reported, as in NF1-associated tumors, in vestibular schwannomas and meningiomas from patients with NF2. In addition, mutations in the *NF2* gene and loss of merlin expression are also seen in 30% to 70% of sporadic meningiomas and nearly all sporadic schwannomas. This suggests that merlin is an indispensable negative growth regulator for leptomeningeal cells and Schwann cells.

ANIMAL MODELS

In an effort to learn more about the molecular pathogenesis of NF-associated clinical features and to develop preclinical models for NF1 and NF2, a number of research groups have generated mice with targeted disruptions of the *Nf1* and *Nf2* genes. Early studies demonstrated that homozygous deletion of the *Nf1* gene resulted in embryonic lethality by gestational day 14. These mice die not of tumors, but of a cardiac developmental abnormality (double outlet right ventricle). Mice heterozygous for a mutation in the *Nf1* gene (*Nf1+/-* mice) exhibit normal development but manifest deficits in specific learning and memory paradigms.[14] By age 18 to 24 months, *Nf1+/-* mice developed two malignancies associated with NF1, myeloid leukemia and pheochromocytoma. *Nf1+/-* mice do not develop neurofibromas or astrocytomas, the two most common tumor types seen in patients with NF1.

To develop more refined models of NF1-associated tumors, several different approaches have been taken. First, mice have been generated by varying the percentage of *Nf1* null embryonic stem cells in the developing blastocyst. These experiments bypassed the inherent lethality of complete absence of neurofibromin during development and ensured the presence of some neurofibromin-expressing cells during development. Some of these chimeric mice developed plexiform neurofibromas that were histologically similar to those of their human counterparts.[15] The initiating event in the pathogenesis of plexiform neurofibromas in these mice therefore appears to be the complete absence of neurofibromin in specific tissues at an early stage of development. Likewise, plexiform neurofibromas in humans are also thought to be congenital lesions, suggesting *NF1* inactivation in specific cells during fetal development.

A second approach involved the generation of mice with exon-specific deletions to study the role of alternative splicing in neurofibromin function and tumorigenesis. Mice that lacked the alternatively spliced exon 23a that lies within the GTPase activating (GAP) domain were viable, phenotypically normal, and did not have increased tumor predisposition.[16] However, these mice had spatial and contextual learning disorders, similar to the standard *Nf1+/-* mice. Since exon 23a-containing neurofibromin is less efficient at RAS regulation, the fact that these mice exhibited learning deficits supports a non-RAS function for neurofibromin in learning and memory.

Other investigators bypassed the known lethality of *Nf1* null mice by selectively ablating the gene in specific cell types. Selective ablation of the *Nf1* gene in neurons using the Cre/loxP system resulted in mutant mice with growth retardation and cerebral astrogliosis, but no tumor formation.[17] Astrocyte-specific *Nf1* conditional knockout mice showed increased astrocyte proliferation, supporting a role for neurofibromin in regulation of astrocyte proliferation.[17a] Further analysis of these mice and other tissue-specific conditional knockout mice should begin to unravel some of the unique functions of neurofibromin in specific tissues during development and in adulthood.

In order to determine what additional genetic events are required for the development of malignant tumors, mice heterozygous for *Nf1* inactivation were mated with mice heterozygous for a targeted mutation in *p53*, another tumor suppressor gene, which is mutated in many sporadic tumors. Depending on the genetic background, these *Nf1+/-; p53+/-* mice developed MPNSTs, high grade sarcomas, or glioblastomas due to loss of heterozygosity at *both* the *p53* and *Nf1* loci.[18] These findings corroborate observations on human tumors, in which some NF1-associated MPNSTs harbor mutations in the *p53* gene. However, compared with the glioblastomas in the mouse model, NF1-associated pilocytic astrocytomas lack *p53* mutations and only rarely become clinically aggressive tumors. Further studies will likely identify the genes responsible for the phenotypic differences seen between mice of different backgrounds with identical *p53* and *Nf1* mutations.

Neurofibromin may also play an important role in learning and memory. It is uncertain at this time whether the cognitive deficits in NF1 result from the effects of neurofibromin dysfunction on brain development, neuronal physiology, or astrocyte proliferation. *Nf1+/-* mice do not develop identifiable central nervous system malformations or tumors, yet they have distinctive deficits in hippocampal-dependent tasks, including spatial memory and contextual discrimination.[14] Further support for a role of neurofibromin in learning derives from studies in *Drosophila*. *Nf1* mutant flies exhibit defects in learning, which can be rescued by re-expression of wild-type neurofibromin.[19] The mechanism by which the *Drosophila* neurofibromin affects learning is incompletely understood, but may involve the regulation of adenylate cyclase and cyclic AMP signaling. Although learning and memory in *Drosophila* might involve non-RAS pathway signaling, circadian rhythm function requires RAS pathway activation.[20] Studies have demonstrated that mammalian neurons also have defects in cyclic AMP activation, suggesting that neurofibromin might have both RAS and cyclic AMP regulatory functions.[21]

Mice in which both copies of the *Nf2* gene are inactivated die by embryologic day 7, owing to failure to complete gastrulation as a result of an abnormal extra-embryologic ectoderm. These findings argue that merlin (like neurofibromin) plays an important role in embryonic development. *Nf2+/-* mice develop highly malignant and metastatic cancers during the second year of life, including malignant sarcomas, hepatocellular carcinomas, and fibrosarcomas.[22] Loss of the wild-type *Nf2* allele was noted in nearly all of these tumors, again indicating that the *Nf2* gene functions as a classic tumor suppressor gene. Similar to *Nf1*+/- mice, the tumors that develop in the *Nf2*+/- mice are not the typical tumors identified in human NF2.

To facilitate development of a more phenotypically accurate mouse model of NF2, mice were created by homozygous disruption of *Nf2* gene only in myelin P_o-expressing cells (Schwann cells). These mice develop tumors characteristic of NF2, including schwannomas, suggesting that loss of merlin is sufficient for schwannoma development.[23] *Drosophila* also expresses a homologue of merlin. Loss of *Nf2* in *Drosophila* leads to increased cellular proliferation without evidence for malignant transformation.

THERAPY

With an improved and detailed understanding of the mechanisms that underlie neurofibromin and merlin growth regulation, the development of targeted and rational therapeutic strategies becomes possible. Although comparatively less is known about how merlin regulates cell proliferation, the identification of the *NF1* gene and the discovery that it may function as a tumor suppressor by inactivating RAS has opened the door to clinical trials aimed at RAS inactivation. Several clinical trials are presently underway using farnesyltransferase inhibitors to block the addition of a farnesyl group to RAS, a post-translational modification required for RAS membrane translocation and activation. Other therapeutic approaches will likely result from additional basic science research.

Presently, the mainstay of NF treatment is anticipatory management.[8] Careful examination of patients at risk for specific age-dependent features and the prompt recognition of specific signs and symptoms suggestive of astrocytomas, neurofibromas, meningiomas, and schwannomas is required in order to identify those patients who require treatment. Multidisciplinary teams including surgeons, ophthalmologists, dermatologists, oncologists, and radiologists with experience with these disorders are mandatory to avoid unnecessary treatment and to identify problems early. Given the natural history of many NF-associated tumors, a conservative approach with close clinical and radiographic surveillance is recommended. The use of radiation and chemotherapy may be indicated for certain tumors, however the potential risk of developing secondary tumors after treatment of patients with tumor suppressor gene syndromes must be considered.

Routine management of patients with NF1 involves annual ophthalmologic assessments to evaluate for visual abnormalities suggestive of a symptomatic optic pathway glioma in children under the age of 10.[4] If deficits are demonstrated on ophthalmologic evaluation, cranial magnetic resonance imaging is indicated. Any other abnormal neurologic symptom, sign, or examination finding should likewise prompt radiographic evaluation. Plexiform neurofibromas should be closely monitored for the development of sudden pain, new neurologic deficit, or rapid growth. Scoliosis should be screened for clinically, and children with tibial bowing should be referred to an orthopedic surgeon. Routine determinations of blood pressure are recommended to recognize potential complications including renal artery stenosis and pheochromocytoma. Growth should be followed and signs of precocious puberty should be identified and further evaluated. A child's school performance should be monitored for signs of learning disabilities.

Management of NF2 patients requires close surveillance for cranial and spinal tumors.[8] Complete cranial and spinal magnetic resonance imaging is indicated at diagnosis. Annual physical examinations and repeat cranial and spinal imaging studies are recommended to identify and follow tumors as clinically indicated. Audiometry and brain stem auditory evoked responses aid in the detection of clinically significant vestibular schwannomas. Patients are best followed in centers that have a multidisciplinary team familiar with NF2. Some individuals may benefit from hearing aids, cochlear implants, or brain stem implants, depending on the particular situation.

FUTURE DIRECTIONS

The ability to design more rational therapies for NF-associated tumors is heavily dependent on an improved basic understanding of the mechanisms by which merlin and neurofibromin regulate cell growth.[24] Although preliminary insights into these mechanisms have been achieved since the 1990s, future targeted therapies will likely derive from a more detailed appreciation of the molecular and cellular biology of the cells involved in NF-associated tumorigenesis and the consequence of *NF* gene loss on these cell types. The combined study of human tumor tissue, preclinical animal models, and tumor cell lines will facilitate these fundamental advances.

REFERENCES

1. Friedman JM, Gutmann DH, MacCollin MM, Riccardi VM: Neurofibromatosis, 3rd ed. Baltimore, Johns Hopkins Press, 1999.

2. King AA, DeBann MR, Riccardi VM, Gutmann DH: Malignant peripheral nerve sheath tumors in neurofibromatosis 1. Am J Med Genet 2000;93:388–392.

3. Ferner RE, Lucas JD, O'Doherty MJ, et al: Evaluation of (18)fluorodeoxyglucose positron emission tomography ([18]FDG PET) in the detection of malignant peripheral nerve sheath tumours arising from within

plexiform neurofibromas in neurofibromatosis 1. J Neurol Neurosurg Psychiatry 2000;68:353–357.

4. Listernick R, Louis DN, Packer RJ, Gutmann DH: Optic pathway gliomas in children with NF1: Consensus statement from the NF1 Optic Pathway Glioma Task Force. Ann Neurol 1997;41:143–149.

5. Ruggieri M, Huson S: The clinical and diagnostic implications of mosaicism in the neurofibromatoses. Neurology 2001;56:1433–1443.

6. DeBella K, Szudek J, Friedman JM: Use of the National Institutes of Health criteria for diagnosis of neurofibromatosis 1 in children. Pediatrics 2000;105:608–614.

7. Parry DM, MacCollin M, Kaiser-Kupfer MI, et al: Germ-line mutations in the neurofibromatosis 2 gene: Correlation with disease severity and retinal abnormalities. Am J Hum Genet 1996;59:529–539.

8. Gutmann DH, Aylsworth A, Carey JC, et al: The diagnostic evaluation and multidisciplinary management of neurofibromatosis 1 and neurofibromatosis 2. JAMA 1997;278:51–57.

9. Kleihues P, Cavenee WK: Tumors of the Nervous System. Lyon, France, IARC Press, 2000.

10. Gutmann DH: The neurofibromatoses: When less is more. Hum Mol Genet 2001;10:747–755.

11. Messiaen LM, Callens T, Mortier G, et al: Exhaustive mutation analysis of the NF1 gene allows identification of 95% of mutations and reveals an increased frequency of unusual splicing defects. Human Mut 2000;15:541–545.

12. Morrison H, Sherman LS, Legg J, et al: The NF2 tumor suppressor gene product, merlin, mediates contact inhibition through interactions with CD44. Genes Dev 2001;15:968–980.

13. Shaw RJ, Paez JG, Curto M, et al: The NF2 tumor suppressor, merlin, functions in Rac-dependent signaling. Dev Cell 2001;1:63–72.

14. Costa RM, Federov NB, Kogan JH, et al: Mechanism for the learning deficits in a mouse model of neurofibromatosis type 1. Nature 2002;415:526–530.

15. Cichowski K, Shih TS, Schmitt E, et al: Mouse models of tumor development in neurofibromatosis type 1. Science 1999;286:2172–2176.

16. Costa RM, Yang T, Huynh DP, et al: Learning deficits, but normal development and tumor predisposition, in mice lacking exon 23a of Nf1. Nat Genet 2001;27:399–405.

17. Zhu Y, Romero MI, Ghosh P, et al: Ablation of NF1 function in neurons induces abnormal development of cerebral cortex and reactive gliosis in the brain. Genes Dev 2001;15:859–876.

17a. Bajenaru ML, Zhu Y, Hedrick NM, et al: Astrocyte-specific inactivation of the neurofibromatosis 1 gene (NF1) is insufficient for astrocytoma formation. Mol Cell Biol 2002;22:5010–5013.

18. Reilly KM, Loisel DA, Bronson RT, et al: Nf1;Trp53 mutant mice develop glioblastoma with evidence of strain-specific effects. Nat Genet 2000;26:109–113.

19. Guo H, Tong J, Hannan F, et al: A neurofibromatosis-1-regulated pathway is required for learning in *Drosophila*. Nature 2000;403:895–898.

20. Williams JA, Su HS, Bernards A, et al: A circadian output in *Drosophila* mediated by neurofibromatosis-1 and Ras/MAPK. Science 2001;293:2251–2256.

21. Tong J, Hannan F, Zhu Y, et al: Neurofibromin regulates G protein-stimulated adenylyl cyclase activity. Nat Neurosci 2002;5:95–96.

22. McClatchey AI, Saotome I, Mercer K: Mice heterozygous for a mutation at the NF2 tumor suppressor locus develop a range of highly metastatic tumors. Genes Dev 1998;12:1121–1133.

23. Giovannini M, Robanus-Maandag E, van der Valk M: Conditional biallelic Nf2 mutation in the mouse promotes manifestations of human neurofibromatosis type 2. Genes Dev 2000;14:1617–1630.

24. MacCollin M, Gutmann DH, Korf B, Finkelstein R: Establishing priorities in neurofibromatosis research: A workshop summary. Genet Med 2001;3:212–217.

The Genetic Epilepsies

Marc A. Dichter

Jeffrey R. Buchhalter

The term *epilepsy* describes a family of neurologic disorders characterized by recurrent, unprovoked seizures. Seizures are paroxysmal, involuntary motor, sensory, or cognitive phenomena due to the abnormal, synchronous discharge of cortical neurons. Some forms of epilepsy may be inherited, and these may occur in a variety of transmission patterns. Other forms may arise secondary to a brain injury or acquired neurologic disorder.

Not everyone with seizures has epilepsy. Provocative factors that can induce a seizure, but not necessarily cause epilepsy, include acute metabolic derangements, head trauma, alcohol ingestion, and high fever (in children).

Epidemiology

A conservative estimate of the overall incidence of epilepsy is between 31 and 57:100,000 cases, which indicates that there are 70,000 to 129,000 new cases per year in the United States.[1] This compares to 3:100,000 for Duchenne muscular dystrophy and 0.4:100,000 for myasthenia gravis. The prevalence of active epilepsy cases, when corrected for under-reporting, is 6.42:1000 using the 1975 Rochester, Minnesota data[2] that calculates to approximately 1.6 million people in the United States, a relatively high proportion of whom are children.

Problems Associated with the Genetic Analysis of the Epilepsies

It should be stated at the outset that the cellular pathophysiology of seizures in humans is unknown. Thus, our current classifications are based upon observation of behavioral manifestations of seizures (e.g., arm jerking, staring) and/or patient's report of internal phenomena (e.g., tingling in an extremity, visual/auditory/gustatory hallucinations) that may be correlated with concurrent electroencephalographic (EEG) activity.

Analysis of the varying manifestations of seizures, EEG patterns, functional impairment, family history, known etiologies, and response to antiepileptic medication strongly suggests that *epilepsy* is a generic term, like *cancer*, and is somewhat misleading due to the implication of a single clinical syndrome and underlying cause. Thus, the *epilepsies* is a more realistic descriptor of this group of disorders that have in common an abnormality in the regulation of neuronal excitability.

Several kinds of problems complicate interpretation of published genetic analyses of the epilepsies. Criteria often are not specified for inclusion as an affected kindred member. These criteria have included seizure type, an EEG finding by itself, or a combination of clinical and EEG features weighted toward either. If an abnormal EEG were an important inclusion criterion for a given syndrome, all kindreds in which EEGs have not been obtained on unaffected and affected family members would be invalid for analysis. Similarly, because some forms of EEG abnormalities are age-dependent (possibly disappearing by age 20 to 25 years), even in studies in which all family members were tested, older adults could not have been adequately assessed. In addition, incomplete as well as age-dependent penetrance is not always taken into account. The statement of "family history of seizures" frequently does not specify if it is the same type of seizure as in the proband or another seizure type. In some cases, this would be important, while in others it might not be. (It is relatively common among families in which multiple members have seizures for there to be multiple seizure types expressed.) Finally, when ascertaining family histories, it is not always recognized that families frequently conceal affected members.

The current state of the genetic analyses of human epilepsies is very heterogeneous. For some forms of epilepsy, epidemiologists are still trying to determine whether there is any familial (hereditary) predisposition. Other forms of epilepsy are known to run in families, but the mode of inheritance and degree of penetrance of the trait are still in doubt. Finally, a number of forms of epilepsy have been localized to specific chromosomes, and several specific genetic mutations have been identified.

As will be discussed in the following section, a variety of cellular processes can lead to a state of heightened excitability, and the determination of the process underlying a specific epilepsy in any given family will provide the basis for future understanding of the epilepsies at the molecular and genetic level. The corollary of this multifactorial causality is that multiple perturbations of brain function can produce common phenomenologic outcomes, thus different genetic mechanisms may produce a relatively homogeneous clinical syndrome in different kindreds.

Classification

In order to investigate the pathophysiology, genetics, treatment, and prognosis of any class of disorders, a rational classification scheme is required. This effort has been particularly difficult in the epilepsies due to the variety of terms used for description. These include terms that relate to presumed brain focus *(frontal, temporal)*, perceived impact *(grand mal, petit mal)*, associated EEG pattern *(spike-wave)*, neurophysiologic system involved *(motor, sensory, autonomic)*, seizure morphology *(motor, sensory, psychic, psychomotor)*, knowledge of etiology *(idiopathic, symptomatic)*, and presumed pattern of onset *(partial/focal/local, generalized)*. Authors have used modifiers such as *simple, complex, minor, major, typical* and *atypical* in an idiosyncratic fashion. These modifiers often had fundamentally different meanings when used by different authors.

Currently, two types of classification systems are in widespread use. The first classification system is based on seizure type, whereas the second is based on epilepsy syndrome (i.e., a constellation of clinical, historical, and electrophysiologic features that describe a patient population).

The International Classification of Epileptic Seizures[3] uses behavioral and electrophysiologic data to classify seizures (Table 38–1). The fundamental difference among seizures as classified by this system is the presumed mode of onset (i.e. partial versus generalized). Thus, behavioral onset demonstrated by jerking of a single extremity or a focal ictal/interictal epileptiform EEG abnormality in the context of a nonlocalizing seizure (e.g.,

TABLE 38–1. International Classification of Epileptic Seizures

Partial seizures (beginning locally)
Simple partial seizures (with no impairment of consciousness)
With motor symptoms
With somatosensory or special sensory symptoms
With autonomic symptoms
With psychic symptoms
Complex partial seizures (with impairment of consciousness)
Simple partial onset followed by impairment of consciousness
With impairment of consciousness at onset
Partial seizures evolving to secondary generalized seizures
Generalized seizures (convulsive or nonconvulsive)
Absence
Typical
Atypical
Myoclonic seizures
Clonic seizures
Tonic seizures
Tonic-clonic seizures
Atonic seizures
Unclassified epileptic seizures

Adapted from Commission on Classification and Terminology of the International League Against Epilepsy. Proposal for revised clinical and electroencephalographic classification of epileptic seizures. Epilepsia 1981; 22:489–501.

tonic-clonic, staring) is sufficient to assign a partial onset to the seizure. Partial seizures are then subdivided into simple, complex, and secondarily generalized. Impairment of consciousness distinguishes a complex partial seizure from a simple partial seizure. A simple partial seizure can have motor, sensory, autonomic, or psychic components. Secondary generalization implies spread from the initiating focus to the remainder of the cortex. The group of generalized seizures is defined by an inability to identify a discrete seizure focus by clinical features or EEG recording. The seizures may take the form of staring, atonic, clonic, tonic, myoclonic, or tonic-clonic activity. Thus, the two most common seizure phenotypes, staring and tonic-clonic convulsions, can be due to either partial or generalized onset. Information regarding family history or prognosis is not part of this classification system.

The other classification system is based upon epilepsy type rather than seizure type. This was not a new concept when the International League Against Epilepsy proposed and subsequently revised[4] its Classification of Epilepsies and Epileptic Syndromes (Table 38–2). This classification scheme also uses localization-related (partial) versus generalized as the first major branch point in the categorization of epilepsy types. A distinction is then made between idiopathic and symptomatic groups. *Idiopathic* is defined by "no known or suspected etiology, other than possible hereditary predisposition," whereas *symptomatic* indicates that a disorder is known or suspected. Originally, epilepsies or epileptic syndromes in which genetic factors were believed to play a role were classified as generalized and idiopathic. However, recently, several types of partial epilepsies with clear genetic components have been identified. As noted in Table 38–2, this classification acknowledges that there are seizures in which the mode of onset is uncertain and that occur under special circumstances (e.g., febrile seizures).

The Electroencephalogram

The electroencephalogram (EEG) is not only the major laboratory means of recording abnormal brain electrical activity, but the nature of abnormalities in the EEG has been used in several classification schemes. Furthermore, EEG "traits" may be present in asymptomatic relatives of patients with epilepsy and have been used to mark disease for pedigree analysis.

The summed excitatory and inhibitory postsynaptic potentials in the superficial layers of cortex underlying the electrode generate the EEG. Although precise mechanisms are unknown, diencephalic structures such as the thalamus stimulate and synchronize cortical neurons. The recorded EEG has a characteristic amplitude and frequency distribution across various regions of cortex. These characteristics change dramatically as a function of state of arousal and age. Thus, identification of abnormal activity must account for these factors. The distribution of abnormalities is defined as "generalized" if the entire brain is simultaneously affected, or "focal" if restricted to one or two EEG contact points. Its amplitude, sharpness, and frequency describe the morphology of the abnormality. Although significant interindividual differences exist,

TABLE 38–2. International Classification of Epilepsies and Epileptic Syndromes

Localization-related (focal, local, partial) epilepsies and syndromes
  Idiopathic with age-related onset
    Benign childhood epilepsy with centrotemporal spike
    Childhood epilepsy with occipital paroxysms
  Symptomatic
    Syndromes of great individual variability that are mainly based on anatomical localization, clinical features, seizure type, and etiological factors (if known)
Generalized epilepsies and syndromes
  Idiopathic, with age related onset, listed in order of age
    Benign neonatal familial convulsions
    Benign neonatal convulsions
    Benign myoclonic epilepsy in infancy
    Childhood absence epilepsy (pyknolepsy)
    Juvenile absence epilepsy
    Juvenile myoclonic epilepsy (impulsive petit mal)
    Epilepsy with grand mal seizures on awakening (GTCS).
  Other generalized idiopathic epilepsies, if they do not belong to one of the above syndromes, can still be classified as generalized idiopathic epilepsies
  Idiopathic and/or symptomatic, in order of age or appearance
    West syndrome (infantile spasms)
    Lennox-Gastaut syndrome
    Epilepsy with myoclonic-astatic seizures
    Epilepsy with myoclonic absences

Symptomatic
  Nonspecific etiology
    Early myoclonic encephalopathy
  Specific syndromes
    Epileptic seizures may complicate many disease states
Epilepsies and syndromes undetermined as to whether they are focal or generalized
  With both generalized and focal seizures
    Neonatal seizures
    Severe myoclonic epilepsy in infancy
    Epilepsy with continuous spike waves during slow-wave sleep
    Acquired epileptic aphasia (Landau-Kleffner syndrome)
  Without unequivocal generalized or focal features
    This heading covers all cases in which clinical and EEG findings do not permit classification as clearly generalized or localization-related, such as in many cases of sleep grand mal
Special syndromes
  Situation-related seizures
    Febrile convulsions
    Seizures related to other identifiable situations such as stress, hormonal changes, drugs, alcohol, or sleep deprivation
  Isolated, apparently unprovoked epileptic events
  Epilepsies characterized by specific modes of seizure precipitation
  Chronic progressive epilepsia partialis continua of childhood

it is clear that the expression of both normal and abnormal patterns is at least partially under genetic control.

The EEG can mark intrinsic hyperexcitability during periods when seizures are not occurring and can provide data about the possible location of abnormal cortical tissue or about a generalized hyperexcitable state. However, even in individuals with well-characterized epilepsy, EEGs may be normal during the interictal period, especially in individuals with localization-related epilepsy. The EEG is usually abnormal during the seizure, and the presence and characteristics of the abnormal discharges can be used to define and localize the seizure. Occasionally, the ictal EEG recorded from the scalp may remain normal, especially during simple partial seizures and some forms of complex partial seizures (e.g., those originating from frontal cortex or deep temporal cortex). Electrographic seizures can be recorded in such patients when electrodes are placed deep in brain structures during presurgical evaluations.

Specific EEG patterns highly correlate with and in some cases define specific types of epilepsy, such as the generalized 3-Hz spike slow-wave discharge in childhood absence epilepsy, the photoconvulsive response (PCR) in primary generalized epilepsies, or the characteristic centro-temporal focal discharge in benign epilepsy of childhood with Rolandic spikes (discussed later). As expected, these abnormalities share the age-related penetrance with the associated epilepsy syndrome. The 3-Hz spike-wave pattern and the PCR are sufficiently closely linked to the clinical epilepsy syndromes that they can be used for identification of asymptomatic relatives. Similarly, studies that have selected patients based on focal spikes or sharp waves in temporal-central regions independent of epilepsy type have indicated a significant familial inheritance of the EEG trait.

CELLULAR AND MOLECULAR MECHANISMS OF EPILEPSY

Many types of cellular changes (e.g., in ion channel function, neurotransmitter receptor regulation, and energy metabolism) can result in an increase in excitability and an epileptic event. The normal vertebrate cortex is composed of individual small cellular networks that are easily perturbed to develop hypersynchronous discharges. To understand how specific genetic alterations in CNS function could lead to a form of epilepsy, it is appropriate to review the pathophysiology of seizures.

A seizure occurs when neurons in a focal area of brain, or throughout the entire brain, become activated in an unusually synchronous manner. Normally, neuronal activity is relatively desynchronized, such that groups of neurons are activated or inhibited sequentially as information passes through the brain. However, under a variety of circumstances, this distributed level of neuronal activation becomes organized into synchronous discharges, and these discharges are readily able to involve nearby and distant neurons in the abnormal activation pattern. The type of seizure that will then occur will depend on the amount and location of the CNS tissue that is included in the abnormal activation and the speed with which the discharge spreads through the brain. If stimulated in a particularly intense and specific manner, the normal anatomic microstructure of the vertebrate cortex and the normal physiology of the local connections appear to be sufficient substrates for development and propagation of hypersynchronous activity. Thus, in many respects, the development of seizure activity in the brain does not necessarily imply anything more than a momentary alteration in CNS physiology. On the other hand, the propensity to recurrent and unprovoked seizures (epilepsy) is usually the result of some anatomic or physiologic abnormality. Since many different disturbances can produce a similar final common outcome (a seizure), it is possible for many different forms of genetic abnormality to produce epilepsy. The genetic epilepsies are not a homogeneous collection of syndromes but represent multiple forms of genetic disturbances in the differentiation and function of different elements within the CNS.

Mechanisms Underlying Focal Epileptiform Activity

One of the hallmarks of hyperexcitable brain is an interictal spike discharge in the EEG. These discharges are manifestations of hypersynchronous activation of a group of pyramidal neurons underlying the area in which the spike is observed. The underlying cellular event that generates the EEG spike is a large depolarizing potential that occurs synchronously in many neurons within the area of hyperexcitability or "epileptic focus." This has been called the paroxysmal depolarizing shift (DS). A large prolonged hyperpolarization (the post-DS HP) that is the cellular correlate of the slow wave that follows EEG spike discharges usually follows the DS. Neurons are alternately excited during the DS and inhibited during the HP. The DS is generated by a combination of synaptic currents (mediated by the excitatory neurotransmitters glutamate and aspartate) flowing through neuronal dendrites arranged perpendicular to the cortical surface, and voltage-dependent depolarizing currents, especially calcium currents. Some neurons in the cortex are able to generate endogenous bursts owing to large voltage-dependent calcium currents, and these may serve as "triggers" or amplifying agents. However, such bursting neurons are not necessary for network hyperexcitability to be sustained.

The neurons become synchronized by several mechanisms. Local recurrent excitatory circuits are enhanced, either chronically because of reorganization of synaptic circuits after a lesion, or acutely because of increases in synaptic efficacy related to high-frequency activation of neurons. The latter may involve the recruitment of NMDA receptors. These glutamate- or aspartate-activated receptor/channel complexes are relatively quiescent during normal synaptic transmission, as they are blocked at normal neuronal resting potentials by ambient concentrations of magnesium. However, as neurons depolarize, the magnesium block becomes less effective, and more depolarizing channels can be activated by a given amount of excitatory neurotransmitter. Thus, both the circuitry and the nature of excitatory synaptic actions establish a positive feedback system. In addition, as neurons depolarize, one or more classes of voltage-dependent calcium channels are activated. The depolarization produced by current flow through these channels can also contribute to the DS. All of these mechanisms are present in normal neurons within the cortex. They presumably are activated at relatively low levels during normal CNS activity, and excessive activation must be kept in check by powerful inhibitory mechanisms. When such inhibition is reduced for any reason, this pattern of regenerative activity occurs, which leads to a focal epileptic discharge. If inhibitory control mechanisms break down further, the excitatory activity can spread to both nearby and distant areas of brain and a generalized seizure can develop.

The hyperpolarization that follows the DS (and which contributes to the "wave" of the "spike-wave complex" in the EEG) is thought to be produced by a variety of mechanisms. Synaptic inhibition, especially that mediated by gamma-amino butyric acid (GABA) via both GABA$_A$ and GABA$_B$ receptors, is very powerful and ubiquitous in cortex, producing both feedforward and feedback inhibition. As pyramidal cells discharge, they activate inhibitory interneurons that relay inhibition back to the neurons discharging and to local surround areas. Thus, synaptic inhibition can shut off the discharge and limit its spread within the cortex. In addition, voltage-dependent hyperpolarizing currents (mostly potassium currents) are activated during the DS that also serve to limit its duration. Finally, the large influx of calcium that occurs during the DS also activates calcium-dependent currents (potassium and possibly chloride) that further limit the duration of the excitatory event.

Neurons can also be synchronized by large currents that flow extracellularly around their dendrites, by changes in their external environment during excessive activity (increases in extracellular potassium and decreases in extracellular calcium), and by electrical coupling, which may be present within some areas of cortex.

Mechanisms Underlying the Transition into Seizures

When inhibitory mechanisms break down, or when excitatory mechanisms become even more enhanced, relatively limited interictal discharges can be converted to a full seizure. This transition involves both an *escape* of the local discharge and the *spread* of the discharge to nearby and distant areas of brain.

Both the development of seizure activity and the spread of seizure activity into normal areas of brain also appear to involve normal synaptic pathways and physiologic mechanisms. Discharges travel down axons, invade projection areas, and are fed back into the actively discharging areas by recurrent excitatory connections. High-frequency discharges produce frequency potentiation of excitatory synapses, both via presynaptic and postsynaptic mechanisms. In addition, as postsynaptic neurons depolarize, more NMDA receptors become active, more depolarization occurs, and more calcium enters the cell. As enhancement of excitatory synaptic efficacy continues, other mechanisms of plasticity may become involved to potentiate these pathways further.

At the same time that excitation is being potentiated, inhibitory circuits may diminish in potency. The actions of GABA can be very powerful, but inhibitory synaptic efficacy appears to be very sensitive to high-frequency activation. Therefore, activation patterns that will enhance excitatory efficacy will also decrease inhibitory potency and lead to the development and spread of epileptic activity.

As excitation enhances and inhibition diminishes, more and more areas will be incorporated into the seizure. In addition to the "downstream" spread, axon terminals in the primary area of discharge can become activated, presumably because of the neurotransmitters being released and the accumulation of extracellular potassium. These axons will fire antidromically, activating areas of brain "upstream" from the focus, and, via their recurrent collaterals, multiple additional areas. Thus, seizure activity can spread very rapidly from a focal area of abnormality to many other areas that are not part of the epileptic focus. The speed and extent of spread will depend on the connections from the primary area of abnormality, the intensity of the primary discharge, and the "receptive" state of other regions of brain.

The last factor may conceptually explain how certain systemic events can cause individuals with a seizure propensity to develop a seizure at a given point in time. For example, some women will have seizures only at specific times in their menstrual cycles. This could be due to the actions of estrogen on the epileptic focus itself, or its actions on the excitability of normal areas of brain into which the primary epileptic focus is projecting. Similarly, stress, illness, or other factors could facilitate seizures via a variety of physiologic changes, related to secretion of stress hormones and cytokines and the interaction between neuronal excitability and the endocrine and immune systems. None of these factors will produce epilepsy on their own, but each may facilitate the development of seizures in someone with an underlying excitable lesion or predisposition.

Development of Epileptogenic Areas

Areas of hyperexcitability can develop acutely, for example in response to drugs that block inhibition or enhance excitation. However, many individuals develop epilepsy after some form of brain injury. Under these circumstances, it appears that injury evokes a reaction in the surviving neurons such that their axons sprout collaterals that "fill in" for missing synapses. These new synapses tend to be excitatory and increase the local recurrent excitatory connections in an area. Moreover, there are alterations in neurotransmitter receptors (including those for NMDA and GABA) and possibly glial cells, in those regions that likely contribute to the hyperexcitability. In addition, under certain circumstances, inhibitory interneurons may be more susceptible to hypoxia or injury, leading to a selective loss of inhibitory elements after some forms of brain injury—again creating a hyperexcitable area of cortex. The mammalian hippocampus appears to be particularly vulnerable to hypoxia and injury, and in addition, is particularly epileptogenic (perhaps owing to the close packing of neurons in this structure). It is not surprising, therefore, that many individuals with complex partial seizures have structural abnormalities in their hippocampi.

Mechanisms Underlying Primary Generalized Seizures

Most forms of primary generalized epilepsy are thought to be genetic, although mode of inheritance and number of genetic factors responsible are not well characterized (discussed later). These forms of epilepsy are generally characterized by bilateral synchronous spike-wave discharges seen diffusely throughout the cortex. The most prominent current hypothesis for the pathophysiology of primary generalized absence seizures relates to alterations in thalamocortical rhythms. Under normal circumstances, the thalamocortical network generates both low- and high-frequency oscillations, the nature of which depend on the arousal state of the individual. These rhythms appear to originate in the reciprocal excitatory circuits that exist between many parts of neocortex and the main thalamic relay nuclei. Axons of cortical pyramidal cells form excitatory synapses with neurons in thalamic relay nuclei; these cells, in turn, make excitatory connections with neurons in ipsilateral cortex. Collaterals from both axon sets synapse on GABAergic, inhibitory neurons in the intralaminar nuclei, and these, in turn, send inhibitory connections to thalamic relay cells, other intralaminar neurons, and widespread areas of neocortex.

Neurons in the thalamus have a form of voltage dependent Ca current, called the T-current, which is unusually large. This current is inactivated at normal resting potentials and becomes de-inactivated, or reset, when the neuron is hyperpolarized. When depolarization triggers T-currents, they produce relatively large and long-lasting depolarizations that secondarily trigger bursts of action potentials. Simultaneously, the depolarization inactivates the T-type Ca channels. Hyperpolarizing afterpotentials (that repolarize the membrane and de-

inactivate the T-channels and activate another intrinsic, voltage-dependent current in these cells that can serve as a pacemaker) follow the bursts of action potentials. It has been hypothesized that either altered inhibitory inputs into the thalamic relay cells or T-currents that have different activation/inactivation kinetics may foster the development of this kind of thalamocortical rhythmicity, producing the 3- to 4-Hz spike-wave activity commonly seen. This could occur by subtle genetic alterations in a receptor, transmitter, or channel.

When the spike-wave discharges become prolonged, more of the normal brain activity can be entrained (probably utilizing mechanisms similar to those regarding the transition to seizures in partial epilepsy) and generalized tonic-clonic seizures will develop. Thus, again, mild perturbations in normal synaptic physiology, especially those related to frequency-dependent changes in synaptic efficacy, can produce dramatic changes in brain electrophysiology and behavior.

ANIMAL MODELS OF INHERITED EPILEPSY

Genetic models of epilepsy are found in numerous species, including mice, rats, gerbils, baboons, chickens, and dogs. Many of these have been well-characterized in relation to seizure morphology, electroencephalography, neuropathology, and responsiveness to antiepileptic drugs. Several single-gene mutations have been identified, and the mechanisms underlying the epilepsy are being elucidated. In addition to spontaneous mutations, a number of transgenic mice have been developed with specific gene knockouts that have spontaneous seizures as part of the phenotypic consequences of the altered gene. It is beyond the scope of this chapter to review all important issues related to the genetic analyses of these varied epilepsy models, and several comprehensive reviews are available.[5,6] However, a number of important principles have emerged from the studies of these models. These principles can be directly applied to the analysis of human genetic epilepsies and will be emphasized. In addition, we will summarize the available data about the nature, pathophysiology, and genetics of some of the important animal models and compare these models to specific forms of human epilepsy. Again, it must be emphasized that epilepsy can be relatively easily produced in all vertebrates by a wide range of perturbations in normal physiology or brain biochemistry. Therefore, it is not surprising that a wide range of genetic alterations can produce epileptic syndromes.

General Principles

The most well-characterized of the animal epilepsies, from the genetic perspective, are those caused by single-gene mutations in the mouse.[5] At least thirteen distinct chromosomal loci are known where mutations can cause spontaneous convulsive seizures, and six additional loci appear to be individually involved in absence-like seizures. All but two of these are inherited as autosomal recessive traits. These mutant mice clearly demonstrate that single-gene mutations can induce an entire epilepsy phenotype and profoundly affect brain excitability. Analyses of seizures produced by these mutations indicate that different genetic defects can produce very similar phenotypes. Moreover, single-gene defects can produce multiple seizure phenotypes in individual mice (e.g., absences and motor seizure in tottering mice). Interactions between specific genes appear to produce intermediate epilepsy syndromes, and interactions between the epilepsy genes and others may mask the epilepsy phenotype.[5] Finally, many of these mice exhibit age-dependent expression of seizure phenotypes and EEG changes, emphasizing the importance of performing developmental studies when examining genetic epilepsy.

Not all mutations that significantly affect brain development produce seizures. As pointed out by Noebels,[5] a number of mutations that cause cortical and cerebellar dysgenesis do not produce seizures or clearly epileptogenic EEGs. Although this may be evidence that *nonspecific* lesions of the nervous system do not always produce epilepsy, the corollary that all mutations that produce epilepsy operate on *epilepsy-specific* processes is not necessarily true. As mentioned previously, many factors that affect brain excitability can produce epilepsy, and it may be inappropriate to identify any one particular genetic abnormality that causes epilepsy as an epilepsy-specific gene.

Analyses of another series of inbred mice that have various levels of susceptibility to audiogenic seizures (AGS) have led to additional conclusions. Again, expression of the epileptiform traits is age-dependent. These animals have been studied extensively with sophisticated crossbreeding paradigms. However, the mode of inheritance of AGS susceptibility remains unclear. Proposals include a single autosomal dominant with minor modifying factors, an autosomal recessive loosely linked to another gene, two unlinked loci with variable degrees of penetrance, or multiple genetic factors.

Single Gene Mutations in Mice That Produce Epilepsy

A very large number of single-gene mutations in inbred mouse strains, arising spontaneously or by induction, are available for phenotypic analysis.[6] Several of these were noted to have an absence-like seizure phenotype, consisting of cessation of motor activity and occasional posturing associated with a spike-wave abnormality in the EEG. The EEG often shows 6- to 7-Hz activity rather than 3-Hz activity seen in humans, although the slow-wave epilepsy (SWE) mouse exhibits 3- to 4.5-Hz activity. Four of these mice, tottering (tg), lethargic (lh), stargazer (stg), and ducky (dky), have been found to have mutations in subunits of voltage-

dependent calcium channels that produce variable abnormalities in function, including decreased and, in one case, apparent increased function. SWE has a mutation in the Na-H exchanger. The specific links between the mutations and the epilepsy have not been completely elucidated (see reference 6 for a detailed review.)

Epileptic Rats

Two strains of rats with genetically determined susceptibility to epilepsy have proved useful as polygenic inheritance and susceptibility genes and as models for studies with antiepileptic agents. Genetically epilepsy-prone rats (GEPRs) are derived from the Sprague-Dawley strain and have increased susceptibility to audiogenic seizures. Genetic absence epilepsy rats (GAERs) are a variant of the Wistar strain that exhibit absence-like seizures that correlate with EEG spike-wave discharges at 7 to 8 Hz and develop during late adolescence (4 to 5 weeks) and continue through adulthood. Many characteristics of the absence seizures in these rats mimic absence seizures in humans. The GAERs also respond to classical antiepileptic drugs in a similar pattern to their human counterparts. Neither the pathophysiology of the seizures nor the genetic abnormality has been elucidated.

INHERITED HUMAN EPILEPSIES: THE GENETICS OF GENERALIZED EPILEPSIES AND SYNDROMES

Benign Familial Neonatal Convulsions (BFNC)

Clinical. BFNC is an epilepsy syndrome characterized by apnea, and focal or generalized clonic or tonic seizures described in multiple families. Onset is usually in the first week of life, but may occur up to 4 months. Seizure frequency is in the range of 1 to 40 per day with duration of 30 seconds to 3 minutes. The EEG usually reveals generalized abnormalities, but focal onset has also been demonstrated. Metabolic studies as well as neuroimaging are normal. The seizures most commonly remit weeks to months following onset. The term *benign* may not be entirely appropriate, as 3% to 16% of children will have neurologic sequelae such as learning disabilities, epilepsy, and developmental delays. Thus, phenotypic heterogeneity exists within this syndrome.

Genetics. BFNC is the first epilepsy syndrome to which a chromosome assignment was made (chromosome 20). In 1998, positional cloning techniques were used to identify the *EBN1* locus as a potassium channel gene (*KCNQ2*).[7] The mutated channel did not produce a measurable current when expressed in frog oocytes. Homology mapping identified a potassium channel (*KCNQ3*) in the family mapping to *EBN2* on chromosome 8q.[8] A variety of mutations, including frameshift, missense, and splice-site mutants, have been identified. The expression of *KCN2* and *KCN3* in mammalian neocortex and hippocampus and the production of an M-type potassium current when co-injected into oocytes suggests that these genes produce a heterodimer that regulates an important channel controlling neuronal excitability. Heterozygous mice in which one of the *KCN2* genes has been knocked out do not have spontaneous seizures, but are more susceptible to pentylenetetrazol-induced convulsions than wild-type mice. This animal model corresponds to the human condition in which one, but not both, potassium channels are affected and a mild epilepsy syndrome results. However, in a study of unrelated individuals with unprovoked motor seizures within the first 4 months of life and a family history of childhood seizures, all or most idiopathic seizures were not due to these voltage-gated potassium channel mutations. There were no detectable mutations in *KCN2*, *KCN3*, or the recently described *KCN5* genes.

Benign Familial Infantile Convulsions (BFIC)

Clinical. Children with this benign idiopathic epilepsy syndrome have seizure onset between 4 and 8 months of age. Seizures usually occur in clusters and are characterized by behavioral arrest, slow horizontal deviation of head and eyes, cyanosis, and generalized hypertonia with unilateral and/or bilateral limb jerks. The interictal EEG is normal whereas the ictal EEG demonstrates parieto-occipital onset with or without secondary generalization. Imaging and metabolic studies have been unrevealing. The prognosis is excellent as seizures stopped in all the probands, and psychomotor decline has not been reported with limited follow-up.

Genetics. Pedigree analysis of the original cohort suggested an autosomal dominant mode of transmission. Because of similarities with the syndrome of BFNC, markers for this syndrome were analyzed, but the results excluded this locus. Linkage to markers on chromosome 19q was reported in five families. However, linkage to this locus was excluded by two further studies using the same criteria. A locus on chromosome 16p was then described that linked to individuals with BFIC who did or did not have choreoathetosis associated with the seizures. These studies indicate that genetic heterogeneity can underlie the BFIC phenotype and that allelism exists to the syndrome associated with choreoathetosis.

Generalized Epilepsy with Febrile Seizures Plus (GEFS+) and Severe Myoclonic Epilepsy of Infancy (SMEI)

Clinical. A number of families have now been described wherein individuals have seizures with fever during early childhood that continue beyond the age of 6 and/or are associated with seizures in the absence of fever. The types of seizures varied, and included myoclonic, atonic, absence, and complex partial seizures. Most seizures ceased by mid-adolescence, and most had normal neurologic development. EEGs often showed generalized spike-wave or polyspike discharges.[9]

Genetics. Two genes responsible for the GEFS+ syndrome have been identified, both of which are part of the voltage-dependent Na channel family. The first gene mapped, *GEFS1*, was found on chromosome 19q and was identified as the β1 subunit of the Na channel *(SCN1B)*.[10] The second, *GEFS2*, was identified on chromosome 2q, as the a1 subunit *(SCN1A)*.[11] Several families have been described with different mutations in both of these subunits. The known mutations in both subunits appear to have as a common physiologic consequence a decreased inactivation of the Na current and the appearance of a persistent Na current that leads to neuronal hyperexcitability. These mutations are similar to those in skeletal muscle Na channels that cause myotonia. Other families have been described with the syndrome of FEBS+ that do not appear to have mutations in either of these two genes, so that other mutations must exist.

Severe myoclonic epilepsy of infancy (SMEI) is a form of epilepsy that develops in infants and is characterized by tonic, clonic, or tonic-clonic seizures that often occur initially in the context of febrile illnesses but then recur without fever. Later, other forms of seizures appear, including myoclonic, absence, and simple and complex partial. Children developing this form of epilepsy usually experience psychomotor retardation in the second year of life. This syndrome has been linked to another mutation in the same *SCN1A* gene that produces the milder forms of GEFS+ discussed above, thus illustrating another example of genetic heterogeneity among the genetic epilepsies.

Generalized Epilepsy with Febrile Seizures and Absence (Gefs+/Absence)

Clinical. Several families have been described in which individuals have febrile seizures, some of whom go on to develop typical absence epilepsy. Some members of the family also develop other forms of nonfebrile seizures, so in many respects these families are similar to the GEFS+, except that absence seizures tend to predominate in the cohort.

Genetics. Several mutations have now been identified in *GABA* receptor complex genes in these families. The first identified was a mutation in the γ2 subunit[12] that produced a loss of benzodiazepine sensitivity. Two other families have been described with mutations in the same subunit that cause complete loss of GABA sensitivity in receptors containing the mutated subunit.[13]

Age-Related Idiopathic Generalized Epilepsies (IGE)

It is estimated that these syndromes account for 30% to 40% of all epilepsy and are composed of several clinical entities with overlapping clinical and electrographic features. They have in common an age-dependent onset (younger than 20 years), normal cognitive development, and absence of abnormalities on neurologic examination. Seizure types include absence, myoclonus, and generalized tonic-clonic seizures. The EEG reveals a normal background and ≥3-hz generalized spike-wave discharges. Syndromes having a prominent familial predisposition include juvenile myoclonic epilepsy (JME), juvenile absence epilepsy (JAE), childhood absence epilepsy (CAE), and generalized tonic-clonic seizures on awakening. Several factors complicate the genetic analysis of these syndromes. The distribution and frequency of seizure types within identified syndromes and pedigrees can be variable, influencing the designation of family members within pedigrees as affected or unaffected. As noted below, this intrafamilial heterogeneity can have a profound effect on genetic linkage studies. The EEG traits used to define syndromes and to include asymptomatic family members as affected may also have an age-dependent occurrence. Recent analyses have emphasized the importance of precise and extensive clinical and electrographic diagnosis for the genetic definition of these related but not uniform, syndromes.

Juvenile Myoclonic Epilepsy (JME)

Clinical. JME is a syndrome occurring in individuals between 8 and 20 years of age with seizures consisting of myoclonic jerks, usually in the morning upon awakening, which may proceed to generalized tonic-clonic seizures (GTCS). Absences occur at a variable rate with the possibility that frequent absences may indicate a genetically distinct syndrome. The most common EEG abnormality is 4- to 6-Hz bilaterally symmetric poly-spike wave complexes or 2- to 3-Hz spike-wave complexes.

Genetics. It is clear that there is a high incidence of JME as well as several other generalized seizure types in families of individuals with JME. There is also a fairly high incidence (approximately 11% to 12% in siblings and parents) of abnormal EEGs (diffuse spike-wave complexes or spike-sharp and slow wave complexes) in family members who do not develop clinical seizures. Several groups have performed genetic linkage analyses on individuals with abnormal EEGs as inclusion criteria, whereas earlier studies employed only phenotypic descriptions of seizures as inclusion criteria.

The mode of inheritance of JME may differ with individual kindreds. A dominant mode with high penetrance (70% to 90%)[14] and a recessive mode have been proposed. More recent analyses of twin, linkage, and segregation studies indicate that a two-locus model provides a better fit for the data on affected individuals than a simple Mendelian dominant or recessive single locus.[15]

As argued by Delgado-Escueta et al., it is possible that at the molecular level different abnormal genes, even at the same locus, could have different modes of expression and appear more or less dominant under different circumstances. (For example, a mutation in one gene causing its coded protein to fail to be expressed may appear to be inherited as an autosomal recessive, as it would require two copies for the individual to be affected.) Alternatively, a mutation in the same gene in a different kindred might cause the production of an altered protein that would interfere with normal functioning in a way that only one copy was needed for phenotypic expression. This mutation would then appear to be inherited as autosomal dominant. Both phenotypes could be the same—seizures. For analysis of the genetic basis of this syndrome (e.g., which gene is involved and what the effects of the mutation are), the mode of inheritance may not be critical.

The importance of precise phenotypic characterization for accurate linkage analysis has been demonstrated in several studies. A large (38-member) and seven smaller families with classical JME (without pyknoleptic absences) were linked to the *EJM1* locus with a combined LOD score of >7. However, when nonclassical JME families in which these absences and 3-Hz spike-wave discharges were screened using the same short tandem-repeat polymorphic markers, the 6p site was excluded. Furthermore, the 6p-locus site could not be confirmed in another independent study of 19 families with JME. Subsequently, a locus of chromosome 15q was found in one group of families, but not in two other samples of families with JME. Another IGE syndrome, adolescent-onset grand mal seizures on awakening, has been linked to *EJM1* using HLA blood-typing markers, whereas a clinically similar syndrome in which adolescent-onset grand mal seizures occur at any time during waking is not linked to this locus.

The manner in which families are ascertained also plays an important role. When the ascertainment is via an individual with other IGE syndromes (CAE, JAE, or idiopathic GTCS) instead of JME, an association with *EJM1* was excluded. However, if the families in which JME was a prominent phenotype were segregated and an AD mode with a high penetrance was assumed, linkage to the *EJM1* locus was suggested.

These studies explicitly assume the importance of syndrome heterogeneity. It is important to perform linkage analysis in families identified with a specific syndrome or subsyndrome, although significant overlap exists between the IGE syndromes with the phenotype of some patients not classifiable by the current scheme. The possibility that common genetic influences underlie the IGE syndromes was tested in a genome scan of 130 IGE multiplex families. Potential susceptibility loci were identified on chromosomes 3q, 2q and 14q. Linkage to chromosome 18 was suggested in a study of 91 multiplex families ascertained based on a proband with adolescent onset IGE. In addition, upon segregation according to seizure type, linkage to chromosome 6 was found for families with myoclonic jerks, chromosome 8 in those without myoclonic jerks, and chromosome 5 in those with absences. Thus, JME provides an excellent example of complex epilepsy syndrome. There is complexity in the significant phenotypic and genetic heterogeneity that may indicate one or more genes is responsible for "susceptibility," whereas other genes determine phenotypic features such as age of onset and seizure type(s).

Childhood and Juvenile Absence Epilepsy

Clinical. Childhood absence epilepsy (CAE or pyknolepsy) is a syndrome of idiopathic generalized epilepsy that occurs predominantly in developmentally normal children between 4 and 10 years of age with females representing approximately 70% of cases.[16] It has been estimated that childhood absence epilepsy is present in 13% to 17% of individuals with epilepsy. Core symptoms include multiple daily absences with significant impairment of consciousness associated with a generalized 3-Hz spike-wave discharge. Phenotypic variations such as myoclonic jerks of the extremities, mouth, and eyelids and irregular, fragmentary or polyspike EEG discharges may be present. The magnitude of these movements and the timing in relation to the appearance of the absence and the EEG findings have been used to include or exclude individuals from a diagnosis of "typical absence." Furthermore, it has been suggested that the clinical course distinguishes subsyndromes with different genetic etiologies. These syndromes include children who will stop having seizures of all types (66%), those with continued absences and generalized tonic-clonic seizures as adults (22%) and those who will develop juvenile myoclonic epilepsy after CAE (12%). The concept of absence seizures as part of individual syndromes as opposed to a biologic phenomenon common to several disorders has been previously discussed in detail.[17] Absence seizures tend to respond well to ethosuximide or valproate, although only valproate is effective against the GTCS. CAE needs to be distinguished from juvenile absence, a related primary generalized epilepsy occurring in a later age group, and atypical absence, which is frequently associated with neurologic lesions and psychomotor retardation.

JAE is an adolescent-onset IGE, presenting at approximately 8 to 10 years of age and overlapping in age, clinical, and electrographic features with CAE. In contrast to CAE, the absences are much less frequent and produce less impairment of consciousness. The majority of children will have GTCS within several years of onset. The EEG may reveal the classic 3-Hz spike-wave of CAE or a faster (4 to 5 Hz) generalized spike-wave more characteristic of JME. Although the cognitive outcome is excellent, these children have more difficulty achieving complete seizure control and a greater likelihood of seizures in adulthood than do those with childhood-onset IGE.

Genetics. Childhood absence epilepsy has a clear genetic predisposition. Complicating the genetic analysis, however, is the observation that among family members of children with this form of epilepsy, generalized spike-wave bursts are common, even in the absence of clinical seizures, and these EEG patterns may disappear in later life.

Concordance rates for monozygotic twins with absence epilepsy have been recorded at 75% if only absence seizures are considered, and as high as 84% if 3-Hz spike wave EEGs are also included in the analysis. This would indicate a high degree of penetrance for those who inherit this particular gene (or set of genes). Several studies have suggested an autosomal dominant mode of inheritance for this form of epilepsy,[18] although the data are somewhat confused by different classification schemes used to define the epilepsy patterns. Studies utilizing DNA markers have failed to demonstrate linkage to the *EJM1* locus on chromosome 6 for CAE and JAE or a site on chromosome 21 associated with progressive myoclonic epilepsy for family members of CAE probands.

Linkage to markers on chromosome 8q24 was found in a large family from India ascertained based on a proband with CAE and persistent GTCs. This finding was then confirmed in five similar families with CAE in the same study. The applicability of this localization to other families with different CAE syndromes and sporadic cases of absence epilepsy remains to be demonstrated. It is apparent that significant phenotypic and genetic heterogeneity exists with the epilepsies primarily associated with absence seizures. Additional susceptibility loci have been suggested in studies of IGE in which families have been further segregated by seizure type (see JME section).

A gene (jerky) that produces absence-like seizures in mice has a human homology on chromosome 8q24. It was excluded from families with CAE and persisting GTCs, but was found in one individual with CAE that evolved into JME.[19] Note that the linkage to jerky was on 8q, but the human CAE that evolves to JME is on 1p.

Other Forms of Myoclonic Epilepsy

The difficulty in classification of epilepsies in which myoclonic seizures are the prominent type has long been recognized, and a variety of schemes have been proposed.[16] The wide variation in the morphology of the "myoclonic seizure" and subsequent developmental out come of the associated epilepsy syndromes raises doubt as to the biologic homogeneity of these syndromes. This is demonstrated most clearly by comparison of the idiopathic JME with the symptomatic infantile spasms (West's syndrome) in which "massive myoclonus" plays a defining role. Historically, investigators have divided these syndromes based upon similar clinical and/or neuropathologic features. As described below for the subgroups termed the "progressive myoclonic epilepsies," both of these approaches can be misleading regarding genetic identification. For the discussions here, we rely on those reports that emphasize the genetic nature of specific syndromes, especially when enough information is available for the inclusion (or exclusion) of specific chromosomal loci.

Severe Myoclonic Epilepsy in Infancy (SME)

This is discussed in GEFS+.

Early Childhood Myoclonic Epilepsy (ECME)

Clinical. Early childhood myoclonic epilepsy (ECME) or epilepsy with myoclonic astatic seizures is rare form of primary generalized epilepsy consisting of atonic drop attacks with or without myoclonic jerks, absences, or generalized tonic-clonic seizures. EEGs show 2- to 3-Hz spike-wave or polyspike-wave complexes and/or 4- to 6-Hz polyspike-wave complexes. These individuals are intellectually and neurologically normal and do not have demonstrable CNS lesions. Seizures are usually, but not always, responsive to valproate.

Genetics. An analysis of families with ECME indicate that 24 of 122 family members (20%) in 14 affected families had one or another form of epilepsy, with idiopathic primary generalized epilepsy occurring in about 80% of those affected. These data are based only on seizures, and EEG data are currently being collected. A more complete description of the inheritance pattern of this form of epilepsy will await determination of how many at-risk individuals without seizures demonstrate abnormal EEGs. Similarly, linkage analyses will depend on clear definitions of the complete syndrome.

Progressive Myoclonus Epilepsy (PME)

The most common disorders considered as progressive myoclonus epilepsies (PME) include Lafora disease, Unverricht-Lundborg (UL) and related syndromes, ceroid lipofuscinosis, the sialidoses, and mitochondria-based disorders. A general neurologic deterioration associated with both sporadic nonepileptic myoclonus and epileptic seizures (myoclonic, clonic, tonic, or generalized tonic-clonic) characterize these syndromes. These syndromes have in common the progressive nature of the neurologic deterioration (e.g., myoclonus, dementia, ataxia) as well as autosomal dominant and recessive modes of inheritance.

PME: Lafora Type
Clinical. This is a rapidly progressive syndrome that often begins in mid-teens with generalized tonic-clonic or myoclonic seizures. This is followed by a relatively rapid deterioration in intellectual function, sometimes accompanied by psychotic symptoms. Muscle atrophy is also seen. These individuals have PAS-positive inclusion bodies (containing acid mucopolysaccharides) throughout the gray matter of the CNS, in skeletal and heart muscle, and in liver. Within the brain, the cerebellum, olives, red nucleus, substantia nigra, thalamus, and cortex are most involved. The course tends to be rapid.

Genetics. It is thought that inheritance is via an autosomal recessive pattern. The gene responsible has been identified as a dual-specificity phosphatase on chromosome 6q24 (see reference 20 for review.)

PME: Unverricht-Lundborg Disease and Related Syndromes
Clinical. The characteristic phenotype includes presentation between 6 and 15 years, progressive (but variable) cognitive decline associated with generalized tonic-clonic seizures. Unverricht-Lundborg disease (ULD) was originally described in the Finnish population but has since been reported in multiple geographic locations and racial groups. In specific, Baltic and Mediterranean PME were distinguished from ULD by slightly different clinical features (e.g., age of onset, rate of progression), whereas all three were differentiated from Lafora disease by absence of the pathologic features present in the latter. Although it is very uncommon, the Baltic myoclonus epilepsy syndrome may be particularly important to recognize, as phenytoin, which is often employed as an antiepileptic drug in these patients, may produce an acceleration in the neurologic deterioration.

Genetics. ULD and related disorders appear to follow an autosomal recessive pattern. In 1991, ULD was mapped to chromosome 21q using linkage analysis,[21] and the locus was designated *EPM1*. Baltic and Mediterranean PME have an identical chromosomal localization. Subsequently, families with Italian, Japanese, Iranian, Turkish, and French-Canadian ancestries mapped to the *EPM1* locus. The gene for ULD has been identified as coding for the enzyme cystatin B, a ubiquitously distributed protease inhibitor. It has not been elucidated how dysfunction of this gene is linked to the seizures and neurologic deterioration.

PME: Northern Epilepsy Syndrome
Clinical. This syndrome was described in 1994 in 11 Finnish families derived from 2 ancestral pedigrees. The

most common age of onset is between 5 and 7 years, although presentation at 9 months has been reported. Generalized tonic-clonic seizures predominate with or without complex partial events. Seizure frequency peaks during puberty then declines as the patient becomes a young adult. Clonazepam is the most effective anticonvulsant. Mental deterioration is a constant feature by 30 years of age in all affected family members and accompanies progressive impairment of fine-motor tasks, equilibrium, and gait. CT examination reveals initial brainstem and cerebellar atrophy followed by generalized cortical atrophy.

Genetics. Linkage analysis has mapped the disease locus, designated *EPMR*, to the short arm of chromosome 8. More recently, this syndrome has been considered as one of the neuronal ceroid lipofuscinoses and the causative gene, designated *CLN8*, encodes a transmembrane protein.

PME: Ceroid Lipofuscinoses
Clinical. The neuronal ceroid lipofuscinoses (NCL) is a group of disorders named for the storage material (lipofuscin) found within neurons and within a variety of other tissues including conjunctiva, liver, rectum, and lymphocytes. The age of onset ranges from the neonatal period to adulthood with a similar variation in seizure type and severity. The syndrome includes cognitive deterioration, associated neurologic symptoms (e.g., blindness, ataxia) and reduced life expectancy. The late infantile, juvenile, and adult forms have myoclonic seizures as a prominent part of the syndrome.

Genetics. It is believed that all types have an autosomal recessive pattern of inheritance, although the adult form may also be transmitted as autosomal dominant. Eight subtypes are currently recognized with genes identified for 6. The juvenile onset form (Batten's disease) presenting at 4 to 10 years of age with severe atypical absence and generalized tonic-clonic seizures has been mapped to a locus on chromosome 16p. The gene, *CLN3*, produces a novel lysosomal transmembrane protein. The infantile form, which is phenotypically distinct from the other PME syndromes, has been linked to chromosome 1p. The gene designated as *CLN1* produces palmitoyl protein thioesterase. The classic late-infantile form is due to a *CLN2* mutation on 11p that results in a defect in tripeptidyl peptidase production. Several late-infantile variants have been described. The Finnish variant has been mapped to 13q and designated CLN5, and it codes for a transmembrane protein like some of the other NCLs. Another type *(CLN6)* has been linked to chromosome 15q, but the gene product is unknown. The Turkish variant of the late infantile form, *CLN7*, has not been mapped. As noted above, Northern myoclonic epilepsy (also known as progressive myoclonic epilepsy with mental retardation) is now considered an NCL subtype, *CLN8*. The NCLs demonstrate how a similar pathologic marker may not be predictive of either phenotypic or genetic homogeneity.

PME: Sialidosis Type 1
Clinical. This syndrome is also referred to as cherry-red-spot myoclonus due to the macular appearance associated with the stimulus-sensitive massive myoclonus. This syndrome presents after age 7 years. Neuraminidase deficiency is associated with both sialidosis types 1 and 2.

Genetics. Mutations in the neuraminidase gene on chromosome 6p21 have been demonstrated in several forms of this disorder.

PME: Myoclonus Epilepsy and Ragged Red Fibers (MERRF)
Clinical. Another form of progressive neurologic deterioration associated with myoclonus, dementia, ataxia, and spasticity has been associated with abnormal mitochondria, first detected as "ragged red fibers" in muscle biopsies. The clinical course is variable, and individuals with this condition, even within single families, may show different levels of dysfunction. In general, however, the disease tends to be progressive. Despite evidence of widespread cortical dysfunction at both the neurologic and electrophysiologic level, postmortem examinations fail to reveal major cortical abnormalities. However, PET scans show decreases in cortical metabolism consistent with abnormalities in the metabolic respiratory chain.

Genetics. Early studies of this condition recognized its familial predisposition. The maternal mode of transmission suggested initially that it might be an X-linked disease, but analysis of larger kindreds allowed elimination of dominant, recessive and X-linked inheritance in favor of a mitochondrial DNA mutation.[22] Initial molecular biologic studies on several individuals indicated that the MERRF phenotype was associated with a single A to G transition mutation at nucleotide pair 8344 in human mitochondrial DNA (mtDNA) coding for the *tRNA(Lys)* gene.[23] As this mutation is not found in 10% to 20% of individuals with MERRF, five cases without the mutation were studied and one was found to have a T to C transition at nucleotide pair 8356. A recent study of 150 individuals with suspected mitochondrial disease revealed that although the majority of cases with the MERRF phenotype had the A to G transition at position 8344, four MERRF patients did not. Furthermore, the A to G transition was found with a variety of other clinical presentations including Leigh's disease, myoclonus/myopathy with lipomas, and proximal myopathy. These data indicate that both phenotypic and genotypic heterogeneity exists with neurologic syndromes associated with mitochondrial mutations.

The A to G mutation in MERRF causes enzymatic defects in the oxidative phosphorylation system of mitochondria. It is not known how the defect in mitochondrial energy metabolism is translated into an epileptic phenotype. Many possibilities exist, as so much of the physiology of the brain is dependent on maintenance of ion gradients, both across cell membranes and between intracellular organelles and the cytoplasm. It is also not yet clear why the disease is progressive, unless the proportion of mitochondria affected increases with time, or the defect in energy metabolism produces secondary abnormalities that can have a cumulative effect on the CNS. Given the precision with which this single-gene mutation is understood and our growing understanding of mitochondrial genetics, this disease could be an interesting model for the study of many of these questions. This disease may also become a model target for gene replacement therapy of mitochondrial genetic diseases.

INHERITED HUMAN EPILEPSIES: THE GENETICS OF LOCALIZATION-RELATED EPILEPSIES

Although an anatomic lesion is commonly assumed to underlie partial seizures, several syndromes (e.g., benign epilepsy of childhood with Rolandic spikes) have long been known to have a positive family history for epilepsy. In the last few years, additional genetic syndromes of partial epilepsy have been identified, chromosomal loci have been assigned and excluded, and a number of mutations have been identified as causes of these syndromes.

Benign Epilepsy of Childhood with Rolandic Spikes (BECRS)

Clinical. BECRS may be the most common identifiable type of childhood epilepsy syndrome. It was found in 25% of epileptic children in a large prospective population study. BECRS is the prototypical benign childhood epilepsy syndrome in that it is defined by normal developmental history and normal neurologic and neuroradiologic examinations. The interictal EEG consistently reveals normal background activity and a characteristic unihemispheric- or bihemispheric-shifting monomorphic epileptiform discharge, usually with amplitude maximum over the inferior Rolandic cortex. This neuroanatomic localization is congruent with the clinical events that are characterized by hemifacial or lingual tingling or twitching, drooling, and a motor-based inability to speak. The seizures are predominantly nocturnal but may be diurnal. In some patients, the focal discharge secondarily generalizes to a hemi-clonic or tonic-clonic seizure. The prognosis is excellent, as most seizures are easily controlled by a single medication, and the epilepsy completely resolves in greater than 95% of cases by age 20 years. Like most of the proposed epilepsy syndromes, cases are reported that may lack one of the defining features indicating "normalcy," but are identical in the electrographic pattern, response to medication, and prognosis.

Genetics. A family history of epilepsy is cited in most series with a range from 9% to 68%. Age-related penetrance is strongly suggested by the appearance of the seizures and the EEG trait at approximately 4 years and by the resolution of the seizures and the EEG abnormality by the end of the teens. A recent study reported 69 siblings of 43 probands. Among the probands, a positive family history for epilepsy was present in 40%. Five siblings had seizures, three of which were febrile, two generalized tonic-clonic, and none with BECRS. The waking and sleep EEG of the siblings revealed epileptic activity in 51%. Only approximately 6% were focal. Generalized spike-wave discharges were present in 32% of siblings with epileptiform abnormalities. This study illustrates several important points. A family history of seizures does not necessarily indicate that the same types of seizures are present in the proband and family. In addition, the EEG may serve as a marker for epileptogenicity in both symptomatic and unaffected family members, but may not have a similar "epileptiform" abnormality in all affected members. In fact, in this partial epilepsy with a characteristic centro-temporal focus, the most common abnormality found in relatives was a generalized spike-wave pattern.

Statistical techniques have been applied to determine the likely pattern of inheritance. An a priori method was used to analyze 19 probands selected based on characteristic clinical and EEG features and having a sibling between 3 and 13 years old. Histories and EEGs were obtained in the majority of parents and siblings of the probands. The histories and EEGs showed that 68% of the probands had a family history of seizures in childhood; 11% and 15% of the parents and siblings, respectively, had seizures; and 34% of the siblings had characteristic centro-temporal spikes. Assumptions of dominant inheritance provided a high correlation between the expected and observed cases. Thus, autosomal dominant inheritance with age-dependent, variable penetrance was deemed likely, although a polygenic basis is also reasonable.

It has been proposed that the EEG trait of centrotemporal spikes has an autosomal dominant inheritance, whereas the expressed phenotype of BECRS is best described by a more complex inheritance pattern. Recent molecular studies have excluded the sites associated with fragile X, juvenile myoclonic epilepsy, and benign neonatal familial convulsions. Linkage to loci on 15q has been described in several isolated families as well as 7q and 1q in developmentally delayed children.[24]

Benign Epilepsy with Occipital Paroxysms

Clinical. Within the group of partial epilepsies localized to the occipital lobes, several subgroups exist. At least one of these is familial and considered a discrete epilepsy syndrome. As will be illustrated, these syndromes can have similar features (clinical or electrographic), yet have very different outcomes and genetic features. In the 1989 ILAE Revised Proposal for Classification of Epilepsies and Epileptic Syndromes, childhood epilepsy with occipital paroxysms (CEOP) is listed as a localization-related, idiopathic syndrome. The features include partial symptomatology involving visual phenomena, and, in addition, hemi-clonic and occasionally, generalized tonic-clinic seizures often followed by a headache. Normal EEG background and bilateral or unilateral occipital spike-wave pattern that attenuates with eye opening are also characteristic. A normal developmental status and absence of lesions on neuroimaging procedures is implied in the "idiopathic" designation.

Although the clinical-electrographic features of CEOP were suggested in the early 1950s, it was not until Gastaut's report of 36 children with "benign epilepsy with occipital spike-waves" (BEOSW) with a mean onset of seizures at 6 years of age that this syndrome began receiving intense attention. The ictal phenomena included visual symptoms (e.g., blindness, phosphenes); hemi-clonic convulsions followed in 44% of patients, and headache followed 36% of events. Anticonvulsant therapy controlled seizures in 53% of cases; 92% of cases resolved by age 19 years. Thus, this group defined the features of what was to be adopted as a syndrome. However, when this group with additional patients (63 total) was updated, the spectrum of clinical features had been expanded to include patients with developmental retardation and hemiparesis. In addition to the ictal visual phenomena and hemiclonic seizures, complex partial and generalized tonic-clonic seizures were noted. Control of seizures with medications was achieved in 60%, and eventually complete resolution of the seizures occurred in 95%, of individuals.

Another occipital epilepsy syndrome originally termed "benign childhood epilepsy with occipital paroxysms" and now referred to as "early-onset benign childhood partial seizures with occipital spikes," as well as "idiopathic photosensitive occipital lobe epilepsy" has been described. This is an age-related syndrome with a mean onset of 4 to 5 years in which seizures are characterized by ictal vomiting, eye deviation, autonomic phenomena, impairment of consciousness, and occasional partial status epilepticus. The vast majority of children will have complete seizure remission within a few years of onset. Development remains normal.

Genetics. A family history of epilepsy was present in 37% of patients in the group with the ictal visual phenomena and hemi-convulsions, but no further information was provided. Another report of occipital lobe epilepsy described two groups of children, one of which corresponded to the ILAE criteria of CEOP and the other with brain lesions. In the first group, a family history of "convulsive disorders" was noted in 44% of first- and second-degree relatives. In the second group, this history was present in only one case. Unfortunately, no further information regarding the transmission pattern is provided.

In the other idiopathic syndrome characterized by nocturnal occurrence, ictal vomiting and eye deviation, a clear inheritance pattern has not emerged although relatives with seizures have been reported. Thus, it is suggested that there are at least two benign occipital lobe epilepsy syndromes that differ in ictal symptomatology and perhaps family history.

Autosomal Dominant Nocturnal Frontal Lobe Epilepsy

Clinical. Autosomal dominant nocturnal frontal lobe epilepsy (ADNFLE) was originally described in 1994 in a group of patients suspected of having a sleep disorder.[25] Cognitive function and neurologic examination were normal in all individuals. Seizures most frequently occurred with drowsiness or during the first few or last few hours of sleep. Age of onset was 2 months to 52 years (median, 8 years), with 88% at younger than 20 years. Seizures have wide variation in severity and recurrence, but tend to occur in clusters. Reports of auras were frequent with a variety of somatosensory, special sensory, psychic, and autonomic phenomena. Motor activity included tonic, clonic, and hyperkinetic movements. The interictal EEG was normal in 84%; abnormalities, when present, consisted of bifrontal, central and unitemporal, and frontotemporal discharges. Ictal EEG recording revealed bihemispheric, frontal predominant spike-wave ($n = 3$), generalized rhythmic 9 Hz ($n = 1$), or no ictal features ($n = 6$). Neuroimaging (CT or MR) was reported as normal in all 14 individuals.

Genetics: Segregation analysis of five original families indicated an autosomal dominant inheritance pattern with 69% penetrance. In one of the multigenerational families selected for analysis to eliminate the possibility of genetic heterogeneity, linkage was found to chromosome 20q13.2. Subsequently, the gene for the α4 subunit of the nicotinic acetylcholine receptor (CHRNA4),[26] was mapped to this locus, providing the first human genetic epilepsy in which an associated gene had been identified. A second acetylcholine (ACh) receptor subunit mutation has also been identified in ADNFLE in the β2 subunit (CHRNB2), thus emphasizing genetic heterogeneity. Of note, these loci have been excluded in other families with the ADNFLE phenotype. The mutations in CHRNA4 appear to produce decreased current in the ACh receptors via decreased permeability to Ca and enhanced desensitization, whereas the mutation in CHRNB2 does not affect desensitization properties but causes a tenfold increase in affinity of the receptor. How each or either of these mutations produces an epileptic phenotype has not yet been determined.

Partial Epilepsy with Auditory Features

Clinical. In 1995 a family was identified in which 11 members had idiopathic/cryptogenic epilepsy in addition to 3 with symptomatic epilepsy and 3 with acute symptomatic seizures. Clinical features of the idiopathic group included: age of onset 8 to 19 years; 10 individuals were cognitively normal; seizures were infrequent and of clear partial onset in 73%; and 55% were associated with auditory phenomena. The family members with symptomatic epilepsy were associated with brain tumor, head injury, and cerebral palsy. The acute symptomatic seizures were associated with fever and alcohol. Subsequently, other families have been identified with similar phenotypes.

Genetics. The inheritance pattern was best fit by assuming autosomal dominant transmission with a penetrance of 71%. Linkage analysis demonstrated a maximum LOD score of 3.99 with markers spanning a 10 cM region on chromosome 10q. The mutated gene was subsequently identified as the leucine-rich, glioma-inactivated 1 gene *(LGI1)*.[27] The expression pattern of mouse *LGI1* is "predominantly neuronal and is consistent with the anatomic regions involved in temporal lobe epilepsy."[27]

Other Partial Epilepsy Syndromes of Genetic Origin

During the past several years, there have been a number of reports on families with clear inheritance patterns of a variety of partial epilepsy syndromes. These include familial temporal lobe epilepsy (FTLE) and familial partial epilepsy with variable foci (FPEVF). To date, no specific gene mutations have been associated with either syndrome.

Acquired Partial (Focal) Epilepsy

Clinical. Several groups have attempted to determine if various forms of acquired or "symptomatic" epilepsy have a genetic predisposition. Many early studies used an older, less reliable classification scheme for characterizing seizures in the index patients. Some included focal seizures in children that we now consider separate syndromes with a strong genetic predisposition (e.g., BECRS) with other forms of focal epilepsy. Most studies relied on historical data about seizure occurrence in families of individuals who present in one way or another with acquired focal epilepsy. Seizure types in family members were often unspecified; the degree of relation between the probands and the family members may not have been indicated; the number of relatives at risk was often not identified; and rarely have EEGs been performed on relatives to use EEG abnormalities in otherwise asymptomatic relatives as a possible identifying characteristic. Despite the many limitations, the data that exist point to a possible genetic predisposition for the development of focal epilepsy after brain tumors, brain trauma, and in children with infantile hemiplegia. For recent reviews of this literature, see Ottman and Treiman.[28,29]

Genetics. Several studies have indicated that relatives of individuals with acquired partial epilepsy have increased prevalence of seizures. Two studies of children with focal motor seizures or psychomotor seizures indicated a positive history of seizures in 14% to 23% (first-degree relatives) and 28% to 55% (all relatives). Other studies of individuals with "temporal lobe epilepsy" indicated that 11%, 13% to 20%, or 30% had a family history of epilepsy. In a large prospective VA cooperative study of antiepileptic drug therapy, careful family histories were obtained from 612 participants. Within this group, 28% had positive family histories of epilepsy, with 9% of the individuals having one or more siblings with seizures. These data collectively suggest that there may be a genetic predisposition for the development of epilepsy, or may indicate that there is a genetic predisposition to develop another neurologic condition that could lead to epilepsy. However, none of these studies is well-controlled for a variety of confounding variables, and none provides information about possible modes of inheritance. Despite these studies, other studies of individuals with intractable focal epilepsy treated surgically (notably those of Penfield and Paine[30] and Andermann and Metrakos[31]) indicated no increased incidence or very slightly increased incidence of epilepsy in family members.

In an excellent review, Ottman[28] focused on three specific questions relating to the genetics of the partial epilepsies: (1) "Do the partial and generalized epilepsies differ on degree of familial aggregation?" (2) "To what extent is genetic susceptibility involved in the etiology of complex partial seizures?" and (3) "Are there focal EEG abnormalities for which genetic susceptibility is important?" Three studies are cited that compare the prevalence of seizures in relatives of individuals with primary generalized and partial epilepsy. All three indicate a higher incidence in the former (ca. 4.5%) than the latter (3%). However, all three indicate a higher incidence in relatives of individuals with focal epilepsy than the incidence rate generally assumed for control populations (approximately 0.5 to 1%). Two other studies compared relatives of partial seizure patients with relatives of controls. Both found prevalence rates in controls of close to 3% (with slightly higher rates in relatives of individuals with partial epilepsy). Thus, it appears from these studies that there may be a small genetic predisposition for partial epilepsy.

When examining patients with complex partial seizures specifically, the data remain unclear. Four studies cited by Ottman indicate an approximate 4% prevalence of seizures in relatives of individuals with CPS compared with approximately 3% prevalence in relatives of controls. The mechanisms by which acquired partial epilepsy could have a genetic component are myriad. Small changes in almost any component of neuronal excitability may be aggravated by a brain injury in a way that promotes the development of epilepsy. Similarly, variations in the response to injury unrelated to any baseline changes in excitability could produce a tendency toward the development of post-injury epilepsy.

Thus, again, the issue of whether genes that might "promote" epilepsy are in any way directly involved in the epileptic event will need to be addressed.

INHERITED HUMAN EPILEPSIES: THE GENETICS OF THE EPILEPSIES THAT OCCUR AS PART OF SPECIAL SYNDROMES

Febrile Convulsions

Clinical. Febrile convulsions (FC) are defined as "seizures accompanied by fever, occurring between the ages of 1 month and 7 years, not symptomatic of recognized acute neurologic illness."[32] FC are called "simple" if the seizures are brief generalized tonic-clonic seizures. FC are called "complex" if prolonged (>30 minutes), focal, or if they recur within 24 hours. Epidemiologic studies have indicated that in patients with simple FC (without additional risk factors such as history of prior neurologic deficit or developmental problem, prior afebrile seizures, family history of afebrile seizures), there appears to be either no higher incidence or only slightly higher incidence of development of epilepsy than in a control population without febrile convulsions.[32] However, this conclusion is partly based on a large prospective study by the National Collaborative Perinatal Project (NCPP)[32] that followed children to only age 7 years. Follow-up through the first 20 to 30 years of life may be necessary to firmly establish this conclusion.

Children with complex FC, on the other hand, are at significantly higher risk for developing epilepsy. For children with focal or prolonged seizures or repeated episodes of febrile convulsions with the same illness, the risks of additional afebrile seizures range from 6% to 8% (with one of these features) to 17% to 22% (with two) to 49% (with three). It should also be noted that the age at which the unprovoked seizures developed ranged from early childhood, after the first febrile convulsion, to well into young adulthood, with several individuals experiencing their first afebrile seizure between ages 20 and 25 years.

Retrospective analyses of adults with complex partial seizures further complicate the issue of the consequences of febrile convulsions. Many such individuals (9% to 38% in several studies) have histories of normal early development and "febrile convulsions." It is often difficult, in a retrospective manner, to determine if these seizures met the criteria for "simple febrile convulsions" or were clearly of the less benign variety. Thus, if one were to analyze only young adults with serious seizure disorders, it would appear that febrile convulsions were a high-risk factor.

Genetics. The syndrome of febrile convulsions represents the most common form of seizures seen in childhood. In the United States and Western Europe, approximately 2% of the population experience FC, whereas in Japan the estimate is approximately 8%.

Males and females are equally affected. It is clear that such seizures have a familial predisposition, although the exact mode of inheritance is not known. The NCPP data[32] indicate a positive family history of seizures in approximately 7% of individuals with FC. Other studies indicate a higher incidence; 12% in parents of children with FC and as high as 25% in siblings. Twin studies have shown somewhat variable incidences of concordance rates for MZ twins, ranging from 31% (with a "case-wise" risk of 44%) to 70%. It is interesting that DZ twins have a concordance rate of about 14% to 18% in all of the above studies.

Given that twin pregnancies are at somewhat higher risk for neonatal problems (especially those occurring in the 1950s and 1960s that supplied data for the Lennox-Buchthal and Schiottz-Christensen studies), it would be expected that some of the "febrile" convulsions included in these studies would have been of the complex variety rather than the simple FC. Thus, there may be an overrepresentation of epilepsy in these studies.

The general population studies can be interpreted to indicate that FC do have a genetic component and that either a partial penetrance for the FC trait or a polygenic pattern of inheritance exists. The limited concordance among MZ twins suggests the former. If FC were inherited as a single gene with a 50% penetrance, then a 25% incidence in siblings would indicate an actual 50% incidence of the gene and would favor an autosomal dominant form of inheritance. Unfortunately, at the present time, the data do not allow firm conclusions to be drawn about the mode of inheritance of febrile convulsions. A complex segregation analysis has indicated that when the probands have single febrile seizures, a polygenic model is most likely. However, if probands with multiple febrile seizures are considered, an autosomal dominant, single-locus model provides the best fit for the data.

Recently, it has become possible to analyze inheritance patterns of FC in greater depth by studying one or a few large kindreds with significant numbers of affected members. However, many biochemical and therefore electrophysiologic aspects of brain function are temperature-dependent, and it is possible or likely that seizures in the presence of fever or of fever-associated events could have multiple etiologies and be influenced by several genes. Linkage analyses of large multigenerational families in which febrile seizures is inherited in an autosomal dominant pattern have been utilized to identify several loci on chromosome 8q designated as *FEB1*, on chromosome19p *(FEB2)* and chromosome 2q *(FEB3)*. A similar approach identified a locus *(FEB4)* on chromosome 5q in a large Japanese family that was then confirmed in 39 nuclear families. (The syndrome of generalized epilepsy with febrile seizures plus (GEFS+) has been described previously.)

Pyridoxine Dependent Seizures

Clinical. Although relatively uncommon, the pyridoxine-dependent seizure disorder is of significant interest as it is the only human epilepsy that is known to be due to a specific biochemical disorder. The seizures are secondary to a greater than normal requirement for pyridoxine by dependent enzymes within the central nervous system. This state is to be distinguished from pyridoxine-deficiency, in which the cofactor is missing because of inadequate dietary intake or impaired gastrointestinal absorption, with consequent effects throughout the body. Diagnosis of both syndromes is made by noting a rapid improvement in epileptiform EEG and consequent seizures in response to intravenous administration of pyridoxine. However, the pyridoxine-dependent individual must then be maintained on a daily oral dose. In these patients, seizures recur days to months after discontinuing the vitamin.

Pyridoxine-dependent seizures were initially described as neonatal convulsions that presented within the first few hours to days of life and were refractory to standard anticonvulsants. Subsequently, it has been recognized that significant clinical heterogeneity exists within this seizure disorder as defined by its responsiveness to supplementation. Schriver hypothesized that the seizures are due to lack of glutamic acid decarboxylase (GAD) activity for which B6 is a cofactor, thereby resulting in lack of GABA production and consequently less inhibition. This has some experimental basis in the autopsy results of one patient that showed a disproportionate loss of GABA in frontal and occipital cortices. It has also been suggested that in the B6-deficient rat, kynurines (tryptophan metabolites) may compete with the endogenous benzodiazepine ligand for binding on the GABA receptor complex.

Genetics. Small pedigrees have been described in which the family history indicated that siblings of the proband either had documented pyridoxine-dependent seizures or a history consisting of a infant who did or did not have fetal distress, but developed refractory seizures and subsequently died. In this form of epilepsy, identification of affected family members is made in clinically affected or suspected individuals. Studies of EEG traits in relatives have not been performed. An autosomal dominant mode of inheritance has been suggested based on data indicating that children of both sexes within a generation could be affected in the absence of parental disease.

Seizures Associated with Other Inherited Metabolic Deficits

Many inherited metabolic conditions that cause an encephalopathy also can result in seizures. However, seizures play a prominent role in a relatively limited number. Inherited, presumably metabolic, disorders that can present with seizures include: ceroid lipofuscinosis (esp. Bielschowsky's, autosomal recessive), polyunsaturated fatty acid lipidosis (autosomal recessive), and Alpers syndrome. Other conditions in which seizures are frequent include: hyperglycinemia, Menke disease (X-linked), infantile GM_2 gangliosidosis (autosomal recessive), Niemann-Pick (autosomal recessive), and GM_1-gangliosidosis (autosomal recessive).

Seizures Associated with Inherited Phacomatoses

A number of congenital conditions present with lesions in the skin and central nervous system and have collectively been called the phacomatoses. Each of these is discussed separately in this volume, but those that can either present as seizures or in which seizures are a primary manifestation are briefly discussed in this section.

Neurofibromatosis

Clinical. Neurofibromatosis (NF) presents in two forms, NF1 (von Recklinghausen's disease) and NF2 (central, bilateral acoustic), which are described in detail in Chapter 51. Thus, only a brief summary with emphasis on seizures will follow.

NF1 is characterized by cafe au lait spots, cutaneous neurofibromas (benign tumors of Schwann cells), hyperplasia of cutaneous tissue, abnormalities of bone, and several different types of intracranial tumors, including neurofibromas, neuromas, gliomas, and meningiomas. In a recent report of a well-characterized cohort of children with NF1, seizures were found in 30%, with partial and generalized morphologies. Symptoms may be related directly to focal lesions or may be due to increased intracranial pressure. Recently, subependymal calcifications have been reported that resemble tuberous sclerosis and may be associated with the development of seizures.

Genetics. NF1 and NF2 are inherited in an autosomal dominant fashion with the genes located on chromosomes 17 and 22, respectively. See Chapter 51 for details.

Tuberous Sclerosis

Clinical. Another condition that manifests itself by lesions in the skin and CNS is tuberous sclerosis. However, the skin lesions (adenoma sebaceum, shagreen patches, or subungual fibromas) may be subtle and the patient may present with either seizures or slow development. Often other family members with normal intelligence and no neurologic problems are diagnosed with TS only after one or more severely afflicted members is recognized.

Genetics. Two different genes for TS have now been identified, and the pathobiology of the disease is currently being elucidated (see Chapter 12).

Sturge-Weber Disease (Encephalotrigeminal Angiomatosis)

Clinical.   Sturge-Weber Disease (SWD) is characterized pathologically by leptomeningeal angiomatosis, frequently over parieto-occipital cortex but occasionally extending to the entire hemisphere. Bihemispheric involvement is also noted. In the classic presentation, a cutaneous angioma in the distribution of one or more components of the trigeminal nerve is present, with ipsilateral to unihemispheric involvement. Similar to the cerebral lesion, the cutaneous "port wine" nevus may extend to the other side of the face, neck, trunk, and extremities. Usual neurologic signs of SWD include hemiparesis, hemianopsia, and hemiatrophy contralateral to the leptomeningeal angioma. Mental retardation is found in 33% to 65% of patients. Seizures occur in 75% to 90% of patients. The interictal EEG reveals decreased background amplitudes, polymorphic delta, decreased response to hyperventilation, and photic stimulation on the side of the cerebral lesion.

Genetics.   It is currently believed that most cases of SWD are sporadic, although it has been suggested that either autosomal dominant with variable penetrance or autosomal recessive modes of inheritance may be operating in several families. In addition, it has been hypothesized that SWD may represent a difficult to detect, partial trisomy.

Cerebelloretinal Angiomatosis (Von Hippel-Lindau Disease)

Clinical.   Angiomas or hemangioblastomas occurring in the retina and the CNS characterize this condition. In the latter case, they are often single but may be multiple. Angiomas in the brain are most often seen in the cerebellum, but have also been reported in cortex and spinal cord. The condition is often associated with polycystic kidney disease, which can progress to renal carcinoma. In fact, in some families, the renal disease is most prominent. Occasionally individuals with cerebelloretinal angiomatosis present with seizures, and the angioma is discovered in the course of the evaluation. More commonly, the angiomas will present by hemorrhaging.

Genetics.   It is thought that cerebelloretinal angiomatosis is inherited as an autosomal dominant condition.

Epilepsy, Paroxysmal Movement Disorders, and Migraine

Most of the mutations identified as causing epilepsy discussed previously are in genes coding for either voltage-gated (e.g., K, Ca) or ligand-gated (ACh or GABA) channels. As such, these groups of disorders have been described as "channelopathies." Similar mutations have been found in the same genes or in related genes encoding channels in several other paroxysmal disorders, especially paroxysmal movement disorders such as the episodic ataxias, paroxysmal dyskinesias, and migraine. Some patients with these conditions have epilepsy, and some do not. Animal models of inherited epilepsies often also show ataxia and/or other movement disorders. It is likely that as more genetic mutations (or even polymorphisms) are identified as underlying any of these conditions, more families with variable phenotypic expressions will be identified where multiple paroxysmal disorders are clustered.

TREATMENT OF EPILEPSY

Seizures can be disabling in many ways. They may damage brain directly, cause injuries secondary to falls, interfere with cognitive function and memory, disturb normal endocrine function, and interfere with the opportunity to have normal educational, psychological, social, and vocational activities. Even infrequent seizures may prevent driving, which in our society can be socially disabling. Thus, for most individuals, seizures need to be treated, and the primary modality at the present time is pharmacotherapy designed to suppress seizures. It is beyond the scope of this chapter to discuss detailed treatments for many forms of epilepsy. The general principles are: make the correct diagnosis; classify the seizures that the individual is having and, if possible, the specific epilepsy syndrome involved; eliminate external causes of the seizure disorder (e.g., intracranial masses, infections); and choose a medication that is effective against the specific seizure involved. It is best to treat individuals with one medication at optimal doses rather than to use polytherapy.

There are 14 commonly used antiepileptic drugs (AEDs). Some have been available since before 1985, and at least eight are new and have been approved for use in the United States only since 1993.[33-35] For partial seizures with or without secondary generalized tonic-clonic seizures, carbamazepine, phenytoin, valproic acid, phenobarbital, gabapentin, lamotrigine, levetiracetam, oxcarbazepine, topiramate, zonisamide, tiagabine, and felbamate are all effective. These drugs differ in side effects, tolerability, drug interactions, and safety more than efficacy. Data indicate that most or all of these drugs will be effective in suppressing seizures in approximately 50% of individuals with new-onset epilepsy. For those who fail the first of these, another 10% to 15% may become seizure-free on a second choice. This leaves approximately 30% to 35% unlikely to achieve a seizure-free state on current medications, either as monotherapy or in combination therapy.[36]

For individuals with primary generalized absence epilepsy, the choices are more limited. Ethosuximide and valproic acid are known to be effective, while topiramate, zonisamide, levetiracetam, and lamotrigine are likely to be effective also. Benzodiazepines can also be used, but with chronic use, some patients develop tolerance. All of these drugs but ethosuximide would be effective for primary generalized tonic clonic seizures.

For some patients whose seizures are not controlled by medication, surgery may provide a "cure" or may significantly reduce seizure frequency. Individuals with intractable complex partial seizures that have a unilateral mesial temporal electrical focus and who have MRI evidence for unilateral hippocampal sclerosis have a greater than 70% chance of becoming seizure free after a temporal lobectomy. Those with similar seizures but with no anatomic evidence for mesial temporal sclerosis and those with neocortical epilepsy have a lower chance of becoming seizure-free after surgery, but may have a major reduction in seizure frequency. Under some circumstances, corpus callosum section can also be useful to prevent frequent generalized seizures that result in frequent falls and injuries.

A newer surgical therapy involves stimulation of one vagus nerve via electrodes placed around the nerves in the neck that are attached to an implanted pacemaker. This form of therapy can produce a seizure-free state in approximately 10% of patients and may reduce seizure frequency significantly in another 30% to 40%.

Finally, some children with very refractory epilepsy can be treated with a special ketogenic diet. It is not known how this diet works, but some children with extremely difficult epilepsy have shown dramatic improvement when adhering strictly to this regimen.

The exact mechanisms of action of AEDs are not clearly known, but many (CBZ, PHT, LTG, OXC, ZON) appear to work by selectively suppressing voltage-dependent sodium currents in a use- and voltage-sensitive manner. Others (PHB, BZs, TGB) work by enhancing inhibitory synaptic transmission mediated by GABA, the main inhibitory neurotransmitter in the brain. Others work by inhibition of voltage-dependent Ca channels (ESM, GBP), while the mechanisms underlying the antiseizure effects of VPA and some of the newer AEDs remains largely unknown. In no case has an AED's mechanism of action been "matched" to a genetic defect in an inherited epilepsy as a form of specific "target-directed" therapy. Whether this will be possible in the future remains to be determined as more becomes known about the genetic susceptibilities underlying more common forms of seizures and the mechanisms by which many AEDs operate.

GENETIC COUNSELING FOR EPILEPSY

Questions about inheritance of epilepsy usually arise in the setting of a parent (or both) with epilepsy, parents of one (or more) children with epilepsy who either are concerned about the unaffected children or who want additional children, or couples with one or more family members with epilepsy. It is beyond the scope of this chapter to include details of genetic counseling that

would be appropriate for all circumstances. Much of the information in this chapter about the inherited characteristics of identified epilepsy syndromes should serve as the basis for providing approximate "risk" analysis.

The following general rules apply:

1. Identify with the best precision available the specific epilepsy syndrome that exists in the affected individual(s). This classification should include seizure phenotype and EEG characteristics.
2. Determine whether there is any other predisposing inherited condition that would affect the risk (e.g., tuberous sclerosis, a metabolic disorder, etc.).
3. Examine as best as possible the specific family tree of the involved individuals, as individual families may have idiosyncratic inheritances that do not conform to the studies cited in this chapter.
4. Recognize what syndromes are "benign" or relatively "benign" and what symptoms are likely to be much more disruptive of normal life. Although there may be a strong likelihood of inheriting a benign form of epilepsy, the effect of such a disorder may be relatively minor and parents should appreciate such considerations when making reproductive decisions.

Table 38-3 summarizes in very approximate terms the likelihood of developing epilepsy (based on family analyses published in the literature, not on the mendelian ratios) if a sibling or one parent has the kind of epilepsy indicated, as well as these authors' judgments as to the relative consequences of this form of epilepsy. This table refers to the more common forms of each syndrome and not to specific families in which inheritance patterns can be more specifically delineated where specific genetic risk determinations can be made.

Another issue, in terms of the risk to children of a mother with epilepsy, relates to the risk of antiepileptic therapy on the developing fetus. Although this is not a genetic risk, per se, the genetics of the epilepsy in the mother add to the effects of AEDs in influencing the outcome of a pregnancy. The risk of epilepsy in the child is directly related to the risks discussed above. However, the risks of malformation will be a combination of the genetic influence as well as the effect of the AEDs. How a mother metabolically "handles" an AED may also be critical in determining whether teratogenic metabolites are formed, and this is likely to be genetically determined.

CONCLUSION

The epilepsies are a family of diverse disorders that have in common an increased excitability of the brain and an

TABLE 38–3. Approximate Genetic Risks for Specific Epilepsy Syndromes

Syndrome	Proposed Mode of Inheritance	One Sibling with Syndrome	One Parent with Syndrome	Comments
Febrile convulsions		Possibly 15%–25%	15%	Usually benign
Benign familial neonatal convulsions	Autosomal dominant	40%–50%	40%–50%	Usually benign
Juvenile myoclonic epilepsy	Unclear inheritance pattern	7%	2%–4% 7%	Intermediate to serious
Childhood absence epilepsy	Unclear inheritance pattern	8%–20%	6% 10%–35%	Intermediate to serious
Benign epilepsy of childhood with Rolandic spikes	Autosomal dominant?, age dependent, variable penetrance	10%–15% 33%	40%–50%	Usually benign
Benign epilepsy with occipital paroxysms	Different forms with positive and negative family histories	Not available	Not available	Usually benign; some forms may be more severe
Acquired partial epilepsy		<5%	<5%	May be severe

increased tendency for neurons in the CNS to become synchronized. There are many types of seizures and many epilepsy syndromes. In both experimental animals and humans, seizures can be produced in absolutely normal individuals by a large variety of perturbations in physiology, and there is not likely to be "one" cause of epilepsy, nor is it necessary, nor likely that all of the epilepsies have a genetic component. However, many forms of epilepsy, both in animals and in humans, are clearly hereditary, and in both mice and man, it has been shown that single-gene mutations can cause epilepsy syndromes.

REFERENCES

1. Hauser WA, Hesdorffer DC: Epilepsy: Frequency, Causes and Consequences. New York, Demos, 1990.

2. Hauser WA, Kurland LT: The epidemiology of epilepsy in Rochester, Minnesota, 1935 through 1967. Epilepsia 1975;16:1–66.

3. Commission on Classification and Terminology of the International League Against Epilepsy: Proposal for revised clinical and electroencephalographic classification of epileptic seizures. Epilepsia 1981;22:489–501.

4. Commission on Classification and Terminology of the International League Against Epilepsy: Proposal for revised classification of epilepsies and epileptic syndromes. Epilepsia 1989;30:389–399.

5. Noebels JL: Mutational analysis of inherited epilepsies. In Delgado-Escueta AV, Ward JR, Woodbury DM, Porter RJ (eds): Advances in Neurology. New York, Raven Press, 1986, pp 97–109.

6. Noebels JL: Single-gene models of epilepsy. Adv Neurol 1999;79:227–238.

7. Charlier C, Singh NA, Ryan SG, et al: A pore mutation in a novel KQT-like potassium channel gene in an idiopathic epilepsy family. Nat Genet 1998;18:53–55.

8. Hirose S, Zenri F, Akiyoshi H, et al: A novel mutation of KCNQ3 (c.925T→C) in a Japanese family with benign familial neonatal convulsions. Ann Neurol 2000;47:822–826.

9. Scheffer I, Berkovic S: Generalized epilepsy with febrile seizures plus: A genetic disorder with heterogeneous clinical phenotypes. Brain 1997;120:479–490.

10. Wallace R, Wang DW, Singh R, et al: Febrile seizures and generalized epilepsy associated with a mutation in the Na-channel β1 subunit gene SCN1B. Nat Genet 1998;19:366–370.

11. Wallace R, Scheffer IE, Barnett S, et al: Neuronal sodium-channel α1 subunit mutations in generalized epilepsy with febrile seizures plus. Am J Hum Genet 2001;68:859–865.

12. Wallace R, Marini C, Petrou S, et al: Mutant GABA(A) receptor gamma 2 subunit in childhood absence epilepsy and febrile seizures. Nat Genet 2001;28:49–52.

13. Harkin L, Bowser D, Dibbens L, et al: Truncation of the GABA(A) gamma 2 subunit in a family with generalized epilepsy with febrile seizures plus. Am J Hum Genet 2002;70:530–536.

14. Panayiotopoulos CP, Obeid T: Juvenile myoclonic epilepsy: An autosomal recessive disease. Ann Neurol 1989;25:440–443.

15. Delgado-Escueta A, Serratosa J, Liu A, et al: Progress in mapping human epilepsy genes. Epilepsia 1994;35:S29–S40.

16. Engel JJ: Seizures and Epilepsy. Philadelphia, FA Davis, 1989.

17. Berkovic SF, Andermann F, Andermann E, Gloor P: Concepts of absence epilepsies: Discrete syndromes or biological continuum? Neurology 1987; 37:993–1000.

18. Serratosa J, Weissbecker K, Delgado-Escueta A: Childhood absence epilepsy: An autosomal recessive disorder? Epilepsia 1990;31:651.

19. Moore T, Hecquet S, McLellann A, et al: Polymorphism analysis of JRK/JH8, the human homologue of mouse jerky, and description of a rare mutation in a case of CAE evolving to JME. Epilepsy Res 2001;46:157–167.

20. Delgado-Escueta A, Ganesh S, Yamakawa K: Advances in the genetics of progressive myoclonus epilepsy. Am J Med Genet 2001;106:129–138.

21. Lehesjoki A, Koskiniemi M, Sistonen P, et al: Localization of a gene for progressive myoclonus epilepsy to chromosome 21q22. Proc Natl Acad Sci U S A 1991;88:3696–3699.

22. Rosing HS, Hopkins LC, Wallace DC, et al: Maternally inherited mitochondrial myopathy and myoclonic epilepsy. Ann Neurol 1985;17:228–237.

23. Silverstri G, Moraes C, Shanske S, et al: A new mtDNA mutation in the tRNA(Lys) gene associated with myoclonic epilepsy and ragged red fibers (MERRF). Am J Hum Genet 1992;51:1213–1217.

24. Neubauer BA: The genetics of Rolandic epilepsy. Epilepsia 2000;41:1061–1062.

25. Scheffer I, Bhatia K, Lopes-Cendes I, et al: Autosomal frontal lobe epilepsy misdiagnosed as sleep disorder. Lancet 1994;343:515–517.

26. Steinlein O, Mulley J, Propiing P, et al: A missense mutation in the neuronal nicotinic acetylcholine receptor a4 subunit is associated with autosomal dominant nocturnal frontal lobe epilepsy. Nat Genet 1995; 11:1–5.

27. Kalachikov S, Evgrafov O, Ross B, et al: Mutations in LGI1 cause autosomal dominant partial epilepsy with auditory features. Nat Genet 2002: 335–341.

28. Ottman R: Genetics of the partial epilepsies: A review. Epilepsia 1989;30:107–111.

29. Treiman DM: Genetics of the partial epilepsies. In Mannagetta GB, Anderson EV, Doose H, Janz D (eds): Genetics of the Epilepsies. Berlin, Springer-Verlag, 1989, pp 73–82.

30. Penfield W, Paine K: Results of surgical therapy for focal epileptic seizures. Can Med Assoc J 1955; 73:515–531.

31. Andermann E, Metrakos J: A multifactorial analysis of focal and generalized cortico-reticular (centrencephalic) epilepsy. Epilepsia 1972;13:348–349.

32. Nelson K, Ellenberg J: Predictors of epilepsy in children who have experienced febrile seizures. N Engl J Med 1976;295:1029–1033.

33. Brodie M, Dichter M: Antiepileptic drugs. N Engl J Med 1996;334:168–175.

34. Dichter MA, Brodie MJ: New antiepileptic drugs. N Engl J Med 1996;334:1583–1590.

35. Brodie MJ, French JA: Management of epilepsy in adolescents and adults. Lancet 2000;356:323–329.

36. Kwan P, Brodie MJ: Early identification of refractory epilepsy. N Engl J Med 2000;342:314–319.

CHAPTER

39

Demyelinating Diseases

Stephen L. Hauser

Jorge R. Oksenberg

Demyelinating diseases are characterized by their high frequency, tendency to strike young adults, and diversity of manifestations. These disorders share features of inflammation and selective destruction of central nervous system (CNS) myelin; the peripheral nervous system (PNS) is spared. No specific tests for the demyelinating diseases exist, and diagnosis is based on recognition of the distinctive clinical patterns of CNS injury they produce. Multiple sclerosis (MS) is the prototypic demyelinating disease in humans. It is the most common cause of acquired neurologic dysfunction arising during early and mid-adulthood and affects more than 1 million people in North America and western Europe. Women are affected twice as often as men, suggesting that gender is a significant risk factor. MS pathogenesis is complex and multifactorial, with a genetic component that is not strictly mendelian and involves the interaction, either programmed or stochastic, of two or more genes, as well as a number of postgenomic DNA changes. In addition, it is likely that interactions with infectious, nutritional, climatic, and/or other environmental influences affect susceptibility considerably. This complex array of factors results in severe disregulation of the immune response, loss of immune homeostasis and self-tolerance, and development of abnormal (i.e., autoimmune) inflammatory pathogenic responses against structural components of the CNS. Myelin loss, gliosis, and varying degrees of axonal pathology culminate in progressive neurologic dysfunction, including sensory loss, weakness, visual loss, vertigo, incoordination, sphincter disturbances, and altered cognition.[1] The autoimmune model of MS pathogenesis has set the tone for immunotherapy in this disease, first by global immunosuppression using anti-inflammatory drugs and more recently by selective tar-geting of specific components of the immune response. The 1990s saw progress in defining additional aspects of the molecular and genetic basis of MS, preparing the stage for new therapeutic approaches based on correction of specific underlying disease mechanisms.

CLINICAL FEATURES AND DIAGNOSTIC EVALUATION

Manifestations of MS vary from a benign illness to a rapidly evolving and incapacitating disease. Onset may be abrupt or insidious. Symptoms may be severe or seem so trivial that a patient may not seek medical attention for months or years. Initial symptoms are commonly one or more of the following: weakness or diminished dexterity in one or more limbs, a disturbance of gait, optic neuritis, sensory disturbance, diplopia, and ataxia. As the disease progresses, bladder dysfunction, fatigue, and heat sensitivity occurs in most patients. Ancillary symptoms include Lhermitte symptom, trigeminal neuralgia, facial weakness and/or myokymia, vertigo, tonic spasms, and other paroxysmal symptoms. Cognitive dysfunction may be recognized early or late in the course of MS. Cognitive deficits most commonly include memory loss, impaired attention, problem-solving difficulties, slowed information processing, and difficulties in shifting between cognitive tasks. Impaired judgment and emotional lability may be evident. These symptoms affect activities of daily living in as many as 20% of patients. Depression is experienced by approximately 60% of patients during the course of the illness. Suicide is 7.5-fold more common than in age-matched controls.

Approximately 85% of patients with MS experience an abrupt onset of symptoms and signs at disease onset. Thereafter, the clinical course may be characterized by acute episodes of worsening (exacerbations or relapses), gradual progression of disability, or combinations of both. Four clinical patterns are recognized by international consensus. Patients with relapsing-remitting MS (RRMS) experience relapses with or without complete recovery and are clinically stable between these episodes. Approximately 50% of patients with RRMS convert to secondary progressive MS (SPMS) within 10 years of disease onset. The secondary progressive phase is characterized by gradual progression of disability with or without superimposed relapses. In contrast, patients with primary progressive MS (PPMS) experience gradual progression of disability from onset without superimposed relapses. Approximately 10% of patients with MS experience this clinical pattern. Patients with progressive relapsing MS experience gradual progression of disability from disease onset, later accompanied by one or more relapses; this clinical pattern affects approximately 5% of patients.

Most patients with MS experience progressive disability. Fifteen years after diagnosis, fewer than 20% of patients with MS have no functional limitation, 50% to 60% require assistance when ambulating, 70% are limited or unable to perform major activities of daily living, and 75% are not employed. In 1998, it was estimated that the total annual economic burden of MS in the United States exceeded 6.8 billion. The following clinical and brain magnetic resonance imaging (MRI) features may confer a more favorable prognosis: presentation with isolated optic neuritis or sensory symptoms, complete recovery from a first attack, age of onset younger than 40 years, female gender, relapsing-remitting clinical course, and fewer than two relapses in the first year of illness. In general, patients who experience minimal neurologic impairment 5 years after the first symptoms are least likely to be severely disabled 10 to 15 years later. By comparison, patients with persistent truncal ataxia, severe action tremor, or a disease course that is progressive from the onset are more likely to experience progression of disability. In patients who experience an initial attack of monosymptomatic optic neuritis, brain stem signs, or myelopathy, brain MRI provides useful prognostic information. If the brain MRI reveals multiple T2-weighted lesions, the risk of developing definite MS within a 10-year period of follow-up is 70% to 80%. Conversely, if the brain MRI is normal, less than 10% of patients experience a second episode of symptoms consistent with MS within 10 years.

Acute MS (Marburg variant) is a rare, acute, fulminant process that generally ends in death from brain stem involvement within 1 year. There are no remissions. Diagnosis can be established only at postmortem examination; widespread demyelination, axonal loss, edema, and macrophage infiltration are characteristic, and discrete plaques may also be seen. It has been suggested that acute MS may be associated with an immature form of myelin that is more susceptible to breakdown.

Neuromyelitis optica (Devic syndrome) is another clinical variant of MS, characterized by separate attacks of acute optic neuritis and myelitis. Optic neuritis may be unilateral or bilateral and precede or follow an attack of myelitis by days, months, or years. Respiratory failure may result from cervical cord lesions. In contrast to patients with MS, patients with Devic syndrome do not experience brain stem, cerebellar, and cognitive involvement, and the brain MRI is normal. Characteristically, MRI demonstrates a transiently enhancing focal region of swelling and cavitation that extends over three or more spinal cord segments. In contrast to MS, histopathology of these lesions may reveal areas of necrosis and thickening of blood vessel walls. This syndrome is unusual in whites but appears to be more common in Asians. It is unclear whether Marburg and Devic variants represent extreme forms of MS or other diseases altogether.

Diagnosis. There is no definitive diagnostic test. Diagnostic criteria for clinically definite MS require documentation of two or more episodes of symptoms and two or more signs that reflect pathology in anatomically noncontiguous white matter tracts of the CNS. Symptoms must last more than 1 day and occur as distinct episodes that are separated by 28 or more days. At least one of the two required signs must be present on neurologic examination. The second sign may be documented as an abnormal paraclinical test, either brain or spinal cord MRI, or visual, auditory, or somatosensory evoked electrical response. In patients who experience gradual progression of disability for 6 or more months without superimposed relapses, documentation of intrathecal immunoglobulin G (IgG) may be used to support the diagnosis. Additional laboratory testing that may be advisable in certain cases includes serum vitamin B_{12} level; human T cell lymphotropic virus type I (HTLV-I) titer; erythrocyte sedimentation rate; rheumatoid factor; antinuclear, anti-DNA antibodies; serum VDRL, angiotensin-converting enzyme (sarcoidosis); *Borrelia* serology (Lyme disease); very-long-chain fatty acids (adrenoleukodystrophy) and serum or cerebrospinal fluid (CSF) lactate; muscle biopsy; or mitochondrial DNA analysis (mitochondrial disorders).

Diagnostic Tests

MRI. Widespread availability of brain and spinal cord MRI has revolutionized the diagnosis and management of MS. Disease-related changes are detected by MRI in more than 95% of patients who otherwise meet diagnostic criteria for definite MS. An increase in vascular permeability, detected by leakage of the intravenous contrast agent gadolinium diethylenetriaminepenta-acetic acid into the brain, appears to be a very early event in the formation of new MS lesions and perhaps is a marker of inflammation. Gadolinium enhancement persists for 2 to 8 weeks; the residual mixture of edema, inflammation, demyelination, axonal loss, and gliosis in the MS plaque remains visible as a focal area of hyperintensity on spin-echo (T2-weighted) and proton-density images. Lesions often appear to extend outward from the ventricular surface, corresponding to a pattern of perivenous demyelination that is observed pathologically in MS (Dawson fingers). Lesions are also commonly found within the brain stem, corpus callosum, cerebellum, and spinal cord. Lesions of the anterior corpus callosum are particularly useful diagnostically because this site is usually spared in cerebrovascular disease. Specific criteria for the use of MRI in support of a diagnosis of MS have been proposed.

The correlation between the total volume of T2-weighted signal abnormality—the "lesion burden"—and the clinical measures of disability is poor. Approximately one third of hyperintense T2-weighted lesions appear hypointense on T1-weighted imaging sequences. These "black holes" provide more specific imaging markers of irreversible demyelination and axonal loss that correlate more robustly with clinical measures of disability. The correlation between MRI measures and clinical status is even stronger with emerging imaging techniques, including magnetization transfer imaging and proton-magnetic resonance spectroscopic imaging, which can distinguish irreversible demyelination and axonal loss from reversible edema and inflammation.

Evoked Responses. Evoked response testing may detect slowed or absent conduction in visual, auditory, somatosensory, or motor pathways. These tests use computer-averaging techniques to record the electrical response evoked in the nervous system after repetitive sensory stimuli. One or several evoked responses are abnormal in 80% to 90% of patients with MS. Abnormalities in evoked responses occur with a variety of neurologic disorders that disrupt pathways being measured; thus, they are not specific to MS. Testing is of diagnostic value when it provides evidence of a subclinical second lesion in a patient who manifests only one abnormality on neurologic examination.

CSF. CSF abnormalities consist of abnormally increased levels of intrathecally synthesized IgG, oligoclonal banding, and mononuclear cell pleocytosis. Various formulas are used to distinguish intrathecally synthesized IgG from serum IgG that may have entered the CNS passively across a disrupted blood-brain barrier (BBB). One formula expresses the ratio of IgG to albumin in the CSF divided by the ratio in the serum ("the CSF IgG index"). Oligoclonal banding of CSF IgG is detected by agarose gel electrophoresis techniques. Two or more oligoclonal bands are found in 75% to 90% of patients with MS. Oligoclonal banding may be absent at the onset of MS, and in individual patients the number of bands present may increase with time. It is important that paired serum samples be studied to exclude a systemic origin of the oligoclonal bands.

Other CSF abnormalities also occur but are less specific for MS. In one large series, CSF mononuclear pleocytosis (>5 cells/μL) was present in 25% of patients with MS. CSF cell counts are generally fewer than 20/μL in patients with MS, and counts higher than 50/μL are unusual but may occur with acute myelopathy. Pleocytosis of more than 75 cells/μL or a finding of polymorphonuclear leukocytes in CSF makes the diagnosis of MS unlikely. Pleocytosis is more common in young patients with RRMS than in older patients with progressive forms of MS. The total CSF protein content is usually normal or only slightly increased. A protein elevation of more than 100 mg/dL is rare and should prompt consideration of alternative diagnosis, such as infection or tumor.

PATHOLOGY

The pathologic hallmark of MS is the plaque, a well-demarcated gray or pink lesion, characterized histologically by inflammation, demyelination, proliferation of astrocytes with ensuing gliosis, and variable axonal degeneration (Fig. 39–1). MS plaques are typically multiple, asymmetric, and clustered in deep white matter near the lateral ventricles, corpus callosum, floor of the fourth ventricle, deep periaqueductal region, optic nerves and tracts, corticomedullary junction, and cervical spinal cord. Plaques vary in size from 1 or 2 mm to several centimeters in diameter. Although the prevalence of cortical lesions is unknown, some observers have suggested that they are greatly under-reported. Motor and sensory cortex lesions may contribute to ambulatory decline and cognitive dysfunction. It is also important to note that pathologic characteristics have been reported in normal-appearing white matter of MS brains when analyzed by imaging or molecular techniques.[2]

Perivascular and parenchymal infiltration by mononuclear cells, both T cells and macrophages, is characteristic of the acute MS lesion. Parenchymal and perivascular T cells consist of variable numbers of CD4+ and CD8+ cells. Although the vast majority bears the common form of the antigen receptor (i.e., the α/β heterodimer), T cells carrying the other form, the γ/δ heterodimer, have also been identified. The observed selective accumulation of activated T cells during certain stages of the plaque cycle indicates a specific pattern in the trafficking of T cells to the lesion and suggests that an immune response to discrete antigenic molecules is present. Although fewer in number, B cells and plasma cells also contribute to the inflammatory response. The role of this inflammatory response in MS pathogenesis is discussed later in this chapter.

At sites of inflammation, the BBB is disrupted, but the vessel wall itself is preserved, distinguishing the MS lesion from vasculitis. In some inflammatory lesions, dissolution of the multilamellated compact myelin sheaths that surround axons occurs. Myelin-specific autoantibodies have been detected bound to the vesiculated myelin

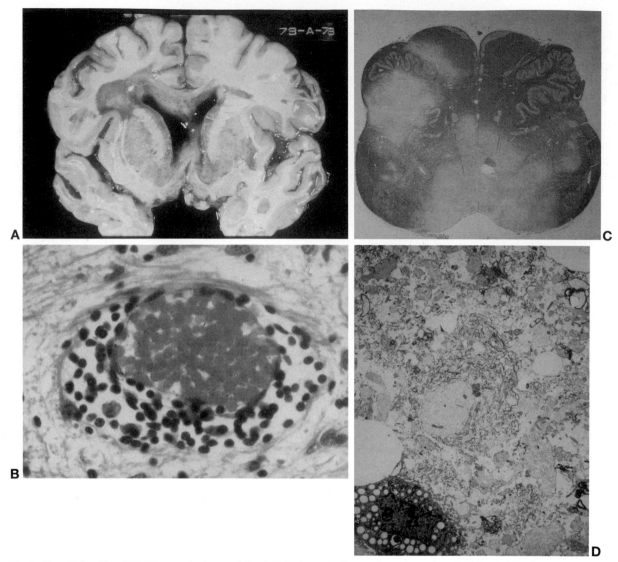

FIGURE 39–1. (See Color Plate IV) Histopathology of the MS lesion. *A*, Coronal section of an MS brain displays an acute periventricular area of demyelination and edema in the left temporal white matter and a smaller, linear plaque in a mirror position. The older plaque is less edematous and therefore is better demarcated. *B*, Low-power horizontal section through the medulla at the level of the inferior olives illustrates multiple asymmetric, sharply outlined areas of myelin loss that appear clear (luxol fast blue). *C*, Microscopic section of a lesion. Lymphocytes and macrophages appear as black, rounded nuclei surrounding a blood vessel. Some inflammatory cells have migrated farther into the brain parenchyma. *D*, Electron micrograph of MS myelin pathology on a biopsy of subcortical white matter. Disintegrating myelin membranes around the axon *(center)* have been transformed into a vesicular network. Fibrous astroglial processes, naked axons, and a reactive ameboid microglial cell *(lower left corner)* can also be identified.

fragments, at least in some patients; these autoantibodies are thought to promote demyelination.[3] As lesions evolve, axons traversing the plaque show marked irregular beading, proliferation of astrocytes occurs, and lipid-laden macrophages containing myelin debris are prominent. Progressive fibrillary gliosis ensues, and mononuclear cells gradually disappear. In some MS lesions, but not others, proliferation of oligodendrocytes appears to be present initially, but these cells are apparently destroyed as the gliosis progresses. In chronic MS lesions, complete or nearly complete demyelination, dense gliosis (more severe than in most other neuropathologic conditions), and loss

of oligodendroglia are found. In some chronic, active MS lesions, gradations in the histologic findings from the center to the lesion edge suggest that lesions expand by concentric outward growth.

The traditional neuropathologic view of MS highlights myelin loss as the prominent event occurring in the plaque, resulting in exposure to ion channels and impaired propagation of action potentials across the demyelinated region of the axon. However, the early literature on MS has already described substantial axonal damage in actively demyelinated lesions.[4] It is not known whether this process is independent or is a consequence of demyelination, but renewed interest in this aspect of MS pathology has focused considerable attention on the neurodegenerative aspects of this disease. Studies confirm that partial or total axonal transection begins early in the disease process and suggest that the cumulative axonal loss may ultimately determine neurologic disability.[5] Histopathologic studies reveal abundant transected and dystrophic axons in sites of active inflammation and demyelination. Axonal loss is perhaps the principal contributor to atrophy in MS, although demyelination may also decrease tissue volume. Axonal loss and cavitation are particularly prominent in the subtype of MS known as neuromyelitis optica or Devic syndrome. Axonal injury, as identified by amyloid precursor protein (APP) accumulation and reduced axonal density, was also observed in inactive and remyelinated lesions, cortical tissue, and normal-appearing white matter. N-acetyl aspartate (NAA), a chemical component of CNS axons involved in energy storage, provides a relatively specific pathologic marker of axonal degeneration. Reduced NAA in acute lesions is partly reversible, indicating that early axonal damage owing to inflammatory demyelination can be reversible, an observation compatible with the observed clinical recovery accompanying remissions.

It is important to emphasize that MS plaques are heterogeneous in their structural and immunopathologic patterns. Lucchinetti and colleagues reported that although most lesions contain an inflammatory reaction, diverse patterns of myelin destruction can be observed.[6] In their series, the majority of active MS lesions were characterized by the deposition of immunoglobulins and complement at sites of myelin breakdown, similar to what has been observed in the animal model of MS—experimental allergic encephalomyelitis (EAE) induced with myelin oligodendrocyte glycoprotein (MOG). Other cases are more suggestive of oligodendrocyte dystrophy, as reflected by loss of myelin associated glycoprotein (MAG) and oligodendrocyte apoptosis. These lesions are more reminiscent of viral, ischemic, or toxin-induced demyelination. These fundamentally different types of lesions appeared to breed true in individual cases; that is, all lesions from the same case are of the same type. The therapeutic implications of such pathologic heterogeneity are considerable because they may reflect fundamentally distinct immunopathogenic mechanisms.

MOLECULAR-GENETIC DATA

An important conceptual development in the understanding of MS pathogenesis has been the compartmentalization of the mechanistic process into two distinct but overlapping and connected phases, inflammatory and neurodegenerative. During the initial state of the inflammatory phase, lymphocytes with encephalitogenic potential are activated in the periphery and then home to the CNS, become attached to receptors on endothelial cells, and proceed to pass across the BBB, through the endothelium and the subendothelial basal lamina, and directly into the interstitial matrix (Fig. 39–2). Remarkably, the presence of immunocompetent cells with autoimmune potential appears to be an embedded characteristic of the (healthy) immune system in vertebrates. These cells may provide important inflammatory signals necessary for wound healing, angiogenesis, neuroprotection, and other maintenance functions. The transition from physiologic to pathologic autoimmunity involves at least two factors: (1) the loss of immune homeostasis, normally maintained through inhibitory signaling pathways, induction of anergy or apoptosis, and anti-idiotypic networks, and (2) the engagement and activation of lymphocytes by adjuvant signals including, conceivably, recurrent exposures to exogenous pathogens. This could occur via nonspecific polyclonal activation of T and B cells by bacterial or viral antigens or, alternatively, as a consequence of structural homology between a self-protein and a protein in the pathogen, a process commonly referred as molecular mimicry. It is notable, for example, that components of the myelin sheath share amino acid homologies with proteins of measles, influenza, herpes, papilloma, adenovirus, and other viruses. These pathogens acquire sufficient homology to engage myelin-specific T cells, with the potential for a misguided response. In addition, amino acid identity may not even be required for cross-reactivity to occur between the autoantigen and the mimic, as long as they share chemical properties at critical residues that allow anchoring to antigen-presenting molecules and interaction with the T cell antigen receptor. An alternative hypothesis proposes that activation of autoimmune cells occurs as a consequence of viral infection of CNS cells; such infections may be asymptomatic but cause cytopathic effects to target cells in the course of an antiviral response. The prolonged release of neural antigens may then induce inflammatory responses that eventually become self-perpetuating and pathologic.

Once activated, T cells express surface molecules called integrins, which mediate binding to the specialized capillary endothelial cells of the BBB (see Fig. 39–2). One such integrin, VLA-4, binds the vascular cell adhesion molecule (VCAM) expressed in the capillary endothelial cells after induction by tumor necrosis factor α (TNF-α) and interferon γ (IFN-γ) during an inflammatory response. As the activated T cells migrate across the BBB to reach the CNS parenchyma, they express gelatinases (matrix metalloproteinases [MMPs]) responsible for lysis of the dense subendothelial basal lamina. The clinical relevance of metalloproteinases is underlined by the observation that some members of this family of molecules are present in the CSF of patients with MS but not in normal controls.[7] It is also noteworthy that the sequence in the putative cleavage of the TNF-α precursor reveals homologies with peptide sequences known to be cleaved by metalloproteinase-like enzymes. Thus metalloproteinases may not only act as mediators of cell traffic across the BBB, but also increase the inflammatory

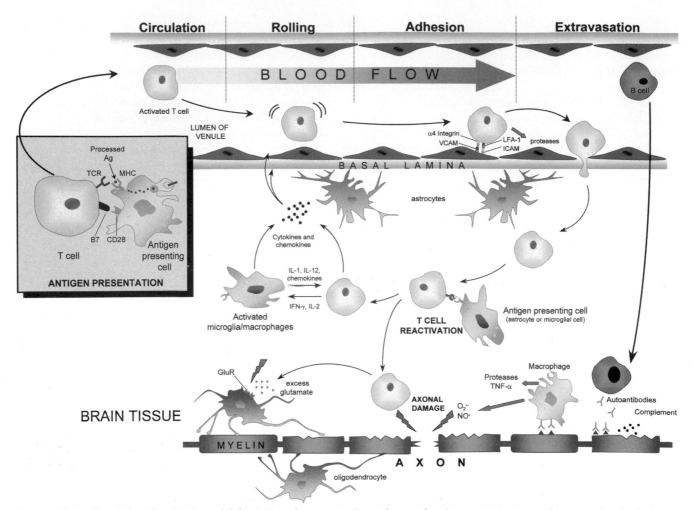

FIGURE 39–2. (See Color Plate V) A model for MS pathogenesis. Crucial steps for disease initiation and progression include peripheral activation of autoreactive lymphocytes, homing to the CNS and extravasation across the blood-brain barrier, reactivation of T cells by exposed autoantigens, secretion of cytokines, activation of microglia and astrocytes, stimulation of the antibody cascade, myelin destruction, and axonal degeneration.

reaction through TNF processing. Furthermore, a direct neurotoxic effect for metalloproteinases has been proposed as well; microinjection of activated MMPs into the cortical white matter of experimental animals results in axonal injury, even in the absence of local inflammation.

A different group of molecules involved in leukocyte homing and extravasation comprises soluble chemoattractants named *chemokines* and their receptors. Chemokines are members of an expanding family of small serum proteins between 7 and 16 kDa in size, primarily involved in selective trafficking and homing of leukocytes to sites of infection and inflammation, leukocyte maturation in the bone marrow, tissue repair and vascularization, and hematopoiesis and renewal of circulating leukocytes. The spatial and temporal expression of chemokines correlates with disease activity in EAE and MS. In addition, chemokine receptors have been shown to mediate entry of microorganisms into target cells and also to participate in the viral-mediated induction of pro-inflammatory (Th-1) cytokines, both potential mediators of the encephalitogenic response. Even though the

chemokine network is remarkably redundant and promiscuous, some investigators have proposed that individual chemokines and receptors might be reasonable targets for therapeutic intervention in MS.

After traversing the BBB, pathogenic T cells are believed to be reactivated by fragments of myelin antigens. Reactivation induces additional release of proinflammatory cytokines that open further the BBB and stimulate chemotaxis, resulting in additional waves of inflammatory cell recruitment and leakage of antibody and other plasma proteins into the nervous system. Pathogenic T cells may not be capable of producing or inducing tissue injury in the absence of the secondary leukocyte recruitment. For example, in EAE mediated by adoptive transfer of myelin-reactive encephalitogenic T lymphocytes, these cells are among the first to infiltrate the CNS but constitute only a minor component of the total infiltrate in the full-blown lesion.

All together, a large body of experimental data has firmly established that myelin-specific T cells in MS patients are present in greater numbers than in healthy

PLATE I

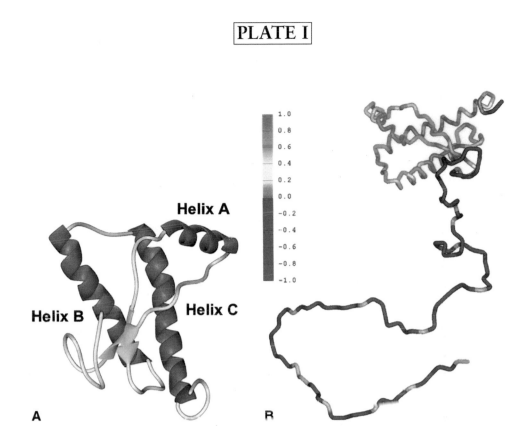

FIGURE 2–3. Structures of the cellular isoform of the prion protein. *A*, NMR structure of recombinant Syrian hamster (SHa) PrP(90–231). Presumably, the structure of the α-helical form of SHaPrP(90–231) resembles that of PrP^C. SHaPrP (90–231) is viewed from the interface where PrP^Sc is thought to bind to PrP^C. α-Helices A (residues 144 to 157), B (172 to 193), and C (200 to 227), strand S1 (residues 129 to 134), and strand S2 (residues 159 to 165) are shown. The arrows span residues 129 to 131 and 161 to 163, as these show a closer resemblance to β-sheet.[95] *B*, Schematic diagram showing the flexibility of the polypeptide chain for PrP(29–231).[96] The structure of the portion of the protein representing residues 90 to 231 was taken from the coordinates of PrP(90–231).[95] The remainder of the sequence was hand-built for illustration purposes only. The color scale corresponds to the heteronuclear {¹H}-¹⁵N NOE data: from red for the lowest (most negative) values, where the polypeptide is most flexible, to blue for the highest (most positive) values in the most structured and rigid regions of the protein. (Reprinted with permission from Proc Natl Acad Sci U S A 1997;94:13452–13457. Copyright 1997 National Academy of Sciences.)

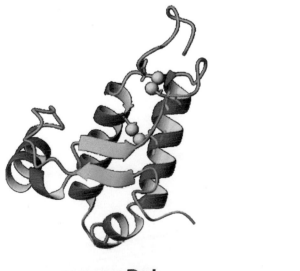

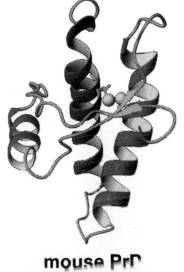

FIGURE 2–4. NMR structures of Dpl and PrP from mice. (Figure prepared by Jane Dyson and Peter Wright.)

mouse Dpl
(Mo et al., 2001)

mouse PrP
(Riek et al., 1996)

PLATE II

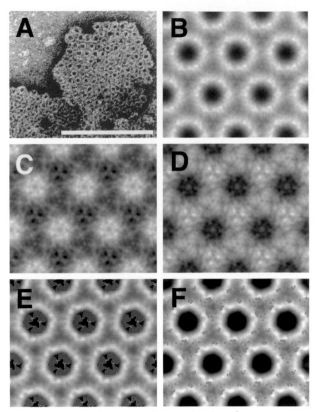

FIGURE 2–5. Two-dimensional crystals of PrP^{Sc}. *A,* A 2D crystal of PrP^{Sc}106 stained with uranyl acetate. Bar = 100 nm. *B,* Image processing result after correlation-mapping and averaging followed by crystallographic averaging. *C and D,* Subtraction maps between the averages of PrP 27–30 and PrP^{Sc}106 *(panel B). C,* PrP^{Sc}106 minus PrP 27–30 and *D,* PrP 27–30 minus PrP^{Sc}106, showing major differences in lighter shades. *E and F,* The statistically significant differences between PrP 27–30 and PrP^{Sc}106 calculated from panels *C* and *D* in red and blue, respectively, and overlaid onto the crystallographic average of PrP 27–30. (Copyright 2002 National Academy of Sciences, USA.)

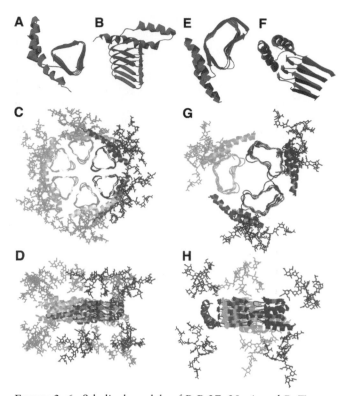

FIGURE 2–6. β-helical models of PrP 27–30. *A and B,* Top and side views, respectively, of PrP 27–30 modeled with a left-handed β-helix. The β-helical portion of the model is based on the *Methanosarcina thermophila* γ-carbonic anhydrase structure. *C and D,* Top and side views, respectively, of the trimer-of-dimer model of PrP 27–30 with left-handed β-helices. *E and F,* Top and side views, respectively, of PrP 27–30 modeled with a right-handed β-helix. The β-helical portion of the model is based on the most regular helical turns of *Bordetella pertussis* P.69 pertactin. *G and H,* Top and side views, respectively, of the trimer model of PrP 27–30 with right-handed β-helices. The structure of the α-helices was derived from the solution structure of recombinant SHaPrP. In the single molecule images (*A, B, E, and F*), residues 141 to 176 that are deleted in PrP106 are colored blue. (Copyright 2002 National Academy of Sciences, USA.)

PLATE III

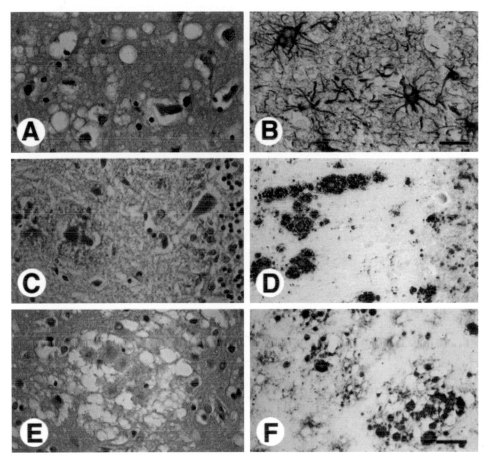

FIGURE 13–2. Neuropathology of human prion diseases. Sporadic Creutzfeldt-Jakob disease (sCJD) is characterized by vacuolation of the neuropil of the gray matter, by exuberant reactive astrocytic gliosis, the intensity of which is proportional to the degree of nerve cell loss, and rarely by PrP amyloid plaque formation (not shown). The neuropathology of familial CJD is similar. GSS(P102L), as well as other inherited forms of Gerstmann-Sträussler-Scheinker disease (not shown), is characterized by numerous deposits of PrP amyloid throughout the central nervous system. Variant CJD (vCJD) has clinical and epidemiological features that suggest it was acquired by infection with bovine spongiform encephalopathy (BSE) prions. The neuropathological features of vCJD are unique among CJD cases because of the abundance of PrP amyloid plaques that are often surrounded by a halo of intense vacuolation. A, sCJD, cerebral cortex stained with hematoxylin and eosin showing widespread spongiform degeneration; B, sCJD, cerebral cortex immunostained with anti-GFAP antibodies demonstrating the widespread reactive astrocytic gliosis; C, GSS, cerebellum with most of the GSS-plaques in the molecular layer (left 80% of micrograph) and many but not all stained positively for the periodic acid–Schiff (PAS) reaction. Granule cells and a single Purkinje cell are seen in the right 20% of the panel; D, GSS, cerebellum at the same location as C with PrP immunohistochemistry after hydrolytic autoclaving reveals more PrP plaques than seen with the PAS reaction; E, vCJD, cerebral cortex stained with hematoxylin and eosin shows that the plaque deposits are uniquely located within vacuoles. With this histology, these amyloid deposits have been referred to as "florid plaques"; F, vCJD, cerebral cortex stained with PrP immunohistochemistry after hydrolytic autoclaving reveals numerous PrP plaques often occurring in clusters as well as minute PrP deposits surrounding many cortical neurons and their proximal processes. Bar in B represents 50 μm and applies also to panels A, C, and E. Bar in F represents 100 μm and applies also to panel D.

PLATE IV

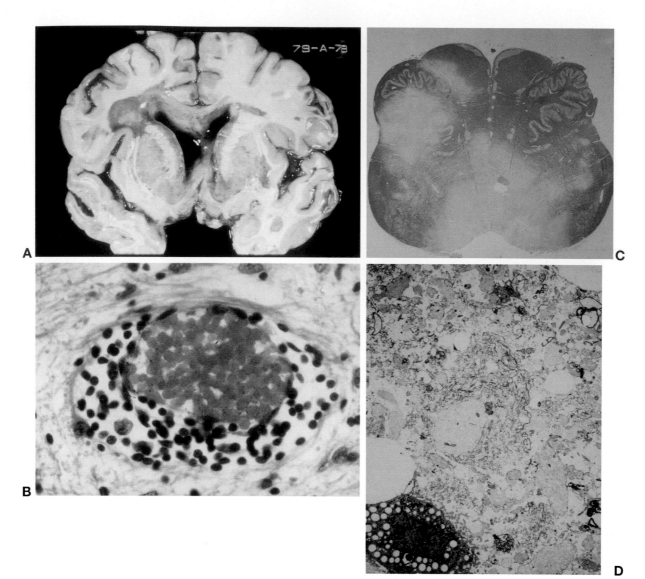

FIGURE 39–1. Histopathology of the MS lesion. *A*, Coronal section of an MS brain displays an acute periventricular area of demyelination and edema in the left temporal white matter and a smaller, linear plaque in a mirror position. The older plaque is less edematous and therefore is better demarcated. *B*, Low-power horizontal section through the medulla at the level of the inferior olives illustrates multiple asymmetric, sharply outlined areas of myelin loss that appear clear (luxol fast blue). *C*, Microscopic section of a lesion. Lymphocytes and macrophages appear as black, rounded nuclei surrounding a blood vessel. Some inflammatory cells have migrated farther into the brain parenchyma. *D*, Electron micrograph of MS myelin pathology on a biopsy of subcortical white matter. Disintegrating myelin membranes around the axon *(center)* have been transformed into a vesicular network. Fibrous astroglial processes, naked axons, and a reactive ameboid microglial cell *(lower left corner)* can also be identified.

PLATE V

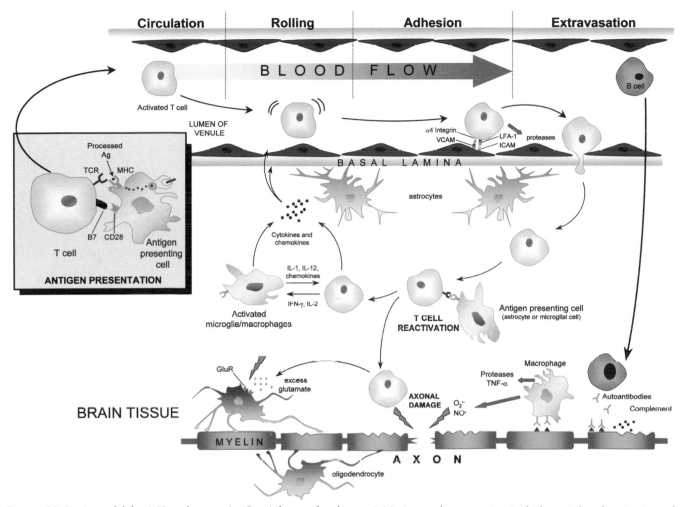

FIGURE 39–2. A model for MS pathogenesis. Crucial steps for disease initiation and progression include peripheral activation of autoreactive lymphocytes, homing to the CNS and extravasation across the blood-brain barrier, reactivation of T cells by exposed autoantigens, secretion of cytokines, activation of microglia and astrocytes, stimulation of the antibody cascade, myelin destruction, and axonal degeneration.

PLATE VI

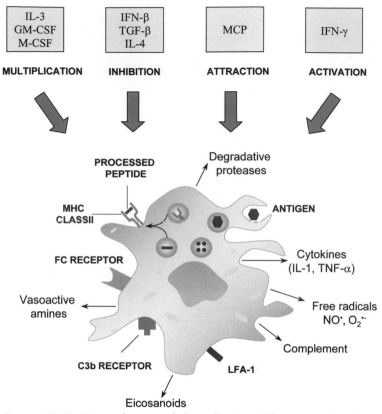

FIGURE 39–3. Macrophages and demyelination. The macrophage is a key participant in the inflammatory response in MS.

PLATE VII

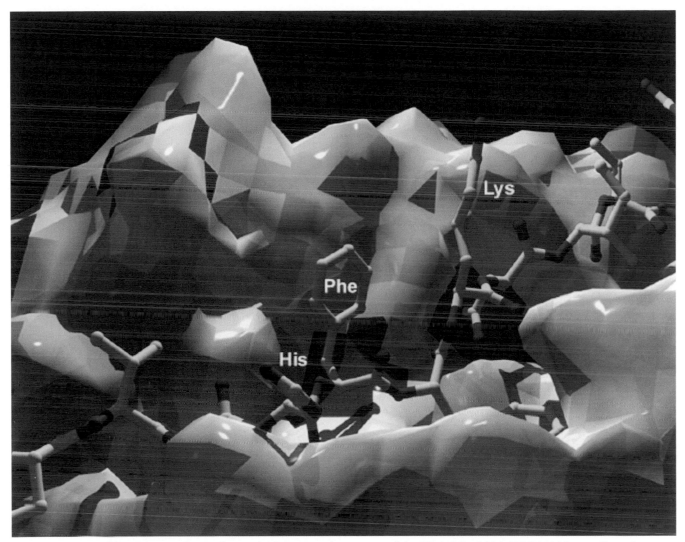

FIGURE 39–4. Graphic representation (side view) of the crystal structure of the HLA-DRα0101, DRβ1501 heterodimer in complex with a putative MS autoantigen, the myelin basic protein peptide 85–99.

PLATE VIII

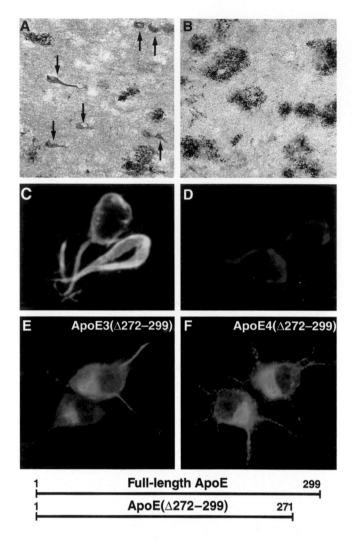

E ApoE3(Δ272–299)
F ApoE4(Δ272–299)

1   Full-length ApoE   299
1   ApoE(Δ272–299)   271

FIGURE 52–2. C-terminal-truncated forms of apoE accumulate in AD brains and NFTs. Immunostaining of AD brain sections with anti–N-terminal apoE (*A*), which identified both amyloid plaques and NFTs (*arrows*), or anti–C-terminal apoE *(B)*, which identified only amyloid plaques. Double immunofluorescence staining of AD brain sections with anti–p-tau (red) and anti–N-terminal apoE (green) (*C*) or anti–p-tau (red) and anti–C-terminal apoE (green) (*D*). *E* and *F*, C-terminal-truncated apoE induces the formation of apoE- and p-tau–immunoreactive intracellular inclusions in N2a cells. N2a cells were transiently transfected with apoE3(Δ272-299) (*E*) or apoE4(Δ272-299) *(F)* cDNA and immunostained with anti-apoE.

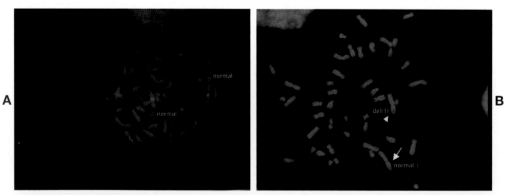

FIGURE 59–2. Fluorescence in situ hybridization (FISH). Metaphase spreads of cultured skin fibroblasts from the Glut1DS patients were probed with a fluorescence labeled DNA probe specific for GLUT1. *A*, Patient #12 carried a heterozygous deletion (1086delG); the two alleles of GLUT1 were indicated by *arrows* with "normal." *B*, Patient #24 was hemizygous for GLUT1 in the short arm of chromosome 1 indicated by *arrows* with "normal 1" and "del(1)."

PLATE IX

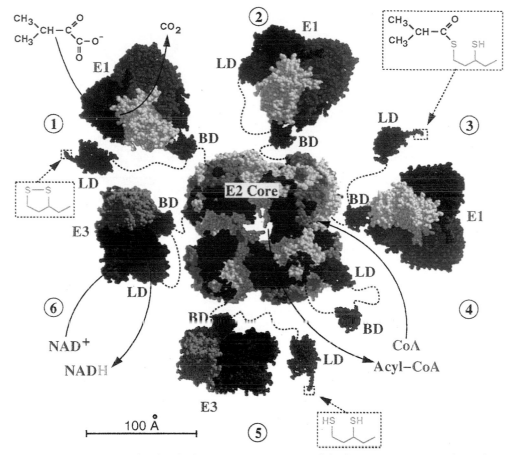

FIGURE 60–1. Structural organization and individual component reactions of the human BCKD complex. The macromolecular structure (4×10^6 Da in size) is organized about a cubic transacylase (E2) core (based on the structure of *Azotobacter* pyruvate dehydrogenase E2), to which a decarboxylase (E1) (based on the *Pseudomonas* BCKD E1 structure), a dehydrogenase (E3) (according to the structure of *Azotobacter* pyruvate dehydrogenase E3) are attached through ionic interactions. E2 of the BCKD complex contains 24 identical subunits with each polypeptide made up of three folded domains: lipoyl (LD), E1/E3-binding (BD), and the E2 core domains that are linked by flexible regions (represented by *dotted lines*). E1 $\alpha_2\beta_2$ heterotetramers or E3 homodimers are attached to BD. The mammalian BCKD kinase and BCKD phosphatase (not shown) presumably bind to LD. E1 catalyzes the TPP-mediated oxidative decarboxylation of α-ketoacids. The TPP-hydroxyacylidene moiety is transferred to a reduced lipoyl prosthetic group *(in the box)* on LD. The flexible LD carries S-acyldihydrolipoamide to the active site in the E2 core to generate acyl-CoA. The reduced lipoyl moiety on LD is oxidized by E3 on BD with a concomitant reduction of NAD$^+$. (From Ævarsson A, Seger K, Turley S, et al: Crystal structure of 2-oxoisovalerate dehydrogenase and the architecture of 2-oxo acid dehydrogenase multienzyme complexes. Nat Struct Biol 1999;6:785–792.)

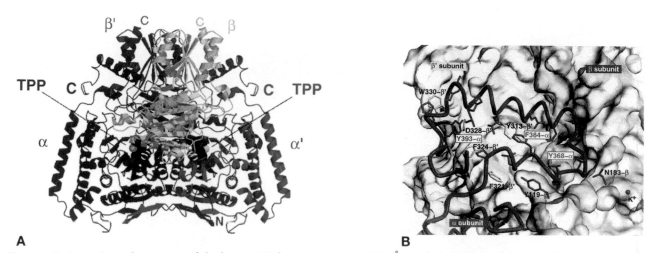

FIGURE 60–2. *A*, Crystal structure of the human E1 heterotetramer at 2.7-Å resolution. Each of the two identical 400-residue α subunits is composed of a large domain containing mostly α helices. The α subunit also shows an extended *N*-terminal tail and a small helical *C*-terminal domain. Each of the two identical β subunits of 346 residues is divided into two domains of similar size. They correspond to the *N*-terminal and *C*-terminal halves of the polypeptide. Each domain of the β subunit comprises four parallel central β strands with several helices packed in variable orientations against the β strands. Interactions between the equivalent $\alpha\beta$ and $\alpha'\beta'$ heterodimeric intermediates result in the assembly of the 167-kDa E1 heterotetramer. Each human E1 binds two TPP molecules, two Mg^{2+} and four K^+ ions. *B*, E1α MSUD mutations in the "Mennonite" region impede interactions of the α subunit with the β or β' subunit. The *C*-terminal domain of E1α subunit shown as a coil backbone is packed against semi-transparent surfaces of the β and β' subunits. Selected side chains are marked and the three aromatic residues Tyr-393-α, Phe-364-α, and Tyr-368-α that are affected in MSUD are boxed. This segment of the E1α chain is called the "Mennonite" region due to the presence of the prevalent Y393N-α mutation in this population. Tyr-393-α is hydrogen-bonded to Asp-328-β', in the β' subunit. Phe-364-α is packed against Tyr-313-β', also in the β' subunit. Tyr-368-α is packed against the β subunit at the α/β subunit interface. (From Ævarsson A, Chuang JL, Wynn RM, et al: Crystal structure of human branched-chain α-ketoacid dehydrogenase and molecular basis of multienzyme complex deficiency in maple syrup urine disease. Structure 2000;8:277–291.)

controls, have lower thresholds of activation, and have different effector profiles. However, whereas the role of CD4+ and CD8+ T cells as initiators and regulators of the CNS inflammatory response is well established, their role as direct effectors of myelin injury remains uncertain. Potential T cell–mediated mechanisms of myelin damage have been established in vitro; TNF-α kills myelinating cells in culture, anti-myelin basic protein (anti-MBP) CD4+ cells can display cytolytic functions, and CD8+ cells induce cytoskeleton breaks in neurites. Interestingly, axonal injury correlates better with the presence of CD8+ T cells and macrophages than with CD4+ T cells. It is clear, however, that the MS lesion is not exclusively T cell mediated; rather, a synergistic cellular and humoral response is required to produce demyelination and axonal damage. The most convincing mechanisms of tissue injury involve antibody binding and complement activation and macrophage/microglia activation followed by myelin phagocytosis and release of toxic factors.

B cell activation and antibody responses are necessary for the full development of demyelination, in both human and experimental disease. In most MS patients, an elevated level of intrathecally synthesized immunoglobulins can be detected in the CSF. Although the specificity of these antibodies is mostly unknown, anti-MBP specificities have been detected. Myelin-specific infiltrating B cells have been detected in the MS brain, and in the CSF and brain of affected individuals there is an elevated frequency of clonally expanded B cells with properties of

postgerminal center memory or antibody-forming lymphocytes. Antibodies may participate in myelin destruction through different mechanisms, such as opsonization that facilitates phagocytosis by macrophages and/or complement fixation. The presence in the serum of MS patients of autoantibodies generally associated with other autoimmune conditions has also been established and may reflect systemic immune disregulation.

A third class of cells, the resident *microglia*, lying within the parenchyma, also become activated as a result of locally released cytokines (Fig. 39–3).[8] Microglia act as scavengers that remove debris and as antigen-presenting cells (APCs) that present processed antigens to T cells, contributing to their local clonal expansion. Mutual interactions between T cells and macrophages induce proliferation of both cell types through mediation of such molecules as interleukin-2 (IL-2) and colony-stimulating factors. Furthermore, endothelia and T cells provide colony-stimulating factors that maintain macrophage activation, and prevent apoptosis and cell death. Microglia are also likely to directly induce myelin damage and killing of oligodendroglial cells through the release of mediators such as free radicals (nitric oxide O_2^- and superoxide anion ^+NO), vasoactive amines, complement, proteases, cytokines (IL-1, TNF-α), and eicosanoids. Excess of glutamate released by microglia and macrophages during inflammation, accompanied by a decrease in glutamate intake and metabolism, activates AMPA (α-amino-3-hydroxy-5-methil-4-isoxazolppropionic acid), which is toxic to oligodendroglial cells

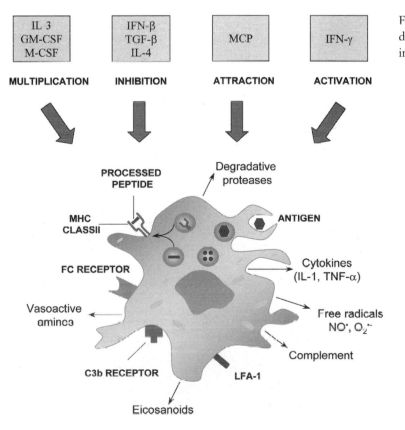

FIGURE 39–3. (See Color Plate VI) Macrophages and demyelination. The macrophage is a key participant in the inflammatory response in MS.

and neurons. Blockade of AMPA-responsive glutamate receptors with AMPA antagonists ameliorates neurologic sequelae in EAE, increases oligodendrocyte survival, and reduces dephosphorylation of neurofilament H, an indicator of axonal damage.

GENETIC BASIS OF MS

Compelling data indicate that susceptibility to MS is inherited. Familial aggregation, recognized by Charcot in the late nineteenth century, is well documented with an increased relative risk (λ_s) of 20–40 to siblings of an affected person compared with the general population. Concordant sibs tend to share age of symptom onset rather than year of onset, and second- and third-degree relatives of MS patients are also at an increased risk for MS. In addition, concordance within multiple-affected families for early (pattern of optic nerve and/or spinal cord manifestations in the first and second attacks) and late (disability and overall late handicap scores) clinical features were reported. Finally, studies of half-siblings and adoptees support the concept that inherited factors distinct from common environmental exposure influence susceptibility.

Genetic studies in MS in the 1990s were influenced by three large, multistage, whole genome screens performed in multiple-affected families ascertained in the United States, the United Kingdom, and Canada.[9–11] A fourth study concentrated on a genetically isolated region of Finland but was based on a small number of families.[12] Follow-up screenings in confirmatory and additional data sets have been completed as well. The studies altogether identified about 60 genomic regions with potential involvement in disease susceptibility, consistent with the long-held view that MS is a polygenic disorder. However, total or even predominant replication between the different screens was absent. This was in part due to the strategy of reporting all "hits" suggestive of linkage, recognizing that false positives are generated along with true positives. It is also possible that the study design in each case underestimated the confounding influence of disease heterogeneity and the limitations of parametric methods of statistical analysis. It should be noted, however, that because each study used a somewhat overlapping but different set of genetic markers and different clinical inclusion criteria, the direct comparison of results is not straightforward.

Nevertheless, a detailed analysis of the composite published data identified 13 overlapping regions of interest among the 4 original genomic scans, including 1p36-p33, 2p23-p21, 3p14-p13, 3q22-q24, 4q31-qter, 5p14-p12, 5q12-q13, 6p21-22, 6q22-27, 7q21-q22, 17q22, 18p11, 19q12-13.[13] In addition, meta-analysis of the raw and published data singled out discrete overlapping MS-susceptibility regions at chromosomes 5, 6, 17, and 19. Although further work is necessary to better define the complete roster of MS loci, these studies represent real progress in mapping the full set of MS-associated genes.

MS1, THE MAJOR HISTOCOMPATIBILITY COMPLEX

The human major histocompatibility complex (MHC) (the human leukocyte antigen [HLA] system) consists of linked gene clusters located at 6p21.3, spanning almost 4 million base pairs. HLA molecules are cell surface glycoproteins whose primary role in an immune response is to display and present short antigenic peptide fragments to peptide/MHC-specific T cells. Many of the *HLA* genes are highly polymorphic, resulting in the generation of enormously diverse numbers of different genotypic combinations or haplotypes. The polymorphic residues that define an *HLA* allele are clustered in the antigen-peptide–binding groove of the molecule. Hence, the ability to respond to an antigen, whether foreign or self, and the nature of that response are to a large extent determined by the unique amino acid sequences of *HLA* alleles, an observation that provided the rationale for focusing on associations between *HLA* genotypes and susceptibility to autoimmune disease.

The *HLA-DR2* haplotype (*DRB1*1501, DQB1*0602*) within the MHC is the strongest genetic effect identified in MS and has consistently demonstrated both linkage and association in family and case-control studies.[14] Using family data, the proportion of the total λ_s explained by the *HLA-DR* locus can be estimated. At the upper end, under a multiplicative genetic model and assuming a λ_s of 15, the HLA-DR association can explain as much as 60% of the genetic etiology of MS. At the lower end, under an additive model and assuming a λ_s of 40, it could explain as little as 17%. The mechanism(s) underlying the genetic association of *HLA-DRB1*1501-DQB1*0602* with MS is not yet fully understood. One possibility is that these MHC molecules fail to negatively select (delete) autoreactive T cells within the embryonic thymic microenvironment. Alternatively, *DRB1*1501* and/or *DQB1*0602* genes may encode antigen recognition molecules with a propensity to bind peptide fragments of myelin and stimulate encephalitogenic T cells. The HLA-DRα0101-DRβ1501 heterodimer binds with high affinity to the myelin basic protein (MBP) 89–98 peptide. X-ray crystallography of the DR-MBP peptide complex reveals a DRβ1501 structure different from other DRβ molecules in that aromatic residues are preferred in the P4 pocket of the peptide binding domain (Fig. 39–4). In addition, it was found that two peptide side chains of the p85–99 MBP immunodominant peptide, Val89 and Phe92, are the primary anchors and account for the high-affinity binding of the MBP peptide to HLA-DRα0101/DRβ1501. The structural analysis also revealed that only two primary T cell receptor contact residues of MBP p85–99 had to be conserved to properly stimulate antigen-specific clones. The data increase the likelihood

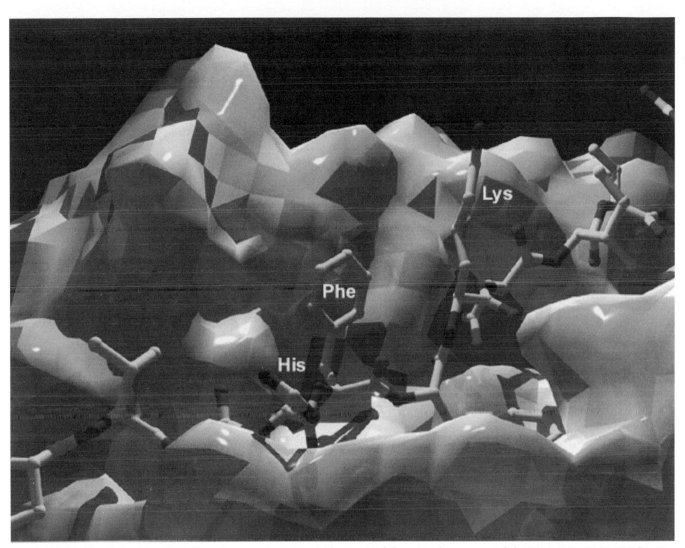

FIGURE 39–4. (See Color Plate VII) Graphic representation (side view) of the crystal structure of the HLA-DRα0101, DRβ1501 heterodimer in complex with a putative MS autoantigen, the myelin basic protein peptide 85–99.

that microbial peptides with only limited sequence identity with a self-peptide could well activate autoreactive T cells.

MS2, CHROMOSOME 19q13

Genomic screens have shown support for linkage to this region, and a meta-analysis of all four genomic screens has identified 19q13 as the second most significant region after the MHC. Additional evidence for this region came from allelic association studies and, more recently, from follow-up analyses by our group.[15] Based on this study, the effect of the 19q13 locus is likely to be small, with an estimated locus-specific λ_s of 1.5, thus accounting for 4% to 6% of the overall genetic component in MS. This region contains many attractive candidate genes. The well-documented involvement of APOE in neurologic disease, for example, makes this gene an interesting candidate for MS studies. The apoE protein has long been associated with regeneration of axons and myelin after lesions of CNS and PNS tissue, and its isoforms have been shown to have differential effects on neuronal growth. Additional suggestive candidate genes include *TGFβ1*, immunoglobulin-like transcripts (ILT), killer cell inhibitory receptors (KIR), the leukocyte-associated inhibitory receptors (LAIR), the Fc receptor, IL-11, the heavy chain of the MHC class I–like Fc receptor, and *APOC4*.

LOCUS HETEROGENEITY

Locus heterogeneity, meaning that different genes can cause identical or similar forms of the disease, is a key element for the understanding of MS pathogenesis. In an analysis of 184 families with more than one affected member, linkage and association to the *HLA-DR* locus and a strong association with the specific *DR2* haplotype were observed.[16] Remarkably, all the linkage information and evidence for association is derived from families in which *DR2* was present in at least one nuclear member. No genetic effect of the *HLA-DR* locus could be discerned in the DR2-negative family set. In fact, our results exclude linkage for at least 20 cM around *HLA-DR* in the DR2-negative families for both autosomal dominant and recessive models. These data provide strong evidence that heterogeneity at the *HLA* locus exists in MS and suggest a fundamentally different disease mechanism in the DR2-negative families without discernible genetic influence of other DR alleles or HLA genes.

Another example of heterogeneity in MS is provided by studies of Japanese patients. In this group, one form of MS is apparently characterized by disseminated CNS involvement and is associated with the *HLA-DR2* haplotype, whereas more restricted forms of disease, in which optic nerve and/or spinal cord involvement predominate and lesions are more severe and necrotizing, are not associated with *HLA-DR2*.[17] The strength of the association between PPMS and *HLA-DR2* is also uncertain. A number of small studies failed to show any association between PPMS and *DR2*, although a more recent, larger study from northern Ireland appeared to show the association. The implications of heterogeneity are considerable because they may reflect fundamentally distinct immunopathogenic mechanisms. The pharmacogenomic consequences of HLA locus heterogeneity in MS are also important and could explain individual differences in treatment response to Glatiramer acetate, a molecular mimic of a region of myelin basic protein that is immunodominant in *HLA-DR2*–positive individuals.[18] Whether the genotype dictates different forms of MS in response to a common causative agent or trigger, or whether the genotype reflects different diseases with different environmental causes, is not known. Clearly, however, clinical and demographic variables will assume critical importance as stratifying elements for genetic studies in MS.

· SUSCEPTIBILITY GENES VERSUS MODIFIERS

Clinical symptoms in MS are extremely variable. The course may be relapsing-remitting or progressive, severe or mild, and may involve the neuraxis in a widespread fashion or predominantly affect spinal cord and optic nerve. Very little is known about the underlying cause of disease variability in MS. The susceptibility *HLA-DRB1*1501-DQA1*0102-DQB1*0602* haplotype has been reported to be associated with lower age at onset; gender; and severe, relapsing-remitting, and mild MS courses, or it has been reported to have no influence. Several studies suggesting the influence of non-*HLA* genes (*IL-1R, TNF, TGFB, APOE, CTLA4*, and *CCR5*, among others) on disease course and severity in MS have been reported and await confirmation.

MS AND OTHER AUTOIMMUNE DISEASES

MS shares several characteristics with other autoimmune disorders, including gender dimorphism, increasing prevalence throughout adult life with peak incidence between ages 20 and 40 years, tendency for remission during pregnancy with transient deterioration or increased incidence of onset in the postpartum period, polygenic inheritance, specific associations with particular HLA alleles within the MHC, and evidence that environmental exposure of some type is involved. Familial clustering of multiple autoimmune diseases and the presence of autoantibodies generally associated with other autoimmune conditions have also been reported. Although the significance of these findings is unclear, they suggest that common genetic susceptibility factors for autoimmunity may exist. A meta-analysis of linkage results from 23 human and experimental immune-mediated diseases, including MS and EAE detected overlapping of susceptibility loci,[19] further supporting the hypothesis that the pathophysiology of clinically distinct autoimmune disorders may be controlled, at least in part, by a common set of genes. In a genome scan of rheumatoid arthritis, several identified linked regions had been previously implicated in studies of MS, systemic lupus erythematosus, or inflammatory bowel disease.[20]

MODEL OF INHERITANCE

A simple model of inheritance for all MS is unlikely and cannot account for the nonlinear decrease in disease risk in families with increasing genetic distance from the proband. As summarized previously, the available data are most compatible with a complex multifactorial etiology, including both genetic and environmental factors. Recurrence risk estimates in multiplex families combined with twin data predict that the MS-prone genotype results from multiple independent or interacting polymorphic genes, each exerting a small or moderate effect. Thus, the abundance of data supports a polygenic model for this disorder, although a mendelian-like genetic etiology cannot be ruled out for a small subset of pedigrees. Equally significant, it is also likely that genetic heterogeneity exists, meaning that specific genes influence susceptibility and pathogenesis in some affected persons but not in others. Results in multiplex families confirm the genetic importance of the MHC region in conferring susceptibility to MS. Susceptibility may be mediated by the class II genes themselves (*DR, DQ*, or both) related to the known function of these molecules in the normal immune response (e.g., antigen binding and presentation, T cell repertoire determination). Data also indicate that although the MHC region plays a significant role in MS susceptibility, much of the genetic effect in MS remains to be explained. Some loci may be involved in the initial pathogenic events, whereas others could influence the development and progression of the disease. Their characterization will help to define the basic etiology of the disease, improve risk assessment, and influence therapeutics.

INTERPLAY OF GENES AND ENVIRONMENTAL FACTORS

Migration studies have been widely used to illustrate potential environmental influences on MS.[21] Children born to parents who have migrated from a high-risk area to a low-risk area for MS appear to have a lower lifetime risk than their parents. Conversely, migration of parents from a low-risk area to a high-risk area may confer a higher risk for MS in the children. Although the interpretation of migration studies has been difficult, in part because of the small number of migrants who develop MS in the individual reports, they have been influential and do suggest the existence of a critical period, between ages 13 and 20 years, for exposure to a putative environmental disease agent. A large number of environmental exposures have been investigated in MS. These include viral and bacterial infections; nutritional and dietary factors; exposure to animals, minerals, or well water; trauma owing to accident or surgery; exposure to chemical agents, metals, or organic solvents; geographical influences; and various occupational hazards.

Reports of clusters or outbreaks of MS, such as those described in the Faroe Islands, although also problematic, underscore the potential role of an infectious agent. Various microbes have been implicated in MS pathogenesis. In the 1920s, spirochetes were claimed to be the cause of MS. This was a reasonable assumption given that syphilis can cause a relapsing/remitting CNS inflammatory disease with synthesis of oligoclonal immunoglobulins in the CSF. Since then, more than 20 infectious agents ranging from retroviruses to mycobacteria have been associated with MS onset or relapses. Viruses are among the most frequently studied and biologically plausible putative infectious agents related to MS pathogenesis, and many have been proposed to be the causative MS agent. One common approach to investigate viral involvement in MS has been to examine serologic titers for specific viruses. Prominent candidates have included measles, rubella, mumps, and the herpesviruses, including Epstein-Barr virus (EBV), herpes simplex virus (HSV) 1 and 2, and varicella zoster virus (VZV). Higher antibody titers against each of these have been detected in the serum and CSF samples of MS patients compared with controls. However, attempts to isolate the causative pathogen have been largely unproductive and have failed to provide major insight into mechanisms of disease susceptibility and pathogenesis. No single infectious agent has proved to have enough specificity and universality to be considered an "MS pathogen."

Climatic factors, such as pollution, solar radiation, temperature, rainfall, and humidity have all been investigated; however, the only consistent effect appears to be due to latitude. MS is, in general, a disease of temperate climates with a population prevalence that decreases with decreasing latitude. High incidence rates are found in Scandinavia, Iceland, and the British Isles (about 1 in 1000). Even within the United States, distinctions exist in the prevalence of MS between populations living north and south of the 37th parallel. MS is uncommon in Japan (2 per 100,000) and other Asian nations, in sub-Saharan Africa, in the Indian sub-continent, and among native populations in Oceania and the Americas. According to some observers, this characteristic geographic distribution implicates in the etiology of MS a pathogen that is not ubiquitously distributed. However, this prevalence pattern can also be explained by the geographic clustering of northern Europeans and their descendants with susceptible genetic profiles. The high occurrence of MS in populations of northern European origin, irrespective of geographic location, and the observation of resistant ethnic groups residing in high-risk regions (e.g., Gypsies in Bulgaria, Japanese in the United States), suggest that the differential risk observed in different population groups results primarily from genetic susceptibility or resistance.

ANIMAL MODELS

EAE (or experimental autoimmune encephalomyelitis) can be induced in a variety of animal species, including nonhuman primates, by immunization with myelin proteins or their peptide derivatives, as well as by adoptive transfer of CD4+ activated cells specific for myelin components. When studied in genetically susceptible animals, immunization induces brain inflammation accompanied by varied signs of neurologic disease, ataxia, and paralysis, first in the tail and hind limbs, then progressing to forelimb paralysis and eventually to death. EAE and MS share common clinical, histologic, immunologic, and genetic features; hence, EAE is widely considered a relevant model of the human disease. The concept of susceptibility versus resistance in EAE is relative rather than absolute, as evidence demonstrates that modifications of the experimental protocol will induce detectable disease in strains previously considered resistant. A second, virally induced animal model for MS uses the Theiler murine virus from the Picorna family of viruses to induce brain inflammation and injury of the myelin sheath. Genetic studies in EAE have been very informative in defining the complex interplay of multiple genes that can result in brain inflammation and demyelination. These studies have also been useful in validating EAE as an MS disease model. The best characterized EAE susceptibility gene resides within the MHC on murine chromosome 17.[22] Induction and full clinical manifestations of EAE are strongly influenced by inherited polymorphisms of MHC class II region genes; certain MHC haplotypes are more permissive for EAE, whereas others are more resistant. The use of classic genetics and whole-genome screening has identified several additional genetic regions that participate in conferring EAE susceptibility, including loci on chromosomes 3, 6, 7, 15, 17 (MHC), 17 (distal to MHC), and X. Other regions, including segments on chromosomes 1 to 5, 7 to 12, and 14 to 18, have been implicated as containing disease-modifying genes. These studies provide compelling evidence for the hypothesis that susceptibility to autoimmune demyelination is in part genetically determined. A multiple-locus model is applicable; each locus may contribute to a specific stage of EAE pathology, although some loci are probably involved in several steps of the autoimmune process.[23] However, no locus seems to be an absolute requirement for the susceptible phenotype (i.e., a susceptible EAE phenotype can be achieved in different crosses by different combinations of genotypes). As the actual roster of genes that contribute to EAE is identified, such genes will represent strong "candidates" for testing in human disease.

THERAPY

Three treatment options for patients with RRMS are approved for use in the United States: (1) IFN-1b (Betaseron), (2) IFN-1a (Avonex), and (3) glatiramer acetate (Copaxone).[24] Each of these treatments is also prescribed for patients with SPMS who experience frequent exacerbations, because this clinical pattern cannot be distinguished reliably from RRMS with incomplete recovery from exacerbations. In phase III clinical trials, recipients of IFN-1b, IFN-1a, and glatiramer acetate experienced approximately 30% fewer clinical exacerbations and significantly fewer new MRI lesions compared with placebo recipients. IFN-1b and IFN-1a also convincingly delayed time to onset of sustained progression of disability. Furthermore, IFN-1a was found to delay the development of clinically definite MS in patients who experienced a single episode of demyelination and had MRI findings indicating prior subclinical disease.

However, none of these reagents has consistently and repeatedly demonstrated a long-term shift in the natural history of MS; a substantial amount of patients are not responders. It is not at all certain how significant the effect and impact on disease progression are and if there are true differences among these three agents. It is also important to note that therapy with IFN-β has been associated with a number of adverse reactions. Frequent side effects include influenza-like symptoms, transient laboratory abnormalities, menstrual disorders, increased spasticity, and dermal reactions. Other possible side effects include autoimmune reactions, capillary leak syndrome, anaphylactic shock, thrombotic-thrombocytopenic purpura, insomnia, headache, alopecia, and depression. In the experimental demyelinating model of MS using the Theiler virus, long-term treatment with type I IFNs actually increased the extent of demyelination. Another distressing occurrence is the presence of neutralizing antibodies (NABs), mainly in IFNβ-1b–treated patients. NAB+ influence in IFN-β therapy is not fully understood. Irrespective of the agent chosen, treatment should probably be discontinued in patients who continue to experience frequent clinical exacerbations or gradual

progression of disability for 6 months. It is unknown whether patients who fail to respond adequately to treatment with any one of these interventions will respond more favorably to another; thus, it is reasonable to try a second agent. The value of combination therapy is also unknown at this time.

IFN-1b and mitoxantrone (Novantrone) were each shown to reduce annual exacerbation rates and MRI activity and delay time to onset of sustained progression of disability in patients with SPMS. No approved therapies for PPMS exist at this time. The results of ongoing trials of IFN-1a, glatiramer acetate, and mitoxantrone in PPMS are awaited. Off-label treatment options for RRMS and SPMS include azathioprine, methotrexate, cyclophosphamide, intravenous immunoglobulin, cladribine, and methylprednisolone. The severity and duration of acute exacerbations are reduced by treatment with glucocorticoids. In one small controlled trial, plasma exchange was effective in some patients with unusually fulminant attacks of demyelination unresponsive to glucocorticoids.

The autoimmune model of MS pathogenesis provides a useful conceptual framework for understanding the mechanisms of action of existing therapies, as well as the failed therapies and the rationale behind drugs currently under development. Beta interferons most likely have pleiotropic effects, including antagonism of IFN-γ mediated MHC upregulation on APCs, altering the profile of cytokine expression to an anti-inflammatory Th2 pattern and blocking migration across endothelia. Glatiramer acetate also affects the cytokine expression pattern and may induce active T cell suppression against MBP and saturate MHC molecules on APC, preventing efficient presentation of autoantigens. Glucocorticoids are also potent inhibitors of antigen presentation function. The chemotherapeutic drug cyclophosphamide is lympholytic and stimulates production of Th2 cytokines. Most experimental therapies focus on interference with antigen presentation to encephalitogenic T cells (altered peptide ligand, intravenous antigen), induction of a Th2 response (oral tolerance), T cell depletion (anti-CD52 or anti-Vβ5), blockade of adhesion molecules (anti-VLA4 antibody), administration of anti-inflammatory cytokines (IL-10, TGF-β), or neutralization of proinflammatory cytokines (type IV phosphodiesterase inhibitors, nerve growth factor, TNFR p55 Ig fusion protein, anti TNF-α IgG1).

Statins that inhibit LFA-1 and block the development of EAE, and antihistamines that engage H1 receptors found in MS brain and can block EAE when given orally, may allow new uses for previously approved drugs. The use of agents that block subtypes of glutamate receptors is a new direction in the development of therapies for stroke and neurodegenerative conditions, and this approach may also prove useful for treatment of the chronic degenerative phase of MS as well. Neuroprotection against glutamate insult was observed by immunizing mice with glatiramer acetate, perhaps as a result of the activation of regulatory T cells. Finally, it is now possible to reverse ongoing paralysis in the EAE model, with vectors encoding regulatory cytokines or inflammatory cytokine inhibitors or by tolerizing the immune system via injection of DNA encoding myelin antigens along with DNA encoding the Th2 cytokine IL-4. DNA vaccination has been taken into the clinic for infectious disease and cancer, and trials are now being organized to apply this approach to autoimmune diseases, including MS. The partial, negligible, or deleterious effects that some of these approaches have demonstrated in the clinic reflect the complex molecular interactions operating in autoimmunity and the limitations of the current working models as a true reflection of MS pathogenesis.

CONCLUSION AND FUTURE DIRECTIONS

Genes play a primary role in determining who is at risk for developing MS, how the disease progresses, and how someone responds to therapy. With the aid of high-capacity technologies, the combined analysis of genomic and transcriptional information will define the full set of genes operating in this disease, providing a reliable conceptual model of pathogenesis, as well as the rationale for novel curative strategies. The use of phenotypic (clinical and paraclinical), epidemiologic, and demographic variables will assume increasing importance as stratifying elements for genetic studies of MS, and to address the fundamental question of genotype-phenotype correlation in autoimmune demyelination. The analysis of non-white patient populations with low and intermediate disease risk, both in their native environment and after migration, will provide important new insights and clues about gene-environment interactions and clinical heterogeneity. These studies will be necessarily linked to the development of novel mathematical formulations designed to identify modest genetic effects, as well as interactions among multiple genes and among genetic, clinical, and environmental factors.

Acknowledgments

The authors are supported by the National Multiple Sclerosis Society, the National Institutes of Health, and the Nancy Davis and Sandler Foundations.

REFERENCES

1. Hauser SL, Goodkin DE: Multiple sclerosis and other demyelinating diseases. In Braunwald E, Fauci AD, Kasper DL, et al (eds): Harrison's Principle of Internal Medicine, 15th ed. New York, McGraw Hill, 2001.

2. Goodkin DE, Rooney WD, Sloan R, et al: A serial study of new MS lesions and the white matter from which they arise. Neurology 1998;51:1689–1697.

3. Genain CP, Cannella B, Hauser SL, Raine CS: Identification of autoantibodies associated with myelin damage in multiple sclerosis. Nature Med 1999;5:170–175.

4. Kornek B, Lassmann H: Axonal pathology in multiple sclerosis: A historical note. Brain Pathol 1999;9:651–656.

5. Trapp BD, Peterson J, Ranshoff RM, et al: Axonal transection in the lesions of multiple sclerosis. N Engl J Med 1998;338:278–285.

6. Lucchinetti C, Bruck W, Parisi J, et al: Heterogeneity of multiple sclerosis lesions: Implications for the pathogenesis of demyelination. Ann Neurol 2000;47:707–717.

7. Leppert D, Ford J, Stabler G, et al: Matrix metalloproteinase-9 (gelatinase B) is selectively elevated in CSF during relapses and stable phases of multiple sclerosis. Brain 1998;121:2327–2334.

8. Sriram S, Rodriguez M: Indictment of the microglia as the villain in multiple sclerosis. Neurology 1997;48:464–470.

9. Ebers GC, Kukay K, Bulman DE, et al: A full genome search in multiple sclerosis. Nature Genet 1996;13:472–476.

10. Multiple Sclerosis Genetics Group: A complete genomic screen for multiple sclerosis underscores a role for the major histocompatibility complex. Nature Genet 1996;13:469–471.

11. Sawcer S, Jones HB, Feakes R, et al: A genome screen in multiple sclerosis reveals susceptibility loci on chromosome 6p21 and 17q22. Nature Genet 1996;13:464–468.

12. Kuokkanen S, Gschwend M, Rioux JD, et al: Genomewide scan of multiple sclerosis in Finnish multiplex families. Am J Hum Genet 1997;61:1379–1387.

13. Oksenberg JR, Baranzini SE, Barcellos LF, Hauser SL: Multiple sclerosis: Genomic rewards. J Neuroimmunol 2001;113:171–184.

14. Multiple Sclerosis Genetics Group: Linkage of the MHC to familial multiple sclerosis suggests genetic heterogeneity. Hum Molec Genet 1998;7:1229–1234.

15. Pericak-Vance MA, Rimmler JB, Martin ER, et al: Linkage and association analysis of chromosome 19q13 in multiple sclerosis. Neurogenetics 2001;3:195–201.

16. Barcellos FL, Oksenberg JR, Green AJ, et al: Genetics basis for clinical expression in multiple sclerosis. Brain 2002;125:150–158.

17. Kira J, Kanai T, Nishimura Y, et al: Western versus Asian types of multiple sclerosis: Immunogenetically and clinically distinct disorders. Ann Neurol 1996;40:569–574.

18. Fusco C, Andreone V, Coppola G, et al: HLA-DRB1*1501 and response to copolymer-1 therapy in relapsing-remitting multiple sclerosis. Neurology 2001;57:1976–1979.

19. Becker KG, Simon RM, Bailey-Wilson JE, et al: Clustering of non-major histocompatibility complex

susceptibility candidate loci in human autoimmune diseases. Proc Natl Acad Sci U S A 1998;95:9979–9984.

20. Jawaheer D, Seldin MF, Amos CI, et al: A genomewide screen in multiplex rheumatoid arthritis families suggests genetic overlap with other autoimmune diseases. Am J Hum Genet 2001;68:927–936.

21. Martyn CN, Gale CR: The epidemiology of multiple sclerosis. Acta Neurol Scand 1997;169:3–7.

22. Encinas JA, Weiner HL, Kuchroo VK: Inheritance of susceptibility to experimental autoimmune encephalomyelitis. J Neurosci Res 1996;45: 655–669.

23. Butterfield RJ, Blankenhorn EP, Roper RJ, et al: Identification of genetic loci controlling the characteristics and severity of brain and spinal cord lesions in experimental allergic encephalomyelitis. Am J Pathol 2000; 157:637–645.

24. Goodin DS, Frohman EM, Garmany GP Jr, et al: Disease modifying therapies in multiple sclerosis: Subcommittee of the American Academy of Neurology and the MS Council for Clinical Practice Guidelines. Neurology 2002;58:169–178.

CHAPTER

40

Peripheral Neuropathies

Steven S. Scherer

Kleopas A. Kleopa

Phillip F. Chance

Merrill D. Benson

The diseases considered in this chapter are listed in Tables 40–1 and 40–2, along with their associated genetic cause and other features. In addition to the topics covered in this chapter, a host of inherited diseases often cause axonal neuropathies. Many of these appear elsewhere in this volume in chapters on mitochondrial diseases, including NARP and multiple symmetric lipomatosis (see Chapter 12), adrenoleukodystrophy (see Chapter 13), Fabry disease (see Chapter 14), some disorders of amino acid and lipid metabolism, including hereditary tyrosinemia type I, maple syrup urine disease, abetalipoproteinemia, analphalipoproteinemia (see Chapter 28), disorders of porphyrin metabolism (see Chapter 30), inherited causes of vitamin E/α-tocopherol or B_{12} deficiency (see Chapter 32), and certain inherited ataxias, including Friedreich ataxia and ataxia telangiectasia (see Chapter 45).Similarly, Refsum's disease (see Chapter 13), metachromatic leukodystrophy, and Krabbe's disease (see Chapter 14) cause demyelinating neuropathy. Finally, inherited axonal neuropathies may be a feature of other rare diseases, such as neuroaxonal dystrophy, in which the genetic causes remain to be determined.

How do such diverse genetic diseases all cause neuropathy? The answers may be equally diverse, and will ultimately provide critical insights into the biology of axons and myelinating Schwann cells.[1,2] The key issues are whether mutations in a given gene have cell autonomous effects, and whether the neuropathy is part of a syndrome. If the expression of an altered gene independent of its expression in neurons causes neuropathy, then it is nonautonomous; this may be particularly common in syndromic diseases. The familial amyloidotic polyneuropathies (FAP) are the examples of this possibil-

ity discussed in this chapter. Most syndromic inherited axonal neuropathies are caused by the effects of mutations in neuronally expressed genes, and all of the syndromic and nonsyndromic inherited demyelinating neuropathies are caused by mutations in genes expressed by myelinating Schwann cells. These generalizations may have exceptions, but provide a robust framework for discussing the cellular and molecular basis of these disorders.

THE BIOLOGY OF MYELINATING SCHWANN CELLS

Myelinating Schwann cells form a specialized sheath around a single axon. In keeping with their unique structure, they express high levels of myelin-related proteins and their cognate mRNAs.[1,3] The maintenance of these features depends on the integrity of axon-Schwann cell interactions. Axonal degeneration leads to Wallerian degeneration, in which previously myelinating Schwann cells dedifferentiate and their myelin sheaths are phagocytosed by macrophages. The expression of myelin-related mRNAs is down-regulated, but if axons regenerate, Schwann cells re-ensheathe them in a manner that is highly reminiscent of development, and re-express high levels of myelin-related mRNAs and proteins. Nearly all myelin-related mRNAs and proteins are affected in this manner, including myelin protein zero (P_0), peripheral myelin protein 22 kD (PMP22), connexin32 (Cx32), myelin-associated glycoprotein (MAG), myelin basic protein (MBP), and periaxin (Prx).

Axons appear to determine whether a Schwann cell will develop a myelinating or nonmyelinating phenotype.[3,4] While the nature of the axonal signal remains to be determined, two unrelated transcription factors,

TABLE 40–1. Nonsyndromic inherited neuropathies

Disease (OMIM)	Locus	Gene	Disease (OMIM)	Locus	Gene
CMT1 (dominant demyelinating)			**Autosomal recessive demyelinating neuropathy (CMT4)**		
HNPP (162500)	17p11	PMP22	CMT4A (214400)	8q13–q21.1	GDAP1
CMT1A (118220)	17p11	PMP22	CMT4B-1 (601382)	11q22	MTMR2
CMT1B (118200)	1q22–23	MPZ/PO	CMT4B-2 (604563)	11p15	
CMT1C (601098)	16p13		CMT4C (601596)	5q32	
CMT1	10q21	EGR2	CMT4D-Lom (601455)	8q24	NDRG1
CMT1X (302800)	Xq13.1	GJB1/Cx32	CMT4E	10q21	EGR2
Intermediate CMT (autosomal dominant)			CMT4F (605260)	19q13	PRX
I-CMT1 (606482)	19p12–13.2		HMSN-R (605285)	10q23.2	
I-CMT2 (606483)	10q24.1–25		**Autosomal recessive axonal neuropathy**		
CMT2 (autosomal dominant axonal/neuronal)			AR-CMT2A (605588)	1q21.2	LMNA
CMT2A (118210)	1p35–36	KIF1Bβ	AR-CMT2B (605589)	19q13.3	
CMT2B (600882)	3q13–22		Early onset (604431)		
CMT2C (606071)			Congenital (no MIM)	5q deletion	
CMT2D (601472)	7p14		**Hereditary sensory and autonomic neuropathies (HSAN)**		
CMT2E (162280)	8p21	NEFL	HSAN-I (dominant) (162400)	9q22.1–22.3	SPTLC1
CMT2F (606595)	7q11–21		HSAN-II (201300)		
CMT2G (604484)	3q13.1		HSAN-III/Riley-Day (recessive) (223900)	9q31	IKBKAP
Severe (dominant or recessive) demyelinating neuropathies			HSAN-IV/CIPA (recessive) (256800)	1q21–q22	TRKA
Dejerine-Sottas	17p11	PMP22	HSAN-V		
Syndrome/HMSN	1p22	MPZ/P0	**Hereditary motor neuropathies (HMN)**		
III/CMT3 (145900)	Xq13.1	GJB1/Cx32	HMN 1 (AD or AR) (182960)		
	10q21	EGR2	HMN 2 (158590)	12q24	
	19q13.1	PRX	HMN 5 (600794)	7p	
Congenital	10q21	EGR2	HMN 7 (158580)	2q14	
hypomyelinating	17p11	PMP22	SMARD1 (604320)	11q13.2–4	IGHMBP2
neuropathy (605253)	1p22	MPZ/P0	HMN-Jerash (605726)	9p21.1–p12	

The neuropathies are classified by MIM, available at http://www.ncbi.nlm.nih.gov/Omim/
References available at http://www.neuro.wustl.edu/neuromuscular/time/hmsn.html and http://molgen www.uia.ac.be/CMTMutations/
DataSource/MutByGene.cfm
See text for abbreviations.

Oct-6 (a POU domain family) and Egr2 (a zinc finger protein), are essential for the normal development of myelinating Schwann cells. Mice lacking either Oct-6 (Oct-6 –/– mice) or Egr2 (Egr2 –/– mice) have drastically reduced numbers of myelinated axons, presumably because myelinating Schwann cells fail to differentiate. There is a surfeit of promyelinating Schwann cells that associate with axons in a 1:1 manner but lack a myelin sheath. These pathologic findings resemble those found in some infants with severe demyelinating neuropathy.

To understand how mutations cause inherited demyelinating neuropathies, consider the structure of myelinated axons.[5] Myelin is a multilamellar spiral of specialized cell membrane that ensheathes axons larger than 1 μm in diameter. By reducing the capacitance and/or increasing the resistance, myelin reduces current flow across the internodal axonal membrane, thereby facilitating saltatory conduction at nodes. Figure 40–1A depicts two internodes; one has been unrolled to reveal its trapezoidal shape. The myelin sheath itself can be divided into two domains—compact and noncompact myelin— each containing a nonoverlapping set of proteins (Fig. 40–1B). Compact myelin forms the bulk of the myelin sheath. It is largely composed of lipids, mainly cholesterol

TABLE 40–2. Syndromic Inherited Neuropathies

Disease (OMIM)	Locus	Gene	Associated features
Demyelinating			
Metachromatic leucodystrophy (250100)	22q13	Arylsulfatase A	optic atrophy, mental retardation
Globoid cell leukodystrophy (Krabbe's disease) (245200)	14q31	Galactosylceramide β-galactosidase	spasticity, optic atrophy, mental retardation
Cockayne's syndrome (216400)	5 loci		dwarfism, hyperpigmentation, optic atrophy, mental retardation
Refsum disease (266500)	10pter-p11.2	Phytanoyl-CoA	deafness, retinitis pigmentosa, ichthyosis, heart failure
	7q21–22	hydroxylase Peroxin-1	infantile (more severe) variant[Au]
Wardeenburg type IV (602229)	22q13	SOX10	CNS and PNS dysmyelination, Hirschsprung disease
Minifascicular neuropathy (605423)	12q12–q13	DHH	mental retardation, hypogonadism
Congenital disorder of glycosylation type Ia	16p13	Phosphomannose isomerase-I	leukodystrophy, abnormal serum glycoproteins, mental retardation, hypotonia, ataxia
(CDG Ia) (212065) merosin-deficiency (156225)	6q22	LAMA2 (Laminin-2)	congenital muscular dystrophy
Deafness and neuropathy (603324)	1p35.1	GJB3/Cx31	hearing loss, chronic skin ulcers
Axonal/neuronal			
FAP-1 and FAP-2 (176300)	18q21–11q23	ATTR	carpal tunnel syndrome (type 2)
FAP-3 ("Iowa" type) (107680)		AApoA1	nephropathy, liver disease
FAP-4 ("Finnish" type) (137350)	9q32–q34	AGel: Gelsolin	corneal lattice dystrophy, cranial neuropathies
NARP (neuropathy, ataxia, retinitis pigmentosa) (551500)	mtDNA mutation 8993	MTATP6 (Complex V-ATPase subunit 6)	ataxia, retinitis pigmentosa, seizures
Multiple symmetric lipomatosis (Madelung syndrome) (151800)	mtDNA	A8344G mutation in mitochondrial tRNA^{lys}	multiple lipomas, hyperuricemia, hyperlipidemia
Adrenoleukodystrophy (300100)	Xq28	ALDP (ATP-binding transporter)	spastic paraparesis, adrenal insufficiency
Fabry disease (301500)	Xq22	α-galactosidase	angiokeratoma, neuropathy, renal failure, cardiomyopathy
Hereditary tyrosinemia type 1 (276700)	15q23–q25	Fumaryl-acetoacetase	hepatic and renal disease, cardiomyopathy
Maple syrup urine disease (248611)	6q22–p21	BCKDHB	intermittent seizures, drowsiness, ataxia
Abetalipoproteinemia (200100)	4q24	MTP (microsomal triglyceride transfer protein)	ataxia, acanthocytosis
Analphalipoproteinemia (205400)	9q31	ABC1 (ATP-binding cassette transporter)	orange tonsils, organomegaly
Acute intermittent porphyria (176000)	11q23.3	Porphobilinogen deaminase	abdominal pain, psychosis, depression, dementia, seizures

(Continued)

TABLE 40–2. (Continued)

Disease (OMIM)	Locus	Gene	Associated features
Coproporphyria (121300)	3q12	Coproporphyrinogen 3 oxidase	skin photosensitivity
Variegate porphyria (176200)	1q22	Protoporphyrinogen oxidase	skin photosensitivity (mainly in South Africa—founder effect)
AVED (Ataxia with selective vitamin E deficiency) (277460)	8q13.1–q13.3	ATTP (a-tocopherol transfer protein) (ATTP)	Similar to Friedreich ataxia, tendon xanthomas, retinitis pigmentosa
Friedreich ataxia, FRDA-1 (229300)	9q13–21.1	Frataxin	ataxia, cardiomyopathy (types 1 and 2 cannot be distinguished clinically)
FRDA-2 (601992)	9p23–p11		
Ataxia telangectasia (208900)	11q22–q23	ATM	ataxia, telangectasias, immune deficiency, endocrinopathy
SCA1 (neuropathy in 40%) (164400)	6p23	Ataxin-1 (CAG expansion)	ataxia, gaze paresis, slow/absent saccades, spasticity
SCA2 (neuropathy in 80%) (183090)	12q24.1	Ataxin-2 (CAG expansion)	ataxia, slow saccades, tremor, myoclonus
SCA3 (neuropathy in 50%) (109150)	14q32.1	Ataxin-3 (CAG expansion)	ataxia, gaze paresis, extrapyramidal, bulging eyes
DRPLA (125370)	12p13.31	DRPLA protein	myoclonus epilepsy, ataxia, chorea, dementia
Giant axonal neuropathy (256850)	16q24	Gigaxonin	mental retardation, spasticity, kinky or curly hair
Andermann's syndrome (218000)	15q13–15		seizures, malformed corpus callosum, mental retardation
Cowchock's syndrome (310490)	Xq24–26		mental retardation (60%), deafness
Infantile neuroaxonal dystrophy (256600)			seizures, dystonia, ataxia, deafness, mutilation
Hereditary neuralgic amyotrophy (HNA) (162100)	17q25		painful episodes of brachial palsy, dysmorphic features
HSMN V (600361)			spastic paraparesis
Congenital sensory and autonomic neuropathy and neurotrophic keratitis—Navajo (256810)			corneal opacification, liver disease, acromutilation, death by 10 years of age
Congenital cataracts, α dysmorphism neuropathy (CCFDN) (604168)	18q23-qter		cataracts, microcornea, facial dysmorphism, skeletal deformities

and sphingolipids, including galactocerebroside and sulfatide. Noncompact myelin is found in the paranodes and incisures. Because mutations in the genes encoding P_0 (MPZ), PMP22 (PMP22), and Cx32 (GJB1) are the most common cause of Charcot-Marie-Tooth disease (CMT1), we will review their biology in this chapter.

P_0 is the most abundant protein in compact myelin. It has a cytoplasmic C-terminus, a transmembrane domain, and an extracellular domain that is similar to an immunoglobulin variable chain, including a disulfide bond. Like other members of the immunoglobulin gene superfamily, P_0 is a cell adhesion molecule. Its crystal structure reveals that P_0 forms tetramer that bind other tetramers both in cis (in the plane of the membrane) and in trans (on the apposed membrane), thereby holding together the extracellular surfaces of the myelin sheath. The positively charged cytoplasmic tail of P_0 likely interacts with the negatively charged phospholipids of the membrane, thereby augmenting the role of MBP in holding together the apposed cytoplasmic surfaces of the membranes. The analysis of mice lacking P_0 (Mpz –/– mice) confirms the importance of P_0, as Schwann cells form a multilamellar spiral of membrane around axons, but the myelin does not compact properly. Mpz-heterozygous (+/–) mice develop a late-onset demyelinating neuropathy, indicating that reducing the amount of P_0 by 50% destabilizes compact myelin.[6]

PMP22 is a small (160 amino acids) intrinsic membrane protein of uncertain function. A structural role seems

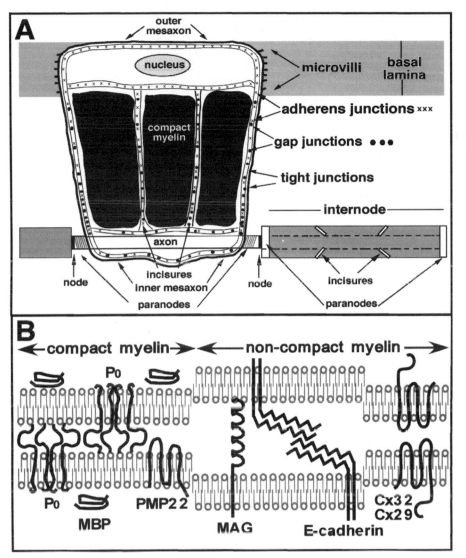

FIGURE 40–1. The architecture of the myelinated axon in the PNS. *A*, One Schwann cell has been "unrolled" to reveal the regions forming compact myelin, as well as paranodes and incisures, regions of noncompact myelin. *B*, P_0, PMP22, and MBP are found in compact myelin, whereas Cx29, Cx32, MAG, and E-cadherin are localized in noncompact myelin.

likely, as PMP22 forms dimers and may interact with P_0. Mice lacking one (*Pmp22* +/– mice) or both (*Pmp22* –/– mice) Pmp22 genes develop a mild or a severe demyelinating neuropathy, respectively.[6] Thus, the correct amount of P_0 and PMP22 in compact myelin is critical, indicating that perturbations in any one component can alter the stability of the whole membrane. Trembler and TremblerJ mice have different missense mutations in PMP22 (Asp150Gly and Leu16Pro, respectively), both of which correspond to human mutations. The key lesson from Trembler mice and their human counterparts is that a missense mutation in one *PMP22* gene causes a much more severe demyelinating neuropathy than does the absence of one copy of the *PMP22* gene. These missense mutations must, therefore, have additional, deleterious effects.

As depicted in Figure 40–1, gap junction-like plaques have been found between tight junction strands in non-compact myelin. Myelinating Schwann cells express Cx32, which belongs to a family of about 20 highly homologous proteins, the connexins. Six connexins form a hemi-channel, and two apposed hemi-channels form a functional channel. Gap junctions mediate the diffusion of ions and small molecules between adjacent cells, but in the myelin sheath they allow diffusion between the layers of the same cell. Such a radial pathway—directly across the layers of the myelin sheath—would be advantageous, as it provides a much shorter pathway (up to 1000-fold) than a circumferential route. Disruption of this radial pathway may be the reason that *GJB1/Gjb1* mutations cause demyelination in humans and in mice. However, the diffusion of small molecules in *Gjb1* –/– mice did not appear to be different than in wild-type mice, implying that another connexin also forms functional gap junctions in myelin sheaths. At least in rodents, this is likely to be Cx29.[7]

CLASSIFYING INHERITED NEUROPATHIES

Inherited neuropathies have been recognized since the late 1800s, when Charcot, Marie, Tooth, Herringham, Dejerine, and Sottas described various forms.[8–11] With an estimated prevalence of 1:2500 persons having a form of CMT, it is collectively one of the most common kinds of neurogenetic diseases.

The classical features of CMT arise from length-dependent axonal loss. The onset is insidious and the rate of progression is slow. Patients most commonly present with signs and symptoms related to weakness, more often involving the lower legs and feet, later progressing to affect the hands and forearms. When weakness is present, a history of abnormal (steppage) gait as well as tripping and falling is frequently elicited. Patients may also present because of foot deformities (pes cavus or hammer toes), which results from weakness of intrinsic foot muscles; more severely affected patients may also have "claw hand" deformities owing to weakness of intrinsic hand muscles. Despite the involvement of the sensory nerves in CMT, patients may not report the presence of limb pain or sensory disturbances. The neurologic findings mainly depend on the severity of the neuropathy. Motor and sensory nerve function are typically symmetrically affected in a length-dependent manner, with distal muscle weakness and atrophy, impaired sensation (particularly "large-fiber" modalities), and diminished or absent deep-tendon reflexes. It has long been recognized that clinical examination alone cannot reliably classify all patients.

The pioneering work of Dyck et al[8] subdivided CMT/hereditary motor and sensory neuropathy (HMSN) according to clinical, electrophysiologic, and histologic features. CMT1/HMSN-I is more common and is characterized by an earlier age of onset (first or second decade of life), nerve conduction velocities (NCVs) less than 38 m/s in upper-limb nerves, and segmental demyelination and remyelination with onion bulb formations in nerve biopsies. CMT2/HMSN-II has a later onset, NCVs greater than 38 m/s, and biopsies mainly show a loss of myelinated axons.

The terms Dejerine-Sottas syndrome (DSS) and HMSN-III have been used to describe children who have a severe neuropathy.[8–11] They have delayed motor development before age 3 years, sometimes extending to infancy. Their motor abilities typically improve during the first decade, followed by progressive weakness to the point that many affected individuals use wheelchairs. Ventilatory failure, presumably caused by phrenic nerve involvement, can occur, even during infancy or childhood. Kyphoscoliosis, short stature, and foot deformities are common in older children. Sensory loss is profound, especially for modalities subserved by myelinated axons, to the point that some children have a severe sensory ataxia. Tendon reflexes are absent. Occasional patients have cranial nerve involvement: miosis, reduced pupillary responses to light, ptosis, facial weakness, nystagmus, and hearing loss. CSF protein may be elevated, and nerve roots may be enhanced by MRI. NCVs are very slow (<10 m/s), with marked temporal dispersion but no conduction block. Nerves are often enlarged, and biopsies reveal a complete absence of axons with normal/thick myelin sheaths. The remaining myelinated axons have inappropriately thin myelin sheaths for the axonal caliber. Onion bulbs are prominent, composed of Schwann cell processes or just their basal laminae. While these clinical, electrophysiologic, and pathologic features distinguish DSS from CMT1, the literature contains many examples of patients who are said to have CMT (often "severe CMT") who could have just as readily been labeled DSS. New dominant mutations in MPZ, PMP22, and EGR2 are the most common causes, but homozygous mutations of MPZ, PMP22, EGR2, or other genes also cause DSS (see Table 40–1). Thus, while DSS is still a meaningful label of a clinical phenotype, its lack of specificity makes it problematic in genetic classifications.

Congenital hypomyelinating neuropathy (CHN) is a term that should be reserved for infants who have hypotonic weakness at birth caused by a severe neuropathy. These infants may even have arthrogryposis caused by a prenatal onset, and swallowing or respiratory difficulties may result in death during infancy or later. NCVs are severely reduced (<5 m/s), and biopsies show similar features as described for DSS. Owing to their overlapping clinical and pathologic features, CHN appears to be a more severe subtype of DSS, consistent with the finding that MPZ, PMP22, and EGR2 mutations can cause CHN or DSS. It is possible that the most severe cases of CHN, associated with arthrogryposis, have different genetic causes, as no MPZ, PMP22, or EGR2 mutations have been shown to cause this phenotype.

PROBLEMS OF CLASSIFICATION

There are several problems in this regard. Neuropathies that are overshadowed by other manifestations of a syndrome are usually not classified with nonsyndromic neuropathies, but in neuralgic amyotrophy and some kinds of inherited amyloidosis the neuropathy predominates. Conversely, at least one form of CMT (CMT4D) appears to be syndromic. Moreover, many advances in our understanding of the molecular basis of inherited neuropathies are difficult to reconcile with the older classification schemes that were well entrenched prior to these discoveries. Older schemes take into account the severity of the clinical phenotypes and even associated stigmata, but do not readily accommodate the diversity of phenotypes caused by different mutations of the same gene or the diversity of genes that can cause the same phenotype. After genetic heterogeneity was discovered by linkage studies, CMT1 was subdivided into CMT1A (chromosome 17), CMT1B (chromosome 1), CMT1X (X chromosome), and CMT1C (chromosome unknown). However, as more loci were discovered, they were not named according to this scheme. For example, individuals with a "CMT1-like phenotype" caused by mutations in EGR2 were not designated CMT1D. The discoveries of more severe phenotypes (DSS) or even milder phenotypes (hereditary neuropathy with liability to pressure palsies; HNPP) caused by mutations in the same genes that cause CMT1 (discussed later), is more problematic. If linkage alone is the criterion, then these individuals should be named according to their linkage to the affected gene, and not according to their phenotypes.

Whether a peripheral neuropathy is axonal or demyelinating is also important. In an axonal neuropathy, the axon (or even the neuron) suffers the primary injury; if myelin sheaths degenerate subsequent to an axonal injury, this is Wallerian degeneration and not demyelination. In contrast, in a demyelinating neuropathy, the myelinating Schwann cells are affected first; even though axons may degenerate subsequent to demyelination, the neuropathy should still be considered as demyelinating. For a variety of reasons, this fundamental concept is frequently misrepresented or even misunderstood. Demyelination invariably causes axonal loss for reasons that are not well understood, and axonal neuropathies can result in secondary demyelination. Further, in a clinical setting, it is often difficult, even impossible, to determine whether a given neuropathy is a primary demyelinating or a primary axonal neuropathy.

Using forearm conduction velocities (greater or less than 38 m/s) for determining whether an inherited neuropathy is demyelinating or axonal has turned out to be inadequate. When this idea was first promulgated, it was a heuristic criterion, as it facilitated the separation of CMT1 and CMT2. It was based on a large number of genetically heterogeneous CMT1 patients whose median motor NCVs ranged from normal to very low. The distribution appeared bimodal, with one peak around 20 m/s (corresponding to CMT1), and another between 40 and 60 m/s (corresponding to CMT2). Although the two groups overlapped, they appeared to intersect at 38 m/s. This imperfect distinction between CMT1 and CMT2 has been useful in the clinical setting, but an uncritical adherence to this criterion has contributed to the misconception that some demyelinating neuropathies are axonal, exemplified by CMT1X. To decide whether demyelination is "primary" or "secondary," we advocate a biologically based analysis, which can be done in genetically authentic animal models. This approach indicates that demyelination is the first manifestation of inherited demyelinating neuropathy.[6]

We have organized our discussion of inherited demyelinating neuropathies according to the genes that cause them. For each gene, we discuss the phenotypic consequences of different mutations. The original references regarding these mutations are available at http://molgenwww.uia.ac.be/CMTMutations/Data Source/MutByGene.cfm

PMP22 DELETIONS CAUSE HNPP

Deletion and duplication of *PMP22* causes HNPP and CMT1A, respectively, establishing a singular genetic mechanism as the cause of the two most common inherited neuropathies.[8-11] Two homologous DNA sequences flanking the PMP22 gene are the molecular basis for its deletion/duplication; their high degree of homology promotes unequal crossing over during meiosis, which simultaneously generates a duplicated and a deleted allele. These homologous regions are found in humans and chimpanzees, so that deletions/duplications have arisen many times during human evolution. When *de novo* deletions and duplications occur, they usually originate in the father. Because most cases of HNPP and CMT1A are inherited from an affected parent, their high prevalence in various ethnic groups indicates that they do not seriously affect reproductive fitness. For example, the prevalence of HNPP in a Finnish population was 16:100,000, likely underestimated because many affected individuals are asymptomatic.

Episodic mononeuropathies at typical sites of nerve compression are the hallmark of HNPP. In order of frequency, they occur in the peroneal nerve at the fibular head, the ulnar nerve at the elbow, the brachial plexus, the radial nerve at the spiral groove, and the median nerve at the wrist. Other nerves may be affected, and atypical presentations have been described. Over half of the patients recover completely, usually within days to months, but deficits may persist. Some patients with HNPP develop a progressive generalized sensory-motor neuropathy, with or without episodes of pressure palsies. Thus, ankle jerks may be absent in over one third of the patients, and 12.5% are areflexic.

During the acute episodes of pressure palsies, electrophysiologic studies may show conduction block. In addition to focal changes at common sites of nerve entrapment, genetically affected individuals with or without episodes of pressure palsies have a mild, sensory-motor polyneuropathy. Sensory velocities and distal latencies are diffusely slowed, especially in the upper extremities. Motor NCVs are minimally slowed, but distal motor latencies are consistently prolonged. Biopsies of unpalsied nerves show focal thickenings (tomaculae) caused by folding of the myelin sheath, as well as segmental demyelination and remyelination. Although it is plausible that severe focal demyelination (causing conduction block) followed by remyelination (restoring conduction) are the cellular alterations associated with the focal neuropathies, this remains to be directly demonstrated.

HNPP is usually caused by deletion of one copy of *PMP22*, but 7 different *PMP22* mutations also cause this phenotype. These mutations, unlike most *PMP22* mutations, mainly cause a simple loss of function. How reduced gene dosage affects myelinating Schwann cells is not known, but there is less *PMP22* mRNA in peripheral nerves from HNPP patients, and PMP22 protein is reduced in the compact myelin from individuals with HNPP. *Pmp22* +/− mice, an animal model of HNPP, also develop a demyelinating neuropathy with many features of HNPP.[6]

PMP22 DUPLICATIONS CAUSE CMT1A

CMT1A, by definition, is CMT1 linked to chromosome 17, and is almost always associated with the 17p11.2

duplication, which includes the *PMP22* gene.[8–11] In one large series,[12] the age at onset ranged from 2 to 76 years, but most patients were affected by the end of the second decade. Weakness, atrophy, and sensory loss in the lower limbs, foot deformities, and areflexia were invariably present. At a mean age of 40 years, functional disability was mild or absent in 35% of the patients, 25% were asymptomatic, 61% had difficulty walking or running but were still independent, and only one patient (less than 1%) required a wheelchair. There is considerable variability in the degree of neurologic deficits within families, and even between identical twins, indicating that stochastic and environmental factors modulate the severity.

In CMT1A patients with duplications, NCVs are abnormally slowed, ranging from 5 to 35 m/s in forearm motor nerves, but most average around 20 m/s.[12] The lack of conduction block or temporal dispersion and the high correlation between the motor NCVs in different nerves are all hallmarks. NCVs are slow in children, even well before the clinical onset of disease. In individual patients, motor NCVs (nerve conduction velocity) do not change significantly even over two decades, whereas the motor amplitudes decrease in most patients, albeit slowly. Conduction velocities, like clinical disability, vary widely within families, but an early age at onset and greatly reduced median NCV are associated with a more severe course. Nevertheless, motor amplitudes and the number of motor units correlate with clinical disability, indicating that axonal loss and not conduction velocity per se, causes weakness.

The pathologic findings in nerve biopsies from CMT1A patients with duplications evolve during the disease. Demyelination is more prevalent in children, and "hypomyelinated" axons (remyelinated axons with myelin sheaths that are inappropriately thin for the axonal caliber) become relatively more numerous with age. Although the data were generated before genetic testing was possible, age-related axonal loss is a feature of CMT1.

How the duplication of *PMP22* causes demyelination is not settled.[2] The amount of *PMP22* protein in compact myelin appears to be increased, which could destabilize the myelin sheath. An alternative view is that the overexpression of *PMP22* results in demyelination because *PMP22* acts like a growth-arrest gene in Schwann cells. Overexpressing *PMP22* in myelinating Schwann cells of rodents leads to dose-dependent alterations in myelination, with nearly complete failure to myelinate in the highest expressing lines.

PMP22 MUTATIONS CAUSE DSS, CMT1A, OR HNPP

Besides gene duplications and deletions, over 40 different *PMP22* mutations have been identified. These mutations cause amino acid substitutions (missense mutations), premature stop (nonsense mutations), or frameshifts. The available clinical information suggests that seven of these mutations cause HNPP, six cause CMT1, four cause "severe CMT" (many of these could have equally well been called DSS), 17 cause DSS, and four are recessive or possible polymorphisms. Except for patients with the HNPP phenotype, most patients with *PMP22* point mutations, including those with a CMT1 phenotype, are more severely affected than those harboring the duplication. They typically have an earlier age of onset, a more severe phenotype at any given age, more slowing of NCVs, and distinctive pathologic changes in biopsies.

Individuals who are heterozygous for one of three *PMP22* mutations, Thr118Met, Arg157Trp, and Arg157Gly, have no discernible phenotype. Homozygosity of Arg157Trp, however, causes DSS. Further, individuals who are compound heterozygotes—possessing a *PMP22* deletion and either a Thr118Met or an Arg157Gly mutation—have a CMT1 phenotype. Thus, demyelination occurs only when these mutant proteins are not combined with wild-type *PMP22*, a situation that has been termed a *recessive gain of function*.[10]

PMP22 mutations causing phenotypes that are more severe than HNPP are not simply null alleles; they have gain of function/toxic effects. The mutant *PMP22* proteins analyzed to date are retained in the endoplasmic reticulum (ER), and do not reach the compact myelin. Interestingly, one of the "recessive" mutations, Thr118 Met, reaches the cell membrane in transfected cells, although not as efficiently as wild-type *PMP22*. In nerve biopsies from patients with *PMP22* point mutations, *PMP22* accumulates in the ER and Golgi. Abnormal trafficking of mutant *PMP22* point mutations was previously demonstrated in myelinating Schwann cells of Trembler and TremblerJ mice, whose human counterparts have DSS and severe CMT, respectively. *PMP22* dimerizes, and mutant *PMP22* may interact abnormally with its wild-type counterpart, forming aggregates that accumulate in the ER, possibly triggering an ER "stress response."

MPZ MUTATIONS CAUSE DSS, CMT1B, OR A CMT2-LIKE PHENOTYPE

Many different *MPZ* mutations have been identified, including missense, nonsense, and frameshift mutations. Of the 83 reported mutations, 37 cause CMT1, 22 cause "severe CMT," 13 cause DSS, 8 cause a CMT2-like phenotype, 2 are recessive or possible polymorphisms, and 1 causes an HNPP-like phenotype. Moreover, the phenotypes of patients labeled CMT1 range from mildly affected individuals to patients who could be called DSS.

How can one make sense of so many mutations and diversity of phenotypes they cause? The lesson from *PMP22* mutations is to compare the effects of *MPZ* mutations to a null allele. Deletion of one MPZ gene in humans has not been described, but the comparable mutation in mice causes a late-onset, demyelinating neuropathy (discussed previously). The Val102 frameshift mutation, however, may be comparable to a *MPZ* deletion, as the protein would not function as a cell adhesion molecule because it lacks its transmembrane domain. It was discovered in two siblings with DSS (who were both homozygous for this mutation), but their heterozygous parents and grandparents were asymptomatic, had normal sensory and motor amplitudes, and only mild NCV slowing (for example, the median motor NCVs ranged from 35 to 42m/s). Thus, given the mild phenotypes of *MPZ* mutations with loss of function, mutations that cause DSS, severe CMT, or even CMT, must have a toxic gain of function.

There are other mildly affected kindreds. Four siblings in their fifties were found to have the Ile99Thr mutation only after one appeared to develop chronic inflammatory demyelinating polyneuropathy. The other three siblings had mildly reduced or normal NCVs; one had a nerve biopsy that showed some thinly myelinated axons as well as clusters of regenerated axons. Kindreds with the Asp35Tyr, Ser51Phe, Phe64del, or Glu71stop also appear to have milder neuropathies than typical CMT1B kindreds; the patient with the Glu71stop mutation has an HNPP-like phenotype.

A few *MPZ* mutations cause a CMT2-like phenotype. The best example is the Ser44Phe mutation, as clinically affected individuals have little or no slowing of NCVs despite significant axonal loss. In contrast, clinically affected individuals with the Thr124Met mutation have median/ulnar motor NCVs that range from "intermediate" slowing (25 to 40 m/s) to normal, whereas those in younger/clinically unaffected individuals tend be normal. As in CMT1X patients (discussed later), the NCVs appear to be nonuniformly slowed, and nerve biopsies show some thinly myelinated axons as well as clusters of regenerated axons. In spite of a late onset, many patients progress relatively rapidly to the point of using a wheelchair. In addition, abnormally reactive pupils (often the first clinical finding), dysphagia, positive sensory phenomena (including painful lacerations), and hearing loss are common. One family with the Glu97Val mutation has a comparable phenotype, with a late onset progressive neuropathy associated with hearing loss and pupillary abnormalities. Two clinically affected individuals had intermediate slowing of their median motor NCVs (29 to 30 m/s), whereas a clinically unaffected boy had a nearly normal NCV (45 m/s). Patients with the Asp75Val mutation have a late-onset neuropathy associated with hearing loss and pupillary abnormalities, and relatively normal motor NCVs; it was not stated whether their weakness progressed rapidly. Patients with Asp61Gly or Tyr119Cys mutations have an adult-onset neuropathy (but without hearing loss or pupillary abnormalities). Their NCVs were mildly slowed (median motor NCVs 39 to 43 m/s), and their biopsies showed decreased numbers of myelinated axons and clusters of regenerated axons. Finally, a Gln141stop mutation was found in two children (11 and 16 years old) who had a mild CMT phenotype and little if any slowing of motor NCVs. In sum, a few *MPZ* mutations cause mild demyelinating neuropathy (Asp35Tyr, Ser51Phe, Phe64del, Glu71stop, Val102frameshift), some cause late-onset neuropathy that does not progress (Asp61Gly, Ile99Thr, Tyr119Cys), and others cause a complicated phenotype with rapid progression, hearing loss, and/or pupillary abnormalities (Asp75Val, Glu97Val, Thr124Met). Ser44Phe and Gln141stop are the only mutations for which there is scant evidence for demyelination.

The range in clinical severity and the large number of *MPZ* mutations gives the appearance of a continuum, so that comparisons are tenuous. At best, the clinical findings can be correlated with the clinical electrophysiology and nerve biopsy findings. DSS patients cannot be separated from patients with DSS caused by mutations in other genes. Patients with "severe CMT1" overlap those with DSS in terms of clinical onset (often before age 3); clinical electrophysiology (forearm motor responses 8 to 15 m/s; advanced distal muscle atrophy; absent sensory responses); and biopsy findings (severe loss of myelinated fibers, hypertrophic changes, and onion bulbs). Most *MPZ* mutations appear to cause a CMT1 phenotype that is more like the one caused by *PMP22* missense mutations than by *PMP22* duplications; in the former, the age of onset is younger, atrophy appears earlier and extends to proximal muscles, and NCVs are slower (typically 10 to 20 m/s).

The report of Bird et al[13] on a large family with a Lys96Glu mutation is particularly instructive. The youngest members were all affected before age 10 years, several before age 3 years. Delayed walking and clumsy running were common early symptoms; absent tendon reflexes followed by distal weakness and atrophy were early clinical findings. Proximal weakness and atrophy developed over time, and motor impairment outweighed sensory findings in most patients. The disease was insidiously progressive but did not affect longevity. The median and ulnar motor NCVs ranged from 6 to 15 m/s, changing little over time, except that distal motor responses became unobtainable, presumably due to the loss of motor axons. An autopsy of a 92-year-old affected woman revealed degeneration of fasciculus gracilis, which is consistent with severe axonal/neuronal loss caused by demyelination. In this family, which we consider to be an example of "severe CMT1," there was some variability in age of onset and disease severity at any given age, but the variability seems less than what has been described for CMT1A caused by *PMP22* duplications.

Nerve biopsies have revealed some possible clues. Uncompacted myelin has been reported with the Ser63del, Glu71stop, Arg98Cys, Arg98His, and Cys127Tyr mutations; other mutations have abnormally folded myelin sheaths (Val32Phe, Asp61Asn, Ile62Phe, Ser78Leu, Asp90Glu, Lys96Glu, Asp109Asn, Lys130Arg,

Asn131Lys, Ile135Leu). All of these mutations are localized in the extracellular domain, which mediates adhesion, but the phenotypes associated with both uncompacted myelin and abnormally folded myelin sheaths range from DSS to mild CMT. Perhaps these histologic abnormalities reflect different disturbances in the way P_0 is assembled into tetramers, and/or the way these tetramers interact in *cis* and *trans* to maintain the structure of the myelin sheath.

How do different *MPZ* mutations result in such different phenotypes? The possibility that P_0 mutants have diminished adhesion has been evaluated in transfected cells. Disrupting the disulfide bond, truncating the cytoplasmic domain, abolishing N-linked glycosylation, or phosphorylation of an intracellular serine all reduced adhesion, sometimes even of a coexpressed wild type *MPZ* allele (a dominant-negative effect). Because all these *MPZ* mutations affect adhesion, it is hard to relate the diverse range of phenotypes to adhesion alone. One suspects that some of these mutations have other important effects, such as on the trafficking. In two cases, the nature of the mutation probably plays a key role. The Ser54Pro mutation, for example, results in a milder (CMT1B) phenotype than the Ser54Cys mutation (which causes DSS). Similarly, the Arg98Pro, Arg98His, and Arg98Ser mutations all cause CMT1B, while the Arg98Cys causes severe CMT/DSS. The substitution by cysteine generates a thiol group, which could act in a dominant manner by forming aberrant disulfide bonds.

GJB1 MUTATIONS CAUSE CMT1X

Shortly after the initial reports of autosomal dominant kindreds of CMT, Herringham reported a family in which only the males had peripheral neuropathy, many years before Morgan's description of X-linked inheritance. Although long under-recognized, CMT1X is the second most common form of CMT1.[8-11] It is considered to be an X-linked dominant trait because it affects female carriers; their clinical involvement varies, likely owing to the proportion of myelinating Schwann cells that inactivate the X chromosome carrying the mutant *GJB1* allele. Affected women usually have a later onset (after the end of the second decade) and a milder version of the same phenotype. In affected males, the clinical onset is between 5 and 20 years. The initial symptoms include difficulty running and frequent ankle sprains; foot drop and sensory loss in the legs develop later. Depending on the tempo of the disease, the distal weakness may progress to involve the gastrocnemius and soleus muscles, even to the point where assistive devices are required for ambulation. Weakness, atrophy, and sensory loss also develop in the hands, particularly in thenar muscles. These clinical manifestations are the result of a chronic, length-dependent neuropathy, and are nearly indistinguishable from those seen in patients with CMT1A. Atrophy, however, particularly of intrinsic hand muscles, positive sensory phe-

nomena, and sensory loss, may be more prominent in CMT1X patients.

Besides the pattern of inheritance, the degree of NCV slowing helps to distinguish CMT1A/B from CMT1X. In affected men, the motor NCVs in the arms show "intermediate" slowing (25 to 40 m/s), which is faster than in typical CMT1A (10 to 30 m/s) but slower than normal (>50 m/s). Some degree of slowing is usually found in female carriers, even asymptomatic ones. As compared to CMT1A, CMT1X patients have more heterogeneous NCVs and more distal axonal loss. The overlap in motor NCVs in CMT1X and CMT2 (discussed later) has led to the erroneous conclusion that *GJB1* mutations can cause CMT2. In all of these cases, however, CMT1X should have been considered, as there was no male-to-male transmission, and the motor NCVs of affected male patients showed intermediate slowing. Nerve biopsies from CMT1X patients show less demyelination and remyelination and more axonal degeneration and regeneration than do those from CMT1A/B patients.

CMT1X is caused by mutations in *GJB1*, the gene that encodes Cx32. An amazing number (more than 240) and variety of mutations have been identified, affecting every domain of the Cx32 protein, the promoter and 3' untranslated region, as well as deletions of the entire gene. The 265–273 deletion and Phe235Cys cause DSS, and several mutations (Arg22stop, Arg22Gln, Val163Ile, 147frameshift) appear to cause a more severe form of CMT1X than typical mutations. Perhaps these mutations have toxic or dominant-negative effects that transcend a simple loss of function. The Asn175Asp and Thr191Ala mutations are associated with a mild phenotype. It remains to be determined whether there is a genotype-phenotype correlation in CMT1X, as most of the kindreds that have been associated with either mild or severe phenotypes are too small. Genotype-phenotype correlations are one of the key issues that will be addressed by analyzing the "CMT database" that has been initiated by Dr. Michael Shy at Wayne State University in collaboration with Indiana University.

Other associated manifestations of CMT1X have been reported. Hearing loss has been found, but only in one of three families with the Arg142Gln mutation. Most patients have electrophysiologic evidence of slowed CNS conduction, but few have been reported to have clinical findings (such as extensor plantar responses; abnormal MRIs) that indicate CNS involvement.

How different *GJB1* mutations cause CMT1X has been analyzed by expressing the mutant proteins in heterologous cells. Most mutants do not form functional gap junctions, indicating the importance of each amino acid in the function of this large but highly conserved gene family. In mammalian cells, most mutants that fail to reach the cell membrane accumulate in the ER or Golgi apparatus and are degraded via endosomal and proteosomal pathways. The Phe235Cys mutation appears to have novel electrophysiologic characteristics; these may cause a more severe phenotype.

EGR2 MUTATIONS CAUSE CMT1 OR DSS

One recessive and 6 dominant *EGR2* mutations have been described. *EGR2* is a transcription factor expressed by myelinating Schwann cells, and *EGR2* mutants likely affect the expression of myelin-related genes.[4] Mutations affecting the zinc finger domain impair DNA binding, and the amount of residual binding directly correlates with disease severity. An R1 domain mutation prevents interaction of *EGR2* with the NAB corepressors and thereby increases transcriptional activity.

NEURONS AND AXONAL NEUROPATHIES

The PNS consists of the neurons whose axons are found outside of the CNS, as well as their associated receptor cells and glial cells. These include the motor, sensory, sympathetic, parasympathetic, and enteric neurons and their axons, as well as most of the special senses. Even though these neurons serve diverse functions, their shared molecular characteristics join them in certain genetic diseases. For example, the relevant sensory and autonomic neurons are absent in individuals with congenital insensitivity to pain with anhidrosis (CIPA; HSAN-IV) because of mutations in the gene encoding the TrkA receptor.[14] TrkA binds nerve growth factor (NGF), which is required for the survival of these neurons during their early development. Similarly, a shared molecular defect affecting different neurons may explain why hearing loss, mental retardation, and/or retinitis pigmentosa are associated with certain inherited neuropathies.

In most neuropathies, the clinical features tend to have a distal predilection, both in terms of first appearance and in ultimate severity. This suggests that axonal length is a factor in determining which neural elements are at risk, but distal distribution does not mean that the defect necessarily lies in the axon. It could just as well represent a primary neuron cell body abnormality. For instance, large doses of pyridoxine promptly kill large primary sensory neurons, whereas smaller doses cause only subtle shrinkage of these neurons and indolent, distal axonal degeneration. Thus, a modest neuronal abnormality may result in distal axonopathy, but a more severe insult of the same type may cause the neuron itself to degenerate as the primary event. The neuropathologic appearance of some inherited axonal neuropathies consists of primary nerve cell body degeneration with secondary anterograde degeneration of the axons. Many inherited axonal neuropathies could be considered as primary neuronopathies (see Chapter 23) rather than primary axonopathies, but it is not yet possible to make this distinction.

It is commonly supposed that the selective vulnerability of PNS neurons that leads to neuropathy is the length of the axons themselves, which are the longest cells in the body. Axons have a prominent cytoskeleton composed of intermediate filaments and microtubules. Neurofilaments are the main neuronal intermediate filament and are composed of three subunits, termed heavy, medium, and light. Dominant mutations in NEFL, the gene encoding the light subunit, cause an axonal neuropathy (CMT2E). Further, recessive mutations in the gigaxonin gene, which encodes a protein that likely interacts with cytoskeleton proteins, cause giant axonal neuropathy. Because axons synthesize little if any protein, these must be transported down the axon after they are synthesized in the cell body. Axonal transport is mediated by microtubule-activated ATPases, known as kinesins, molecular motors that use microtubules as tracks. Kinesins form a large gene family, and each kinesin transports a specific organelle. A mutation in the gene encoding kinesin KIF1Bβ, which transports synaptic vesicles to the axon terminals, causes CMT2A.[15]

DOMINANTLY INHERITED AXONAL NEUROPATHIES (CMT2)

The dominantly inherited forms, CMT2/HMSN-II, are distinguished from CMT1/HMSN-I as described above. There are rare recessive forms (see Table 40–1), and many forms that are part of inherited syndromes (see Table 40–2). Patients with CMT2 usually present in the second decade, but one third of patients present up to decades later, so that some affected individuals have few signs, even in the sixth and seventh decades, and may be unaware that they have the disorder. Nevertheless, few cases of chronic idiopathic ataxic neuropathy are diagnosed as CMT2, even with long-term follow-up. Positive sensory symptoms, including dysesthesias, are uncommon. Sensory ataxia due to loss of large primary sensory neurons subserving proprioception is common, and manifests as unsteadiness of gait, particularly on walking in the dark or on rough ground. Areflexia, of ankle jerks first and knee jerks later, reflects dysfunction mainly of neurons subserving the afferent limb of the myotatic reflex arc. Autonomic function can be mildly affected, with diminished sudomotor function in the limbs, and occasional impotence in men. Cardiovascular reflex control mechanisms, including those regulating blood pressure and heart rate, are normal.

The pathologic picture in CMT2 is primarily that of loss of axons and nerve cell bodies. Large myelinated fibers, both motor and sensory, are most affected. Surprising numbers of clusters of regenerating axons are seen in roots and proximal nerves, but this fades in distal nerves where most axons are missing. Quite extensive neuronal loss is seen in lumbar and cervical dorsal root ganglia and in the anterior horns of the cervical and lumbar enlargements. Correspondingly, there is severe loss of central processes of primary sensory neurons in the posterior columns (the gracile column more than the cuneate), resulting in a distinctive pattern of pallor on myelin stains of the posterior columns.

Like CMT1, CMT2 is genetically heterogeneous, with at least seven loci (see Table 40–1). The gene defects have been described for CMT2A (*KIF1Bβ*) and CMT2E (*NEFL*). Two large kinships with vocal cord, intercostal muscle, and diaphragm weakness in addition to the expected axonal motor-sensory findings in the limbs have been reported. Onset may occur in infancy or childhood, and life expectancy may be shortened due to respiratory insufficiency. This phenotype has been classified as CMT2C, and does not map to other CMT2 loci. The relationship, if any, between the two North American families labeled CMT2 and the two large kinships in Wales with autosomal dominant distal spinal muscular atrophy with vocal cord paralysis remains uncertain.

CMT2A patients have a typical axonal phenotype. The Gln98Leu mutation in kinesin1Bβ (*KIF1B*), a molecular motor for transporting synaptic vesicles, affects a highly conserved ATP-binding region and results in a loss of function. Haplotype insufficiency can account for the dominant phenotype in humans, as mice that are heterozygous for a null *Kif1B* allele develop neuropathy, and the levels of synaptic vesicle proteins are selectively decreased in peripheral axons. The function of kinesin1Bβ explains why CMT2A is length-dependent: a relative reduction in this molecular motor leads to axonal impairment starting at the most remote part of the neuron.

The CMT2B patients described in three reports appear to be clinically similar. In addition to length-dependent weakness and severe sensory loss, distal ulcerations in the feet are common, often leading to toe amputations. A similar, ulceromutilating neuropathy has been reported in an Austrian family, which did not link to the CMT2B locus, indicating further genetic heterogeneity in this phenotype.

CMT2E is caused by mutations in the gene that encodes the neurofilament light subunit (*NFEL*). In a large Russian kindred, clinical manifestations of CMT2E become apparent in the second or third decades, with difficulty walking, distal weakness, diminished sensation (including pain sensation), and absent reflexes in the legs, followed by slow progression. In a smaller kindred, distal weakness progresses to paresis by the fourth decade. In the Russian kindred, the median motor NCVs were mildly reduced or normal (38 to 52 m/s), whereas in the other kindred they were considerably slowed (median motor NCV 25 to 39 m/s; ulnar motor NCV 30 to 42 m/s). In animal models, neurofilament mutations have profound effects on axonal caliber, potentially accounting for the slowed NCVs seen in CMT2E patients. Alternatively, expression of mutant NFL in Schwann cells may contribute to the disease.

CMT2F was described in one multigenerational Russian family and linked to 7q11-21. The onset is in the second or third decade, with typical CMT2 features. Weakness may progress to foot drops; fasciculations have been described in elderly family members. The CMT2G kindreds from Okinawa (Japan) map to chromosome 3, but to a different region (3q13.1) than CMT2B. These patients have a distinct phenotype: painful muscle cramps and progressive weakness in proximal more than distal muscles. Although myelinated sensory axons are affected, distal ulcerations do not develop. The disorder was named "proximal CMT2" (CMT2-P), although it has features of a neuronopathy, including loss of anterior horn cells.

Diagnosis of CMT2 depends on finding affected family members in other generations as well as among siblings. The propositus should demonstrate a long-standing, usually adult-onset, motor and sensory neuropathy, distal and symmetric in its distribution, with normal or minimally slowed conduction velocities, few or no positive sensory symptoms, but often positive motor symptoms, particularly cramping. The clinical and electrophysiologic picture coupled with the pattern of inheritance establishes the diagnosis. The outlook is for continued, slow progression that rarely reaches the stage of confinement to a wheelchair. Management is symptomatic.

In summary, just as mutations in genes expressed by myelinating Schwann cells cause CMT1, the CMT2 mutations identified to date affect genes expressed by neurons. The axonal loss in CMT2A and CMT2E is likely to be cell autonomous. The finding that CMT2 patients can have NCV below 38 m/s makes the distinction between CMT1 and CMT2 even more problematic. A neurobiologic approach, based on the molecular and cellular biology of myelinated axons, will potentially provide a more meaningful classification.

RECESSIVELY INHERITED DEMYELINATING NEUROPATHIES (CMT4)

Rare, autosomal recessive forms of demyelinating CMT, usually in inbred populations, have been collectively designated CMT4 (see Table 40–1). CMT4A was found in Tunisian families and mapped to the 8q13 locus. It is characterized as a severe neuropathy starting in the first 2 years of life, causing delayed motor development, progressing to involve proximal muscles by the end of the first decade to the point that many patients become wheelchair-dependent. Motor NCVs average 29 m/s in the arms, and nerve pathology includes hypomyelination, basal lamina onion bulbs, and loss of large caliber axons. Recently, mutations in the gene encoding the ganglioside-induced differentiation-associated protein 1 (*GDAP1*) have been shown to cause CMT4A, and, surprisingly, the axonal variant with vocal cord paralysis linked to the same locus.

CMT4B has been found in Italian and Saudi Arabian families and causes a similar phenotype, although early motor milestones are usually achieved, in contrast to CMT4A. Motor NCVs are uniformly slow (14 to 17 m/s in the arms), and nerve biopsies show distinct features: irregular folding and redundant loops of myelin. Mutations in the myotubularin-related protein-2 gene, *MTMR2*, which belongs to the family of myotubularin-related dual specific phosphatases, causes CMT4B. *MTMR2* is expressed by Schwann cells, and by a variety of other cell types. After two Tunisian families with the same phenotype, including focally folded myelin sheaths, were linked to a different locus (11p15) and designated CMT4B2, CMT4B caused by *MTMR2* mutations is now called CMT4B1.

CMT4D could be considered a syndromic neuropathy, as it is associated with hearing loss and dysmorphic features. It was initially described in gypsies from Lom, Bulgaria, but has been subsequently found in gypsies living elsewhere. The onset is in childhood, with foot deformities and abnormal gait, and progresses to severe disability by the fifth decade. Motor NCVs are severely reduced and become unobtainable after age 15, indicating severe axonal loss. Biopsies show demyelination, onion bulb formation, and cytoplasmic inclusions in Schwann cells. Mutations in N-myc downstream-regulated gene-1 (*NDRG1*), which is expressed by Schwann cells, cause CMT4D.

A large Lebanese family defined CMT4F. Affected members have a DSS phenotype, with delayed motor milestones and progressing to severe distal weakness, areflexia, sensory loss, and even sensory ataxia. NCVs are severely slowed (<5 m/s) or undetectable, and biopsies show thinly myelinated axons, onion bulbs, and severe axonal loss. Mutations in the periaxin gene (*PRX*) were identified in this family, and in unrelated cases of Dejerine-Sottas syndrome. The *PRX* gene encodes periaxin, a PDZ domain protein that is expressed by myelinating Schwann cells, in which it links dystroglycan to the actin cytoskeleton and possibly compact myelin.[16]

HEREDITARY SENSORY AND AUTONOMIC NEUROPATHIES (HSAN)

These diseases are considerably less frequent than the CMT, and are probably as diverse both clinically and genetically. Dyck has designated this sundry group as hereditary sensory and autonomic neuropathy (HSAN) types I to V.[17]

For the dominant form (HSAN-I, also called HSN1) the onset of the acral sensory loss is postnatal and progressive. The main clinical features are insidious loss of cutaneous sensation, mainly pain and temperature sensibility with variable degrees of hypesthesia to touch, predominantly in the feet and lower legs but also later in the hands. In some families, spontaneous, severe lancinating pain may accompany progression but eventually sub-

sides. At times when distal cutaneous sensation may be grossly deficient, proprioception and ankle jerks may still be relatively normal, although the sural nerve trunk at the ankle may show very few remaining myelinated fibers. This suggests that the muscle spindle and joint position afferents are affected less severely and later in the course than the smaller cutaneous afferents. In addition to sensory neurons, HSAN-I affects other kinds of neurons. One postmortem study showed extensive cell loss and gliosis in the thalamus, red nuclei, inferior olivary nuclei and claustrum, all outside of the somatosensory and auditory pathways, suggesting a multi-system degeneration of neurons.[18]

Recently, mutations in the gene encoding the long-chain base subunit 1 of serine palmitoyl transferase (*SPTLC1*) were shown to cause HSAN-I.[19] Lymphoblast cell lines from the mutations of affected individuals have increased synthesis of glucosyl ceramide, which has been shown to mediate non-neuronal cell death. Whether affected neurons have increased ceramide, and how this produces the appearance of a length-dependent axonal neuropathy, remains to be determined.

In the recessively inherited, HSAN-II to HSAN-V, sensory abnormalities often seem to be present at birth, although secondary changes due to unheeded trauma may not be evident until late infancy or childhood. In many children, the neurologic deficit does not appear to be progressive, although secondary complications may give that appearance. The frequently congenital nature of the neurologic deficit suggests that a specific and selective failure of neuronal development may have occurred during fetal life. This possibility has been demonstrated for HSAN-IV/CIPA syndrome, which is caused by mutations in the *TRKA*.[14] Nevertheless, the issue of static versus progressive deficit is not entirely settled for the other congenital sensory neuropathies.

HEREDITARY MOTOR NEUROPATHIES (HMN)

This group of disorders, also known as distal spinal muscular atrophy (SMA), predominantly affects motor axons. Several types (HMN 1 to HMN 7) have been described based on their clinical phenotypes and modes of inheritance, and some have been mapped (see Table 40–1). The onset is usually in childhood or early adulthood, with distal weakness typically affecting the extensor muscles of the toes and feet. In the HMN 5 linked to chromosome 7p, however, upper-limb predominance is characteristic. Cranial nerves are usually not affected, but vocal cord weakness is a hallmark of HMN 7. Sensory nerves are normal, although mild axonal loss is evident in the sural nerve biopsy. Motor responses are reduced, with normal or moderately reduced NCVs. Needle electromyography demonstrates chronic denervation. In the autosomal recessive form of HMN found in consanguineous families from Jordan (Jerash type), younger patients also have findings of a myelopathy, but these progressively disappeared owing to the predominance of motor axon loss. Whether the myelopathy is caused by a neuronopathy or a length-dependent degeneration of CNS axons remains to be determined. Clinical findings of CNS involvement have also been described in some patients with distal HMN 5.

Autosomal recessive SMA with respiratory distress (SMARD) is clinically distinguished by predominant distal muscle weakness and diaphragm paralysis. At least two genetically distinct forms have been identified, and mutations in the gene encoding immunoglobulin μ-binding protein 2 (*IGHMBP2*) on chromosome 11q13.2 causes SMARD type 1 (infantile onset). Like the *SMN1* gene product (see Chapter 23 on SMA), IGHMBP2 co-localizes with the RNA-processing machinery in both the cytoplasm and the nucleus, and may share common functions with the *SMN* gene product, which is required for motor neuron survival. This first gene identified in the HSN group establishes the close relationship of these disorders to SMA, although different mechanisms of selective motor neuron and/or motor axon degeneration may be present in the other HMN types.

THE DIAGNOSIS AND TREATMENT OF CMT AND RELATED DISORDERS

Before genetic testing is considered, an accurate diagnosis of an inherited peripheral neuropathy should be established by the family history, as well as the patient's history, physical exam, and clinical electrophysiology (Figure 40–2). It is particularly important to perform median and ulnar motor NCVs, as the degree of slowing and its uniformity should confirm or refute the clinical diagnosis and even suggest a specific kind of inherited neuropathy. Because the pattern of inheritance is of paramount importance, it is important to examine multiple family members for subtle signs of neuropathy, and to perform clinical electrophysiology on all probands, persons at risk, and parents, if possible. This is especially important in evaluating a male who appears to have an inherited neuropathy, as the neuropathy could be acquired, auto-

somal dominant (representing either a *de novo* mutation or false paternity), X-linked, or even autosomal recessive. In our opinion, a nerve biopsy should not be part of the initial diagnostic evaluation except in problematic cases or for research purposes.

The findings that should suggest CMT1A, CMT1B, CMT1X, CMT2, HNPP, HSAN, or a hereditary motor neuropathy have already been described, including their electrophysiologic features. An accurate assessment of the phenotype of individual patients—their age of onset, historical progression, as well as their current physical findings—will usually distinguish between inherited and acquired causes. On occasion, it may be difficult or impossible to exclude an acquired chronic axonal neuropathy or chronic inflammatory demyelinating polyneuropathy.

We suggest a strategy for genetic testing that is depicted in Figure 40–2. In cases of suspected HNPP, testing for the *PMP22* deletion should be performed first, as this is by far the major cause; if this is negative, then both alleles of *PMP22* should be sequenced. In CMT patients with uniform slowing of motor NCVs between 10 and 35 m/s, testing for the *PMP22* duplication should be performed, as this the major cause of CMT1. If the patient does not have the duplication, then *PMP22, MPZ, GJB1*, and *EGR2* should be sequenced. In DSS with appropriately slowed NCVs, testing for the duplication will usually be negative, and sequencing of the *PMP22, MPZ, GJB1, EGR2*, and *PRX* genes should be included in the initial evaluation. In cases where CMT1X is the most likely diagnosis (intermediate slowing of NCVs, no male-to-male transmission), sequencing *GJB1* alone is the appropriate initial test; if negative, consider sequencing *MPZ* and *NEFL*. In cases of suspected CMT2, it is probably premature to test for *MPZ* and *NFEL* mutations alone (the only commercially available tests), but a more comprehensive battery should be available in the future as more genetic causes are found. Discovering these causes depends on the participation of referring physicians and affected families. Testing for mutations of these genes can be done at several laboratories. More information is available at http://www.genetests.org/.

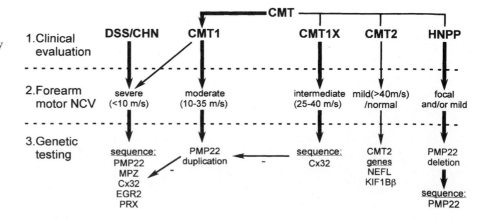

FIGURE 40–2. A workup for nonsyndromic inherited neuropathies. Updated information on the availability of new genetic testing is available at http://www.genetests.org.

Treatment for HNPP is largely supportive. Patients should avoid activities that cause nerve compression. Surgical decompression of nerves is controversial and must be decided on an individual basis. There is some evidence that surgical repair of carpal tunnel syndrome in HNPP is of little benefit and transposition of the ulnar nerve at the elbow may produce poor results because the nerves are especially sensitive to manipulation and minor trauma. No treatment for HNPP, CMT, or DSS reverses or slows the progression of the neuropathy. Multicenter clinical trials should be possible, as homogeneous patient groups can be identified. Further, excellent animal models for different kinds of inherited neuropathy have been created, and therapeutic interventions could be studied first in these models.[6] There is still much to be learned before rational treatments can be devised.

Current treatment for inherited neuropathies is symptomatic, involving neurologists, physiatrists, orthopedic surgeons, and physical and occupational therapists, according to the needs of the patient. Daily heel cord stretching exercises can prevent shortening of the Achilles tendon, and special shoes, including those with good ankle support, may be needed. Patients often require ankle/foot orthoses (AFOs) to correct foot drop and aid walking and occasionally orthopedic surgery to correct deformities. Forearm crutches or canes may be required for gait stability, but fewer than 5% of patients need wheelchairs. Avoiding obesity and exercising within the patient's capability are desirable. The disease may affect career and employment options, and this should be discussed with the patient. When pain is present, the cause should be identified as accurately as possible. Musculoskeletal pain may respond to acetaminophen or nonsteroidal antiinflammatory agents, whereas neuropathic pain may respond to tricyclic antidepressants, carbamazepine, or gabapentin.

Chemotherapeutic agents known to affect peripheral nerves should be used with great caution in patients with inherited neuropathies. In the case of vincristine, total avoidance is strongly advised, as serious consequences have been documented following the administration of standard oncologic dosages in patients with CMT, including CMT1A and CMT2. Complications ranged from precipitation of severe neuropathies in clinically asymptomatic at-risk individuals to degrees of marked clinical worsening or death due to respiratory collapse.

Two organizations that support clinical and scientific aspects of inherited neuropathies are the Charcot-Marie-Tooth Association, available at http://www.charcot-marie-tooth.org, and the Muscular Dystrophy Association, available at http://www.mdausa.org/disease/cmt.html.

AMYLOID NEUROPATHY

Neuropathy may be a part of several kinds of amyloidosis, systemic diseases in which soluble plasma proteins are transformed into β-structured fibrils that are deposited in various organs and apparently cause dysfunction by their presence and magnitude.[20,21] While each kind of amyloidosis is characterized by the specific protein that contributes the subunit of the fibrils, the pathologic processes leading to amyloid deposition are similar. A normally soluble protein exits the circulation, is partially proteolysed by cell-associated mechanisms, and then assembled into proteolytically resistant β-structured fibrils in extravascular spaces. These fibril deposits progressively enlarge, displacing normal structures including cells, basement membrane, and connective tissue. The degree and distribution of organ function impairment dictates the clinical manifestations. The types of amyloidosis that may cause neuropathy as part of the disease are immunoglobulin (AL) amyloidosis and the hereditary amyloidoses associated with mutants of plasma transthyretin (TTR), gelsolin, apolipoprotein AI (ApoAI) genes (see Table 40–2). Neuropathy is not a feature of reactive (secondary) amyloidosis nor of the hereditary amyloidoses caused by mutations in fibrinogen Aα chain, lysozyme, apolipoprotein AII genes, and most of the variant forms of ApoAI. Only the inherited forms of amyloid that cause neuropathy are considered here; all are dominant disorders.

TRANSTHYRETIN AMYLOIDOSIS (FAP 1 AND 2)

The most common type of hereditary amyloid neuropathy is caused by mutations in the TTR gene. At least 80 mutations that are associated with amyloidosis have been identified. All are caused by a single nucleotide change that results in an amino acid substitution, except for one mutation that deletes a codon, resulting in the loss of a valine (ΔVal122). TTR mutations have been described in most countries and in many ethnic groups. In the United States, the majority of mutations are found in families of European ancestry, and, in many cases, the mutations have been traced to the country of origin. The Val30Met mutation was probably present in Portugal by 1400 AD. It was then brought to Sweden and later to Japan and Brazil. The Thr60Ala mutation originated in Northern Ireland and was brought to the United States before 1800. The Leu58His mutation came with German migrants to Pennsylvania in the late 1700s. Many mutations that have been found associated with amyloidosis have been assumed, but not proven, to be the definitive cause of the genetic disease because of insufficient data. The associations with well-characterized mutations or well-studied families of inherited amyloidosis are probably valid. Only two cases of de novo mutations have been verified—one in Japan (Gly47Arg) and one in the United States (Ala25Ser).

The typical neuropathy of Val30Met amyloidosis was described by Andrade in his 1952 report on kindreds from northern Portugal,[22] later designated FAP 1. It starts with dysesthesias in the lower extremities with or without small fiber findings such as decreased temperature sensation. Sensory loss usually progresses over several years, and may eventually involve the trunk. When sensory loss has reached the level of the knees, similar loss occurs in the upper extremities and motor loss in the lower extremities declares itself by footdrop. Progression of motor impairment may span 10 to 20 years and often leads to use of braces, canes, crutches, and finally a wheelchair. Autonomic dysfunction (constipation, diarrhea, or impotence) often occurs early in the disease and may be the first symptom. Orthostatic hypotension occurs later, and while probably partly caused by autonomic dysfunction, it is most prominent in individuals who also have restrictive cardiomyopathy. Heart failure caused by restrictive cardiomyopathy has replaced neuropathy as the major direct cause of death. Leg ulcers, osteomyelitis, and malnutrition took their toll before antibiotics and improved levels of supportive care were developed. A smaller number of patients have renal failure and a few patients die from loss of gastrointestinal function.

The TTR gene (18q23) has four exons. No mutations have been found in exon 1, which encodes a signal peptide and the first three residues of the mature protein. Exons 2 (amino acid residues 4 to 47), 3 (residues 48 to 92), and 4 (residues 93 to 127) each have similar proportion of mutations that cause amyloidosis (n=80) and mutations that do not cause amyloidosis (n=10). To date, neither the position of the altered amino acid nor the type of amino acid substitution has been implicated in amyloid formation. Nevertheless, there are many variations on the clinical theme of amyloidosis, and some may be related to specific mutations. Many affected individuals have carpal tunnel syndrome, and in some the disease starts with this entity, especially in the Maryland/German (Leu58His) and Indiana/Swiss (Ile84Ser) kindreds; this was the justification for naming this clinical variant FAP 2. Amyloid deposition in the vitreous of the eye is a variable feature, occurring in about one fourth of the kindreds, and may be the only manifestation of the disease in some individuals. The recurrent laryngeal nerve and facial nerve are uncommonly affected. Spinal claudication due to amyloid deposition in structures around the cord and nerve roots may occur, and magnify the deficits in patients who only have moderate neuropathy. Leptomeningeal amyloid deposition may be a major manifestation of TTR amyloidosis due to a number of variants (Leu12Pro, Asp18Gly, Val30Gly, Leu55Arg, Phe64Ser, Tyr114Cys, ΔVal122). This may present as intracerebral hemorrhage, seizures, headaches, and in some cases, dementia. Many TTR variants that cause leptomeningeal deposition also cause vitreous opacities (Val30Gy, Tyr69His, Tyr114Cys).

The incidence of TTR amyloidosis is difficult to determine, but is high in certain populations. In Skelleftea and Lulea (in northern Sweden) and among the fishermen of Pavoa de Varzim (in northern Portugal), 3% to 5% of inhabitants have the Val30Met mutation. A rare disease in most of the world, the large number of TTR mutations adds to a sizable total of affected individuals. The Val122Ile is the most prevalent, but does not cause neuropathy. It affects approximately 3% African Americans, but is underappreciated because it causes clinically significant disease only after age 60 years, manifesting primarily as congestive heart failure that is often attributed to other more common diseases such as hypertension.

TTR is a plasma protein that is synthesized almost exclusively by the liver, and has a plasma half-life of only 1 to 2 days. There is some synthesis by the choroid plexus of the brain and by the retinal pigment epithelium. The former site probably provides TTR for the cerebral spinal fluid and the latter for the vitreous of the eye, both known sites for amyloid deposition. In plasma, TTR is a tetramer composed of four identical monomers, each of which is composed of a single polypeptide chain of 127 amino acids. Each monomer has extensive β-structure (four β-strands in each of two planes), which must be an important factor in the formation of amyloid fibrils, as even wild type TTR is amyloidogenic, providing the fibrils in senile cardiac amyloidosis. It is not known how the various inherited mutations promote amyloid formation. It has been suggested that mutations in the protein destabilize the tetramer, thereby favoring the aggregation of subunits and fibrillogenesis. Changes in structure and protein stability may increase the metabolic turnover of TTR, as individuals with amyloid-associated TTR mutants have reduced plasma TTR levels (but equal amounts of normal and variant TTR mRNA in the liver). Persistent mysteries in the pathogenesis of amyloidosis are the reason for delay of fibril deposition until adulthood and the variation of onset between individuals with different or even the same mutation. The TTR tetramer has a central channel with two binding sites for thyroxin. Retinol/vitamin A–saturated retinol-binding protein binds to the outside of the tetramer. Although TTR was assumed to serve as a transporter of these two important metabolic moieties, mice lacking TTR have very low plasma levels of retinol, but normal fecundity and development.[23] Thus, it is unlikely that the altered ability of TTR mutants to bind thyroxin and retinol-saturated retinol-binding protein plays an important role in the pathogenesis of the amyloidosis.

Although TTR amyloidosis is an autosomal dominant disease, penetrance is variable and obscured by the late onset of manifestations in many kindreds. Even when the manifestations are present, it is often not diagnosed, thereby obscuring the family history and misleading the clinician. The availability of DNA testing, however, has greatly enhanced the ability to diagnose suspected cases of amyloidosis.[24] When the specific TTR mutation is known, DNA analysis can be accomplished for any individual in the kinship. For some mutations, the single strand conformation polymorphism (SSCP) gel pattern allows large numbers of individuals to be screened in one procedure. If a *TTR* mutation is suspected, but no specific mutation is being considered, it is necessary to sequence all of the coding regions or screen for mutations with SSCP. Each exon can be amplified by PCR and then analyzed by SSCP, with approximately 80% sensitivity. If an abnormal gel pattern is seen for one exon, this can be sequenced.

Liver transplant is the only specific therapy for *TTR* amyloidosis. After the transplant, plasma levels of mutant *TTR* fall rapidly. Several hundred individuals have received liver transplants for this disease. Disease progression stops for many patients, although few have had definite evidence of disease regression. Individuals with certain mutations (e.g., Val30Met) may have better results than those with other mutations (e.g., Glu42Gly); this difference may be related to the degree of cardiac involvement at the time of transplant. After amyloid deposition has progressed to a certain degree (still unknown), normal *TTR* may continue to form cardiac amyloid. Normal *TTR* accounts for 40% of cardiac amyloid before transplant, but may increase to 60% at the time of death from heart failure in patients who survived for more than 3 years after liver transplant.

Other therapies can prolong the life and function of individuals with *TTR* amyloidosis. These include treatment of painful dysesthesias, diarrhea, and heart failure. Avoidance of drugs that impair contractility (including most antiarrhythmics) can reduce the incidence and degree of heart failure. Cardiac pacing is often necessary. Renal dialysis may benefit some patients. Surgical decompression of carpal tunnel syndrome should be thorough because amyloid deposition is progressive, and recurrence is possible. Spinal claudication due to infiltration of ligamentum flavum, dural tissues, and spinal blood vessels can be partially relieved by multilevel laminectomy.

GELSOLIN AMYLOIDOSIS (FAP 4)

Gelsolin amyloidosis is an autosomal dominant disease with odd features.[25] Its main manifestations are lattice corneal dystrophy and facial paralysis, but it is unknown why these are the sites of amyloid deposition. Corneal deposits appear first, usually at about age 20 years. These appear as linear branching structures and usually do not cause serious loss of vision for several years. Progressive cranial neuropathy develops about age 40, causing bilateral facial palsies, which can be quite disfiguring and can cause corneal damage owing to the failure of the upper and lower lids to close. Amyloid is deposited in trigeminal and facial nerve roots, often sparing other cranial nerves, both in the endoneurium and in the blood vessels. Amyloid is also deposited in other organs, including the heart, intestines, and kidneys, but usually does not shorten longevity. In some individuals who are homozygous for the mutant gelsolin, renal and cardiac disease is accelerated and life-threatening.

Gelsolin is a plasma protein, and by analogy to its intracellular form, it is assumed to be important in cleavage and catabolism of intravascular actin. A mutation in plasma gelsolin (Asp to Asn change at position 187 of the 755 amino acid residue mature protein) causes amyloidosis. The fibril subunit is a 71 residue peptide that contains the variant residue and, unlike *TTR*, no normal gelsolin peptide is found in the amyloid fibrils. Thus, the normal and variant proteolytic fragments go their separate ways prior to fibril formation. The crystal structure of gelsolin is known, but the degree of β-structure in the resultant amyloid forming proteolytic peptide and its contribution to fibrillogenesis are unknown. In addition to the well-characterized disease that originated in Finland, a similar disease caused by an Asp to Tyr mutation at the same site in gelsolin has been reported from kindreds in Denmark and the Czech Republic. Haplotype analysis suggests that the Asp to Asn mutation has occurred more than once.

The gelsolin gene is on chromosome 9 (9q32-34) and has at least 14 exons. The exact genomic position of the mutations that cause amyloidosis has not yet been determined, but genetic testing for the Finnish mutation is available by PCR/RFLP technique. The test uses a "mutagenesis primer" that creates a MunI restriction site in the presence of the G to A mutation. Individuals with systemic amyloidosis with corneal lattice dystrophy should consider DNA analysis, since the clinical course and prognosis are different from other forms of amyloidosis.

There is no specific therapy for gelsolin amyloidosis. If vision is impaired by corneal dystrophy, corneal transplant is an accepted and successful procedure. As with other corneal dystrophies, the condition can recur after several years and may require repeat corneal transplant. Skeletal muscle synthesizes plasma gelsolin in large part. Therefore, unlike *TTR*, organ transplant is not a therapeutic option. In the unusual patients with symptomatic renal, gastrointestinal, or cardiac amyloidosis, therapy is similar to that described for *TTR* amyloidosis.

APOLIPOPROTEIN AI AMYLOIDOSIS (FAP 3)

ApoAI amyloidosis was first described by Van Allen et al.[26] They documented a progressive axonal neuropathy involving sensory, motor, and autonomic neurons. Sensory loss in the legs was usually the first sign of neuropathy, and motor impairment followed. Impotence was common, but gastrointestinal motility problems, as seen with *TTR* amyloidosis, did not occur. In the original family described by Van Allen et al.,[26] several affected individuals developed deafness. CSF protein levels were elevated in the four patients who had spinal fluid analysis. This family was found to have an arginine for glycine substitution at position 26 of the *ApoAI*. Subsequently, other families with this mutation have been identified; some have renal amyloidosis but no clinical evidence of neuropathy, while others have both the nephropathy and neuropathy. Studies of members of the next generation of the Iowa family reveal renal and hepatic amyloidosis, but as yet, no evidence of neuropathy.

ApoAI is part of plasma high-density lipoprotein (HDL) and is believed to be important in reverse cholesterol transport. The complete absence of a functional *ApoAI* gene causes severe, early-onset atherosclerosis. How *ApoAI*, which has little β-structure, is altered to form β-amyloid fibrils is not clear. This property is shared with serum amyloid A (SAA), which is also an apolipoprotein constituent of HDL, and gives rise to the subunit (AA) amyloid fibrils in reactive amyloidosis. Only the mutant Gly26Arg protein is incorporated into amyloid fibrils, suggesting that *ApoAI* is dissociated from HDL before the mutant protein enters the pathway to fibril formation. The organ distribution of *ApoAI* amyloid is similar to that seen with SAA (kidney, liver, adrenal). However, only the amyloid formed by *ApoAI* Gly26Arg mutant (and not by other HDL apolipoproteins SAA and *ApoAII*) causes neuropathy.

ApoAI amyloidosis is an autosomal dominant disease. The *ApoAI* gene is on chromosome 11 (11q23). Nine mutations in *ApoAI* have been identified. All cause renal, hepatic, or cardiac amyloidosis, but only the Gly26Arg mutation is associated with neuropathy. Kindreds with the Gly26Arg mutation have been identified in the United Kingdom, continental Europe, and the United States; whether the Gly26Arg mutation arose separately in these families is not known. DNA analysis for the Gly26Arg mutation (which is the result of a guanine to cytosine transversion in the first position of codon 26) is available by PCR/RFLP.

Gly26Arg amyloidosis is slowly progressive, with survival for 15 to 20 years after clinical presentation. Renal dialysis is the major supportive therapy since renal failure is the major cause of death. Hypertension (probably related to the renal disease) is common and should be treated early. Although not all circulating *ApoAI* is of hepatic origin, several patients have had liver transplants, and early results are encouraging. Thus, increasing the relative amount of normal to variant *ApoAI* may favorably affect the disease.

DIAGNOSIS OF AMYLOID NEUROPATHY

Diagnosis of systemic amyloidosis is not difficult, especially if neuropathy is part of the clinical presentation. Amyloidosis typically affects multiple organ systems, so even if it starts with neuropathic symptoms, this will not remain the sole feature for long. The greatest deterrent to a timely diagnosis is a lack of familiarity with the disease and, therefore, the failure to search for more extensive involvement. Neurologists, like most subspecialists, tend not to look far beyond their organ system of special interest. For the patient with an axonal neuropathy, or even signs of autonomic neuropathy alone (e.g., impo-

tence), it is essential to look for renal disease (proteinuria, elevated serum creatinine), cardiac disease (anginal-type pain, EKG, echocardiogram), and gastrointestinal dysfunction (constipation, diarrhea, early satiety).

A definitive diagnosis is made by demonstrating amyloid deposits. A nerve biopsy is usually not needed because biopsies of rectal mucosa or minor salivary glands, or an abdominal fat aspirate will reveal the amyloid deposits in approximately 80% of cases. After biopsy diagnosis, determining the exact type of amyloidosis is essential for both counseling and treatment. A family history of amyloidosis effectively excludes *AL* amyloidosis, which is probably the most common cause of amyloid neuropathy. The absence of a family history, however, does not exclude inherited amyloidosis. The clinical syndromes of *AL*, *TTR*, and *ApoAI* neuropathies are similar and distinct from gelsolin neuropathy. The availability of DNA analysis has significantly improved the ability to counsel the patient and family about inheritance, prognosis, and treatment, and a limited number of laboratories offer comprehensive genetic testing for amyloid-associated mutations. Expertise in this area is available from the Amyloid Research Group at Indiana University School of Medicine at http://www.iupui.edu/~amyloid/ and the Amyloid Treatment and Research Program at Boston University Medical Center at http://medicine.bu.edu/amyloid/amyloid1.htm. Testing for these mutations is available at http://www.genetests. org/.

REFERENCES

1. Kamholz J, Menchella D, Jani A, et al: Charcot Marie Tooth disease type 1: Molecular pathogenesis to gene therapy. Brain 2000;123:222–233.

2. Berger P, Young P, Suter U: Molecular cell biology of Charcot-Marie-Tooth disease. Neurogenetics 2002;4:1–15.

3. Scherer SS, Salzer J: Axon-Schwann cell interactions in peripheral nerve degeneration and regeneration. In Jessen KR, Richardson WD (eds): Glial Cell Development. Oxford, Oxford University Press, 2001, pp 299–330.

4. Nagarajan R, Svaren J, Le N, et al: EGR2 mutations in inherited neuropathies dominant-negatively inhibit myelin gene expression. Neuron 2001;30: 355–368.

5. Arroyo EJ, Scherer SS: On the molecular architecture of myelinated fibers. Histochem Cell Biol 2000; 113:1–18.

6. Martini R: Animal models for inherited peripheral neuropathies. J Anat 1997;191:321–336.

7. Altevogt BM, Kleopa KA, Postma FR, et al: Distinct expression of Cx29 by myelinating glial cells of the central and peripheral nervous system. J Neurosci 2002;22:6458–6470.

8. Dyck PJ, Chance P, Lebo R, Carney JA: Hereditary motor and sensory neuropathies. In Dyck PJ,

Thomas PK, Griffin JW, et al (eds): Peripheral Neuropathy. Philadelphia, WB Saunders, 1993, pp 1094–1136.

9. Keller MP, Chance PF: Inherited neuropathies: From gene to disease. Brain Pathol 1999;9:327–341.

10. Lupski JR, Garcia CA: Charcot-Marie-Tooth peripheral neuropathies and related disorders. In Scriver CR, Beaudet AL, Sly WS, Valle D (eds): The Metabolic and Molecular Basis of Inherited Disease. New York, McGraw-Hill, 2001, pp 5759–5788.

11. Wrabetz L, Feltri ML, Hanemann CO, Muller HW: The molecular genetics of hereditary demyelinating neuropathies. In Jessen KR, Richardson WD (eds): Glial Cell Development. Oxford, Oxford University Press, 2001, 331–354.

12. Birouk N, Gouider R, Le Guern E, et al: Charcot-Marie-Tooth disease type 1A with 17p11.2 duplication: Clinical and electrophysiological phenotype study and factors influencing disease severity in 119 cases. Brain 1997;120:813–823.

13. Bird TD, Kraft GH, Lipe HP, et al: Clinical and pathological phenotype of the original family with Charcot-Marie-Tooth type 1B: A 20-year study. Ann Neurol 1997;41:463–469.

14. Indo Y: Molecular basis of congenital insensitivity to pain with anhidrosis (CIPA): Mutations and polymorphisms in TRKA (NTRK1) gene encoding the receptor tyrosine kinase for nerve growth factor. Hum Mutat 2001;18:462–471.

15. Zhao C, Takita J, Tanaka Y, et al: Charcot-Marie-Tooth disease type 2A caused by mutation in a microtubule motor KIF1Bb. Cell 2001;105:587–597.

16. Sherman DL, Fabrizi C, Gillespie CS, Brophy PJ: Specific disruption of a Schwann cell dystrophin-related protein complex in a demyelinating neuropathy. Neuron 2001;30:677–687.

17. Dyck PJ: Neuronal atrophy and degeneration predominantly affecting peripheral sensory and autonomic neurons. In Dyck PJ, Thomas PK, Griffin JW, et al (eds): Peripheral Neuropathy. Philadelphia, WB Saunders, 1993, pp 1065–1093.

18. Horoupian DS: Hereditary sensory neuropathy with deafness: A familial multisystem atrophy. Neurology 1989;39:244–248.

19. Dawkins JL, Hulme DJ, Brahmbhatt SB, et al: Mutations in SPTLC1, encoding serine palmitoyltransferase, long chain base subunit-1, cause hereditary sensory neuropathy type I. Nat Genet 2001;27:309–312.

20. Costa PP, Figuera AS, Bravo FR: Amyloid fibril protein related to prealbumin in familial amyloidotic polyneuropathy. Proc Natl Acad Sci U S A 1978;75:4499–4503.

21. Benson MD: Amyloidosis. In Scriver CR, Beaudet AL, Sly WS, et al (eds): The Metabolic and Molecular Bases of Inherited Disease, 4th ed. New York, McGraw Hill, 2001, pp 5345–5378.

22. Andrade C: A peculiar form of peripheral neuropathy. Familial atypical generalized amyloidosis with special involvement of the peripheral nerves. Brain 1952;75:408–427.

23. Episkopou V, Maeda S, Nishiguchi S, et al: Disruption of the transthyretin gene results in mice with depressed levels of plasma retinol and thyroid hormone. Proc Natl Acad Sci U S A 1993;90:2375–2379.

24. Nichols WC, Benson MD: Hereditary amyloidosis: Detection of variant prealbumin genes by restriction enzyme analysis of amplified genomic DNA sequences. Clin Genet 1990;37:44–53.

25. Meretoja J: Familial systemic paramyloidosis with lattice dystrophy of the cornea, progressive cranial neuropathy, skin changes and various internal symptoms. A previously unrecognized heritable syndrome. Ann Clin Res 1969;1:314–324.

26. Van Allen MW, Frolich J, David JR: Inherited predisposition to generalized amyloidosis. Neurology 1969;19:10–25.

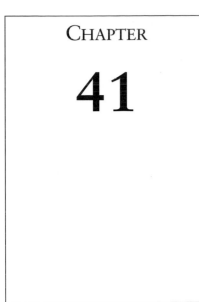

CHAPTER

41

The Molecular Genetic Basis of Spinal Muscular Atrophies

Ching H. Wang

Spinal muscular atrophy (SMA) is a neuromuscular disorder characterized by degeneration of the spinal cord motor neurons and muscle weakness. SMA is phenotypically heterogeneous and has been classified into three clinical subtypes according to the age of onset and disease severity. The gene for the three types of autosomal recessive SMA was mapped to chromosome 5q13 in 1990. Further progress in the field led to the identification of the *SMN* (survival of motor neuron) gene in 1995. The *SMN* gene is presented in two highly homologous copies: the telomeric *SMN1* and the centromeric *SMN2*. More than 95% of SMA patients harbor a homozygous deletion or mutation of *SMN1* but retain at least one intact copy of *SMN2*. SMA severity is correlated with the copy number of *SMN2*. Milder SMA phenotypes are also associated with the higher amounts of intact *SMN* mRNA and protein. The *SMN* protein plays an important role in the assembly and regeneration of a spliceosomal complex and in pre-mRNA splicing. A mouse model of SMA has been generated using a combination of knocking out the mouse *SMN* and knocking in a human *SMN2* to the mouse genome. These SMA-like mice exhibit both clinical and pathologic resemblance to human SMA. Therapeutic emphasis of recent SMA research has concentrated on applying the molecular genetic findings to identify a way to augment the production of intact *SMN* protein by the *SMN2* gene retained in SMA patients. Several transcription factors have been identified that can induce the production of intact *SMN* protein by interacting with a splicing enhancer sequence on exon 7 of the *SMN2* gene. Large-scale drug screening has been started in an attempt to identify pharmacologic compounds that can stimulate in vivo production of intact *SMN* protein. So far, two compounds have been identified that can aug-

ment the production of full-length *SMN* transcript in both SMA cell lines and SMA-like mice. This progress has made gene therapy a possibility through clinical therapeutic trial. This could revolutionize patient care in the near future.

CLINICAL SYMPTOMS

SMA is a motor neuron disease characterized by degeneration of spinal cord anterior horn cells and muscular atrophy.[1,2] The childhood-onset autosomal recessive SMA affects about 1:10,000 live births with a carrier frequency of 1:40 to 1:60.[3–5] SMA is the most common fatal genetic disorder of infancy and is the second most common childhood neuromuscular disease following Duchenne muscular dystrophy. Before the identification of the *SMN* gene, electromyography (EMG) and muscle biopsy were standard procedures for clinical diagnosis. The EMG shows frequent spontaneous activities such as positive sharp wave, fasciculation, and fibrillation. The motor-unit potentials display high amplitude and long duration along with a decreased recruitment. The muscle biopsy is characterized by group atrophy with islands of hypertrophic fibers typical of a neurogenic pathology. SMA is classified into three clinical subtypes according to severity and age of onset (types I, II, and III).[6] Type I SMA (severe/infantile/acute/Werdnig-Hoffman disease) is the most severe phenotype. The onset of symptoms is within the first 6 months of life. Some multiparous mothers report decreased fetal movement during pregnancy compared with their previous pregnancy with a healthy child. Profound hypotonia with absence of deep tendon reflexes are early presenting signs. Intercostal muscle weakness and lack of airway protection lead to respiratory insufficiency and aspiration pneumonia, often resulting in early infant death. Type II SMA (intermediate type) has its onset in early childhood (before age 18 months) and is characterized by failure to stand or walk unassisted. These children often succumb to the disease before adolescence due to respiratory insufficiency. Individuals with type III SMA (mild or Kugelberg-Welander disease) typically develop symptoms after age 18 months and display a wide range of clinical heterogeneity. The clinical spectrum ranges from rapid progressive weakness resulting in wheelchair dependence in late childhood to the ability to walk and live a productive and independent lifestyle for the majority of their lives. Types II and III SMAs are sometimes referred to as "chronic SMA."

Although this review is limited to the childhood-onset autosomal recessive forms of SMA, related forms of SMA also occur, often as adult-onset or X-linked disorders. Distal SMA occurs as autosomal dominant, autosomal recessive, and sporadic forms, with onset in childhood or adult life.[7,8] In distal SMA, the weakness is predominantly in the distal limb muscles, and progression is usually slow. The genetic heterogeneity of distal SMA was supported by the identification of at least 4 gene loci linked to chromosomes 2, 7, 11, and 12.[9–12] Segmental or focal SMA is usually sporadic and briefly progressive, with the patient sustaining a fixed, localized deficit. The shoulder and hands are common targets (monomelic amyotrophies), but other muscle groups are susceptible as well. Monomelic SMA is not associated with a deletion or mutation of the SMN gene.[13] The gene for the X-linked form of SMA with bulbar involvement and gynecomastia (spinal and bulbar muscular atrophy or Kennedy's disease) has been isolated and is associated with the expansion of CAG trinucleotide repeat in the first exon of the androgen receptor gene.[14] Another gene for a lethal form of X-linked SMA with arthrogryposis has been mapped to Xp11.[15]

POSITIONAL CLONING OF THE SMN GENE

In 1990, the gene locus for all three forms of childhood-onset SMA was mapped to chromosome 5q13.[16–18] Initially, a region of approximately 10 centimorgans (cM) genetic interval was identified by linkage analysis. Subsequent studies, using meiotic recombinant mapping, narrowed the disease locus to a region of 1 cM to 2 cM.[19–23] The next stage of research focused on constructing a high-resolution physical map of the SMA gene region. By 1994, multinational research efforts led to the high resolution mapping and cloning of the SMA region via a series of overlapping genomic clones harbored within yeast artificial chromosomes (YACs).[22,24–26] Closer inspection of the YAC clones spanning the SMA region revealed a relatively unusual and confounding feature of this chromosomal region. The disease gene region is characterized by an abundance of low-copy repeat

sequences. Both microsatellite markers and protein-coding sequences in this region are present as multiple copies.[22,23,27,28] In some cases, the homologous gene copies are also present elsewhere on chromosome 5 or on another chromosome.[29] These low-copy repeat sequences stymied the search for the SMA gene. They made the physical mapping extremely difficult. These low-copy repeats probably also contributed to the genomic instability in the region. This genomic instability is reflected by the tendency of YAC clones to contain rearranged or shortened genomic sequences.

In 1994, Melki et al reported that several of the multicopy microsatellite markers from the SMA region, including C272, were preferentially deleted in SMA patients (Fig. 41–1).[30] At the same time, researchers in MacKenzie's lab showed that an individual copy (CATT-40G1) of the multicopy microsatellite locus (CATT1) detects significant linkage disequilibrium with SMA.[31] Guided by the microsatellite deletion and linkage disequilibrium data, these two groups reported detailed physical maps that further pinpointed the disease gene locus. Melki's group identified a large genomic inverted repeat sequence in the disease gene region wherein each repeat spans about 500 kb and are composed of other low-copy repeat elements. Although the repeat sequences are highly homologous, the group used Southern blot hybridization to show that a small, 11-kb Hind III restriction enzyme fragment unique to the "telomeric" repeat sequence was preferentially missing in SMA patients. This data helped to narrow the SMA gene to a region of approximately 140 kb within the telomeric repeat. Using the genomic DNA from this region as a hybridization probe, a human fetal brain cDNA library was screened to identify a candidate gene—the survival motor neuron (SMN) gene.[32]

One copy of this gene was isolated from the telomeric repeat (SMN1), and a second highly homologous copy was mapped to the centromeric repeat (SMN2). These two SMN gene copies contain sequences that are extremely homologous. Only two single-base-pair differences exist in the entire 1.7-kb coding region. The SMN1 gene contains 9 exons with a genomic span of about 20 kb. The open reading frame predicts a 294 amino acid protein product. The SMN protein is a 40-Kd molecule that is part of a large spliceosomal complex (discussed later in "Subcellular Localization and Biochemical Function of the SMN Protein"). The SMN1 copy is homozygously missing in over 90% of SMA patients, whereas at least one copy of SMN1 is present in the vast majority of normal controls.[33–35] SMN2 is homozygously deleted in about 5% of normal control samples, but all SMA patients retain at least one copy of the SMN2 gene. Several microdeletions, frame-shift mutations, and missense mutations have also been reported.[36–39]

Simultaneous to Melki's report of the SMN gene, MacKenzie's group reported a second candidate gene for SMA.[40] This group focused on a microsatellite sublocus

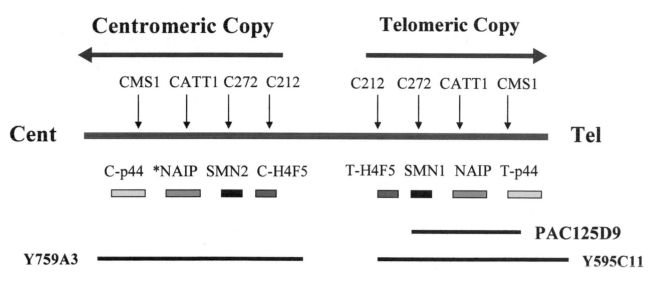

FIGURE 41-1. Schematic physical map of the SMA critical genetic region. Two inverted repetitive fragments of the genomic DNA are marked as centromeric and telomeric copies (*horizontal arrows*). Genomic clones YACs and PAC (*horizontal lines*) and gene copies (*short horizontal bars*) are not drawn to scale. YAC 595C11 contains the telomeric repeat sequence, YAC 759A3 contains the centromeric repeat, and YAC 920C9 contains both repeat copies. Two copies of the multilocus microsatellite markers (C212, C272, CATT1, and CMS1) are shown (*arrows*). Each of these markers is found within one of the corresponding genes. The PAC (P1 artificial chromosome) 125D9 contains *SMN1, NAIP,* and a portion of *T-p44*. The copy of *NAIP* in the centromeric repeat is missing several exon sequences and likely represents a pseudogene.

CATT-40G1 that showed linkage disequilibrium to the disease locus. They constructed a very detailed "contig" across the region around this sublocus (and all other subloci of the multicopied microsatellite marker CATT1) using many genomic clones. One PAC clone (125D9) was especially interesting since it not only contained CATT-40G1 but also another multicopy microsatellite marker *(CMS1),* one of whose subloci defined a border of the SMA genetic region.[22] A cosmid clone bearing the CATT-40G1 locus was used to screen a human fetal brain cDNA library. This search led to the identification of the 3'-end of a novel gene, the neuronal apoptosis inhibitory protein *(NAIP),* which contained DNA sequence homologous to a previously characterized baculoviral apoptosis inhibitory protein.[40] Exon trapping and further cDNA library screening was used to isolate the entire *NAIP* gene. The *NAIP* is also preferentially deleted in SMA samples when compared with those of controls. Although roughly half of all SMA individuals appear to be missing both *SMN* and *NAIP* genes, it is now clear that *SMN* is the only SMA determining gene and that *NAIP* is a very close innocent bystander that is also deleted in many SMA patients (see Fig. 41-1).

Further work in other laboratories lead to the identification of other genes in this region that were reported as possible modifier genes.[41,42] Gilliam's laboratory identified a third gene, the p44 subunit of basal transcription factor II *(BTF2p44).* This multicopy gene maps immediately adjacent to *SMN* and *NAIP* and is preferentially

deleted in SMA patients.[41] An assay of a single base pair difference in exon 7 of the two homologues copies of *BTFTp44* showed that one copy (T-p44) mapped to the telomeric repeat region containing *SMN1,* and the other copy (C-p44) mapped to the centromeric repeat containing *SMN2.* Another proposed SMA modifier gene in the region was reported by Kunkel's laboratory.[42] This novel transcript, *H4F5,* mapped 6.5 kb upstream of exon 1 of both *SMN* gene copies and contains the multicopy microsatellite marker C212 that is deleted in 90% of type I SMA chromosomes. The schematic physical map of the genes and markers in the SMA genetic region is shown in Figure 41-1.

FUNCTIONAL ANALYSIS OF THE *SMN* GENE

One purpose of identifying the SMA determining gene was to study the physiologic function of the gene in order to understand the pathogenesis of SMA. After the identification of the gene, several research groups devoted their efforts to studying the cellular function of the *SMN* gene. Others attempted to correlate the *SMN* gene mutations with the clinical phenotypes of SMA.

Genotype-Phenotype Correlation

While it is established that all three types of SMA are caused by the defect of *SMN1,* it is puzzling that a dysfunction of the same gene could result in such a wide range of phenotypic variation. Therefore, studying genotype-phenotype correlation seemed to be a logical way to provide an answer for this important question. Unfortunately, since the *SMN1* gene is missing in the majority of SMA patients, it was difficult to correlate directly between the genotypes of the *SMN1* mutations and the clinical severities in a large number of SMA patients. However, in our lab, we noticed that in addition to the deletion of the *SMN1* gene, the copy numbers of other genes in the *SMN* gene region were also decreased on type I SMA chromosomes compared with those of the milder phenotypes or normal controls. This suggested that the extent of genomic DNA deletion occurring in the *SMN* gene region might be correlated with SMA phenotypic severity. We performed several studies to confirm this hypothesis.[43] Using human-hamster hybrid haploid cell lines (CHO), we were able to identify the extent of DNA deletion on a single SMA chromosome and correlate the size of these deletions with the hosts' clinical phenotype. We studied a multigenerational family in which the mother of the propositus was affected with type III SMA and her child was affected with type I SMA. We performed genotyping on the haploid cell lines constructed from the mother and the child. We also performed genotyping on several other family members using total genomic DNA. We found that one of the mother's chromosomes contained a large deletion (designated as a severe allele), and her other chromosome contained a small deletion, only affecting the *SMN* gene (designated as a mild allele). She married a carrier who contributed another severe allele on his mutant chromosome. The severely affected child inherited a severe allele from each of the two parents and was homozygous for the severe allele. This study showed that the extent of DNA deletion is positively correlated with disease severity. The result of this study is illustrated in Figure 41–2.

The molecular pathogenesis of SMA continued to be an active topic of investigation. Several groups proposed that a gene conversion phenomenon rather than deletion might have been the molecular basis for a milder phenotype. They observed that in milder SMA patients there is a high frequency of "gene conversion,"[44–47] in that the patient did not lose the entire copy of the *SMN1* gene. Instead, one of the *SMN1* copies underwent sequence conversion at exons 7 and 8, changing it from the *SMN1* signatures to the *SMN2* signatures. This gene conversion significantly compromised the normal *SMN1* gene function and resulted in the onset of the disease. Why then, would this gene conversion result in milder phenotypic severity? It is now known that this gene conversion on its own does not directly correlate with a milder phenotype,[48] but that it probably resulted in the increased copy number of the *SMN2* gene. It had been proposed that the increased *SMN2* gene copy is correlated with the milder phenotype.[49] In our laboratory, we were interested in studying the *SMN2* gene expression

and how its expression patterns correlate with the phenotypic variation. Unlike the *SMN1* gene, which is transcribed into mostly full-length mRNA, the *SMN2* produces only a small amount of full-length but a large amount of truncated RNA transcripts, lacking either exon 5 or 7, or both.[50] Consequently, in the cells of normal subjects (retaining both *SMN1* and *SMN2* copies), we measured more full-length transcript than the truncated transcripts. However, in the cells of SMA patients, the ratio is reversed because the spared *SMN2* gene produced more truncated transcripts than the full-length transcript. We found that the ratio of the full-length to truncated RNA transcript is correlated with disease severity; the higher the ratio (approaching that of normal subjects), the milder the disease phenotype.[50] Other groups have studied the *SMN* gene expression in human central nervous system, both in mRNA transcript and in full-length *SMN* protein levels. They found that the level of intact *SMN* protein is significantly decreased in the severe SMA phenotype.[51–53]

Subcellular Localization and Biochemical Function of the *SMN* Protein

One of the most intriguing progresses in SMA research is the subcellular localization of the *SMN* protein and its apparent biologic functions. The *SMN* gene encodes a novel protein that is ubiquitously expressed and is found in the cytoplasm and the cellular nucleus. *SMN* is co-localized with the intranuclear coilins named "gem," which stands for the gemini of the coil bodies.[54] *SMN* is tightly associated with a novel protein named SIP1 (*SMN* interacting protein-1, which is now named Gemin2). The *SMN* and SIP1/Gemin2 interact with several small nuclear ribonuclear proteins (snRNPs), including the Sm core proteins, and form a protein complex. It appears that the *SMN* protein functions as a platform, onto which the SIP1/Gemin2 binds to its N-terminus and the Sm proteins bind to its C-terminus.[55–56] The *SMN* protein plays an important role in the biogenesis of snRNPs. The *SMN* protein is required for the assembly of the snRNPs in the cytoplasm and the pre-mRNA splicing in the nucleus. A mutant protein lacking 27 amino acids in the N-terminus *(SMNΔN27)* prevents the assembly of the snRNPs in the cytoplasm and also inhibits pre-mRNA splicing in the nucleus. On the contrary, the wild-type *SMN* protein would stimulate pre-mRNA splicing in the same setting.[57–58] This suggests that the *SMN* protein plays an important role in the assembly of the cytosolic snRNPs, facilitating their transport into the nucleus, and allowing them to be regenerated into functional spliceosomal complex, which is required for the pre-mRNA splicing. Mutations in the exon 6 homo-oligomerization domain of the *SMN1* gene result in defects in self-association of the *SMN* protein. The degree of defects in *SMN* protein oligomerization is correlated with the severity of SMA

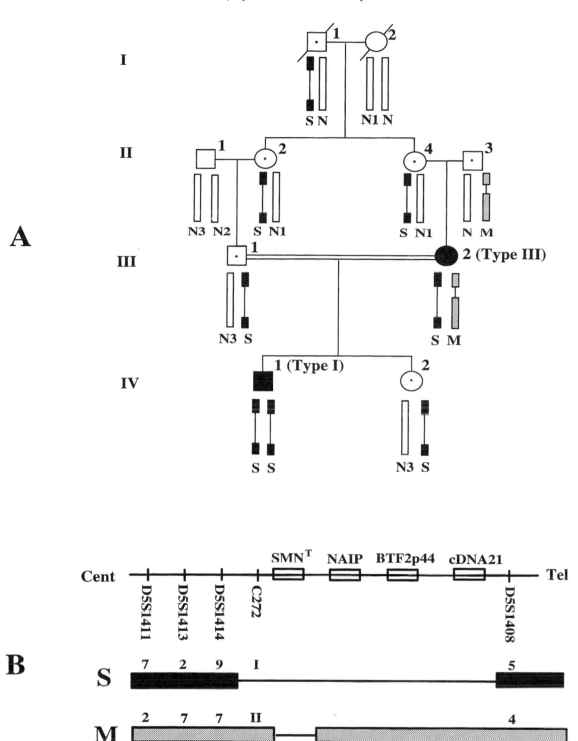

FIGURE 41–2. SMA phenotypic variation correlates with the degree of gene deletion. *A,* First-cousin marriage SMA family with SMA type III and SMA type I in two generations. Microsatellite and gene deletion analysis identified four unique normal chromosomal homologues *(unfilled bars N1, N2, N3)* and two disease homologues *(S and M)* in this multigenerational SMA family. The filled interrupted bars and the hatched interrupted bars represent a severe, or "S" homologue, and a mild or "M" homologue, respectively *(panel B).* Haplotype analysis confirms linkage to the chromosome 5q13 SMA gene locus. *B,* Genotyping of severe and mild chromosomal homologues. Human:hamster somatic cell hybrid techniques were used to separate the two chromosome 5 homologues from individual III-2. Human:hamster hybrid cell lines, haploid for each of the chromosome 5 homologues, were genotyped with microsatellite markers and gene-specific assays for markers and genes spanning the SMA region. The unique alleles identified by each microsatellite marker are indicated below each marker. The narrow bar indicates loss of the corresponding gene sequence. The filled or hatched bar indicates presence of the marker or gene sequence. The multilocus microsatellite marker C272 detected one allele on the severe and two alleles on the mild homologues. Deletion screen of *SMN* exons 7 and 8, *NAIP* exon 5, *BTF2p44* exon 7, and *cDNA21* sequences show the severe homologue S lacks all four gene-coding sequences, while the mild homologue M only lacks the *SMN* gene.

symptoms.[59] Mutation on exon 3 in the tudor domain results in defect in binding of *SMN* with other snRNPs.[60] Although these findings provide direct evidence that mutation of the *SMN* gene results in impairment of very important cellular functions such as pre-mRNA splicing, it is currently not known how this functional impairment affects specifically the spinal cord motor neurons.

CLINICAL IMPLICATION OF THE *SMN* GENE DISCOVERY

The identification of the *SMN* gene in 1995 represented a major breakthrough in SMA research. This discovery prompted a dramatic change in the clinical protocols used for the diagnosis of SMA, enabling us to detect mutant gene carriers and to perform direct and accurate prenatal diagnosis. More importantly, it provided us with the understanding of the molecular pathogenesis of SMA and allowed us to start thinking along the line of therapeutic interventions. This section will address some of these clinical implications of the identification of the *SMN* gene.

Molecular Diagnosis of SMA

Before the identification of the *SMN* gene, EMG and muscle biopsy were standard procedures needed for the diagnosis of SMA. After the initial identification of the gene locus in 1991, linkage analysis became available for the diagnosis of symptomatic relatives or prenatal diagnosis after one family member was diagnosed with SMA. This DNA diagnostic tool prevented the second affected family member from painful procedures such as EMG and muscle biopsy. However, this linkage method can be applied only after one affected member is diagnosed using conventional methods. The linkage analysis requires the availability of DNA samples from the affected persons and their parents and/or grandparents. This could be difficult if the first affected member expired early and the patient's blood or tissue was not preserved. Also, performing linkage analysis requires genotyping of several markers within the SMA genetic interval. This is somewhat laborious. With the identification of the *SMN* gene, more than 90% of SMA patients can be detected directly using a combined PCR-enzyme digestion assay[61] or an

allele-specific PCR (polymerase chain reaction) method.[62] This molecular diagnosis is rapid and specific. It eliminates the need for painful procedures such as EMG and muscle biopsy. The cost of the DNA mutation screen is much lower than that of the other diagnostic procedures. Compared with the molecular diagnostic tests for other known genetic disorders, *SMN* gene mutation screen is one of the most accurate diagnostic tests for a genetic disorder. In our laboratory, we have screened more than 200 SMA families using SSCP (single-stranded conformation polymorphism) method. The detection rate is over 90%, as shown in Table 41-1.

Carrier Detection

Carrier detection in SMA is complicated by the genomic duplication in the *SMN* gene region. The extreme sequence homology between the two *SMN* gene copies has made the screening of mutant gene carriers very difficult. While most SMA patients retain two mutant chromosomes, each with a DNA deletion flanking the *SMN1* gene, asymptomatic carriers retain only one mutant chromosome with the other being normally intact. In other monogenic disorders in which there is no gene duplication, detecting the carrier of a deleted gene can normally be done by quantitative measurement of one versus two gene copies in the genome. However, because of the duplication of the *SMN* genes, detecting a mutant *SMN1* gene carrier is much more complicated because PCR amplification of the *SMN1* fragment would often amplify the *SMN2* copies. This confounds the assessment of the *SMN1* gene copies. Since the presence of the *SMN2* gene does not determine the disease state, specific amplification and quantified measurement of the *SMN1* gene is needed. Thomas Prior's laboratory first developed a careful quantitative method of *SMN1* gene dosage using the PCR-densitometry method, which achieved a relatively high specificity and accuracy.[63] However, this method is fairly laborious and involved radioactive material for labeling the probes. Our lab developed an allele-specific PCR that can specifically amplify the *SMN1* gene copy. We utilized the sequence variation on the sixth base pair on exon 7 of the *SMN* genes (C for *SMN1* and T for *SMN2*) and added a second base-pair mismatch on the adjacent sequences to

TABLE 41-1.   SSCP Analysis of Exons 7 and 8 of SMN1

Exons	Type I (N = 62a)	Type II (N = 36)	Type III (N = 34)	Total SMA (N = 132*)	Control (N = 48)
7-/8-[b]	56[c](90%)	32 (89%)	23 (68%)	111 (84%)	0 (0%)
7+/8+	4 (6.4%)	1 (2.8%)	5 (15%)	10 (7.6%)	48 (100%)
7-/8+	2 (3.2%)	3 (8.3%)	6 (18%)	11 (8.3%)	0 (0%)
7+/8-	0 (0%)	0 (0%)	0 (0%)	0 (0%)	0 (0%)

*all cases are diagnosed with EMG and muscle biopsy.
[a]number of families studied.
[b]absence (-) or presence (+) of exons 7 or 8 of SMN1.
[c]number of families observed to have such genotype.

design allele-specific primers that allow specific amplification of the *SMN1* copy. The PCR primers are designed according to the diagram in Figure 41–3.

We then applied a TaqMan technology (a real-time quantitative PCR method using fluorescent labeling) to quantify the *SMN1* gene copy. This method has allowed a fairly accurate prediction of the mutant gene carriers.[64] Recently, other laboratories have also developed similar techniques for carrier detection.[65–67] This is an area in SMA research that will need continuing improvements in order to achieve a wide applicability in the clinical setting.

Prenatal Diagnosis and Genetic Counseling

Without accurate prenatal diagnosis, parents of an SMA child were often hesitant to have another child prior to the identification of the *SMN* gene. With a 25% chance of having another affected child, many parents opted not to take the chance. With the identification of the *SMN* gene, it is now possible to perform an accurate and rapid diagnosis of SMA prenatally. Both chorionic villi sampling (CVS) and amniocentesis can be performed in early gestational age and the affective status of the fetus determined. This provides the parents with an option of whether or not to continue the pregnancy. For those parents who do not want to face the possibility of having to terminate a pregnancy, pre-implantation assay is now available. Using in vitro fertilization (IVF) technique, the fertilized ovum is allowed to grow through a few cellular divisions in cultured media. The embryos are then biopsied and a few cells within the blastomeres are collected. The cells within the blastomeres are tested for the *SMN1* gene mutation. After completion of the mutation assay, the embryos are then implanted using a single-cell allele-specific PCR method. This procedure is highly technical and is available only in certain research centers.

CREATING A MOUSE MODEL FOR SMA

Another exciting progress in SMA research is the success of creating a mouse model for SMA. With the availability of a mouse model, we can now ask many questions that are otherwise impossible. Creating the mouse model for SMA was an intriguing process due to a unique feature of the mouse *SMN* that is not seen in human *SMN*. We will discuss this process in this section.

The Mouse *SMN* Gene

Unlike the human *SMN*, which is present in duplicated copies on chromosome 5, the mouse genome contains only a single copy of *SMN* in a syntenic region on chromosome 13.[69] The mouse *SMN* also contains 9 exons and

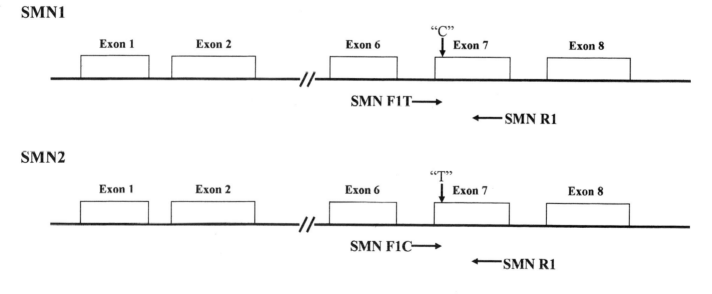

SMN F1C: 5' CTTCCTTTATTTTCCTTACAGGGCTT**C 3'**

SMN F1T: 5' CTTCCTTTATTTTCCTTACAGGGCTT**T 3'**

SMN R1: 5' CAAACCATAAAGTTTTACAAAAGTAAGATTCAC 3'

FIGURE 41–3. Allele Specific PCR. The allele-specific primers *SMN F1C* and *SMN F1T* were designed by utilizing the gene-specific *SMN* exon 7 polymorphism (nucleotide C for SMN1 and T for *SMN2*). The polymorphic site was used at the 3' end of the forward primers. Furthermore, a second base-pair mismatch (nucleotide C) was created at 4 bp from this polymorphic site to promote specific annealing and extension. These primers enable a specific amplification of either *SMN1* or *SMN2* gene copy.

is 83% homologous to the human *SMN1* in its open reading frame. There appears to be no alternative splicing in the mouse because only a full-length transcript of ~1.4 kb is observed in all tissues. The predicted mouse *SMN* protein is 82% identical to human *SMN*.[69] It is proposed that, in the evolutionary timetable, the duplication of the *SMN* gene in primates occurred after the splitting of the rodents and primates. But the human *SMN2* gene appears only after the splitting of the nonhuman primates and *Homo sapiens*. This is because the signatures of the human *SMN2* gene copies are not seen in nonhuman primates such as chimpanzees, despite the existence of multiple copies of the *SMN* gene in their genome.[70]

The Mouse Model for SMA

Initial attempts to create an SMA mouse model were met with surprises. The homozygous knockout of the *SMN* gene (*SMN−/−*) resulted in early embryonic lethality.[71] The embryo underwent massive cell death and degeneration at 4 to 5 days gestational age. On the contrary, the heterozygous *SMN+/−* mice were phenotypically normal. This finding suggested that the mouse *SMN* gene is essential for early embryonic development. However, a 50% reduction of the gene dosage is not enough to cause measurable symptoms. This finding also suggested that different strategies other than the conventional knockout procedure would be needed in order to create a mouse model for human SMA. On further comparison of the genomic structure between the human and mouse *SMN* genes, it is clear that the human *SMN2* gene (which is missing in the mouse genome) must have played an important role in sustaining early human embryonic development. This is because human SMA patients, who are homozygously missing the *SMN1* gene but retain at least one copy of the *SMN2* gene, survive through the embryonic stage. Yet mouse *SMN−/−* embryos lacking the *SMN2* gene are not viable. Therefore, in order to create a mouse model with symptoms resembling human SMA, one would need to provide *SMN−/−* mouse embryos with at least a copy of human SMN2 gene. This would enable the survival of the *SMN−/−* mouse embryos, yet produce symptoms of human SMA because the human *SMN2* would produce only mostly truncated transcript and an insufficient amount of intact *SMN* protein. Indeed, using this new strategy, researchers in Taiwan were able to establish the first mouse model for SMA.[72] They first generated the transgenic knocked-in lines with a genomic fragment containing one to three copies of human *SMN2* gene. These founder lines were then crossed with the *SMN+/−* line to produce the *SMN+/−SMN2* lines. These F1 progenies were then allowed to intercross or backcross with the *SMN+/−* line to produce the *SMN−/−SMN2* progenies. These *SMN−/−SMN2* progenies exhibit human SMA symptoms both clinically and histopathologically. Interestingly, the severity of the symptoms is closely correlated with the number of *SMN2* gene copies retained in

the mouse genome. The less the gene copy the more severe the phenotype. The severe phenotype resembles human type 1 SMA in both early onset of symptoms and the paucity of the *SMN* protein in both skeletal muscle and spinal cords. Using similar strategy, two other research groups also generated mouse models with clinical symptoms and histopathology resembling human SMA.[73,74]

CURRENT PROGRESS TOWARD SMA GENE THERAPY

Another exciting aspect of SMA research is the possibility of designing therapeutic protocols using the unique features of the *SMN* gene. The genomic duplication of the human *SMN* gene offers an excellent opportunity for therapeutic intervention using molecular genetic techniques. This section will discuss progress in these areas.

Regulation of the *SMN2* Gene Expression

Unlike most monogenic disorders in which a single gene defect is responsible for the disease onset, the SMA pathogenesis involves two gene copies—the *SMN1* and *SMN2*. While most SMA patients are homozygously missing the functional *SMN1* gene, all of them retain at least one copy of the *SMN2* gene. The presence of this "spared" *SMN2* gene in all SMA patients provides a unique opportunity for us to design a therapeutic protocol utilizing this spared *SMN2* gene. In normal individuals, the *SMN1* gene is responsible for the production of a sufficient amount of intact *SMN* protein. However, in SMA patients, the retained *SMN2* gene is able to produce only a small amount of the *SMN* protein. This is not sufficient to sustain the survival and normal functioning of the spinal cord motor neurons. Therefore, a logical strategy would be to augment the production of intact *SMN* protein by the retained *SMN2* gene in order to restore the normal function of the motor neurons in SMA patients.

In order to restore the *SMN2* gene expression, it is crucial to identify the regulatory mechanism that distinguishes the expression patterns between the *SMN1* and *SMN2* genes. Researchers have shown that a single base-pair difference on the +6 position of the exon 7 between the two *SMN* copies is sufficient to distinguish the two expression patterns.[75] The nucleotide at the +6 position of exon 7 on the *SMN1* gene is a crucial component of a short exon splicing enhancer (ESE) sequence.[76] This ESE, recognized by the splicing factors, facilitates the active inclusion of exon 7 during *SMN1* pre-mRNA splicing. Disruption of this ESE sequence, as in the case of *SMN2* that harbors a C to T change (C6T) at this position, results in skipping this exon. Further studies showed that this ESE was recognized by a splicing factor SF2/ASF during mRNA splicing.[77] These investigators introduced a second mutation at the +11 position of exon 7 (A to G transition) in order to recreate a high-score motif for the

SF2/ASF recognition. This resulted in restoration of the exon 7 splicing and the production of an intact transcript by the *SMN2* gene. These studies convincingly demonstrated that the C to T change on the +6 position of exon 7 results in exon skipping of *SMN2* during its transcription.

Progress in the Search for Therapeutic Agents for SMA

The identification of a crucial splicing enhancer sequence (ESE) on exon 7 of the *SMN1* gene provided an ideal substrate for therapeutic strategy. The next logical step was to identify splicing factors that interact with this splicing enhancer sequence, hoping that increasing the availability of these splicing factors may enable enhancement of intact protein production during the *SMN2* gene expression. One group of researchers used a minigene construct to screen for a series of splicing factors that could augment the production of a full-length *SMN*. They found that overexpression of the human β_1 isoform of the Tra2 splicing factor (Htra2-β1) stimulated inclusion of exon 7 during mRNA splicing and was able to restore the production of a full-length *SMN* transcript in cells containing only the *SMN2* gene.[78] This finding provided the first hope that the transcription of the *SMN2* gene could be modified. The Htra2-β1 is an endogenous splicing factor and is known to be active in vivo. However, increasing the level of Htra2-β1 activity in a living organism is relatively difficult. Alternatively, screening for exogenous compounds that can stimulate the inclusion of exon 7 during *SMN2* gene transcription would be more direct and efficient. Two research groups have identified two compounds that stimulate the production of full-length *SMN* protein by the *SMN2* gene.[79,80] Andreassi et al screened a library of chemicals and identified aclarubicin, a compound that induced incorporation of exon 7 into the *SMN2* transcript in fibroblast from type I SMA patients. Treatment of aclarubicin also restored production of full-length *SMN* protein in motor-neuron–like cells.[79] Chang et al reported another compound, sodium butyrate, which modified the *SMN2* expression and effectively increased the production of full-length *SMN* protein in SMA lymphoid cell lines.[80] This group also used their SMA mice to conduct in vivo therapeutic trials of sodium butyrate. They reported that oral sodium butyrate treatment decreased the birth rate of severe SMA-like mice by the homozygous $SMN^{-/-}$ mothers who retain variable copies of the human *SMN2* gene. Oral treatments of type II and type III mice with sodium butyrate resulted in milder symptoms and longer life spans. Sodium butyrate appears to stimulate the inclusion of exon 7 in *SMN2* transcription via increasing the production of splicing-factor SR proteins (Ser-Arg proteins).[80]

Considerations for Future Gene Therapy in SMA

The rapid progress in recent SMA research provided us with good insight into the molecular pathogenesis of this disorder. This wealth of knowledge also enabled us to design a therapeutic approach that is scientifically based and likely to be successful. The fact that the *SMN2* gene can be modified to simulate the *SMN1* gene function in cultured SMA cells and in SMA-like mice has enlightened a high hope for clinical applications of this knowledge. The two chemical compounds, aclarubicin and sodium butyrate, which have been shown to modify the *SMN2* gene expression, are obviously the prime candidates for use in clinical trials. In the case of sodium butyrate, oral ingestion of moderate dose in SMA-like mice did not seem to create any obvious adverse effect. As both cell lines and animal models are now available for drug screening using high throughput technology, more compounds will surely be identified in the near future. These compounds will soon be ready for human clinical trials. As this is sure to happen in the near future, we should think about the directions and issues that may rise in this next stage of SMA research.

The first issue is when to start the treatment. It may seem obvious that we should start as soon as a child is diagnosed. However, in the case of a prenatal diagnosis, can we treat patients prenatally, and since we do not know the clinical phenotype, how do we measure the outcome of the treatment? The second issue is how long the patient should receive treatment. It seems likely that any compound will have to be used on a long-term basis. The endogenous *SMN2* gene will need a continuous "reminder" for it to produce the full-length *SMN* protein in order to sustain the cellular function of the spinal cord motor neurons. How long should we observe to be sure there are no significant side effects from long-term usage of the compound? The third issue is how we measure clinical efficacy and outcome. In the case of type I SMA, it seems obvious that survival would be one indicator for clinical efficacy. However, survival should not be the only indicator of clinical efficacy in these patients. We should also consider their quality of life. Will it be possible that once *SMN* gene function is restored that type I SMA patients will not merely survive but also gain adequate strength to perform their activities of daily living? In all three clinical subtypes of SMA patients, an objective measurement of motor functions will be needed in order to obtain and compare quantitatively the efficacy of the various compounds. A standardized device will be needed for this purpose that can be used by multicenter research groups.

In conclusion, researchers in SMA have made very impressive progress over the last decade. Many exciting breakthroughs have taken us from identifying the SMA gene locus to cloning the *SMN* gene, from identifying the subcellular localization of the *SMN* protein to elucidating its putative functions in pre-mRNA splicing and spliceosomal regeneration, and from identifying the SMA mouse model to localizing the crucial enhancer-splicing sequence on exon 7 of the *SMN1* gene. Several reagents have been identified and have been shown to modify the

SMN2 gene expression. These discoveries have prepared us for a very exciting stage of SMA research—the clinical therapeutic trials. It is foreseeable that care for SMA patients will be drastically improved within the next decade because we can improve their quality of life as well as sustain their lives.

REFERENCES

1. Pern JH: Infantile motor neuron diseases. In Rowland LP (ed): Advances in Neurology. New York, Raven Press, 1982, pp 121–130.

2. Roy L, Dubowitz V, Wolman L: Ultrastructure of muscle in infantile spinal muscular atrophies. J Neurol Sci 1971;12:219–232.

3. Pearn JN: The gene frequency of acute Werdnig-Hoffmann disease (SMA type I): A total population survey in northeast England. J Med Genet 1973;10: 260–265.

4. Pearn JN, Wilson J: Acute Werdnig-Hoffmann disease, acute infantile spinal muscular atrophy. Arch Dis Child 1973;48:425–430.

5. Pearn JN, Gardner-Medwin D, Wilson J: A clinical study of chronic childhood spinal muscular atrophy: A review of 141 cases. J Neurosci 1978;37:227–248.

6. Munsat TL, Davies KE: Workshop report: International SMA Consortium meeting. Neuromuscul Disord 1992;2:423–428.

7. Richieri-Costa A, Rogatko A, Levisky R, et al: Autosomal dominant late adult spinal muscular atrophy, type Finkel. Am J Med Genet 1981;9:119–128.

8. Meadows JC, Marsden CD: A distal form of chronic spinal muscular atrophy. Neurology 1969;19: 53–58.

9. McEntagart M, Norton N, William H, et al: Localization of the gene for distal hereditary motor neuronopathy VII (dHMN-VII) to chromosome 2q14. Am J Hum Genet 2001;68:1270–1276.

10. Christodoulou K, Kyriakides T, Hristova AH, et al: Mapping of a distal form of spinal muscular atrophy with upper limb predominance to chromosome 7p. Hum Mol Genet 1995;4:1629–1632.

11. Viollet L, Barois A, Rebeiz JG, et al: Mapping of autosomal recessive chronic distal spinal muscular atrophy to chromosome 11q13. Ann Neurol 2002;51: 585–592.

12. Van der Vleuten AJW, Van Ravenswaaij-Arts CMA, Frijns CJM, et al: Localisation of the gene for a dominant congenital spinal muscular atrophy predominantly affecting the lower limbs to chromosome 12q23–q24. Eur J Hum Genet 1998;6:376–382.

13. Guglielmo GD, Brahe C, Di Muzio A, Uncini A: Benign monomelic amyotrophies of upper and lower limb are not associated to deletions of survival motor neuron gene. J Neurosci 1996;141:111–113.

14. La Spada AR, Wilson EM, Lubaha DB, et al: Androgen receptor gene mutations in X-linked spinal and bulbar muscular atrophy. Nature 1991,352:77–79.

15. Kobayashi H, Baumbach L, Matise TC, et al: A gene for a severe lethal form of X-linked arthrogryposis (X-linked infantile spinal muscular atrophy) maps to human chromosome Xp11.3-q11.2. Hum Mol Genet 1995;4:1213–1216.

16. Brzustowicz LM, Lehner T, Castilla LH, et al: Genetic mapping of chronic childhood-onset spinal muscular atrophy to chromosome 5q11.2-13.3. Nature 1990;344:540–541.

17. Gilliam TC, Brzustowicz LM, Castilla LH, et al: Genetic homogeneity between acute and chronic forms of spinal muscular atrophy. Nature 1990;345:823–825.

18. Melki J, Abdelhak S, Sheth P, et al. Gene for chronic proximal spinal muscular atrophies maps to chromosome 5q. Nature 1990;344:767–768.

19. Brzustowicz LM, Kleyn PW, Boyce FM, et al: Fine-mapping of the spinal muscular atrophy locus to a region flanked by MAP1B and D5S6. Genomics 1992;13:991–998.

20. Soares VM, Brzustowicz LM, Kleyn PW, et al: Refinement of the spinal muscular atrophy locus to the interval between D5S435 and MAP1B. Genomics 1993;15:365–371.

21. Clermont O, Burlet P, Burglen L, et al: Use of genetic and physical mapping to locate the spinal muscular atrophy locus between two new highly polymorphic DNA markers. Am J Hum Genet 1994;54:687–694.

22. Kleyn PW, Wang CH, Lien LL, et al: Construction of a yeast artificial chromosome contig spanning the spinal muscular atrophy disease gene region. Proc Natl Acad Sci USA 1993;90: 6801–6805.

23. Wang CH, Kleyn PW, Vitale E, et al: Refinement of the spinal muscular atrophy locus by genetic and physical mapping. Am J Hum Genet 1995;56:202–209.

24. Carpten JD, DiDonato CJ, Ingraham SE, et al: A YAC contig of the region containing the spinal muscular atrophy gene: Identification of an unstable region. Genomics 1994;24:51–356.

25. Francis MJ, Morrison KE, Campbell L, et al: A contig of non-chimaeric YACs containing the spinal muscular atrophy gene in 5q13. Hum Mol Genet 1993; 2:1161–1167.

26. Wirth B, Voosen D, Rohig D, et al: Fine mapping and narrowing of the genetic interval of the spinal muscular atrophy region by linkage studies. Genomics 1993,15:113–118.

27. Burghes AHM, Ingraham SE, McLean M, et al: A multicopy dinucleotide marker that maps close to the spinal muscular atrophy gene. Genomics 1994;21: 394–402.

28. Theodosiou AM, Morrison KE, Nesbit AM, et al: Complex repetitive arrangements of gene sequence in the candidate region of the spinal muscular atrophy gene in 5q13. Am J Hum Genet 1994,55:1209–1217.

29. Selig S, Bruno S, Scharf JM, et al. Expressed cadherin pseudogenes are localized to the critical region of

the spinal muscular atrophy gene. Proc Natl Acad Sci U S A 1995;92:3702–3706.

30. Melki J, Lefebvre S, Burglen L, et al: De novo and inherited deletions of the 5q13 region in spinal muscular atrophies. Science 1994;264:1474–1477.

31. McLean MD, Roy N, MacKenzie AE, et al: Two 5q13 simple tandem repeat loci are in linkage disequilibrium with type I spinal muscular atrophy. Hum Mol Genet 1994;3:1951–1956.

32. Lefebvre S, Burglen L, Reboullet S, et al: Identification and characterization of a spinal muscular atrophy-determining gene. Cell 1995;80:155–165.

33. Rodrigues NR, Owen N, Talbot K, et al: Deletions in the survival motor neuron gene on 5q13 in autosomal recessive spinal muscular atrophy. Hum Mol Genet 1995;4:631–634.

34. Cobben JM, van der Steege G, Grootscholten P, et al: Deletions of the survival motor neuron gene in unaffected siblings of patients with spinal muscular atrophy. Am J Hum Genet 1995;57:805–808.

35. Hahen E, Forkert R, Merke C, et al: Molecular analysis of candidate genes on chromosome 5q13 in autosomal recessive spinal muscular atrophy: Evidence of homozygous deletions of the SMN gene in unaffected individuals. Hum Mol Genet 1995;4.1927–1933.

36. Bussaglia E, Clermont O, Tizzano F, et al: A frame-shift deletion in the survival motor neuron gene in Spanish spinal muscular atrophy patients. Nat Genet 1995;11:335–337.

37. Wang CH, Xu J, Carter TA, et al: Characterization of survival motor neuron (SMN^T) gene deletions in asymptomatic carriers of spinal muscular atrophy. Hum Mol Genet 1996;5:359–365.

38. Wang CH, Bruinsma P, Papendick BD, et al: Identification of a novel mutation of the SMN^T gene in two siblings with spinal muscular atrophy. Neurogenetics 1998,1.273–276.

39. Lefebvre S, Burglen L, Frezal J, et al: The role of the SMN gene in proximal spinal muscular atrophy. Hum Mol Genet 1998;7:1531–1536.

40. Roy N, Mahadevan MS, McLean M, et al: The gene for neuronal apoptosis inhibitory protein is partially deleted in individuals with spinal muscular atrophy. Cell 1995;80:167–178.

41. Carter TA, Bonnemann CG, Wang CH, et al: A multicopy transcription-repair gene, BTF2p44, maps to the SMA region and demonstrates SMA associated deletions. Hum Mol Genet 1997;6:229–236.

42. Scharf JM, Endrizzi MG, Wetter A, et al: Identification of a candidate modifying gene for spinal muscular atrophy by comparative genomics. Nat Genet 1998;20:83–86.

43. Wang CH, Carter TA, Das, K, et al: Extensive DNA deletion associated with severe disease alleles on SMA homologues. Ann Neurol 1997;42:41–49.

44. van der Steege G, Grootscholten PM, Cobben JM, et al: Apparent gene conversions involving the SMN gene in the region of the spinal muscular atrophy locus on chromosome 5. Am J Hum Genet 1996;59:834–838.

45. Hahnen E, Scholing J, Rudnik-Schoneborn S, Wirth B. Hybrid survival motor neuron genes in patients with autosomal recessive spinal muscular atrophy: New insights into molecular mechanisms responsible for the disease. Am J Hum Genet 1996;59:1057–1065.

46. DiDonato CJ, Ingraham SE, Mendell JR, et al: Deletion and conversion in spinal muscular atrophy patients: Is there a relationship to severity? Ann Neurol 1997;41:230–237.

47. Campbell L, Potter A, Ignatius J, et al: Genomic variation and gene conversion in spinal muscular atrophy: Implications for disease process and clinical phenotype. Am J Hum Genet 1997;61:40–50.

48. Talbot K, Rodrigues NR, Ignatius J, et al: Gene conversion at the SMN locus in autosomal recessive spinal muscular atrophy does not predict a mild phenotype. Neuromuscul Disord 1997;7:198–201.

49. Velasco E, Valero C, Valero A, et al: Molecular analysis of the SMN and NAIP genes in Spanish spinal muscular atrophy (SMA) families and correlation between number of copies of cBCD541 and SMA phenotype. Hum Mol Genet 1996,5.257–263.

50. Gavrilov DK, Shi X, Das K, et al: Differential SMN2 expression associated with SMA severity. Nat Genet 1998;20:230–231.

51. Lefebvre S, Burlet P, Liu Q, et al: Correlation between severity and SMN protein level in spinal muscular atrophy. Nat Genet 1997;6:265–269.

52. Battaglia G, Princivalle A, Forti F, et al: Expression of the SMN gene, the spinal muscular atrophy determining gene, in the mammalian central nervous system. Hum Mol Genet 1997;6:1961–1971.

53. Burlet P, Huber C, Bertrandy S, et al: The distribution of SMN protein complex in human fetal tissues and its alteration in spinal muscular atrophy. Hum Mol Genet 1998;12:1927–1933.

54. Liu Q, Dreyfuss G: A novel nuclear structure containing the survival of motor neurons protein. EMBO J 1996;15:3555–3565.

55. Liu Q, Fischer U, Wang F, Dreyfuss G: The spinal muscular atrophy disease gene product, SMN, and its associated protein SIP1 are in a complex with spliceosomal snRNP proteins. Cell 1997;90:1013–1021.

56. Fischer U, Liu Q, Dreyfuss G: The SMN-SIP1 complex has an essential role in spliceosomal snRNP biogenesis. Cell 1997;90:1023–1029.

57. Pellizzoni L, Kataoka N, Charroux B, Dreyfuss G: A novel function for SMN, the spinal muscular atrophy disease gene product, in pre-mRNA splicing. Cell 1998;95:615–624.

58. Pellizzoni L, Charroux B, Rappsilber J, et al: A functional interaction between the survival motor neuron complex and RNA polymerase II. J Cell Biol 2001;152:75–85.

59. Lorson CL, Strasswimmer J, Yao JM, et al: SMN oligomerization defect correlates with spinal muscular atrophy severity. Nat Genet 1998;19:63–66.

60. Pellizzoni L, Charroux B, Dreyfuss G: SMN mutants of spinal muscular atrophy patients are defective in binding to snRNP proteins. Proc Nat Acad Sci U S A 1999;96:11167–11172.

61. Van der Steege G, Grootscholten PM, van der Vlies P, et al: PCR-based DNA test to confirm clinical diagnosis of autosomal recessive spinal muscular atrophy. Lancet 1995;345:985–986.

62. Ichikawa S, Wang, CH: Differential amplification of the SMN gene copies by allele-specific PCR: A new method for rapid diagnosis of spinal muscular atrophy. Am J Hum Genet 1998;63:A232.

63. McAndrew PE, Parsons DW, Simard LR: Identification of proximal spinal muscular atrophy carriers and patients by analysis of SMN^T and SMN^C gene copy number. Am J Hum Genet 1997;60:1411–1422.

64. Ichikawa S, Chen X, Kwok PY, Wang CH: A rapid and accurate detection of the SMA gene carriers using real-time quantitative PCR. Am J Hum Genet 1999;65:216.

65. Scheffer H, Cobben JM, Mensink RG, et al: SMA carrier testing—validation of hemizygous SMN exon 7 deletion test for the identification of proximal spinal muscular atrophy carriers and patients with a single allele deletion. Euro J Hum Genet 2000;8:79–86.

66. Saugier-Veber P, Drouot N, Lefebvre S, et al: Detection of heterozygous SMN1 deletions in SMA families using a simple fluorescent multiplex PCR method. J Med Genet 2001;38:240–243.

67. Feldkotter M, Schwarzer V, Wirth R, et al: Quantitative analyses of SMN1 and SMN2 based on real-time lightCycler PCR: Fast and highly reliable carrier testing and prediction of severity of spinal muscular atrophy. Am J Hum Genet 2002;70:358–368.

68. Moutou C, Gardes N, Rongieres C, et al: Allele-specific amplification for preimplantation genetic diagnosis (PGD) of spinal muscular atrophy. Prenat Diagn 2001;21:498–503.

69. DiDonato CJ, Chen XN, Noya D, et al: Cloning, characterization, and copy number of the murine survival motor neuron gene: Homolog of the spinal muscular atrophy-determining gene. Genome Res 1997;7:339–352.

70. Rochette CF, Gilbert N, Simard LR: SMN gene duplication and the emergence of the SMN2 gene occurred in distinct hominids: SMN2 is unique to *Homo sapiens*. Hum Genet 2001;108:255–266.

71. Schrank B, Götz R, Gunnersen JM, et al: Inactivation of the survival motor neuron gene, a candidate gene for human spinal muscular atrophy, leads to massive cell death in early mouse embryos. PNAS 1997;94:9920–9925.

72. Hsieh-Li HM, Chang JG, Jong YJ, et al: A mouse model for spinal muscular atrophy. Nat Genet 2000;24:66–70.

73. Monani UR, Sendtner M, Coovert DD, et al: The human centromeric survival motor neuron gene *(SMN2)* rescues embryonic lethality in $Smn^{-/-}$ mice and results in a mouse with spinal muscular atrophy. Hum Mol Genet 2000;9:333–339.

74. Jablonka S, Schrank B, Kralewski M, ct al: Reduced survival motor neuron *(Smn)* gene dose in mice leads to motor neuron degeneration: An animal model for spinal muscular atrophy type III. Hum Mol Genet 2000;9:341–346.

75. Lorson CL, Hahnen E, Androphy EJ, Wirth B: A single nucleotide in the SMN gene regulates splicing and is responsible for spinal muscular atrophy. Proc Nat Acad Sci U S A 1999;96:6307–6311.

76. Lorson CL, Androphy EJ. An exonic enhancer is required for inclusion of an essential exon in the SMA-determining gene SMN. Hum Mol Genet 2000;9:259–265.

77. Cartegni L, Krainer AR: Disruption of an SF2/ASF-dependent exonic splicing enhancer in SMN2 causes spinal muscular atrophy in the absence of SMN1. Nat Genet 2000;30:377–384.

78. Hofmann Y, Lorson CL, Stamm S, et al: Htra2-beta 1 stimulates an exonic splicing enhancer and can restore full-length SMN expression to survival motor neuron 2 (SMN2). Proc Nat Acad Sci U S A 2000;97:9618–9623.

79. Andreassi C, Jarecki J, Zhou J, et al: Aclarubicin treatment restores SMN levels to cells derived from type I spinal muscular atrophy patients. Hum Mol Genet 2001;10:2841–2849.

80. Chang JG, Hsieh-Li HM, Jong YJ, et al: Treatment of spinal muscular atrophy by sodium butyrate. Proc Nat Acad Sci U S A 2001;98:9808–9813.

42

Dystrophinopathies

Eric P. Hoffman

Dystrophinopathies are the most common of the muscular dystrophies. The high incidence in all world populations is the result of a very high de novo mutation rate (1:10,000 sperm and oocytes in all individuals sustain new mutations of the 2.5 million base pair dystrophin gene). The dystrophin gene is X-linked. Mutations can cause complete loss of dystrophin and result in Duchenne muscular dystrophy (DMD) in males; partial loss of function resulting in milder variants in males (Becker muscular dystrophy, cardiomyopathies, restricted muscle involvement, asymptomatic elevations of serum creatine kinase); or mosaic expression in females, typically resulting in asymptomatic carrier state. However, a range of clinical symptoms can occur due to preferential use of the abnormal X chromosome. Dystrophin is a major component of the membrane cytoskeleton, where the dystrophin/sarcoglycan/dystroglycan/laminin complex is partially redundant with the vinculin/integrin/laminin complex. The dystrophin membrane complex imparts structural integrity to the myofiber plasma membrane, but it also has direct and indirect signal transduction roles. While dystrophin deficiency is manifested biochemically from fetal life, typically it takes many years before patients show overt weakness, after which progression to an early death often takes 15 or more years. The pathophysiologic cascades downstream of dystrophin-deficiency are complex, and include ischemia, immune cell infiltration, fibrosis, and failure of regeneration. Aspects of these cascades appear species-specific, with dystrophin-deficient dogs, cats, and mice showing different phenotypes. Experimental therapeutics is rapidly expanding, with promising results in animal models in both gene delivery and interventional pharmacology. A key to progress in therapeutics will be to enter all children into clinical trials upon diagnosis.

DUCHENNE MUSCULAR DYSTROPHY

Clinical and Diagnostic Features

The most common and devastating of the muscular dystrophies is DMD, named after a French physician who wrote extensively about the disease in the late 1800s. Recent research into the history of the disease, however, has established that a British physician, Meryon, elegantly described the disorder and its inheritance pattern some years earlier, and in fact brought the disease to Duchenne's attention.[1] The disease is one of the most common inherited lethal disorders of humans (1:3500 males, although incidence has been decreasing in developed countries due to recent preventive measures) and affects all world populations equally. Owing to the very high mutation rate of the gene, many cases are sporadic. When inherited, the disease shows an X-linked recessive pattern, with approximately half the male offspring of a carrier mother being affected.

Typically, affected boys present at age 4 to 5 years with proximal muscle weakness and calf hypertrophy. It is possible to detect patients earlier due to delay in motor milestones and elevated muscle enzyme concentrations in serum. Proximal weakness manifests as difficulty keeping up with peers, awkward running, and difficulty climbing stairs. The classic Gowers maneuver is typical: in rising from the floor, the child uses the hands on his or her knees to push the body to a standing position. Progressive proximal weakness then leads to excessive lordosis and a waddling gait. Progression is relatively stereotypical: boys have increasing difficulty ambulating and become confined to a wheelchair between ages 7 and 15 years (usually around age 11 years). The hip-girdle weakness is initially more dramatic, although weakness of the shoulder girdle soon follows. Many muscles, particularly those of the calves, appear unusually large and can have a doughy consistency early in the disease progression. This enlarged muscle mass has traditionally been dubbed *pseudohypertrophy* due to the concomitant muscle weakness and to the connective tissue proliferation seen in muscle biopsies. However, correlations with animal models suggest that this represents true hypertrophy of muscle fibers, at least in the early stage of the disease.

Strength is continuously lost, and mobility is gradually restricted due to muscle wasting and contractures, although facial musculature and speech are spared. Contractures can be more disabling than weakness, with Achilles tendon contractures leading to toe walking and instability. Physical therapy and tendon releases attempt to compensate for the contractures. Wheelchair-bound patients continue to develop disabling contractures, and spinal fusions are often indicated to correct scoliosis. Patients usually succumb to respiratory failure by the end of the second decade, although age 30 to 40 years is attainable if the patient is mechanically ventilated.

Patients can show other symptoms in addition to skeletal muscle involvement. The heart is affected: there is first hypertrophic, then dilated cardiomyopathy, and progressive fibrosis is most pronounced in the basolateral free wall of the left ventricle. A minority of Duchenne dystrophy patients die of overt heart failure, although the progressive weakness decreases the demands on the compromised heart muscle. It is conceivable that preservation of skeletal muscle function would lead to a higher incidence of heart failure in adolescent males. Approximately 30% of patients show nonprogressive mental retardation that affects verbal more than other functions. The mental retardation may result from hypersensitivity of the central nervous system to ischemic insults, which are most likely to happen in the perinatal period.[2] Smooth muscle dysfunction is present, but it is only rarely symptomatic.

All patients show grossly elevated serum CK levels from birth (more than 50 times the upper limit of normal), and transaminases and lactate dehydrogenase are also elevated. Although the transaminases almost certainly derive from muscle tissue, occasionally these elevated serum enzyme levels mislead clinicians to investigate liver dysfunction in still asymptomatic patients. Neonatal screening for DMD is highly efficient at detecting all patients at birth,[3] but the current lack of effective therapy has made screening programs controversial and generally frowned upon (despite the value of genetic counseling for the family, and avoidance of multiple affected siblings born before the oldest is detected clinically).

Pathology

Muscle biopsy shows features consistent with a dystrophic myopathy, including fiber size variation, eosinophilic hypercontracted fibers, increased endomysial connective tissue (fibrosis), and occasional areas of overt necrosis with macrophage infiltration (Fig. 42–1A, B). The histopathology changes as a function of age, with young patients showing less fibrosis and less dramatic changes in muscle, whereas end-stage muscle shows large numbers of very small fibers that have failed to fully regenerate, extensive endomysial fibrosis, and a few remaining hypertrophic fibers (see Fig. 42–1A, B). No histopathologic feature is diagnostic for DMD, but muscle biopsies can be tested for dystrophin protein content, which is considered diagnostic.[4] DMD is caused by absence, or near absence, of dystrophin, a component of the myofiber membrane cytoskeleton[5] (Fig. 42–1C, D). In the past, electromyography (EMG) was a standard diagnostic tool, but the findings are relatively nonspecific, and EMG is less commonly employed today.

BECKER MUSCULAR DYSTROPHY

Clinical and Diagnostic Features

Becker muscular dystrophy (BMD) derives its eponym from Emil Becker, a contemporary German physician who described extensive X-linked pedigrees with a form of muscular dystrophy that was less severe than DMD. Unlike DMD, the disease was often compatible with reproduction, and all daughters of affected males were carriers of the disease. The distribution of weakness was similar to that of the more severe DMD, although the progression was slower. It is now clear that both disorders are the result of dystrophin abnormalities: DMD is due to absence of dystrophin, whereas BMD is caused by dystrophin that is abnormal in molecular weight, quantity, or both (Fig. 42–2).[4]

In the absence of contributory family history, the differential diagnosis of BMD from autosomal recessive limb-girdle dystrophy was difficult or impossible using clinical or histopathologic data. The problems in differential diagnosis of BMD were underscored with the first reports of dystrophin gene and protein studies in neuromuscular disease patients: Of all isolated male patients carrying a diagnosis of BMD or limb-girdle muscular dystrophy, fully 50% were found to be incorrectly classified.[6,7] As molecular testing became routine in the diagnostic workup of muscular dystrophy patients, the clinical spectrum of BMD widened dramatically. Presentations of BMD now include proximal weakness starting at nearly any age, myoglobinuria, hyperCKemia, muscle cramps, muscle pain, weakness limited to quadriceps, and heart failure.[8] Progressions are as variable as presentations. Some patients show progressive weakness affecting both limb girdles, whereas others can remain quite static. Intrafamilial variability is common. The car-

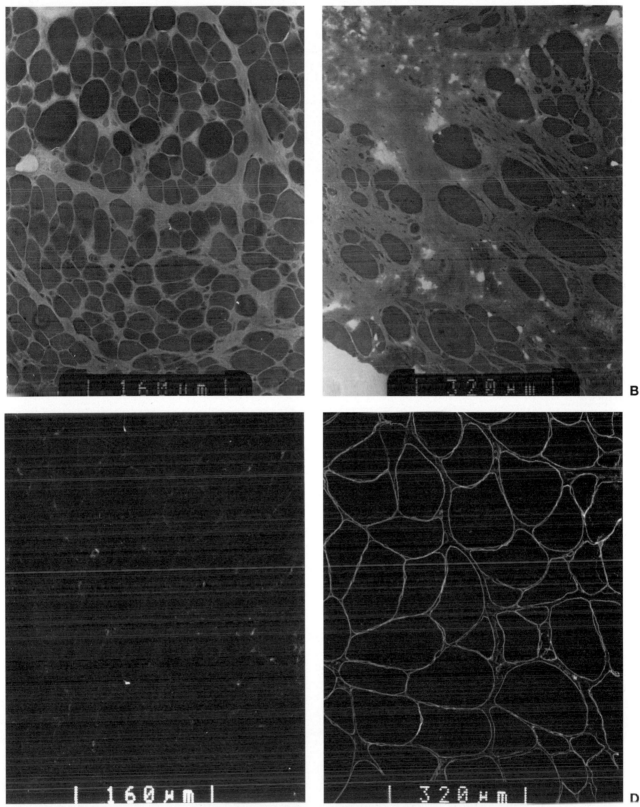

FIGURE 42–1. Histopathologic and immunohistochemical findings in Duchenne muscular dystrophy. *A,* Hematoxylin-eosin histopathology of a 6 month-old boy with Duchenne muscular dystrophy (dystrophin deficiency). Fiber size variation is evident, with endomysial fibrosis. *B,* Muscle biopsy from a 9-year-old boy with Duchenne muscular dystrophy, showing dramatic replacement of the muscle by fibrotic tissue, wide variation in fiber size, and evidence of failed regeneration of myofibers embedded in dense connective tissue. *C,* Dystrophin immunostaining in a Duchenne muscular dystrophy patient with dystrophin antibody (d10) showing complete deficiency. *D,* Dystrophin immunostaining in a patient with an unrelated disease showing dystrophin at the plasma membrane of each muscle fiber.

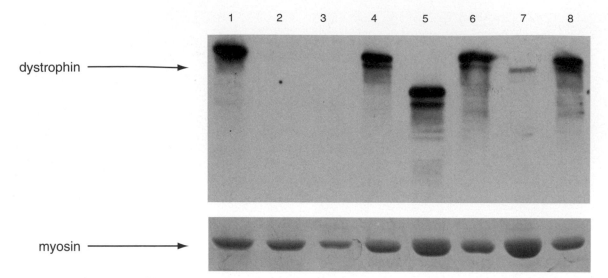

FIGURE 42–2. Dystrophin immunoblot analysis of muscle samples from Duchenne and Becker muscular dystrophy patients. Shown is immunoblot (Western blot) analysis of solubilized muscle samples from fetuses *(lanes 1–3)*, and patients *(lanes 4–8)*. Shown are the dystrophin signal *(top panel)* and muscle content control *(Coomassie blue staining of post-transfer gel, lower panel)* for each sample. Normal fetal heart *(lane 1)* shows an intense dystrophin signal of expected size (427 kd), consistent with the expected expression of dystrophin at high levels in normal fetal heart and skeletal muscle. Heart muscle samples from two fetopsy specimins *(lanes 2 and 3)* show no detectable dystrophin despite muscle content of the lanes indicated by myosin staining. This result is diagnostic of Duchenne muscular dystrophy, and this analysis is often used to confirm the diagnosis of fetuses after genetic mutation and linkage studies are complete. Normal adult skeletal muscle *(lanes 4, 6, and 8)* shows the expected full-length dystrophin at normal levels. Dystrophin analysis of two male muscular dystrophy patients is shown *(lanes 5 and 7)*. The first patient *(lane 5)* was biopsied at age 6 years and was an isolated case who presented with delayed motor development; motor function, however, seemed to improve with advancing age. At 9 years old, he shows very mild proximal weakness. Dystrophin analysis of his muscle *(lane 5)* shows dystrophin of abnormal molecular weight (350 kd; normal = 427 kd), with very high levels (100% of normal). This result is diagnostic of Becker muscular dystrophy and is consistent with the clinical phenotype. The second patient *(lane 7)* was biopsied at age 12 years and was an isolated case who presented with progressive weakness and difficulty climbing stairs and running since age 6 years. Currently 15 years old, he shows obvious proximal weakness but is still ambulatory. Dystrophin analysis *(lane 7)* shows dystrophin of abnormal molecular weight (380 kd) and very reduced quantities (5% of normal). This result is diagnostic of severe Becker muscular dystrophy and is consistent with the clinical phenotype. (Patients referred by Corrado Angelini, MD, and Elena Pegoraro, MD, University of Padova Neuromuscular Clinic, Padova, Italy.)

diomyopathy present in all dystrophinopathy patients is often more pronounced in BMD, presumably because the preservation of strength relative to DMD puts greater demands on the compromised cardiac musculature.[9]

The term *Becker muscular dystrophy* has gradually become defined by molecular rather than clinical features. Any patient in whom dystrophin is present but abnormal is now diagnosed as BMD. The biochemical definition of BMD can occasionally be problematic: Rare patients with abnormal dystrophin can remain completely asymptomatic their entire lives and yet carry the diagnosis of muscular dystrophy. On the other hand, severe BMD patients can become wheelchair-bound by age 20 years.[6] Abnormal dystrophin is likely to remain associated with the term *Becker muscular dystrophy*, but care should be taken to explain the clinical range of the disorder to patient and family.

Pathology

Histopathology of the muscle biopsy shows a dystrophic myopathy of variable severity. Biopsy findings can be quite similar to DMD or nearly normal, with only mild fiber size variation and increased central nuclei. The severity of histopathology generally reflects clinical severity. EMG shows a myopathic pattern, mixed myopathic and neurogenic features (rarely), or neurogenic features alone.

FEMALE CARRIERS

Clinical and Diagnostic Features

Girls and women in families with DMD are at risk of being carriers. Carriers only rarely show clinical symptoms. When they do, it is usually the result of skewed X inactivation. A disproportionately high percentage of myonuclei in women's muscle uses the mutant dystrophin gene and inactivates the normal gene. Thus, in a female carrier showing skewed X inactivation, as many as 90% of muscle nuclei cannot make dystrophin and only 10% can. Female carriers with X:autosome translocations involving a breakpoint in the dystrophin gene *(Xp21)* show complete skewing of X inactivation, thus keeping the mutant dystrophin gene active in most or all cells. These girls often show a clinical picture as severe as DMD in boys.

Dystrophin protein testing of muscle biopsies by immunofluorescence has made it possible to visualize X inactivation patterns indirectly in female muscle. Muscle fibers (or fiber segments) with nuclei harboring active normal X showed normal dystrophin immunostaining, whereas nuclei containing active abnormal X showed dystrophin deficiency. Thus, most carrier muscle shows a mosaic pattern of dystrophin-positive and dystrophin-negative muscle fibers in cross-section. It became apparent that isolated female muscular dystrophy patients without family history of DMD in male relatives may also have dystrophin mosaicism (female carrier state) as the underlying cause of their disease.[7] Nearly all of these isolated female cases were diagnosed as limb-girdle muscular dystrophy before dystrophin testing became available. Large collaborative studies have shown that approximately 10% of female limb-girdle patients are instead female carriers of DMD.[10]

The clinical presentation of dystrophinopathy in isolated female patients is as varied as BMD in males.[10] Female patients can show asymmetric weakness due to varied X inactivation patterns in different muscles. Also, the disease in female patients is generally less rapidly progressive than in male patients with similar presentations. The reason for the slower progression is the tendency of female muscle to become more dystrophin-normal with age (genetic and biochemical normalization).[11]

Pathology

Histopathology of muscle biopsies from female carriers is extremely variable between patients and often in the same patient or even in the same biopsy. This variability is the result of varying X inactivation patterns in different patients and occasionally even in the same patient. Indeed, some carriers show weakness localized to a single arm or leg, presumably due to variations in the percentage of mutant dystrophin genes being used in that limb. Often, muscle biopsy shows regions that appear quite normal next to other regions that appear highly dystrophic. EMG is usually reported as myopathic.

DYSTROPHINOPATHIES

Clinical and Molecular Genetics

DMD was the first human inherited disorder to be clarified at the molecular level by positional cloning, with no prior knowledge of the biochemical defect. The identification of the causative gene was aided by a number of early observations that narrowed the regions of the genome requiring analysis. First, it was known that the disease was X-linked, which limited the search to the 10% of the genome in the X chromosome. Second, some girls with muscular dystrophy clinically indistinguishable from DMD in boys had X:autosome translocations involving *Xp21*. Third, a boy affected with multiple X-linked recessive diseases, including DMD, was found to harbor a small but microscopically visible deletion of the *Xp21* region of the X chromosome.[12] Genomic DNA from this boy was used to isolate small fragments of genetic material from the *Xp21* region, and one of these *(pERT87)* led to the identification of neighboring coding sequence (exons) of the gene that was eventually characterized: its protein product was dubbed *dystrophin*.[13,14]

The dystrophin gene consists of 80 exons, with multiple spliced isoforms and multiple tissue-specific promoters; internal promoters lead to smaller isoforms including only a subset of the 80 exons. Lack of one particular transcript appears responsible for most muscle abnormalities and clinical symptoms: the prototypical "full length muscle dystrophin" transcript that encodes a dystrophin isoform of 427 kd.[15] Lack of other isoforms cause subclinical abnormalities of the tissues in which they are expressed. For example, a specific dystrophin isoform is expressed in the retina, and DMD patients show abnormal electroretinograms.[16]

The dystrophin gene is by far the largest gene identified to date in any species. At about 2.5 million base pairs (2.5 Mbp), it is nearly 10 times larger than the next largest gene (see http://www.genome.ucsc.edu). It takes 16 hours to produce a single mRNA from this enormous gene.[17] Whereas other proteins are as large or larger than dystrophin, few genes have as many exons and introns, and few have such a high proportion of seemingly useless intron sequences relative to coding exons: There are approximately 200 bp of intron for every base of exon. The reasons underlying the apparently inefficient evolutionary development of this gene are not yet understood.

The most common type of gene mutation in both DMD and BMD is a deletion encompassing one or more exons of the enormous gene. Because introns are so much larger than exons, nearly all deletion mutations begin and end in intron sequences. There are two deletion hot spots, one in the region of exons 44 to 50, and another near the beginning of the gene (exons 2 to 13).[14] The most important feature of a deletion regarding prognosis is the resulting reading frame[18]: If the remainder of the gene can still be spliced together into an RNA that avoids a frame-shift "nonsense" codon (in-frame deletion mutation), then a milder phenotype (BMD) is usually observed. Deletion mutations that result in new neighboring exons (junction) that do *not* share the same reading frame show a frame-shift mutation, loss of dystrophin protein, and clinically severe DMD. However, approximately 8% of deletion mutations are exceptions to the reading frame rule (e.g., out-of-frame deletion in a milder BMD patient). These exceptions occur primarily at the 5' end of the gene, where the transcriptional machinery can override the frameshift by use of a different initiator methionine codon (ATG) or can make use of alternative splicing.[19] If the boundaries of a deletion mutation can be precisely identified, there is a 92% accuracy for distinguishing DMD from BMD based on the reading frame alone.

The carboxyl terminus of the dystrophin protein, where the syntrophins and dystroglycan proteins bind, seems particularly important for dystrophin function. If this domain is lacking, a severe Duchenne phenotype usually results. In general, little or no truncated dystrophin protein is seen in DMD patients with frameshift deletions. This is due to the instability of both truncated RNA and truncated protein. In rare patients, truncated protein accumulates to some level, but these patients still show a DMD phenotype, consistent with the apparent critical importance of the carboxyl terminus of dystrophin. The amino-terminal actin-binding domain also appears important. Many patients lacking this domain have a particularly severe BMD phenotype, although the remainder of the protein is intact. Most deletion mutations occur in the large central rod domain, which fortunately appears to be the least critical for dystrophin function: some mild Becker dystrophy patients had most of this region either deleted or duplicated. The amount of abnormal protein that accumulates can affect clinical severity, an important feature in BMD. However, there is interpatient variability, even when dystrophin gene and protein findings are similar.

Approximately 45% of Duchenne patients and 30% of Becker patients do not have deletion mutations, but instead have duplications or point mutations.[20] Duplications follow the same in-frame/out-of-frame rule as deletion mutations, and approximately 5% of Duchenne or Becker patients show this type of mutation. Point mutations are particularly difficult to identify given the size and complexity of the gene, but about 100 point mutations have been characterized to date.[20] Given the high mutation rate of the gene, each patient has a different point mutation, making it impossible to screen for common point mutations, as is done in other disorders, such as cystic fibrosis. Most point mutations affect splicing or translation of the protein, and only a few putative missense (single amino acid change) mutations have been identified to date. It is difficult to prove causality of missense mutations because there is no defined functional test for mutant dystrophin proteins.

Biochemistry

Dystrophin was found to be associated with the plasma membrane both by subcellular fractionation studies and by immunostaining of muscle biopsy cryosections.[21,22]

Immunoelectron microscopy studies showed dystrophin to be at the intracellular face of the plasma membrane, with some periodicity suggesting a network.[23] Dystrophin associates with the membrane via a series of "dystrophin-associated proteins"; the carboxyl-terminal region of dystrophin binds to the transmembrane beta-dystroglycan.[24] Both the sarcoglycan complex (four proteins in stoichiometric tetrameres), and α-dystroglycan stabilize the association of dystrophin with β-dystroglycan, and α-dystroglycan in turn binds to the myofiber basal lamina via the laminin α2 component (also called merosin).[25] Dystrophin binds to filamentous actin at multiple sites along the molecule, with the strongest interacting sites in the amino-terminal "actin binding" domain of the protein. In linking the intracellular actin network to the plasma membrane and to the extracellular basal lamina, the dystrophin-based membrane cytoskeleton likely protects the membrane from contraction-induced damage (Fig. 42–1). Both sarcoglycans and dystroglycans are decreased when dystrophin gene mutations cause primary dystrophin deficiency. Mutations in any of the four sarcoglycan genes cause autosomal recessive dystrophies that are clinically similar to DMD.

Much is known about the structure and function of the many dystrophin-associated proteins (including the syntrophins, actin, nNOS, aciculin, and others). nNOS appears particularly important, because it regulates vascular perfusion, mitochondrial function, calcium trafficking, necrosis, and myofibrillar contractility. nNOS usually associates indirectly with dystrophin via syntrophin, but when dystrophin is lost, nearly all nNOS immunostaining at the plasma membrane is secondarily lost. The loss of nNOS is probably responsible for the functional ischemia seen in dystrophin-deficient muscle. The reader is referred to other reviews of these proteins.[26]

There is a second membrane cytoskeleton system in myofibers: the vinculin/integrin/laminin cytoskeleton, which is partially redundant with the dystrophin/dystroglycan/laminin cytoskeleton. Overexpression of components of muscle integrin can rescue the dystrophin-deficient *dmdx* mice.[27]

Pathophysiology and Animal Models

A series of in vivo and in vitro studies have shown that dystrophin-deficient muscle membranes are more fragile than normal myofiber membranes. First, cultured dystrophin-negative myotubes are considerably more susceptible than normal myotubes to damage by cell volume changes caused by osmotic shock.[28] Second, dystrophin is concentrated at specialized sites on the membrane that are subjected to the greatest stress, including the myotendinous junction,[29] costameres,[30] and the neuromuscular junctions. Third, membrane instability has been directly measured in dystrophin-deficient cells, and dystrophin-deficient *mdx* myotubes showed a fourfold decrease in membrane stiffness.[31] Fourth, electron microscopic studies of human muscle biopsies have demonstrated overt breaks of the plasma membrane in dystrophin-deficient muscle.[32] Finally, dystrophin-deficient myofibers are more susceptible to damage by proteases in vivo.[33] There may be similarities between the cues signaling muscle hypertrophy in normal muscle and the hypertrophy seen in young patients with DMD: Sublethal damage of the myofiber membrane may be the normal physiologic signal for subsequent muscle hypertrophy. Thus, the fragility of the plasma membrane in Duchenne muscle may lead to miscued hypertrophy early in the disease, and necrosis and weakness later in the disease.

It is tempting to conclude that any disruption of the membrane cytoskeleton causes myofiber death and hence a muscular dystrophy phenotype. Considerable evidence suggests, however, that the pathophysiology of DMD is much more complicated than a simple cause-and-effect relationship between membrane instability and muscle weakness. Dystrophin and its associated proteins are fully expressed at birth, and dystrophin deficiency can be biochemically detected from fetal life onward. Thus, the static biochemical defect stands in marked contrast to the progressive clinical course. Although many animal models of DMD have dystrophin deficiency and dystrophin gene mutations, clinical progression in these animals is quite distinct from the human disease. Dystrophin-deficient *mdx* mice have elevated serum CK concentrations soon after birth but do not show overt histopathology until 3 to 4 weeks of age. A remarkable histopathologic feature is that large groups of fibers die synchronously (grouped necrosis) at 3 to 6 weeks, with subsequent degeneration or regeneration occurring at a much slower pace. Mice do in fact show a 50% reduction in lifespan but show little evidence of clinical weakness earlier than 1 year of age.[34] Sporadically occurring dystrophin-deficient cats found in all corners of North America show a similar phenotype, which is quite different from that of other dystrophin-deficient species.[35] Affected cats show progressive muscle hypertrophy, which can become lethal (one cat died from esophageal constriction secondary to dramatic hypertrophy of the diaphragm, and another went into renal failure owing to inefficient water intake secondary to hypertrophied lingual musculature). Histopathologically, the muscle looks similar to that of the *mdx* mouse, with degeneration and regeneration of myofibers, but there is little overt fibrotic replacement. In dogs, dystrophin deficiency has been documented in golden retrievers, wire-haired fox terriers, rottweilers, and shelties.[36] All dogs show a severely progressive muscular dystrophy, often resulting in death by 6 months of age. Both clinically and histopathologically, the dog's disease is very similar to the human disease, including relative age of onset and speed of progression.

Many pathogenetic models have attempted to explain the enigmatic progression of DMD and the differences in phenotypes of the different animal models. One theory suggests that other proteins can compensate for dystrophin to some extent, and it is the variability in these compensatory proteins that conditions the progression and species differences. Utrophin (also a dystrophin-related protein) is a 420-kd protein that looks much like dystrophin at the primary amino acid sequence level, but has a very different tissue distribution and temporal expression pattern. One therapeutic avenue being pursued is to induce excess production of utrophin in patient muscle (upregulation) through pharmacologic means (see dystrophinopathies section).[37] Another theory places the burden of disease progression on the mitotic capabilities of the stem cells that are responsible for regenerating damaged myofibers (variably called myoblasts, muscle precursor cells, or satellite cells). It is possible that human and dog myoblasts simply exhaust their mitotic capability, leading to muscle regeneration failure, muscle atrophy, and early death. A third pathogenetic model invokes involvement of the immune system and muscle tissue microenvironment. The grouped necrosis may be best explained by a bystander effect mediated by inflammatory cells,[38] and the progressive connective tissue proliferation may be a species-specific response to chronic cytoplasm efflux from dystrophin-deficient myofibers. The latter theory has the support of the well-documented interspecies variability in tissue repair and inflammatory cell biology. The recent advent of genomewide transcriptional analyses (expression profiling) has enabled a global-scale comparison of human DMD muscle, and the *mdx* mouse muscle; this has pointed out specific differences in transcriptional profiles that begin to explain interspecies differences in pathophysiology.[39,40] It is becoming increasingly likely that all of the pathophysiologic pathways discussed have a component role in the complex downstream consequences of dystrophin deficiency. It also follows that therapeutics targeted at slowing disease progression may need pharmacologic approaches to address multiple pathophysiologic pathways at the same time.

THERAPY

There is currently no true therapy for DMD or related dystrophinopathies. Patients must be managed to compensate for the gradual loss of muscle tissue and strength. Tendon contractures affect the comfort and mobility of the patient. Achilles tendon contractures often lead to toe walking; stretching of these and other involved tendons via physical therapy can slow or alleviate contractures. Night splints and other forms of bracing are often recommended in young patients (age 4 to 5 years) to prevent leg contractures. Surgical lengthening of the Achilles tendon is frequently done if toe walking begins to limit mobility. More aggressive and earlier surgical intervention, with release of multiple tendons in the hip girdle, has been proposed.[41]

Knee-foot orthoses assist in stabilizing standing, thereby preserving strength and bone density. Use of braces often requires iliotibial band release. Braces are generally effective for only a limited time because patients often become wheelchair-bound soon after braces are required. Standard care includes use of electric wheelchairs because upper girdle weakness prevents easy use of manual wheelchairs.

Spinal involvement includes lordosis as a compensatory mechanism for maintaining balance in the presence of proximal weakness. Later in the disease process, weakness of paraspinal muscles leads to contractures of the spine, which presents as scoliosis. Scoliosis can be a significant clinical complication if unchecked: Severe curvature leads to decreased vital capacity and respiratory problems. Customized wheelchair design is important to slowing the progression of scoliosis. When scoliosis begins to limit vital capacity, surgical placement of Harrington rods is often considered. Respiratory function and heart involvement should be monitored late in the disease progression.

Corticosteroids slow the progression of DMD to some extent.[42] Prednisone administered at 0.75 mg/kg per day increases strength and, if administered relatively early in the disease process, can prolong ambulation for 3 years or longer. A derivative of prednisone, deflazacort, also shows efficacy in slowing the disease, and has fewer side effects than prednisone.[43] The strength gained by prescription of immunosuppressive agents for long periods must be weighed against the side effects associated with such treatment regimens.

FUTURE RESEARCH DIRECTIONS

Therapeutics for DMD address the primary genetic and biochemical defect (Fig. 42–3) and the multiple "downstream" pathways causing disease progression. Pharmacologic trials addressing the downstream pathophysiology of dystrophin-deficiency, and/or compensatory pathways, have been done in the *mdx* mouse model. IGF-1, carnitine, creatine, pentoxifylline, glutamine, oxatamide, integrins, myostatin inhibitors, green tea extract, nNOS, increase in glycosylation via GalNAc transferase expression, utrophin upregulation, have all been shown to improve the strength and/or histopathology of *mdx* mice.[44–49] Cooperative International Neuromuscular Research Group (CINRG), an international clinical trial network, has been established to test such agents in human patients,[50] although no drug trial data is yet available. Although the dog model of DMD simulates more closely the human disease, the clinical variability of individual dogs, and the higher cost of conducting drug trials in this species, has limited the use of this model in drug screening. It is anticipated that cocktails of agents will significantly slow the progression of DMD, and that these will become standard care. The definition of pharmacologic approaches is absolutely dependent on clinical trials, and it is important to have many, if not all, newly diagnosed patients entered into randomized clinical trials to expedite progress.

While pharmacologic approaches are likely to slow the progression of the disorder, hope for a true "cure" relies on replacement of the dystrophin protein in patient muscle and heart using molecular approaches. If dystrophin is effectively delivered to a myofiber and cardiocyte, then all proteins showing secondary deficiencies will be reinstated in the membrane cytoskeleton and the cell will be rescued from future necrosis. It is commonly believed that it is difficult or impossible to deliver the dystrophin *protein* in purified form to a patient's muscle. Dystrophin is a very large cytoskeletal protein that must be delivered to the intracellular face of the myofiber plasma membrane, and there are currently no techniques that can accomplish such a delivery. Instead, most efforts have focused on delivering the normal dystrophin gene to patient muscle, or on repairing the patient's endogenous dystrophin gene using mRNA correction, or genomic DNA correction.

One method to replace the defective gene in DMD patients is transplant of either muscle tissue or muscle stem cells (myoblasts). Whole muscle groups in a DMD patient could conceivably be transplanted, but all muscles are eventually involved in the disease process, and whole-body muscle transplantation is not envisioned as a possible therapy for DMD. Another approach is to introduce normal muscle cells from a donor into DMD patient muscle. Cellular transplantation is being tried in many disorders and has also been attempted in DMD. Although this approach, known as *myoblast transfer*, showed some success in mice, relatively few cells survive after injection, and immunologic barriers appear daunting. An additional hurdle is the very limited spread of cells from the site of injection; cells migrate only a few millimeters from the injection site. Recent attention has been focused on systemic delivery of "muscle stem cells." However, the frequency of cells reaching muscle and participating in myofiber regeneration is vanishingly small, and likely clinically insignificant.[51]

The second method of introducing normal dystrophin genes in dystrophin-deficient muscle is via gene delivery (AKA "gene therapy"). The goal of gene delivery (see Chapter 6) is to supply therapeutic genes into cells via recombinant viruses or other delivery systems. Human trials in gene therapy are currently under way in many universities for disorders such as adenosine deaminase deficiency, cystic fibrosis, and cancer. Despite the early discovery of the dystrophin gene, there are no human gene therapy clinical trials for DMD. The reasons for the seemingly slow pace of DMD gene therapy are many. First, the gene is extremely large, and it is difficult for viruses to contain this gene within their genome without disrupting the packaging of the viral DNA or RNA into infectious particles. Second, mature muscle is refractory to infection by the viruses used in many other gene therapy protocols (retrovirus, adenovirus). Third, delivery of

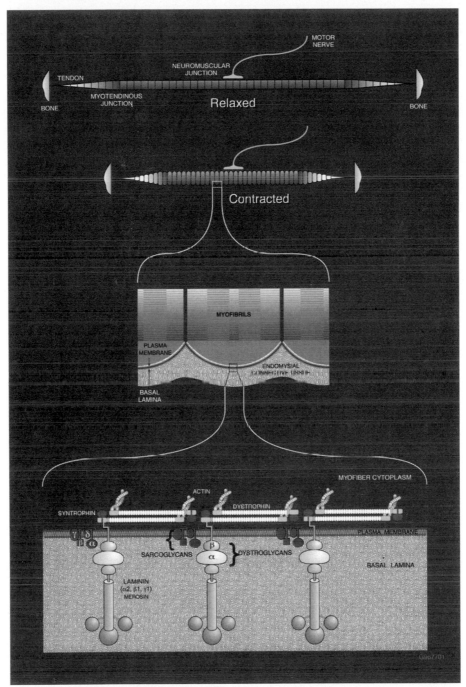

FIGURE 42–3. Location and organization of dystrophin and dystrophin-associated proteins in the myofiber. Shown is a schematic representation of a myofiber *(top)* which is a syncytial cell stretching from tendon to tendon in the muscle tissue. Contraction of the myofiber through stimulation by the motor nerve causes a shape change in the cell, with redistribution of cytoplasm. This causes bulging of the plasma membrane from regions of attachment to the myofibril line (costameres), giving a scalloped appearance to the surface of the cell. The changes in cell shape and the transduction of force from the contracting intracellular myofibrils to the extracellular matrix presumably require a specialized membrane cytoskeleton. The dystrophin membrane cytoskeleton includes dystrophin as a major structural component on the intracellular face of the plasma membrane, where it is thought to form a meshlike oligomeric structure. A series of dystrophin-associated proteins interact with dystrophin and mediate its attachment to the membrane and other proteins. Three groups of dystrophin-associated proteins have been identified to date. The sarcoglycan complex includes four distinct transmembrane proteins (α-, β-, γ- and δ-sarcoglycan. Primary deficiencies of each protein have been shown to cause cases of inherited muscular dystrophies with a clinical phenotype similar to Duchenne or Becker muscular dystrophy. The dystroglycan complex is formed by the proteolytic cleavage of a single polypeptide into a transmembrane β-dystroglycan, and a larger extracellular α-dystroglycan. The dystroglycans mediate the attachment of dystrophin to the major component of the myofiber basal lamina, laminin 2. Laminin 2 is a heterotrimer consisting of a large central protein ($\alpha 2$ laminin, also called merosin), and two smaller subunits ($\beta 1$ and $\gamma 1$ laminin) *(outer arms of molecule)*. Deficiency of $\alpha 2$ laminin causes approximately 30% of congenital muscular dystrophy cases.

the gene to muscle continues to be problematic: The target tissue is 30% of body mass and has a unique cellular structure. Finally, most estimates suggest that at least 20% of normal levels of dystrophin must be delivered to muscle before the clinical phenotype is abrogated; this would require a large number of dystrophin genes in a considerable amount of muscle tissue.

To overcome the size barrier for delivering dystrophin genes by viral vectors, the size of the dystrophin coding sequence has been reduced so that it can be contained in both adenoviral viral vectors, and adeno-associated viral vectors.[52] These so-called "mini-genes" or "micro-dystrophins" lack large sections of the central rod domain of dystrophin, and often some of the carboxyl-terminal sequence, which seem less important for its function.[53,54]

The most promising animal studies to date have used a recombinant adeno-associated virus (AAV) containing a dystrophin mini-gene.[52] AAV is, in many ways, ideally suited for gene delivery to muscle. AAV is a naturally occurring, helper-dependent virus that appears to infect most people by 2 years of age and lies latent in muscle and the female reproductive tract. Naturally occurring AAV produces no known pathology. In fact, it may protect us from more harmful viruses by parasitizing them. Little immune response is observed against transgenes delivered to normal muscle (although dystrophic muscle is likely to promote immune surveillance and rejection of novel proteins). In animal models of sarcoglycan-deficient muscular dystrophy, recombinant AAV vectors have been shown to fully rescue muscle for over 2 years post-injection.[55] Recent delivery of mini-dystrophin genes using AAV in *mdx* mice have shown similar success in rescuing muscle histologically and functionally.[52] It is likely that human clinical trials using AAV-mediated delivery of dystrophin mini-genes will take place in the near future. It will be critical to establish the functional efficacy of Becker-like mini-genes in human DMD muscle. It remains challenging to deliver adequate therapeutic doses of virus to sufficiently large regions of muscle to obtain functional benefit to patients.

Promising alternative approaches to genetic complementation employ repairing the gene mutation using chimeric oligonucleotide (chimoligo) approaches,[56] or forcing the translational machinery to skip over the mutation by antisense mRNA approaches.[57]

REFERENCES

1. Emery AEH, Emery MLH: The History of a Genetic Disease. Duchenne Muscular Dystrophy, or Meryon's Disease. London, Royal Society of Medicine Press, 1995.

2. Mehler MF, Haas KZ, Kessler JA, Stanton PK: Enhanced sensitivity of hippocampal pyramidal neurons from *mdx* mice to hypoxia-induced loss of synaptic transmission. Proc Natl Acad Sci U S A 1992;89:2461.

3. Naylor EW, Hoffman EP, Paulus-Thomas J, et al: Neonatal screening for Duchenne/Becker muscular dystrophy: Reconsideration based on molecular diagnosis and potential therapeutics. Screening 1992;1:99.

4. Hoffman EP, Fischbeck KH, Brown RH, et al: Dystrophin characterization in muscle biopsies from Duchenne and Becker muscular dystrophy patients. N Engl J Med 1988;318:1363.

5. Hoffman EP, Brown RH, Kunkel LM: Dystrophin: The protein product of the Duchenne muscular dystrophy locus. Cell 1987;51:919.

6. Hoffman EP, Kunkel LM, Angelini C, et al: Improved diagnosis of Becker muscular dystrophy by dystrophin testing. Neurology 1989;39:1011.

7. Arikawa E, Hoffman EP, Kaido M, et al: The frequency of patients having dystrophin abnormalities in a limb-girdle patient population. Neurology 1991; 41:1491.

8. Doriguzzi C, Palmucci L, Mongini T, et al: Exercise intolerance and recurrent myoglobinuria as the only expression of Xp21 Becker type muscular dystrophy. J Neurol 1993;240:269.

9. Nigro G, Comi LI, Politano L, et al: Evaluation of the cardiomyopathy in Becker muscular dystrophy. Muscle Nerve 1995;18:283.

10. Hoffman EP, Arahata K, Minetti C, et al: Dystrophinopathy in isolated cases of myopathy in females. Neurology 1992;42:967.

11. Pegoraro E, Schimke RN, Garcia C, et al: Genetic and biochemical normalization in female carriers of Duchenne muscular dystrophy: Evidence for failure of dystrophin production in dystrophin competent myonuclei. Neurology 1995;45:677.

12. Kunkel LM, Monaco AP, Middlesworth W, et al: Specific cloning of DNA fragments absent from the DNA of a male patient with an X chromosome deletion. Proc Natl Acad Sci U S A 1985;82:4778.

13. Monaco AP, Neve RL, Colletti-Feener C, et al: Isolation of candidate cDNAs for portions of the Duchenne muscular dystrophy gene. Nature 1986;323:646.

14. Koenig M, Hoffman EP, Bertelson CJ, et al: Complete cloning of the Duchenne muscular dystrophy (DMD) cDNA and preliminary genomic organization of the DMD gene in normal and affected individuals. Cell 1987;50:509.

15. Koenig M, Monaco AP, Kunkel LM: The complete sequence of dystrophin predicts a rod-shaped cytoskeletal protein. Cell 1988;53:219.

16. Pillers DM, Bulman DE, Weleber RG, et al: Dystrophin expression in the human retina is required for normal function as defined by electroretinography. Nat Genet 1993;4:82.

17. Tennyson CN, Klamut HJ, Worton RG: The human dystrophin gene requires 16 hours to be transcribed and is cotranscriptionally spliced. Nat Genet 1995;9:184.

18. Monaco AP, Bertelson CJ, Liechti-Gallati S, et al: An explanation for the phenotypic differences between patients bearing partial deletions of the DMD locus. Genomics 1988;2:90.

19. Winnard AV, Mendell JR, Prior TW, et al: Frameshift deletions of exons 3–7 and revertant fibers in Duchenne muscular dystrophy: Mechanisms of dystrophin production. Am J Hum Genet 1995; 56: 158–166.

20. White S, Kalf M, Liu Q, et al: Comprehensive detection of genomic duplications and deletions in the DMD gene by use of multiplex amplifiable probe hybridization. Am J Hum Genet 2002;71:365–374.

21. Zubrzycka-Gaarn EE, Bulman DE, Karpati G, et al: The Duchenne muscular dystrophy gene product is localized in the sarcolemma of human skeletal muscle fibres. Nature 1988;333:466.

22. Bonilla E, Samitt CE, Miranda AF, et al: Duchenne muscular dystrophy: Deficiency of dystrophin at the muscle cell surface. Cell 1988;54:447.

23. Watkins SC, Hoffman EP, Slayter HS, Kunkel LM: Immunoelectron microscopic localization of dystrophin in myofibres. Nature 1988;333:863.

24. Ozawa E, Yoshida M, Hagiwara Y, et al: Dystrophin-associated proteins in muscular dystrophy. Hum Mol Genet 1995;4:1711.

25. Cote PD, Moukhles H, Carbonetto S: Dystroglycan is not required for localization of dystrophin, syntrophin, and neuronal nitric-oxide synthase at the sarcolemma but regulates integrin alpha 7B expression and caveolin-3 distribution. J Biol Chem 2002 Feb 15;277:4672–4679.

26. Rando TA: Role of nitric oxide in the pathogenesis of muscular dystrophies: A "two hit" hypothesis of the cause of muscle necrosis. Microsc Res Tech 2001;55:223–235.

27. Burkin DJ, Wallace GO, Nicol KJ, et al: Enhanced expression of the alpha7 beta1 integrin reduces muscular dystrophy and restores viability in dystrophic mice. J Cell Biol 2001;152:1207–1218.

28. Menke A, Jockusch H: Decreased osmotic stability of dystrophin-less muscle cells from the *mdx* mouse. Nature 1991;349:69.

29. Tidball JG, Law DJ: Dystrophin is required for normal thin filament-membrane associations at myotendinous junctions. Am J Pathol 1991;138:17.

30. Minetti C, Bentrame F, Marcenaro G, Bonilla E: Dystrophin at the plasma membrane of human muscle fibers shows a costameric localization. Neuromuscul Disord 1992;2:99.

31. Pasternak C, Wong S, Elson EL: Mechanical function of dystrophin in muscle cells. J Cell Biol 1995;128:355.

32. Mokri B, Engel AG: Duchenne dystrophy: Electron microscopic findings pointing to a basic or early abnormality in the plasma membrane of the muscle fiber. Neurology 1975;25:1111.

33. Gorospe JRM, Tharp MD, Demitsu T, Hoffman EP: Dystrophin-deficient myofibers are vulnerable to mast cell granule-induced necrosis. Neuromuscul Disord 1994;4:325.

34. Pastoret C, Sebille A: *mdx* Mice show progressive weakness and muscle deterioration with age. J Neurol Sci 1995;129:97.

35. Gaschen FP, Hoffman EP, Gorospe JRM, et al: Dystrophin deficiency causes lethal muscle hypertrophy in cats. J Neurol Sci 1992;110:149.

36. Gorospe JRM, Nishikawa BK, Hoffman EP: Pathophysiology of Duchenne muscular dystrophy: A clinical and biological enigma. In Lucy JA, Brown SC (eds): Dystrophin: Gene, Protein and Cell. London, Cambridge University Press, 1997, pp 201–232.

37. Tinsley JM, Davies KE: Utrophin: A potential replacement for dystrophin? Neuromuscul Disord 1993;3:537.

38. Spencer MJ, Tidball JG: Do immune cells promote the pathology of dystrophin-deficient myopathies? Neuromuscul Disord 2001;11:556–564.

39. Tseng BS, Zhao P, Pattison JS, et al: Regenerated mdx mouse skeletal muscle shows differential mRNA expression. J Appl Physiol 2002;95:537.

40. Chen YW, Zhao P, Borup R, Hoffman EP: Expression profiling in the muscular dystrophies: Identification of novel aspects of molecular pathophysiology. J Cell Biol 2000;151:1321–1336.

41. Manzur AY, Hyde SA, Rodillo E, et al: A randomized controlled trial of early surgery in Duchenne muscular dystrophy. Neuromuscul Disord 1992;2:379.

42. Griggs RC, Moxley RT, Mendell JR, et al: Duchenne dystrophy: Randomized, controlled trial of prednisone (18 months) and azathioprine (12 months). Neurology 1993;43:520.

43. Angelini C, Pegoraro E, Turella E, et al: Deflazacort in Duchenne dystrophy: Study of long term effect. Muscle Nerve 1994;17:386.

44. Granchelli JA, Pollina C, Hudecki MS: Pre-clinical screening of drugs using the mdx mouse. Neuromuscul Disord 2000;10:235–239.

45. Barton ER, Morris L, Musaro A, et al: Muscle-specific expression of insulin-like growth factor I counters muscle decline in mdx mice. J Cell Biol 2002;157:137–148.

46. Buetler TM, Renard M, Offord EA, et al: Green tea extract decreases muscle necrosis in mdx mice and protects against reactive oxygen species. Am J Clin Nutr 2002;75:749–753.

47. Wehling M, Spencer MJ, Tidball JG: A nitric oxide synthase transgene ameliorates muscular dystrophy in mdx mice. J Cell Biol 2001;155:123–131.

48. Nguyen HH, Jayasinha V, Xia B, et al: Overexpression of the cytotoxic T cell GalNAc transferase in skeletal muscle inhibits muscular dystrophy in mdx mice. Proc Natl Acad Sci U S A 2002;99: 5616–5621.

49. Rybakova IN, Patel JR, Davies KE, et al: Utrophin binds laterally along actin filaments and can couple costameric actin with sarcolemma when overexpressed in dystrophin-deficient muscle. Mol Biol Cell 2002;13:1512–1521.

50. Escolar DM, Henricson EK, Mayhew J, et al: Clinical evaluator reliability for quantitative and manual muscle testing measures of strength in children. Muscle Nerve 2001;24:787–793.

51. Partridge TA: Cells that participate in regeneration of skeletal muscle. Gene Ther 2002;9:752–753.

52. Wang B, Li J, Xiao X: Adeno-associated virus vector carrying human minidystrophin genes effectively ameliorates muscular dystrophy in mdx mouse model. Proc Natl Acad Sci U S A 2000;97:13714–13719.

53. Roberts ML, Wells DJ, Graham IR, et al: Stable micro-dystrophin gene transfer using an integrating adeno-retroviral hybrid vector ameliorates the dystrophic pathology in mdx mouse muscle. Hum Mol Genet 2002;11:1719–1730.

54. Harper SQ, Hauser MA, DelloRusso C, et al: Modular flexibility of dystrophin: Implications for gene therapy of Duchenne muscular dystrophy. Nat Med 2002;8:253–261.

55. Dressman D, Araishi K, Imamura M, et al: Delivery of alpha- and beta-sarcoglycan by recombinant adeno-associated virus: Efficient rescue of muscle, but differential toxicity. Hum Gene Ther 2002;13: 1631–1646.

56. Bertoni C, Rando TA: Dystrophin gene repair in mdx muscle precursor cells in vitro and in vivo mediated by RNA-DNA chimeric oligonucleotides. Hum Gene Ther 2002 Apr;13(6):707–718.

57. De Angelis FG, Sthandier O, Berarducci B, et al: Chimeric snRNA molecules carrying antisense sequences against the splice junctions of exon 51 of the dystrophin pre-mRNA induce exon skipping and restoration of a dystrophin synthesis in Delta 48–50 DMD cells. Proc Natl Acad Sci U S A 2002;99:9456–9461.

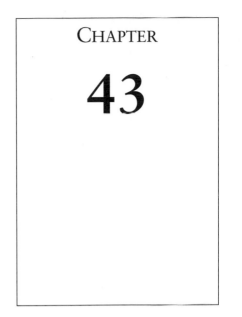

Limb-Girdle Muscular Dystrophies

Rita Barresi

Kevin P. Campbell

The limb-girdle muscular dystrophies (LGMD) are a heterogeneous group of genetically determined myopathies characterized by progressive weakness and atrophy involving predominantly proximal muscle groups.[1,2] These diseases affect populations worldwide, and have widely variable age of onset, rate of progression, and severity. Both autosomal recessive and dominant forms are recognized. LGMDs were initially identified as a separate group to differentiate them from X-linked or facioscapulohumeral muscular dystrophies. However, genetic studies and other advanced diagnostic tools have documented that LGMD encompasses many distinct myopathies with different inheritance patterns and pathogenetic mechanisms. Therefore, differential diagnosis of the different types of LGMD is not achievable with clinical evaluation alone, and requires the support of DNA and protein analyses. Exclusion diagnostic criteria for LGMD are also useful, such as evidence of abnormal staining or deficiency of dystrophin on muscle biopsies, or evidence of metabolic or neurogenic abnormalities. Furthermore, as many of the proteins involved interact, the primary defect of one of these proteins is often associated with the loss of others, presenting a challenge where the diagnosis is based on immuno and biochemical findings only.

After the discovery that components of the dystrophin-glycoprotein complex (DGC) are implicated in the pathogenesis of LGMD,[3] within a relatively short time a large number of genes have been identified as responsible for different forms of LGMD. Currently, 15 types can be recognized, and the present classification of LGMD is based both on mode of inheritance and gene involved (Table 43–1).

AUTOSOMAL DOMINANT LIMB-GIRDLE MUSCULAR DYSTROPHIES (LGMD1)

Only a relatively small percentage of LGMD (approximately 10%) is transmitted by autosomal dominant inheritance. Common features of this class of disease are late onset, relatively mild phenotype, and slow progression. The serum creatine kinase (CK) levels are also lower than in the recessive forms of LGMD. Five genes have already been mapped, but genetic exclusion studies suggest that others may exist.

LGMD1A

Mutations in the myotilin gene (5q22–q34) have been identified in one North American family of German descent with LGMD1A (Hauser et al, 2000). This late-onset, slowly progressive disease is characterized by weakness of the hip and shoulder girdles and dysarthric speech. CK levels are elevated 1.6- to 9-fold. Affected muscles show a large number of autophagic vesicles with rimmed vacuoles. Z-line streaming similar to that seen in nemaline myopathy is also observed.

Myotilin is a sarcomeric protein that binds to α-actinin and is associated with the Z-line.[4] In muscle biopsies from affected individuals, myotilin appears correctly localized to the Z-line, but it is not clear whether the protein is a product of the normal or the mutated allele. Failure to link to α-actinin is probably not the cause of the muscle pathology, since the mutant myotilin binds α-actinin as well as the wild-type protein. Myotilin may play a role in anchoring the myofibrils to the plasma membrane through its interaction with γ-filamin, which,

TABLE 43–1.   Limb-Girdle Muscular Dystrophies: Gene Location and Proteins Involved

Autosomal Dominant Limb-Girdle Muscular Dystrophies

Disease	Gene Location	Gene (protein)	References
LGMD1A	5q22–q34	MYOT (myotilin)	Speer et al. *Am J Hum Genet* 1992;50:1211–1217
			Hauser et al. *Hum Mol Genet* 2000;9:2141–2147
LGMD1B	1q11–q21	LMNA (lamin A/C)	Muchir et al. *Hum Mol Genet* 2000;9:1453–1459
LGMD1C	3p25	CAV3 (caveolin 3)	Minetti et al. *Nat Genet* 1998;18:365–368
			McNally et al. *Hum Mol Genet* 1998;7:871–877
LGMD1D	6q23	?	Messina et al. *Am J Hum Genet* 1997;61:909–917
LGMD1E	7q	?	Speer et al. *Am J Hum Genet* 1999;64:556–562

Autosomal Recessive Limb-Girdle Muscular Dystrophies

Disease	Gene Location	Gene (protein)	References
LGMD2A	15q15.1–q21.1	CAPN3 (calpain 3)	Beckmann et al. *CR Acad Sci III* 1991;312:141–148
			Young et al. *Genomics* 1992;13:1370–1371
			Richard et al. *Cell* 1995;81:27–40
			Richard et al. *Am J Hum Genet* 1997;60:1128–1138.
LGMD2B	2p13	DYSF (dysferlin)	Bashir et al. *Hum Mol Genet* 1994;3:455–457
			Bashir et al. *Nat Genet* 1998;20:37–42
			Liu et al. *Nat Genet* 1998;20:31–36
LGMD2C	13q12	SGCG (γ-sarcoglycan)	Ben Othmane et al. *Nat Genet* 1992;2:315–317
			Azibi et al. *Hum Mol Genet* 1993;2:1423–1428
			Noguchi et al. *Science* 1995;270:819–822
			McNally et al. *Am J Hum Genet* 1996;59:1040–1047
			Piccolo et al. *Hum Mol Genet* 1996;5:2019–2022
LGMD2D	17q12–q21.33	SGCA (α-sarcoglycan)	Roberds et al. *Cell* 1994;78:625–633
			Piccolo et al. *Nat Genet* 1995;10:243–245
			Passos-Bueno et al. *Hum Mol Genet* 1995;4:1163–1167
			Ljunggren et al. *Ann Neurol* 1995;38:367–372
			Carrié et al. *J Med Genet* 1997;34:470–475
LGMD2E	4q12	SGCB (β-sarcoglycan)	Lim et al. *Nat Genet* 1995;11:257–265
			Bonnemann et al. *Nat Genet* 1995;11:266–273
LGMD2F	5q33–q34	SGCD (δ-sarcoglycan)	Passos-Bueno et al. *Hum Mol Genet* 1996;5:815–820
			Nigro et al. *Nat Genet* 1996;14:195–198
LGMD2G	17q11–q12	TCAP (telethonin)	Moreira et al. *Am J Hum Genet* 1997;61:151–159
			Moreira et al. *Nat Genet* 2000;24:163–166
LGMD2H	9q31–q34.1	TRIM32 (TRIM32)	Weiler et al. *Am J Hum Genet* 1998;63:140–147
			Frosk et al. *Am J Hum Genet* 2002;70:663–672
LGMD2I	19q13.3	FKRP (fukutin-related protein)	Driss et al. *Neuromuscul Disord* 2000;10:240–246
			Brockington et al. *Hum Mol Genet* 2001;10:2851–2859
LGMD2J	2q	TTN (titin)	Haravuori et al. *Neurology* 2001;56:869–877

Adapted from Neuromuscul Disord 2002;12:82–100.

in turn, may bind to γ- and δ-sarcoglycans. Mutations in α-tropomyosin, another protein that localizes to the Z-line, have been shown to cause nemaline myopathy (NEM2). Interestingly, α-tropomyosin also binds α-actinin, and missense mutations in the gene result in autosomal dominant nemaline myopathy with disruption of the Z-line.[5] The similarity between these two disorders raises the possibility that LGMD1A might have been misdiagnosed as late-onset nemaline myopathy. Although the locus for LGMD1A overlaps with a distinct clinical disorder characterized by velopharyngeal weakness and involvement of the distal musculature (VCPDM), genetic analysis of VCPDM patients did not reveal mutations in the myotilin gene (Hauser et al, 2000).

LGMD1B

LGMD1B is a slowly progressive disorder characterized by weakness of proximal leg muscles, mild or late contractures, and atrioventricular cardiac conduction disturbances that worsen with time. CK levels are normal or slightly elevated. The disease is caused by mutations in the *LMNA* gene on chromosome 1q11–1q21. The gene encodes two proteins of the nuclear envelope, lamins A and C (lamin A/C), which are organized in dimers and interact with chromatin and integral proteins of the inner nuclear membrane.[6] Thus, perturbation of the nuclear architecture may be what triggers muscle pathology. Mutations in the *LMNA* gene are also associated with autosomal dominant Emery-Dreifuss muscular dystrophy (AD-EDMD). This disorder differs from LGMD1B because of the presence of early elbow and ankle contractures, predominant humeroperoneal muscle wasting, and severe cardiomyopathy with conduction defects that may be present at the onset or occur at any age. Furthermore, the *LMNA* gene is implicated in cardiomyopathies with conduction defect (DCM-CD), Dunningan-type familial partial lipodystrophy (FPLD), axonal Charcot-Marie-Tooth type 2 (AR-CMT2A),[7] and mandibuloacral dysplasia (MAD).[8] Further analysis of the phenotype-genotype correlation will be necessary to clarify the varying phenotypes observed in these allelic diseases.

LGMD1C

Mutations in the caveolin-3 gene associated with significant reduction of protein expression cause LGMD1C (McNally et al, 1998; Minetti et al, 1998). A number of missense mutations have also been reported in patients with LGMD, where neither the expression nor the localization of caveolin-3 were altered. As the same sequence variations were found in normal controls, these amino acid substitutions represent polymorphisms and are not likely to cause autosomal dominant muscular dystrophy.[9] Patients with mutations in the *CAV3* gene have normal motor milestones, but develop myopathy during childhood, with calf hypertrophy and mild to moderate proximal muscle weakness. A characteristic feature of LGMD1C is the occurrence of muscle cramps after exercise. CK levels are elevated 4- to 25-fold. The progression of the disease is variable.

Caveolin-3 is the muscle-specific member of a family of proteins localized at small invaginations of the plasma membrane (caveolae) that are believed to be involved in signal transduction.[9] Mutations in caveolin-3 give rise to unstable high molecular mass aggregates composed of normal and mutated protein that are retained in the Golgi complex. Although caveolin-3, like dystrophin, localizes at the sarcolemma, it is not an integral part of the DGC. However, caveolin-3 has been shown to interact with the dystrophin-binding site of β-dystroglycan, suggesting that it may regulate the interaction of β-dystroglycan with dystrophin.[10] Caveolin-3 also interacts with neuronal nitric oxide synthase (nNOS), and binding results in loss of nNOS activity. Severe reduction in the number of caveolae has been described at the sarcolemma of LGMD1C patients. This demonstrates that caveolin-3 plays an important role in the formation of these structures in skeletal muscle. Furthermore, the T-tubule system is profoundly altered in LGMD1C muscle fibers.[11]

Mutations in *CAV3* have been demonstrated in LGMD1C, but also in hyperCKemia, distal myopathy, and rippling muscle disease. The same mutations are associated with different phenotypes in the same families, but there are few large families with caveolin-3 mutations. Caveolin-3 may also have a role in the pathogenesis of other muscular dystrophies, as muscle from patients with Duchenne muscular dystrophy (DMD) shows overexpression of caveolin-3 along with increased number of caveolae.[9] In addition, abnormal localization of dysferlin has been reported in muscle from patients with LGMD1C, suggesting a structural or functional interaction between these proteins.[12]

LGMD1D (FDC-CDM)

LGMD1D is an autosomal dominant adult-onset disorder linked to chromosome 6q23 (Messina et al, 1997). Features include proximal weakness and dystrophic changes in the muscle biopsy, such as variable fiber size and increased connective tissue. CK levels are elevated twofold to fourfold, and the clinical progression is slow. Cardiac involvement is significant, with a high frequency of arrhythmia and congestive heart failure. Sudden death without prior cardiac symptoms has also been reported. In the single French-Canadian family described, males were more severely affected with both skeletal and cardiac disease. A candidate gene is currently being investigated.

LGMD1E

A new locus for LGMD has been identified on chromosome 7q in two families with autosomal dominant inheritance (Speer et al, 1999). Affected individuals present in early adulthood with proximal weakness involving primarily the lower limbs. Serum CK levels are normal to elevated threefold. Linkage analysis to candidate genes is currently ongoing.

AUTOSOMAL RECESSIVE LIMB-GIRDLE MUSCULAR DYSTROPHIES (LGMD2)

Ten different loci have been linked to autosomal recessive LGMD (LGMD2), and the genes have been identified. However, linkage analysis in a number of families still excludes all known loci, indicating that other genes must be responsible for the disease. The recessive LGMDs are more frequent than the dominant forms and usually have earlier onset. LGMD2A is probably the most common, accounting for about 30% of cases, whereas LGMD2G, 2H, and 2J have been described in only a few families. Genes responsible for LGMD2C–F encode components of the sarcoglycan complex, and the recently identified gene for LGMD2I encodes a putative glycosyltransferase involved in posttranslational processing of α-dystroglycan. Thus, many of the LGMD2 types involve members of the DGC.

LGMD2A

LGMD2A is caused by mutations in the gene coding for the muscle-specific calcium-dependent protease calpain 3 located on chromosome 15 (Richard et al, 1995). Mutations in the gene were originally identified in families of French descent on La Réunion Island and subsequently found in numerous individuals worldwide. Calpainopathy is characterized by variable onset that ranges from 2 to 40 years, but is most common in the early teens. The progression of the disease is slow, and muscle impairment is highly selective, affecting more severely the lower extremities and sparing the hip abductors. CK levels are elevated 7- to 80-fold.

Calpain 3 has three unique regions (NS, IS1, and IS2) that confer its muscle specificity. The protein interacts with titin via one of these muscle-specific sequences, IS2, which also contains a nucleus translocation signal-like sequence. A study of muscle biopsies from calpainopathy patients showed more apoptotic nuclei than in biopsies from patients with other muscular dystrophies. This was associated with a perturbation of the IκBα/NF-κB pathway.[13] At present, several hypotheses have been formulated for the function of calpain 3 in skeletal muscle, and the mechanism that generates muscular dystrophy in the absence of this protein could be a combination of a number of factors. As calpain 3 is found in both nucleus and cytoplasm, it may play a role in the control of the expression of muscle-specific transcription factors, thereby regulating muscle differentiation. Furthermore, the secondary reduction of calpain 3 in muscle biopsies from LGMD2B patients[14] suggests that this protein may be involved in the process of membrane resealing and repair.

LGMD2B

Dysferlin, the gene mutated in LGMD2B, is located at chromosome 2p13 (Bashir et al, 1998; Liu et al, 1998).

Mutations in the dysferlin gene are also responsible for Miyoshi myopathy, a distal muscular dystrophy.[15] As the same mutations have been associated with proximal and distal phenotypes, modifier genes may produce the observed clinical heterogeneity. Patients have normal motor development and function early in life. Onset of LGMD2B is in the late childhood to early adult age. Serum CK can be very high (elevated 10- to 72-fold), but the rate of progression is slow. After most of the lower-limb muscles become involved, the upper extremities also exhibit weakness. Dystrophic signs and inflammatory infiltrates are observed both in muscle from LGMD2B patients and from the SJL mouse, a naturally occurring model of dysferlinopathy. It is not clear whether the inflammation contributes to the pathology or is merely a secondary phenomenon.[16]

Dysferlin is a member of the FER-1-like protein family. It is characterized by a C-terminus transmembrane domain and multiple C2 domains, which are predicted to play a role in transduction pathways and membrane trafficking. The homologous FER-1 has been identified in *Caenorhabditis elegans,* where it is involved in spermatogenesis. In humans, dysferlin is more widely distributed, although it predominates in skeletal muscle, where it localizes at the sarcolemma and in intracellular vesicles. A dysferlin point mutation responsible for muscular dystrophy was expressed in cultured cells where it reduced the calcium-sensitive phospholipid-binding ability of dysferlin.[17] These data indicate that dysferlin may play a role in regeneration and repair. Caveolin-3 potentially interacts with dysferlin, suggesting that one function of dysferlin may be to maintain the signaling functions of caveolae.

SARCOGLYCANOPATHIES

Involvement of the α, β, γ, and δ components of the sarcoglycan complex is responsible for LGMD2C–F.[3] The sarcoglycans (SGs) are members of a group of proteins associated with dystrophin, the protein affected in Duchenne and Becker muscular dystrophies. The DGC is organized in three subcomplexes: the cytoskeletal proteins, dystrophin, and syntrophins; the dystroglycans (α and β); and the sarcoglycan-sarcospan subcomplex.[18] Many other proteins have recently been shown to associate with the DGC, including dystrobrevin and neuronal nitric oxide synthase. The interaction of the DGC with the extracellular matrix provides a structural scaffold that may protect the muscle fibers from damage caused by contraction. Transmembrane glycoproteins α-, β-, γ- and δ-SG share a number of features: They all contain a small intracellular domain, a single transmembrane domain, and a large extracellular domain that contains potential N-glycosylation sites. Expression of α-SG is limited to striated muscle, while β-, γ-, and δ-SG are also expressed in smooth muscle in association with ε-SG, a glycoprotein homologous to α-SG.[19] Recent evidence suggests that the vascular smooth muscle SG complex is involved in the cardiac muscle pathology observed in δ-, β-, and γ-, but not α-sarcoglycanopathies.[20] Mutations in α-sarcoglycan (2D) are the most common, whereas mutations in δ-sarcoglycan (2F) are rare. LGMD2C–F present a number of common characteristics: The clinical phenotype is characterized by progressive skeletal muscle weakness, with intra- and interfamilial variability in age of onset, rate of progression, and severity. Symptoms at onset include weakness, toe walking, and muscle pain, with severe involvement of shoulder girdle and hamstrings. CK levels are very high. When there is a mutation in one of the SG genes, there is also a secondary reduction of the other SGs, accompanied in some cases by less severe reduction of dystrophin. Immunostaining of muscle biopsies with specific antibodies may be suggestive of the gene primarily involved, but correct diagnosis requires genetic analysis.

LGMD2C (γ-Sarcoglycan)

Previously labeled "Duchenne-like muscular dystrophy" or "severe childhood autosomal recessive muscular dystrophy," LGMD2C was first described in North Africa, and in the European gypsy population (Azibi et al, 1993; Ben Othmane et al, 1992; Piccolo et al, 1996). The gene responsible for this disorder was localized to chromosome 13, and the defective protein recognized as γ-SG (Noguchi et al, 1995). Patients exhibit predominantly early onset with proximal lower-limb weakness (often sparing the quadriceps muscles) and normal intelligence. Loss of ambulation develops in the early teens, and respiratory failure occurs in the third decade. Cardiac involvement may be present in the later stages of the disease.

LGMD2D (α-Sarcoglycan)

The most common form of sarcoglycanopathy has been mapped on chromosome 17q21, and the protein involved is α-SG (Roberds et al, 1994). The original description of this disorder was in Algerian families, with subsequent identification in Brazilian families; however, α-sarcoglycanopathy occurs worldwide (Passos-Bueno et al, 1993; Piccolo et al, 1995). The most commonly reported mutation, independent of ethnicity, is Arg77Cys (Carrié et al, 1997). This form of muscular dystrophy has variable severity, ranging from early onset with rapidly progressive weakness to late onset with ambulation preserved throughout life. A correlation exists between type of mutation, levels of α-SG expression, and disease severity. Null mutations result in complete loss of the protein and a Duchenne muscular dystrophy–like phenotype. Progression of the disease is usually faster in patients with early onset, and they are usually confined to a wheelchair by age 15 years.

LGMD2E (β-Sarcoglycan)

Defects in the β-SG gene are responsible for LGMD2E (Bonnemann et al, 1995; Lim et al, 1995). A missense mutation in this gene was originally described in northern and southern Indiana Amish families. Mutations in the β-SG gene are now reported in other populations worldwide. A wide range of clinical severity has been observed in LGMD2E patients. The age of onset varies from early childhood to adult life with proximal weakness and enlarged calves. Wheelchair dependence may occur in the early teens, but some patients maintain independent ambulation into their sixth decade. Intrafamilial variability for age of onset and progression has been reported as a common feature of LGMD2E.

LGMD2F (δ-Sarcoglycan)

The gene coding for δ-SG is located on chromosome 5q33–34 (Nigro et al, 1996). Mutations in this gene were first identified in families of African-Brazilian descent. Patients with LGMD2F show a severe clinical course with onset within the first decade, loss of independent ambulation in the early teens, and death between 9 and 19 years. Cardiac abnormalities are frequent. Patients carrying dominant mutations in the δ-SG gene may show dilated cardiomyopathy without skeletal muscle involvement. The same gene is spontaneously mutated in the BIO14.6 Syrian hamster, an animal model of cardiomyopathy that displays only minor involvement of skeletal muscle, suggesting the δ-SG gene is a candidate for familial and idiopathic dilated cardiomyopathies as well as LGMD.[21]

LGMD2G

Mutations of the human telethonin gene have recently been shown to cause LGMD2G in three Brazilian families (Moreira et al, 1997, 2000). Besides severe involvement of the proximal muscles in the upper and lower limbs, these patients have early involvement of distal muscles, foot drop, mildly elevated serum CK levels (3- to 30-fold), and rimmed vacuoles in muscle biopsies. Age of onset ranges from 9 to 15 years, and 40% of patients become nonambulatory in the third or fourth decade of life. Cardiac involvement may be present.

Telethonin is a sarcomeric protein expressed at the Z-line in skeletal and cardiac muscle.[4] Telethonin is a substrate of the serine kinase domain of titin, which phosphorylates the carboxy-terminal domain of telethonin in early differentiating myocytes. The transcript in mouse is developmentally regulated in both cardiac and skeletal muscle and is downregulated after denervation. Telethonin may be involved in myofibril assembly and turnover; however, further studies are required to clarify the pathogenetic mechanisms of LGMD2G.

LGMD2H

Originally described in the Hutterite population of Manitoba (Weiler et al, 1998), LGMD2H has late onset and a mild, slowly progressive course. In addition to weakness of proximal limb muscles, patients may present weakness of facial muscles as the disease progresses. The gene has been mapped on chromosome 9q31–q34.1 and encodes TRIM32, a putative E3 ubiquitin ligase highly expressed in heart and skeletal muscle (Frosk et al, 2002). The role of E3 ligases involves the labeling of target proteins with ubiquitin, so that the proteins may be tagged for degradation by the proteasome pathway. Mutations in this gene may cause failure to recognize the target proteins, and their accumulation can lead to muscle disease. At present, there is no evidence for protein accumulation in muscle; however, further studies may clarify this issue.

LGMD2I

The gene for fukutin-related protein (FKRP), responsible for LGMD2I, maps on chromosome 19q13.3 (Brockington et al, 2001; Driss et al, 2000). FKRP was identified through homology to fukutin, the putative glycosyltransferase involved in the pathogenesis of Fukuyama congenital muscular dystrophy. Mutations in the *FKRP* gene were first found in a form of congenital muscular dystrophy (MDC1C) with secondary reduction in laminin $\alpha2$ and abnormal glycosylation of α-dystroglycan (α-DG).[22] The features of MDC1C are severe weakness, wasting of the shoulder girdle musculature, and hypertrophy and weakness of other muscles such as calf and thigh. Macroglossia has also been reported. Several patients show progressive respiratory failure and cardiomyopathy. Individuals with LGMD2I present a similar, though milder, phenotype. The age of onset varies between 0.5 to 27 years, and progression is slow with a large range of phenotypic severity. A significant number of families have mutations in the *FKRP* gene, and many other patients unlinked to the known LGMD loci may carry mutations in this gene.

FKRP is a ubiquitous protein expressed at highest levels in skeletal muscle, heart, and placenta. The aminoterminus sequence targets FKRP to the Golgi complex, where it colocalizes with α-mannosidase II. The homology to fukutin strongly suggests an enzymatic role for FKRP in the glycosylation pathway. Analysis of muscle from patients affected with mild LGMD2I has revealed a selective deficit of higher molecular weight α-DG, and loss of its laminin-binding properties. The dystroglycan complex in muscle forms an axis that connects the intracellular cytoskeleton to the extracellular matrix through direct binding of α-DG to laminin and β-DG to dystrophin.[23] Dystroglycan is the product of the *Dag1* gene, which, through posttranslational processing generates two noncovalently linked proteins: the extracellular heavily glycosylated α-DG, and the transmembrane β-DG. The nature of the carbohydrate moiety of α-DG has not been clarified, but it is clear that altered glycosylation results in loss of laminin binding. A selective reduction in α-DG staining was also observed in patients with MDC1C and LGMD2I, indicating that mutations in the

FKRP gene may affect glycosylation of α-DG. These findings underscore the existence of a common pathogenetic mechanism in MDC1C/LGMD2I, Fukuyama congenital muscular dystrophy, and MEB, in which the affected genes are putative glycosyltransferases. Mutations in different genes coding for enzymes involved in the glycosylation pathway of α-DG may render the protein unable to interact with its ligands, thereby perturbing the central link between extracellular matrix and cytoskeleton and leading to sarcolemmal instability and muscular dystrophy.[24]

LGMD2J

Tibial muscular dystrophy is a mild autosomal dominant disease involving mostly distal muscles and caused by mutations in the titin gene.[25] However, homozygous patients have also been described, presenting proximal early-onset limb-girdle muscular dystrophy with high serum CK levels and secondary deficiency of calpain 3 (Haravuori et al, 2001).

Titin is a large sarcomeric protein that may play a role in the sarcomere assembly and in keeping the myosin filaments in place during contraction cycles.[4] Several ligand-binding sites are present along the protein. Two of the ligands are calpain 3 and telethonin, which are responsible for two other types of LGMD2. The observation that calpain 3 is reduced in heterozygous patients and absent in homozygous LGMD2J suggests that in heterozygotes the binding activity of titin is partially preserved. The loss of activity in homozygous patients results in a phenotype similar to a primary calpainopathy. In support to this hypothesis, apoptotic myonuclei with altered distribution of NF-κB and IκBα are often observed in muscle samples of LGMD2J patients. It is possible that the disease in other LGMD patients with a secondary deficiency of calpain 3 may be due to mutations in titin, and the disease is unnoticed in heterozygous parents due to the mild phenotype.

CONCLUSION

Mutations in the genes involved in LGMD produce allelic heterogeneity and a broad array of phenotypes. The different characteristics of the proteins involved in LGMD (Fig. 43–1) are suggestive of diverse pathogenetic mechanisms. Perturbations of the components of the DGC affect the link between the cytoskeleton and the extracellular matrix, leading to loss of sarcolemmal integrity, and muscular dystrophy. Impaired membrane repair and resealing of damaged muscle fibers may be related to the pathogenesis of LGMD due to dysferlin and calpain 3 mutations. The identification of a group of sarcomeric proteins involved in dystrophic changes indicates that disturbance of the myofibril assembly may be responsible for LGMD. Finally, the linkage of the putative ubiquitin ligase TRIM32 to an LGMD locus may suggest that protein degradation abnormalities

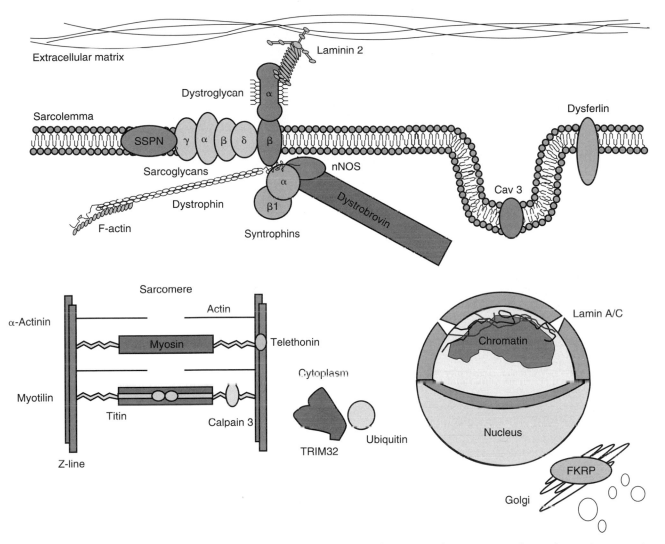

FIGURE 43–1. Schematic representation of the proteins involved in the pathogenesis of LGMD. Sarcolemmal proteins comprise sarcoglycans, caveolin 3, and dysferlin. Titin, telethonin, and myotilin are sarcomeric proteins. Lamin A/C is found at the nuclear envelope. FKRP localizes in the Golgi complex. TRIM32 may be involved in the ubiquitination pathway.

may also lead to muscular dystrophy. Although advances have been significant, much remains to be learned about the functions of these proteins and the pathologic consequences of their deficiency. The analysis of spontaneous mutants and the generation of animal models lacking proteins affected in the various LGMD pathologies are shedding light on the pathogenetic mechanisms involved and providing insight on future therapies for the treatment of these diseases.

REFERENCES*

1. Bushby KM: Making sense of the limb-girdle muscular dystrophies. Brain 1999;122:1403–1420.

2. Piccolo F, Moore SA, Mathews KD, Campbell KP: Limb-girdle muscular dystrophies. Adv Neurol 2002;88:273–291.

3. Cohn RD, Campbell KP: Molecular basis of muscular dystrophies. Muscle Nerve 2000;23: 1456–1471.

4. Faulkner G, Lanfranchi G, Valle G: Telethonin and other new proteins of the Z-disc of skeletal muscle. IUBMB Life 2001;51:275–282.

5. Laing NG, Wilton SD, Akkari PA, et al: A mutation in the alpha tropomyosin gene TPM3 associated with autosomal dominant nemaline myopathy. Nat Genet 1995;9:75–79.

6. Moir RD, Spann TP: The structure and function of nuclear lamins: Implications for disease. Cell Mol Life Sci 2001;58:1748–1757.

7. De Sandre-Giovannoli A, Chaouch M, Kozlov S, et al: Homozygous defects in LMNA, encoding lamin A/C nuclear-envelope proteins, cause autosomal recessive axonal neuropathy in human (Charcot-Marie-Tooth disorder type 2) and mouse. Am J Hum Genet 2002;70: 726–736.

*Parenthetical reference citations may be found in Table 43–1.

8. Novelli G, Muchir A, Sangiuolo F, et al: Mandibuloacral dysplasia is caused by a mutation in LMNA-encoding lamin A/C. Am J Hum Genet 2002;71:426–431.

9. Galbiati F, Razani B, Lisanti MP: Caveolae and caveolin-3 in muscular dystrophy. Trends Mol Med 2001;7:435–441.

10. Sotgia F, Lee JK, Das K, et al: Caveolin-3 directly interacts with the C-terminal tail of β-dystroglycan. Identification of a central WW-like domain within caveolin family members. J Biol Chem 2000;275: 38048–38058.

11. Minetti C, Bado M, Broda P, et al: Impairment of caveolae formation and T-system disorganization in human muscular dystrophy with caveolin-3 deficiency. Am J Pathol 2002;160:265–270.

12. Matsuda C, Hayashi YK, Ogawa M, et al: The sarcolemmal proteins dysferlin and caveolin-3 interact in skeletal muscle. Hum Mol Genet 2001;10: 1761–1766.

13. Baghdiguian S, Richard I, Martin M, et al: Pathophysiology of limb girdle muscular dystrophy type 2A: Hypothesis and new insights into the IκBα/NF-κB survival pathway in skeletal muscle. J Mol Med 2001; 79:254–261.

14. Anderson LV, Harrison RM, Pogue R, et al: Secondary reduction in calpain 3 expression in patients with limb girdle muscular dystrophy type 2B and Miyoshi myopathy (primary dysferlinopathies). Neuromuscul Disord 2000;10:553–559.

15. Bushby KM: Dysferlin and muscular dystrophy. Acta Neurol Belg 2000;100:142–145.

16. Gallardo E, Rojas-Garcia R, de Luna N, et al: Inflammation in dysferlin myopathy: Immunohistochemical characterization of 13 patients. Neurology 2001;57:2136–2138.

17. Davis DB, Doherty KR, Delmonte AJ, et al: Calcium-sensitive phospholipid binding properties of normal and mutant ferlin C2 domains. J Biol Chem 2002;277:22883–22888.

18. Ervasti JM, Campbell KP: Membrane organization of the dystrophin-glycoprotein complex. Cell 1991;66:1121–1131.

19. Barresi R, Moore SA, Stolle CA, et al: Expression of γ-sarcoglycan in smooth muscle and its interaction with the smooth muscle sarcoglycan-sarcospan complex. J Biol Chem 2000;275:38554–38560.

20. Coral-Vazquez R, Cohn RD, Moore SA, et al: Disruption of the sarcoglycan-sarcospan complex in vascular smooth muscle: A novel mechanism for cardiomyopathy and muscular dystrophy. Cell 1999;98:465–474.

21. Tsubata S, Bowles KR, Vatta M, et al: Mutations in the human δ-sarcoglycan gene in familial and sporadic dilated cardiomyopathy. J Clin Invest 2000; 106:655–662.

22. Brockington M, Blake DJ, Prandini P, et al: Mutations in the fukutin-related protein gene (FKRP) cause a form of congenital muscular dystrophy with secondary laminin alpha2 deficiency and abnormal glycosylation of α-dystroglycan. Am J Hum Genet 2001;69: 1198–1209.

23. Henry MD, Campbell KP: Dystroglycan inside and out. Curr Opin Cell Biol 1999;11:602–607.

24. Cohn RD, Henry MD, Michele DE, et al: Disruption of the Dag1 in differentiated skeletal muscle reveals a role for dystroglycan in muscle regeneration. Cell 2002;110:639–648.

25. Hackman P, Vihola A, Haravuori H, et al: Tibial muscular dystrophy is a titinopathy caused by mutations in TTN, the gene encoding the giant skeletal-muscle protein titin. Am J Hum Genet 2002;71:492–500.

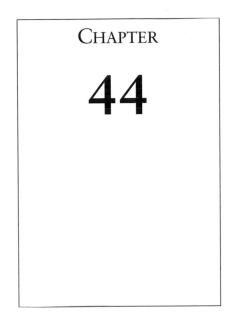

CHAPTER

44

The Congenital Myopathies

Heinz Jungbluth

Caroline A. Sewry

Francesco Muntoni

The structural congenital myopathies are a heterogeneous group of neuromuscular disorders with characteristic histopathologic findings on muscle biopsy. The concept of the congenital myopathies was established following the introduction of new histochemical techniques to the investigation of diseased muscle tissue in the 1950s and 1960s. Central core disease,[1] nemaline myopathy,[2] myotubular (centronuclear) myopathy,[3] and minicore myopathy (or multicore disease)[4] were the major conditions identified.

Mutations in several genes have recently been identified in a proportion of the congenital myopathies, advancing our understanding of their molecular basis. Genetic advances suggest that the boundaries between conditions defined according to histopathologic and clinical criteria are often indistinct and do not necessarily reflect underlying molecular mechanisms. It is now accepted that mutations in the same gene can give rise to diverse clinical and histopathologic phenotypes, and that a similar phenotype can arise from mutations in a variety of genes due to functional association of the respective gene products.

Recognition of clinical and histopathologic phenotypes remains essential for an informed consideration of possible genetic mechanisms. This chapter will therefore follow the traditional histopathologic and clinical classification of the congenital myopathies and discuss underlying genetic defects in close relation to their phenotypic expression.

CENTRAL CORE DISEASE

Central core disease (CCD) is characterized by core-like areas devoid of oxidative enzyme activity (Fig. 44–1A).

Genetics

CCD is commonly transmitted as an autosomal-dominant trait with variable penetrance; many sporadic cases have also been reported. Initial linkage studies assigned a locus to chromosome 19q13.1, and dominant mutations in the skeletal muscle ryanodine receptor gene (*RYR1*) were subsequently detected.[5] Linkage to the *RYR1* locus has been established in most pedigrees without confirmed mutation. Malignant hyperthermia susceptibility (MHS) is an allelic condition but shows marked locus heterogeneity.

The *RYR1* gene contains 106 exons and encodes for a protein of 5037 amino acids, composing the skeletal muscle ryanodine receptor (RyR1), a giant tetrameric structure located in specialized junctional parts of the sarcoplasmic reticulum between the terminal cisternae and transverse tubules. RyR1 is a ligand-gated release channel for Ca^{2+} stored in the terminal cisternae and plays a crucial role in excitation-contraction coupling by regulating cytosolic calcium levels.

RyR1 calcium release is primarily triggered by voltage-induced conformational changes of the abutting dihydropyridine receptor (DHPR), and secondarily by a number of exogenous and endogenous effector molecules. The predicted structure of the ryanodine receptor suggests that the calcium release channel is located in the C-terminal part of the protein, whereas the N-terminal portion interacts with the DHPR. The complex genotype-phenotype correlations associated with mutations in the *RYR1* gene may be partly explained by the degree of functional differentiation within this large protein. More than 30 different mutations have been identified in *RYR1* to date.[5] The first mutations identified predominantly gave rise to the MHS phenotype and affected mainly two

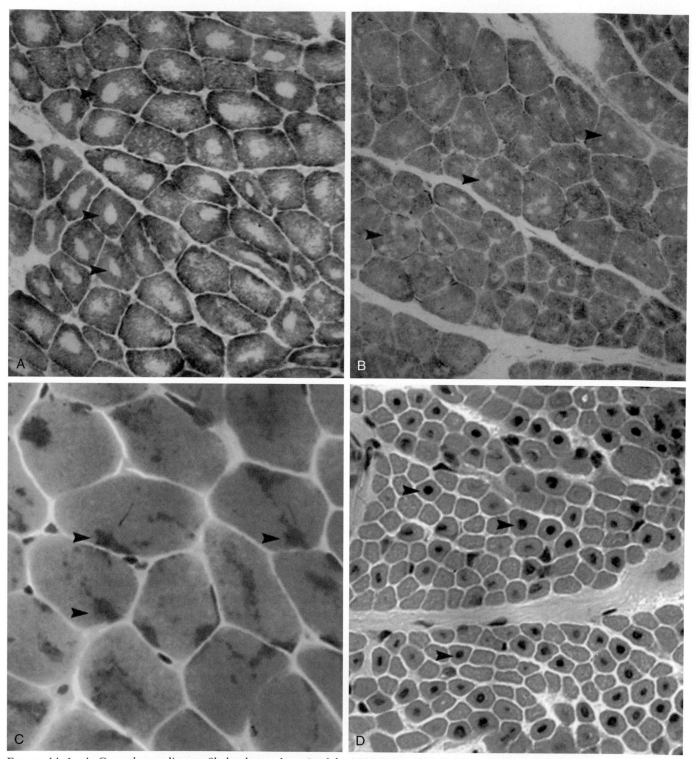

FIGURE 44–1. *A,* Central core disease. Skeletal muscle stained for NADH-TR showing large and predominantly central cores devoid of staining *(arrows)* in most fibers. Associated fiber-type uniformity with all fibers shows high oxidative activity. *B,* Minicore myopathy (multicore disease). Skeletal muscle stained for NADH-TR showing multiple focal areas devoid of staining *(arrows)* in most fibers. Associated fiber-type uniformity with all fibers shows high oxidative activity. *C,* Nemaline myopathy. Skeletal muscle stained with the Gomori trichrome method showing multiple nemaline rods *(arrows)* in most fibers. *D,* Myotubular myopathy. Skeletal muscle stained with hematoxylin and eosin (H & E) showing many fibers with prominent central nuclei *(arrows).*

regions of the protein: the cytoplasmic N-terminal domain (MHS/CCD region 1, amino acids 35 to 614), and the cytoplasmic central domain (MHS/CCD region 2, amino acids 2163 to 2458). Few patients with the CCD phenotype were found to have mutations in these regions. More recently, there has been increasing evidence that mutations affecting the C-terminal portion of the receptor molecule (MHS/CCD region 3, amino acids 4550 to 4940) are common in patients with CCD.[6-7] Some of these patients may also show nemaline rods on muscle biopsy.[8]

The vast majority of mutations in the *RYR1* gene are missense mutations, although small deletions have been reported.[7] De novo dominant mutations have also been documented and probably account for the majority of sporadic cases. A few recessive pedigrees have been reported; we have recently identified a homozygous missense mutation in exon 101 of the *RYR1* gene in one consanguineous family with a congenital myopathy characterized by cores and few additional nemaline rods.[9]

The effect of individual *RYR1* mutations on *RyR1* function has been studied both in homologous and heterologous cell systems. When expressed in heterologous cell cultures, mutant forms of the ryanodine receptor associated with both MHS and CCD have been shown to release calcium in response to lower levels of added caffeine or halothane compared to the normal receptor. Studies on mutant *RyR1* expressed in muscle of *RYR1* knockout mice suggested disturbance of excitation contraction coupling as another pathogenetic mechanism.[10] Abnormalities of calcium homeostasis have been reported in lymphoblastoid cell lines from patients with *RYR1* mutations.[6]

Histopathology

While central accumulation of stain with the modified Gomori trichrome technique was the first abnormality identified,[1] the name CCD was introduced later reflecting the characteristic central absence of oxidative enzyme activity.

The degree of histologic changes can be variable and sampling and age of the patient have to be taken into account. The cores typically affect type 1 fibers, and marked type 1 predominance or uniformity may be the only abnormal feature at an early age. The cores may be central or peripheral, single or multiple. Differentiation from the histopathologic appearance of minicore myopathy may sometimes be difficult. Cores are not specific to CCD, and similar (targetoid) lesions can be induced by denervation or tenotomy, and have been described in hypertrophic cardiomyopathy secondary to mutations in the β-myosin gene. Core length can be variable, but they typically extend down an appreciable length of a fiber. The cores represent areas of sarcomeric disorganization. Electron microscopy shows mitochondrial depletion and variable degrees of disintegration of the contractile apparatus.

Immunohistochemical studies have demonstrated abnormal expression of various sarcomeric and intermediate filament proteins.[11]

Clinical Features

CCD is characterized by a variable degree of hypotonia and axial and proximal muscle weakness predominantly affecting the hip girdle. Presentation is usually in infancy or early childhood. Facial involvement is mild, and lack of complete eye closure may be the only finding. Orthopedic problems such as congenital dislocation of the hips, scoliosis and talipes, and ligamentous laxity are common. Serum creatine kinase (CK) activity is usually normal or only moderately elevated. Most affected individuals achieve the ability to walk, although severe variants are on record. The natural course is static or only slowly progressive. In contrast to other congenital myopathies, cardiac involvement is not a feature and respiratory involvement is rare. MHS is a common complication, and all cases should be considered at risk.

Muscle ultrasound can help in the assessment of individuals from CCD families, as it often shows a striking increase in echogenicity even in paucisymptomatic individuals. We have reported a specific pattern of selective muscle involvement using magnetic resonance imaging.[9]

MINICORE MYOPATHY (MULTICORE DISEASE)

Multicore disease[4] is characterized by multifocal areas of myofibrillar disruption (see Fig. 44–1*B*). The term *minicore myopathy* was introduced later to distinguish the condition from central core disease with multiple cores.

Genetics

It has become obvious that minicore myopathy represents a syndrome with different underlying genetic abnormalities and considerable overlap with other neuromuscular disorders. Most published cases have been either sporadic or compatible with autosomal-recessive inheritance. Recessive mutations in the *selenoprotein N (SEPN1)* gene, implicated in congenital muscular dystrophy with early rigidity of the spine (RSMD1), have also been identified in a subset of patients with minicores on muscle biopsy and characteristic clinical features.[12] In addition, the identification of recessive mutations in the *RYR1* gene in another clinically distinct group provided the genetic basis for the suspected clinical and histopathological continuum between CCD and minicore myopathy.[9,13] Other cases of minicore myopathy not linked to either the *RYR1* or the *SEPN1* locus suggest further heterogeneity and await genetic resolution.

Histopathology

Multifocal lesions characterized by absence of oxidative enzyme stain activity are the histopathologic hallmark of minicore myopathy (see Fig. 44–1B). Ultrastructurally, these are focal areas with absence of mitochondria and variable disruption of myofibrils affecting only a few sarcomeres. Minicores occur in both type 1 and type 2 fibers. Other features such as type 1 predominance and hypotrophy and increase in central nuclei are common. While a degree of histopathologic overlap with CCD was already acknowledged in early reports,[4] minicores may occur to a limited extent as an additional feature in several other neuromuscular disorders.

Immunohistochemical studies in minicore myopathy have suggested sarcoplasmic reticulum and desmin abnormalities similar to those observed in central core disease.[11]

Clinical Features

Clinical findings of minicore myopathy are highly variable, and at least four different clinical phenotypes have been described.[14,15] The most common phenotype is associated with recessive mutations in the SEPN1 gene[12] and features marked axial weakness with spinal rigidity, scoliosis, and respiratory failure. Early respiratory failure is a frequent finding in this group of patients, and regular sleep studies are recommended. The second largest group is characterized by partial or complete external ophthalmoplegia. The phenotype in a third group is similar to CCD while marked distal weakness and wasting are observed in only a small number of patients. The two latter phenotypes appear to be associated with mutations in the RYR1 gene.[9,13]

NEMALINE MYOPATHY

Nemaline myopathy is characterized by an abundance of rodlike structures in muscle that stain red with the modified Gomori trichrome technique (see Fig. 44–1C).[2]

Genetics

Nemaline myopathy exists in both autosomal recessive and autosomal dominant forms. Five genes have been implicated in nemaline rod formation as of this writing: the gene for slow α-tropomyosin (TPM3),[16] nebulin (NEB),[17] skeletal muscle α-actin (ACTA1),[18] β-tropomyosin (TPM2),[19] and, more recently, muscle Troponin T (TNNT1).[20]

Mutations in the nebulin gene (NEB) are most commonly involved in the classical autosomal recessive congenital form, but severe neonatal cases have also been reported. The majority of mutations in the NEB gene are nonsense or frame shifting.[17]

Mutations in the skeletal muscle α-actin (ACTA1) gene are predominantly autosomal dominant and only rarely recessive.[18] There is a high rate of de novo mutations. Mutations in this gene are the second most-common known cause of nemaline myopathy. Mutations in the tropomyosin gene are a rare cause of nemaline myopathy. A dominant mutation in the TPM3 gene has been identified in a mild form,[16] while recessive mutations have been implicated in one homozygous case with early severe presentation.[21] Mutations in the TPM2 gene have also been identified in a mild form of nemaline myopathy.[19] Nemaline myopathy due to mutations in the muscle TNNT1 gene[20] appears to be limited to the Amish population in North America. Further genetic heterogeneity is expected, as some families show no linkage to any of the known loci. All genes identified in nemaline myopathy as of this writing code for thin-filament—associated proteins. This suggests disturbed assembly or interplay of these structures as a pivotal mechanism in the evolution of rod pathology.

Histopathology

Nemaline rods are the hallmark of nemaline myopathy. There may be associated type 1 predominance or uniformity, with or without type 1 hypotrophy. Nemaline rods are often subsarcolemmal but may occur intranuclearly in severe cases with ACTA1 mutations. Nemaline rods are not specific and have been described in tenotomy, inflammatory disease, and even normal muscle. The occurrence of nemaline rods and cores in the same patient has been repeatedly described and was recently attributed to mutations in both the RYR1[8,9] and ACTA1[22] genes.

Both the structure and composition of nemaline rods suggest a close relationship with the Z-disk. On electron microscopy, nemaline rods are often in continuity with the Z lines and show a similar lattice structure. Immunohistochemical studies have demonstrated that the Z line component α-actinin is also a component of nemaline bodies. Immunohistochemical studies with different polyclonal antibodies in cases with NEB gene mutations have shown residual expression of the protein; in individual cases, absence of staining with one antibody but not others might help in targeting mutation analysis to specific regions of the gene.[23] In many patients with confirmed mutations in the ACTA1 gene, immunohistochemical labeling of actin is normal; however, unevenness or accumulation of staining may occur.

Clinical Features

The clinical spectrum of nemaline myopathy is wide and ranges from severe cases with antenatal onset to only mildly affected adults. The most common classical form of nemaline myopathy is tightly associated with recessive mutations in the NEB gene and characterized by onset in infancy or childhood with hypotonia and general weakness predominantly affecting facial and axial muscles.[24] Disproportionate feeding difficulties are very common and often require tube feeding and gastrostomy insertion later in life. Severe respiratory impairment requires nighttime ventilation in many ambulant cases. Skeletal involvement comprising scoliosis, spinal rigidity, and foot deformities is frequent, while an associated cardiomyopathy has been occasionally described. The course is typically static or only slowly progressive, and the degree of cardiorespiratory involvement is the main prognostic factor.

Dominant mutations in the *ACTA1* gene account for both severe neonatal cases and cases of later onset, and there is significant clinical overlap with the form due to mutations in the *NEB* gene.[18,22]

MYOTUBULAR (CENTRONUCLEAR) MYOPATHY

Myotubular (centronuclear) myopathy is characterized by numerous centrally placed nuclei with a surrounding central zone devoid of oxidative enzyme activity or oxidative enzyme accumulation (see Fig. 44–1*D*).

Genetics

X-linked, autosomal recessive, and dominant inheritance have all been reported, but not all of these cases have been genetically characterized.

Deletions, missense, and nonsense mutations in the myotubularin gene (*MTM1*) on chromosome Xq28 have been identified in more than 90% of affected males with the X-linked recessive form of myotubular myopathy.[25] Disease manifestations in carriers have been described, occasionally associated with a deletion in the Xq27-q28 region or skewed X inactivation. This latter phenomenon can lead to girls being as severely affected as boys. Therefore, screening of the *MTM1* gene should also be considered in females with suggestive clinical and histologic features (personal observation).

Myotubularin belongs to a family of dual-specific phosphatases, playing a role in the epigenetic regulation of signaling pathways involved in growth and differentiation. A specific role of myotubularin in dephosphorylating phosphatidylinositol 3-phosphate [PI(3)P], a lipid second messenger with a crucial role in membrane trafficking, has recently been reported.[26]

The autosomal recessive and autosomal dominant forms remain genetically unresolved.

Histopathology

Numerous centrally located internal nuclei (see Fig. 44–1*D*) surrounded by a perinuclear halo devoid of myofilaments are the hallmark of myotubular myopathy.

Oxidative enzyme staining may show a dark central area, or there may be a pale peripheral halo. Type 1 hypotrophy may precede or accompany the appearance of central internal nuclei, and the number of central nuclei may vary between muscles and with age. Multiple minicores may be an associated finding. Congenital myotonic dystrophy can be a histopathologic phenocopy and must be excluded.

While the term myotubular myopathy was suggested to describe a possible developmental abnormality, some immunohistochemical studies[11] and recent in vitro studies do not support this. Monoclonal antibodies against myotubularin are not suitable for immunohistochemical studies, but have been successfully applied in radioimmunoassays.

Clinical Features

The clinical phenotype of myotubular (centronuclear) myopathy is highly variable depending on the mode of inheritance. The X-linked form gives rise to a severe phenotype in males presenting with polyhydramnios, reduced fetal movements, marked hypotonia, a variable degree of external ophthalmoplegia, respiratory failure at birth, and an often fatal course. Severely affected infants who are entirely ventilator-dependent in the neonatal period may survive if receiving continuous invasive ventilation, but they show almost complete lack of motor developmental progress. A small proportion of less severely affected males not requiring immediate ventilation may survive into their teens or beyond and may suffer from other medical complications.[27] Genotype-phenotype correlation studies are complicated by often marked intrafamilial phenotypic variability. Autosomal-dominant forms are milder and of later onset, while the phenotype in the autosomal recessive forms can range from early presentation with marked proximal weakness and inability to walk, to milder variants characterized by generalized weakness and a variable degree of external ophthalmoplegia. Additional features may comprise facial dysmorphism, scoliosis, and foot deformities. Respiratory involvement may be severe, and an associated cardiomyopathy has been described in a few cases. In the absence of significant cardiorespiratory involvement, the prognosis is favorable.

CONCLUSION

The understanding of the genetic bases of the congenital myopathies is rapidly advancing. While a confident histopathologic diagnosis can be established in several of the conditions described, it is not unusual to find cases in which the histopathologic hallmarks are atypical or only incompletely expressed. These cases represent diagnostic challenges, and only a combined histopathologic and clinical approach will enable an accurate genetic diagnosis.

REFERENCES

1. Shy GM, Magee KR: A new congenital nonprogressive myopathy. Brain 1956;79:610–621.

2. Shy GM, Engel WK, Somers JE, Wanko T: Nemaline myopathy. A new congenital myopathy. Brain 1963;86:793–810.

3. Spiro AJ, Shy GM, Gonatas NK: Myotubular myopathy. Arch Neurol 1966;14:1–14.

4. Engel AG, Gomez MR, Groover RV: Multicore disease: A recently recognized congenital myopathy associated with multifocal degeneration of muscle fibers. Mayo Clin Proc 1971;46:666–681.

5. McCarthy T, Quane KA, Lynch PJ: Ryanodine receptor mutations in malignant hyperthermia and central core disease. Hum Mut 2000;15:410–417.

6. Tilgen N, Zorzato F, Halliger-Keller B, et al: Identification of four novel mutations in the C-terminal membrane spanning domain of the ryanodine receptor 1: Association with central core disease and alteration of calcium homeostasis. Hum Mol Genet 2001;10: 2879–2887.

7. Monnier N, Romero NB, Lerale J, et al: Familial and sporadic forms of central core disease are associated with mutations in the C-terminal domain of the skeletal muscle ryanodine receptor. Hum Mol Genet 2001;15: 2581–2592.

8. Monnier N, Romero NB, Lerale J, et al: An autosomal dominant congenital myopathy with cores and rods is associated with a neomutation in the RYR1 gene encoding the skeletal muscle ryanodine receptor. Hum Mol Genet 2000;9:2599–2608.

9. Jungbluth H, Müller CR, Halliger-Keller B, et al: Autosomal-recessive inheritance of RYR1 mutations in a congenital myopathy with cores. Neurology 2002;59:284–287.

10. Avila G, O'Brien JJ, Dirksen RT: Excitation contraction uncoupling by a human central core disease mutation in the ryanodine receptor. Proc Natl Acad Sci U S A 2001;98:4215–4220.

11. Sewry CA: The role of immunocytochemistry in the congenital myopathies. Neuromuscul Disord 1998;8:394–400.

12. Ferreiro A, Quijano-Roy S, Pichereau C, et al: Mutations of the *selenoprotein* N gene, which is implicated in rigid spine muscular dystrophy, cause the classical phenotype of multiminicore disease. Am H Hum Genet 2002;71:739–749.

13. Ferreiro A, Monnier N, Romero NB, et al: A recessive form of central core disease, transiently presenting as multi minicore disease, is associated with a homozygous mutation in the ryanodine receptor type 1 gene. Ann Neurol 2002;51:750–759.

14. Jungbluth H, Sewry C, Brown SC, et al. Minicore myopathy in children: A clinical and histopathological study of 19 cases. Neuromuscul Disord 2000;10:264–273.

15. Ferreiro A, Estournet B, Chateau D, et al: Multi minicore disease—searching for boundaries: Phenotype analysis of 38 cases. Ann Neurol 2000;48:745–757.

16. Laing NG, Wilton SD, Akkari PA, et al: A mutation in the alpha tropomyosin gene TPM3 associated with autosomal dominant nemaline myopathy. Nat Genet 1995;9:75–79.

17. Pelin K, Hilpela P, Donner K, et al: Mutations in the nebulin gene associated with autosomal-recessive nemaline myopathy. Proc Natl Acad Sci U S A 1999;96:2305–2310.

18. Nowak KJ, Wattanasirichaigoon D, Goebel HH, et al: Mutations in the skeletal muscle alpha actin gene in patients with actin myopathy and nemaline myopathy. Nat Genet 1999;23:208–212.

19. Donner K, Ollikainen M, Ridanpaa M, et al: Mutations in the beta-tropomyosin (TPM2) gene: A rare cause of nemaline myopathy. Neuromuscul Disord 2002;12:151–158.

20. Johnston JJ, Kelley RI, Crawford TO, et al: A novel nemaline myopathy in the Amish caused by a mutation in troponin T1. Am J Hum Genet 2000;67:814–821.

21. Tan P, Briner J, Boltshauser E, et al: Homozygosity for a nonsense mutation in the alpha-tropomyosin gene TPM3 in a patient with severe nemaline myopathy. Neuromuscul Disord 1999;9:573–579.

22. Jungbluth H, Sewry CA, Brown SC, et al: Mild phenotype of nemaline myopathy with sleep hypoventilation due to mutation in the skeletal muscle alpha-actin (ACTA1) gene. Neuromuscul Disord 2001;11:35–40.

23. Sewry CA, Brown SC, Pelin K, et al: Abnormalities in the expression of nebuline in chromosome-2 linked nemaline myopathy. Neuromuscul Disord 2001;11:146–153.

24. Wallgren-Pettersson C, Pelin K, Hilpela P, et al: Clinical and genetic heterogeneity in autosomal-recessive nemaline myopathy. Neuromuscul Disord 1999;9: 564–572.

25. Laporte J, Biancalana V, Tanner SM, et al: MTM1 mutations in X-linked myotubular myopathy. Hum Mutat 2000;15:393–409.

26. Blondeau F, Laporte J, Bodin S, et al: Myotubularin, a phosphatase deficient in myotubular myopathy, acts on phosphatidylinositol 3-kinase and phosphatidylinositol 3 phosphate pathway. Hum Mol Genet 2000;9:2223–2229.

27. Herman GE, Finegold M, Zhao W, et al: Medical complications in long-term survivors with X-linked myotubular myopathy. J Pediatr 1999;134:206–214.

Appendix

Muscle and nerve are joined by a complex structural and functional apparatus, the neuromuscular junction, which allows electrical impulses to be transmitted from the motor nerve terminal to acetylcholine receptors (AChR) on the synaptic folds of the neuromuscular junction as discrete packets (quanta) of acetylcholine (ACh). Although a lot of work has been done on the acquired autoimmune disorders of neuromuscular transmission (myasthenia gravis and Eaton-Lambert syndrome), relatively little was known until recently about the variety of inherited defects that affect different components of the neuromuscular junction and result in a clinically and genetically heterogeneous group of disorders known as *congenital myasthenic syndromes* (CMSs). As most of these disorders affect infants, it seems appropriate to summarize them here, as an appendix to the chapter on congenital myopathies.

The table that follows, kindly provided by Dr. Andrew G. Engel (Mayo Clinic), classifies the CMSs on the basis of the site of the lesion. Functionally, the common feature of all CMSs is a reduced safety margin of neuromuscular transmission, a function of the relationship between the depolarization caused by activation of AChRs (endplate potential, EPP) and the depolarization needed to activate voltage-dependent sodium channels of the $Na_v1.4$ type. A pathologic decrease of the safety margin can be due to genetic defects in presynaptic factors, in the synaptic basal lamina, or in postsynaptic factors. The clinical, structural, functional, and molecular features of these disorders can be found in the review article from which the table is reproduced (Engel AG, Ohno K, Sine SM: Sleuthing molecular targets for neurological diseases at the neuromuscular junction. Nature Rev Neurosci 2003;4:14.)

TABLE 1.   Classification of the Congenital Myasthenic Syndromes Based on Site of Defect[*]

Site of Defect	Index Cases
Presynaptic Defects (7%)	
Choline acetyltransferase deficiency[†]	7
Paucity of synaptic vesicles and reduced quantal release	1
Lambert-Eaton–like syndrome	1
Other presynaptic defects	4
Synaptic Basal Lamina–Associated Defects (14%)	
Endplate AChE deficiency[†]	25
Postsynaptic Defects (79%)	
Kinetic abnormality of AChR with/without AChR deficiency[†]	45
AChR deficiency with/without minor kinetic abnormality[†]	83
Rapsyn deficiency[†]	17
Kinetic defect in $Na_v1.4$[†]	1
Plectin deficiency	1
Total (100%)	**185**

[*]Classification based on a cohort of patients with a congenital myasthenic syndrome investigated at the Mayo Clinic between 1988 and 2003.
[†]Gene defects identified.
AChE, acetylcholinesterase; AChR, acetylcholine receptor; ChAT, choline acetyltransferase.

CHAPTER 45

The Distal Myopathies

Ami K. Mankodi
Robert C. Griggs

Distal myopathies are a group of inherited or sporadic primary muscle disorders characterized by predominant distal muscle weakness and atrophy in hands, forearms, lower legs, and feet. In this chapter we emphasize progress in understanding disease mechanisms and describe some novel forms of distal myopathies.

Advances in immunohistochemical and molecular diagnostic techniques have clarified the genetic basis and potential pathophysiology of distal myopathies. Specific chromosomal localization is now known for all major disorders. The gene product has been identified for Miyoshi myopathy[1] and hereditary inclusion body myopathy.[2] A candidate gene has been suggested for Markesbery-Griggs-Udd myopathy.[3] Interestingly, it is now known that mutations in the same gene (dysferlin) can cause either limb girdle muscular dystrophy (*LGMD2B*) or Miyoshi myopathy.[1] In addition, Nonaka myopathy, hereditary inclusion body myopathy, and quadriceps sparing-vacuolar myopathy are all linked to the same genetic locus on chromosome 9p indicating that these are indeed allelic disorders.[4] Thus, future classifications of distal myopathies may be based on the gene protein product or gene mutation rather than on the distribution of weakness. However, the current classification based on age at onset, pattern of muscle involvement, and mode of inheritance is clinically useful and facilitates further diagnostic procedures (Table 45-1).

LATE ADULT ONSET DISTAL MYOPATHIES

Type 1: Welander Myopathy

Clinical Features. Inheritance is autosomal dominant. Most reported families are of Scandinavian descent.

Symptom onset is usually in the fifth decade, although some patients first notice weakness as late as in their seventies. Onset before age 30 years is unusual. Patients usually develop symptoms in distal upper extremities, typically finger and wrist extensors. Marked atrophy of thenar and intrinsic hand muscles becomes manifest after several years of disease. In 85% of patients, the weakness is asymmetric. With time the finger and wrist flexors become affected as well. Symptoms gradually extend to the lower extremities, with weakness predominantly in toe and ankle extensors. Proximal weakness is uncommon. Muscle stretch reflexes are preserved except for ankle reflexes, which may be lost later in the disease. Sensory system examination is usually normal. The progression of disease is typically slow, and most patients continue full activities and have normal life span. Cardiomyopathy does not occur. Rare homozygous patients have more severe disease with early age at onset, proximal muscle weakness, and wheelchair dependency.

Laboratory Findings. Serum creatine kinase (CK) level is normal or twofold to threefold elevated. Needle electromyography (EMG) reveals small, brief motor unit potentials with early recruitment. Fibrillations and myotonic discharges have been observed. Although routine nerve conduction studies are normal, mild abnormalities in sural nerve biopsies and deficits in vibration and temperature examination by quantitative sensory testing suggest underlying asymptomatic, length-dependent, predominantly sensory small-fiber neuropathy. Muscle biopsy shows dystrophic features with fiber size variability, increase in connective and fat tissue, central nuclei, and split fibers. Rimmed vacuoles and 15- to 18-nm cytoplasmic and nuclear filaments are

TABLE 45–1. Classification of Distal Myopathies

Type	Description	Inheritance	Locus/Gene	Onset age (yr)	Early symptoms	CK	Pathology
Definite entities							
Welander myopathy	Welander 1951	AD	2p13	>40	hands, finger extensors	1–3x	Dystrophic, rimmed vacuoles
Tibial muscular dystrophy	Markesbery and Griggs 1974; Udd 1994	AD	2q24-31 ?titin	>35	anterior lower leg	1–4x	Dystrophic, rimmed vacuoles, calpain3 defect
Nonaka myopathy	Nonaka 1981	AR	9p1-q1 ?GNE	15–30	anterior lower leg	3–4x	Dystrophic, prominent rimmed vacuoles
Miyoshi myopathy	Miyoshi 1985	AR	2p13 Dysferlin	15–30	posterior lower leg, calf	20–150x	Dystrophic, dysferlin defect
Laing myopathy (MPDI)	Laing 1995[14]; Voit 2001[15]	AD	14q	3–25	anterior lower leg	1–3x	Mild to moderate dystrophic
Myofibrillar myopathies							
Desmin-related myopathy	Dalakas 2000	AD/sporadic	2q35 Desmin	variable	distal and proximal weakness, cardiomyopathy	1–4x	Dystrophic, rimmed vacuoles, desmin bodies
Desmin-related myopathy	Vicart 1998[23]	AD/sporadic	11q αB-crystallin	variable	distal leg and hands, cardiomyopathy	–	Dystrophic, rimmed vacuoles, desmin bodies
Myofibrillar myopathy with arrhythmogenic right ventricular cardiomyopathy	Melberg 1999[24]	AD	10q22.3	30–60	axial weakness, anterior lower leg	–	Dystrophic, rimmed vacuoles, desmin bodies
Scapuloperoneal myopathy	Wilhelmsen 1996[20]	AD	12q				
Single families							
Adult-onset myopathy	Felice 1996	AD	2, 9, 14 excluded	20–40	anterior lower leg	2–6x	Mild nonspecific changes
Distal myopathy with respiratory failure	Chinnery 2001[7]	AD anticipation	2, 9, 14 excluded	32–75	anterior lower leg	1–2x	Dystrophic, rimmed vacuoles, amyloid + desmin inclusions
Distal anterior compartment myopathy	Illa 2001[13]	AR	2p13 Dysferlin	14–28	anterior lower leg, rapid progression	20–150x	Dystrophic, dysferlin defect
Distal myopathy with vocal cord and pharyngeal weakness (MPD2)	Feit 1998[17]	AD	5q31	35–60	anterior lower leg, dysphonia	1–8x	Rimmed vacuoles
Distal myopathy with pes cavus and areflexia	Servidei 1999[18]	AD	19p13	15–50	lower leg, dysphonia, dysphagia	2–6x	Dystrophic, rimmed vacuoles

seen in patients with moderate to severe weakness. Absence of inflammation helps distinguish Welander myopathy from inclusion body myositis.

Molecular Genetics. Welander myopathy has been linked to chromosome 2p13.[5] The locus of the proposed gene is close to dysferlin. Mutation screening of the dysferlin gene may help clarify whether Welander myopathy is allelic to Miyoshi myopathy, *LGMD2B*, and to distal anterior compartment myopathy.

Type 2: Markesbery-Griggs-Udd Distal Myopathy (Tibial Muscular Dystrophy)

Clinical Features. This form of late-onset, dominantly inherited distal myopathy has been reported in English, French, and Finnish families. Symptoms usually begin after age 40 years. Weakness begins in the anterior compartment of the legs. This condition is often referred to as tibial muscular dystrophy (TMD). As the disease progresses, finger and wrist extensors may be affected. Much later in life, proximal weakness may also occur. Non-Finnish patients were reported to progress rapidly. The ability to walk may be lost after 15 or 20 years of disease, progressing to complete incapacity after 30 years. One English patient had cardiomyopathy with heart block requiring a pacemaker. In contrast, Finnish patients had much slower progression, upper extremities were rarely affected, and most of them remained ambulatory. However, eight individuals from a Western Finland (Larsmo) pedigree exhibited an *LGMD* phenotype ascribed to a homozygous dominant mutation. Facial, bulbar, and respiratory muscles are not affected.

Laboratory Findings. Serum CK levels can be normal or threefold to fourfold elevated. EMG reveals small, brief-duration motor-unit potentials with early recruitment in the tibialis anterior muscle. Muscle biopsy showed prominent rimmed vacuoles in addition to dystrophic process in non-Finnish patients. However, vacuoles were inconsistently seen in Finnish patients, in whom 15 to 20nm tubulofilaments were occasionally observed in the cytoplasm adjacent to rimmed vacuoles. Immunohistochemical stains for desmin, dystrophin, laminins, spectrin, tau, and beta-amyloid were negative.

Molecular Genetics. The disease has been linked to chromosome 2q31 in both Finnish and non-Finnish families. All Finnish patients carry an identical core haplotype for the 2q13 region, suggesting that they share one ancestral mutation. Patients in the Larsmo kindred with severe *LGMD* phenotype are indeed homozygous for the disease haplotype, but those with milder *LGMD* syndrome are heterozygotes, signifying phenotypic heterogeneity.[3]

A spontaneous mutation in a mouse chromosome 2 region syntenic to human chromosome 2 causes severe autosomal recessive degenerative muscle disease, "muscular dystrophy with myositis" (MDM).[3] These mice develop abnormal gait, weight loss, and have shortened life span. Similar to patients with TMD, these mice show pronounced signs of skeletal muscle degeneration in the tibialis anterior muscle. The titin gene *Ttn* may co-localize with the mouse locus and hence is considered a candidate gene in TMD patients.[3]

Titin is a giant structural protein of the sarcomere with molecular weight of more than 3000 Kd. A single molecule of titin spans half of a sarcomere, from Z discs to M line, extending 2 μm in vivo. Titin may be a "molecular ruler," keeping the myosin filament at the center of the sarcomere during muscle contraction cycles and regulating the ultrastructure of the vertebrate thick filament. Several ligand-binding sites exist along the length of the titin molecule; calpain3 and telethonin are ligands of special interest because they are mutated in *LGMD2A* and *LGMD2G*. No mutations have been detected in a limited sequence analysis of the titin gene targeted to regions that are differentially expressed in heart and skeletal muscle. Immunohistochemistry on frozen muscle sections from patients using antibodies against titin has revealed normal distribution of titin protein in TMD as well as in *LGMD* with homozygous core haplotype. Interestingly, calpain3 protein was significantly reduced in skeletal muscle from patients with *LGMD* phenotype and in WMDM mice by western blot analysis.[3] Results were variable in heterozygotes with TMD phenotype: Calpain3 levels were decreased in some but not all. Similar to *LGMD2A*, perturbations of IκBα/NF-κB pathway leading to myonuclear apoptosis were observed in TMD patients and in MDM mice, related to secondary calpain3 deficiency.[3] The large size of the titin gene makes sequence analysis quite laborious. Because of the evidence that there is secondary deficiency of calpain3, a ligand for titin, studies are currently focusing on sequence analysis of calpain3-binding sites on the titin gene.

Single Families with Clinical/Genetic Heterogeneity. Felice et al[6] described an autosomal dominant distal myopathy resembling Markesbery-Griggs-Udd myopathy that does not localize to chromosome 2, 9, or 14 loci, which have been linked to other distal myopathies.

Chinnery et al[7] reported on 24 individuals, spanning three generations, with tibialis anterior weakness beginning in mid-adult life. The second generation of patients had an earlier age at onset and more rapid progression than the first generation. In contrast to Markesbery-Griggs-Udd myopathy, early respiratory failure was a prominent symptom. All known candidate gene loci for distal myopathies on chromosomes 2, 5, 9, and 14 have been excluded in this family.

EARLY ADULT-ONSET DISTAL MYOPATHIES

Type 1: Nonaka Distal Myopathy

Clinical Features. Initial reports of this disease came from Japan. However, subsequently the disease has been reported in patients from North America, South America, and possibly Italy. Inheritance is autosomal recessive. Symptoms begin late in the second or third decade, and average age at onset is 26 years. Weakness initially involves ankle dorsiflexors and toe extensors, causing foot drop and a steppage gait. Mild distal upper-extremity weakness may be present earlier in the illness. At later stages, patients may develop proximal weakness, although the quadriceps muscles remain relatively spared. Most patients lose ambulation 10 to 15 years after disease onset. Neck flexors may be affected. Cranial muscles are not involved. Cardiac arrhythmia necessitating pacemaker implant has been reported.

Laboratory Findings. Serum CK level is elevated threefold to fourfold. EMG shows small, brief motor-unit potentials and fibrillation potentials. Muscle biopsy reveals prominent vacuoles and dystrophic changes. Vacuoles are lined with granular material that is basophilic with hematoxylin and eosin (H & E) staining and purple red with modified Gomori trichrome staining. The vacuoles exhibit acid phosphatase activity. Electron microscopy reveals 15- to 18-nm filamentous inclusions in the nucleus and cytoplasm, in addition to the vacuoles.

Similar clinical presentation has been reported in families from Middle Eastern countries, North America, and India with the diagnosis of hereditary inclusion body myopathy or quadriceps-sparing myopathy. These patients differ from those with sporadic inclusion body myopathy by their earlier age at onset, initial symptom of foot drop, autosomal recessive inheritance, and absence of inflammation on muscle biopsy.

Molecular Genetics. Like quadriceps-sparing myopathy, Nonaka myopathy is a hereditary inclusion body myopathy linked to chromosome 9p12-13.[4] The candidate gene has been identified in patients with hereditary inclusion body myopathy.[2] Forty-seven Jewish families from Middle Eastern countries were homozygous for missense mutation (2186T→C, M712T) in the kinase domain of UDP-N-acetylglucosamine 2 epimerase/N-acetyl mannosamine kinase (GNE).[2] In addition, three families of different ethnic origins (Asian Indian, North American, and Caribbean) were heterozygous for distinct missense mutations in the kinase and epimerase domains of the GNE.[2] GNE is a bifunctional enzyme that catalyzes the first two steps in the biosynthesis of N-acetylneuraminic acid or sialic acid. Interestingly, dominant mutations in the epimerase domain of the gene cause sialuria. None of the patients with hereditary inclusion body myopathy had elevated sialic acid levels. GNE is exclusively shared by vertebrates and bacteria. There is no GNE ortholog in Drosophila melanogaster, Caenorhabditis elegans, or yeast. The two enzymatic activities of GNE are carried out by separate proteins in bacteria. GNE is a ubiquitous molecule, encoded by a single gene. GNE has been shown to be the rate-limiting enzyme in the sialic acid biosynthetic pathway. Sialic acid modification of glycoproteins and glycolipids expressed at the cell surface is crucial for their function in many biologic processes, including cell adhesion and signal transduction. It would be of interest to check sialic acid levels and extent of sialylation of proteins in normal and affected muscles. The GNE gene is currently being studied for mutations in patients with Nonaka myopathy.

Type 2: Miyoshi Distal Myopathy

Clinical Features. Early reports of Miyoshi myopathy came from Japan. Subsequently, the disease has been reported in many ethnic groups. Symptoms begin between ages 15 and 25 years. Inheritance is autosomal recessive. Initial symptoms are in the distal lower extremities (gastrocnemius). Patients complain that they cannot walk on their toes or climb stairs. Aching or discomfort in the calves is common. The gastrocnemius muscles become atrophic, and ankle reflexes are lost. The anterior compartment muscles are spared initially but later become involved. The predilection for early involvement of the posterior compartment in Miyoshi myopathy distinguishes it from other distal myopathies. At presentation, calf involvement may be asymmetric, and in a small number of patients symptoms may remain confined to one leg. As the disease progresses, proximal muscles in legs and arms may also be affected. Progression of the disease appears to correlate better with disease duration than with age at onset. About one third of patients are confined to a wheelchair within 10 years of symptom onset.

Laboratory Findings. Miyoshi myopathy is characterized by a marked increase in CK levels compared to other distal myopathies. Serum CK levels range from 20 to 150 times normal. Indeed, elevated CK levels (hyperCKemia) are often detected prior to symptoms or signs in these patients. EMG shows small, brief myopathic motor-unit potentials and early recruitment. Very weak and atrophic gastrocnemius muscles may show long duration polyphasic motor-unit potentials with reduced recruitment. Muscle biopsy in severely affected gastrocnemius muscle may show "end-stage" disease with widespread fibrosis, fatty replacement, and loss of most muscle fibers. The ideal muscles to biopsy are the hamstrings, as they provide most information on muscle histology. Rimmed vacuoles are not common in these patients. With identification of the gene dysferlin (*DYSF*),[1] characterization of its protein product, and development of antibodies, the diagnosis of Miyoshi myopathy can now be confirmed by a simple immunohistochemical technique. Dysferlin normally localizes to the plasma membrane of muscle fibers. In patients with Miyoshi myopathy and *LGMD2B*, dysferlin is absent in the plasma membrane, whereas scattered granular staining in the cytoplasm or nuclear membrane may be observed.

Molecular Genetics. The first gene causing any distal myopathy was identified in patients with Miyoshi myopathy. Interestingly, identical mutations in the dysferlin gene on chromosome 2p13 can cause Miyoshi myopathy, *LGMD2B*, or distal myopathy with onset in anterior tibial muscles.[1] In a single pedigree, the same mutation can cause Miyoshi myopathy in one sibling and *LGMD2B* in another. The only clinical features shared by these diseases are early age at onset, recessive inheritance, and marked rise in serum CK levels. The patterns of muscle involvement in these allelic phenotypes are quite distinct, as their names suggest. At present, the reason for such diverse phenotypes caused by similar gene defects (phenotypic heterogeneity) is not known.

Dysferlin is a novel protein without homology to other known mammalian proteins. However, it shows homology throughout its length to the *C. elegans* spermatogenesis factor *fer-1*. In fact, the name dysferlin comes from dystrophy-associated *fer-1–like* protein. Dysferlin is expressed in many tissues, including heart, skeletal muscle, kidney, stomach, liver, spleen, lung, uterus and, to a lesser extent, brain and spinal cord.[8] Dysferlin is expressed in the embryonic tissues from the earliest time point examined.[8] As mentioned earlier, it is localized to the plasma membrane. However, dysferlin does not interact with dystrophin, sarcoglycans, or dystroglycans.

The presence of C2 domains in dysferlin suggests that it may play an important role in signaling pathway. C2 domains are believed to bind calcium and thereby trigger signal transduction and membrane trafficking events. Immunoprecipitation studies revealed that dysferlin interacts with caveolin-3.[9] (Mutations in caveolin-3 cause *LGMD1C* and a new form of distal myopathy.[10]) Dysferlin staining was abnormal in two *LGMD1C* muscles. However, caveolin-3 expression was normal in *LGMD2B* muscles. Thus, caveolin-3 deficiency causes secondary dysferlin deficiency but not vice versa.[9] Possible caveolin-3 binding domains have been identified in dysferlin. Indeed, structural abnormalities of the sarcolemma, including subsarcolemmal vacuoles and papillary projections, have been reported in patients with Miyoshi myopathy.[11] Further studies are needed to define the mode of interaction between these proteins and its potential role in muscle degeneration.

A mouse model for dysferlin deficiency (SJL-Dysf)[12] is due to spontaneous mutations in the fourth C2 domain. These mice develop muscle weakness, atrophy, and histologic changes identical to *LGMD2B*. This animal model may help understand the mechanism of muscle degeneration due to dysferlin deficiency, and will be useful for the development of therapeutic rescue strategies.

A Novel Phenotype of Dysferlin Deficiency. Rapidly progressive distal and proximal symmetric weakness with onset in anterior tibial muscles (distal myopathy with anterior tibial onset, or distal anterior compartment myopathy) has been reported in a Spanish Mediterranean family.[13] Inheritance is autosomal recessive. Symptoms begin between 14 and 28 years of age. Patients are wheelchair bound 11 to 22 years from onset of symptoms. A frameshift mutation has been identified in the dysferlin gene, and dysferlin staining is abnormal in skeletal muscle.

Type 3: Laing Distal Myopathy (MPD1)

Clinical Features. Symptoms begin between the ages of 2 and 25 years. Inheritance is autosomal dominant. Since Laing's report of an English-Welsh family in 1995,[14] at least three more families have been identified. Two were from Germany[15] and one from Austria.[16] Weakness begins in ankle dorsiflexors, toe extensors, and neck flexors. Finger extensors and shoulder muscles are affected later in the disease. Hypomyelinating neuropathy has been reported in one German family. The course is protracted, and most patients remain ambulatory.

Laboratory Findings. Serum CK level is normal or mildly elevated (up to threefold). EMG shows short, brief myopathic potentials, and muscle biopsy reveals moderate myopathy. Vacuoles are not prominent.

Molecular Genetics. The disease has been linked to chromosome 14q11.[14,15] The gene has not been identified.

DISTAL MYOPATHY WITH VOCAL CORD AND PHARYNGEAL WEAKNESS (MPD2)

Clinical Features. Feit et al[17] described a large pedigree with an autosomal dominantly inherited myopathy characterized by distal upper and lower extremity weakness and development of vocal cord and pharyngeal weakness. Symptoms begin between ages 35 and 60 years with weakness in ankle dorsiflexors and toe extensors. Sometimes finger extensors may be affected before leg muscles. The weakness may be asymmetric at the onset.

Laboratory Findings. Serum CK levels ranged from normal to up to eightfold increased. Nerve conduction studies showed mild slowing of velocities. EMG showed myopathic potentials. Muscle biopsy revealed a myopathy with rimmed vacuoles.

Molecular Genetics. MPD2 has been linked to a region on chromosome 5q overlapping the locus for *LGMD1A*. A mutation in myotilin has been reported in one pedigree with *LGMD1A*, making it also the candidate gene for MPD2.

In an Italian pedigree with distal muscle atrophy, dysphonia, dysphagia, pes cavus, and areflexia (unusual in distal myopathies) were also described. The disease has been linked to chromosome 19p13.[18] The gene product has not been identified.

MYOFIBRILLAR MYOPATHIES WITH ABNORMAL FOCI OF DESMIN (DESMIN-RELATED MYOPATHIES)

Myofibrillar myopathies are a heterogenous group of severe distal myopathies, often associated with cardiomyopathy. As the name suggests, these myopathies are characterized by the pathologic finding of abnormal accumulation of myofibrillar proteins like desmin, dystrophin, vimentin, gelsolin, and β-spectrin. Of these proteins, desmin has been the one most consistently and most abundantly present in muscle from patients. Indeed, pathogenic mutations have now been identified in the desmin gene in some families.

Clinical Features. Amato et al[19] have reviewed the wide clinical spectrum of these disorders. The pattern of inheritance is autosomal dominant, but sporadic cases (and rarely X-linked recessive inheritance) have been reported. Most patients develop weakness between ages 25 and 45 years. However, there are reports of onset in infancy, as well as later in life. In some kindreds, weakness begins in the hands and, in others, in the distal lower extremities, primarily the anterior compartment. Progression to proximal muscles usually occurs, and some patients develop respiratory failure requiring mechanical ventilation. A scapuloperoneal distribution was reported in one large pedigree.[20] In many cases, there is cardiomyopathy with arrhythmias, heart block, and congestive heart failure. Cardiac symptoms may precede skeletal muscle weakness. Muntoni et al[21] described a family with distal muscle weakness, cardiac/respiratory involvement, and mental retardation. Children can have diffuse, primary proximal or distal weakness. Several children with giant axonal neuropathy had desmin accumulations in heart and skeletal muscle.

Laboratory Findings. Serum CK level is modestly elevated, up to fivefold. EMG shows short, small amplitude motor-unit potentials and fibrillation potentials. Complex repetitive discharges are common. Muscle biopsy reveals nonspecific myopathic features: variability in fiber size, fiber splitting, increase in central nuclei, increase in connective tissue, and occasional rimmed vacuoles. The two major structural abnormalities in light as well as electron microscopy are: non-hyaline lesions consisting of foci of myofibrillar destruction, and hyaline lesions composed of compacted and degraded myofibrillar elements (cytoplasmic or spheroid bodies). The nonhyaline lesions appear as irregular, lobulated dark green areas of amorphous material with the modified Gomori trichrome stain. These lesions include desmin, dystrophin, neural cell adhesion molecule, gelsolin, and β-amyloid precursor protein but do not contain myosin, actin, or α-actinin. The hyaline lesions are spherical, serpentine, or pleomorphic cytoplasmic inclusions, usually eosinophilic with the H & E stain and dark blue or purple-red with the modified Gomori trichrome stain. These lesions react variably to antibodies against desmin, whereas they react strongly to antibodies against dystrophin, gelsolin, β-amyloid precursor protein, titin, nebulin, actin, myosin, and α-actinin. They do not react to antibodies against neural cell adhesion molecule.

Focal accumulation of desmin is, however, a nonspecific finding. It can be seen in many neuromuscular diseases, including spinal muscular atrophy, congenital myotonic dystrophy, myotubular myopathy, and nemaline myopathy, as well as in regenerating muscle fibers of any etiology.

Molecular Genetics. More than one genetic defect can induce the clinical and histologic pattern of myofibrillar myopathy. At least seven missense mutations and two distinct deletions have been reported in the desmin gene (*DES*) on chromosome 2q35. Desmin is a muscle protein consisting of intermediary filaments and is located at Z discs and in subsarcolemmal regions of skeletal, cardiac, and smooth muscle, where it serves as a major scaffold structure. It appears to play an important role in maintaining the structural and functional integrity of muscle fibers by linking the Z discs to the plasma membrane. *DES* knockout mice develop normally and are fertile. Overexpression of mutant desmin protein (L385P) in cultured cells formed intracytoplasmic *DES*-positive aggregates quite similar to the accumulations seen in muscle biopsy specimens. The majority of cells with cytoplasmic desmin aggregates died within 72 hours by apoptosis, suggesting a direct toxic effect of the mutant *DES* protein.[22] In addition, a mutation in the αB crystallin gene on chromosome 11q21-23 was identified in a pedigree with dominantly inherited myofibrillar myopathy.[23] αB crystallin is a molecular chaperone and is believed to interact with DES in the assembly of intermediary filaments. The pedigree with scapuloperoneal weakness and cardiomyopathy has been linked to chromosome 12q.[20] A large Swedish pedigree with autosomal dominant, predominantly distal weakness and arrhythmogenic right ventricular cardiomyopathy has been linked to chromosome 10q22.3.[24] It is expected that many more genetic defects causing myofibrillar myopathies will be identified in the future.

DISTAL MYOPATHY DUE TO CAVEOLIN-3 MUTATION

Mutations in the caveolin-3 gene cause various forms of myopathies (caveolinopathies) including *LGMD1C*, hyperCKemia, rippling muscle disease, and a novel form of distal myopathy.[10] Tateyama et al[10] reported a sporadic patient with hyperCKemia (diagnosed at age 12 years, twentyfold increase), atrophy, and moderate weakness of small muscles in hands and feet. EMG at age 12 years revealed myopathic potentials in hand muscles, and muscle biopsy from the biceps brachii showed mild myopathy. Immunoreactivity for caveolin-3 and dysferlin was markedly reduced in muscle while it was normal for dystrophin, merosin, α-sarcoglycan, and β-dystroglycan. By Western blot, caveolin-3 was absent whereas dysferlin was normal in size and amount. Sequence analysis of the caveolin-3 gene revealed a previously reported mutation (80 G→A substitution).

CONCLUSION

Although distal myopathies were initially reported in Scandinavian and Japanese populations, they are now recognized in all ethnic groups. Molecular definition has helped increase awareness of these diseases. With identification of gene products, including dysferlin, calpain3, and caveolin-3, it is now feasible to diagnose some of these myopathies by immunohistochemistry or Western blotting. Characterization of pathologic findings has helped define the heterogenous group of myofibrillar myopathies and has facilitated molecular diagnosis in families and in sporadic patients. With better understanding of disease mechanisms, we have begun to define targets for gene replacement strategies in the distal myopathies.

REFERENCES

1. Liu J, Aoki M, Illa I, et al: Dysferlin, a novel skeletal muscle gene, is mutated in Miyoshi myopathy and limb girdle muscular dystrophy. Nat Genet 1998;20:31–36.
2. Eisenberg I, Avidan N, Potikha T, et al: The UDP-N-acetylglucosamine 2-epimerase/N-acetylmannosamine kinase gene is mutated in recessive hereditary inclusion body myopathy. Nat Genet 2001;29:83–87.
3. Haravuori H, Vihola A, Straub V, et al: Secondary calpain3 deficiency in 2q-linked muscular dystrophy: Titin is the candidate gene. Neurology 2001;56:869–877.
4. Askanas V: New developments in hereditary inclusion body myopathies. Ann Neurol 1997;41:421–422.
5. Ahlberg G, Tell D, Borg K, et al: Genetic linkage of Welander distal myopathy to chromosome 2p13. Ann Neurol 1999;46:399–404.
6. Felice K, Meredith C, Binz N, et al: Autosomal dominant distal myopathy not linked to the known distal myopathy loci. Neuromuscul Disord 1999;9:59–65.
7. Chinnery P, Johnson M, Walls T, et al: A novel autosomal dominant distal myopathy with early respiratory failure: Clinico-pathologic characteristics and exclusion of linkage to candidate genetic loci. Ann Neurol 2001;49:443–452.
8. Anderson L, Davison K, Moss J, et al: Dysferlin is a plasma membrane protein and is expressed early in human development. Hum Mol Genet 1999;8:855–861.
9. Matsuda C, Hayashi Y, Ogawa M, et al: The sarcolemmal proteins dysferlin and caveolin-3 interact in skeletal muscle. Hum Mol Genet 2001;10:1761–1766.
10. Tateyama M, Aoki M, Nishino I, et al: Mutation in the caveolin 3 gene causes a peculiar form of distal myopathy. Neurology 2002;58:323–325.
11. Selcen D, Stilling G, Engel A: The earliest pathologic alterations in dysferlinopathy. Neurology 2001;56:1472–1481.
12. Bittner R, Anderson L, Burkhardt E, et al: Dysferlin deletion in SJL mice (SJL-Dysf) defines a natural model for limb girdle muscular dystrophy 2B. Nat Genet 1999;23:141–142.
13. Illa I, Serrano-Munuera C, Gallardo E, et al: Distal anterior compartment myopathy: A dysferlin mutation causing a new muscular dystrophy phenotype. Ann Neurol 2001;49:130–134.
14. Laing N, Laing B, Meredith C, et al: Autosomal dominant distal myopathy: Linkage to chromosome 14. Am J Hum Genet 1995;56:422–427.
15. Voit T, Kutz P, Leube B, et al: Autosomal dominant distal myopathy: Further evidence of a chromosome 14 locus. Neuromuscul Disord 2001;11:11–19.
16. Zimprich F, Djamshidian A, Hainfellner J, et al: An autosomal dominant early adult onset distal muscular dystrophy. Muscle Nerve 2000;23:1876–1879.
17. Feit H, Silbergleit A, Schneider L, et al: Vocal cord and pharyngeal weakness with autosomal dominant distal myopathy: Clinical description and gene localization to 5q31. Am J Hum Genet 1998;63:1732–1742.
18. Servidei S, Capon F, Spinazzola M, et al: A distinctive autosomal dominant vacuolar neuromyopathy linked to 19p13. Neurology 1999;53:830–837.
19. Amato A, Kagan-Hallet K, Jackson C, et al: The wide-spectrum of myofibrillar myopathy suggests a multifactorial etiology and pathogenesis. Neurology 1998;51:1646–1655.

20. Wilhelmsen K, Blake D, Lynch T, et al: Chromosome 12-linked autosomal dominant scapuloperoneal muscular dystrophy. Ann Neurol 1996;39:507–520.

21. Muntoni F, Catani G, Mateddu A, et al: Familial cardiomyopathy, mental retardation and myopathy associated with desmin-type intermediate filaments. Neuromuscul Disord 1994;4:233–241.

22. Sugawara M, Kato K, Komatsu M, et al: A novel de novo mutation in the desmin gene causes desmin myopathy with toxic aggregates. Neurology 2000;55:986–990.

23. Vicart P, Caron A, Guicheney P, et al: A missense mutation in the αB-crystallin chaperone gene causes a desmin-related myopathy. Nat Genet 1998;20: 92–95.

24. Melberg A, Oldfors A, Blomstrom-Lundqvist C, et al: Autosomal dominant myofibrillar myopathy with arrhythmogenic right ventricular cardiomyopathy linked to chromosome 10q. Ann Neurol 1999;46:684–692.

Hereditary Inclusion Body Myopathies

Valerie Askanas

W. King Engel

SPORADIC INCLUSION-BODY MYOSITIS (s-IBM)

In 1971, the term *inclusion-body myositis* (IBM) was introduced by Yunis and Samaha to designate a subset of chronic polymyositis patients whose biopsies showed, in addition to lymphocytic inflammation, vacuolated muscle fibers containing characteristic filamentous inclusions in the cytoplasm and nuclei (reviewed in reference 1). Several years later, very intriguing aspects of the IBM muscle-fiber phenotype were discovered, namely that (1) both the vacuolated muscle fibers and their inclusions contain accumulations of a complex of proteins characteristic of Alzheimer disease (AD) brain (reviewed in references 1–3), most of which were previously considered "specific" to neuronal tissue and foreign to skeletal muscle; and (2) some of those proteins formed the intra-muscle-fiber congophilic amyloid[1,2] (i.e., they were misfolded). Note that *amyloid* is a general term for any aggregated protein that has acquired congophilia (i.e., that is in a β-pleated sheet configuration).

The various proteins abnormally accumulated within s-IBM vacuolated muscle fibers include: (1) amyloid-β-precursor protein (AβPP) and its proteolytic product amyloid-β (Aβ) (the latter is in the form of ultrastructural 6- to 10-nm amyloid-like fibrils, often clustered into plaquette-like inclusions); (2) phosphorylated tau in the form of ultrastructural paired-helical filaments (PHFs), corresponding to intraneuronal clusters of PHFs in AD brain (usually clustered into squiggly amyloid inclusions); (3) presenilin 1; (4) apolipoprotein E; and (5) several other Alzheimer-characteristic proteins. Cellular prion protein is also abnormally accumulated, as part of both the clustered 6- to 10-nm filaments and the PHF protein assembly.[1,2] Increased accumulation of AβPP and of cellular prion results, at least partially,

from their increased synthesis evidenced by the increase of their mRNAs.[1,2] (To our knowledge, IBM is the only human disease in which increased synthesis of cellular prion protein has been demonstrated.)

Although s-IBM is the most common progressive muscle disease, beginning at age 50 years and leading to severe disability, it is not the focus of this article. Its clinical and molecular pathologic features have been reviewed elsewhere.[1,2]

HEREDITARY INCLUSION-BODY MYOPATHIES (h-IBMs)

In 1993, we introduced the term *hereditary inclusion-body myopathies* (h-IBMs)[3] to designate hereditary muscle diseases with pathologic features strikingly resembling those of s-IBM, except for lack of lymphocytic inflammation (and other features discussed later). Therefore, we used the term *myopathy* instead of *myositis*.[3] The h-IBMs encompass several autosomal recessive and autosomal dominant syndromes of progressive muscle weakness with similar pathologic features in the muscle biopsy, but with various clinical presentations.[2–4]

Because the characteristic pathologic phenotype of the h-IBMs is now well-defined, we consider all hereditary muscle diseases whose muscle biopsies contain the characteristic vacuoles and IBM-type inclusions, and other features (discussed later), to be forms of h-IBM. The h-IBMs can be classified on the basis of their mode of inheritance and genetic mutation (Table 46–1). The rather imprecise term, *distal myopathy*, in relation to h-IBM syndromes is undesirable because it has included several syndromes with pathologic phenotypes different from that of the h-IBMs. Several muscle diseases previously designated as "distal myopathies" are indeed h-IBMs, based on their

TABLE 46–1. Hereditary Inclusion Body Myopathies (h-IBMs)

Autosomal Recessive, AR-IBM	Gene/Linkage
1. AR1-IBM, Quadriceps Spared	
• Persian (Iranian) Jews	GNE*
• Persian (Iranian) Jewish pseudo-dominant (presumed two-allele one-allele intermarriage)	9p12-13
• Afghani Jews	9p1-q1
• Indian family	9p1-q1
• Japanese distal myopathy with rimmed vacuoles	9p1-q1
• Mexican family	GNE†
• Tunisian family with leukoencephalopathy	GNE‡
• Others	?
2. AR2-IBM, Quadriceps Not Spared	
• French-Canadian family with central nervous system abnormality	?
• Others	?
Autosomal Dominant, AD-IBM	
• Swedish	Myosin heavy chain IIa
• Welander distal myopathy	2p13
• Finnish tibial muscular dystrophy	2q13
• Chicago family	?
• Pennsylvania family	?
• Denver family	?
• Los Angeles Mexican family	?
• Others	?

*GNE = UDP-N-acetylglucosamine-2 epimerase/N acetylmannosamine-kinase.
†S Mitrani-Rosenbaum and V Askanas, unpublished, 2002.
‡F Hentati, personal communication, 2002.

morphologic phenotype and the new genetic studies (details follow). There are some discrepancies in the literature regarding h-IBMs because diagnostic morphologic criteria are differently applied in various laboratories. When the diagnostic criteria of h-IBMs are firmly established, h-IBMs will be diagnosed more accurately and more often.

THERAPEUTIC IMPLICATIONS OF THE STRONG SIMILARITIES BETWEEN s-IBMs AND h-IBMs

We have suggested that these striking similarities may result from similar or identical steps in the midstream and downstream pathogenic cascade of cellular disturbances within the affected muscle fibers.[1,2] A treatment found effective in one form of IBM might benefit both forms in preventing muscle fiber destruction, although the upstream step might be different (i.e., genetic mutation or virus). There is still no specific treatment for the h-IBMs. However, research that unveils the pathogenetic steps will provide the best basis for formulating treatments.

DIAGNOSTIC CRITERIA OF h-IBM MUSCLE BIOPSIES

Light-Microscopic Histochemistry and Immunocytochemistry and the Immunoreactivities of Various Proteins on h-IBM PHFs

Characteristic light-microscopic pathologic features of h-IBMs on the Engel-Gomori trichrome reaction are muscle fibers with one or several irregular and various-sized vacuoles on a 10 μm thick cross-section.[2] Although some vacuoles are rimmed, many in the h-IBMs are not. Within the vacuoles, there is usually sparse reddish and sometimes greenish gray material.

In s-IBM, 60% to 80% of vacuolated muscle fibers (VMFs) on a given section contain amyloid foci positive with Congo-red, thioflavine-s, and crystal violet.[1,2] In h-IBM VMFs, there is usually minimal amyloid deposition, and it is more evident in older patients (Askanas and Engel, unpublished data). One exception is an autosomal dominant form of h-IBM with prominent muscle-fiber congophilia.[5] In the h-IBMs, vacuoles can be very small and sometimes present in only a few muscle fibers. Amyloid deposits can easily be missed if sought only by Congo red staining visualized through polarizing filters, thioflavine-s, or crystal violet. Our fluorescence-enhanced Congo red technique readily identifies amyloid deposits.[6] This paucity of amyloid suggests that intracellular amyloid depositions per se are not essential destructive aspects in the h-IBMs (and perhaps by analogy not even in s-IBM), but possibly they are mildly aggravating when they do appear. We suggest that the proteins, whose abnormal (probably pathologically unfolded) state led to their becoming aggregated as β-pleated-sheet amyloid, may destructively impair essential cellular molecular processes in their pre-amyloid dysconfigurative state.

To diagnose h-IBM, we recommend (1) Engel-Gomori trichrome staining[7] to visualize lack of lymphocytic inflammation, vacuolated muscle fibers, and other abnormal structures such as occasional ragged-red fibers (which contain abnormal mitochondria) and cytoplasmic bodies present in some patients; (2) fluorescence-enhanced Congo-red stain; and (3) light microscopic immunocytochemical staining for PHFs, using SMI-31 monoclonal antibody (originally made to react with the phosphorylated heavy-chain of neurofilaments), which recognizes the phosphorylated tau of PHFs in s-IBM and in the h-IBMs.[8] If SMI-31 antibody is not available, ubiquitin immunoreactivity can be used.[9]

Ragged-red fibers and cytochrome-c-oxidase (COX)–negative muscle fibers, both indicating mitochondrial abnormality, are present in older patients in some forms of h-IBM,[2] but they are not diagnostic. Multiple mitochondrial DNA deletions occur in s-IBM muscle and in some older h-IBM patients' muscle,[10] but their contribution to muscle-fiber malfunction and degeneration is yet undefined. We propose that overexpression of AβP/Aβ may contribute to the mitochondrial abnormalities.

Small angular muscle fibers that are histochemically dark with the pan-esterase and/or NADH-tetrazolium-reductase reactions generally indicate a recent-denervation component. Some are characteristically present in both s-IBM and h-IBM muscle biopsies. We conclude that there is an important denervation component contributing to the weakness in both s-IBMs and h-IBMs, possibly more so in distal lower-limb muscles.[1-3] On the basis of our data, we have suggested that the dysinnervation of the IBMs muscle may be mainly myogenous owing to the postsynaptic abnormality at the neuromuscular junction.[1,2,11]

Ultrastructural Abnormalities of h-IBM Vacuolated and Some Nonvacuolated Muscle Fibers

As in s-IBM, PHFs in h-IBM fibers (often in clusters) occur in the cytoplasm and occasionally in nuclei. They are essentially identical to PHFs of AD brain (15 to 21 nm in diameter and containing phosphorylated tau).[1,2,8] The ultrastructural appearance of IBM PHFs depends on the tissue preparation[2]; sometimes they appear as tubulofilaments. In h-IBM muscle nuclei, there are clusters (inclusions) of 15- to 21-nm tubulofilaments, which in favorable sections look like paired-helical filaments like those in the cytoplasm. They occur usually in 2% to 4% of the nuclei, but in one autosomal-dominant form, they were in about 40% of the nuclei[5] (Askanas and Simmons, unpublished data). The h-IBM VMF cytoplasm also contains Aβ positivity in collections of 6- to 10-nm filaments[2]; fine flocculomembranous material; and amorphous material.[2] Myelin-like whorls and other lysosomal debris are also in the VMFs. In older patients, abnormal mitochondria containing paracrystalline inclusions are occasionally present, but are not diagnostic.[2] The pathologic phenotype of h-IBM muscle biopsy is summarized in Table 46–2.

Specificity of the IBM Phenotype

The unusual assembly of proteins within VMFs is characteristic of s-IBM and h-IBMs. It does not occur in: (1) vacuolated fibers of other muscle diseases (e.g., acid maltase deficiency, periodic paralysis); (2) the "empty" vacuoles of polymyositis and dermatomyositis; or (3) other non-IBM vacuolar myopathies. The only exception is oculopharyngeal muscular dystrophy (OPMD), which we propose to consider as a form of h-IBM (discussed later). The occasional vacuoles and tubulofilaments reported in rare muscle fibers in a few other muscle diseases (e.g., myotonic dystrophy) and in older patients (Askanas and Engel, unpublished observation, 1998) are very sparse and are probably not pathogenetically significant for those diseases.

DIFFERENT FORMS OF HEREDITARY IBM

Our new classification of the h-IBM syndromes is presented in Table 46–1.

Autosomal Recessive Forms

Autosomal Recessive "Quadriceps Sparing" Myopathy (AR1-IBM)

Persian (Iranian) Jews. These comprise a distinct subgroup of h-IBM patients, with clinical onset usually in the second or third decade, characterized by progressive lower- and upper-limb muscle weakness.[2,4,12] Distal lower limb muscles are affected early, followed by proximal weakness involving the iliopsoas, hamstring, adductor, and gluteal muscles. The most characteristic feature is relative sparing of the quadriceps muscles.[2,12] Lower limbs are affected more severely than upper limbs. Cranial-nerve muscles are not usually involved, but one of our otherwise typical patients had unilateral ptosis. His ptosis and hand weakness responded somewhat to edrophonium and pyri-

TABLE 46–2. Pathologic Phenotype and Immunoreactivities of Proteins on Paired Helical Filaments of h-IBM

Pathological Phenotype		Ultrastructural Immunoreactivities of Proteins on PHFs	
Around muscle fibers		**Protein**	
Inflammation, lymphocytic	–	Phosphorylated tau with antibodies [†]	
Within muscle fibers		SMI-31	+
Vacuolation	+	AT8	+
Congo red-positive amyloid	–/+	SMI-310	–
Ubiquitin [†]	+	PHF-1	–
Amyloid β-precursor protein [†]	+	Ubiquitin [†]	+
Amyloid β-precursor protein mRNA	+	Prion protein [†]	+
Phosphorylated tau with antibodies [†]		Neuronal NO synthase [†]	+
SMI-31	+	Inducible NO synthase [†]	+
AT8	–/+	Amyloid β-precursor protein [†]	–
SMI-310	–/+	Apolipoprotein E [†]	–
PHF-1	– d	Nitrotyrosine [†]	–
Prion protein [†]	+		
Prion protein mRNA	+		
Neuronal NO synthase [†]	+		
Inducible NO synthase [†]	–/+		
Nitrotyrosine [†]	+m		
Apolipoprotein E [†]	+d		
Ragged-red fibers	–/+ §		
COX-negative muscle fibers	–/+ §		

mRNA, messenger RNA; NO, nitric oxide; COX, cytochrome c oxidase
[†], immunoreactivity; d, diffuse; m, multiple dots; §, more in older patients.
These data from our studies of the h-IBM in Persian-Jews and other patients.

dostigmine treatment, although other tests for myasthenia gravis were negative.[2] Some patients with non-quadriceps-sparing h-IBMs have facial muscle weakness.[13] Parents of Persian Jewish h-IBM patients are often related (frequently first cousins). Sometimes there is a "pseudo-dominant" pattern, such as when affected children issue from an affected person married to a cousin or other close relative who is a carrier, a presumed 2-allele 1-allele marriage (Engel and Askanas, unpublished data). There are also seemingly sporadic Persian Jewish patients, but their disease could be autosomal recessive; muscle biopsies of such patients can have features typical of AR1-IBM.

The abnormal gene was initially linked to chromosome 9 p1-q1.[14] It was later narrowed to 9p1 by two groups, who also reported that patients of other ethnic groups had the same linkage.[15,16] More recently, the genetic locus was modified to 9p12-13,[17] followed by the very important identification of missense mutations in the UDP-N-acetylglucosamine-2 epimerase/N-acetyl-mannosamine-kinase (GNE) gene by the Mitrani-Rosenbaum group.[18] That finding will facilitate analysis of the pathogenic cascade in this and possibly other forms of h-IBM, as well as in s-IBM.

GNE is a bifunctional enzyme catalyzing the first two steps in the synthesis of N-acetylneuraminic (sialic) acid.[19–21] In h-IBMs, missense mutations were found in the kinase (amino-terminus) and epimerase (carboxyl-terminus) domains.[18] GNE modulates the structure of many protein complexes in virtually all organs.[19–21] GNE-dependent synthesis of sialic acid occurs in the cytoplasm. In addition, some sialic acid can be derived from several other sources, including cell-surface glycoproteins and lipids cleaved in the lysosomal compartment. Sialic acid is a terminal component of glycan structures bound to proteins and gangliosides. It is considered to play important roles in several cellular processes including cellular adhesion; formation of and/or marking recognition-sites for toxins and other pathogenic agents; stabilization of glycoprotein structures; signal transduction; and cell-mediated immune responses.[19–21] Because of the important cellular functions of sialic acid, dysregulation of its biosynthesis and distribution can lead to severe abnormalities of glycoconjugates biosynthesis.[22]

In the AR1-IBM of Persian Jews (see Table 46–1), seven mutations in the GNE gene have been found.[18] It has been proposed that there is only partial loss of GNE enzymatic functions because there is a high proportion of missense mutations, all patients having at least one and often two.[18] Since GNE modulates many proteins in virtually all tissues, it will be important to determine why only skeletal muscle is involved in AR1-IBM. Speculatively, h-IBM mutations may especially influence sialation/glycation of one or several important muscle proteins, perhaps one that regulates other proteins. If some of the AßPP and/or tau protein molecules are abnormally glycated in h-IBMs, this could be pathogenically important and fit with our data. Of possible relevance is that tau in AD brain contains large amounts of truncated glycans, which may contribute to its pathologic assembly and stabilization in the AD PHFs.[23]

Japanese Patients. Similar to the h-IBM of Persian Jews, in Japanese patients originally reported as having "distal myopathy with rimmed vacuoles," the quadriceps muscles were relatively spared, and the gastrocnemius muscles also were less affected than other muscles.[24] Onset was in the second or third decade, manifested by weakness mainly of distal leg muscles. An autosomal-recessive pattern was evident in 37% of patients. In 11% of patients without a family history, consanguinity was reported, suggesting that their disease might also be autosomal recessive.[24] Muscle biopsies have the characteristic h-IBM pathology, including vacuoles, nuclear and cytoplasmic tubulofilamentous inclusions, lack of inflammation, and what we consider "IBM-characteristic" proteins accumulated in the vacuoles.[25] In addition, muscle biopsies of two Japanese patients studied in our laboratory with a variety of IBM markers were indistinguishable from biopsies of the quadriceps-sparing h-IBM of Persian Jews (Askanas and Nonaka, unpublished data, 1997). The Japanese patients were also reported to link to the 9p1-q1 locus.[26] Because we postulated several years ago that both ethnic groups have the same form of h-IBM,[27] we anticipate that the Japanese patients will have mutations in the same *GNE* gene. (*Note:* Two papers describing GNE mutations in Japanese distal myopathy with rimmed vacuoles [Japanese quadriceps sparing h-IBM] have been published by Tomimitsu H et al [2002] and Arai A et al [2002].)

Other Autosomal Recessive Forms. Two Mexican brothers of Spanish heritage, whose parents were first cousins, have autosomal-recessive quadriceps-sparing h-IBM, with muscle biopsies typical of h-IBM and linkage to 9p1.[15] In one, a mutation in the GNE gene was recently found (Mitrani-Rosenbaum and Askanas, unpublished data, 2002); his brother's genes have not yet been studied.

In a Tunisian kindred with quadriceps-sparing h-IBM and symptomatic leukoencephalopathy (reviewed in references 2, 4, and 27), mutations in the *GNE* gene were recently found (Hentati, personal communication, 2002).

Other forms were also reported (reviewed in references 2, 4, and 27). In a kindred without quadriceps spar-

ing and with asymptomatic leukodystrophy, there was no linkage to chromosome 9p1.[13]

Autosomal Dominant Forms of h-IBM

Swedish h-IBM with Missense Mutation (Glu-706→Lys) in the Myosin-Heavy-Chain-IIa Gene. A large Swedish family with 19 affected persons had the following clinical features: congenital joint contractures that normalize during early childhood, external ophthalmoplegia, and predominantly proximal limb-muscle weakness.[28] In childhood and adolescence, myopathy was mild and patients had only minor morphologic abnormalities in muscle biopsies. Several patients developed progressive limb-muscle weakness and the h-IBM muscle phenotype (consisting of vacuoles and SMI-31-positive tubulofilaments) between 30 and 50 years of age.[28] A missense mutation in the myosin-heavy-chain-IIa gene was recently reported.[28] The mechanisms by which that mutation causes the myopathy are not yet known.

The fact that significant clinical weakness and the full IBM pathologic phenotype both developed after age 30 years harmonizes with our previously proposed correlation between aging and provocation of the IBM pathogenesis (discussed later).

Welander Distal Myopathy. This myopathy occurs in Sweden. The clinical onset most commonly is in the third or fourth decade, with symmetric distal weakness of forearm muscles, especially the finger extensors (reviewed in references 2, 4, and 27). Eventually the lower limbs also become involved, especially distally. Muscle biopsies have features typical of the h-IBMs, namely vacuoles and intracytoplasmic and intranuclear tubulofilaments (PHFs). Whether their muscle biopsies contain accumulations of IBM-characteristic proteins awaits evaluation. The disease has been linked to a 2p13 locus (reviewed in reference 4), but the abnormal gene is not yet known.

Finnish Tibial Muscular Dystrophy. These patients have onset of muscle weakness in the third decade, manifesting as pronounced foot-drop due to weakness of the tibialis anterior (reviewed in references 2, 4, and 27). Red-rimmed vacuoles were described in 28% of the 32 muscle biopsies, but tubulofilaments (or PHFs) were not reported. Finding tubulofilaments/PHFs during routine electronmicroscopic examination is often quite difficult, especially when sparse. We suggest that they be searched for more extensively by using the light-microscopic SMI-31 immunocytochemical technique.[8] Linkage to chromosome 2q31 was reported (reviewed in reference 4).

Other Examples Of Autosomal Dominant Forms. Three Chicago siblings have had progressive lower- and upper-limb muscle weakness.[29] Their father also had a similar neuromuscular disorder clinically but was not biopsied. The siblings' muscle biopsies had an h-IBM pattern of vacuoles, lack of inflammation, some degree of congophilia, and tau-positive PHFs, as well as aspects of oxidative stress as in other h-IBMs and s-IBM.[29]

In two generations of a Denver family there was mainly proximal muscle weakness of both lower and upper limbs (reviewed in references 2, 4, and 27). The weakness began in the second or third decade, and the typical h-IBM muscle-biopsy pathology was present.

A Pennsylvania family involving several generations with late-onset progressive muscle weakness and h-IBM features in muscle biopsies had two unusual features. They had very frequent muscle nuclei containing congophilic tau-positive PHFs and large areas of "apoptotic-like" fibers (Askanas and Simmons, unpublished data).

Other patients in the United States with distal myopathy of probable autosomal-dominant inheritance and vacuolated muscle fibers were described (reviewed in references 2, 4, and 27). It will be important to re-evaluate their muscle biopsies to seek PHFs.

Oculopharyngeal muscular dystrophy (OPMD) may be considered a form of late-onset autosomal-dominant h-IBM. OPMD is caused by short expansions of the GCG trinucleotide repeat encoding the polyalanine tract of poly(A)-binding protein 2 (PABP2).[30] Clinically, there is ptosis, dysphagia, and proximal limb-muscle weakness, all becoming more evident after age 50. About 2% of the skeletal muscle nuclei contain 5- to 8-nm tubulofilamentous Tomé inclusions characteristic for OPMD.[31] Otherwise the muscle-fiber pathologic phenotype is like that of h-IBM muscle.[32] Similar to GNE, PAB2 is ubiquitously expressed, but the clinical and pathologic phenotypes of both quadriceps-sparing h-IBM and OPMD are restricted to skeletal muscle. PABP2 in skeletal muscle induces transcription of the myogenic factor MyoD, by itself and in association with SKIP (the protein that interacts with both the cellular and viral forms of the oncoprotein Ski).[33] In OPMD, perhaps a mutated PABP2 alters MyoD synthesis. This leads to aspects of the IBM pathologic phenotype and clinical weakness later in life when the effects of other myogenic factors are putatively decreased.

SPECULATIONS ON PATHOGENIC MECHANISMS

General Considerations

The pathogenic cascade is not well understood in either s-IBM or the h-IBMs. The several forms of h-IBM have different genetic transmissions, chromosomal linkages, and abnormal genes, most of which are not yet identified. (The etiology of s-IBM with its typical lymphocytic inflammatory aspect is presumably different, but still unknown; a viral etiology is an unconfirmed possibility.[1]) These multigenetic and multifactorial disorders have specific muscle-fiber pathologic features in common, including vacuolar degeneration; filamentous inclusions composed of PHFs containing phosphorylated tau; increased transcription and accumulation of AβPP epitopes, including the proteolytic fragment Aβ; and accumulated presenilin1, ApoE, and other Alzheimer characteristic proteins.[1,2] We previously postulated that in various IBMs different etiologies lead to a downstream common pathogenic cascade that is ultimately responsible for the characteristic vacuolar degeneration. This would be the same principle as in AD, in which at least five genes (and other unknown factors) lead to the same pathologic phenotype in the brain.[34,35]

Our Current Concepts on the Pathogenesis of the IBMs

Putative Key Pathogenic Role of Intracellular Accumulation of AβPP/Aβ in IBM Muscle Fibers

We have proposed a key upstream or midstream role of increased intracellular AβPP/Aβ in the pathogenesis of both s-IBM and h-IBMs by its causing abnormal signal-transduction, modulation of other genes, induction of oxidative stress, mitochondrial malfunction, and other abnormalities.[1] Our hypothesis is supported by tissue-culture studies that show that (1) experimental overexpression of AβPP through direct AβPP gene transfer (via adenovirus vector) into human normal, rather mature, cultured muscle fibers induced several aspects of the IBM pathologic phenotype, including vacuolation, intracellular congophilia, nuclear PHFs, and abnormal mitochondria[1]; (2) in cultured h-IBM muscle fibers, an AβPP overexpression, presumably genetically determined, preceded other IBM-like abnormalities (reviewed in references 1 and 2); and (3) in contrast to normal-control cultured human muscle, both experimentally and genetically AβPP-overexpressing cultured muscle fibers had abnormal neuromuscular junctions (NMJs) and could not become innervated by cocultured fetal-rat spinal-cord neurons.[11] This led us to propose that in IBM muscle, AβPP overexpression may be responsible for postulated "myogenous denervation"[11] and for the more recently reported NMJ abnormalities in IBM biopsies.[1]

Additional support for our hypothesis of an *intracellular* role of AβPP and Aβ in the IBM pathogenesis was provided by two transgenic mouse models overexpressing AβPP within muscle fibers (reviewed and referenced in reference 1). In both models, some aspects of the human IBM pathology were produced, including fiber vacuolation, intracellular accumulation of AβPP, and intracellular amyloid deposits.[1] These muscle-fiber abnormalities were evident only in *aging* transgenic mice, supporting our idea that an aging cellular environment is important for development of IBM.

Oxidative Stress Has a Possible Role in the Pathogenic Cascade of the IBMs

There is increasing evidence that free-radical toxicity may participate in IBM pathogenesis. Indicators of oxidative stress, as well as enzymes participating in the cellular defense against oxidative stress, are accumulated in h-IBM and s-IBM muscle fibers.[1,2,29] Direct causes of intra-cellular oxidative stress in the IBMs are not known. Because Aβ can induce oxidative stress in several experimental models, and accumulation of AβPP/Aβ seems to precede other abnormalities within IBM muscle fibers,[1,11] we have proposed that overproduction of AβPP and accumulation of AβPP/Aβ can cause cellular disturbances leading to increased generation of free radicals, which result in oxidative stress. Potential therapeutic avenues for the IBMs could be to reduce free radicals or prevent their formation within muscle fibers.

Aging of Muscle Fibers Possibly Contributes to Development of the IBMs

s-IBM typically becomes clinically manifest after age 50 years, and more often in the sixties and seventies. Among sporadic inflammatory myopathy patients, the previously described specific vacuolar degeneration of muscle fibers occurs only in s-IBM; it is not part of the polymyositis (PM) or dermatomyositis muscle-fiber phenotype. However, it occurs in the h-IBMs, which typically lack an inflammatory component. It is rare to see a patient older than 50 years with what could be considered "pure PM"; virtually all older patients with lymphocytic myositis have s-IBM. We have suggested that in s-IBM the milieu of the aging muscle fiber might modify the provocation of, and response to, the lymphocytic inflammation (reviewed in reference 1) and promote development of the IBM-characteristic progressive vacuolar degeneration.[1] In the h-IBMs, the causative gene abnormality exists from conception but does not produce clinically evident muscle damage until the second, third, or fourth decade of life. We postulate that a specific h-IBM genetic defect, combined with the adult "early-aging" muscle fiber milieu, leads to the h-IBM-characteristic vacuolar degeneration. Aging changes may predispose to the muscle-fiber mitochondrial abnormalities in s-IBM and older h-IBM patients, provoking a vicious circle between mitochondrial malfunctions and the oxidative stress evident in the fiber.

Thus, in the aging muscle-fiber cellular milieu, there may be diminished cellular homeostatic mechanisms caused by either underexpression of "youthful" genes encoding beneficial cellular factors or overexpression of yet-unknown genes encoding toxic cellular factors. Such aging mechanisms may predispose to, or underlie, the mus-cle-fiber vacuolar-degeneration, atrophy, and cell death in the h-IBMs (and in s-IBM). Knowledge of the mechanisms and the non-IBM genes governing aging should aid our understanding of the pathogenic cascade destroying the IBM muscle fibers. Such collateral genes presumably influence the different age of onset and severity of h-IBM in patients who have an identical mutation of GNE.

Possible Relevance of Morpho-Chemical Similarities between IBM Muscle and Alzheimer-Disease (AD) Brain

The same proteins that accumulate within sporadic and hereditary IBM muscle fibers also accumulate in the brain of sporadic and hereditary forms of AD. Therefore, the muscle and the brain diseases might share certain steps in their pathogenic cascade, and knowledge of one disease might help elucidate the other. Both cellular aging and evidence of oxidative stress are associated with the IBMs and ADs (reviewed in reference 1). The IBMs and ADs (including sporadic and hereditary forms of both groups) are multifactorial and polygenetic. Within both the IBM and AD categories, the pathologic phenotypes of sporadic and hereditary forms are very similar, despite the different direct causes being mainly nongenetic versus mainly genetic. Therefore, in each disease category it has been proposed by us in the IBMs and by others in the ADs (reviewed in reference 1) that different etiologies, including different genetic defects in hereditary forms, lead to the same upstream step. This then promotes a midstream and downstream final common pathogenic cascade of events resulting in the specific cellular deterioration. However, each disease category remains organ-specific, involving postmitotic-muscle fibers or postmitotic-neurons. The tissue affected in the sporadic forms, muscle versus brain, may be influenced by etiologic agent (? a virus), previous exposure to an environmental factor(s), and/or the patient's genetic background (the cellular microclimate).

Involvement and Sparing of Selective Muscles in the h-IBMs Have Therapeutic Implications

In the autosomal-recessive h-IBM of Persian Jews and some other groups, the relative sparing of the quadriceps is a remarkable feature. Learning the reason might lead to a medical treatment that would make susceptible muscles behave like the quadriceps, which (because of its specific cellular environment) might be less dependent on the function of normal GNE, or less susceptible to a function perturbed by mutated GNE. Understanding the cellular functions dependent on GNE and leading to the molecular/biochemical disturbances we have demonstrated in h-IBM muscle should uncover steps susceptible to therapeutic intervention.

Acknowledgments

Our studies as described in this chapter were supported in part by the National Institutes of Health (grants NS31836, NS34103, and AG16768), Muscular Dystrophy Association, Alzheimer Foundation, and the Helen Lewis, Sheldon Katz, and Ron Stever Research Funds. We are grateful to our research and clinical colleagues and staff for their participation in the various aspects of our studies.

REFERENCES

1. Askanas V, Engel WK: Inclusion-body myositis: Newest concepts of pathogenesis and relation to aging and Alzheimer disease. J Neuropathol Exp Neurol 2001;60:1–14.

2. Askanas V, Engel WK: Newest approaches to diagnosis and pathogenesis of sporadic inclusion-body myositis and hereditary inclusion-body myopathies, including molecular-pathologic similarities to Alzheimer disease. In Askanas V, Serratrice G, Engel WK (eds): Inclusion-body Myositis and Myopathies. United Kingdom, Cambridge University Press, 1998, pp 3–78.

3. Askanas V, Engel WK: New advances in inclusion-body myositis. Curr Opin Rheumatol 1993;5:732–741.

4. Tomé FMS, Fardeau M: Hereditary inclusion body myopathies. Curr Opin Neurol 1998;11:453–459.

5. Alvarez RB, Simmons Z, Engel WK, Askanas V: New autosomal-dominant inclusion-body myopathy (AD-IBM) with many congophilic muscle nuclei that contain paired-helical filaments (PHFs) composed of phosphorylated tau. Neurology 1998;50:204.

6. Askanas V, Engel WK, Alvarez RB: Enhanced detection of Congo-red-positive amyloid deposits in muscle fibers of inclusion-body myositis and brain of Alzheimer disease using fluorescence technique. Neurology 1993;43:1265–1267.

7. Engel WK, Cunningham GG: Rapid examination of muscle tissue and improved trichrome method for fresh-frozen biopsy sections. Neurology 1963;13:919–923.

8. Askanas V, Alvarez RB, Mirabella M, Engel WK: Use of anti-neurofilament antibody to identify paired-helical filaments in inclusion-body myositis. Ann Neurol 1996;39:389–391.

9. Askanas V, Serdaroglu P, Engel WK, Alvarez RB: Immunolocalization of ubiquitin in muscle biopsies of patients with inclusion body myositis and oculopharyngeal muscular dystrophy. Neurosci Lett 1991;130:73–76.

10. Jansson M, Darin N, Kyllerman M, et al: Multiple mitochondrial DNA deletions in hereditary inclusion body myopathy. Acta Neuropathol 2000;100:23–28.

11. McFerrin J, Engel WK, Askanas V: Impaired innervation of cultured human muscle overexpression βAPP experimentally and genetically: Relevance to inclusion-body myopathies. Neuroreport 1998;9:3201–3205.

12. Argov Z, Mitrani-Rosenbaum S: Hereditary inclusion-body myopathy with quadriceps sparing: Epidemiology and genetics. In Askanas V, Serratrice G, Engel WK (eds): Inclusion-Body Myositis and Myopathies. United Kingdom, Cambridge University Press, 1998, pp 200–210.

13. Argov Z, Sadeh M, Eisenberg I, et al: Facial weakness in hereditary inclusion body myopathies. Neurology 1998;50:1925–1926.

14. Mitrani-Rosenbaum S, Argov Z, Blumenfeld A, et al: Hereditary inclusion body myopathy maps to chromosome 9p1-q1. Hum Mol Genet 1996;5:159–163.

15. Christodoulou K, Papadopoulou E, Tsingis M, et al: Narrowing of the gene locus for autosomal quadriceps sparing inclusion-body myopathy (ARQS-IBM) to chromosome 9p1. Acta Myol 1998;2:7–9.

16. Eisenberg I, Thiel C, Levi T, et al: Fine-structure mapping of the hereditary inclusion body myopathy locus. Genomics 1999;55:43–48.

17. Eisenberg I, Hochner H, Shemesh M, et al: Physical and transcriptional map of the hereditary inclusion body myopathy locus on chromosome 9p12-p13. Eur J Hum Genet 2001;9:501–509.

18. Eisenberg I, Avidan N, Potikha T, et al: The UDP-N-acetylglucosamine 2-epimerase/N acetylmannosamine kinase gene is mutated in recessive hereditary inclusion body myopathy. Nat Genet 2001;29:83–87.

19. Stäschet, Hinderlich S, Weise C, et al: A bifunctional enzyme catalyzes the first two steps in N-acetyl-neuraminic acid biosynthesis of rat liver. J Biol Chem 1997;272:24319–24324.

20. Lucka L, Krause M, Danker K, et al: Primary structure and expression analysis of human UDP-N-acetyl-glucosamine-2-epimerase/N-acetylmannosamine kinase, the bifunctional enzyme in neuraminic acid biosynthesis. FEBS Lett 1999;454:341–344.

21. Keppler OT, Hinderlich S, Langner J, et al: UDP-GlcNAc 2-epimerase: A regulator of cell surface sialylation. Science 1999;284:1372–1376.

22. Yarema KJ, Goon S, Bertozzi CR: Metabolic selection of glycosylation defects in human cells. Nat Biotechnol 2001;19:553–558.

23. Sato Y, Naito Y, Grundke-Iqbal I, et al: Analysis of N-glycans of pathological tau: Possible occurrence of aberrant processing of tau in Alzheimer's disease. FEBS Lett 2001;496:152–160.

24. Sunohara N, Nonaka I, Kamei N, Satoyoshi E: Distal myopathy with rimmed vacuole formation: A follow-up study. Brain 1989;112:65–83.

25. Murakami N, Ihara Y, Nonaka I. Muscle fiber degeneration in distal myopathy with rimmed vacuole formation. Acta Neuropathol 1995;89:29–34.

26. Ikeuchi T, Aska T, Saito M, et al: Gene locus for autosomal recessive distal myopathy with rimmed vacuoles maps to chromosome 9. Ann Neurol 1997;41:432–437.

27. Askanas V, Engel WK: Newest advances in the understanding of sporadic inclusion-body myositis and hereditary inclusion-body myopathies. Curr Opin Rheumatol 1995;7:486–496.

28. Martinsson T, Oldfors A, Darin N, et al: Autosomal dominant myopathy: Missense mutation (Glu-706 → Lys) in the myosin heavy chain lla gene. Proc Natl Acad Sci U S A 2000;97:14614–14619.

29. Yang CC, Alvarez RB, Engel WK, et al: Nitric-oxide induced oxidative stress in autosomal recessive and dominant inclusion-body myopathies. Brain 1998;121:1089–1097.

30. Brais B, Bouchard JP, Xie YG, et al: Short GCG expansions in the PABP2 gene cause oculopharyngeal muscular dystrophy. Nat Genet 1998;18:164–167.

31. Tomé FM, Fardeau M: Nuclear inclusions in oculopharyngeal dystrophy. Acta Neuropathol (Berl) 1980;49:85–87.

32. Askanas V, Alvarez RB, Sarkozi E, et al: Partial expression in oculopharyngeal muscular dystrophy (OPMD) muscle fibers of the intracellular phenotype of sporadic inclusion-body myositis (s-IBM). Neurology 1997;48:331.

33. Kim Y-J, Noguchi S, Hayashi Y, et al: The product of an oculopharyngeal muscular dystrophy gene, poly (A)-binding protein 2, interacts with SKIP and stimulates muscle-specific gene expression. Hum Mol Genet 2001;10:1129–1139.

34. Lippa CF, Saunders AM, Smith TW, et al: Familial and sporadic Alzheimer's disease neuropathology cannot exclude a final common pathway. Neurology 1996;46:406–412.

35. Hyman BT: Alzheimer's disease or Alzheimer's diseases? Clues from molecular epidemiology. Ann Neurol 1996;40:135–136.

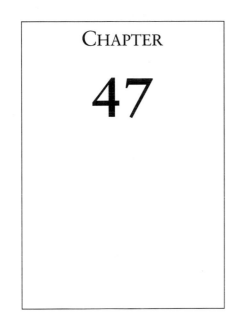

CHAPTER

47

The Myotonic Dystrophies

Richard T. Moxley, III

Giovanni Meola

Following the discovery in 1992 that classical myotonic dystrophy, Steinert's disease, DM-1, results from an unstable CTGn repeat expansion on chromosome 19q13.3,[1–3] investigators in 1994 identified a group of related disorders labeled myotonic dystrophy type-2, DM-2,[4] and proximal myotonic myopathy, PROMM,[5] that are similar to but distinct from Steinert's disease (Table 47–1). Since the early 1990s, our knowledge of these "myotonic dystrophy–like" or "Steinert disease–like" disorders has increased considerably.[6–8] Individuals with PROMM do not have an unstable CTGn repeat expansion on chromosome 19q13.2 at the DM-1 locus. They do not show linkage to the loci on chromosomes 7 and 17 for the skeletal muscle chloride and sodium channel genes. Mutations in these genes lead to chloride or sodium channel myotonia, respectively. Recently, investigators have found that DM-2/PROMM[9] results from an unstable CCTGn repeat expansion on chromosome 3q21.[10] This exciting discovery indicates that at least two types of nucleotide repeat expansions (CTGn for DM-1 and CCTGn for DM-2) can lead to similar disorders. This observation raises the possibility that other mutations producing the PROMM syndrome (PROMM phenotype) may result from unstable nucleotide repeat expansions. Because of the identification of this new group of "Steinert disease–like" disorders, a new classification has been established. It refers to the entire group as the *myotonic dystrophies*.[11] Table 47–1 lists these disorders. Myotonic dystrophies share certain core features: (1) autosomal dominant inheritance; (2) myotonia; (3) muscle weakness; (4) posterior capsular iridescent cataracts; and (5) multisystem complications, often involving the heart, brain, and endocrine system. Each of these disorders has variable phenotypes. However, despite the vari-

ability and the similar characteristics, it is usually possible to identify clinical and laboratory features that establish the diagnosis.

CLINICAL FEATURES AND DIAGNOSTIC EVALUATION

Classical Myotonic Dystrophy, Steinert's Disease, Myotonic Dystrophy Type 1, DM-1

Clinical Features. DM-1 has the most variable clinical manifestations of the myotonic dystrophies. It can present in late life with only cataracts, baldness, or occasionally with heart block. Weakness and myotonia may be absent or very mild. In the second and third decades, DM-1 can present with grip myotonia, trouble holding items, ankle weakness, or slurring of speech. Weakness of face, finger flexors, intrinsic hand muscles, and foot dorsiflexors is usually present, as is myotonia. The myotonia typically occurs following a strong grip or after percussion of the thenar and forearm extensor muscles. Dysarthria, difficulty swallowing, hypersomnia, sleep apnea, decreased vital capacity, and cardiac conduction disturbances develop over subsequent years. Respiratory failure, pneumonitis, and cardiac conduction block are usual causes of death. Patients may be limited to a wheelchair at the time these life-threatening complications occur. Myotonia along with muscle weakness contributes to difficulties with speech, swallowing, respiration, and smooth muscle function (including intestinal dismotility and uterine dysfunction). Myotonia is not present early in life in DM-1, and it is often difficult to detect on clinical examination in the late stages of the disease. In newborns, DM-1 can present as a severe illness, congenital

TABLE 47–1. The Myotonic Dystrophies

Disease	Genetic Abnormality
Classic myotonic dystrophy, Steinert's disease, myotonic dystrophy type-1, DM-1	Dominant. Unstable CTG repeat expansion on chromosome 19q13.3 in the noncoding region of a serine-threonine protein kinase (DMPK) gene. DM-1 patients have CTG repeat sizes from 50 to >2000 repeats. Normal patients have 5 to 37 repeats.
Proximal myotonic dystrophy syndromes (PROMM)	
1. Myotonic dystrophy type 2, DM-2/PROMM	Dominant. Unstable CCTGn repeat expansion on chromosome 3q21 in intron 1 of the zinc finger 9 protein gene (ZNF9). DM-2 patients have 75 to 11,000 CCTG repeats. Normal patients have <75 repeats.
2. Proximal myotonic dystrophy PDM/DM-2/PROMM	Dominant. Identical locus to DM-2. Range of CCTG repeat sizes remains to be established.
3. Myotonic dystrophy type 3, DM-3/PROMM	Dominant. Not linked to 3q21 or 19q13.3. Locus (or loci) to be identified.

myotonic dystrophy. Congenital DM-1 causes generalized weakness and hypotonia, respiratory failure, feeding difficulty, and talipes. No myotonia is apparent in these infants. Most of these severely afflicted infants are born from mothers who have mild or moderate DM-1. Careful clinical examination of the mother is often necessary to detect myotonia and weakness.

Electromyographic evaluation of the mother is helpful. Without careful examination of the mother, the cause for the illness in the infant may be ascribed to perinatal factors, including matrix hemorrhage in the brain or eventration of the diaphragm, both of which occur in congenital DM-1. If babies with congenital DM-1 survive the newborn period, they typically have mental retardation, learning disabilities, toilet training difficulties, and slowed motor development. However, they usually show consistent improvement in all these areas throughout childhood and the early teens. In the second and third decades, congenital DM-1 patients begin to develop adult-onset, classical DM-1 symptoms and have slowly progressive weakness and complications as noted earlier.

PROXIMAL MYOTONIC DYSTROPHY SYNDROMES (PROMM)

Myotonic Dystrophy Type-2, DM-2/PROMM

Clinical Features. DM-2/PROMM typically presents in adult life, usually with myotonic stiffness or weakness (proximal legs or long finger flexors).[4–10] Patients complain of muscle stiffness, fluctuating myotonia of grip, thigh muscle stiffness, or muscle pain.[6] The muscle pain is independent of exercise or the severity of myotonia on clinical examination. The pain varies in severity over days to weeks. The cause for the variation is unknown. In the initial stages of DM-2/PROMM, there is often

mild weakness of long finger flexors, thigh flexors, and hip extensors along with grip myotonia. The myotonia is most apparent following percussion of forearm extensor and thenar muscles. The myotonia that occurs after a powerful grip, often has a jerky, tremulous quality that differs from the grip myotonia observed in DM-1. Facial weakness and the wasting of face, forearm, and distal leg muscles that are typical for DM-1 are not observed in DM-2. Even in the late stages, typical DM-2/PROMM patients have relatively mild muscle wasting. Occasionally, patients with DM-2/PROMM have calf muscle hypertrophy.[4–6,9] Early-onset of cataracts that require surgery is common. Later in life, patients may present with complaints of difficulty climbing stairs or arising from a squat. Myotonia and muscle pain are less prominent when onset is late. Patients typically ascribe their complaints to "old age" or arthritis. In contrast to DM-1, respiratory failure, difficulty swallowing, and gastrointestinal dysfunction are uncommon in DM-2/PROMM. Cardiac conduction disturbances occur in DM-1, DM-2/PROMM, and DM-3/PROMM.[6,7] Frequency and severity appear to be less in DM-2/PROMM and DM-3/PROMM.[6,7] Childhood forms of DM-2/PROMM or DM-3/PROMM have not been clearly identified. However, anticipation (earlier onset of more severe symptoms in successive generations) occurs in both DM-2/PROMM and DM-1.[6,12] For this reason, it seems likely that cases of childhood-onset DM-2/PROMM will become apparent once DNA testing for the expanded CCTG-repeat becomes routinely available.

Proximal Myotonic Dystrophy, PDM/DM-2/PROMM

Clinical Features. PDM/PROMM/DM-2[13] results from the same mutation in the zinc finger protein 9 (ZNF9) gene that causes DM-2/PROMM.[6,8,10] This is a rare type of PROMM syndrome. Clinical features are based mainly on the detailed report of a large kindred from Borko Islands off the coast of Finland.[6,13] Patients develop slowly progressive weakness and wasting of scapulohumeral, pelvifemoral, and neck muscles. Onset is in the second to fourth decade of life. There are no clinical signs of myotonia, which is detected only on electromyographic study. Facial weakness is mild, and patients can walk on their heels and tiptoes until knee extensor muscle wasting and weakness prevent weight bearing. Muscle pain, swallowing difficulty, respiratory failure, and cardiac conduction disturbances are not typical features. Disability results mainly from severe wasting and weakness of shoulder and hip girdle muscles. More information is necessary to define the natural history and to determine the prevalence of this form of the PROMM syndrome.

Myotonic Dystrophy Type-3 (or More), DM-3/PROMM

Clinical Features. In kindreds with dominantly transmitted myotonia and weakness not linked to the 3q21 locus, some patients have clinical features that are indistinguishable from those described above for DM-2/PROMM. These patients with DM-3/PROMM do not show linkage to the DM-2 or DM-1 loci.[6,8] The existence of DM-3/PROMM reveals the genetic heterogeneity of the PROMM syndrome. However, it is interesting that at least three different mutations can lead to the same PROMM phenotype. Until the clinical spectrum and manifestations of the DM-3 and DM-2 forms of PROMM will be further defined, it seems appropriate to use the clinical features described under DM-2/PROMM above to also identify patients with DM-3/PROMM. In the immediate future, DNA testing will permit separation of DM-1 and DM-2/PROMM from DM-3/PROMM. For a more detailed description of the clinical features of DM-3/PROMM and other families without definite linkage to the ZNF9 locus on chromosome 3q21, we recommend a recent review of the different PROMM syndromes.[6]

Diagnostic Evaluation of the Myotonic Dystrophies

The major problem in making the diagnosis of one of the myotonic dystrophies is the tendency of clinicians to ignore these entities in their practice. Common complaints, such as trouble seeing, gait instability, dropping items, muscle stiffness, muscle pain, or trouble swallowing, may be symptoms of one of the myotonic dystrophies. Patients with DM-1 and DM-2/PROMM may also present with one or more of the multisystem manifestations of these diseases. Cardiac arrhythmias and early cataracts (typically, iridescent posterior capsular cataracts) are examples. In contrast, patients with other

hereditary myotonic disorders, such as chloride or sodium channel myotonias, do not have cardiac arrhythmias or cataracts. DM-1 patients occasionally present with prolonged apnea after general anesthesia, while DM-2/PROMM patients may infrequently develop rhabdomyolysis with renal failure after general anesthesia.[6,14] These complications can occur in individuals with only mild clinical signs. Endocrine abnormalities are common for DM-1, DM-2/PROMM, and DM-3/PROMM.[6,14,15] There is testicular atrophy, gonadal failure, decreased testosterone, and impotence in males. Such problems in a patient who complains of muscle stiffness or weakness should suggest one of the myotonic dystrophies. Hypothyroidism and pregnancy can unmask myotonia and weakness, specifically in DM-2/PROMM.[16,17] In DM-1, DM-2/PROMM, and DM-3/PROMM, there is increased frequency of insulin resistance. Patients will often have a history of abnormal glucose tolerance and hyperlipidemia.[6,14,15] In addition to endocrine dysfunction, patients with DM-1, DM-2/PROMM, and DM-3/PROMM may have brain manifestations. Recent investigations have shown that there are prominent neurobehavioral alterations in association with decreased frontal and temporal cortical blood flow on PET scan in the myotonic dystrophies.[18] Other alterations, such as mild elevation in serum creatine kinase and gamma glutamyl transferase levels, are common findings.[6,14,15] Figure 47–1 proposes a diagnostic flowchart to identify myotonic dystrophy in an individual with muscle weakness, stiffness, or pain but without clear diagnostic findings on examination. The gold standard to establish the diagnosis of DM-1 and DM-2/PROMM is the presence of abnormal expansions of CTG repeats in the 19q13.3 DMPK locus for DM-1, and of CCTG repeats in the 3q21 ZNF9 locus for DM-2/PROMM. The CTG repeat sizes in the *DMPK* gene isolated from circulating leucocytes range from 5 to 37 repeats in normal individuals.[1–3,14,15] In late-onset, mild DM-1, CTG sizes typically range from 50 to 150 repeats, while in moderately severe patients with onset in second or third decade, CTG sizes often range from 300 to 1000 repeats.[14,15] Severe, congenital DM-1 patients have CTG sizes ranging from 800 to over 2000 repeats.[14,15] Standard DNA testing is available for DM-1.

DNA testing for DM-2/PROMM has become available. CCTG repeat sizes in alleles containing the ZNF9 gene isolated from circulating leucocytes are less than 75 repeats in individual subjects. In DM-2/PROMM patients, CCTG repeat sizes range from 75 to over 11,000 repeats. We anticipate that in the near future standardized DNA analysis will become routine for DM-2/PROMM.

Standardized testing for the large number of point mutations that cause chloride and sodium channel myotonia is not yet available but may become available in the near future. Only selected screening for a few of the known mutations in these genes is available at present.

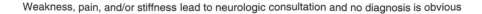

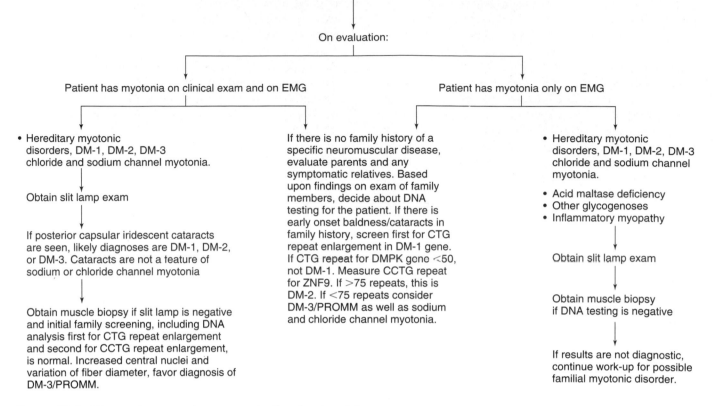

FIGURE 47–1. Diagnostic approach to myotonic disorders in adults.

More comprehensive screening for the chloride and sodium channel myotonias is needed to distinguish patients with mild DM-3/PROMM from those with other nondystrophic myotonic disorders and to establish a specific diagnosis for the chloride or sodium channel myotonias. The gene locus or loci responsible for DM-3/PROMM remain unknown, and specific genetic testing is not yet available.

PATHOLOGY

DM-1, DM-2/PROMM, and DM-3/PROMM have similar pathologic changes on muscle biopsy.[6,14,15] There are increased central nuclei, atrophy of type 1 fibers (mainly in DM-1), ringed fibers, and subsarcolemmal masses. Early in the course of PDM/PROMM/DM-2, the findings on biopsy resemble those seen in DM-2/PROMM and DM-3/PROMM. In patients with advanced weakness, there are more severe changes. For example, there are pronounced dystrophic changes in the quadriceps femoris muscle, with increased internal nuclei, hypertrophied fibers, and increased fibrous tissue.

MOLECULAR GENETICS AND ANIMAL MODELS

DM-1 results from an unstable CTG repeat expansion in the 3′ noncoding region of a gene that encodes a serine/threonine kinase, DMPK.[1–3] The specific alteration that leads to the unstable expansion of the CTG repeat in DM-1 remains a mystery. One clue is that alleles containing CTG sizes of 19 to 30 repeats have a predilection to become unstable, although they are within the normal range for repeat expansion (5 to 37 repeats).[14] More research is needed to investigate the mechanism underlying this predisposition to instability. One interesting feature of the repeat instability in DM-1 is the variation in the size of mutated alleles isolated from different tissues. There is a pronounced tissue mosaicism of repeat sizes.[14,15] Skeletal muscle, myocardium, and certain regions of the brain have CTG repeat expansions severalfold larger than circulating leucocytes.[14,15] It is tempting to propose that tissue mosaicism accounts for the variation in severity of clinical symptoms and that severity is greatest in those target tissues containing larger repeat expansions. Clinical studies show that DM-1 patients with larger repeat expansions in leucocyte DNA have earlier onset and more severe muscle weakness.[14,15] However, caution is needed before stating that the size of the CTG repeat in the *DMPK* gene can reliably predict severity of disease manifestations. Studies describing various cognitive deficits, alterations in cerebral blood flow, and cardiac conduction defects in patients with DM-1 have failed to demonstrate a direct relationship between size of the CTG repeat expansion measured in leucocyte DNA and severity of brain or heart manifestations.[14,18]

It is conceivable that CTG repeat sizes in alleles from the specific target tissues involved (brain and heart) might have demonstrated a direct relationship between the repeat size, tissue pathology, and degree of altered function in these studies. However, studies of postmortem skeletal muscle, brain, and cardiac tissue are needed to explore more fully this hypothesis.

It seems likely that most of the disease manifestations of DM-1 are due to factors other than a haploinsufficiency of *DMPK*. The function of *DMPK* is unknown, but mouse knockout models of *DMPK* and overexpression models have failed to produce findings that resemble human DM-1.[14,15] Other studies have raised the possibility that the manifestations of DM-1 result from an effect on flanking genes, because increasing the size of the CTG repeat expansion in the DM-1 gene reduces the expression of the flanking genes, *SIX5* and *DMWD*.[14,15,19–21] Another study has demonstrated that SIX5 knockout mice develop cataracts typical of DM-1.[20] Thus, if the CTG repeat expansion in the *DMPK* gene can alter the expression of a flanking gene, it might cause at least one of the manifestations observed in DM-1.

MOLECULAR PATHOLOGY

One of the most attractive pathogenetic hypotheses for DM-1 is that it may result from a toxic accumulation of *DMPK* mRNA.[22–24] Transcripts generated from the mutant *DMPK* allele, although fully processed and polyadenylated, remain in the cell nucleus in multiple discrete foci. Evidence that these accumulations of RNA may mediate disease manifestations comes from investigations of transgenic mice. Investigators have generated lines of mice that contain a human skeletal muscle actin transgene with a DNA insert that is comprised exclusively of 250 CTG repeats. The transgene has none of the other DNA in DM-1 *DMPK* gene. They have compared their findings to strains of mice with the actin transgene containing a normal CTG repeat size of 5 repeats. LR-mice, with the long 250 CTG repeat transgene, develop a DM-like phenotype, including myotonia, histopathologic changes similar to those in DM-1, and multifocal accumulations of expanded transcripts with CUG repeats in the nucleus.[22] Additional studies have shown that similar accumulations of *DMPK* mRNA transcripts with expanded CUG repeats are present in the nuclei of muscle biopsy samples from patients with DM-1 (n = 9) and DM-2/PROMM (n = 9). Such accumulations do not occur in disease controls or healthy individuals (n = 23). Muscleblind, a nuclear regulatory protein that interacts with expanded CUG repeats, localizes to intranuclear foci in muscle biopsy samples from patients with DM-1 and DM-2/PROMM. This finding raises the possibility that the abnormally expanded CUG-containing transcripts contribute to the pathogenesis of DM-1 and DM-2/PROMM by impairing nuclear function.[23] More recent investigations of the LR-mice indicate that the accumulation of transcripts with the expanded CUG repeats leads to abnormal splicing of the mRNA for the skeletal muscle chloride channel (ClC-1),[24] which, in turn, causes a severe decrease in chloride conductance.[24] This decreased chloride conductance appears to be the basis for the myotonia in mice. It also seems likely that abnormal splicing of mRNA for the ClC-1 occurs in patients with DM-1 and DM-2/PROMM. Antibody staining for the ClC-1 protein in muscle biopsies from patients with DM-1 and DM-2/PROMM as well as from the LR-mice shows a marked decrease in membrane associated ClC-1 protein. It is logical to propose that myotonia in DM-1 and DM-2/PROMM also results from a decrease in chloride conductance, as it does in the LR-mice. Taken together, these findings support a disease model for DM-1 and DM-2/PROMM in which nuclear accumulation of mRNA transcripts containing expanded CUG or CCUG repeats causes aberrant splicing of ClC-1 mRNA, loss of ClC-1 protein, and reduced chloride conductance, and results in hyperexcitability of the muscle membrane.[24]

THERAPY

Despite recent progress in molecular genetics of the myotonic dystrophies, the pathomechanism responsible for muscle wasting, especially the marked wasting in DM-1 and in PDM/PROMM/DM-2 remains unclear. The primary approach to treatment is symptomatic for all myotonic dystrophies. Typical components of symptomatic therapy are: bracing, motorized scooters, wheelchairs, serial monitoring of ECG with pacemaker placement as necessary, careful perioperative management (special caution concerning respiratory depression with opiates, barbiturates, general anesthetics), serial monitoring of forced vital capacity, consultations with physical therapy, orthopedics, cardiology, ophthalmology, and pulmonary medicine. Myotonic stiffness and grip myotonia occasionally become so persistent that a trial with antimyotonic drugs seems warranted. Antimyotonia treatment has not received careful evaluation in these conditions, especially in DM-2/PROMM and DM-3/PROMM, but medications, such as mexiletine, phenytoin, and acetazolamide, all merit consideration. Frequent serial monitoring of ECG is necessary during treatment with mexiletine. Cataracts also require serial monitoring and at some point may require surgical removal.[6,14] There is no specific treatment for the very troublesome, intermittent muscle pain that occurs in DM-2/PROMM and DM-3/PROMM. Presently, treatment with nonsteroidal anti-inflammatory drugs, carbamazepine, or short-term corticosteroid therapy deserves consideration. Occasionally, opiates are necessary to control the pain.

A limited number of randomized controlled trials of specific treatments have occurred in the myotonic dystrophies, and almost all of them have been in DM-1. The results have not identified a standardized effective treatment for the skeletal muscle manifestations of DM-1. For a more detailed review of these completed therapeutic trials, we recommend recent publications.[14,15] Following is a brief review of selected treatment trials that have occurred since the early 1990s.

Treatment Trials for Muscle Wasting and Weakness

Gonadal failure and a deficiency of testosterone are common in men with DM-1. Testosterone is one of the principal anabolic hormones for skeletal muscle. For years, it was suspected that lack of testosterone accounted for much of the muscle wasting and weakness in DM-1. To determine if maintaining a high physiologic level of testosterone can increase muscle mass and function, investigators have performed a 12-month, double-blind, randomized, controlled study of men with DM-1. They compared weekly intramuscular injections of testosterone enanthate (3 mg/kg per week) to placebo. After 12 months of treatment, patients receiving testosterone had significantly greater muscle mass, but no significant improvement in strength or function. Testosterone had the net effect of increasing noncontractile muscle protein without increasing muscle function. Testosterone also made these patients more insulin resistant. This insulin resistance may have counteracted some of the beneficial actions of testosterone. At present, testosterone therapy in the myotonic dystrophies is primarily indicated to restore normal blood levels and to treat impotence.

Another hormonal abnormality that may contribute to muscle wasting in DM-1 relates to altered circulating levels of the anabolic hormone, growth hormone. Many DM-1 patients have impaired release of growth hormone during sleep and after certain provocative stimuli. To determine if a consistent, high physiologic level of growth hormone can enhance muscle anabolism, investigators carried out a 16-week open trial of daily intramuscular recombinant human growth hormone in 10 men with classical DM-1 (reviewed in reference 14). Growth hormone therapy produced a 10% increase in lean body mass and a 28% increase in muscle protein synthesis. Unfortunately, despite the improvement in protein anabolism, there was no significant increase in strength or muscle function. As with testosterone, an increase in noncontractile muscle protein was not accompanied by an increase in contractile protein and muscle function. Growth hormone therapy also increased basal insulin levels and raised the concern that testosterone maintenance of high physiologic levels of growth hormone may cause insulin resistance. As with testosterone, the insulin resistance may counteract some of the beneficial effects of growth hormone.

To bypass the insulin resistance side effect of growth hormone while preserving its anabolic actions, investigators completed a study using the product of growth hormone, insulin-like growth factor-1 (IGF-1).

IGF-1 enhances, rather than antagonizes, insulin action, and it exerts broad anabolic effects on skeletal muscle metabolism. In the study, investigators gave subcutaneous 5-mg injections of recombinant human IGF-1 (n = 7) or placebo (n = 9) twice daily for 16 weeks to patients with typical DM-1. A subgroup of four DM-1 patients showed improvement both in strength and in function. The dosage of IGF-1 in these four patients was greater than 70 μg/kg, which appears to represent a threshold dosage to achieve a beneficial effect on muscle function. All seven patients receiving IGF-1 showed an increased rate of protein synthesis and increased sensitivity to insulin. Overall, the results of this trial of IGF-1 are promising, but further investigations are necessary to extend and reproduce these observations and to establish the optimal dosage.

In addition to gonadal insufficiency, one of the most common endocrine alterations in DM-1 is insulin resistance.[14,15] Insulin is the primary anabolic hormone in humans. Loss or decline in its anabolic actions may contribute to muscle wasting and weakness. Therapeutic trials to reverse the skeletal muscle insulin resistance that occurs in DM-1 are in progress. One trial is using the thiazolidinedione derivative, troglitazone. Other thiazolidinediones have also become available. Studies using these medications will help to determine if reversing or lessening the insulin resistance in DM-1 can limit disease manifestations.

Another potentially useful hormonal therapy in DM-1 involves treatment with the androgenic hormone, dehydroepiandrosterone sulfate (DHEAS), which the adrenal gland produces in declining amounts throughout life. The precise function of DHEAS remains unclear, but it appears to act both on skeletal muscle and on the brain. Past studies have demonstrated that patients with DM-1 have markedly decreased blood levels of DHEAS. To test whether a deficiency of DHEAS may contribute to the muscle wasting and weakness, investigators have initiated therapeutic trials using daily intravenous infusions of 200 mg of DHEAS. The results of these open trials are encouraging. Patients have shown increased muscle function and decreased myotonia. More studies are in progress.

Trials to Treat Myotonia

Only a few small-scale controlled studies have evaluated the effects of antimyotonia therapy in the myotonic dystrophies, and they all have occurred in DM-1. The most encouraging of these studies has demonstrated that in 9 DM-1 patients, the lidocaine derivatives mexiletine (400 to 600 mg/day) and tocainide (1200 mg/day) are significantly more effective than phenytoin (300 mg/day) or disopyramide (300 mg/day) in ameliorating myotonia. Mexiletine and tocainide have comparable efficacy, but the investigators recommend mexiletine as a first choice because of the increased risk of bone marrow suppression associated with tocainide. Further large-scale trials of mexiletine in DM-1, DM-2/PROMM, and DM-3/PROMM deserve consideration.

Trial of Treatment of Hypersomnia

Investigators have conducted an open-label trial of modafinil (200 to 400 mg/day) for an average of 16.4 weeks in nine patients with DM-1.[25] There were no major side effects. Modafinil appears to offer a new, possibly more effective alternative to methylphenidate or pemoline as a treatment for daytime somnolence. Future large-scale controlled trials of modafinil are necessary to confirm these initial encouraging findings.

CONCLUSIONS AND FUTURE RESEARCH DIRECTIONS

Fundamental similarities among the myotonic dystrophies (dominant inheritance, distinctive cataracts, myotonia, muscle weakness, and multisystem alterations affecting the heart, brain, and endocrine systems) suggest that there are common final pathways in DM-1, DM-2/PROMM, PDM/DM-2/PROMM, and DM-3/PROMM. The variable manifestations that occur in DM1 may represent a composite phenotype that results from several distinct but interacting pathogenic mechanisms, such as loss of *DMPK* function, silencing of the flanking gene *SIX5*, and gain of function by mutant mRNA. This view is supported by the appearance of partial DM-like phenotypes in various animal models, such as delayed cardiac conduction and reduced muscle force generation in *DMPK* knockout mice, cataracts in *SIX5* knockout mice,[20] and myotonia and myopathy in LR mice that overexpress the actin transgene containing the expanded 250 CUG repeats.[22] However, this view of DM-1 as a pathogenically complex, multigenic disease is difficult to reconcile with the observation that many of its manifestations are reproduced in DM-2/PROMM and DM-3/PROMM, which result from mutations in loci without any obvious homology or functional relationship with the DM-1 locus. One interesting genetic similarity of the myotonic dystrophies, at least of DM-1 and DM-2/PROMM, is that both disorders result from unstable nucleotide repeat expansions. DM-1 has CTG repeats at the *DMPK* locus at 19q13.3 and DM-2/PROMM has CCTG repeats at *ZFP9* locus at 3q21. The only common features are the repeat expansions. There is no apparent connection between the gene products or the flanking genes. It is interesting to hypothesize that the accumulations of CUG- or CCUG-containing transcripts that appear in the nuclei of patients with DM-1 and DM-2/PROMM may set the stage for a shared pathomechanism. In both diseases, RNA-mediated toxicity may alter nuclear function. In turn, this alteration may lead to specific muscle and nonmuscle manifestations. Future research is necessary to address this hypothesis and to determine if DM-3/PROMM is also due to an unstable nucleotide repeat expansion. There is optimism that future investigations will produce new ideas about the genetic pathomechanism of the myotonic dystrophies, and studies in patients and animal models will improve understanding of the pathophysiology that underlies the different disease manifestations. The knowledge to be gained from these studies will lead to more effective treatment for the many and varied problems that occur in patients with the myotonic dystrophies.

REFERENCES

1. Brook JD, McCurrach ME, Harley HG, et al: Molecular basis of myotonic dystrophy: Expansion of a trinucleotide (CTG) repeat at the 3' end of a transcript encoding a protein kinase family member. Cell 1992;68: 799–808.

2. Fu YH, Pizzuti A, Fenwick RG, et al: An unstable triplet repeat in a gene related to myotonic muscular dystrophy. Science 1992;255:1256–1258.

3. Mahadevan M, Tsilfidis C, Sabourin L, et al: Myotonic dystrophy mutation: An unstable CTG repeat in the 3' untranslated region of the gene. Science 1992; 255:1253–1255.

4. Thornton CA, Griggs RC, Moxley RT: Myotonic dystrophy with no trinucleotide repeat expansion. Ann Neurol 1994;35:269–272.

5. Ricker K, Koch MC, Lehmann-Horn F, et al: Proximal myotonic myopathy: A new dominant disorder with myotonia, muscle weakness, and cataracts. Neurology 1994;44:1448–1452.

6. Moxley RT, Meola G, Udd B, Ricker K: Report of the 84th ENMC Workshop: PROMM (Proximal Myotonic Myopathy) and Other Myotonic Dystrophy-Like Syndromes: 2nd Workshop. 13th–15th October 2000. Loosdrecht, The Netherlands. Neuromuscul Disord 2002;12:306–317.

7. Meola G, Sansone V, Marinou K, et al: Proximal myotonic myopathy: A syndrome with a favourable prognosis? J Neurol Sci 2002;93:89–96.

8. Meola G: Clinical and genetic heterogeneity in myotonic dystrophies. Muscle Nerve 2000;23:1789–1799.

9. Day JW, Roelofs R, Leroy B, et al: Clinical and genetic characteristics of a five-generation family with a novel form of myotonic dystrophy (DM2). Neuromuscul Disord 1999;9:19–27.

10. Liquori CL, Ricker K, Moseley ML, et al: Myotonic dystrophy type 2 caused by a CCTG expansion in intron 1 of ZNF9. Science 2001;293:864–867.

11. The International Myotonic Dystrophy Consortium (IDMC): New nomenclature and DNA testing guidelines for myotonic dystrophy type 1. Neurology 2000;54:1218–1221.

12. Schneider C, Ziegler A, Ricker K, et al: Proximal myotonic myopathy: Evidence for anticipation in families with linkage to chromosome 3q. Neurology 2000;55: 383–388.

13. Udd B, Krahe R, Wallgren-Pettersson C, et al: Proximal myotonic dystrophy—a family with autosomal dominant muscular dystrophy, cataracts, hearing loss and hypogonadism: Heterogeneity of proximal myotonic syndromes? Neuromuscul Disord 1997;7:217–228.

14. Moxley RT, Meola G. Myotonic dystrophy. In Deymeer F (ed): Neuromuscular Diseases: From Basic Mechanisms to Clinical Management. Basel, S Karger AG, 2000, pp 61–78.

15. Harper PS: Myotonic Dystrophy. Philadelphia, WB Saunders, 2001.

16. Sansone V, Griggs RC, Moxley RT: Hypothyroidism unmasking proximal myotonic myopathy. Neuromuscul Disord 2000;3:165–172.

17. Newman B, Meola G, O'Donovan DG, et al: Proximal myotonic myopathy (PROMM) presenting as myotonia during pregnancy. Neuromuscul Disord 1999; 3:144–149.

18. Meola G, Sansone V, Perani D, et al: Reduced cerebral blood flow and impaired visual-spatial function in proximal myotonic myopathy. Neurology 1999;53: 1042–1050.

19. Timchenko NA, Iakova P, Cai ZJ, et al: Molecular basis for impaired muscle differentiation in myotonic dystrophy. Mol Cell Biol 2001;21:6927–6938.

20. Klesert TR, Cho DH, Clark JI, et al: Mice deficient in Six5 develop cataracts: Implications for myotonic dystrophy. Nat Genet 2000;25:105–109.

21. Frisch R, Singleton KR, Moses PA, et al: Effect of triplet repeat expansion on chromatin structure and expression of DMPK and neighboring genes, SIX5 and DMWD, in myotonic dystrophy. Mol Genet Metab 2001;74:281–291.

22. Mankodi A, Logigian E, Callahan L, et al: Myotonic dystrophy in transgenic mice expressing an expanded CUG repeat. Science 2000;289:1769–1773.

23. Mankodi A, Urbinati CR, Yuan QP, et al: Muscleblind localizes to nuclear foci of aberrant RNA in myotonic dystrophy types 1 and 2. Hum Mol Genet 2001;10:2165–2170.

24. Mankodi A, Takahashi M, Jiang H, et al: Expanded CUG repeats in myotonic dystrophy trigger aberrant splicing of ClC-1 chloride channel pre-mRNA and hyperexcitability in skeletal muscle. Mol Cell 2002;10:1–20.

25. Damian MS, Gerlach A, Schmidt F, et al: Modafinil for excessive daytime sleepiness in myotonic dystrophy. Neurology 2001;56:794–796.

Facioscapulohumeral Dystrophy

Rabi Tawil

Facioscapulohumeral muscular dystrophy (FSHD) is the third most common form of muscular dystrophy, with an estimated prevalence of 1:20,000.[1] It is characterized by an initially restricted regional distribution of muscle weakness, slow progression, and relatively benign course seldom affecting life expectancy. Inheritance is autosomal dominant with a high frequency of sporadic cases.[2] Penetrance is virtually complete with greater than 95% of affected individuals expressing the disease by age 20 years. There is, however, extraordinary variability in disease severity in terms of age of onset, side-to-side symmetry, rate of progression, and distribution of affected muscles. This variability occurs both within and between kindreds.

GENETICS

In 1990, FSHD was linked to chromosome 4q35, where subtelomeric rearrangements were identified.[3] These rearrangements consist of deletions of an integral number of copies of a 3.3-kb DNA repeat named *D4Z4*. Whereas normal individuals have 15 or more 3.3-kb repeats, individuals with FSHD have 12 or fewer repeats (Fig. 48–1). However, the deletions do not appear to disrupt an expressed gene, as no transcribed gene sequences have been identified within the 3.3-kb repeat elements.[4] Analysis of the repeat sequences show high homology to a family of repeats in heterochromatin, which is highly compacted DNA that is transcriptionally inactive.[5] This finding has led to the hypothesis that deletion of a critical number of repeats brings the FSHD gene(s) closer to heterochromatic telomeric DNA, thus interfering with gene expression, a mechanism referred to as position effect variegation.[5] The search for genes centromeric to the

D4Z4 repeats, whose expression may be altered by the FSHD-associated deletion, is hampered by the complexity of the 4q35 region, which has high density of repetitive sequences and high homology to regions on other chromosomes.

The vast majority of kindreds with clinical FSHD have a demonstrable deletion on 4q35. There are rare, but well documented, kindreds whose clinical picture is identical to classic FSHD but who are unlinked to the 4q35 locus. No alternative locus has yet been identified for these kindreds.[6]

CLINICAL FEATURES

FSHD is defined by a characteristic distribution of weakness with a generally descending pattern of involvement, starting with usually asymptomatic facial weakness followed sequentially by scapular fixator, humeral, truncal, and lower extremity weakness. The rate of progression is generally slow and steady. Many patients report a relapsing course with long periods of quiescence interrupted by periods of rapid deterioration involving a particular muscle group, and sometimes heralded by pain in the affected limb. Eventually, 20% of patients become wheelchair-bound.[1] A subpopulation of patients with infantile onset FSHD is severely disabled at an early age.

The most common presenting symptom is scapular winging secondary to weakness of the scapular fixators, specifically the serratus, rhomboid, supraspinatus, and infraspinatus muscles. Facial weakness is almost invariably present but typically without perceived symptoms. Although the initial symptoms are often described as recent in onset, a history of long-standing difficulties climbing rope, doing push-ups, whistling, or drinking

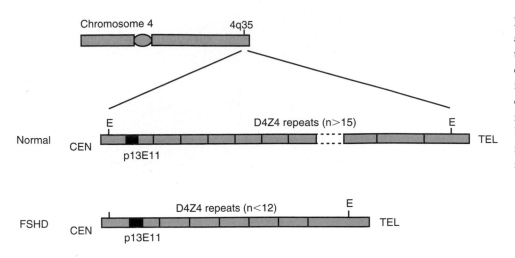

FIGURE 48–1. The FSHD-associated deletion is at the telomeric end of the long arm of chromosome 4. Normal individuals have greater than 15 copies of the 3.3-kb (D4Z4) repeat on 4q35. FSHD is caused by a rearrangement that results in a reduction in number of repeats to less than 12.

through a straw can often be elicited. Parents often describe their children as having always slept with their eyes partially open indicating long-standing unnoticed facial weakness. Striking bifacial weakness can be the presenting symptom in infantile FSHD and may be misdiagnosed as Möbius syndrome. Some patients first present with footdrop. These individuals invariably have coexisting, asymptomatic facial and scapular fixator weakness. Leg involvement is initially distal, but proximal weakness is present in many patients and can be more severe than distal weakness. Indeed, the availability of specific molecular diagnostic testing for FSHD is leading to an expansion of the clinical spectrum of the disease, as some, usually sporadic, patients with limb-girdle patterns of weakness are found to have the characteristic 4q35 FSHD deletion.[7]

On inspection, FSHD patients have widened palpebral fissures and decreased facial expression. The lips are pouted and dimples are often evident at the corners of the mouth. Examination confirms bifacial, typically asymmetric, weakness with a transverse smile, inability to purse lips, and inability to bury eyelashes (Fig. 48–2C, D). Extraocular, eyelid, and bulbar muscles are spared. Neck flexors remain strong and are relatively spared compared to the neck extensors. The anterior view of the shoulders shows a typical appearance with straight clavicles, forward sloping, and rounding. The pectoral muscles are atrophied and occasionally absent. Pectoralis atrophy results in the appearance of an axillary crease (Fig. 48–2B). The scapulae are laterally displaced, and winging is evident either at rest or with attempted forward arm flexion or abduction (Fig. 48–2A). The selective involvement of the lower trapezius muscles results in a characteristic upward jutting of the scapulae when the arms are abducted. The biceps and triceps muscles are typically involved with remarkable sparing of the deltoid. With exception of the wrist extensors, the forearm and hand muscles are spared early in the course of FSHD. This pattern of intact deltoids, forearm muscles, and wasted arm muscles results in a "Popeye" arm appearance.

Abdominal muscle weakness is prominent, resulting in a protuberant abdomen and secondary lumbar lordosis. The lower (occasionally upper) abdominal wall muscles are selectively involved causing a striking upward movement of the umbilicus on neck flexion (Beevor's sign), a sign uncommon in other myopathic conditions. In the lower extremities, the peroneal muscles are involved with foot dorsiflexor weakness usually sparing the calf muscles. Although proximal leg muscles are thought to become involved only late in the disease, studies with quantitative myometry have shown early involvement of knee extensors and flexors. Muscle stretch reflexes are often reduced in FSHD, and sensory examination is normal. Contractures are rarely present even in profoundly weak muscles.

One of the striking features of FSHD is the degree of side-to-side asymmetry in muscle weakness. One study showed that the dominant limb was weaker, suggesting that overuse may accelerate progression. Another study, however, failed to show a relationship between handedness and degree of weakness, suggesting that other factors contribute to this asymmetry.[8]

The most common, though usually asymptomatic, extramuscular manifestations of FSHD are high-frequency hearing loss and retinal telangiectasias.[9] Systematic evaluation of FSHD kindreds shows mild high-frequency hearing loss in most. Hearing loss can be occasionally severe enough to require the use of hearing aids, especially in infantile FSHD. Similarly, screening an FSHD kindred with fluorescein angiography reveals peripheral retinal telangiectasis in a majority of affected individuals. Occasionally, these vascular malformations can result in exudative retinopathy and retinal detachment or Coat's syndrome.

Until the late 1990s, symptomatic cardiac involvement in FSHD was not clearly documented. Cases of atrial standstill, a cardiac manifestation typical of Emery-Dreifuss syndrome, were reported in four patients with FSHD. However, the clinical description of these patients was insufficient to exclude Emery-Dreifuss, and these

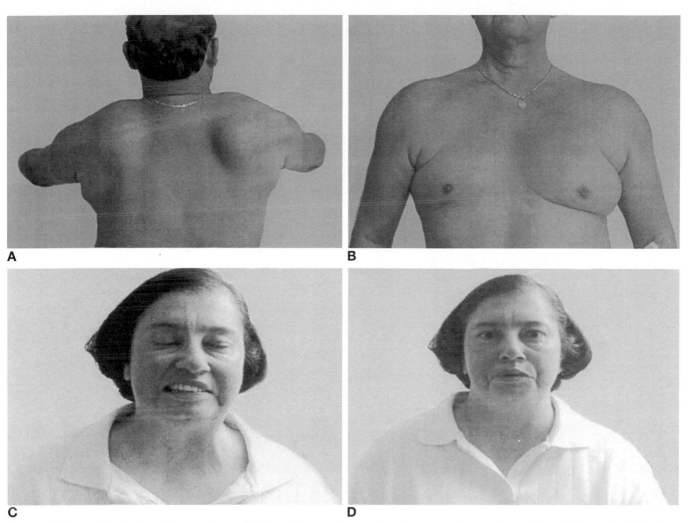

FIGURE 48–2. *A*, Limitation of forward arm flexion with scapular winging due to weakness of scapular stabilizers; *B*, Typical appearance of shoulders with straight clavicles and bilateral axillary creases indicative of wasting of pectoral muscles; *C*, Weakness of forced eye closure and asymmetric lower facial muscle weakness with a transverse smile; *D*, Asymmetric weakness of orbicularis oris muscle demonstrated by inability to pucker lips and whistle.

reports were published at a time when molecular diagnostic confirmation was unavailable. More systematic studies, however, described other, usually asymptomatic, atrial abnormalities on surface ECG and a tendency to develop inducible atrial arrhythmias in FSHD. These findings were confirmed in a study of molecularly documented cases of FSHD, in which about 5% had cardiac involvement with conduction abnormalities and a predilection for supraventricular tachyarrhythmias.[10]

The spectrum of extramuscular manifestations in FSHD has now been expanded to include the central nervous system. A survey of Japanese patients with molecularly confirmed FSHD showed that 8 of 20 patients with early-onset FSHD were mentally retarded, and 4 of these also suffered from seizures.[11]

PATHOPHYSIOLOGY

While the molecular lesion for FSHD is known, the gene or genes that mediate the effects of this deletion remain unknown. Consequently, the pathophysiology of FSHD

is also unclear. The nonspecific histologic changes seen in FSHD muscle biopsies give no clues to possible metabolic or structural abnormalities. The role of the inflammatory infiltrates seen in some FSHD biopsies is more likely to be reactive to muscle injury than to be of fundamental pathogenic significance. The presence of inflammation does not correlate with either disease duration or activity and seems to be characteristic of certain kindreds. Although the latter finding suggests locus or allelic heterogeneity in FSHD, there is no evidence that FSHD patients with inflammation represent a genetically distinct group. The association of retinal abnormalities, hearing loss, cardiac abnormalities and, rarely, central nervous system manifestations suggests that either the responsible gene has pleiotropic effects or, as the position effect hypothesis would suggest, several genes are involved.[9]

Although the pathophysiology of FSHD remains unclear, clues are emerging from molecular studies as well as from genotype-phenotype studies. A case report of an individual with a chromosomal aberration resulting in a single copy (haploinsufficiency) of 4q35 but showing no signs of FSHD suggests that mutations within *D4Z4* in FSHD result in a deleterious gain of function.[12] It has also become clear that the larger the deletion (i.e., the smaller the residual restriction fragment), the more severe the clinical manifestations.[8,13] This correlation appears to hold true for the extramuscular manifestations of FSHD as well. Thus, patients with mental retardation and seizures have the largest deletions reported thus far.[11] These findings support the position-effect hypothesis suggesting that larger deletions may affect the expression of a larger number of genes. Deletion size, however, is clearly not the only determinant of severity. Affected members of the same kindred, who share the same size deletion, can differ vastly in the severity of their disease. Further support to the position-effect hypothesis in FSHD comes from the observation that it is the number of *D4Z4* repeats on 4q35 rather than the actual sequence of the repeats that is associated with FSHD. Thus, translocation between 4q35 and a homologous region on 10q26 results in FSHD only when the exchange results in less than 12 repeats on 4q35, regardless of the origin of the repeats.[14]

Despite the stability of the mutation within a kindred, several clinical studies based on age at disease onset or disease severity measured by quantitative myometry suggested the presence of anticipation.[8,13] This view has been challenged by Zatz et al, who suggested that the apparent "anticipation" is seen mostly in cases of maternal transmission to male offspring and can be explained by the fact that women, as a whole, are less severely affected with FSHD.[15]

Because of the difficulty in identifying genes within the 4q35 locus, research into the molecular pathophysiology of FSHD has now shifted toward looking for aberrant message expression in FSHD skeletal muscle as clues to identifying the causative gene or genes responsible for the disease.[16] Using these techniques, Gabellini et al demonstrated that three 4q35 genes *(FRG1, FRG2, and ANT1)* are overexpressed in FSHD muscle samples as compared to normal muscle, a pattern not seen in disease control muscle samples.[17] This overexpression is muscle-specific, as it was not seen in lymphocytes from FSHD patients. Moreover, the degree of overexpression is inversely related to the number of *D4Z4* repeats. Gabellini et al go on to demonstrate the presence of a 27-bp sequence within *D4Z4* that binds a multiprotein complex that acts as a transcriptional repression element.[17] This study, for the first time, provides proof for a potential mechanism through which a position effect can be mediated. However, it still does not resolve the issue as to which gene(s) are causally related to FSHD. *FRG1* and *FRG2* lack homologies to other proteins. *ANT1* is a potential candidate gene. The gene encodes a component of the mitochondrial permeability transition pore complex and is expressed mostly in skeletal and cardiac muscle. *ANT1* mutations have been implicated in some forms of dominantly inherited progressive external ophthalmoplegia.[18]

However, this condition, presumably resulting from reduced *ANT1* activity, is clinically and pathologically distinct from FSHD. Overexpression of *ANT1* can produce apoptosis, which has been demonstrated in many dystrophies, but is not particularly prominent in FSHD.

DIAGNOSIS

In the majority of cases, FSHD remains a fairly straightforward clinical diagnosis if the examining physician recognizes the characteristic pattern of muscle involvement. Molecular diagnosis is helpful in confirming the diagnosis, especially in atypical cases.

Clinical Diagnosis

The bedside diagnosis of FSHD is based on the characteristic distribution of weakness. The presence of prominent contractures and weakness of respiratory or bulbar muscles excludes the diagnosis of FSHD. In typical FSHD, disease progression occurs in a descending fashion. Therefore, shoulder girdle muscles are typically more severely involved than leg muscle in the early stages. This gradient becomes less obvious in more advanced cases. To confirm the diagnosis in individuals with atypical presentations, careful examination of other family members is essential. Laboratory studies, other than molecular diagnostic testing, are helpful only in ruling out other conditions. Creatine kinase (CK) levels are normal to slightly elevated (three to five times normal); CK levels elevated more than ten times normal suggest an alternative diagnosis. Electromyography shows nonspecific changes of active and chronic myopathy. The presence of myotonia or changes of chronic denervation rule out the diagnosis of FSHD. Muscle biopsy in FSHD shows nonspecific myopathic changes. As many as one third of biopsies have variable degrees of inflammation. If molecular confirmation cannot be obtained or molecular testing does not show a typical FSHD-associated deletion, a muscle biopsy should be performed. Several conditions can mimic the clinical presentation of FSHD but have characteristic muscle histopathology. These include: desmin storage (myofibrillar) myopathy, polymyositis, late-onset acid maltase deficiency, inclusion body myositis, mitochondrial myopathy, and congenital nemaline and centronuclear myopathy.[4]

Molecular Genetic Diagnosis

Molecular diagnosis of FSHD is now readily available in the United States, Canada, and Europe. Molecular diagnosis of FSHD is performed by conventional gel electrophoresis with leukocyte DNA using probe p13E-11 following digestion with *Eco*RI. However, p13E-11 also hybridizes to a region on 10q26 homologous to 4q35 and detects fragments in the size range diagnostic for FSHD (potentially complicating molecular diagnosis).[19] The

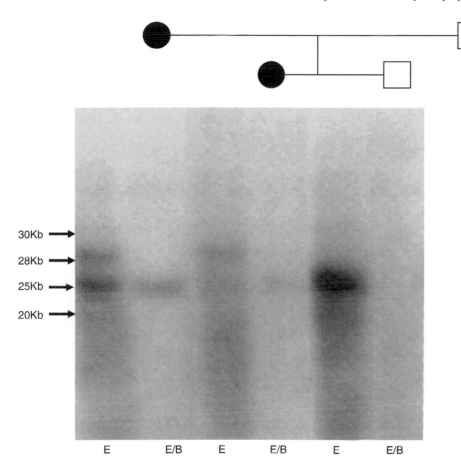

FIGURE 48–3. Double digestion with *Eco*RI/*Bln*I enhances the accuracy of FSHD molecular diagnosis. Pulse field gel electrophoresis (PFGE) with *Eco*RI digestion *(lanes labeled E)* suggest the presence two fragments in the range associated with FSHD (28 kb and 25 kb). Double digestion with *Eco*RI/*Bln*I *(lanes labeled E/B)* shows 28-kb fragment reduced to 25 kb with double digestion, indicating chromosome 4q origin; the 25kb fragment is totally digested, indicating chromosome 10q origin (nonpathogenic).

accuracy of FSHD molecular diagnosis was significantly improved with the finding of a restriction site (*Bln*I) that is unique to the 3.3-kb repeats of 10q26 origin.[20] Double digestion with *Eco*RI/*Bln*I results in complete digestion of 10q26 alleles and confirms the 4q35 origin of the remaining alleles (Fig. 48–3). Molecular diagnosis using the double digestion technique identifies the FSHD-associated 4q35 deletion in more than 95% of cases with the disease. Normal individuals have two alleles of 50 kb to 300 kb, whereas affected individuals have one allele in the normal range and one containing the deletion and ranging from 10 kb to 35 kb.[21] Thus, the detection of a deletion in affected family members or its appearance de novo in sporadic cases confirms a diagnosis of FSHD. Translocations between 4q35 and 10q26 creating hybrid 3.3-kb repeats can at times complicate the interpretation of the results of conventional molecular diagnosis. Analysis of such cases requires the characterization of all four (4q and 10q) alleles. This cannot be achieved with conventional gel electrophoresis because the normal alleles are large (>50 kb) and would require the use of pulse field gel electrophoresis (PFGE) or field inversion gel electrophoresis (FIGE). Further refinement in FSHD molecular diagnostics will help enhance the sensitivity and specificity of the test.[22] There remains some ambiguity about the upper limit of the fragment size (i.e., minimal number of deleted repeats) associated with FSHD. Although a cutoff of 35 kb will detect more than 95% of patients, there are clearly some patients with clinical features of FSHD that have fragments of 38 kb.[21,23]

THERAPY

In the absence of knowledge about the pathologic mechanism of FSHD, treatment remains supportive by necessity. In general, because FSHD is slowly progressive, affected individuals develop effective adaptive strategies to compensate for their disabilities, often without necessitating assistive devices. Ankle-foot orthoses are useful for foot drop, particularly early in the course of the disease. If significant quadriceps weakness sets in, however, ankle-foot orthoses can hinder ambulation. Surgical scapular fixation, in a select group of patients, can significantly enhance arm mobility.[24] Several factors must be considered before recommending surgery. One is whether fixation will actually result in greater arm movement in a given patient. This is easily tested at the bedside by assessing the degree of functional gain when the examiner manually fixes the scapula. The second factor is the rate of progression in the individual patient. If the disease is rapidly progressive, the benefit of surgery may be short-lived. Finally, although scapular fixation can improve arm abduction, shoulder range of motion becomes more restricted. Consequently, bilateral fixation should be discouraged.

Pharmacologic treatments aimed at slowing disease progression have been tried in FSHD. Because of the presence of inflammation in FSHD muscle, prednisone was tried and reported to be at least transiently effective in individual case reports. However, a prospective 3-month open-label trial of prednisone failed to show any benefit in either strength or lean body mass.[25] More recently, an open label trial of slow-release albuterol, a β_2 agonist, demonstrated a significant increase in both lean body mass and in strength measured by quantitative isometric myometry. The β_2-adrenergic agonists demonstrate significant anabolic potential in animal models of muscle wasting, including the mdx mouse, an animal model for Duchenne muscular dystrophy. A 1-year randomized controlled trial of albuterol in FSHD has been completed. The results failed to show improvement in strength, although lean body mass increased significantly at 1 year.[26] More recently, creatine has received much attention in the treatment of muscle-wasting diseases. Two small studies, which included a variety of neuromuscular conditions including FSHD, have demonstrated improvement in overall strength following short-term supplementation with creatine monohydrate.[27] Creatine-P is the immediate source of energy during vigorous muscle contraction. How it can improve strength in long-standing dystrophic conditions remains unclear. Creatine supplementation in normal athletes, at best, slightly enhances performance during high-intensity, short-term exercise.

REFERENCES

1. Padberg GW: Facioscapulohumeral Disease. Leiden, The Netherlands, University of Leiden, 1982.

2. Padberg GW, Frants RR, Brouwere OF, et al: Facioscapulohumeral muscular dystrophy in the Dutch population. Muscle Nerve 1995;2:S81–S84.

3. Wijmenga C, Hewitt JE, Sandkuijl LAX, et al: Chromosome 4q DNA rearrangements associated with facioscapulohumeral muscular dystrophy. Nat Genet 1992;2:26–30.

4. Tawil R, Figlewicz DA, Griggs RC, Weiffenbach B: Facioscapulohumeral dystrophy: A distinct regional myopathy with a novel molecular pathogenesis. Ann Neurol 1998;43:279–282.

5. Winokur ST, Bengtsson U, Feddersen J, et al: The DNA rearrangement associated with facioscapulohumeral muscular dystrophy involves a heterochromatin-associated repetitive element: Implications for a role of chromatin structure in the pathogenesis of the disease. Chromosome Res 1994;2:225–234.

6. Tim RW, Gilbert JR, Stajich JM, et al: Clinical studies in non-chromosome 4-linked facioscapulohumeral muscular dystrophy. J Clin Neuromusc Dis 2001;1:1–7.

7. Felice KJ, Moore SA: Unusual clinical presentations in patients harboring the facioscapulohumeral dystrophy 4q35 deletion. Muscle Nerve 2001;24:352–356.

8. Tawil R, Forrester J, Griggs RC, et al: Evidence for anticipation and association of deletion size with severity of facioscapulohumeral muscular dystrophy. Ann Neurol 1996;39:744–748.

9. Padberg G, Brouwer OF, de Keizer RJ, et al: On the significance of retinal vascular disease and hearing loss in facioscapulohumeral muscular dystrophy. Muscle Nerve 1995;2:S73–S80.

10. Laforet P, de Toma C, Eymard B, et al: Cardiac involvement in genetically confirmed facioscapulohumeral muscular dystrophy. Neurology 1998;51:1454–1456.

11. Funakoshi M, Goto K, Arahata K: Epilepsy and mental retardation in a subset of early onset 4q35-associated facioscapulohumeral muscular dystrophy. Neurology 1998;50:1791–1794.

12. Tupler R, Berardinelli A, Barbierato L, et al: Monosomy of distal 4q does not cause facioscapulohumeral muscular dystrophy. J Med Genet 1996;33:366–370.

13. Lunt PW, Jardine PE, Koch MC, et al: Correlation between fragment size at D4F104S1 and age of onset or at wheelchair use, with a possible generational effect, accounts for much phenotypic variation in 4q35-facioscapulohumeral muscular dystrophy (FSHD). Hum Mol Genet 1995;4:951–958.

14. Lemmers RJLF, van der Maarel S, van Deutekom JCT, et al: Inter- and intrachromosomal subtelomeric rearrangements on 4q35: Implications for facioscapulohumeral muscular dystrophy (FSHD) etiology and diagnosis. Hum Mol Genet 1998;7:1207–1214.

15. Zatz M, Marie SK, Cerquiera A, et al: The facioscapulohumeral muscular dystrophy gene affects males more severely and more frequently than females. Am J Med Genet 1998;77:155–161.

16. Tupler R, Perini G, Pellegrino MA, Green MR: Profound misregulation of muscle-specific gene expression in facioscapulohumeral muscular dystrophy. PNAS 1999;96:12650–12654.

17. Gabellini D, Green MR, Tupler R: Inappropriate gene activation in FSHD: A repressor complex binds chromosomal repeat deleted in dystrophic muscle. Cell 2002;110:339–348.

18. Kaukonen J, Juselius JK, Tiranti V, et al: Role of adenine nucleotide translocator 1 in mtDNA maintenance. Science 2000;289:782–785.

19. Bakker E, Wijmenga C, Vossen RH, et al: The FSHD-linked locus D4F104S1 (p13E-11) on 4q35 has a homologue on 10qter. Muscle Nerve 1995;2:S39–S44.

20. Deidda G, Cacurri S, Piazzo N, et al: Direct detection of 4q35 rearrangements implicated in facioscapulohumeral muscular dystrophy (FSHD). J Med Genet 1996;33:361–365.

21. Orrell RW, Tawil R, Forrester J, et al: Definitive molecular diagnosis of facioscapulohumeral dystrophy. Neurology 1999;52:1822–1826.

22. Van der Maarel SM, Lemmers RJ: A new dosage test for subtelomeric 4;10 translocations improves con-

ventional diagnosis of facioscapulohumeral muscular dystrophy (FSHD). J Med Genet 1999;36:823–828.

23. Vitelli F, Villanova M, Malandrini A, et al: Inheritance of a 38-kb fragment in apparently sporadic facioscapulohumeral muscular dystrophy. Muscle Nerve 1999;22:1437–1441.

24. Bunch WH, Siegel IM: Scapulothoracic arthrodesis in facioscapulohumeral muscular dystrophy: Review of seventeen procedures with three to twenty-one-year follow up. J Bone Joint Surg Am 1993; 75:372–376.

25. Tawil R, McDermott MP, Pandya S, et al: A pilot study of prednisone in facioscapulohumeral muscular dystrophy. Neurology 1997;48:46–49.

26. Kissel JT, McDermott MP, Mendell JR, et al: Randomized, double-blind, placebo-controlled trial of albuterol in facioscapulohumeral muscular dystrophy. Neurology 2001;57:1434–1440.

27. Walter MC, Lochmuller H, Reilich P, et al: Creatine monohydrate in muscular dystrophies: A double-blind placebo-controlled clinical study. Neurology 2000;54:1848–1850.

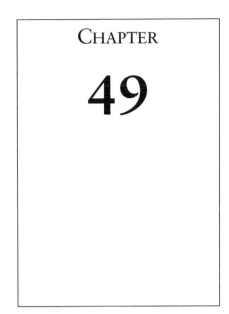

CHAPTER 49

Ion Channel Disorders

Kleopas A. Kleopa
Robert L. Barchi

Ion channels are complex proteins that span the lipid bilayer of the cell membrane where they orchestrate the electrical signals necessary for normal function of the central nervous system, peripheral nerves, and both skeletal and cardiac muscle. The role of ion channel defects in the pathogenesis of numerous disorders has become increasingly apparent over the last decade. Progress in molecular biology has allowed cloning and expression of genes that encode channel proteins, whereas comparable advances in biophysics, including patch-clamp electrophysiology and related techniques, have made the study of expressed proteins at the level of single channel molecules possible.

During normal muscle contraction, electrical signals spread from the motor nerve at the neuromuscular junction over the surface of each muscle fiber and into the T-tubular system before the contractile elements can be activated following calcium-induced calcium release from the sarcoplasmic reticulum (SR). In this setting, abnormal ion channel activity may translate into either high or low levels of excitability in the muscle membrane. Muscle membrane hyperexcitability can lead to repetitive action potentials and inappropriately sustained muscle contraction following brief physiologic stimuli. Clinically, this is expressed as myotonia, the persistent contraction of skeletal muscle in response to a brief voluntary activation. In the electrodiagnostic laboratory, this appears as sustained trains of muscle action potentials, the myotonic discharge. Inappropriate release of calcium from the SR into the myoplasm can cause prolonged muscle contraction with potentially serious manifestations of hypermetabolism and hyperthermia. Conversely, abnormally low levels of muscle membrane excitability will produce failure of contraction, leading to weakness or paralysis. Neuromuscular syndromes caused by defects in ion channels are usually characterized by one or the other of these clinical features.

All ion channel diseases discussed here have been recognized for more than a century on the basis of their distinctive clinical presentation. Knowledge of the major clinical phenotypes that fall into this area, as well as the physiologic principles that govern skeletal muscle function, is essential for the understanding of the molecular mechanisms that underlie ion channel disorders.

CLINICAL MANIFESTATIONS OF ION CHANNEL DISORDERS

Myotonia Congenita

In both dominant (Thomsen) and recessive (Becker) myotonia congenita, the predominant symptom is muscle stiffness due to persistent bursts of spontaneous action potentials arising at the level of individual muscle fibers. The myotonia is most severe during initial voluntary muscle activity after a period of rest and can be worsened by stress and fatigue. Repeated muscle contraction results in progressive diminution of the myotonic stiffness, the so-called warm-up phenomenon.

The autosomal dominant form of myotonia congenita was originally described in 1876 by Dr. Thomsen, a physician who noticed the associated symptoms in four generations of his own family. The disease typically appears in infancy or early childhood and remains mild throughout life, without progression to muscle weakness. Milder cases may remain undiagnosed until late childhood and penetrance may be variable. The myotonia is generalized, although the legs are usually most affected, causing frequent falls in children. Muscle hypertrophy is

527

common, especially in the lower extremities, and often gives these patients an athletic appearance. Muscle strength and tendon reflexes are normal.[1,2]

In the autosomal recessive form of myotonia congenita, onset is usually later, in the first or second decade of life. Men appear to be more frequently affected than women; however, family studies have shown that women are affected at the same frequency, although less severely. Recessive myotonia congenita is much more common than the dominant form, with an estimated prevalence between 1 in 23,000 and 1 in 50,000. The clinical presentation resembles that of the dominant form, although the myotonia tends to be more severe and causes more disability in recessive myotonia congenita. Moreover, patients with recessive myotonia occasionally develop permanent weakness later in life. As in the dominant form, baseline muscle strength and stretch reflexes are usually normal, and hypertrophy of leg and gluteal muscles can be seen. In recessive myotonia congenita, however, shoulder and arm muscles are often less well developed.[1,2]

Serum creatine kinase (CK) levels are normal or mildly elevated in myotonia congenita. Electromyography (EMG) shows typical myotonic discharges triggered by needle insertion or percussion. They may also be found in asymptomatic family members, especially male carriers. These repeated spikes, which wax and wane in amplitude (10 µV to 1 mV) and frequency (50 to 150 Hz), represent recurrent single muscle fiber potentials and can take two forms: either a run of positive sharp waves, or a train of negative spikes resembling fibrillations. Histologic evaluation of the muscle shows nonspecific changes, usually limited to increased variability in fiber size, increased numbers of internalized nuclei, and absent type IIB fibers.[1]

Potassium-Aggravated Myotonia

Certain clinical phenotypes that resemble myotonia congenita have been described with different names in the literature, including myotonia fluctuans, myotonia permanens, and acetazolamide-responsive myotonia. The common feature in all these variants of myotonia is a tendency for symptoms to be worsened by potassium. Therefore, they have been grouped under the name potassium-aggravated myotonia.[2,3] This disorder is characterized by childhood-onset with typical myotonia, in which "warming up" relieves symptoms. In some families, the myotonia may be aggravated by cold, but this is not a constant feature. Muscle stiffness may also be provoked by exercise, and often occurs during rest after heavy exercise. There is no associated weakness or episodic paralysis. Involvement of the extraocular muscles, in addition to the trunk and limbs, is characteristic. The myotonia may fluctuate on a day-to-day basis or be constant, often associated with hypertrophy of neck and shoulder muscles. Occasionally aggravation of the myotonia by intake of

potassium-rich food causes hypoventilation due to stiffness of thoracic muscles, especially in children. Patients with acetazolamide-responsive myotonia have muscle stiffness that may persist even in a warm environment, as well as exercise-induced muscle pain. Both stiffness and pain are alleviated by acetazolamide. Other clinical variants of potassium-aggravated myotonia, including a particularly painful form of myotonia and a milder phenotype presenting with familial cramps, have been reported.[1,2,3]

Paramyotonia Congenita

Paramyotonia congenita was first described by Eulenburg in 1886 and is characterized by paradoxical myotonia that appears after the onset of muscle activity and worsens with repetitive exercise, in contrast to the "warm-up" phenomenon seen with myotonia congenita. The symptoms of paramyotonia begin at birth or in early childhood and usually do not improve with age.[1,3] Paramyotonia congenita is transmitted as a dominant trait with complete penetrance. When exposed to cold, patients with this disorder develop muscle stiffness, which has a predilection for the face, tongue, eyelid, neck and distal upper extremity muscles. The legs are generally less affected, and there is usually no muscle pain, atrophy, or hypertrophy. Weakness may occur after prolonged exercise and exposure to cold. Episodic attacks of flaccid paralysis are common and may be induced by oral potassium intake. The attacks may be accompanied by myotonia, resembling hyperkalemic periodic paralysis. In various members of the same family, intermittent paralysis may occur without myotonia, or vice versa. Similar to myotonia congenita, the EMG in patients with paramyotonia can show myotonic discharges, even at normal temperature. Serum CK is often mildly elevated.

The Inherited Periodic Paralyses

The inherited periodic paralyses are rare disorders of skeletal muscle that present with recurrent episodes of muscle weakness. The weakness is often generalized, but the arms or legs may be preferentially affected in a particular attack. They are transmitted as an autosomal dominant trait, with onset in the first or second decade. Clinical variants have been distinguished according to the precipitating factors, serum potassium levels during the attack, frequency and duration of the attacks, and associated myotonia.

Hyperkalemic Periodic Paralysis

Hyperkalemic periodic paralysis (HyperPP) is characterized by frequent attacks of weakness that may occur one or more times daily and usually last only 20 minutes to an hour. Paralysis may occur at any time during the day, especially after a period of rest following prior exercise, cold exposure, or fasting. Potassium intake often provokes an attack, and potassium loading has been used for diagnostic confirmation. Many patients with HyperPP have either clinical or electrophysiologic manifestations of myotonia between paralytic episodes. When present, clinical myotonia is usually very mild and causes stiffness only of the hands and face. Similar to paramyotonia, paradoxical myotonia of the eyelids also occurs in HyperPP. Sometimes patients experience paresthesias or a sensation of muscle tension before the attack.[1] HyperPP shows complete penetrance affecting both sexes equally and the first attack usually occurs in infancy or early childhood.

Serum potassium level is often elevated up to 5 to 6 mEq/L during paralysis, but may remain within the upper normal range, or may even transiently fall at the end of the episode. Water diuresis, elevation of muscle enzymes, and myalgias often accompany the HyperPP attack. EMG between episodes of HyperPP may be normal, but occasionally shows typical myotonic discharges with increased insertional activity. During the onset of paralysis, muscle irritability and myotonia may increase, which may explain the sensation of muscle tension. However, when paralyzed, the muscle remains unexcitable to electrical stimulation. The frequency of paralytic attacks tends to decline in the second half of life, but some patients may develop a progressive myopathy with permanent proximal weakness.

Hypokalemic Periodic Paralysis

Hypokalemic periodic paralysis (HypoPP) is the most common of the inherited periodic paralyses, with an estimated prevalence of 1 in 100,000. Onset of the autosomal dominant inherited HypoPP is usually in adolescence, although in severe cases patients may present in early childhood. Penetrance is complete in men but variable in women, resulting in higher prevalence in men. An acquired form of the disease may occur in the setting of hyperthyroidism, typically in individuals of Asian descent. The frequency of paralytic episodes varies widely, from once daily to once or twice in a lifetime, and each episode may last hours to days. The episodes appear usually in the early morning after a preceding day of vigorous exercise, or a carbohydrate-rich or salty meal the previous evening. Stress can also provoke or worsen the attacks, whereas light physical activity can sometimes prevent or delay them. Serum potassium decreases during the attacks, but not always below the normal range. Proximal lower extremity weakness may progress to involve all four limbs and the trunk. As in HyperPP, bulbar, respiratory, and cardiac muscles are typically spared.[1]

Although the HypoPP attacks tend to remit after the fourth decade, the proximal weakness often becomes permanent later in life, affecting mainly pelvic girdle and lower extremity muscles. The development of a progressive vacuolar myopathy cannot be predicted from either the severity or the frequency of the paralytic episodes. Similar to HyperPP, serum CK is usually normal or slightly increased between the attacks, but may increase transiently after a major attack. However, in contrast to HyperPP, the electromyogram (EMG) in HypoPP does not show myotonia between the attacks. In cases where a vacuolar myopathy and chronic weakness have developed, a myopathic pattern may be seen. During the paralytic episodes, there is decreased muscle excitability with lack of insertional activity.

Malignant Hyperthermia

Malignant hyperthermia (MH) is an anesthetic-induced syndrome that results in a hypermetabolic state. The disease was first recognized over a century ago and the name was coined because of the rapid rise in temperature and the high mortality in untreated patients during anesthesia. Following reports of anesthetic deaths in families it became clear that MH susceptibility is inherited as an autosomal dominant trait. The association between inherited muscle diseases and increased risk of MH has also been recognized.[4] The incidence of serious MH events is estimated at around 1:50,000 to 100,000, but it may be as high as 1:15,000 in the pediatric age group. MH crises develop most commonly between 3 and 30 years of age, with slightly higher incidence among males. Patients who eventually develop MH often had prior uneventful anesthetic events. Additional environmental factors besides exposure to anesthesia may therefore play a role in the development of MH in a susceptible individual.

MH attacks are typically precipitated by potent inhalational anesthetics including all halogenated ethers and halothane, and by depolarizing muscle relaxants, most commonly succinylcholine. Rising end-tidal pCO_2 is an early sign of hypermetabolism. Muscle rigidity, tachycardia, cyanosis, and hypoxemia occur during or immediately after anesthesia. Hyperthermia is usually present, but in some cases it may be only mild or a late sign. Moreover, MH is often recognized and treated before the temperature elevation occurs. Further complications include lactic acidosis, cardiovascular instability, and cellular damage causing elevation of serum potassium and calcium. Myofibrillar damage may lead to myoglobinuria. If untreated, MH can cause death due to ventricular fibrillation, pulmonary edema, coagulopathy, renal failure, or anoxic brain injury.[4]

Atypical clinical presentations of MH have been recognized, including less severe reactions such as localized masseter spasm or low-grade fever. Such mild reactions may be more common than serious events. Masseter spasm after anesthetic exposure appears to be most common in children, and about 50% of these patients exhibit a positive contracture test suggesting true MH susceptibility.[4] Occasionally, the first indication of MH may be cardiac arrest or arrhythmia precipitated by hyperkalemia, and sometimes evolution is fulminant with rapid death. MH events can also occur without exposure to anesthetics. There are reports of MH after viral infections, exertion, or neuroleptics. Heat stroke, chronically elevated CK, myalgias, and sudden infant death syndrome have been associated with MH susceptibility based on positive contracture tests and family history of MH. MH-susceptible individuals may present with nonspecific musculoskeletal anomalies such as kyphoscoliosis, pectus deformities, dislocated patella, crowed teeth, cryptorchidism, hernias, and cramps.

Several musculoskeletal disorders have been associated with increased risk for MH, most frequently King-Denborough syndrome and central core disease (CCD). CCD is a congenital nonprogressive myopathy with central cores in the biopsy, and patients present in infancy with hypotonia, proximal weakness, and musculoskeletal abnormalities. King-Denborough syndrome is characterized by autosomal dominant inheritance, nonspecific myopathy, dysmorphic features such as short stature, micrognathia, scoliosis, low-set ears, cryptorchidism, and skeletal abnormalities. Increased risk of MH and MH-like anesthetic events has also been recognized among patients with dystrophinopathies, myotonia congenita, myotonic dystrophy, and congenital muscular dystrophy, as well as non-neuromuscular disorders such as osteogenesis imperfecta and myelomeningocele.[4]

Neuromyotonia and Myokymia

In contrast to all disorders described earlier, which arise at the level of the muscle fiber, neuromyotonia and myokymia originate in the peripheral nerve. In contrast to myotonic discharges, the repetitive muscle activity in neuromyotonia can often be abolished by nerve block and always by neuromuscular blocking agents. Neuromyotonia is usually a sporadic disorder characterized by fasciculations, exercise-induced myokymia, and muscle cramps, with onset ranging from childhood to adult life. The characteristic stiffness is initially brought on by exercise, but later may occur at rest or even during sleep. Excessive sweating and laryngeal spasms have also been described. Rare familial cases have been reported often with an associated peripheral neuropathy.[5] Some patients with acquired neuromyotonia may develop autonomic, sensory, or even central nervous system manifestations. The latter is also called Morvan fibrillary chorea and is characterized by confusion, anxiety, agitation, delirium, and insomnia. Muscle hypertrophy can be seen with both generalized myokymia and neuromyotonia, usually involving the calves bilaterally, and sometimes the proximal arm and thigh. Unless the neuromyotonia is secondary to another neuromuscular disorder, there is no associated weakness.

Clinical myokymia is characterized by spontaneous, brief, but repetitive contractions that involve narrow muscle bands and last for several seconds, causing a continuous quivering of muscle fibers visible through the skin as a vermiform movement. Myokymia can be either focal or generalized and is usually sporadic, secondary to motor neuron or peripheral nerve injury, although in some cases no obvious cause can be found, as in the myokymia-cramp syndrome. Rarely, myokymia is inherited, as in episodic ataxia type-1/myokymia syndrome or other related phenotypes.[6,7,8]

EMG in neuromyotonia is characterized by bursts of prolonged, irregular single motor unit potentials reaching a frequency of 40 to 400 Hz, with decremental amplitude. Electrical myokymia consists of spontaneous grouped motor unit potentials that recur regularly, with a short period (a few seconds) of firing at a uniform rate (2 to 20 Hz), followed by a short period of silence. Clinical neuromyotonia may be associated with both myokymic and neuromyotonic discharges in EMG, whereas clinical myokymia is usually associated with myokymic discharges only.[2]

Episodic ataxia type 1 (EA1) is an autosomal dominant inherited paroxysmal central nervous system disorder characterized by brief attacks of cerebellar ataxia and continuous interictal myokymia of peripheral nerve origin.[6] Sudden episodes of ataxia last from seconds to minutes and are usually precipitated by movement, startle, or emotion. The myokymia may be detectable only by EMG. When clinically evident, patients usually present with fine rippling in perioral or periorbital musculature, and lateral finger movements when the hands are held in a relaxed, prone position. Variations of this phenotype, including isolated neuromyotonia without episodic ataxia and myokymia with epilepsy as the only central manifestation, have been reported.[7] Increased incidence of epilepsy has also been recognized among families with the typical EA-1/myokymia syndrome.

Long QT Syndrome and Idiopathic Ventricular Fibrillation

Long QT syndrome is a disorder of cardiac muscle characterized by delayed repolarization leading to a prolonged QT interval on the surface electrocardiogram. Clinical manifestations include ventricular arrhythmias, syncope, and sudden death, usually in young, otherwise healthy individuals.[9] Syncope and sudden death often occur during exercise or emotion, although an important minority of attacks occurs during sleep. The associated ventricular tachyarrhythmia, torsades de pointes, is usually self-terminating, causing a syncopal episode from which the patient recovers quickly, but may rarely be persistent and fatal if immediate cardioversion is not available. Sudden death may be the first manifestation of the disease, a fact supporting the recommendation that asymptomatic patients should be treated prophylactically. Long QT syndrome is estimated to affect 1 in 7000 persons and may cause as many as 3000 unexpected deaths in children and young adults every year. The transmission of the inherited form is autosomal dominant with variable penetrance, although in a rare form of the disease associated with severe congenital hearing loss the deafness is transmitted as a recessive trait. Acquired long QT syndrome is more common than the inherited form and is often caused by the administration of drugs that block cardiac ion channels.

MOLECULAR ARCHITECTURE AND PHYSIOLOGY OF VOLTAGE-GATED ION CHANNELS

Voltage-gated ion channels control membrane excitability in peripheral nerve and both skeletal and cardiac muscle by modulating conductance to ions that are actively maintained in concentration gradients across the cell surface. Typically, K^+ ions are at higher concentration in the cytoplasm than in extracellular fluid, whereas Na^+, Cl^-, and Ca^{2+} ions exhibit the opposite distribution. The resting membrane potential (RMP) results from asymmetrical distribution of these ions across the cell membrane combined with unequal permeability of the membrane to the various ionic species. The usual range of RMP in muscle cells is −60 to −90 mV, with the intracellular compartment at a more negative potential than the extracellular space. Although all permeant ions contribute to the resting membrane potential, K^+ is the most permeant cation. The RMP is therefore closer to the equilibrium potential for potassium and is most sensitive to changes in the transmembrane concentration gradient for this ion.

Muscle and nerve cells are characterized by the ability to generate and propagate brief regenerative action potentials along their surface membranes. During an action potential, the membrane potential rapidly shifts from the negative resting potential through zero to a positive internal potential of +20 to +30 mV before returning to the normal resting level. Although the membrane potential can be altered through modification of either ion concentration gradient, or conductance, the action potential is mainly the result of changes in relative conductance of the membrane to Na^+ and K^+. Because the membrane equilibrium potential is typically +20 to +30 mV, opening of Na^+ channels and increasing the membrane conductance for this ion relative to K^+ causes depolarization. The action potential is terminated by the inactivation of Na^+ channels and subsequent opening of K^+ channels, allowing return to the resting relation between cation conductances. The actual net movement of these two cations that occurs during a single action potential is small and has a negligible effect on the concentration gradient of either ion across the membrane.

Ion channels provide permeation pathways that are highly specific for a particular ion species. For most channels, however, these pathways are not always available for ion movement; they are "gated" by transitions between conducting (open) and nonconducting (closed) conformations. Although the single channel conductance, the ease of current flow for a particular ion through an open channel, is usually a fixed property of a particular channel protein, gating between open and closed states may be modulated by voltage changes across the membrane. Other classes of channels are gated by interaction with a specific ligand. Extracellular ligands, second messengers and metabolites, protein-protein interactions, phosphorylation, and other factors can all influence the channel gating.[10]

The first complete account of the voltage-dependent ionic mechanisms that underlie the action potential was provided by Hodgkin and Huxley, who developed the voltage clamp technique in the squid giant axon preparation. Their early view of Na^+ and K^+ channels as continuously modulated conductance pathways that open and close in a smooth, graded fashion in response to triggering stimuli was based on recordings from large areas of the membrane surface containing thousands of channel molecules. With the introduction of the patch-clamp technique, tiny regions of membrane that may contain only a few channels could be isolated, permitting the analysis of currents through single ion channels. Using this method, it became apparent that single channels open in an all-or-none fashion, to an activated state with a characteristic single channel conductance. After remaining open for a brief period, individual channels close abruptly, usually to a discrete inactivated state. The continuously increasing and decreasing currents seen with macroscopic voltage clamp techniques actually represent the statistical summation over time of stochastic events occurring at the single channel level.

Sodium Channels

In both nerve and muscle, Na^+ ions are maintained in a concentration gradient across the surface membrane that is far from equilibrium by the action of the Na^+-K^+-ATPase. At normal resting potentials, voltage-gated Na^+ channels are closed but are available for activation. When the muscle membrane is depolarized slightly, Na^+ channels open, producing a rapid increase in Na^+ conductance and further membrane depolarization. This change in conductance is responsible for the rapid rising phase of the membrane action potential. Normally, Na^+ channel opening is brief (1 to 2 ms) and is terminated by a fast inactivation process. This consists of conformational changes involving the D3-4 intracellular loop of the α-subunit (see later), which moves in to block the cytoplasmic opening of the channel pore.[11] A slow inactivation mode, which develops over seconds to minutes, has also been recognized, although less is known about the underlying molecular mechanism. Slow inactivation is independent from fast inactivation, is more important in skeletal than in cardiac muscle, and is modulated by all four domains of the α-subunit. Inactivated Na^+ channels enter a refractory state and cannot reopen until they are repolarized and the inactivation process is reversed.

Voltage-gated Na⁺ channels were first isolated and characterized biochemically from eel electroplax and subsequently purified from mammalian muscle and brain.[11] These Na⁺ channels contain a large, heavily glycosylated α-subunit that includes all the elements necessary to form the basic channel pore with its voltage-sensitive gates and ion selectivity filter. In the membrane, the α-subunit is associated with one or two smaller β-subunits.

The family of Na⁺ channel α-subunit proteins includes SCN1A to SCN11A, with several isoforms expressed mostly in the brain (SCN1A, SCN2A1 and SCN2A2, SCN3A, and SCN8A), whereas the SCN4A is found at high levels in the skeletal and the SCN5A in the cardiac or denervated skeletal muscle. In the peripheral nerve, initial segments and nodes of Ranvier contain SCN2A1 during development and mostly SCN6A thereafter, forming the $Na_v1.6$ Na⁺ channels (Fig. 49–1). Novel Na⁺ channel genes may be specifically expressed in individual classes of neurons with specialized functions.

The skeletal muscle Na⁺ channel α-subunit (SCN4A) is a heavily glycosylated protein of ~260 kDa. Within the ~2000 amino acid residues of the primary sequence are four internally homologous repeat domains, each encompassing about 300 amino acids and containing six predicted transmembrane segments, designated S1 through S6 (Fig. 49–2A). In the fourth transmembrane helix of each domain (S4), a positively charged lysine or arginine is found at every third position, separated by two nonpolar residues. These charged helices comprise a

major part of the voltage-sensing mechanism of the channel protein. In the tertiary structure of the protein, the four repeat domains are organized symmetrically around a central aqueous pore, each contributing key elements to the pore. The peptide segment linking S5 and S6 (H5 or P loop) in each domain folds into the membrane from the external surface and forms a portion of the ion channel pore lining, influencing both ion selectivity and conductance. Mutations in this region alter the permeation properties of the channel. The amino and carboxy termini, as well as the peptide segments linking the repeat domains, lie on the cytoplasmic surface of the membrane. This basic structural organization of the Na⁺ channel protein is also found in Ca²⁺ and K⁺ channels (see Fig. 49–2B and C).

The gene encoding the human skeletal muscle isoform (hSkm1) of the Na⁺ channel α-subunit (*SCN4A*) is located on chromosome 17 at q23.1-25.2. The *SCN4A* gene contains 24 exons, distributed over approximately 30 kb. *SCN4A* is expressed only in skeletal muscle, and its product, the tetrodotoxin-sensitive hSkm1, is the only Na⁺ channel detectable in innervated adult muscle tissue.[12]

The β-subunits in nerve and muscle share a common basic structure, encompassing a large, glycosylated extracellular region, a single transmembrane segment, and a small intracellular domain.[11] The interaction between β-subunits and the pore-forming α-subunit is of functional importance, modulating channel gating.

Calcium Channels

Voltage-gated Ca²⁺ channels regulate a number of biological functions, including the generation of action

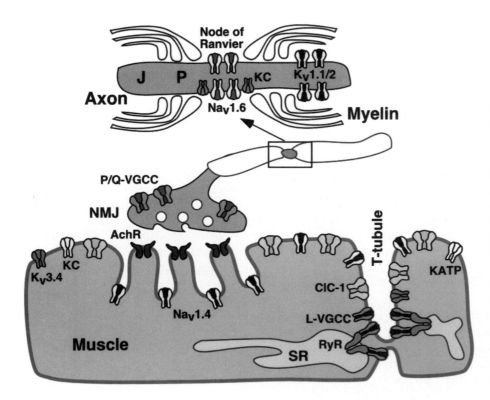

FIGURE 49-1. Diagram of peripheral nerve and skeletal muscle showing the localization of ion channels discussed in this chapter. AchR, acetylcholine receptor; ClC-1, skeletal muscle chloride channel; J, juxtaparanode; KATP, ATP-sensitive potassium channels; KC, other potassium channels; K_v, voltage-gated potassium channels; Na_v, voltage-gated sodium channels; NMJ, neuromuscular junction; P, paranode; RyR, ryanodine receptor; SR, sarcoplasmic reticulum. VGCC, voltage-gated calcium channels. (Reproduced with permission from: Kleopa KA, Barchi RL: Genetic disorders of neuromuscular ion channels. Muscle Nerve 2002;26:299–325.)

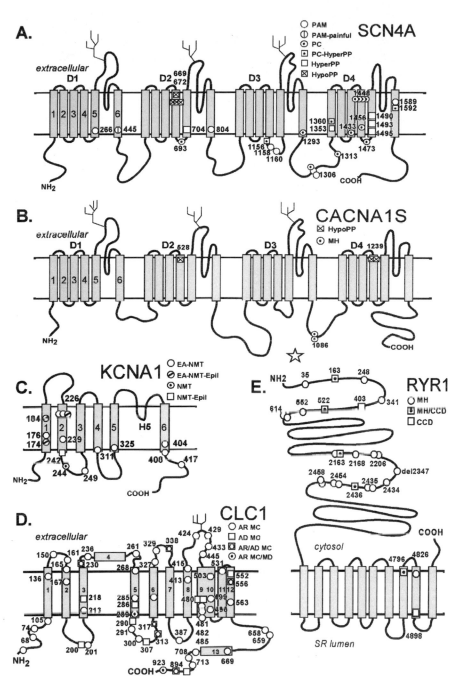

FIGURE 49–2. Mutations in ion channels causing neuromuscular disorders: *A,* Skeletal muscle sodium channel α-subunit (SCN4A) mutations associated with potassium-aggravated myotonia (PAM), paramyotonia congenita (PC), hyperkalemic periodic paralysis (HyperPP), or hypokalemic periodic paralysis (HypoPP). Many mutations are located in domains 3 and 4, and in the intracellular loop connecting them. *B,* Mutations in the L-type skeletal muscle calcium channel α-subunit (CACNA1S) causing HypoPP and malignant hyperthermia (MH). Note the homology between the S4/D2 R528H mutation with both the S4/D4 R1239H/G mutation within the same molecule and with the S4/D2 R672H/G/S mutations in SCN4A. The MH mutations are located in the D3-D4 intracellular loop, which interacts directly or indirectly with the ryanodine receptor *(star).* *C,* Mutations in the Kv1.1 potassium channel α-subunit (KCNA1) associated with episodic ataxia (EA-1), neuromyotonia (NMT), or epilepsy (Epil). *D,* Approximate location of mutations reported in the skeletal muscle chloride channel (ClC-1) associated with either dominant (AD MC) or recessive (AR MC) myotonia congenita, or both. *E,* Mutations in the ryanodine receptor/Ca^{2+}-release channel (RYR1) associated with MH or central core disease (CCD), or both. Note the clustering of mutations in three regions of the protein (MH/CCD regions 1 to 3).

potentials in dendrites, initiation of neurotransmitter release, and a variety of intracellular regulatory processes. Ca^{2+} channel subtypes differ in their voltage dependence, inactivation rate, ionic selectivity, and pharmacology. Specific subtypes, designated L, N, P/Q, R, or T, were initially defined by the kinetics and voltage dependence of inactivation, but have now been cloned and associated with specific genes.[13]

Each Ca^{2+} channel is composed of five subunits (α1, α2/δ, β, and γ). The large α1-subunit, which is homologous in structure to the Na$^+$ channel α-subunit, contains the voltage sensing and ion selectivity elements and forms the channel pore (see Fig. 49–2B). The α1-subunit of the

L-type channel also contains a characteristic receptor for dihydropyridine. The diversity of genes encoding α1-subunits produces Ca^{2+} channels with different properties and cell-specific expression. The L-type Ca^{2+} channel is prominently expressed in skeletal muscle, where the channel protein is concentrated at the transverse tubular-sarcoplasmic reticulum (SR) junction known as the triad (see Fig. 49–1). During the process of excitation-contraction coupling, the conformational change associated with voltage-dependent activation of this Ca^{2+} channel is transmitted through direct protein to protein interaction with the underlying Ca^{2+} release channel of the SR, also known as the ryanodine receptor. This interaction is mediated by the intracellular loop between domains two and three of the Ca^{2+} channel α1-subunit. Using intragenic microsatellite as a marker, the *CACNA1S* gene has been mapped to 1q31-q32. The gene spans 90 kb and consists of 44 exons.[1,13]

The four accessory subunits, α2/δ, β, and γ are usually associated with the pore-forming α1-subunit in a 1:1 to 1:1 ratio. The skeletal muscle L-type Ca^{2+} channel α1-subunit (CACNA1S, previously known as CACNL1A3) has a molecular weight of 190 kDa and consists of an 1873 amino acid chain. The auxiliary cytoplasmic β-subunit (55 kDa) and the transmembrane α2/δ-subunits (170 kDa), which are linked by a disulfide bridge, as well as an additional transmembrane γ1-subunit with a size of 33 kDa, modulate channel activity.

The predominant Ca^{2+} channel present in the SR of skeletal muscle is not related to the voltage-dependent Ca^{2+} channel family. The skeletal muscle Ca^{2+} release channel or ryanodine receptor is a transmembrane protein of ~560 kDa and 5038 amino acids, which forms a tetrameric structure. Although the tetramer spans the SR membrane, large regions of each subunit bridge the gap between the SR and the T-tubular system (see Fig. 49-1). At this location it allows excitation-contraction coupling through the interaction with the voltage dependent L-type calcium channel. Activation of this L-type channel by the T-tubular depolarization initiates conformational changes that induce the opening of the ryanodine receptor channel through direct protein to protein interactions, allowing the release of Ca^{2+} from the lumen of the SR into the sarcoplasm. The ryanodine receptor is also closely associated with other proteins within the SR, including the F-506 binding protein, calmodulin, triadin, and calsequestrin. The C-terminus makes up 20% of the molecule and forms the transmembrane Ca^{2+}-release channel, whereas the N-terminal domain extends into the cytoplasm and forms a large "foot" region that contains most ligand binding sites (see Fig. 49-2E). The *RYR1* cDNA is 15,117 base pairs long, whereas the actual gene encompasses 158,000 base pairs and contains 106 exons, two of which are alternatively spliced to create different isoforms.[14]

Potassium Channels

Voltage-gated potassium (Kv) channels are the most ubiquitous and diverse group of voltage-dependent ion channels found in the body. They regulate the RMP and modulate the shape and frequency of action potentials. In skeletal muscle, several K^+ channel isoforms are present in the sarcolemmal membrane and the T-tubular system. In contrast to other tissues, only a small part of the muscle fiber resting membrane conductance is attributed to K^+ ions. Because of the restricted diffusion pathway available in the T-tubular system, K^+ efflux during action potentials can transiently elevate the local K^+ concentration in this narrow space, resulting in surface membrane

depolarization. In normal muscle, this depolarizing effect is minimized by the high resting conductance to Cl^- ions (discussed later). In comparison, Kv1.1 and Kv1.2 channels in myelinated nerves are concentrated at the juxtaparanodes under the myelin sheath (see Fig. 49-1). They are mainly responsible for the repolarization of the axolemmal membrane following an action potential, which is generated by the opening of Na^+ channels that are highly concentrated in the nodal axolemma.[15]

Functional Kv channels are formed by homotetramers or heterotetramers of four α-subunits. Each α-subunit is comparable in size and structure to one of the internal repeat domains in a Na^+ or Ca^{2+} channel α-subunit (see Fig. 49-2). When 4 K^+ channel α-subunits form a functional channel in the membrane, the resulting tetramer is structurally homologous to a single Na^+ or Ca^{2+} channel α-subunit. The tetramer of K^+ channel α-subunits is often associated with an auxiliary β-subunit, which can modify the gating properties of the heteromultimeric channel complex. This leads to a high degree of diversity in the neuronal K^+ channel population, depending on the subtypes of α- and β-subunits expressed in different tissues and cell types. Heteromeric K^+ channels of different subunit stoichiometry may be localized to different subcellular compartments, presumably because their channel properties are better suited for the physiologic requirements of those locations. Kv channels are subdivided into Kv1 to 4, of which the Kv1 (or "Shaker") class includes at least 10 different subtypes, according to their α-subunits, designated KCNA1 to 10.[16] They are found in the peripheral nerves and brain (KCNA1, 5 and 6), as well as in the cardiac muscle (KCNQ1 or KCNA8). Most of these channels have delayed rectifier properties, determined by their kinetics of activation and inactivation. The Kv3 subclass includes Kv3.4, another delayed rectifier K^+ channel, which is involved in the regulation of the RMP in skeletal muscle.[17]

The *KCNA1* gene product, a well-studied prototype of Kv α-subunits, is a glycoprotein of about 55 kDa, containing 495 amino acids, and 6 transmembrane segments at positions structurally homologous to the S1-S6 helices in one repeat domain of a Na^+ or a Ca^{2+} channel α-subunit (see Fig. 49-2). As with Na^+ and Ca^{2+} channels, the S4 segment of each KCNA1 monomer serves as the voltage sensor, containing positively charged amino acids at every third position.[16] In K^+ channels, however, the voltage-dependent inactivation process involves conformational changes in the amino terminus of any one of the four subunits, which then moves in to occlude the centrally located permeation pathway at the cytoplasmic mouth of the channel pore, blocking ion movement.

Chloride Channels

Chloride channels (ClC) are found in a variety of cell types from the epithelium to neurons, where they perform important roles in regulation of cellular excitability, transepithelial transport, cell volume regulation, and acidification of intracellular organelles. The ClC family of chloride channels has nine known members in mammals that show a differential tissue distribution and function, designated ClC-0 to ClC-7, ClC-Ka and ClC-Kb.[18]

In mammalian muscle, Cl⁻ conductance accounts for about 70% of the resting muscle membrane permeability, whereas most of the remaining resting conductance is attributed to K⁺ ions. Chloride ions are asymmetrically distributed across the muscle fiber membrane, with a predicted equilibrium potential close to the resting potential. This large conductance to Cl⁻ ions serves to stabilize the surface membrane potential during the fluctuations in T-tubular potassium concentration that occur with normal muscle activity (see earlier). Chloride channels are normally inactivated by hyperpolarization. They are open at the resting potential and close on a time scale of tens of milliseconds after voltage shifts in the hyperpolarizing direction, producing inward rectification properties.[18]

The initial biophysical studies of Cl⁻ channels were done in *Torpedo* electroplax, where the presence of two independent conduction pathways (i.e., two pores), was demonstrated for each functional channel unit. The first chloride channel cloned (ClC-0) was obtained from this species. The homologous chloride channel subunit of mammalian skeletal muscle cells (ClC 1) is a protein of 988 amino acids with a predicted molecular weight of 110 kDa. Initially, 13 potential transmembrane domains (D1–D13) were suspected on the basis of sequence analysis, but studies showed that the putative D4 and D13 helices do not span the cell membrane (see Fig. 49 2D). ClC-1 is expressed almost exclusively in skeletal muscle and is activated by depolarization. The human *CLCN1* gene is located on chromosome 7q35 and contains a coding sequence organized into 23 exons, spanning at least 40 kb.[18,19]

Analogous to the torpedo chloride channel, ClC-1 is also predicted to be a homodimer with an unusual "double-barrel" structure, in which each subunit contains a separate pore with identical conductance levels and a common gate that acts on both pores.[20] Strong evidence for dual independent pores in the chloride channels has been obtained from two-dimensional crystallographic images of a prokaryotic ClC channel protein. These images have clearly shown a dimeric structure and the presence of two pores in the dimeric channel that are far enough apart to be electrostatically independent.[21]

MOLECULAR PATHOLOGY OF ION CHANNEL DISORDERS

Sodium Channel Defects in Paramyotonia Congenita, Potassium-Aggravated Myotonia, and Periodic Paralysis

Mutations in the skeletal muscle voltage-gated Na⁺ channel gene can produce the clinical phenotypes of hyperkalemic periodic paralysis (HyperPP), paramyotonia congenita, and potassium-aggravated myotonia (Table 49–1; see also Fig. 49–2A).[2,22] The common pathophysiologic feature of the muscle Na⁺ channelopathies is the depolarization of the muscle membrane during an attack. In muscle from patients with HyperPP and paramyotonia congenita, the presence of a noninactivating Na⁺ current was demonstrated experimentally before the identification of specific channel mutations. This abnormal Na⁺ conductance could be blocked by tetrodotoxin, a ligand that is highly specific for the voltage-gated Na⁺ channel. A small noninactivating Na⁺ current was subsequently demonstrated in voltage-clamped single muscle fibers from patients with HyperPP.

Using the candidate locus approach, a number of laboratories demonstrated linkage of HyperPP to the skeletal muscle Na⁺ channel α-subunit gene (*SCN4A*). Subsequently, using exon-flanking sequences for PCR screening of the *SCN4A* coding region, point mutations were identified that cosegregated with the HyperPP or paramyotonia congenita phenotype. Mutations in *SCN4A* gene have also been demonstrated in families with PAM, where myotonia is potassium sensitive, may be painful, or have other unusual features. All mutations found in the *SCN4A* gene consist of single amino acid substitutions in the primary channel structure. A disproportionate number of these mutations are located in the S4-S5 intracellular loop of the D3 and D4 domains, a region that plays a direct role in channel fast inactivation (see Fig. 49–2A).[1,2]

Expression studies of a number of SCN4A mutations causing paramyotonia, HyperPP, and potassium-aggravated myotonia, using oocytes or mammalian cells in culture, have shown that the mutant channels are able to function but have abnormal inactivation kinetics. With a few exceptions, activation kinetics and ion selectivity are not affected. Mutants causing the paramyotonia congenita phenotype show a marked slowing in the major component of fast inactivation, and the inactivation process appears in some cases to be uncoupled from the voltage-dependent events associated with activation. The V1293I mutant causing paramyotonia without weakness alters both activation and fast inactivation. Furthermore, some mutants also appear to cause slowing of deactivation, the process that reflects the reversible closure of the channel during activation, as opposed to the sustained closure produced by inactivation.

Phenotypes caused by different SCN4A mutations may have variable severity for reasons that are not clear. Comparison of the R1448P and R1448C mutants at the same position that cause a severe and a moderate paramyotonia phenotype, respectively, suggested initially that in addition to defects in fast inactivation, R1448P also slowed deactivation. However, subsequent studies showed that the effect on fast inactivation was greater for R1448P than for R1448C. Quantitative kinetic analysis demonstrated that only 38% of the channels contributing to the Na⁺ current in paramyotonia congenita muscle

Table 49–1. Molecular Genetic Classification of Neuromuscular Channelopathies

Disease*	Ion channel gene, location and gene product	Common mutations
Chloride Channel Disorders		
Myotonia congenita (Thomsen)	CLCN1-7q35 (ClC-1)	G200R, G230E, I290M, R317Q, P480L, R894x
Myotonia congenita (Becker) (recessive)	CLCN1	D136G, F167L, F413C, R496S
Sodium Channel Disorders		
Paramyotonia congenita	SCN4A-17q23-25 ($Na_v1.4$ α subunit)	V1293I, G1306V, T1313M, L1433R, R1448C/H
Potassium-aggravated myotonia	SCN4A	S804F, I1160V, G1306A, G1306E, V1589M
Hyperkalemic periodic paralysis	SCN4A	T704M, M1592V
Hypokalemic periodic paralysis type II	SCN4A	R672H/G/S, R669H
Long QT syndrome-LQT3/IVF	SCN5A-3q21-24 ($Na_v1.5$ α subunit)	Del 1505-1507, R1623Q, R1644H, E1784K
Calcium Channel Disorders		
Hypokalemic periodic paralysis type I	CACNA1S-1q31 (L-type Ca^{2+} channel α subunit)	R528H, R1239H/G
Central core disease (± malignant hyperthermia-1)	RYR1-19q13.1 (ryanodin Ca^{2+}-release channel)	R163C, I403M, Y522S, R2163H
Malignant hyperthermia-1	RYR1	G341R, R614C, V2168M
Malignant hyperthermia-5	CACNA1S	R1086H, R1086C
Potassium Channel Disorders		
Episodic ataxia type 1/myokymia syndrome	KCNA1-12p13 ($K_v1.1$ α subunit)	V174F, F184C, T226R, E325D, V408A
Periodic paralysis (hypo-/hyperkalemic)	KCNE3-11q13-14 (MiRP2-$K_v3.4$ β subunit)	R83H
Andersen syndrome	KCNJ2-17q23 (Kir2.1)	R218W, G300V
BFNC/myokymia syndrome	KCNQ2-20q13.3	R207W
Long QT syndrome-LQT1 (dominant or recessive)	KCNQ1-11p15.5 (I_{ks} α-subunit)	G168R, G314S, A341V
Long QT syndrome-LQT2	HERG-7q35-36 (I_{kx} α-subunit)	A561T/V, T613M, A614V
Long QT syndrome-LQT5 (dominant or recessive)	KCNE1-21q22.1 (I_{ks} β-subunit (MinK)	D76N, W87R
Long QT syndrome-LQT6	KCNE2-21q22.1 (I_{kr} β-subunit (MiRP1)	Q9E, M54T, I57T

*All disorders are autosomal dominant unless noted otherwise.
BFNC, benign familial neonatal convulsions; IVF, idiopathic ventricular fibrillation.
Updated information on new mutations affecting ion channels can be found at different websites, including Online Mendelian Inheritance in Man.
(http://www.ncbi.nlm.nih.gov/Omim/searchomim.html) and the Washington University Neuromuscular Disease Center (http://www.neuro.wustl.edu/neuromuscular).

were of the mutant type, suggesting that variability in the expression of the mutant channel may also contribute to the clinical severity, in addition to the magnitude of the inactivation defect.

Several expression studies have addressed the issue of temperature sensitivity, a clinical hallmark, in mutations that cause paramyotonia congenita. The mutants showed increased persistent sodium current compared with wild-type channels throughout the temperature range studied, suggesting that the sensitivity to cold seen in this disorder is not due to a temperature dependent variation in the impact of the channel mutation on channel kinetics. Cold environment may rather be an independent factor that in conjunction with the genetic defect allows the threshold of channel inactivation failure to be reached and clinical manifestations such as myotonia or paralysis, or both, to occur.

SCN4A mutations causing potassium-aggravated myotonia show similar electrophysiologic changes in channel kinetics as the mutations that cause paramyotonia. The potassium-aggravated myotonia mutations L266V, V445M, S804F, I1160V, G1299E, G1306E, and V1589M cause an increased rate of recovery from inactivation and an increased frequency of late channel openings and open bursts. Slow inactivation is not altered in most mutants analyzed, and is actually enhanced by the V445M mutation causing the painful variant of myotonia.

Slow inactivation is not altered in most mutations that cause paramyotonia or potassium-aggravated myotonia. This is in contrast to the mutations associated with a paralytic or a combined paramyotonia/HyperPP phenotype, such as T704M and M1592V, which impair both fast and slow inactivation.[2] Some HyperPP mutations also cause small shifts in the voltage dependence of channel activation. It has been hypothesized that disruption of slow inactivation leading to stable abnormal depolarization of the RMP may be a common feature of Na+ channel mutations causing periodic paralysis. However, the association of impaired slow inactivation and paralytic phenotype does not hold for all mutations that produce paralysis. Slow inactivation is normal in other HyperPP-associated mutations, such as M1353V, confirming that a defect in this process is not an absolute requirement for the expression of the paralytic phenotype. Moreover, expression studies of some paralysis-associated mutations localized in the D4/S5 segment (F1490L, M1493I, I1495F) demonstrate enhanced slow inactivation without an effect on fast inactivation, which may lead to paralysis by prolonging the channel refractory period. These studies also demonstrate the importance of the D4/S5 segment for the slow inactivation mechanism.

Mutations causing HyperPP and paramyotonia produce intermolecular-dominant negative effects. Unlike the intramolecular-dominant negative effects within a single dimer observed in chloride channel disorders (see later), a small number of Na+ channels containing HyperPP and paramyotonia mutations can produce intermolecular effects on the remaining Na+ channel population through the dependence of normal channel inactivation on the membrane potential. The persistent inward current produced by a subset of slowly inactivating or noninactivating channels results in a slight but long-lasting membrane depolarization. Because of the high sensitivity of normal channels to voltage alterations near the resting potential, even this slight depolarization is sufficient to cause progressive inactivation of normal Na+ channels. There appears to be a fine line between hyperexcitability causing myotonia and hypoexcitability causing paralysis associated even with mutations at the same residue. Electrophysiologic models suggest that mild depolarization (10 to 20 mV) due to impaired channel inactivation will render the membrane hyperexcitable. When the depolarization is slightly greater (20 to 30 mV), both the normal and mutant Na+ channels become inactivated, causing paralysis. Fortunately, the heart muscle uses an Na+ channel isoform produced by a different gene, and the diaphragm, which uses the same gene as skeletal muscle, appears refractory to attacks. Therefore, HyperPP attacks are not life threatening in humans. Patients with recessively inherited Na+ channelopathies have not been described. It is likely that complete loss of function of the muscle Na+ channel is not compatible with life.

Although most cases of hypokalemic periodic paralysis (HypoPP) are associated with mutations in the voltage-dependent Ca^{2+} channel (see later), a family with the typical HypoPP phenotype has been found to harbor the Na+ channel mutation R669H. This arginine substitution in the membrane-spanning D2/S4 segment of the channel alters the outermost positive charge in a critical helix involved in voltage sensing. Functional analysis of the R669H mutation shows enhancement of the Na+ channel slow inactivation, and a 6-fold to 5-fold prolongation of recovery time after depolarization. This genotype is referred to as HypoPP type 2. Subsequently, three further Na+ channel mutations, R672H, R672G, and R672S have been identified in other HypoPP families. These mutations are also localized in the D2/S4 segment, affecting another highly conserved arginine, similar to the R669H. These mutants produced a left shift of the steady-state fast inactivation curve, leading to enhanced inactivation and reduced Na+ currents. Na+ currents are reduced even at potentials where inactivation has been removed, suggesting that decreased expression of the channel protein and low channel density may be contributing to the phenotype.[2] Thus, unlike the mechanism underlying HyperPP, paramyotonia, and potassium-aggravated myotonia, Na+ channel mutations associated with HypoPP result in loss of function.

The Na+ channel α-subunit expressed in adult cardiac muscle (SCN5A) is closely related to, but distinct from, the SCN4A channel isoform found in innervated skeletal muscle. The cardiac SCN5A isoform, however, does appear in immature skeletal muscle, and is potentially expressed in adult skeletal muscle after denervation. Mutations in SCN5A do not affect normal adult skeletal muscle, but have been implicated in a small number of families expressing the long QT syndrome phenotype involving cardiac muscle.[9] Several mutations that have been expressed in vitro show impairment of channel inactivation, similar to their skeletal muscle counterparts. The mutant channels fail to inactivate completely, reopen during prolonged depolarization, and delay myocyte repolarization. Other mutations impair the interaction with the β-subunits that normally modify channel gating. *SCN5A* mutations have been identified in families with another cardiac phenotype, idiopathic ventricular fibrillation, and cause similar alterations in channel kinetics as do the SCN4A mutants associated with paramyotonia or HyperPP.

Calcium Channel Defects in Hypokalemic Periodic Paralysis

In most families with the HypoPP phenotype, expression of the disease is caused by mutations in the gene encoding the α-subunit of the dihydropyridine-sensitive L-type Ca^{2+} channel, designated CACNA1S. The disorder resulting from mutations in this gene is designated HypoPP type 1. Among several unrelated probands, mutations were found in one of two adjacent nucleotides within the same codon, resulting in substitution of a highly conserved arginine in the S4 segment of domain 4 (R1239H/G). A third mutation affects a similarly located arginine in the S4 segment of domain 2 (R528H) (see Fig. 49–2B). At least two thirds of all HypoPP families screened carry the R528H or R1239H mutations.[23]

Although most families with HypoPP harbor a Ca^{2+} channel mutation (HypoPP type 1), about 10% of cases result from Na^+ channel mutations (HypoPP type 2, see earlier).[23] Certain clinical features that may distinguish type 2 families include myalgias following the paralytic attacks, worsening of symptoms with acetazolamide, and the presence of tubular aggregates instead of vacuoles in the muscle biopsy. In 22% of HypoPP index cases, no mutation in either the Ca^{2+} or Na^+ channel gene S4 segment coding regions could be found, indicating that mutations in other regions of CACNA1S or SCN4A or in other genes may cause HypoPP. Another periodic paralysis syndrome sharing clinical features of the congenital myasthenic syndromes has been described in an Australian family and mapped to Xp22.3.

Because of difficulties encountered in the expression of human CACNA1S mutations in vitro, the functional effects of these mutations remain controversial. However, based on analyses of homologous mutations in the rabbit cardiac L-type Ca^{2+} channel, several groups have suggested that a loss-of-function mechanism may predominate in HypoPP-1, as has been shown for SCN4A mutations causing HypoPP-2.

In addition to their loss-of-function effects on the Ca^{2+} channel, HypoPP-1 mutations may alter the function and expression of other channels, especially K^+ channels, perhaps because of alteration of intracellular Ca^{2+} homeostasis. Analysis of HypoPP muscle fibers harboring the R528H mutation show reduced sarcolemmal ATP-sensitive K^+ channel currents that could explain the depolarization and paralysis. Moreover, in the K^+-deficient diet rat model of HypoPP, acetazolamide prevents insulin-induced depolarization and paralysis by stimulating a Ca^{2+}-activated K^+ channel.[24] The discovery of mutations in a K^+ channel β-subunit in patients with either HyperPP or HypoPP-like phenotypes (see later)

also suggests that K^+ channel dysfunction plays a role in the pathophysiology of periodic paralysis.[17]

SR Ca^{2+}-Release Channel Defects in Malignant Hyperthermia and Central Core Disease

More than 50% of all autosomal dominant MH kindreds harbor mutations in RYR1 on chromosome 19q12-13.2, the gene encoding the SR Ca^{2+}-release channel or ryanodine receptor.[4,14] At least 30 different RYR1 mutations have been reported. Most of the mutations segregate with the MH susceptibility trait, whereas a much smaller number is associated with central core disease (CCD). The majority of the mutations cluster in the N-terminal amino acid residues 35 to 614 (referred to as the MH/CCD region-1) and the centrally located residues 2163 to 2458 (MH/CCD region-2) corresponding to the exons 2 to 18 and 39 to 45, respectively. Another group of mutations has been identified outside of these two mutation hot spots in the C-terminus (MH/CCD region-3) encoded by exons 100 to 104 (see Fig. 49–2E). Although most RYR1 mutations result in amino acid substitutions, a single amino acid deletion affecting a conserved glutamic acid at position 2347 has been found in two unrelated MH-susceptible families.[25] Many RYR1 mutations have been detected only in single families, whereas others are more common but their frequency varies among different ethnic groups.[14]

Mutations in RYR1 may cause MH, CCD, or both. The likely deciding factors in determining whether a particular RYR1 mutation results in MH susceptibility or CCD are the sensitivity of the RYR1 mutant proteins to agonists; the level of abnormal channel-gating caused by the mutation; the consequential decrease in the size of the releasable calcium store and increase in resting concentration of calcium in the cytoplasm; and the level of compensation achieved by the muscle with respect to maintaining calcium homeostasis.[14] MH mutations appear to selectively increase the sensitivity of the receptor to stimulators of opening, resulting in more frequent and prolonged opening of the Ca^{2+} release channel, so called *hypersensitive gating*. This gain-of-function in electromechanical coupling causes uncontrolled Ca^{2+}-induced Ca^{2+} release and results in increased myoplasmic calcium level, which lowers contracture threshold, enhances metabolism, and leads to depletion of ATP, glucose and oxygen, as well as excess production of CO_2, lactate, and heat, characteristic of MH. The elevation of Ca^{2+} and the cascade of resulting biochemical abnormalities manifesting as MH appear to be a final common pathway shared by other disorders with increased risk for MH, such as Duchenne muscular dystrophy, in which baseline myoplasmic calcium is abnormally elevated. Anesthetics trigger MH in a susceptible individual by further increasing the already abnormal Ca^{2+} release from the SR, allowing the threshold for a clinical MH event to be reached.[4,14]

The human *RYR1* mutations associated with MH include R614C that corresponds to the recessive R615C mutation in the swine *RYR1* gene causing porcine MH. Affected humans are, however, heterozygous for the same mutation, in keeping with the dominant inheritance in man. The R614C mutant has been well characterized because of the availability of the animal model. Purified ryanodine receptors from MH swine that were reconstituted into lipid bilayers showed prolonged open times and shortened closed times compared with controls. Expression of the R614C mutant in muscle cells and COS-7 cells caused hypersensitive gating of Ca^{2+} release in transfected cells, with Ca^{2+} release in response to lower levels of added caffeine or halothane compared with the normal channel.[4,14]

CCD appears to be genetically homogeneous and has been associated only with *RYR1* mutations.[14] The effects of mutations causing CCD are unclear but may result in loss rather than gain of function. In contrast to the hypersensitive gating characteristic of MH mutations, mutations causing CCD impair excitation-contraction coupling. This mechanism may explain the pathologic changes seen in the SR and the T-tubules in CCD muscle, because the ryanodine receptor bridges the SR and the T tubules at the terminal cisterna. Diminished excitation-contraction coupling in CCD may result in muscle weakness. A mutation that causes both hypersensitive gating and diminished excitation-contraction coupling could cause both MH and CCD phenotypes in the same individual. These mutations cluster in the N-terminal region of the protein, which appears critical for regulation of channel gating and excitation-contraction coupling. In addition to different effects of mutations on RYR1 function, phenotypic variability in CCD and MH may also be explained in part by allelic variants of other proteins that interact with the ryanodine receptor.

The C-terminus mutation I4898T has been identified in a family with severe CCD.[14] Coexpression of normal and mutant *RYR1* cDNAs in a 1:1 ratio, as well as expression of the analogous mutation I4897T in skeletal myotubes derived from *RyR1*-knockout mice, resulted in reduced maximal Ca^{2+} release from the SR, suggesting diminished excitation-contraction coupling as a likely cause of muscle weakness.[26] Another C-terminus mutation, Y4796C causes both severe CCD with rods in muscle fibers and MH susceptibility. Expression studies revealed increased caffeine sensitivity of the channel. Whereas maximal Ca^{2+} release from the SR was reduced, resting cytoplasmic Ca^{2+} levels were elevated, suggesting an increased rate of Ca^{2+} leakage through the mutant channel.[27] Chronic elevation of myoplasmic Ca^{2+} concentration may be responsible for the severe myopathic phenotype. The combination of hypersensitive gating and reduced maximal Ca^{2+} release may explain the coexistence of CCD and MH susceptibility.

In several families, expression of the MH phenotype has been linked to a region near chromosome 17q11 that contains the *SCN4A* gene, and in one of these families both MH and HyperPP were coinherited as autosomal dominant traits. Both traits showed linkage to polymorphic markers within the *SCN4A* gene, suggesting that mutations in the *SCN4A* gene may cause MH. Another group of MH families have mutations in *CACNA1S* encoding the α1-subunit of the voltage-dependent L-type calcium channel. These mutations, R1086H and R1086C, affect an arginine residue in the cytoplasmic loop between domains 3 and 4, a region that is thought to interact with the ryanodine receptor, affecting electromechanical coupling (see Fig. 49–2*B* and *E*). Thus, MH linked to this locus is allelic to HypoPP-1 (see Table 49–1). Further MH susceptibility loci have been identified on chromosome 7q21, which contains the *CACNL2A* gene encoding the α2-subunit of the voltage dependent L-type calcium channel; on chromosome 3q13 found in a single German family; and on chromosome 5p.

Disorders Caused by Potassium Channel Defects

Neuromyotonia and Episodic Ataxia Type 1/Myokymia Syndrome

Voltage-gated K^+ (Kv) channels contribute to the rapid repolarization of muscle and nerve after an action potential. In nerve, loss of K^+ channel function causes impaired repolarization between action potentials, resulting in the repetitive, high frequency discharges and nerve hyperexcitability characteristic of neuromyotonia. Neuromyotonia and neuromyotonic discharges have been described in isolation, as well as in association with a number of other disorders, including acquired and hereditary polyneuropathies, amyotrophic lateral sclerosis, bone marrow transplantation, and paraneoplastic syndromes. Alteration of K^+ channels on a genetic or autoimmune (including paraneoplastic) basis has been shown to play a major role in the pathogenesis of both myokymia and neuromyotonia.[5] Thus, neuromyotonia is a general expression of nerve hyperexcitability that can result from either genetic or acquired modulation of Kv channel function in the peripheral nerve.

The autoimmune form of neuromyotonia is caused by antibodies to voltage-gated K^+ channels, which are at the juxtaparanodes of motor nerves.[5] The anti-Kv antibodies are heterogeneous and bind to different K^+ channel isoforms, as well as different binding sites on the same channel. This variability in target specificity may provide a molecular explanation for the clinical diversity of the syndrome. Whether these antibodies have a blocking effect, alter the kinetics, or accelerate K^+ channel turnover remains unclear.

Primary involvement of peripheral nerve leading to the expression of a form of myokymia has been reported in the episodic ataxia-type 1/myokymia syndrome (EA1/myokymia). This syndrome has been linked to point mutations in the *KCNA1* K$^+$ channel gene on chromosome 12p13.[6] Mutations causing EA-1/myokymia have been found throughout the KCNA1 sequence (see Table 49–1 and Fig. 49–2C). Most cause the typical phenotype of EA-1/myokymia, although some family members with the V174F, F184C, and T226R mutations also have seizures. Almost all *KCNA1* mutations that have been expressed in *Xenopus* oocytes display reduced K$^+$ currents and variable degrees of shift in the voltage dependence of activation toward positive potentials. When mutants are coexpressed with wild-type channel subunits, they exert dominant-negative effects on the wild-type subunits resulting in reduced K$^+$ currents through heteromeric channels.[7]

The functional consequences of *KCNA1* mutations in vivo appear to correlate with the severity of the clinical phenotype. The P244H mutation associated with isolated neuromyotonia causes a mild shift in voltage dependence of activation with normal K$^+$ currents, as opposed to reduced currents in most other K$^+$ mutations studied that cause both neuromyotonia and CNS manifestations. In contrast, the R417 stop mutation, associated with a severe drug-resistant phenotype, causes the most profound reduction of K$^+$ currents and has a dominant-negative effect on the wild-type channel current when heteromeric channels are expressed.[7] For the R239S and F249I mutants, the amount of expressed protein is reduced. Moreover, R239S subunits do not form functional channels when expressed either alone or with wild type channels, suggesting possible rapid degradation or trafficking abnormalities, or both, resulting in haplotype insufficiency. Overall, the location of the mutation in the KCNA1 protein does not reliably predict the type or severity of the clinical manifestations.

Although mutations in two other potassium channel genes, *KCNQ2* and *KCNQ3*, usually cause benign familial neonatal convulsions, the R207W *KCNQ2* mutation can cause both neonatal convulsions and myokymia. This mutation affects a conserved arginine residue within the voltage-sensing S4 segment and results in more severe impairment of the channel activation compared with other mutations that cause convulsions alone. This mutant also exerts dominant-negative effects when it is coexpressed with either wild type KCNQ2 or KCNQ3. KCNQ2 and KCNQ3 mRNAs have been detected in the spinal cord and may be expressed by motor neurons.[8] Whether these K$^+$ channels are also present in the peripheral axons remains to be determined.

Periodic Paralysis

Potassium channels also influence membrane repolarization in skeletal and cardiac muscle. Although few skeletal muscle disorders involve K$^+$ channels, a mutation in a K$^+$ channel β-subunit known as MiRP2 causes either HypoPP or HyperPP phenotypes. MiRP2 belongs to the family of small β-subunit proteins that combine with tetramers of larger α-subunits to form K$^+$ channels in the heart (see later) or skeletal muscle. MiRP2, encoded by the *KCNE3* gene, forms K$^+$ channels in skeletal muscle with the Kv3.4 α-subunit.[17] The MiRP2-Kv3.4 channels have a direct role in setting the RMP in the muscle, thereby modulating excitability. Two families with somewhat atypical HypoPP and HyperPP phenotypes were found to harbor the R83H mutation in MiRP2. In expression studies the mutated MiRP2 reduces MiRP2-Kv3.4 current density causing depolarization of muscle cells. Similar to other K$^+$ channel mutants, it also exerts a dominant-negative effect on coexpressed wild-type channels.

Andersen Syndrome

Andersen syndrome is the first disorder to demonstrate a predicted link between electrical phenotypes of skeletal and cardiac muscle, and is characterized by periodic paralysis, cardiac arrhythmias, and dysmorphic features. The disease results from mutations in *KCNJ2*, located on chromosome 17q23, which encodes the inward rectifying potassium channel Kir2.1, expressed in heart, brain, and skeletal muscle.[28] In several families with Andersen syndrome, seven missense mutations and two deletions have been identified, located throughout the channel protein. Expression of several mutations in oocytes reveals loss of function and a dominant negative effect on Kir2.1 current.

Cardiac Arrhythmias and Hearing Loss

K$^+$ channel mutations that affect skeletal muscle function appear to be rare, whereas mutations in different types of K$^+$ channels are a major source of pathology in cardiac muscle. Among over 180 mutations in five different cardiac ion channel genes that cause long QT syndrome, more than 95% affect K$^+$ channels. Most of these K$^+$ channel mutations affect membrane repolarization, leading to re-entrant arrhythmias.[9] The same mutations can cause deafness in addition to long QT syndrome in homozygous or compound heterozygous conditions due to associated loss of function in the inner ear (Jervell-Lange-Nielsen syndrome), whereas in simple heterozygous conditions they cause isolated long QT syndrome (Romano-Ward syndrome) due to a dominant effect in the heart.

The cardiac slowly inactivating delayed rectifier K$^+$ channel (I_{ks}) is formed by the α-subunit encoded by *KCNQ1*, similar in structure to the isoform found in peripheral nerve encoded by *KCNA1*, and the much smaller β-subunit MinK, encoded by *KCNE1*. The related rapidly inactivating delayed rectifier K$^+$ channel (I_{kr}) is formed by the α-subunit encoded by *HERG* and the MiRP1 β-subunit, encoded by *KCNE2*. Mutations in any of these 4 genes can cause long QT syndrome (see Table 49–1).[9,29] Over 70, mostly missense mutations localized throughout the protein sequence have been identified in each of the two α-subunit genes *KCNQ1* and *HERG*. Mutations in the pore lining S5, S6, and P segments are likely to disrupt K$^+$ ion movement, whereas mutations in the amino or carboxy termini may cause defects in gating and tetramerization. Only about 2% of the known long QT syndrome mutations occur in *KCNE1* and only three missense mutations have been identified in *KCNE2*, two of which caused a mild phenotype and the third predisposed to drug-induced long QT syndrome. Most families with Jervell-Lange-Nielsen syndrome harbor mutations in *KCNQ1*, expressed both in the heart and the stria vascularis of the inner ear. Long QT syndrome mutations associated with Jervell-Lange-Nielsen syndrome produce a less severe I$_{ks}$ channel defect than those causing the Romano-Ward syndrome. Therefore, the heterozygotes in families with Jervell-Lange-Nielsen syndrome have lesser degrees of QT prolongation and fewer cardiac symptoms than do patients with Romano-Ward syndrome. They are nevertheless at high risk for cardiac events. One normal allele in a long QT syndrome gene is sufficient to rescue the deafness phenotype, but the cardiac abnormalities are still present.

Similar to the KCNA1 mutants in peripheral nerve, long QT syndrome mutations causing Romano-Ward syndrome have dominant-negative effects on wild type channel subunits. Several KCNQ1 mutants fail to form functional tetramers, or produce channels with altered gating properties. Other mutations affect the interaction between α- and β-subunits. When coexpressed with wild type KCNQ1, long QT syndrome mutants produce a dominant-negative inhibition of K$^+$ current density. In contrast, carboxy terminus mutations truncate the protein and abolish homotetramer channel function, without affecting wild type α-subunits in heterotetramers. Similarly, S2-S3 mutants produce simple loss of function without significantly changing the biophysical properties of expressed I$_{ks}$ channels.[9,29]

A truncated form of HERG reduces wild type HERG expression by a dominant-negative mechanism possibly affecting the presumed association domain. Other HERG mutations cause faster channel inactivation. The LQT2 mutation A561V reduces wild-type HERG expression. This effect was partially reversible with proteosomal inhibition, or incubation at a lower temperature, suggesting increased turnover and proteolysis of misfolded mutants oligomerized with wild type monomers. Another HERG mutant, G601S, is retained in the rough endoplasmic reticulum, causing reduced K$^+$ currents without alteration of channel kinetics.

Mutations in the two β-subunits MinK and MiRP1 that cause about 5% of long QT syndrome also alter the biophysical properties of the corresponding K$^+$ channels. In addition, one MiRP1 mutant involved in clarithromycin-induced arrhythmia increases channel blockade by the antibiotic. Whereas the majority of patients with long QT syndrome have mutations in cardiac K$^+$ channel genes, several mutations of the cardiac Na$^+$ channel α-subunit gene *SCN5A* have been reported (see earlier). These account for about 8% of long QT syndrome cases (LQT3).[9,29]

Chloride Channel Defects in Myotonia Congenita

Most forms of dominant and recessive myotonia congenita are caused by an abnormality in the skeletal muscle chloride channel. The association of myotonia congenita with a reduction in sarcolemmal Cl$^-$ conductance was first recognized in the myotonic goat and subsequently in humans. Physiologic studies demonstrated that a reduction in membrane Cl$^-$ conductance to less than 20% of normal levels would lead to myotonic activity in otherwise normal muscle. However, not until the 1990s was the causal relationship between genetic defects in the skeletal muscle Cl$^-$ channel (ClC-1) and myotonia confirmed, following the linkage of both the dominant and recessive forms of myotonia congenita to the human *CLCN1* locus and the identification of mutations in the *CLCN1* chloride channel gene of the myotonic mouse.[19] Analysis of a large number of pedigrees has shown that numerous mutations at a variety of locations within the same channel sequence can cause either the dominant or the recessive form of myotonia. Over 50 mutations causing myotonia congenita have been reported to date (see Table 49–1 and Fig. 49–2D).[2]

The descendants of Dr. Thomsen with the dominant form of myotonia congenita share a common P490L mutation affecting a proline that is absolutely conserved in all known Cl$^-$ channel genes. Other mutations that produce the dominant myotonia phenotype include single amino acid substitutions located throughout the channel protein, predominantly in exons 5, 8, and 15, and a stop mutation in exon 23 that causes truncation of the carboxy terminus. More variability has been found in the mutations that produce the recessive form of myotonia. They include point mutations, frame shifts, deletions, and premature transcription terminations.[19,30] Among these, the F413C, R894x, and a deletion in exon 13 were the most frequent in a large study of several families and unrelated individuals with myotonia congenita. Further genetic studies of myotonia congenita families have shown that certain ClC-1 mutations can cause either recessive myotonia or a benign form of dominant myotonia with incomplete penetrance.[19,30]

Not all patients with the recessive myotonia congenita phenotype have an identified mutation in the *CLCN1* gene. In several mutation screenings, less that 50% of the families fulfilling clinical criteria for myotonia congenita had an identifiable mutation, presumably reflecting either technical limitations of the screening process, or genetic heterogeneity.[30] Only 25% of the mutation-positive cases had mutations in both *CLCN1* alleles.[19] The latter group included both individuals homozygous for a single mutation and compound heterozygotes for two different mutations. All other patients with recessive myotonia and only one mutated *CLCN1* allele are thought to have an unidentified mutation on their other gene. Moreover, some presumed disease-causing amino acid substitutions have subsequently been found in normal individuals, raising the question of whether these are harmless polymorphisms or actual pathogenic mutations that cause disease when combined with other base changes.

How different mutations in the same gene can produce dominant or recessive effects is not yet completely understood. Early expression studies of mutant ClC-1 in *Xenopus* oocytes showed abnormally low Cl⁻ currents, suggesting a loss of function mechanism in myotonia congenita. Because pathologic effects are not seen until membrane Cl⁻ conductance falls below 20%, a single abnormal allele should not be symptomatic because the normal gene product from the unaffected allele should produce sufficient channel dimers to ensure normal muscle function. However, ClC-1 channel mutations may have dominant-negative effects on coexpressed wild-type ClC-1. Because ClC-1 proteins exist as dimers in vivo,[18] channels containing mixtures of both normal and mutant proteins may be formed, resulting in abnormal function of the heteromeric channels.

The nature and localization of the mutation is the most important factor in determining the functional changes that result. Most dominant and recessive ClC-1 mutations cause a positive shift of the activation curve, whereas only dominant mutations appear to have a dominant-negative effect on coexpressed wild-type channel monomers. The mechanism of this dominant-negative effect has been studied using fluctuation analysis to characterize the double-gate behavior of a ClC-1 mutant/wild-type heterodimer harboring dominant or recessive mutations. The recessive mutations affected the gating of the mutant homodimers only, whereas dominant mutations modified both the mutant homodimers and the mutant/wild-type heterodimers, possibly by affecting a common intersubunit regulatory surface or gate.[20] The magnitude of this dominant-negative effect in expression studies seems to correlate with the severity of the clinical phenotype.

A shift in voltage dependence of mutant/wild-type heteromeric dimers through alterations of a shared gate appears to be the most common mechanism by which mutations in Thomsen disease exert a dominant-negative effect. However, other dominant mutations have been shown to reduce Cl⁻ currents without gating alterations. For example, the R894x mutation does not affect voltage dependence,[30] but may instead reduce protein stability or trafficking to the membrane because of the truncation after domain D13. Abnormal intracellular trafficking and retention in the cytoplasm is a common theme for other mutant membrane proteins that fail to reach the cell membrane (see Chapter 39).

Expression studies with ClC-1 mutations have shown a variety of functional effects; this range explains in part why myotonia congenita can be transmitted as either a dominant or a recessive trait. In all cases, reduction of Cl⁻ conductance is the final common pathway, allowing after-depolarizations to reach threshold easily and repetitive potentials to develop, which, in turn, causes muscle membrane instability and leads to the electrical and clinical manifestations of myotonia.

THERAPY AND PREVENTION OF ION CHANNEL DISORDERS

Many patients with neuromuscular channelopathies have mild symptoms and prefer to manage their disorder without specific medications. Avoiding exacerbating factors, such as cold exposure in paramyotonia, or carbohydrate rich meals in HypoPP, can be of great help. Those who avail themselves of medical therapy often report variable response to a given modality even though they share a common phenotype. The genetic heterogeneity of the ion channel disorders may explain some of this response variability. Knowledge of the molecular pathophysiology is also a necessary step for the development of more rational, specific, and effective therapies that target the channels with abnormal function.

In myotonia congenita, muscle hyperexcitability results from loss of chloride channel function. There are currently no medications available that directly target the defective chloride channels. However, myotonic symptoms may respond to medications such as phenytoin, carbamazepine, tocainide, and mexiletine, which reduce membrane excitability and suppress myotonic discharges by modifying the kinetics of Na⁺ channels. Acetazolamide is usually effective only in patients with Na⁺ channel myotonia.[1,2,3] Among Na⁺ channel blockers the antiarrhythmic drugs mexiletine and tocainide may be the most effective in preventing myotonic stiffness both in typical myotonia and in paramyotonia caused by Na⁺ channel mutations, although these medications also carry the most significant level of risk. The painful variant of atypical myotonia may respond better to flecainide treatment. Among patients with paramyotonia congenita associated with periodic paralysis, a combination of mexiletine and hydrochlordiazide has been used to prevent stiffness and weakness induced by cold, as well as paralytic attacks. However, in all cases, the potential benefits of these drugs must be carefully weighed against their potential risks, given the benign nature of the disease itself.

In patients with HyperPP, acetazolamide or low-dose diuretics such as hydrochlordiazide and frequent meals rich in carbohydrates and low in potassium may prevent hyperkalemia and the associated paralytic episodes. Prolonged fasting, strenuous exercise, and exposure to cold should be avoided. During the attack, prompt intake of a diuretic such as hydrochlordiazide or calcium gluconate, 0.5–2.0 g given intramuscularly, may attenuate or terminate the paralysis, probably by lowering the serum potassium level. Beta-adrenergic inhalational agents have also been successful in aborting attacks of HyperPP, perhaps because of their stimulating effect on the sodium-potassium pump. The mechanism underlying the beneficial effect of acetazolamide both in preventing and attenuating HyperPP episodes is not completely understood, but activation of K^+ channels is likely, based on studies in HypoPP (see earlier).[24]

As with the other ion channel disorders, mild and rare paralytic attacks in HypoPP may not merit continuous treatment. Acute episodes causing weakness should be treated with potassium, usually in the form of oral potassium chloride 2 to 10 g in aqueous solution. Frequency of the paralytic episodes is reduced by potassium supplements, a low sodium diet, and avoidance of carbohydrate-rich meals and strenuous exertion.[1,2,3] Acetazolamide may be an effective preventive therapy in many, but not all, patients with HypoPP. The lowest possible dose should be used, because serious side effects such as nephrolithiasis may occur, in addition to the common paresthesias. Individuals who initially respond to acetazolamide may become refractory after months of successful treatment. These refractory patients may respond favorably to dichlorphenamide, another carbonic anhydrase inhibitor. It has been recognized that patients with HypoPP-2 caused by Na^+ channel mutations experience worsening of their attacks under acetazolamide treatment,[23] suggesting that response to therapy may be predicted and directed by knowledge of the genetic defect in HypoPP.

Similar to the situation with Cl^- channels and myotonia congenita, in neuromyotonia there are no drugs that restore the function of K^+ channels. Phenytoin and carbamazepine are often effective in suppressing myokymic and neuromyotonic discharges due to their use-dependent inhibitory effect on Na^+ channels.[5] This is also true for the EA-1/myokymia phenotype, as well as for the epileptic manifestations of K^+ channel dysfunction. Immunomodulating agents may be considered for the autoimmune cases of neuromyotonia.

Dysregulation of Ca^{2+} in skeletal muscle is the central mechanism in MH. Excessive release of Ca^{2+} from the SR through the calcium release channel/ryanodine receptor results in prolonged muscle contraction, hypermetabolism, heat production, and rhabdomyolysis. In addition to withdrawing the offending agent, dantrolene is an effective therapy if given early. Dantrolene specifically inhibits the release of calcium from the SR. The usual dose is 2 to 3 mg/kg intravenously, repeated as needed every 5 minutes, up to a total of 10 mg/kg. Further measures to reverse the abnormalities that occur in MH include hyperventilation with oxygen, administration of sodium bicarbonate, and cooling. Urine output is maintained at 2 ml/kg/hr and calcium, calcium antagonists, or beta-blockers are avoided. Early recognition of the disorder by anesthetists and administration of dantrolene, as well as intensive care, have reduced MH mortality from approximately 70% to less than 10%.[4,14]

CONCLUSION AND FUTURE DIRECTIONS

Progress in molecular genetics and electrophysiology in the last decade has shown that a number of nerve and muscle disorders, including myotonia, paramyotonia, neuromyotonia, periodic paralyses, and malignant hyperthermia are caused by structural defects in membrane ion channels. This growing group of ion channel disorders also encompasses cardiac muscle leading to arrhythmias, and central neurons producing paroxysmal brain diseases such as epilepsy, migraine, and ataxia. Clinically, all these disorders share features of intermittently decreased or increased membrane excitability.

The new tools of genetic linkage, gene analysis, and functional expression provide insight into the molecular and pathophysiologic mechanisms underlying the clinical and electromyographic manifestations of these disorders, whose clinical descriptions, in most cases, have been available for decades. Mutations within a critical voltage sensor sequence may alter sensitivity to membrane potential, whereas mutations elsewhere in the structure may impair inactivation mechanisms and cause prolonged channel opening with aberrant currents. Alterations in pore forming segments may affect ion selectivity and conductance. Mutant channel subunits may affect the function and gating of normal subunits, with which they oligomerize. A subgroup of abnormal channels may indirectly modify the function of normal channels through alterations in the membrane potential or in the level of a critical ion. Other pathophysiologic mechanisms include decreased expression and rapid degradation, or improper targeting of misfolded ion channel proteins, ultimately affecting channel distribution and density.

The diversity of phenotypes among the ion channel disorders reflects both the spectrum of ion channels involved and the fact that, within a single channel, the location of a mutation profoundly affects the impact on channel function. The variability in the type and severity of clinical manifestations among individuals harboring the same mutation remains puzzling. Also unexplained is the fact that identical mutations may exhibit either recessive or dominant behavior, or show incomplete penetrance. Clearly, the status of other independent factors that modulate ion channel activity in vivo, such as associated subunits, phosphorylation, and interaction with second messengers, contribute to this phenotypic variability. These factors still await investigation. Developing a fuller understanding of the molecular mechanisms at play in each case will eventually lead to rational diagnostic categories, more focused clinical trials, and more specific and effective therapy for these disorders.

REFERENCES

1. Rüdel R, Hanna MG, Lehmann-Horn F: Muscle channelopathies: Malignant hyperthermia, periodic paralyses, paramyotonia, and myotonia. In Shapira AHV, Griggs RC (eds): Muscle Diseases. Boston, Butterworth-Heinemann, 1999, pp 135–175.

2. Kleopa KA, Barchi RL: Genetic disorders of neuromuscular ion channels. Muscle Nerve 2002;26:299–325.

3. Moxley RT: Myotonic disorders in childhood. J Child Neurol 1997;12:116–129.

4. Heiman-Patterson TD: Malignant hyperthermia. In Rose M, Griggs R (eds): Channelopathies of the nervous system. Oxford, Butterworth-Heinemann, 2001, pp 167–178.

5. Newsom-Davis J: Autoimmune neuromyotonia (Isaac syndrome): An antibody mediated potassium channelopathy. Ann NY Acad Sci 1997;835: 111–119.

6. Browne DL, Gancher ST, Nutt JG, et al: Episodic ataxia/myokymia syndrome is associated with point mutations in the human potassium channel gene, KCNA1. Nat Genet 1994;8:136–140.

7. Eunson LH, Rea R, Zuberi SM, et al: Clinical, genetic, and expression studies of mutations in the potassium channel gene KCNA1 reveal new phenotypic variability. Ann Neurol 2000;48:647–656.

8. Dedek K, Kunath B, Kananura C, et al: Myokymia and neonatal epilepsy caused by a mutation in the voltage sensor of the KCNQ2 K$^+$ channel. Proc Natl Acad Sci USA 2001;98:12272–12277.

9. Vincent GM; Long QT syndrome. Cardiol Clin 2000;18:309–325.

10. Armstrong CM, Hille B: Voltage-gated ion channels and electrical excitability. Neuron 1998;20:371–380.

11. Catterall WA: From ionic currents to molecular mechanisms: The structure and function of voltage-gated sodium channels. Neuron 2000;26:13–25.

12. George AL, Ledbetter DH, Kallen RG, Barchi RL: Assignment of the human skeletal muscle sodium channel α-subunit gene (SCN4A) to 17p23.1–25.3. Genomics 1991;9:555–556.

13. Catterall WA: Structure and regulation of voltage-gated Ca^{2+} channels. Annu Rev Cell Develop Biol 2000a;16:521–555.

14. McCarthy TV, Quane KA, Lynch PJ: Ryanodine receptor mutations in malignant hyperthermia and central core disease. Hum Mutat 2000;15:410–417.

15. Arroyo EJ, Scherer SS: On the molecular architecture of myelinated fibers. Histochem Cell Biol 2000;113:1–18.

16. Jan LY, Jan YN: Voltage-gated and inwardly rectifying potassium channels. J Physiol 1997;505:267–282.

17. Abbott GW, Butler MH, Bendahhou S, et al: MiRP2 forms potassium channels in skeletal muscle with Kv3.4 and is associated with periodic paralysis. Cell 2001;104:217–231.

18. Jentsch TJ, Friedrich T, Schriever A, Yamada H: The CLC chloride channel family. Pflügers Archiv 1999;437:783–795.

19. Koch MC, Steinmeyer K, Lorenz C, et al: The skeletal muscle chloride channel in dominant and recessive myotonia. Science 1992;257:797–800.

20. Saviane C, Conti F, Pusch M: The muscle chloride channel ClC-1 has a double-barreled appearance that is differentially affected in dominant and recessive myotonia. J Gen Physiol 1999;113:457–468.

21. Mindell JA, Maduke M, Miller C, Grigorieff N: Projection structure of a ClC-type chloride channel at 6.5Å resolution. Nature 2001;409:219–223.

22. Ptácek LJ, Tawil R, Griggs RC, et al: Sodium channel mutations in acetazolamide-responsive myotonia congenita, paramyotonia congenita, and hyperkalemic periodic paralysis. Neurology 1994;44:1500–1503.

23. Sternberg D, Maisonobe T, Jurkat-Rott K, et al: Hypokalemic periodic paralysis type 2 caused by mutations at codon 672 in the muscle sodium channel gene SCN4A. Brain 2001;124:1091–1099.

24. Tricarico D, Barbieri M, Camerino DC: Acetazolamide opens the muscular K$_{Ca}$2+ channel. A novel mechanism of action that may explain the therapeutic effect of the drug in hypokalemic periodic paralysis. Ann Neurol 2000;48:304–312.

25. Sambuughin N, McWilliams S, de Bantel A, et al: Single-amino-acid deletion in the RYR1 gene, associated with malignant hyperthermia susceptibility and unusual contraction phenotype. Am J Hum Genet 2001;69:204–208.

26. Avila G, O'Brien JJ, Dirksen RT: Excitation-contraction uncoupling by a human central core disease mutation in the ryanodine receptor. Proc Nat Acad Sci U S A 2001;98:4215–4220.

27. Monnier N, Romero NB, Lerale J, et al: An autosomal dominant congenital myopathy with cores and rods is associated with a new mutation in the RYR1 gene encoding the skeletal muscle ryanodine receptor. Hum Molec Genet 2000;9:2599–2608.

28. Plaster NM, Tawil R, Tristani-Firouzi M, et al: Mutations in Kir2.1 cause the developmental and episodic electrical phenotypes of Andersen syndrome. Cell 2001;105:511–519.

29. Splawski I, Shen J, Timothy K, et al: Spectrum of mutations in long-QT syndrome genes: KVLQT1, HERG, SCN5A, KCNE1, KCNE2. Circulation 2000;102:1178–1185.

30. Meyer-Kleine C, Steinmeyer K, Ricker K, et al: Spectrum of mutations in the major human skeletal muscle chloride channel gene (CLC1) leading to myotonia. Am J Hum Genet 1995;57:1325–1334.

CHAPTER

50

The Phakomatoses

Mia MacCollin

The phakomatoses are a diverse group of diseases charac terized by skin lesions in early childhood followed by tumor development in multiple other organs. Most phakomatoses have a genetic element and are considered to be tumor suppressor gene syndromes. This chapter primarily focuses on the most common of the phakomatoses, neurofibromatosis 1 (NF1) and tuberous sclerosis complex (TSC).

NEUROFIBROMATOSIS 1

Clinical Features and Diagnostic Evaluation

NF1 is an extremely variable disease, with age-dependent development of dermatologic, neurologic, and other system manifestations. Multiple hyperpigmented macules termed café au lait (CAL) spots (Fig. 50–1A) are nearly always the first finding. CAL may be apparent at birth and increase in number, size and conspicuousness until the time of puberty; in some persons they may be better visualized using an ultraviolet or Wood's lamp. Small numbers of CAL (five or fewer) may also be seen in genetically normal people. Nearly all NF1 patients develop cutaneous tumors (Fig. 50–1B, C). Cutaneous tumors begin to appear before puberty and increase in number throughout life. About 25% of patients will find these tumors cosmetically burdensome and request their removal, although their potential for malignant transformation is nil. In 33% of patients, one or more plexiform neurofibromas will develop (Fig. 50–2). Unlike cutaneous tumors, these complex masses are nearly always congenital and carry a lifetime risk of malignant transformation. Many plexiform tumors will have trophic effects

on surrounding tissues with resulting overgrowth or malformation. About 25% of plexiform tumors will require surgical intervention for biopsy, subtotal resection, or removal. T2-weighted changes on cranial MRI scan (unidentified bright objects or "UBOs") are very common in NF1 affected children, especially in the brain stem, cerebellum, and basal ganglia (Fig. 50–3A) and have little clinical significance. About 15% of patients have similar lesions in the optic nerve, chiasm, or tract. In most cases, such disease is limited to nonprogressive enlargement of the structure, but 2% to 5% of patients have progressive optic nerve glioma that leads to visual impairment (Fig. 50–3B).

The most common nontumorous manifestation of NF1 is learning disability with or without attention deficit disorder, which affects nearly half of patients. Rarely, patients may have seizure disorder or psychiatric manifestations such as personality disorder or schizophrenia. Other nontumorous manifestations include headache, pseudarthrosis, disorders of growth and development (most commonly short stature and precocious or delayed puberty), aqueductal stenosis, and hypertension.

The clinical course of NF1 varies widely. Many major manifestations, such as severe mental disability, seizure disorder, and plexiform tumors are obvious in early childhood. Cutaneous tumors usually appear around the time of puberty, but do not usually become burdensome until well into adulthood. Malignancy is rarely encountered before the third decade. NF1 is an autosomal dominant disorder with full penetrance and a birth incidence of 1:3000 individuals. About 50% of affected patients are due to new mutations with clinically unaffected parents. NF1 shows great intrafamilial heterogencity.

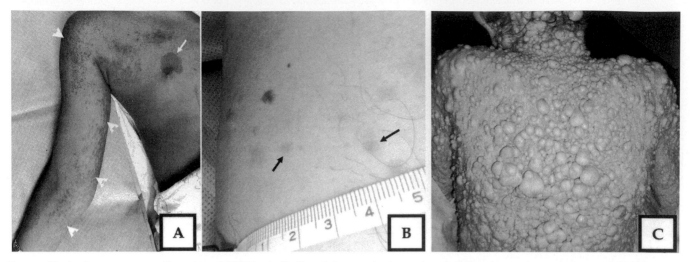

FIGURE 50–1. Cutaneous manifestations of NF1. *A*, Café au lait macule *(arrow)* and diffuse hyperpigmentation and freckling *(arrowheads)*. *B*, Multiple skin tumors *(arrows)* in a young adult. Cutaneous neurofibromas such as these often have a purplish hue. *C*, Nearly contiguous involvement by cutaneous tumors in an older adult. Many of the tumors are pedunculated.

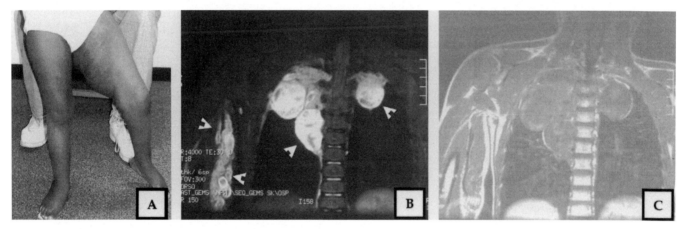

FIGURE 50–2. Plexiform neurofibroma in NF1. *A*, Child with a large plexiform tumor of the pelvis extending down into the left thigh. Note overgrowth of the left leg compared to the right. *B*, T2-weighted MRI scan showing extensive tumor formation in the chest with extension through the right brachial plexus into the right arm *(arrowheads)*. *C*, Contrast-enhanced T1-weighted image of the same area shown in *B*. Plexiform tumors are frequently poorly and inhomogenously contrast-enhancing, as seen in this lesion.

Initial evaluation of a patient known or suspected of having NF1 should include a detailed developmental history, review of growth charts in children, and family history of all first-degree relatives. Physical examination should include measurements of growth and blood pressure, detailed skin inspection using a Wood's lamp, and age-appropriate neurologic examination. Diagnosis using the NIH clinical criteria (Table 50–1) is possible by age 1 year in some patients, and by age 5 years in almost all patients. Once a diagnosis is established, patients with NF1 should undergo a complete neurologic evaluation and blood pressure evaluation annually. Children should also have a developmental assessment and review of growth and sexual development. An annual ophthalmologic exam should be done from ages 2 to 7 years. Routine laboratory investigations are not needed for NF1

TABLE 50–1. Diagnostic Criteria for Neurofibromatosis 1 (NF1*)

Diagnostic criteria for NF1 are met in an individual if TWO or more of the following are found:

1. Six or more café au lait macules of significant size
2. Two or more neurofibromas
3. Freckling in the axillary or inguinal regions
4. Optic glioma
5. Two or more Lisch nodules
6. A distinctive osseous lesion
7. A first-degree relative with NF1

*Adapted from Gutmann, DH, Aylsworth A, Carey JC, et al: The diagnostic evaluation and multidisciplinary management of neurofibromatosis 1 and neurofibromatosis 2. JAMA 1997; 278:51–57.

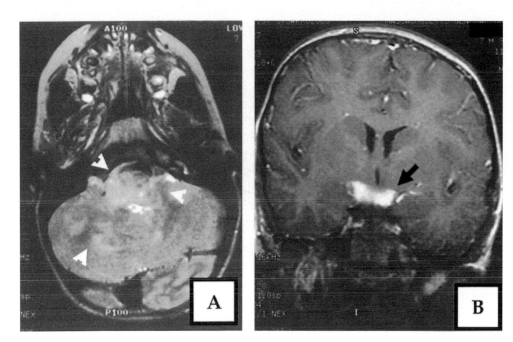

FIGURE 50–3. Cranial imaging in NF1. *A*, T2-weighted axial image in a 7-year-old boy showing signal abnormalities of the pons and cerebellum *(arrowheads)*. These nonenhancing lesions had no clinical correlate despite their extensive anatomic effect. *B*, Contrast-enhanced T1-weighted coronal image of a symptomatic optic chiasm glioma showing intense enhancement *(arrow)*.

patients. Specifically, imaging studies of the brain and spine can be reserved for those with unexplained or progressive symptoms.

Pathology

The hallmark tumor of NF1 is the neurofibroma. Several classification systems have been proposed for neurofibromas.[1] Neurofibromas are heterogeneous nonmalignant tumors derived from the nerve sheath, which contain Schwann cells, perineural fibroblasts, other cellular components, and large quantities of extracellular matrix and collagen. Unlike schwannomas, which grow eccentrically to the nerve itself and are usually well encapsulated, neurofibromas grow within the nerve bundle and do not usually have a surrounding capsule. Plexiform neurofibromas are composed of multiple fascicles of tumor, and often take the gross pathologic appearance of a "bag of worms." Plexiform tumors often infiltrate normal adjacent structures and may cause bony erosion or malformation and somatic overgrowth of an affected limb. Malignant peripheral nerve sheath tumors (MPNST, previously known as malignant schwannomas or neurofibrosarcomas) are highly cellular neoplasms in which mitotic figures, necrosis, and pseudopalisading are common. MPNST may frequently be found embedded within benign plexiform tumors, which presumably represent malignant degeneration of a single portion of the tumor. Schwannomas are rarely seen in NF1 patients, and the finding of a schwannoma by an experienced pathologist should be a reason for diagnostic re-evaluation.

Pilocytic astrocytomas, though less commonly seen in NF1 patients than neurofibromas, are also closely associated with NF1. Elongated fusiform cells with coarse fibrillary cytoplasmic processes characterize pilocytic astrocytomas. Although they may appear in any part of the brain, pilocytic astrocytomas show a preference for the optic nerve, chiasm, and tract and the adjacent hypothalamus. NF1 patients are also at risk for higher-grade gliomas of the brain stem and cortex, pheochromocytoma, and chronic myelogenous leukemia in childhood. The pathology of these tumors is not known to differ from that of the sporadic forms.

Molecular Genetics

The *NF1* locus on chromosome 17 is large, covering 335 kilobase pairs of genomic DNA on 60 exons. Numerous *NF1* homologous loci scattered throughout the human genome are considered to represent unprocessed pseudogenes.[2,3] More recently, a complex tandem duplication of a portion of the NF1 locus was detected adjacent to the gene itself, further complicating the molecular biology of NF1.[4] The *NF1* message has an open reading frame of 8454 base pairs. Based on sequence similarity and functional studies, the NF1 protein product has a GTPase activating domain (GAP) that functions to silence the proto-oncogene RAS. In addition, at least 85% of highly conserved *NF1* sequence lies outside of the GAP-related domain and may have other roles, including modulation of adenyl cyclase activity and microtubule binding. To date, there is no evidence of locus heterogeneity among patients meeting clinical criteria for NF1.

Several investigators have reported the mutational basis of NF1 in typical NF1 patients. In general, the large size and unwieldy structure of the *NF1* gene have hampered these studies. Studies using exon scanning technology complemented by a tiered approach of fluorescent in-situ hybridization, Southern blot analysis, and chromosomal analysis have shown that it is technically possible to detect truncating mutations in 80% to 90% of patients meeting clinical criteria.[5,6] These and other studies show that *NF1* has no hot spot of mutability and that most unrelated kindreds carry private mutations. Mutational studies have not identified any genotype-phenotype relationships for NF1, with the single exception that deletions of the entire gene are associated with a more severe phenotype. Specifically, large-deletion patients have more cutaneous neurofibromas at any given age, and a higher degree of dysmorphism, mental retardation, and cardiovascular anomalies than NF1 patients in general.[7] It is not yet clear if deletion of flanking elements causes this phenotype, or if other intragenic factors play a role.

The demonstration of *NF1* mutations or "second hits" in NF1-related tumors is essential to prove that *NF1* is a true tumor-suppressor gene. Like the detection of germline mutations, this work has been technically difficult.[8] A complicating factor in mutational analysis of these benign tumors is their heterogeneous pathologic composition, including Schwann cells, fibroblastic elements, vascular structures, and mast cells. This wide histologic spectrum seems unlikely to arise from a single progenitor cell. Several workers have thus hypothesized that NF1 acts as a tumor suppressor in a single cell, which then both proliferates and recruits other heterozygous or wild-type elements into the tumor. Supporting this hypothesis, when the Schwannian and fibroblastic components of benign tumors are cultured separately, loss of NF1 can be demonstrated at a genomic, messenger RNA, or protein level in the Schwann cells, but not in the fibroblasts.[9]

Animal Models

Two groups have explored an NF1 mouse model in detail (reviewed in reference 10). Mice heterozygous for null *NF1* mutations are predisposed to a number of malignancies including pheochromocytomas and myeloid leukemia, but they do not develop neurofibromas or other nerve sheath tumors. Interestingly, they also display specific learning deficits that can be rescued by genetic and pharmacologic manipulations that decrease Ras function.[11] Mice homozygous for null *NF1* mutations die at gestational day 14. A number of provocative models to facilitate nerve sheath tumor formation have been created. In the first model, chimeric mice were created by the injection of null *NF1* embryonic stem cells into wild-type blastocysts. These mice uniformly developed neurofibromas in the NF1-/-subpopulation of cells, many of which arose from the dorsal root ganglia and had a prominent schwannian NF1-/-component. In the second model, mice heterozygous for null *NF1* alleles were crossed with mice heterozygous for null alleles at the *p53* tumor suppressor gene. Because *p53* and *NF1* lie on the same mouse chromosome, this model could be created in a trans or cis configuration. As would be expected, the double heterozygous mice showed a greater predisposition to

tumors and shortened life span then either single heterozygote alone. In addition, the cis double heterozygote was affected to a greater degree then the trans, and frequently developed malignant peripheral nerve sheath tumors similar to those seen in human NF1 patients. In a third approach, a conditional (cre/lox) allele confirmed that loss of *NF1* in the Schwann cell lineage is a key event in the generation of tumors, but also demonstrated the need for a permissive haploinsufficient environment to allow expression of the neurofibroma phenotype.[12] These mouse models will undoubtedly prove invaluable in the development of therapeutics for NF1-related tumors.

Therapy

Therapy for NF1 remains primarily surgical. Biopsy can be reserved for lesions that are rapidly growing or otherwise suspicious for malignancy. PET scan may be helpful in defining areas of malignant degeneration within large plexiform lesions.[13] Spinal tumors should be resected only when they produce progressive neurologic symptoms, with or without radiographic progression. Many patients request plastic surgery intervention for cutaneous tumors, especially in later adulthood. Plastic surgery may also be helpful for large deforming plexiform tumors. Complex and repeated surgical interventions are often best accomplished in a multidisciplinary neurofibromatosis center. Two excellent patient-support groups exist, providing educational brochures, patient-to-patient contact, and lay and professional conferences (the National Neurofibromatosis Foundation, available at http://www.nf.org/ and NF, Inc, available at http://www.nfinc.org//).

TUBEROUS SCLEROSIS COMPLEX

Clinical Features and Diagnostic Evaluation

Tuberous sclerosis complex (TSC) is an extremely variable disease, with frequent involvement of skin and nervous system, and less consistent involvement of lung, kidneys, and other organ systems. Patients often come to attention on the basis of cutaneous lesions (Fig. 50–4). Facial angiofibromas (adenoma sebaceum) are hamartomatous nodules with vascular and connective tissue elements and are seen in 75% of patients. Typically, the lesions begin during the preschool years as a few small red papules on the malar region, which may be confused with acne. The lesions gradually become larger and more numerous, sometimes extending down the nasolabial folds or onto the chin. Similar lesions may be seen in multiple endocrine neoplasia type I, leading to diagnostic confusion.[14] The Shagreen patch, usually found on the back or flank area, is an irregularly shaped, slightly raised or textured skin lesion measuring several centimeters in

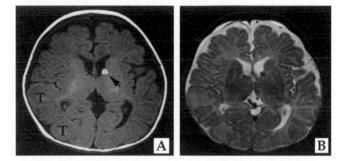

FIGURE 50–5. Cranial imaging in TSC. Typical imaging findings, including subependymal nodules *(arrow)* and cortical tubers *(T)*. *A,* Contrast enhanced T1-weighted image. *B,* T2-weighted image. (From MacCollin M: Tuberous sclerosis complex. In Aminoff M, Daroff R [eds]: Encyclopedia of the Neurological Sciences. San Diego, Academic Press, in press).

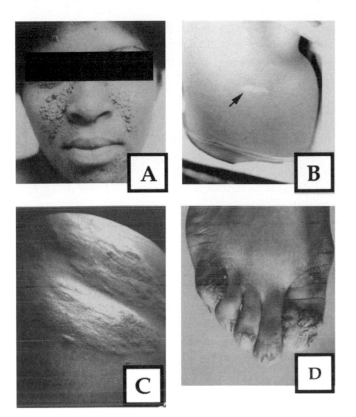

FIGURE 50–4. Cutaneous manifestations of TSC. *A,* Facial angiofibromas (adenoma sebaceum). *B,* Hypomelanotic macule *(ash leaf spot)* best seen with ultraviolet illumination. *C,* Shagreen patch. *D,* Ungual fibromas. (From ES Roach: Diagnosis and management of neurocutaneous syndromes. Semin Neurol 1988;8:83.)

diameter and is seen in about 25% of patients. Similar lesions may be found on the scalp or forehead. Ungual fibromas are nodular or fleshy lesions that arise adjacent to or from underneath the nails in about 20% of adult patients.

Neurologic involvement frequently is the cause of greatest morbidity in TSC patients. About 80% of patients have seizures at some point in their lives, most commonly infantile spasms (often progressing to Lennox Gastaut syndrome) and tonic-clonic seizures. Frequently, older children and adults evolve into a pattern of complex partial or other focal seizures. Slightly over 50% of TSC patients have significant developmental delay and mental retardation. Additionally, 50% of patients have autism or autism spectrum disorder with or without mental retardation. Other frequent neurologic and psychiatric manifestations include hyperactivity, aggressiveness, sleep disturbance, and frank psychosis. Since many mildly affected TSC patients may not be identified and thus included in natural history studies of the disease, the true frequency of these problems may be overestimated in the medical literature.

Neuroimaging studies are frequently abnormal in TSC patients (Fig. 50–5). Imaging findings include subependymal glial nodules (seen in 90% of patients) and cortical or subcortical tubers (seen in 70% of patients). Most lesions are nonprogressive, but subependymal giant cell astrocytomas (SEGA) develop de novo or from existing subependymal nodules in 6% to 14% of patients. Interestingly, despite the extent of brain involvement with TSC, spinal cord lesions are rarely encountered.

A wide variety of other organ systems are affected by TSC. Renal lesions are a major cause of morbidity and mortality, with 80% of patients developing benign angiomyolipomas or cysts. Less then 1% of such lesions progress to malignancy, but hemorrhage in benign lesions and replacement of normal renal tissue may lead to fatal renal failure even without transformation. Cardiac rhabdomyomas are present in about 50% of patients at or before birth, but regress spontaneously in the neonatal period. Lymphangiomyomatosis of the lung is a rare but potentially fatal complication, which affects women between ages 20 and 40 years. Because sudden pneumothorax and chylothorax may occur, screening of asymptomatic women should be considered. Finally, ocular lesions may be of diagnostic utility, but are rarely symptomatic and include hamartomas and achromatic patches.

TSC is an autosomal dominant disorder with variable expressivity and a birth prevalence of about 1:12,000. Although the issue of incomplete penetrance has not been totally resolved, it is unlikely to find a completely asymptomatic full carrier of mutation. More than 50% of cases are due to new mutations and patients have clinically unaffected parents, who are molecularly normal. TSC shows great intrafamilial heterogeneity, with relatives having widely different clinical courses.

Initial evaluation of a patient known or suspected to have TSC should include detailed skin and neurologic examination, ophthalmologic evaluation with slit lamp, cranial imaging study (either contrast-enhanced CT or MRI), and renal ultrasound. Chest x-ray or CT may be performed in young adult women and cardiac ultrasound in neonates if symptoms are present. Neuropsychiatric evaluation is indicated for children with developmental delay, school performance problems, or a history of behavioral difficulties in home or school. Because TSC may be extremely variable within families, and because some patients have very few manifestations, it is often necessary to screen parents and other relatives of an infant or child with known TSC to determine their status and genetic risks. Criteria for the diagnosis of TSC have been formulated, based on natural history studies and imaging findings in large numbers of patients (Table 50–2). Because TSC is extremely variable in its manifestations, diagnosis may be difficult in mild cases, leaving patients with the uncomfortable label of "probable or possible TSC." Once a diagnosis is established, subsequent follow-up should include anticipatory guidance and genetic counseling for families at all stages of disease. Children with TSC should have an annual neurologic and developmental assessment. Cranial imaging to exclude the development of SEGA should be repeated every 12 to 18 months to age 18 years. Renal ultrasound should be performed annually throughout life. Symptomatic patients may require additional follow-up, including ocular examination, renal function tests, chest CT, or other imaging studies. Neurologically, many patients will have difficult-to-control seizure disorders, or behavioral problems, which may be best managed in a multidisciplinary TSC clinic.

Pathology

Several types of brain lesions characterize TSC. Cortical tubers are composed of astroglial elements and small stellate neurons and are best categorized as hamartomas. Subependymal nodules of TSC are most often found in the anterior portions of the lateral ventricles. These nodules are made up of glial and vascular elements and in time accumulate the dense calcium deposits that identify them radiographically. Some of the lesions contain large cells similar to those of the less common giant-cell astrocytoma. Many patients have grossly visible defects in the cerebral cortex, lesions that probably result from failure of neuronal migration during neocortical formation. Sometimes, islands of heterotopic gray matter or areas with little myelin formation underlie these cortical lesions. The appearance of the cortex between the cortical defects and tubers is generally normal, but subtle changes in the organizational pattern of the neurons and gliosis can often be demonstrated even in parts of the brain that are grossly normal.

Molecular Genetics

TSC exhibits locus heterogeneity with two causative loci on chromosome 9p34 *(TSC1)* and 16p13 *(TSC2)*. The *TSC1* gene codes for the protein hamartin, which is implicated in the organization of the actin cytoskeleton and the rho pathway of GTPase signaling. The *TSC2* gene codes for the protein tuberlin, which plays a role in rap1 and rab5 GTPase signaling. Hamartin and tuberlin have no significant sequence similarity, but have been shown to interact physically in vivo. It is not yet clear if these two loci account for all cases of TSC, or if other loci may cause a small number of cases.

TABLE 50–2. Diagnostic Criteria for Tuberous Sclerosis Complex (TSC)*

Major Features	Minor Features
Facial angiofibromas or forehead plaque	Dental pits
Nontraumatic ungual or periungual fibroma	Hamartomatous rectal polyps
Hypomelanotic macules (more then three)	Bone cysts
Shagreen patch	Cerebral white matter migration lines[†]
Multiple retinal nodular hamartomas	Gingival fibromas
Cortical tubers[†]	Nonrenal hamartoma
Subependymal nodule	Retinal achromatic patch
Subependymal giant-cell astrocytoma	"Confetti" skin lesions
Cardiac rhabdomyoma	Multiple renal cysts
Lymphangiomyomatosis[‡]	
Renal angiomyolipoma[‡]	

Definite TSC requires either two major features or one major and two minor features.

Probable TSC requires one major feature and one minor feature.

Possible TSC requires either one major feature or two or more minor features.

*Adapted from Roach ES, Gomez MR, Northrup H: Tuberous Sclerosis Complex Consensus Conference: Revised clinical diagnostic criteria. J Chil Neurol 1998; 13:624–628.
†When cortical tubers and cerebral white matter migration tracts occur together, they are counted as one feature.
‡When lymphangiomyomatosis and renal angiomyolipoma occur together, they are counted as one feature.

Several studies have explored the spectrum and frequency of mutations in *TSC1* and *TSC2*.[15] *TSC2* mutations account for about 85% of all cases, and appear to cause slightly more severe disease than *TSC1* mutations. Mosaicism is relatively common in expressing founders, many of whom do not meet clinical criteria and most of whom do not have mental retardation.[16] Low-level mosaicism may also contribute to the 10% of TSC patients in whom no mutation can be identified in unaffected tissues such as blood. The finding of "second hits" in TSC-derived kidney lesions has confirmed that the *TSC* genes act as true tumor suppressors.[17] However, equivalent studies have not consistently documented second inactivating events in cortical lesions, leaving open the possibility that haploinsufficiency may not be a sufficient genetic determinant for these lesions. Mutations in the *TSC2* gene in the LAM cells of sporadically affected patients (without TSC) have been documented, and comparison with angiomyolipomas suggest that LAM results from migration of smooth muscle cells from renal angiomyolipomas to the lung.[18]

Animal Models

In addition to the long-standing Eker rat model of TSC2, two independently derived knockout mice have been developed.[19,20] Mice null for either locus die around embryonic day 10. Heterozygotes develop a wide range of predominantly benign renal and extrarenal tumors, similar to human patients with TSC. Recapitulation of the CNS phenotype is less clear. *Drosophila melanogaster* homologues of both *TSC1* and *TSC2* have been identified. Homozygous null mutations in *TSC2* cause lethality in embryos and a phenotype termed *gigas* in the eye in which eye cells differentiate normally but continue to replicate their DNA without cell division, resulting in enlarged cells.

Therapy

Therapy for TSC remains symptomatic. The cutaneous lesions may cause great cosmetic discomfort. Laser ablation of facial angiofibromas and forehead plaques may be of benefit. Most retinal lesions are also asymptomatic, and only rarely require intervention. Management of seizure disorders and personality and behavioral disturbances often become the major issue for TSC patients and families. Multidisciplinary clinics that include specialists in epilepsy, behavior management, and family dynamics are often needed. The National Tuberous Sclerosis Foundation (http://www.tsalliance.org/) is an excellent patient support group providing educational brochures and patient-to-patient contact.

OTHER PHAKOMATOSES

Von Hippel-Lindau Disease

Patients with von Hippel-Lindau disease (VHL) develop a number of histologically similar tumors throughout life; neurologic involvement includes the central nervous system, eye, and inner ear. Central nervous system hemangioblastomas are seen in approximately 66% of patients. These benign tumors of mixed cell type primarily occur in the spinal cord and cerebellum (Fig. 50–6). Criteria for the diagnosis of VHL have been formulated, based on natural history observations and molecular studies of at-risk families (Table 50–3). VHL is an autosomal dominant disorder with variable expression that has a birth prevalence of about 1:36,000. Mutational analysis of the VHL gene has allowed detection of a wide range of germline and somatic alterations in typical patients and patient-derived tumor material, and has confirmed its action as a true tumor-suppressor gene. About 20% of patients carry large germline deletions, and most remaining patients have point mutations detectable using exon scanning methods.[21] The pVHL tumor-suppressor protein participates in an intracellular multiprotein complex that targets substrate proteins for ubiquitination and proteasome-dependent degradation.

Xeroderma Pigmentosum

Xeroderma pigmentosum (XP) is a recessive family of conditions involving cellular defects in the ability to process DNA damage. Clinical manifestations include skin photosensitivity, irregular pigmentation of skin, skin cancer (squamous cell carcinoma, basal cell carcinoma, and malignant melanoma), conjunctival scarring, and exposure keratitis. Neurologically, patients exhibit a neurodegenerative phenotype that includes ataxia, choreoathetosis, spasticity, and progressive dementia. XP is due to mutations in nucleotide excision repair genes, which also causes Cockayne syndrome.[22]

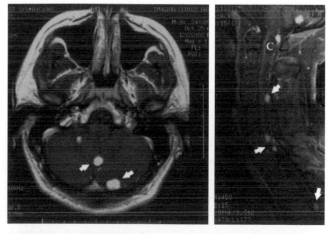

FIGURE 50–6. Imaging findings in VHL. Typical imaging findings in a patient with VHL include both cysts (C) and enhancing tumors in the cerebellum and cervical spine (*arrows*). Contrast-enhanced T1-weighted images. (From MacCollin M: Von Hippel-Lindau disease. In Aminoff M, Daroff R [eds]: Encyclopedia of the Neurological Sciences. San Diego, Academic Press, in press).

TABLE 50–3. Diagnostic Criteria for von Hippel-Lindau Disease (VHL)*

Without Family History of VHL	*With Family History of VHL*
Two or more hemangioblastomas	Single hemangioblastoma
OR	OR
Single hemangiomblastoma	Two of the following:
AND	Renal cell carcinoma
one of the following:	
Multifocal renal cyst	Pheochromocytoma
Renal cell carcinoma	Pancreatic carcinoma
Pheochromocytoma	Epididymal cystadenoma†
	Pancreatic or renal cysts

*Adapted from Seizinger BR, Smith DI, Filling-Katz MR, et al: Genetic flanking markers refine diagnostic criteria and provide insights into the genetics of von Hippel–Lindau disease. Proc Natl Acad Sci USA 1991; 88: 2864–2868 (Strict application of these criteria will not identify all patients/kindreds with VHL, for example, those with familial pheochromocytoma alone).
†Requires pathological diagnosis

Sturge Weber Syndrome

Sturge Weber syndrome consists of a malformation of the capillaries and venules of the leptomeninges (Fig. 50–7). Overlying facial involvement is limited to the area supplied by the first branch of the trigeminal nerve, termed a "port wine stain." Seizures, mental retardation, hemiparesis, glaucoma, and homonymous hemianopia are common. The molecular genetic basis of the disease is unknown, and patients are always sporadic.

Neurofibromatosis 2

Neurofibromatosis 2 (NF2) is an uncommon autosomal dominant disorder that causes benign nervous system tumors, including schwannomas, meningiomas, ependymomas, and astrocytomas. All NF2 patients develop bilateral vestibular schwannomas and become deaf if not treated. Ocular manifestations include cataract and retinal hamartoma. NF2 patients develop cutaneous schwannomas that may be quite subtle and can be easily distinguished from the cutaneous neurofibromas of NF1

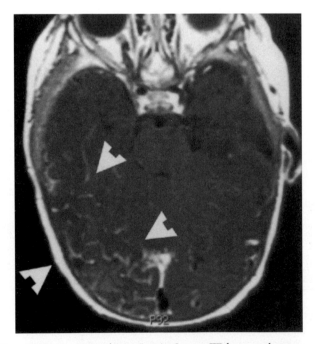

FIGURE 50–7. Cranial imaging in Sturge Weber syndrome. Abnormal leptomeningeal enhancement in the right occipital lobe extending into the right temporal lobe (arrowheads). T1-weighted contrast-enhanced image.

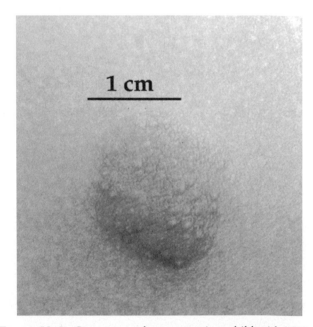

FIGURE 50–8. Cutaneous schwannoma in a child with NF2. Cutaneous tumors can be an important diagnostic clue in children at risk for NF2 as they may be seen well before age 5 years. As contrasted with the cutaneous neurofibromas seen in Figure 50–1B, cutaneous schwannomas are often quite subtle.

patients (Fig. 50–8). The *NF2* gene on chromosome 22 has been shown to act as a true tumor suppressor with "second hits" in both sporadic and NF2-associated schwannomas, meningiomas, and ependymomas. The NF2 protein product is a member of the protein 4.1 family of cytoskeletal elements, and likely functions in communication of extracellular growth signaling pathways to the spectrin/actin cytoskeleton.[24]

REFERENCES

1. Woodruff JM: Pathology of tumors of the peripheral nerve sheath in type 1 neurofibromatosis. Am J Med Genet 1999;89:23–30.

2. Luijten M, Redeker S, Minoshima S, et al: Duplication and transposition of the NF1 pseudogene regions on chromosomes 2, 14, and 22. Hum Genet 2001; 109:109–116.

3. Cummings LM, Trent JM, Marchuk DA: Identification and mapping of type 1 neurofibromatosis (NF1) homologous loci. Cytogenet Cell Genet 1996;73: 334–340.

4. Gervasini C, Bentivegna A, Venturin M, et al: Tandem duplication of the NF1 gene detected by high-resolution FISH in the 17q11.2 region. Hum Genet 2002; 110:314–321.

5. Fahsold R, Hoffmeyer S, Mischung C, et al: Minor lesion mutational spectrum of the entire NF1 gene does not explain its high mutability but points to a functional domain upstream of the GAP-related domain. Am J Hum Genet 2000;66:790–818.

6. Messiaen LM, Callens T, Mortier G, et al: Exhaustive mutation analysis of the NF1 gene allows identification of 95% of mutations and reveals a high frequency of unusual splicing defects. Hum Mutat 2000; 15:541–555.

7. Riva P, Corrado L, Natacci F, et al: NF1 microdeletion syndrome: Refined FISH characterization of sporadic and familial deletions with locus-specific probes. Am J Hum Genet 2000;66:100–109.

8. Serra E, Ars E, Ravella A, et al: Somatic NF1 mutational spectrum in benign neurofibromas: mRNA splice defects are common among point mutations. Hum Genet 2001;108:416–429.

9. Rutkowski JL, Wu K, Gutmann DH, et al: Genetic and cellular defects contributing to benign tumor formation in neurofibromatosis type 1. Hum Mol Genet 2000;9:1059–1066.

10. Gutmann DH, Giovannini M: Mouse models of neurofibromatosis 1 and 2. Neoplasia 2002;4: 279–290.

11. Costa RM, Federov NB, Kogan JH, et al: Mechanism for the learning deficits in a mouse model of neurofibromatosis type 1. Nature 2002;415:526–530.

12. Zhu Y, Ghosh P, Charnay P, et al: Neurofibromas in NF1: Schwann cell origin and role of tumor environment. Science 2002;296:920–922.

13. Ferner RE, Lucas JD, O'Doherty MJ, et al: Evaluation of (18) fluorodeoxyglucose positron emission tomography [(18) FDG PET] in the detection of malignant peripheral nerve sheath tumors arising from within plexiform neurofibromas in neurofibromatosis 1. J Neurol Neurosurg Psychiatr 2000;68: 353–357.

14. Darling TN, Skarulis MC, Steinberg SM, et al: Multiple facial angiofibromas and collagenomas in patients with multiple endocrine neoplasia type 1. Arch Dermatol 1997;133:853–857.

15. Dabora SL, Jozwiak S, Franz DN, et al: Mutational analysis in a cohort of 224 tuberous sclerosis patients indicates increased severity of TSC2, compared with TSC1, disease in multiple organs. Am J Hum Genet 2001;68:64–80.

16. Verhoef S, Bakker L, Tempelaars AM, et al: High rate of mosaicism in tuberous sclerosis complex. Am J Hum Genet 1999;64:1632–1637.

17. Niida Y, Stemmer-Rachamimov AO, Logrip M, et al: Survey of somatic mutations in tuberous sclerosis complex (TSC) hamartomas suggests different genetic mechanisms for pathogenesis of TSC lesions. Am J Hum Genet 2001;69:493–503.

18. Yu J, Astrinidis A, Henske EP: Chromosome 16 loss of heterozygosity in tuberous sclerosis and sporadic lymphangiomyomatosis. Am J Respir Crit Care Med 2001;164:1537–1540.

19. Onda H, Lueck A, Marks PW, et al: Tsc2(+/-) mice develop tumors in multiple sites that express gelsolin and are influenced by genetic background. J Clin Invest 1999;104:687–695.

20. Kobayashi T, Minowa O, Sugitani Y, et al: A germ-line Tsc1 mutation causes tumor development and embryonic lethality that are similar, but not identical to, those caused by Tsc2 mutation in mice. Proc Natl Acad Sci U S A 2001;98:8762–8767.

21. Stolle C, Glenn G, Zbar B, et al: Improved detection of germline mutations in the von Hippel-Lindau disease tumor suppressor gene. Hum Mutat 1998;12; 417–423.

22. Cleaver JE, Thompson LH, Richardson AS, States JCA: Summary of mutations in the UV-sensitive disorders: Xeroderma pigmentosum, Cockayne syndrome, and trichothiodystrophy. Hum Mutat 1999;14:9–22.

23. Gusella JF, Ramesh V, MacCollin M, Jacoby LB: Merlin: The neurofibromatosis 2 tumor suppressor. Biochem Biophys Acta 1999;1423:M29–M36.

24. Gautreau A, Louvard D, Arpin M: ERM proteins and NF2 tumor suppressor: The Yin and Yang of cortical actin organization and cell growth signaling. Curr Opin Cell Biol 2002;14:104–109.

25. Gutmann DH, Aylsworth A, Carey JC, et al: The diagnostic evaluation and multidisciplinary management of neurofibromatosis 1 and neurofibromatosis 2. JAMA 1997;278:51–57.

26. Roach ES, Gomez MR, Northrup H: Tuberous sclerosis complex consensus conference: Revised clinical diagnostic criteria. J Child Neurol 1998;13: 624–628.

27. Seizinger BR, Smith DI, Filling-Katz MR, et al: Genetic flanking markers refine diagnostic criteria and provide insights into the genetics of von Hippel Lindau disease. Proc Natl Acad Sci U S A 1991;88: 2864–2868.

CHAPTER

51

Lipoprotein Disorders

Mary J. Malloy

John P. Kane

The system of lipoproteins that transports lipids in plasma also interacts with neural tissue. The transport of antioxidant tocopherols is critically dependent on lipoproteins of intestinal and hepatic origin that contain the B apolipoproteins (apoproteins). Severe impairment of absorption of tocopherols by the intestine occurs in disorders including abetalipoproteinemia (ABL), and in chylomicron retention disease in which intestinal apo B-48 cannot be secreted normally. The second phase of tocopherol transport, from liver to peripheral tissues, is impaired in disorders in which hepatic secretion of apo B-100 is defective. In recessive ABL resulting from mutations in the microsomal triglyceride transport protein, little or no apo B-100–containing lipoprotein is secreted, reflecting defects in the assembly and movement of nascent lipoproteins within the hepatocyte. Hypobetalipoproteinemia (HBL) frequently results from mutations that lead to truncation of the apo B-100 protein. Truncated products, less than apo B-31 in length, cannot be secreted. The neuropathologic features common to these disorders are attributable to the accumulation of oxidized lipids in myelin, leading to peripheral neuropathy and degeneration of posterior columns and spinocerebellar tracts.

Other disorders of lipoproteins that lead to impairment of the centripetal movement of cholesterol and phospholipids with accumulation of abnormal lipoproteins in plasma, including Tangier disease and deficiency of lecithin-cholesterol acyl transferase (LCAT), can cause peripheral neuropathy. In Tangier disease, a syringomyelia-like syndrome has also been observed.

Several apoproteins are synthesized in the CNS, and others distribute there passively. Some of these play important roles in the sequestration and retrieval of lipids during the regeneration of injured neural tissue. Beta amyloid protein is associated with high-density lipoprotein (HDL) complexes in cerebrospinal fluid and in plasma.

The relationships so far identified between disorders of lipoprotein metabolism and dysfunction of nerve tissue are chiefly the consequences of alterations in lipid constituents of the neuron and its intimate environment. Notable among these are disorders in which an increase in oxidative modification of lipids takes place owing to impaired transport of tocopherol to nerve tissue. Also recognized are disorders of cholesteryl ester metabolism and of the normal centripetal flux of free cholesterol and certain phospholipids. Several apoproteins and the Lp(a) protein are found in CNS tissue or in cerebrospinal fluid. Apoproteins E, D, J, H, and L are expressed in brain in substantial quantities, and the E, D, and J proteins play important roles in the response of nerve tissue to injury. Apoproteins A-I and A-IV that passively enter the CNS may also contribute to lipid transport and remyelination of nerves. Circulating lipoproteins also play a role in the delivery of omega-3 fatty acids to brain. As the complexities of the lipoprotein system unfold, it is likely that further disorders will be revealed in which alterations of apoprotein or lipoprotein metabolism affect the functions of the central or peripheral nervous system.

LIPOPROTEIN STRUCTURE AND METABOLISM

The lipid components of most plasma lipoproteins are organized as spherical microemulsions, with varying proportions of the relatively hydrophobic triglycerides and cholesteryl esters in the cores and the amphipathic phospholipids and unesterified cholesterol arrayed in mixed surface monolayers. The protein constituents of lipoproteins, consisting of a number of discrete apoprotein species, are primarily located at the amphipathic monolayer.

The proteins of the lipoprotein system fall into several distinct groups. These include high molecular weight B apoproteins. Apo B-100, found in very-low-density lipoproteins (VLDL) and lipoproteins derived from VLDL (intermediate- and low-density lipoproteins, IDL and LDL) has a molecular weight of 512 kDa. Apo B-48, secreted by the intestine in chylomicrons, is a product of the apo B gene but is truncated by RNA editing to yield the N-terminal 48% of apo B sequence. Other apoproteins are much smaller, and transfer among lipoprotein particles.

The B apoproteins contain clusters of basic amino acids that bind to heparin, and a ligand domain for the LDL receptor. A number of naturally occurring truncations of apoprotein B are recognized that produce abnormal lipoproteins and that frequently lead to abnormally low levels of VLDL and LDL.[1]

Among the small exchangeable apoproteins, apo A-I is the chief protein of HDL; apo E has affinity for heparin and for the LDL receptor; others modulate lipoprotein metabolism.

Transport of Dietary Lipid

Ingested triglycerides are hydrolyzed in the intestine by pancreatic lipase in the presence of a protein colipase and bile acids. The β monoglycerides and free fatty acids thus formed are absorbed, and triglyceride resynthesis takes place within the enterocyte. Some of the cholesterol absorbed, along with some synthesized de novo, is esterified in the enterocyte by an acylCoA acyltransferase (ACAT). Apo B-48 is synthesized within the enterocyte. Association of B-48 with developing microemulsion particles in the endoplasmic reticulum is mediated by a heterodimeric protein that includes the triglyceride transport protein and a protein disulfide isomerase (MTT-PDI).[2] These particles are secreted via the Golgi apparatus into the lymph spaces. Lipoprotein lipase, situated on capillary endothelium, hydrolyzes up to 80% of the triglyceride content of the particles. As hydrolysis progresses, surface components, including apoproteins A-I, A-II, A-IV, and the C proteins, plus some of the surface lipids, move from the particles to HDL. The apo B-48-containing particle that results is termed a remnant. Chylomicron remnants are removed quantitatively by interaction with LDL receptors and LRP receptors on hepatocytes.

Transport of Endogenous Triglycerides

Triglycerides are formed in the liver from fatty acids derived from lipolysis in adipose tissue and from de novo

synthesis. One copy of apo B-100, synthesized in the rough endoplasmic reticulum, joins a growing microemulsion particle as it progresses through the smooth endoplasmic reticulum to the Golgi, catalyzed by MTT-PDI. Small amounts of C apoproteins, apo E, and (probably) A-I and A-II are added before the particle is secreted from the Golgi to the blood. Again, lipolysis mediated by lipoprotein lipase produces remnants. In this case, they contain apo B-100 and apo E but have lost most of the smaller apoproteins and surface lipid to HDL.[1] This transfer appears to require the activity of phospholipid transfer protein. In normal humans, about 50% of VLDL remnants are endocytosed in the liver by a receptor-mediated process involving interaction of apo E with the LDL receptor. The remaining remnants lose more triglycerides, via the action of hepatic triglyceridase, and also lose apo E, evolving into LDL. During lipolysis, a conformational change occurs in apo B-100, in which the ligand domain for the LDL receptor is conformed. LDL catabolism then proceeds through endocytosis via the LDL receptor and endosomal hydrolysis of cholesteryl esters.

Formation of High-Density Lipoproteins and Centripetal Transport

HDL are formed from lipids effluxed from cell membranes and from lipids of the surface monolayers of triglyceride-rich lipoproteins that are shed during lipolysis. Efflux of phospholipid and cholesterol from cell membranes is effected by the ATP-dependent transporter ABCA-1, with a small HDL particle (prebeta-1 HDL) as acceptor (Fig. 51–1). The cholesterol is esterified by LCAT (which is also found in CSF). The particles organize into large complexes of 250 to 450 kDa. Cholesteryl esters are transferred from mature HDL to liver by two mechanisms: (1) they are transferred to apo-B–containing lipoproteins for eventual uptake in liver, mediated by cholesteryl ester transfer protein (CETP), and (2) they can be taken up directly from HDL by SR-BI receptors on hepatocytes.

Apoproteins in the Nervous System

The realization that apoproteins play direct roles in the sequestration and intercellular transfer of lipid in the CNS and in peripheral nerves presented itself with the discovery that apo E is expressed in brain. Furthermore, the content of apo E in cerebrospinal fluid is higher than would be expected for an ultrafiltered protein. Apo E has been detected immunochemically in association with all forms of astrocytes[3] in a perinuclear distribution, associated with the Golgi, and with cell processes that end on the pia or at blood vessels. Apo E is associated with the glia of peripheral nerves, including visceral nerves. It is absent from neurons, oligodendroglia, and other cell types. Astrocytes and microglia

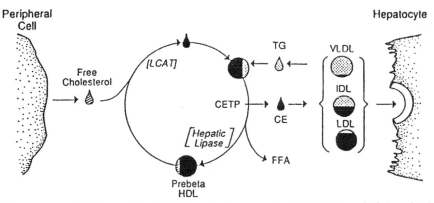

FIGURE 51–1. Centripetal transport of cholesterol by high-density lipoproteins (HDL). Free cholesterol *(shaded areas)* is acquired from cells by pre-β HDL species and is esterified by lecithin:cholesterol acyl transferase. Passage of cholesteryl esters *(black areas)* to acceptor lipoproteins is mediated by cholesteryl ester transfer protein. The liver takes up a portion of remnant (intermediate-density) lipoproteins and low-density lipoproteins (LDL). Some triglycerides *(stippled areas)* transfer from very low-density lipoproteins (VLDL) and intermediate-density lipoproteins (IDL) to HDL species, where they are hydrolyzed in part by hepatic lipase. Some HDL particles deliver cholesterol to the liver directly via the SR-BI receptor.

secrete apo E.[4–6] During experimental demyelination, apo E appears to be secreted by macrophages that enter the tissue. Several classes of lipoprotein complexes exist in CSF. Apo D, apo J, and apo H (β 2 glycoprotein I) are synthesized in the brain in addition to apo E.[7–10] Apo A-I, A-II, and A-IV enter the CSF by a process of transcytosis that is poorly understood. The total lipid content of CSF is between 1 and 2 mg/dL, primarily cholesterol and phospholipids. The principal species of CSF lipoprotein contains apoproteins E, A-I, D, H, and J, possibly functioning in the redistribution of lipids.[11] A minor particle population contains all of these except apo A-I. Another contains only apo A-I and A-II. Beta amyloid binds to apo E containing lipoprotein complexes in CSF. The E2 and E3 isoforms appear to form these complexes more readily than does E4. A number of enzymes and transfer proteins that can modify lipoproteins are found in the brain and may play important roles in lipid transfer there.[12] Lipoprotein lipase (LPL) is among these.[13,14] Though fatty acids are not an energy substrate in brain, LPL may be critical to the delivery of omega-3 fatty acids to the CNS. The bulk of apo A-IV is carried on larger particles. The quantity of apo A-IV in CSF increases after a fat-rich meal where it appears to function as a satiety signal. When infused into rat brains, even without associated lipids, it results in decreased food intake. It also appears to influence gastric acid secretion. LDL receptors have been identified on pial cells of the arachnoid and on astrocytes. The LRP receptor has been identified on the cell bodies and proximal processes of cerebral cortical neurons.[15] These findings support the potential importance of apoprotein-mediated lipid transport in the CNS. The apo E in the CSF was found to be in a more highly sialated state than that in plasma, which is chiefly of hepatic origin. In contrast to the small apoproteins, virtually no apo B is normally detectable in CSF. The

mRNA for apoprotein(a) has been detected in the CNS of Rhesus monkeys. It is not yet known whether this protein exists in complexes or in a molecular dispersion in the nervous system.

Studies on regenerating and remyelinating peripheral nerves have revealed a massive increase in local synthesis of apo E.[3] Synthesis of apo D also takes place in injured nerves. It appears to originate from astrocytes and oligodendrocytes in the CNS and from neurolemma in peripheral nerves.[10,16] Both apo A-I and A-IV appear in increased amounts in injured nerves. A model is emerging that involves apoproteins in the stabilization and intercellular transfer of lipids derived from degenerating nerve membranes and nerve sheaths. It is likely that apo E is involved in the storage of lipids, via the LDL receptor, in anticipation of remyelination.

Tocopherols

Tocopherols as Biologic Antioxidants

Tocopherols (vitamin E) have been shown to break free radical chains efficiently because the tocopheroxyl radical is extremely stable. This radical can then annihilate another peroxyl radical. Free radical chain reactions in biologic systems are promoted by iron and copper, as is the oxidation of LDL. Pathologic states attributed to free radicals have been described in individuals suffering from iron overload. Antioxidant activity is attributable to species of HDL that contain transferrin and ceruloplasmin, respectively. These complexes inhibit the oxidation of LDL much more effectively than transferrin alone.

Other natural defenses against free radical chains include catalase, superoxide dismutases, paraoxonase, and glutathione peroxidase, which destroys hydroperoxides of fatty acids. Paraoxonase is carried partially in plasma as a lipoprotein complex with apo A-I and apo J.

Tocopherol Metabolism

Natural tocopherols differ with respect to substituents on the chromanol ring. The different arrays are termed α, β, γ, and δ. Of eight possible stereoisomeric arrangements of the isoprenoid side chain, the (2R, 4′R, 8′R) configuration is most potent. The side chain intercalates in lipid monolayers leading to accumulation in cell membranes and plasma lipoproteins.

    Bile acids and pancreatic enzymes are necessary for tocopherol absorption in the intestine. Ingested tocopherol appears rapidly in chylomicrons. Although some is transferred to tissues during lipolysis, most is endocytosed by liver in chylomicron remnants. It then appears in newly secreted VLDL. All isomers of tocopherol appear in chylomicrons, but the liver discriminates via a tocopherol transfer protein in favor of d,α-tocopherol when it secretes VLDL. Defects in the transfer protein lead to specific deficiency of tocopherol. During hydrolysis of VLDL triglycerides by lipoprotein lipase, transfer of tocopherol to HDL is mediated by phospholipid transfer protein. LDL formed by lipolysis of VLDL retains the bulk of the tocopherol. Residual tocopherol in LDL then enters cells as LDL is endocytosed. The decay of tocopherol in LDL corresponds with the disappearance of LDL protein. The tocopherol content of peripheral nerves and brain is depleted more slowly than that of other tissues. During depletion, tocopherol levels are partially sustained by efflux from adipocytes via the ABCA-1 transporter. Tissue levels of tocopherols are normal in rabbits lacking LDL receptors, probably attributable to transport of tocopherol from HDL to cells via the SR-B1 receptor. A tocopherol-binding protein widely distributed among tissues may play a critical role in uptake. Familial isolated vitamin E deficiency, a genetic disorder resulting in low tocopherol levels in plasma and tissues, appears to be caused by an inability of liver to secrete α-tocopherol efficiently in VLDL.[17]

Tocopherol Deficiency and Neurologic Disease

Tocopherol deficiency is restricted to conditions in which the transport of the vitamin is interrupted at some point between the intestine and affected tissues. Defects in lipid absorption at the intestinal level, owing to failure of secretion of apo B-48 (ABL) or other defects leading to steatorrhea, are predominant causes of deficiency. The appearance of tocopherol deficiency in normotriglyceridemic ABL in which chylomicron production is normal, and in the syndrome of isolated tocopherol deficiency,[18] indicates that defects farther along in the transport pathway can also result in deficiency.

    The neuropathology of ABL is generally representative of that encountered in tocopherol deficiencies of diverse etiology such as cholestasis and severe fat malabsorption. It includes axonal dystrophy in the posterior columns and in the dorsal and ventral spinocerebellar tracts.[19] Loss of large-caliber myelinated axons is widespread in peripheral sensory nerves (Fig. 51–2). In keeping with excess free radical generation, there is an accumulation of lipofuscin in the Schwann cell cytoplasm of peripheral nerves and in dorsal neurons. Positron emission tomography has demonstrated impaired binding of dopa to both the putamen and caudate in ABL, resembling that observed in Parkinson's disease. Also, studies of mazindol binding reveal a decrease in dopamine terminals in the striatum of tocopherol-deficient rats, further supporting

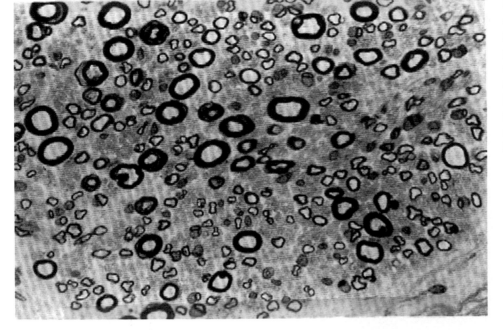

FIGURE 51–2. Abetalipoproteinemia. Section of a sural nerve from a 14-year-old patient with homozygous abetalipoproteinemia showing a marked decrease in the numbers of large-caliber myelinated neurons. (From Sokol R: Vitamin E and neurologic function in man. Free Radic Biol Med 1989;6:189.)

an impact on nigrostriatal function. Electrophysiologic studies demonstrate diminished amplitudes of sensory nerve action potentials with little delayed conduction velocity. Somatosensory-evoked potential studies reveal a central delay in sensory conduction consistent with deficits in function of the posterior columns. A parallel defect is observed in visual evoked potentials. Tocopherol may play a vital role in the embryologic development of the nervous system in addition to maintenance of nerve tissue. This is indicated by the finding that tocopherol, delivered in native lipoproteins, is able to extend considerably the period in which rat brain explants develop in culture.

DISORDERS OF LIPOPROTEINS CONTAINING APOPROTEIN B

Abetalipoproteinemia

Clinical Features and Diagnostic Evaluation

The manifestations of ABL, resulting from the absence of the plasma lipoproteins that contain apo B, include fat malabsorption, acanthocytosis, retinopathy, and progressive neurologic disease. Malabsorption of fat has been noted as early as the neonatal period with diarrhea, vomiting, and failure to gain weight. Somatic underdevelopment may persist. Malabsorption results from failure of the intestinal cells to secrete chylomicrons. Endoscopy reveals yellowish discoloration of the duodenal mucosa, and biopsy reveals normally formed villi engorged with lipids. Although chylomicrons are not secreted, some essential fatty acids are apparently absorbed and transported to liver as free fatty acids. In adults with ABL, loss of fatty acids in stool may be as little as 20% of the ingested amount, but this is enough to induce oxalate urolithiasis in some.

Deficiencies of the fat-soluble vitamins A, E, and K result from the malabsorption of lipid. Vitamin D has its own transport protein, and hence absorption is unimpaired by the lack of chylomicron formation. Vitamin A is normally esterified in the enterocyte. Chylomicrons carry its esters into blood via the intestinal lymphatics and thoracic duct. Levels of vitamin A in the plasma of patients with ABL are low, but normal levels are achieved with supplementation. Low levels of vitamin K in plasma resulting in prothrombin deficiency can occur in ABL, and gastrointestinal bleeding has been observed in early childhood. As is the case with vitamin A, modest supplementation of vitamin K maintains normal levels. In contrast, even massive doses of vitamin E do not raise plasma levels to the normal range in some patients.

Acanthocytes account for half or more of circulating erythrocytes in patients with ABL but are not seen in bone marrow. Low sedimentation rates are observed because their structure inhibits rouleaux formation. The red cell envelope has an abnormally high sphingomyelin-to-lecithin ratio, and total phospholipid and cholesterol content is greater than in normal erythrocytes. Maldistribution of lipids between the bilayer leaflets apparently accounts for the acanthocytosis. Erythroid hyperplasia, reticulocytosis, hyperbilirubinemia, and decreased red cell survival have been described. Severe anemia observed in a number of children with ABL probably reflects deficiencies of some nutrients, including iron, folate, and vitamin E, secondary to fat malabsorption.

Pigmentary retinal degeneration, resembling retinitis pigmentosa, which is not associated with lipoprotein deficiency, is prominent in ABL. The most severe degeneration occurs in patients who also have severe neurologic symptoms. There is loss of pigment epithelium and photoreceptors, with relative preservation of submacular pigment epithelium. These and other pathologic changes, including abundance of lipofuscin pigment, resemble those of experimental deficiency of tocopherol. The retinopathy of ABL may also be related to deficiency of vitamin A, since partial improvement in electrophysiologic behavior of the retina and in dark adaptation has been noted when some patients receive vitamin A supplements. Vitamin A deficiency, however, is not thought to be a key factor in the retinal degeneration in ABL. Loss of night vision is frequently the earliest symptom. A decrease in visual acuity has occurred in the first decade, but many patients have maintained normal vision until adulthood. Ultimately, blindness can occur. Some patients have nystagmus, probably reflecting loss of visual acuity. Others are unaware of progressing retinal disease because it may involve slowly enlarging annular scotomas with macular sparing. Lenticular opacities, often seen with other forms of retinitis pigmentosa, have not been noted frequently in ABL.

Although some patients with ABL do not develop serious neurologic sequelae until later in life, most experience the onset of symptoms before the end of the second decade. Since the advent of early tocopherol therapy, many patients are remaining free of debilitating symptoms.

The large sensory neurons of the spinal ganglia and their myelinated axons that enter the cord lateral to the posterior funiculus are characteristic sites for the degenerative process. Axonopathy is the pathologic description, and demyelination of the fasciculus cuneatus and fasciculus gracilis has been described.[20,21] Striatonigral involvement has also been recognized.[22]

Deep tendon reflexes may decrease in the first decade, probably reflecting loss of function in posterior columns and spinocerebellar pathways. Ataxic gait and loss of proprioception and vibratory sense are usually progressive. The Romberg sign is often present. Before the advent of vitamin E therapy, patients were frequently unable to stand by the third decade, and had severe dysmetric movements and dysarthria. Muscle contractures resulting in equinovarus, pes cavus, and kyphoscoliosis were common. Babinski responses in some patients have been related to pyramidal tract disease, but spastic paralysis has not been described. Head tremor has been reported.

Mental retardation, a feature in some cases, cannot be attributed to the basic metabolic defect of ABL, and evidence of cerebral cortical disease is lacking. Consanguineous matings are frequent, and therefore other rare alleles may be responsible. Steatorrhea and attendant multiple nutritional deficiencies may be related to the general growth failure and slow neuromuscular development noted in some infants with ABL.

Peripheral neuropathy is an infrequent finding, but hypesthesia in the stocking-glove distribution has been described[23] with diminished response to local anesthetics. Abnormalities of somatosensory conduction with normal brain stem-evoked potentials were seen in 9 of 10 patients studied.[21] Decreased amplitude of sensory potentials with slow conduction velocity has been found in tibial and sural nerves, and evidence of skeletal muscle denervation has been noted on electromyograms.[24] Although denervation of the tongue and oculomotor nerve involvement have been seen, the cranial nerves are generally spared. A loss of large myelinated fibers is found in sural nerves, whereas unmyelinated fibers are relatively unaffected.[24] Paranodal demyelination correlates with age and severity of disease. The lesions bear a striking resemblance to those seen in other malabsorption syndromes that involve vitamin E deficiency.

The denervative neuropathy would tend to obscure the myopathy that may be present. The latter was described in a 26-year-old man in whom ceroid pigment was noted in the muscle fibers, resembling that observed in tocopherol-deficient animals. A 10-year-old girl died as a result of cardiomyopathy, the pathologic appearance again suggesting tocopherol deficiency. The muscle weakness that is a common feature of ABL is probably most often secondary to the denervative neuropathy.

Genetic Data

All patients studied have had normal structural genes for apo B, but carry mutations in the microsomal triglyceride transport protein (MTP) that plays a critical role in the formation of chylomicrons and VLDL.[2,25]

Hypobetalipoproteinemia

Clinical Features and Diagnostic Evaluation

Patients heterozygous for familial hypobetalipoproteinemia (HBL) have cholesterol levels ranging from 40 to 180 mg/dL and triglycerides ranging from 15 mg/dL up to the normal range. Lipid composition of the lipoproteins is normal, and patients generally have no symptoms of their disease, with only modest abnormalities in laboratory tests. One patient whose presentation was compatible with heterozygous familial HBL, however, had neurologic findings that resembled olivopontocerebellar atrophy. Homozygous patients resemble those with ABL and

generally have no detectable apo-B–containing lipoproteins. Chylomicrons do not appear after fat feeding. The acanthocytosis, gastrointestinal features, retinitis, and neuromuscular manifestations described in ABL are usually present. In one case, a homozygous truncation resulting in an apo B-50 protein sheds further light on the potential effects of truncations. As would be expected, chylomicron secretion appears to be normal. Although a VLDL-like particle is secreted from the liver, LDL are virtually absent from plasma. This patient had almost undetectable levels of tocopherols in plasma and had ataxia.

Genetic Data

HBL, characterized by very low levels of apo B and LDL cholesterol in plasma, is caused by mutations in the apo B gene that interfere with translation of complete apo B-100, or apo B alleles that produce reduced amounts of normal apo B-100. A number of different mutations leading to truncations of apo B proteins have been identified. Truncated B proteins shorter than B-31 apparently cannot be secreted from hepatocytes or enterocytes. Longer truncations are secreted in lipoproteins. Because the ability to incorporate lipid into lipoprotein complexes appears to be a monotonic function of the length of the apo B chain, many of the secreted lipoproteins have abnormal densities. Apo B chains longer than B-50 are able to organize triglyceride-rich VLDL-like particles, whereas shorter products may appear as hyperdense LDL or may even be found in the HDL density interval. All of the truncations described to date involve the deletion of linear sequence from the carboxyl end of the protein and are attributable to mutations leading to the formation of premature stop codons. Truncated proteins shorter than B-70 would be expected to lack the ligand domain for the LDL receptor. In addition, HBL that cosegregates with the apo B locus but that is not associated with truncations has been observed. These may involve regulatory elements for the gene. An additional distinct mechanism for HBL is suggested by a kindred in which the B-48 protein is secreted into plasma but no B-100 is found.[26] Haplotyping studies have established that, unlike most cases of HBL, this disorder is not linked to the apo B gene locus. It is possible that this represents a tissue-specific defect in B-100 secretion or perhaps complete editing of B-100 mRNA in liver and intestine.

Chylomicron Retention Disease

Anderson and colleagues[27] described an infant with fat malabsorption, fat-laden intestinal epithelial cells, and low levels of LDL, HDL, and fat-soluble vitamins. Postprandial chylomicronemia was absent. Subsequently, similar patients who had severe diarrhea and varying degrees of growth retardation have been reported. One patient had mild acanthocytosis, and three developed neurologic symptoms in the second decade that included diminished deep tendon reflexes and vibratory sense. These three also were considered to have low or low-normal intelligence. Four of five tested had mildly abnormal retinal function. Results of studies of in vitro explants of intestinal biopsy material suggest that apo B-48 synthesis is normal, but formation and secretion of chylomicrons are impaired.[28] The absence of vertical transmission of this phenotype, its frequency among siblings, and consanguineous relationships in families of affected persons suggest an autosomal recessive inheritance. Abnormalities of the apo B gene locus have been excluded as a cause of this disorder.

Therapy

The intestinal symptoms of ABL and the homozygous form of familial HBL correlate with the amount of dietary fat. Restriction of triglycerides containing long-chain fatty acids therefore is key in management of these patients and those heterozygous for familial HBL who have evidence of malabsorption or oxalate urolithiasis. Medium-chain triglycerides should be used sparingly, if at all, because cirrhosis of the liver has been described with their prolonged use.

Supplementation with tocopherol inhibits progression of neurologic sequelae and should be instituted as soon as the diagnosis of ABL or homozygous familial HBL is made. Natural vitamin E is preferred over synthetic preparations or those restricted to α-tocopherol. This is because γ-tocopherol can reduce the peroxynitrite radical and the alpha form cannot. In patients heterozygous for familial HBL, supplementation is advised because they, too, rarely develop neurologic disease. Retinopathy may be prevented or stabilized once it appears if vitamin E is given early. Myopathy has also been reversed with tocopherol. Very large doses are well-tolerated, and concentrated preparations allow a convenient dosage of 1000 to 2000 mg/day for infants and up to 10,000 to 20,000 mg/day for older children or adults. Supplementation with water-soluble preparations of vitamin A are indicated whenever plasma levels are low. Vitamin K should be given if the patient exhibits bleeding or hypoprothrombinemia. Treatment of patients with chylomicron retention disease should include restriction of dietary fat and supplementation with vitamin E and perhaps also vitamin A.

DISORDERS OF HIGH-DENSITY LIPOPROTEINS

Tangier Disease

Clinical Features and Diagnostic Evaluation

Tangier disease is associated with very low levels of HDL and of apo A-I and A-II in plasma, with lipid-filled histocytes in many organs. Large, orange-colored tonsils and orange pigment in the rectal mucosa are hallmarks of this disorder. Deposits of cholesteryl esters are also observed in the cornea, thymus, Schwann cells, spinal ganglia, smooth muscle cells of the intestine, ureters, heart valves, bone marrow, and pulmonary arteries. Patients frequently have lymphadenopathy and splenomegaly, with associated thrombocytopenia and increased hemolysis. Cholesterol levels average about 70 mg/dL in homozygotes and about 160 mg/dL in heterozygotes; however, triglycerides tend to be elevated as high as 400 mg/dL. Fasting chylomicronemia is frequent. Levels of apo A-I and A-II are very low, reflecting increased catabolism.

Neurologic consequences present most commonly as relapsing multiple mononeuropathies, or a syringomyelia-like disorder involving loss of pain and temperature sense.[29] Acute, disabling sensorimotor polyneuropathy has been described.[30] Patients may have loss of corneal sensation and orbicular muscle weakness that may lead to ectropion. Sural nerve biopsy reveals lipid droplets in Schwann cells and interstitial cells, which do not appear to be membrane-enclosed. In the syringomyelia-like presentation, lipid inclusions resembling lipofuscin granules have been observed within neurons of the spinal ganglia and cord.[29] In patients who have neuropathies, demyelination and remyelination occur. In the syringomyelia-like syndrome, there is axonal degeneration of both small myelinated and unmyelinated fibers. Spinal cord neurons contain osmiophilic lipid inclusions 1 to 3 mm in diameter (Fig. 51–3). No specific treatment is known for Tangier disease.

Genetic Data

The underlying defect is a marked decrease in the efflux of cholesterol from cells to form HDL, resulting from mutations in the cell membrane ATP cassette transporter ABCA1.[31]

Familial Lecithin: Cholesterol Acyl Transferase Deficiency

Clinical Features and Diagnostic Evaluation

This is a rare recessive disorder characterized by extremely low levels of activity of LCAT.[32] The content of unesterified cholesterol in plasma and all lipoprotein classes is very high, and that of cholesterol esters is low with a preponderance of palmityl and oleyl esters. Cholesterol-rich lipoproteins with multilamellar and discoidal structures are found in the LDL density interval. Some very large spherical particles appear to be modified chylomicrons. These and a population of large lamellar particles in the LDL density interval, which appear to be modified remnants, diminish when a fat-free diet is consumed. Some LDL of normal diameter but enriched in triglycerides are present. Abnormal HDL particles

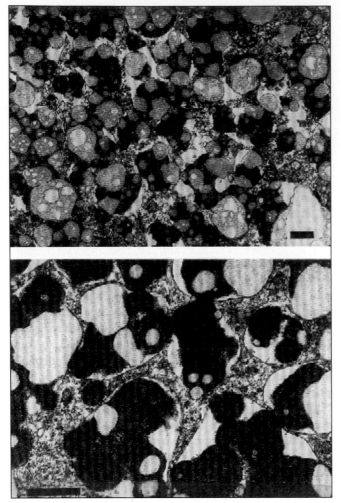

FIGURE 51–3. Tangier disease. Electron micrographs of a dorsal root ganglion cell. *Top:* Low magnification demonstrates the packing of inclusions. *Bottom:* High magnification demonstrates the presence of an electron-dense granular substance and electron-lucent vacuoles. A distinct membrane surrounds inclusions. *Bar:* 1 μm. (From Schmalbruch H, Stender S, Boysen G: Abnormalities in spinal neurons and dorsal root ganglion cells in Tangier disease presenting with a syringomyelia-like syndrome. J Neuropathol Exp Neurol 1987;46:533–543.)

include at least two discoidal forms containing apo A-I and apo E, respectively, and spherical particles of abnormally small diameter (circa 60 Å). The structural abnormalities are attributable to two amphipathic lipid species: free cholesterol and lecithin, both substrates for LCAT. Normalization of the morphology of HDL particles in LCAT-deficient plasma occurs with the addition of recombinant enzyme. Erythrocytes in LCAT deficiency contain excess free cholesterol and phosphatidylcholine, and they assume the configuration of target cells. Several functional abnormalities of red cells are present, and they tend to hemolyze, causing anemia.

A variant form of LCAT deficiency known as fish-eye disease has been identified in which the pathophysio-logic expression is limited to corneal opacity. Esterification of cholesterol in HDL is blocked, but it does proceed in VLDL and LDL, thus mitigating the accumulation of amphipathic lipids.

Most patients develop nephrosis, based on accumulation of lamellar lipid in glomerular capillaries, which often progresses to renal failure. Deposits of C3 complement have been detected in the mesangium. There is a moderately increased incidence of premature atherosclerosis. Though uncommon, peripheral neuropathy occurs in LCAT deficiency, associated with cutaneous xanthomatosis.

Genetic Data

Virtually all cases result from mutations in the structural gene for LCAT. Several mutations causing fish eye disorder have been identified in a specific region of the gene.[32]

Therapy

Treatment for LCAT deficiency involves minimizing the dietary fat intake to reduce the production of lamellar lipoproteins that are derived from chylomicrons.

CONCLUSION

Overt neurologic consequences are recognized in disorders of lipoprotein metabolism that involve deficiency of tocopherol and disorders that perturb the lipid composition of nerve tissue. The important roles played by apoproteins in the regeneration and remyelination of nerves suggest that abnormalities of these elements may affect the recovery of injured nerve tissue. As knowledge of the function of individual cell populations in the nervous system develops, it is likely that more subtle relationships between lipoproteins and neurologic function will emerge.

REFERENCES

1. Kane JP, Havel RJ: Disorders of the biogenesis and secretion of lipoproteins containing the B-apolipoproteins. In Scriver CR, Beaudet AL, Sly WS, Valle D (eds): The Metabolic and Molecular Bases of Inherited Disease. New York, McGraw-Hill, 2001, pp 2705–2716.

2. Wetterau JR, Aggerbeck LP, Bouma LP, et al: Absence of microsomal triglyceride transfer protein in individuals with abetalipoproteinemia. Science 1992; 258:999–1001.

3. Boyles JK, Pitas RE, Wilson E, et al: Apolipoprotein E associated with astrocytic glia of the central nervous system and with nonmyelinating glia of the peripheral nervous system. J Clin Invest 1985; 76:1501–1513.

4. Krul ES, Tang J: Secretion of apolipoprotein E by an astrocytoma cell line. J Neurosci Res 1992; 32:227–238.

5. Pitas RE, Boyles JK, Lee SH, et al: Lipoproteins and their receptors in the central nervous system. J Biol Chem 1987;262:14352–14360.

6. Nakai M, Kawamata T, Taniguchi T, et al: Expression of apolipoprotein E mRNA in rat microglia. Neurosci Lett 1996;211:41–44.

7. Koch S, Donarski N, Goetze K, et al: Characterization of four lipoprotein classes in human cerebrospinal fluid. J Lipid Res 2001;42:1143–1151.

8. Caronti B, Calderaro C, Alessandri C, et al: Beta2-glycoprotein I (beta2-GPI) mRNA is expressed by several cell types involved in anti-phospholipid syndrome-related tissue damage. Clin Exp Immunol 1999; 115:214–219.

9. Danik M, Chabot JG, Hassan-Gonzalez D, et al: Localization of sulfated glycoprotein-2/clusterin mRNA in the rat brain by in situ hybridization. J Comp Neurol 1993;334:209–227.

10. Patel SC, Asotra K, Patel YC, et al: Astrocytes synthesize and secrete the lipophilic ligand carrier apolipoprotein D. Neuroreport 1995;6:653–657.

11. Messmer-Joudrier S, Sagot Y, Mattenberger L, et al: Injury-induced synthesis and release of apolipoprotein E and clusterin from rat neural cells. Eur J Neurosci 1996;8:2652–2661.

12. Demeester N, Castro G, Desrumaux C, et al: Characterization and functional studies of lipoproteins, lipid transfer proteins, and lecithin: Cholesterol acyltransferase in CSF of normal individuals and patients with Alzheimer's disease. J Lipid Res 2000;41:963–974.

13. Ben-Zeev O, Doolittle MH, Singh N, et al: Synthesis and regulation of lipoprotein lipase in the hippocampus. J Lipid Res 1990;31:1307–1313.

14. Bessesen DH, Richards CL, Etienne J, et al: Spinal cord of the rat contains more lipoprotein lipase than other brain regions. J Lipid Res 1993;34:229–238.

15. Wolf BB, Lopes MB, VandenBerg SR, Gonias SL: Characterization and immunohistochemical localization of alpha 2-macroglobulin receptor (low-density lipoprotein receptor-related protein) in human brain. Am J Pathol 1992;141:37–42.

16. LaDu MJ, Gilligan SM, Lukens JR, et al: Nascent astrocyte particles differ from lipoproteins in CSF. J Neurochem 1998;70:2070–2081.

17. Traber MG, Sokol RJ, Burton GW, et al: Impaired ability of patients with familial isolated vitamin E deficiency to incorporate alpha-tocopherol into lipoproteins secreted by the liver. J Clin Invest 1990;85:397–407.

18. Harding AE, Matthews S, Jones S, et al: Spinocerebellar degeneration associated with a selective defect of vitamin E absorption. N Engl J Med 1985; 313:32–35.

19. Rosenblum JL, Keating JP, Prensky AL, Nelson JS: A progressive neurologic syndrome in children with chronic liver disease. N Engl J Med 1981;304:503–508.

20. Sobrevilla LA, Goodman MI, Kane CA: Demyelinating central nervous system disease, macular atrophy and acanthocytosis (Bassen-Kornzweig syndrome). Am J Med 1964;37:821.

21. Brin MF, Nelson MS, Roberts WC, et al: Neuropathology of abetalipoproteinemia: A possible complication of the tocopherol (vitamin E) deficient state. Neurology 1983;33:142.

22. Dexter DT, Brooks DJ, Harding AE, et al: Nigrostriatal function in vitamin E deficiency: Clinical, experimental, and positron emission tomographic studies. Ann Neurol 1994;35:298–303.

23. Schwartz JF, Rowland LP, Eder H, et al: Bassen-Kornzweig syndrome: Deficiency of serum beta-lipoprotein. Arch Neurol 1963;8:438.

24. Wichman A, Buchthal F, Pezeshkpour GH, Gregg RE: Peripheral neuropathy in abetalipoproteinemia. Neurology 1985;35:1279–1289.

25. Ricci B, Sharp D, O'Rourke E, et al: A 30-amino acid truncation of the microsomal triglyceride transfer protein large subunit disrupts its interaction with protein disulfide-isomerase and causes abetalipoproteinemia. J Biol Chem 1995;270:14281–14285.

26. Naganawa S, Kodama T, Aburatani H, et al: Genetic analysis of a Japanese family with normotriglyceridemic abetalipoproteinemia indicates a lack of linkage to the apolipoprotein B gene. Biochem Biophys Res Comm 1992;182:99–104.

27. Anderson CM, Townley RRW, Freeman JP: Unusual causes of steatorrhea in infancy and childhood. Med J Aust 1961;11:617.

28. Levy E, Marcel Y, Deckelbaum RJ, et al: Intestinal apo B synthesis, lipids and lipoproteins in chylomicron retention disease. J Lipid Res 1987;28:1263.

29. Schmalbruch H, Stender S, Boysen G: Abnormalities in spinal neurons and dorsal root ganglion cells in Tangier disease presenting with a syringomyelia-like syndrome. J Neuropathol and Exp Neurol 1987; 46:533–543.

30. Fazio R, Nemni R, Quattrini A, et al: Acute presentation of Tangier polyneuropathy: A clinical and morphological study. Acta Neuropathol 1993;86:90–94.

31. Oram JF, Lawn RM: ABCA1: The gatekeeper for eliminating excess tissue cholesterol. J Lipid Res 2001;42:1173–1179.

32. Santamarina-Fojo S, Hoeg JM, Assman G, Brewer HBJ: Lecithin cholesterol acyltransferase deficiency and fish eye disease. In Scriver CR, Beaudet AL, Sly WS, Valle D (eds): The Metabolic and Molecular Bases of Inherited Disease. New York, McGraw-Hill, 2001, pp 2817–2833.

Apolipoprotein E: Structure and Function in Lipid Metabolism and Neurobiology

Robert W. Mahley

Yadong Huang

Apolipoprotein E (apoE) plays a key role in both lipid metabolism and neurobiology. A major function of apoE is to mediate the binding of lipoproteins or lipid complexes in the plasma or interstitial fluids to specific cell-surface receptors (the low density lipoprotein receptor family) that internalize them; thus, apoE participates in the distribution of lipids among various cells of the body. In addition, direct intracellular effects of apoE may modulate various cellular processes, including cytoskeletal assembly and stability. Elucidation of the functional domains within this protein and of the three-dimensional structure of the receptor binding region of the three major isoforms of apoE (apoE2, apoE3, and apoE4) has contributed significantly to our understanding of its biologic roles at a molecular level. The tremendous body of knowledge concerning this protein has laid the groundwork for the explosion of research attempting to unravel the role of apoE4 in the pathogenesis of Alzheimer disease (AD). It is likely that apoE is involved more widely in processes within the nervous system, possibly encompassing a variety of disorders of neuronal repair, remodeling, and protection.

ApoE is a 34-kDa, 299–amino acid protein that functions as a component of plasma lipoproteins in the transport of lipids among cells of different organs and within specific tissues. Discovered in the early 1970s, it is one of several apolipoproteins associated with very low density lipoproteins (VLDL), intermediate density lipoproteins, chylomicron remnants, and certain subclasses of high-density lipoproteins (HDL). ApoE plays a key role in regulating the clearance of these lipoproteins from the plasma by serving as the ligand for binding to specific cell-surface receptors, including the low density lipoprotein (LDL) receptor and other members of the LDL receptor gene family.[1,2]

There are three major isoforms of apoE that occur in humans: apoE2, apoE3, and apoE4. ApoE3 is considered to be the "normal" form of apoE, whereas apoE2 and apoE4 are variants that occur less frequently, differing from apoE3 by single amino acid substitutions. Investigators established the amino acid and structural differences among the various apoE isoforms and advanced our understanding of the roles of apoE in various metabolic pathways. Understanding of the role of apoE in lipid metabolism was further advanced by the discovery that apoE2 is defective in lipoprotein receptor binding and is associated with the genetic disease type III hyperlipoproteinemia.[1-6] The genetic linkage of apoE4 to the pathogenesis of AD[7,8] has refocused attention on the importance of this apolipoprotein in neurobiology.

Synthesis of ApoE

ApoE is synthesized and secreted from a variety of tissues and several cell types and is abundant in the interstitial fluid and lymph, as well as in the plasma.[1,2,4,6] ApoE may be secreted by cells in a lipid-poor form; however, because of its avidity for lipids (especially phospholipids), apoE almost certainly always exists in association with lipids and most likely acquires them from cell surfaces or from secretory vesicles as it is secreted. In lymph and plasma, it always appears to be associated with lipids and occurs on lipoprotein particles or phospholipid discs.

ApoE mRNA quantification in rats, marmosets, and humans reveals that hepatocytes are major sites of apoE synthesis. ApoE production is also readily detected in the brain (second to the liver in quantity), adrenal, testis, skin, kidney, and spleen and in macrophages in a variety of tissues. In both human and rat brains, apoE mRNA is abundant in the cerebral cortex, cerebellum, and medulla, as well as other regions that have been examined.

In the central nervous system (CNS), astrocytes are primarily responsible for the production of apoE; however, specialized astrocytic cell types also synthesize apoE (e.g., Bergmann glia of the cerebellum, tanycytes of the third ventricle, pituicytes of the neurohypophysis, Müller cells of the retina). ApoE is also produced by some populations of human neurons under specific conditions.[9,10] In the peripheral nervous system, apoE is present in glia surrounding sensory and motor neurons. It is also present in nonmyelinating Schwann cells but not in myelinating Schwann cells. Macrophages are responsible for apoE synthesis and secretion in injured peripheral nerves. Resident macrophages and monocyte-macrophages recruited to the site of injury produce large quantities of apoE that accumulate in the extracellular matrix of the degenerating stump and the regenerating nerve.[1,2,5,6]

BIOCHEMICAL FINDINGS

Structure and Function of ApoE Isoforms in Lipid Metabolism

A major function of apoE is to transport lipids among various cells and tissues of the body.[1,2,6] ApoE is a key regulator of plasma lipid levels and participates in the homeostatic control of plasma and tissue lipid content. This is accomplished in part because apoE binds with high affinity to cell-surface lipoprotein receptors. ApoE mediates the interaction of apoE-containing lipoproteins and lipid complexes to the LDL receptor, the LDL receptor-related protein (LRP), the VLDL receptor, the apoE receptor-2, and gp330. The apoE isoforms differ in their ability to interact with these receptors. In addition, apoE binds to heparin and heparan sulfate proteoglycans (HSPG), again with isoform-specific differences in binding affinity. Interaction with HSPG appears to attract and sequester apoE-containing lipoproteins at cell surfaces and to facilitate their interaction with the LRP and possibly other receptors. Furthermore, the distribution of apoE among the various lipoproteins is isoform specific and reflects the lipid-lipoprotein binding activities of apoE2, apoE3, and apoE4.

Receptor Binding Activity

ApoE possesses two structural domains that are connected by 20 to 30 amino acids that may serve as a hinge between the two domains. The N-terminal two thirds of apoE contains the receptor binding region. Six to eight critical arginine and lysine residues and a histidine residue in the region of amino acids 136–150 mediate the interaction of apoE with the ligand binding domain of the LDL receptor.[1,2,4–6] Arginine 158 appears to be involved in modulating the conformation of the 136–150 region

and is involved only indirectly in receptor binding activity. ApoE3 and apoE4, which display normal receptor binding activity, have arginine at residue 158, whereas apoE2, which is defective in receptor binding activity, has cysteine.

Several naturally occurring mutants of apoE have helped to define the receptor binding region.[1,2,6] Amino acid substitutions at residues 136, 142, 145, and 146 result in defective receptor binding and are associated with the development of dominant type III hyperlipoproteinemia. The mutations at residues 136, 142, and 145 involve the substitution of a neutral amino acid for arginine. The mutations at residue 146 involve the substitution of neutral (glutamine) or acidic (glutamate) amino acids for lysine. The substitution of cysteine at residue 158 for the normally occurring arginine results in the common apoE2 variant, which is defective in LDL receptor binding and is associated with the recessive form of type III hyperlipoproteinemia. For a complete discussion of dominant versus recessive type III hyperlipoproteinemia.[6]

The three-dimensional structure of the receptor binding region of apoE has shed light on the mechanism whereby these specific residues are involved in receptor binding. As shown by X-ray crystallography, the N-terminal two thirds of the apoE molecule (composed of residues 1–191) is a four-helix bundle.[2,4–6] Helix 4 (residues 130–164) contains the receptor binding region. The basic amino acids in the 136–150 region are largely solvent-exposed, extend away from the backbone of the molecule, and form a 20-Å basic field of charge that could be available to interact directly with the receptor. Residue 158 (arginine) lies outside this highly basic region and is involved in receptor binding indirectly, as confirmed by comparison of the crystal structures of apoE2 and apoE3.[2,4,6]

Heparin and Heparan Sulfate Proteoglycan Binding Activity

It is now envisioned that cell-surface HSPGs play an important role in the binding and uptake of apoE-containing lipoproteins either by the LRP and other lipoprotein receptors or directly by HSPG. It appears that interaction of apoE with HSPG is a necessary first step for the LRP-mediated uptake of chylomicron remnants by hepatocytes. This is referred to as the HSPG-LRP pathway. In the absence of cell-surface HSPG, the apoE-containing remnant lipoproteins do not bind and are not internalized by the LRP in in vitro studies. The HSPG-LRP pathway is not restricted to hepatocyte uptake of lipoproteins, but is also operative in other cells (including neurons) and mediates the uptake of lipoproteins enriched in apoE. The concept is that apoE is secreted from the cells, enriching the environment with extracellular apoE and facilitating high-affinity binding of lipoproteins to HSPG. This process has been termed the secretion-capture role for apoE. ApoE-enriched lipoproteins are captured by binding to HSPG, brought into the environment of the LRP, and then transferred to the LRP for actual internalization by the cells. Alternatively, HSPG-LRP may form a complex that is internalized.[2,6,11]

Lipid-Lipoprotein Binding Activity

The isoforms of apoE display preferences for specific classes of lipoproteins.[2,4,5] Examination of the distribution of apoE among the various plasma lipoproteins has shown that apoE4 has a preference for large, triglyceride-rich VLDL particles, whereas apoE3 and apoE2 associate preferentially with the small, phospholipid-rich HDL.

The C-terminal one third of the apoE molecule is critical in mediating lipid binding.[4] In fact, residues in the 244–272 region of apoE form amphipathic α-helices that mediate the ability of apoE to interact with lipoproteins. A truncated segment of apoE encompassing residues 1–244 possesses markedly reduced ability to bind to lipoproteins, whereas a segment encompassing residues 1–272 possesses full lipid-lipoprotein binding activity. (The full-length apoE molecule consists of 299 amino acids.)

Domain Interaction Modulating Molecular Conformation May Explain ApoE Isoform-Specific Activities

The isoform differences in lipoprotein preference illustrate an important point that very likely extends beyond this activity of apoE (i.e., conformational differences modulated by domain interactions alter functional activity). The residues that distinguish the apoE isoforms are in the N-terminus (apoE4, arginine 112; apoE3 and apoE2, cysteine 112). However, the lipid-binding region is in the C-terminus (residues 244–272). This suggests that the N- and C-terminal domains interact to determine the preference of apoE4 for VLDL and of apoE3 and apoE2 for HDL.

Comparison of the three-dimensional structures of the N-terminal domains of apoE3 and apoE4 and site-directed mutagenesis have provided insights into the functional differences among the isoforms and have defined how domain interaction in apoE4 might occur.[2,4,5] The only major differences between the crystallographic structures of apoE3 and apoE4 are in the local environment of residue 112. In apoE3, cysteine 112 is in close proximity to glutamic acid 109 in helix 3 and arginine 61 in helix 2. However, in apoE4, with arginine at residue 112, there is a markedly different orientation for glutamic acid 109 and arginine 61. A salt bridge forms between arginine 112 and glutamic acid 109, and the side chain of arginine 61 is reoriented away from the helix and presumably more available for interaction with other residues, including those in the C-terminal domain. In fact, the exposed side chain of arginine 61 in apoE4, but not in the other isoforms, interacts through a salt bridge with the side chain of glutamic acid 255 within the critical lipoprotein binding region of the C-terminal domain. This so-called "domain interaction" undoubtedly profoundly alters the protein conformation and somehow directs the preference of apoE4 for binding to VLDL, as mutation of either arginine 61 or glutamic acid 255 changes the lipoprotein preference of apoE4 from VLDL to HDL.[4-6] Domain interaction occurs only in apoE4 and is probably responsible for several apoE4-specific roles (Fig. 52–1). The other isoforms do not show domain interaction.

As stated earlier, arginine 61 is one feature of human apoE that distinguishes it from apoE in lower species, which possesses threonine 61.[4] Despite having arginine 112, apoE in lower species associates preferentially with HDL. This further suggests that arginine 61 (in the presence of arginine at residue 112) preferentially directs apoE to the large VLDL particles. The importance of domain interaction extends beyond the isoform-specific roles of apoE in lipid binding and eventually may

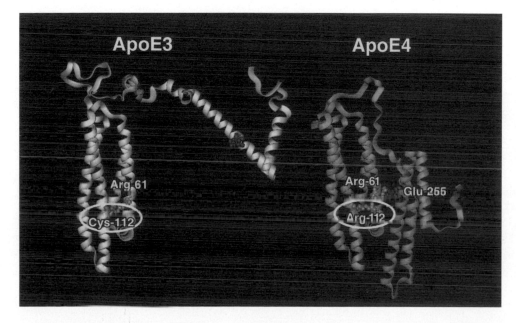

FIGURE 52–1. ApoE domain interaction. In apoE4 *(right)*, arginine 112 orients the side chain of arginine 61 into the aqueous environment where it can interact with glutamic acid 255, resulting in interaction between the N- and C-terminal domains. In apoE3 *(left)*, arginine 61 is not available to interact with residues in the C-terminal domain, resulting in a very different overall conformation.

help us to understand the isoform-specific roles of apoE in AD.

Structure and Function of ApoE in Alzheimer Disease

Several lines of evidence have linked apoE and neurobiology. By the mid-1980s, clues had begun to surface that apoE plays an important role in neurologic diseases. ApoE is produced in abundance in the brain and serves as the principal lipid transport vehicle in cerebrospinal fluid (CSF). It is induced at high concentration in peripheral nerve injury and appears to play a key role in repair by redistributing lipids to regenerating axons and to Schwann cells during remyelination. It modulates neurite outgrowth in either cultured rabbit dorsal root ganglion cells or neuroblastoma (N2a) cells.[1,3,5] The stage was set for the discovery by Roses and associates that apoE is a major susceptibility gene associated with 40% to 65% of cases of sporadic and familial AD and increases the occurrence and lowers the age of onset of the disease.[7,8]

Interactions of ApoE with Amyloid β Peptides

ApoE is associated with neuritic amyloid plaques in vivo, and lipid-free apoE3 and apoE4 in vitro can form a sodium dodecyl sulfate (SDS)- and guanidine hydrochloride-stable complex with amyloid β (Aβ), with apoE4 complexes forming more rapidly and effectively.[17] Interestingly, reducing agents, such as dithiothreitol or β-mercaptoethanol, prevent the formation of SDS-stable complexes, suggesting that oxidation of apoE may be required. Residues 244–272 of apoE are responsible for binding to the Aβ peptide as well as to lipoprotein particles. However, when incubated with Aβ peptide, lipidated apoE3 or apoE4 isolated from stably transfected apoE-expressing cells yielded different responses.[18] Lipidated apoE3 bound with a 20-fold greater affinity to the Aβ peptide than lipidated apoE4. The avid binding of apoE3 to the Aβ peptide may enhance clearance of the complex, preventing the conversion of Aβ into a neurotoxic species. The physiologic relevance of these observations to AD pathology awaits further in vivo studies.

Prolonged incubation (several days) of apoE with Aβ peptide results in insoluble, high-molecular-weight complexes that precipitate as fibers. Again, apoE4 forms a denser, more extensive matrix of amyloid monofibrils and does so more rapidly and effectively than apoE3.[19] ApoE associates with these fibrils along their full length, suggesting that it may help to form a hybrid fibril.[19] This observation has been confirmed in studies in which the formation of fibrils associated with either apoE3 or apoE4 was quantified by fibril counting or by thioflavin fluorescence.[20,21] The increased amyloid fibril formation associated with apoE4 probably triggers or exacerbates the development of AD. Studies in apoE-deficient mice expressing amyloid precursor protein (APP) with the V717F mutation demonstrated that apoE is actually required for amyloid plaque formation.[22]

Effects of apoE on Aβ Neurotoxicity

The neurotoxicity of Aβ appears to be important in the pathogenesis of AD.[23,24] Aβ-induced neuronal death results partially from apoptotic pathways and is related to the activation of several caspases and the Jun-N-terminal kinase (JNK) pathway. The effects of apoE isoforms on Aβ-induced neurotoxicity are controversial and confusing, and the reported differences likely reflect differences in the source and physical state of both Aβ and apoE and in the origin and handling of the cells. ApoE3 may protect against Aβ-induced cell death and apoptosis by enhancing the clearance and degradation of Aβ or by reducing the interaction of Aβ with cell-surface membranes. Alternatively, apoE4 may potentiate $A\beta_{1-42}$–induced lysosomal leakage, cell death, and apoptosis, with apoE3 having little or no protective effect.

Isoform-Specific Effects of ApoE on Aβ-Induced Lysosomal Leakage

Aβ has been shown to induce lysosomal leakage.[25] We have demonstrated an isoform-specific difference in the susceptibility of apoE3- or apoE4-transfected N2a cells to Aβ-induced lysosomal leakage and apoptosis.[26] Lysosomal leakage into the cytosol after treatment of the cells with $A\beta_{1-42}$ was monitored by observing the intracellular pattern of lysosomal staining with Lucifer Yellow or by measuring the lysosomal enzyme β-hexosaminidase in the cytosol. The cells synthesizing and secreting apoE4 showed a significant potentiation of lysosomal leakage compared with apoE3- or neo-transfected cells, which showed a similar degree of lysosomal leakage.

In addition, apoE4 has been demonstrated to enhance Aβ-induced destabilization of lipid bilayer membranes.[26] ApoE4 added to phospholipid vesicles sensitized the artificial bilayer membranes to $A\beta_{1-42}$–induced disruption of the membrane structure, whereas apoE3 in the context of $A\beta_{1-42}$ resulted in less membrane destabilization. Thus, apoE4 may enhance the Aβ-induced disruption of lysosomal membranes, resulting in the release of lysosomal enzymes into the cytosol and initiating apoptosis and cell death.

ApoE Fragmentation and Alzheimer Disease

ApoE has been shown to undergo proteolytic processing within neurons to generate C-terminal truncated fragments (~29–30 kDa and ~14–20 kDa), with apoE4 being more susceptible to cleavage than apoE3.[29] These fragments enter the cytosol and interact with the cytoskeletal components, resulting in the formation of neurofibrillary tangle (NFT)–like inclusions in neurons. Truncated apoE4, which can be generated in cultured neurons and is present in the brains of AD patients, has a greater ability to induce NFT-like inclusions than truncated apoE3.

C-terminal-truncated forms of apoE have been demonstrated to accumulate in AD brains and to be associated with NFTs.[29] AD brain sections were immunostained with antibodies reacting against various regions of apoE. Anti–N-terminal apoE (amino acids 1–271) identified both amyloid plaques and NFTs (Fig. 52–2A), whereas anti–C-terminal apoE (amino acids 272–299) identified only amyloid plaques (Fig. 52–2B). The NFTs were double-immunolabeled with anti-phosphorylated (p)-tau and anti–N-terminal apoE (Fig. 52–2C) but not with anti–C-terminal apoE (Fig. 52–2D). These results suggest that apoE exists in NFTs as C-terminal-truncated form(s).

In in vitro cell culture studies, the approximately 29- to 30-kDa C-terminal-truncated apoE could be detected in lysates of mouse N2a cells expressing apoE3 or apoE4, with more being generated from apoE4 than from apoE3. Furthermore, treatment of the transfected cells with $A\beta_{1-42}$ significantly increased the amount of the C-terminal-truncated forms of both apoE3 and apoE4, but more so with apoE4. These results suggest that $A\beta_{1-42}$ activates an unknown proteolytic enzyme that cleaves apoE, especially apoE4, at its C-terminus.

C-terminal-truncated apoE also induced intracellular NFT-like inclusions in N2a cells transfected with apoE3 or apoE4 constructs possessing C-terminal truncations.[29] Expression of apoE4 lacking the last 28 amino acids of the C-terminus [apoE4(Δ272-299)] resulted in intracellular NFT-like inclusions in 78 ± 8% of transfected N2a cells (Fig. 52–2F). The inclusions were recognized by anti–p-tau, which colocalized with apoE, and anti-phosphorylated neurofilaments of high molecular weight (p-NF-H). Expression of apoE3(Δ272-299) also induced intracellular inclusions, but they were smaller (Fig. 52–2E) and occurred in significantly fewer cells (32 ± 5% versus 78 ± 8% for apoE4, $p < 0.001$). Importantly, exogenous apoE4(Δ272 to 299) that had been complexed with β-VLDL as a lipid transport vehicle and incubated with N2a cells also induced NFT-like structures (data not shown). Importantly, the addition of exogenous full-length apoE to neurons in culture did not result in the formation of C-terminally truncated fragments of apoE. Thus, it appears that the fragments are generated as they traverse the secretory pathway in neurons. Therefore, both endogenously expressed and exogenously added apoE4(Δ272-299)] induced NFT-like inclusions in N2a cells. The truncated apoE probably escapes the secretory or the endosomal-lysosomal internalization pathway, enters the cytosol, and interacts with p-tau and p-NF-H. There is evidence that apoE can appear in the cytosol of various cells,[30] although another study failed to show this.[31]

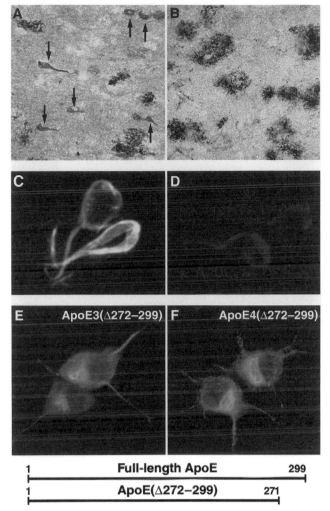

FIGURE 52–2. (See Color Plate VIII) C-terminal-truncated forms of apoE accumulate in AD brains and NFTs. Immunostaining of AD brain sections with anti–N-terminal apoE (A), which identified both amyloid plaques and NFTs (*arrows*), or anti–C-terminal apoE (B), which identified only amyloid plaques. Double immunofluorescence staining of AD brain sections with anti–p-tau (red) and anti–N-terminal apoE (green) (C) or anti–p-tau (red) and anti–C-terminal apoE (green) (D). E and F, C-terminal-truncated apoE induces the formation of apoE- and p-tau–immunoreactive intracellular inclusions in N2a cells. N2a cells were transiently transfected with apoE3(Δ272-299) (E) or apoE4(Δ272-299) (F) cDNA and immunostained with anti-apoE.

It has also been reported that the N-terminal 22-kDa thrombin-cleavage fragment (amino acids 1–191) of apoE4 is more neurotoxic than that of apoE3.[32] This neurotoxicity may be mediated by lipoprotein receptors on the cell surface and by high levels of intracellular calcium. Because the N-terminal 22-kDa fragment of apoE does not contain amino acids 224–260, which are responsible for the interaction with p-tau and p-NF-H that causes the formation of NFT-like inclusions, it is unlikely that the neurotoxic effects of the 22-kDa fragment and the effect of C-terminal-truncated apoE involve the same mechanism.

Effects of ApoE3 and ApoE4 on Cytoskeletal Function and Neurite Extension

In the presence of a lipid source, apoE3 and apoE4 have markedly different effects on neurite extension.[2,3,5] Specifically, apoE3 plus β-VLDL stimulates significant neurite extension, whereas apoE4 plus β-VLDL markedly inhibits neurite branching and extension in both dorsal root ganglion neurons and N2a cells in culture. Furthermore, apoE3-transfected N2a cells grown in medium containing β-VLDL or HDL isolated from CSF showed greater neurite extension than apoE4-transfected N2a cells.

ApoE4-associated inhibition of neurite extension is probably due to its effect on microtubule stability.[2,3,5] When incubated with N2a cells in the presence of β-VLDL, apoE4 yields significantly more monomeric tubulin and less polymerized tubulin than apoE3. Immunocytochemical analysis reveals more diffuse tubulin staining and fewer well-organized microtubules in the cells incubated with apoE4 than in those incubated with apoE3. These results suggest that apoE4 depolymerizes or destabilizes microtubules, disrupting cytoskeletal structure and impairing neurite extension.

Interestingly, the isoform-specific effects of apoE on neurite extension can be abolished by an antibody against the receptor-binding domain of apoE or by reductive methylation of critical lysine residues. These findings suggest that the effect of apoE is mediated by cell-surface lipoprotein receptors. Treatment of cells with heparinase to remove cell-surface HSPG blocked both apoE3-induced neurite extension and apoE4-induced inhibition of neurite extension. Likewise, treatment of cells either with the 39-kDa receptor-associated protein, which blocks the binding of ligands to LRP, or with an anti-LRP antibody abolished the isoform-specific effects. Thus, it appears that the HSPG-LRP pathway is responsible for the isoform-specific effects of apoE3 and apoE4 on neurite extension.[2,3,5]

Interactions of ApoE with Tau

ApoE3 and apoE4 interact differently with tau protein in vitro.[27] ApoE3 forms an SDS-stable complex with tau in a 1:1 ratio, whereas apoE4 does not interact significantly. Phosphorylation of tau by a crude brain extract inhibited the interaction of apoE3 with tau, suggesting that apoE3 binds to nonphosphorylated tau. Furthermore, the N-terminal domain of apoE3 is responsible for binding to tau. In fact, apoE3 irreversibly binds to the microtubule-binding repeat regions of the tau protein.

In neurons, tau normally stimulates the assembly of microtubules by polymerizing tubulin, and it also binds to and stabilizes microtubular structures.[27,28] Microtubules are necessary for neurite extension and for transporting materials along axons and dendrites. In AD brains, tau is abnormally hyperphosphorylated through an unknown mechanism and self-assembles into pathologic paired helical filaments, thereby forming NFTs. Thus, the binding of apoE3 to tau may protect it from hyperphosphorylation, which inhibits tau's ability to stabilize the microtubules. Likewise, the association of apoE4 with the development of AD may be due to the lack of this protective function of apoE3, because apoE4 does not bind well to tau and thus would not protect it from hyperphosphorylation.

MOLECULAR-GENETIC DATA

ApoE Polymorphism

ApoE arises from three common alleles at a single gene locus (chromosome 19), referred to as ε2, ε3, and ε4. The corresponding gene products (protein isoforms) are termed apoE2, apoE3, and apoE4. Thus, there are six common phenotypes: apoE2/2, apoE3/3, and apoE4/4 (homozygous), and apoE3/2, apoE4/2, and apoE4/3 (heterozygous). This genetically determined polymorphism is accounted for by amino acid substitutions at two sites in the protein (positions 112 and 158). ApoE2 differs from apoE3 by a single amino acid difference: apoE2 has cysteine whereas apoE3 has arginine at residue 158. Similarly, apoE4 differs from apoE3 only at residue 112, where apoE4 has arginine and apoE3 has cysteine. These substitutions explain the charge differences that distinguish the three isoforms.[1-6]

A second type of polymorphism is conferred by post-translational glycosylation. Sialylation of apoE gives rise to minor acidic isoforms. The glycosylation occurs at a single site, threonine 194. In the plasma, approximately 80% of apoE circulates as an asialylated form that is devoid of all carbohydrate moieties; however, in the CSF, most of the apoE is sialylated.[2,6]

Human apoE isoforms are distinguished from the apoE of other animals by an interesting amino acid sequence difference. The apoE of most lower animals, including the baboon, cynomolgus monkey, rat, mouse, dog, guinea pig, and sea lion, is "apoE4-like," possessing arginine at a site equivalent to residue 112. The apoE in rabbits and cows is "apoE3-like," possessing cysteine at residue 112. However, unlike human apoE, which has arginine at residue 61, all animals in which the apoE sequence is known have threonine at the corresponding position. Arginine 61 appears to play a critical role in determining the three-dimensional structure of apoE4 and in mediating important interactions between the N- and C-terminal domains of this protein.[2,4,5]

Allelic Frequency Distribution in Different Populations

The apoE3/3 phenotype is the most common, occurring in about 50% to 70% of most populations, and at least one ε3 allele occurs in 70% to 80% of most peoples in the world.[2,6] The ε4 and ε2 alleles nevertheless contribute significantly to the gene pool (ε4, typically 10% to 15%; ε2, 8% to 10%). Different racial groups have different allelic frequencies. For example, Europeans and white Americans have a predominance of ε3 (except for the Finnish, in whom apoE4 is predominant). The Japanese and Turks have the highest prevalence of ε3 and the lowest occurrence of ε4. Africans and African-Americans have a relatively high occurrence of ε4 (25% to 30% compared with 10% to 15% in white Americans). Certain tribal peoples, such as the Huli in Papua New Guinea, have an ε4 allele frequency approaching 50%.

Impact of Allelic Frequency on Lipid Metabolism and Atherogenesis

An apoE polymorphism is one of the common genetic factors that influence inter-individual variation in lipids and plasma lipoproteins. The ε2 allele is associated with lower levels of plasma cholesterol, LDL cholesterol, and apoB. Conversely, ε4 is associated with high plasma cholesterol and LDL cholesterol levels. The effects of apoE on triglyceride and HDL levels are less consistent.[2,6] Studies of the effects of apoE isoforms on coronary artery disease have yielded conflicting results. However, the presence of ε2 (in the absence of type III hyperlipoproteinemia) appears to decrease the risk of atherosclerosis, whereas the ε4 allele appears to be a risk factor for atherosclerosis.[2,6]

Impact of Allelic Frequency on Alzheimer Disease

The disease-related gene for late-onset familial and sporadic AD has been mapped to the apoE locus on chromosome 19. Specifically, Roses and associates have demonstrated a marked overrepresentation of apoE4 in AD patients.[7,8] As stated, apoE4 occurs in 10% to 15% of the general population. However, in the AD patient group, apoE4 occurs with a frequency of 40% to 65%. Whereas apoE4 has been associated with accelerated development of AD, apoE2 has been considered to be protective.

Genetic Linkage of ApoE and Alzheimer Disease

The first evidence that apoE might be involved in the pathogenesis of AD was the observation that apoE colocalized with two neuropathologic lesions of AD—extracellular amyloid deposits and intracellular NFTs.[12] Simultaneously, it was also demonstrated that the apoE4 allele was overrepresented in late-onset familial AD patients (0.50) compared with age- and sex-matched controls (0.16).[13,14] The association of the apoE4 allele with the development of late-onset familial AD was confirmed in several populations[15] and was expanded to late-onset sporadic AD.[13,14] Furthermore, apoE4 has a gene dose

effect on the risk and age of onset of AD.[13] As the number of apoE4 alleles increases from 0 to 2, the risk of developing late-onset familial AD increases from 20% to 90%, and the mean age of onset decreases from 84 to 68 years.[13] Thus, the apoE4 allele is a major risk factor or a susceptibility gene for the development of late-onset AD. The apoE4 allele is also associated with poor clinical outcome in patients with acute head trauma and stroke. In contrast, the apoE2 allele seems to delay the age of onset and decreases the risk of AD, possibly indicating a protective effect. Controversial epidemiologic studies suggested that some apoE gene promoter polymorphisms are associated with increased risk for AD.[16]

ANIMAL MODELS

Transgenic Mouse Models in Alzheimer Disease Research

The first successful transgenic mouse model of AD was generated by using a platelet-derived growth factor-β promoter to drive the expression of a human APP (hAPP) minigene that encodes the AD-linked APP-V717F mutation.[33] The brains of the transgenic mice showed diffuse Aβ deposits and mature plaques associated with astrocytes.[33,34] Subsequently, transgenic mice expressing another AD-linked APP mutant, APP-695swe, showed elevated levels of $A\beta_{40}$ and $A\beta_{42}$, dystrophic neurites, and Aβ deposits in the hippocampus and cortex.[35] The APP-695swe mice also showed impairments in several memory tests.[35] However, none of these mutant APP transgenic mice displayed the other pathologic hallmark of AD, intracellular NFTs.

Transgenic mice expressing human three-repeat or four-repeat tau were generated.[36,37] These mice developed intraneuronal inclusions containing p-tau and had motor neuron deficits but did not develop classic NFTs. However, NFTs composed of straight filaments were generated in neurons of transgenic mice expressing a mutant human tau (P301L), suggesting that other factors, in addition to p-tau, are required to induce NFTs.[38] When the transgenic hAPP mice were crossed with human mutant tau mice, NFT formation increased significantly, indicating that Aβ enhances neurofibrillary pathology.[38]

We have used the neuron-specific enolase (NSE) promoter to express human apoE3 or apoE4 at similar levels in neurons of transgenic mice lacking endogenous mouse apoE.[39] Compared with NSE-apoE3 mice and wild-type controls, NSE-apoE4 mice showed impairments of learning in a water-maze test and in vertical exploratory behavior that increased with age. The impaired behavior was observed primarily in female apoE4 transgenic mice. These results suggest that human apoE isoforms have differential effects on brain function in vivo and that the susceptibility to apoE4-induced deficits is critically influenced by age and gender. Morphologic studies of these transgenic mouse lines demonstrated that human apoE3 prevents the age-dependent neurodegeneration seen in apoE-null mice and prevents kainic acid-induced neurodegeneration.[40] Human apoE4 was not protective.[40] In addition, expression of human apoE3 or apoE4 decreased Aβ deposits in the brains of hAPP-V717F transgenic mice, suggesting that apoE stimulates Aβ clearance.[41] However, apoE3 clears more Aβ from these mice than does apoE4.[41] It has been reported that expression of apoE4 in neurons stimulates tau phosphorylation, but expression of apoE4 in astrocytes does not.[42]

As reviewed earlier, none of the mouse models fully displays a phenotype of AD, and all lack intracellular NFTs in the presence of wild-type tau. However, it is reasonable to speculate that generation of C-terminal-truncated apoE4 within neuronal cells in the context of other factors (e.g., overexpression of human wild-type tau) may induce the formation of NFTs.

The isoform-specific effects of apoE on CNS function have also been examined in transgenic mice.[39] These functional studies included examinations of spatial learning and memory in different water-maze tests and of exploratory activity and curiosity in an open-field test. Transgenic mice expressing human apoE4 in CNS neurons on the apoE-null background were markedly impaired in performing the water-maze tasks, whereas apoE3 mice resembled wild-type control mice. Interestingly, the impairments in spatial learning and memory in the apoE4 mice were more severe in older mice (>6 months of age) and in females. In addition, female apoE4 mice were less curious and displayed less exploratory activity (fewer and shorter rearing events) than apoE3-expressing mice or wild-type mice, which were similar. The detrimental apoE4 effects on CNS function were dominant because apoE3/4 hemizygous mice were impaired to the same degree as apoE4 homozygous mice.[43]

CONCLUSION

Numerous hypotheses have been advanced to explain the association of apoE4 with the risk for AD and other neuropathologic disorders, but clearly our understanding is incomplete. It is reasonable to suggest that apoE affects neurobiology through multiple processes and pathways, depending on specific physiologic or pathologic stimuli or conditions.

Acknowledgments

This work was supported in part by program project grant HL47660 and R01 grant HL64162 from the National Institutes of Health. We thank Sylvia Richmond and Catharine Evans for manuscript preparation, Gary Howard and Stephen Ordway for editorial assistance, John C.W. Carroll and Jack Hull for graphics, and Stephen Gonzales and Chris Goodfellow for photography.

REFERENCES

1. Mahley RW: Apolipoprotein E: Cholesterol transport protein with expanding role in cell biology. Science 1988;240:622–630.

2. Mahley RW, Rall SC Jr: Apolipoprotein E: Far more than a lipid transport protein. Annu Rev Genomics Hum Genet 2000;1:507–537.

3. Mahley RW, Huang Y: Apolipoprotein E: From atherosclerosis to Alzheimer's disease and beyond. Curr Opin Lipidol 1999;10:207–217.

4. Weisgraber KH: Apolipoprotein E: Structure-function relationships. Adv Protein Chem 1994;45:249–302.

5. Weisgraber KH, Mahley RW: Human apolipoprotein E: The Alzheimer's disease connection. FASEB J 1996;10:1485–1494.

6. Mahley RW, Rall SC Jr: Type III hyperlipoproteinemia (dysbetalipoproteinemia): The role of apolipoprotein E in normal and abnormal lipoprotein metabolism. In Scriver CR, Beaudet AL, Sly WS, et al (eds): The Metabolic and Molecular Bases of Inherited Disease, 8th ed, Vol 2. New York, McGraw-Hill, 2001, pp 2835–2862.

7. Roses AD: Apolipoprotein E alleles as risk factors in Alzheimer's disease. Annu Rev Med 1996;47:387–400.

8. Roses AD: Apolipoprotein E and Alzheimer's disease. The tip of the susceptibility iceberg. Ann N Y Acad Sci 1998;855:738–743.

9. Dekroon RM, Armati PJ: Synthesis and processing of apolipoprotein E in human brain cultures. Glia 2001;33:298–305.

10. Xu PT, Gilbert JR, Qiu HL, et al: Specific regional transcription of apolipoprotein E in human brain neurons. Am J Pathol 1999;154:601–611.

11. Mahley RW, Ji ZS: Remnant lipoprotein metabolism: Key pathways involving cell-surface heparan sulfate proteoglycans and apolipoprotein E. J Lipid Res 1999;40:1–16.

12. Namba Y, Tomonaga M, Kawasaki H, et al: Apolipoprotein E immunoreactivity in cerebral amyloid deposits and neurofibrillary tangles in Alzheimer's disease and kuru plaque amyloid in Creutzfeldt-Jakob disease. Brain Res 1991;541:163–166.

13. Corder EH, Saunders AM, Strittmatter WJ, et al: Gene dose of apolipoprotein E type 4 allele and the risk of Alzheimer's disease in late onset families. Science 1993;261:921–923.

14. Saunders AM, Strittmatter WJ, Schmechel D, et al: Association of apolipoprotein E allele ε4 with late-onset familial and sporadic Alzheimer's disease. Neurology 1993;43:1467–1472.

15. Farrer LA, Cupples LA, Haines JL, et al: Effects of age, sex, and ethnicity on the association between apolipoprotein E genotype and Alzheimer disease. A meta-analysis. J Am Med Assoc 1997;278:1349–1356.

16. Smith JD: Apolipoprotein E4: An allele associated with many diseases. Ann Med 2000;32:118–127.

17. Strittmatter WJ, Weisgraber KH, Huang DY, et al: Binding of human apolipoprotein E to synthetic amyloid β peptide: Isoform-specific effects and implications for late-onset Alzheimer disease. Proc Natl Acad Sci U S A 1993;90:8098–8102.

18. LaDu MJ, Lukens JR, Reardon CA, Getz GS: Association of human, rat, and rabbit apolipoprotein E with β-amyloid. J Neurosci Res 1997;49:9–18.

19. Sanan DA, Weisgraber KH, Russell SJ, et al: Apolipoprotein E associates with β amyloid peptide of Alzheimer's disease to form novel monofibrils. Isoform apoE4 associates more efficiently than apoE3. J Clin Invest 1994;94:860–869.

20. Ma J, Yee A, Brewer HB Jr, et al: Amyloid-associated proteins α1-antichymotrypsin and apolipoprotein E promote assembly of Alzheimer β-protein into filaments. Nature 1994;372:92–94.

21. Wisniewski T, Castaño EM, Golabek A, et al: Acceleration of Alzheimer's fibril formation by apolipoprotein E in vitro. Am J Pathol 1994;145:1030–1035.

22. Bales KR, Verina T, Cummins DJ, et al: Apolipoprotein E is essential for amyloid deposition in the APP^{V717F} transgenic mouse model of Alzheimer's disease. Proc Natl Acad Sci U S A 1999;96:15233–15238.

23. Selkoe DJ: Alzheimer's disease: A central role for amyloid. J Neuropathol Exp Neurol 1994;53:438–447.

24. Yankner BA: Mechanisms of neuronal degeneration in Alzheimer's disease. Neuron 1996;16:921–932.

25. Yang AJ, Chandswangbhuvana D, Margol L, Glabe CG: Loss of endosomal/lysosomal membrane impermeability is an early event in amyloid Aβ-42 pathogenesis. J Neurosci Res 1998;52:691–698.

26. Ji Z-S, Miranda RD, Newhouse YM, et al: Apolipoprotein E4 potentiates amyloid β peptide-induced lysosomal leakage and apoptosis in neuronal cells. J Biol Chem 2002;277:21821–21828.

27. Strittmatter WJ, Weisgraber KH, Goedert M, et al: Hypothesis: Microtubule instability and paired helical filament formation in the Alzheimer disease brain are related to apolipoprotein E genotype. Exp Neurol 1994;125:163–171.

28. Goedert M, Sisodia SS, Price DL: Neurofibrillary tangles and β-amyloid deposits in Alzheimer's disease. Curr Opin Neurobiol 1991;1:441–447.

29. Huang Y, Liu XQ, Wyss-Coray T, et al: Apolipoprotein E fragments present in Alzheimer's disease brains induce neurofibrillary tangle-like intracellular inclusions in neurons. Proc Natl Acad Sci U S A 2001;98:8838–8843.

30. Lovestone S, Anderton BH, Hartley K, et al: The intracellular fate of apolipoprotein E is tau dependent and apoE allele-specific. Neuroreport 1996;7:1005–1008.

31. DeMattos RB, Thorngate FE, Williams DL: A test of the cytosolic apolipoprotein E hypothesis fails to detect the escape of apolipoprotein E from the endocytic pathway into the cytosol and shows that direct expression of apolipoprotein E in the cytosol is cytotoxic. J Neurosci 1999;19:2464–2473.

32. Tolar M, Keller JN, Chan S, et al: Truncated apolipoprotein E (apoE) causes increased intracellular calcium and may mediate apoE neurotoxicity. J Neurosci 1999;19:7100–7110.

33. Games D, Adams D, Alessandrini R, et al: Alzheimer-type neuropathology in transgenic mice overexpressing V717F β-amyloid precursor protein. Nature 1995;373:523–527.

34. Masliah E, Sisk A, Mallory M, et al: Comparison of neurodegenerative pathology in transgenic mice overexpressing V717F β-amyloid precursor protein and Alzheimer's disease. J Neurosci 1996;16:5795–5811.

35. Hsiao K, Chapman P, Nilsen S, et al: Correlative memory deficits, Aβ elevation, and amyloid plaques in transgenic mice. Science 1996;274:99–102.

36. Holcomb L, Gordon MN, McGowan E, et al: Accelerated Alzheimer-type phenotype in transgenic mice carrying both mutant amyloid precursor protein and presenilin 1 transgenes. Nat Med 1998;4:97–100.

37. Ishihara T, Hong M, Zhang B, et al: Age-dependent emergence and progression of a tauopathy in transgenic mice overexpressing the shortest human tau isoform. Neuron 1999;24:751–762.

38. Lewis J, Dickson DW, Lin W-L, et al: Enhanced neurofibrillary degeneration in transgenic mice expressing mutant tau and APP. Science 2001;293:1487–1491.

39. Raber J, Wong D, Buttini M, et al: Isoform-specific effects of human apolipoprotein E on brain function revealed in ApoE knockout mice: Increased susceptibility of females. Proc Natl Acad Sci U S A 1998;95:10914–10919.

40. Buttini M, Orth M, Bellosta S, et al: Expression of human apolipoprotein E3 or E4 in the brains of Apoe$^{-/-}$ mice: Isoform-specific effects on neurodegeneration. J Neurosci 1999;19:4867–4880.

41. Holtzman DM, Bales KR, Tenkova T, et al: Apolipoprotein E isoform-dependent amyloid deposition and neuritic degeneration in a mouse model of Alzheimer's disease. Proc Natl Acad Sci U S A 2000;97:2892–2897.

42. Tesseur I, Van Dorpe J, Spittaels K, et al: Expression of human apolipoprotein E4 in neurons causes hyperphosphorylation of protein tau in the brains of transgenic mice. Am J Pathol 2000;156:951–964.

43. Raber J, Wong D, Yu GQ, et al: Apolipoprotein E and cognitive performance. Nature 2000;404:352–354.

Cerebrotendinous Xanthomatosis

Vladimir M. Berginer

Gerald Salen

Shailendra Patel

Cerebrotendinous Xanthomatosis (CTX) is a rare, recessively inherited lipid storage disease caused by defective bile acid synthesis. If untreated, CTX is slowly progressive and often lethal. The clinical phenotype includes tendon xanthomas, juvenile cataracts, and nervous system dysfunction. The latter presents as dementia, mental retardation, behavioral and psychiatric problems, pyramidal tract paresis, cerebellar ataxia, and peripheral neuropathy. Consistent features are epileptic seizures; pathologic electroencephalograms (EEGs) and evoked potentials; and abnormal neuroimaging scans. Osteoporosis, bone fractures, chronic diarrhea in children, and premature atherosclerosis also occur frequently. The underlying cause of CTX is a block in bile acid synthesis resulting in incomplete oxidation of the cholesterol side chain. This is due to inherited mutations of the mitochondrial enzyme sterol 27-hydroxylase (CYP27), located on human chromosome 2. Major biochemical findings are: increased concentrations of cholestanol (the 5α-dihydro derivative of cholesterol) in every tissue, with special enrichment in nervous tissues, cerebrospinal fluid, xanthomas, and bile; low to normal plasma cholesterol levels, with enhanced expression of LDL receptors; abnormal biliary bile acid composition with absence of chenodeoxycholic acid (CDCA) in the bile; and presence of large amounts of C-27 bile alcohols as glucuronides (bile acid precursors) in bile, plasma, and urine. Replacement therapy with CDCA (750 mg/day orally) inhibits defective bile acid synthesis leading to a decline in the production of aberrant bile alcohols and cholestanol and a normalization of biochemical abnormalities. In many cases, this leads to an improvement of neurologic function.

HISTORICAL PERSPECTIVE AND EPIDEMOLOGY

The first description of an affected patient with neurologic disease (dementia and ataxia), cataracts, and xanthomas of the tendons and central nervous system with normal serum cholesterol levels was published in 1937 by van Bogaert, Scherer, and Epstein.[1] Thirty-one years later, Menkes, Schimschock, and Swanson discovered increased amounts of cholestanol, the 5α-dihydro derivative of cholesterol (Fig. 53–1) in the central nervous system.[2] In 1971, Salen reported that biliary bile acid composition was abnormal with no chenodeoxycholic acid but with large amounts of bile alcohols (bile acid precursors) in the bile.[3] Later studies confirmed markedly reduced primary bile acid (cholic acid and chenodeoxycholic acid) synthesis in combination with enhanced cholesterol formation.[4] The bile acid synthetic defect was further elucidated by Setoguchi et al, who noted that the excreted biliary bile alcohols contained 27 carbons, indicative of incomplete cleavage of the 8 carbon steroid side-chain in the conversion of cholesterol to cholic acid.[5] As a result, large quantities of these bile alcohols were produced and excreted as glucuronides and appeared in plasma, bile, feces, and urine.[6–8]

In 1984, Berginer et al reported that long-term replacement therapy with CDCA (see Fig. 53–1), the most deficient biliary bile acid, down-regulated the abnormal bile acid synthesis pathway and eliminated bile alcohols from plasma and urine.[7–9] Elevated cholestanol levels in plasma and cerebrospinal fluid decreased, and neurologic function improved such that dementia cleared and the progression of other incapacitating neurologic symptoms slowed in most CTX subjects.[7]

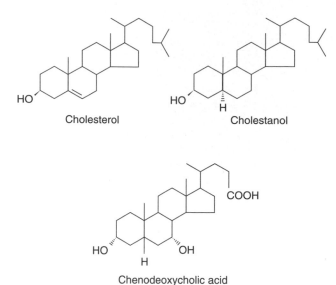

FIGURE 53–1. Structures of cholesterol (5-cholesten 3β ol), cholestanol (5α-cholestan-3β-ol), and chenodeoxycholic acid (3α,7α-dihydroxy 5β-cholestanoic acid).

TABLE 53–1. Clinical Manifestations in Cerebrotendinous Xanthomatosis

Neurologic manifestations
Dementia
Cerebellar syndrome
Pyramidal: paresis, bulbar palsy
Epileptic seizures
Peripheral neuropathy
Diffuse slow activity on electroencephalogram
Brain and spine atrophy and white matter hypodensity on magnetic resonance imaging and computed tomography scans
Psychiatric disorders
Myopathic-like facies
Juvenile cataracts
Xanthomata
Achilles and other tendons
Brain, lung, and skin
Osteoporosis and bone fractures
Large paranasal sinuses
Chronic diarrhea in children

More than 250 CTX subjects have been detected throughout the world. Affected families with the disease have been found in many countries. Most patients have been reported from Japan, the United States, Israel, the Netherlands, and Italy. The disease is inherited as an autosomal recessive trait that affects all races. Based on the varied clinical presentation, we believe that CTX may be more prevalent, with many subjects still undiagnosed.

Cali et al have reported that mutations of the sterol 27-hydroxylase *(CYP 27)* gene located on the long arm of human chromosome 2 underlie CTX.[10]

CLINICAL PRESENTATION

The clinical features develop slowly and may present irregularly in variable combinations in homozygous subjects. Table 53–1 shows the clinical findings in patients with CTX. Tendon xanthomas located in the Achilles tendons were the most common feature. It was noteworthy that the xanthomas often enlarged asymmetrically, especially after injury or biopsy. Neurologic dysfunction was the next most frequent feature followed by cataracts. As the patients grow older, progressive coronary atherosclerosis, including myocardial infarction, may develop. Severe osteoporosis that predisposes to bone fractures is present in all subjects.[14]

Central nervous system abnormalities can be detected early in childhood associated with gradual deterioration of intellectual function. Most patients cannot complete high school. The mental retardation progresses into dementia. In about 5%, intelligence remains normal and can be preserved with long-term CDCA treatment. One subject, age 76 years, has been treated with CDCA since 1972 and her intellectual function remains intact.

Behavior and psychiatric abnormalities are common and may be the presenting symptoms in some subjects. Pyramidal tract signs occur in more than 90% of patients and include increased deep-tendon reflexes, pathologic reflexes, and spastic paraplegia. Cerebellar signs, particularly ataxia, dysarthria, and nystagmus are frequently noted. Parkinsonism (spasticity and resting tremors) was observed in few CTX patients.

Epileptic seizures have been observed in half of symptomatic subjects. In some, the seizure disorder has been the presenting symptom. When juvenile cataracts and or xanthomas are detected in a young person with seizures, cholestanol and bile alcohol glucuronide levels should be measured in plasma, bile, and urine to establish the diagnosis of CTX.

Peripheral neuropathy due to cholestanol deposition and demyelination has been detected in CTX subjects. Nerve conduction velocity and visual, auditory, and sensory-motor–evoked potentials were abnormally slowed, but improved with CDCA treatment.

EEG abnormalities were found in up to 95% of CTX patients. Diffuse slowing of background activity presented as poorly organized theta and delta waves and frequent bursts of spikes and high-voltage slow-delta activity. The abnormal electrical activity improved significantly during treatment with CDCA. However, because abnormal electrical activity can be observed in other lipid storage encephalopathies, the findings are not specific for CTX.

Neuroimaging scans including cranial CT and MRI in patients with CTX demonstrated diffuse brain and spinal atrophy, with brain white matter hypodensity above and especially below the tentorium. The findings were attributed in part to sterol infiltration with secondary demyelination. However, they emphasize the possibility that the neurologic symptoms, no matter how long-standing, may result from metabolic encephalopathy rather than irreversible destruction of the brain by xanthomas.[7] More than 30 patients with CTX were investigated by CT scans, and focal hypodense lesions resembling true xanthomas were detected in only 3. MRI-demonstrated focal brain lesions were located mainly in the basal ganglia and mesencephalon areas. In all examinations, neither surrounding edema nor a significant midline shift was observed, and this was consistent with the absence of symptoms relating to increased intracranial pressure. Treatment with CDCA does not significantly improve neuroimaging (atrophy), although in one 13-year-old girl, the focal hypodense area (presumed xanthoma) seen by CT scan in the cerebellar hemisphere disappeared after 1 year of therapy. Intracranial calcifications are infrequently observed in CTX patients.

The cerebrospinal fluid (CSF) in CTX subjects is colorless with a normal opening pressure. Cholesterol and cholestanol levels in CSF from untreated patients with CTX were almost 1.5 to 20.0 times higher than those in control subjects.[12] In CSF from untreated patients with CTX, immunoreactive apolipoprotein B or apolipoprotein B fragments were increased about 100-fold and albumin about 3.5-fold. These results suggest that the blood-brain barrier is defective and may lead to the entry of cholestanol and LDL from the plasma. During CDCA treatment, the concentration of albumin and apolipoprotein B in the CSF declined and cholestanol levels diminished. It is hypothesized that the high levels of circulating plasma bile alcohols damage the blood-brain barrier to increase permeability with the subsequent rise in brain cholestanol levels and neural damage.

Juvenile cataracts are present in at least 90% of CTX patients. Zonular cortical lens opacities can appear at age 5 to 6 years or younger, but are almost invariably present by the second or third decade of life.

Xanthomas are almost essential features of CTX. They are most often located in the Achilles tendons, but may be present in other extensor tendons and the dermis (tuberous). Interestingly, Achilles tendon xanthomas develop in the proximal portion of the tendon where they attach to the gastrocnemius muscle and first appear in the second or third decade of life. Similar xanthomas have been observed in familial hypercholesterolemia and sitosterolemia, but in these disorders neither juvenile cataracts nor neurologic symptoms are a feature. Although cholestanol is elevated in sitosterolemia, only traces are detectable in the brains of sitosterolemia patients. Conversely, elevated plasma and tissue phytosterols are not found in CTX.

Osteoporosis was present in the majority of CTX patients and may increase the risk of bone fractures.[11] The long bones and vertebrae were particularly vulnerable. However, in CTX patients with osteoporosis, serum calcium, inorganic phosphorus, alkaline phosphatase, parathyroid hormone, calcitonin, and 1,25-dihydroxy vitamin D_3 levels were normal. Serum concentrations of 25-hydroxy vitamin D_3 and 24-25-dihydroxy vitamin D_3 tend to be low, but not subnormal.[11]

Myopathic-like elongated face with slightly open mouth and protuberant tongue and prominent paranasal sinuses were commonly observed in CTX patients who often showed serious dental problems.

BIOCHEMICAL ABNORMALITIES

The major biochemical features that distinguish CTX from other conditions with xanthomas include (1) increased plasma and tissue cholestanol concentrations with particularly large deposits in brain, xanthomas, and bile; (2) low or normal plasma cholesterol concentrations associated with increased expression of LDL receptors; (3) defective primary bile acid synthesis with decreased formation of CDCA and a reduced proportion of biliary CDCA relative to cholic acid; (4) increased quantities of C-27 bile alcohols, with intact 8 carbon side chains appearing as glucuronides in bile, feces, urine, and plasma; and (5) disruption of the blood-brain barrier with increased amounts of cholestanol and apolipoprotein B in CSF.

Increased deposits of cholestanol in the brain of CTX subjects were first discovered by Menkes et al.[2] As discussed, cholestanol is the 5α-dihydro derivative of cholesterol and is normally present in very small amounts in association with cholesterol in all tissues and plasma. However, in CTX, cholestanol accounts for 2% of the plasma sterols, 10% of the biliary and xanthoma sterols, and up to 50% of the brain sterols.[3] Normally, cholestanol represents 0.1% of tissue sterols. Cholestanol is transported with cholesterol in the plasma by low-density and high-density lipoproteins. Despite enhanced production of cholesterol and cholestanol,[4] LDL and HDL sterol levels were diminished in CTX; however, LDL formation was increased. LDL catabolism was accelerated due to increased expression of LDL receptors that contributed to low plasma concentrations. HDL cholesterol levels were subnormal in many CTX subjects, which may account for the accelerated atherosclerosis and xanthoma formation by hindering reverse sterol transport.

Increased cholestanol and apolipoprotein B concentrations have been found in the cerebrospinal fluid of CTX subjects.[12] Apolipoprotein B is neither produced nor catabolized in the central nervous system, so damage to the blood-brain barrier must account for high concentrations in CSF. In addition, cholestanol is produced solely in the liver; therefore, the abnormal sterol deports in the brain likely arise from plasma lipoproteins. Cholestanol formation begins with cholesterol and is markedly increased in CTX.[4] Two pathways have been identified in CTX. The classic mechanism involves the conversion of cholesterol to 4-cholesten-3-one followed by 5α-reduction to cholestanol. Microsomal 3β-hydroxy-steroid-dehydrogenase-isomerase activity is three-fold higher in CTX liver microsomes than controls. An alternative mechanism, proposed by Skrede et al[13] showed that 7α-hydroxycholesterol, a key intermediate in bile acid synthesis that is overproduced in CTX, is partially transformed to cholestanol.

ABNORMAL BILE ACID SYNTHESIS

An important early observation in CTX subjects was the absence of chenodeoxycholic acid in the bile.[3] This suggested that bile acid synthesis may be disturbed and was confirmed by the demonstration of diminished formation combined with the excretion of large amounts of C-27 bile alcohol glucuronides in the bile, urine, and feces of CTX subjects.[4,5]

Defective bile acid synthesis is the primary inherited biochemical defect.[14] Two enzymatic mechanisms seem responsible for the incomplete oxidation of the cholesterol side chain and subnormal production of bile acids in CTX. Molecular analysis indicated that inherited mutations of sterol 27-hydroxylase, a mitochondrial P-450 enzyme that catalyzes multiple oxidation reactions in bile acid synthesis, underlie CTX.[10] However, CYP27 knockout mice with no mitochondrial CYP27 hydroxylase activity do not show any typical CTX-related pathologic or biochemical abnormalities.[15] In recently reported studies, Honda et al. showed that side-chain hydroxylations in bile acid synthesis catalyzed by microsomal CYP3A (alternative 25-hydroxylation pathway) were markedly up-regulated in CYP27 knockout mice but not in CTX.[16,17] Thus, deficient mitochondrial CYP27 activity due to an inherited mutation and the inability to increase alternative side-chain C-25 hydroxylations due to decreased microsomal CYP3A activity results in diminished bile acid production and the excretion of excessive quantities of C-27 bile alcohols with intact side chains.

Experimental attempts to reproduce the CTX phenotype in mice, rabbits, and rats by feeding cholestanol-enriched diets increased levels in liver, heart, and aorta, but did not accumulate much in brain. Damage to the blood-brain barrier presumably by circulating bile alcohol glucuronides is necessary to facilitate the uptake of cholestanol and cholesterol in brain from plasma LDL.

Diagnosis

The clinical diagnosis of CTX in symptomatic patients is based on the demonstration of xanthomas (usually located in the Achilles tendons), juvenile cataracts, and neurologic abnormalities that include behavioral prob-

lems, mental retardation and dementia, pyramidal and cerebellar insufficiency, epileptic seizures, and peripheral neuropathy. Electrophysiologic studies reveal abnormal EEG with diffuse slow waves and sometimes bursts of high-voltage activity, slowness of nerve conduction velocity, and evoked potentials. Neuroimaging (CT and MRI) scans demonstrate cerebral, cerebellar, and spinal atrophy and rarely circumscribed areas of low-density (xanthomas). X-rays of bones often show osteoporosis and large paranasal sinuses of the skull.

Variants of the typical presentation include predominant parkinsonism and, rarely, spinal xanthomatosis. In addition, several CTX patients presented with symptomatic coronary atherosclerosis.

In patients with classic phenotypic characteristics, demonstration of an elevated plasma cholestanol level and barely or undetectable phytosterols is sufficient to confirm a CTX diagnosis. In asymptomatic patients and patients with absent classical features, in addition to an elevated plasma cholestanol level, confirmation of the diagnosis relies on detection of C-27 bile alcohols as glucuronides in bile, plasma, and urine. If the diagnosis remains uncertain, bile acid malabsorption induced by feeding (e.g., administering 12 g/day of cholestyramine for 5 days) stimulates bile acid synthesis and increases plasma cholestanol levels and output of bile alcohols in the urine of CTX patients and, to a much smaller extent, of carriers.[4] Other conditions with xanthomas, such as familial hypercholesterolemia and sitosterolemia (also known as phytosterolemia), can be distinguished from CTX by the demonstration in blood samples of only increased cholesterol levels in the former and elevation of phytosterols in the latter. More recently, knowing the genetic defect(s) in CTX may allow for a molecular diagnosis, especially in identifying new cases in existing families where minimal sampling such as check scrapping for DNA only is available, as well as for antenatal screening. This modality for diagnosis has been reported.[18]

Therapy

The hypothesis that underlies the treatment of CTX is that increased formation of cholestanol and cholesterol that deposit in the brain, blood vessels, and xanthomas results from the inherited defect in bile acid synthesis.[4,5] It further suggests[11] that metabolic encephalopathy due to deposition of cholestanol and cholesterol in nervous tissues is potentially reversible before a critical mass of accumulated sterols and stanols permanently destroys nervous tissues.[7] Therefore, it is important to promptly begin replacement therapy with CDCA. Long-term treatment with CDCA at a dose of 750 mg/day (calculated to be 33% greater than normal daily bile acid production) suppressed abnormal bile acid synthesis. This is evidenced by the almost total replacement of CDCA in the enterohepatic pool and the disappearance of bile alcohol glucuronides from the bile, plasma, and urine.[9] Plasma and CSF cholestanol levels declined gradually, associated with a rise in plasma cholesterol concentrations that reestablished the normal cholestanol/cholesterol ratio. Selective permeability of the blood-brain barrier returned, as noted also by the marked decrease in CSF apolipoprotein B concentrations. The rise in plasma cholesterol with treatment was attributed to decreased expression of LDL receptors with diminished LDL catabolism. The clinical neurologic response to CDCA treatment in CTX subjects was impressive. After 1 year, dementia cleared, erratic behavior in many patients improved, and pyramidal and extrapyramidal cerebellar signs and epileptic seizures disappeared or diminished. EEG became normal or showed fewer abnormalities. Nerve conduction velocities and evoked potentials improved. The neurologic improvement was better when treatment with CDCA was started early to prevent the development of neurologic dysfunction in clinically unaffected but biochemically abnormal subjects with CTX.[7]

It is important to emphasize that treatment with CDCA is lifetime replacement therapy. No untoward effects have been encountered, although some patients have been treated for more than 20 years. Moreover, treatment with CDCA is highly specific, as treatment with ursodeoxycholic acid (its 7β-hydroxy epimer) is totally ineffective.[7]

A brief word of caution about combining CDCA with a statin drug that inhibits HMG-CoA reductase is in order. These statin inhibitors of cholesterol synthesis do not produce additional biochemical benefits when compared with CDCA alone, and clinical benefits have not been forthcoming.[19] Statin drugs may actually enhance LDL receptor expression to increase the uptake of LDL sterols (cholestanol, cholesterol, and bile alcohols) in tissues, which may be counterproductive. LDL-apheresis is another suggested treatment that was reported to reduce the levels of cholestanol in CTX. However, it cannot be recommended for treatment of CTX patients.

MOLECULAR DEFECTS

Following the purification and sequencing of the rabbit sterol 27-hydroxylase, Cali and colleagues isolated the human cDNA and showed that in two patients with CTX, point mutations of the coding of this gene were associated with the disease.[10] The previously purified enzyme protein was known to be a cytochrome P-450 with a high heme content that required the presence of two cofactors for maximal activity: ferredoxin and ferredoxin reductase. Characterization of the cDNA for sterol 27-hydroxylase (CYP 27) showed that it contained a leader signal peptide that would allow its targeting and import to the mitochondrion, and comparison of the protein sequence to known cytochrome P-450 proteins showed it to have 33% amino acid homology.

The *CYP27* gene was localized to chromosome 2q33-ster by somatic cell hybridization and has been sub-

sequently fine-mapped to lie between microsatellite markers D2S1371 and D2S424.[18] Interestingly, the mRNA for *CYP27* is widely expressed with comparable amounts in liver, lung, duodenum, and adrenal gland. Its expression has also been subsequently detected in monocytes and in atherosclerotic lesions. However, expression in the brain is limited.[21] Thus, almost all cells in the body are capable of converting cholesterol to 27-hydroxy cholesterol. However, only the liver is capable of forming bile acids; thus, these metabolites are transferred into the circulation and cleared by the liver. Bjorkhem et al. proposed that this pathway may be important in "reverse" cholesterol transport, and thus *CYP27* may also play a beneficial role in prevention or delay of atheroclerosis.[21]

Leiterdorf et al characterized the human *CYP27* gene and showed in a larger cohort of CTX probands that *CYP27* was mutated in all of these cases.[20] Subsequently, various groups have described mutations in probands drawn from almost every part of the world.[18,22] These are summarized in Figure 53–2. (Mutations are indicated below the gene; missense mutations that may potentially lead to the synthesis of a full-length polypeptide are indicated above the gene. For simplicity, complex mutations such as large genomic deletions are not depicted.) Most mutations result in introduction of a stop codon, frameshift and premature chain termination, or aberrant splicing. Based on three-dimensional modeling, all but two of the missense mutations that are predicted to lead to translation of a peptide map to the critical heme—or adrenodoxin-binding domains—and are thus likely to lead to inactive enzymes.[18] However, two of these mutations affecting peptides Arg 127 and Lys 259 map to domains outside of these and may indicate other potential function domains of the enzyme.[18] Some of the missense mutations (affecting *R395, R405, R474,* and *R479*) have been shown to lead to an almost complete absence of functional enzyme (either in mutant fibroblasts or by heterologous expression). To date, there does not appear to be a direct relationship between the type of genetic defect and the clinical or biochemical severity of CTX.[18,20,22]

MOUSE MODELS AND FUTURE RESEARCH

In 1998, Rosen et al reported on knockout mice with a disrupted *CYP27* gene.[15] However, the *CYP27*$^{-/-}$ mice do not manifest any of the CTX phenotype seen in humans. Moreover, there was no accumulation of cholestanol in the liver or plasma. In bile and feces, only trace amounts of 25-hydroxylated bile alcohols were detected. CDCA, muricholic acid, and cholic acid in bile were reduced when compared to wild-type mice. The only finding resembling human CTX was increased plasma and tissue 7α-hydroxycholesterol concentrations. Thus, neither the clinical nor biochemical features of CTX were reproduced in the *CYP27*$^{-/-}$ mice. Livers from *CYP27*$^{-/-}$ mice produce less 7α-hydroxycholesterol than livers from

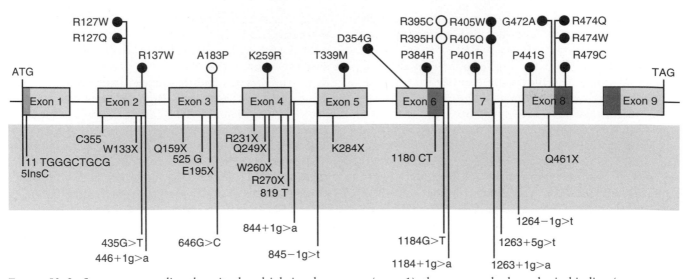

FIGURE 53-2. Sequences encoding the mitochondrial signal sequence (exon 1), the conserved adrenodoxin-binding (or ferredoxin-binding) domain (exon 6), and the heme-binding domain (exons 8 and 9). Missense mutations that may lead to translation of a full-length protein product are shown *(dark circles above gene structure)*. Three point mutations *(R137W, R395C, and R395S)* may not lead to protein, as they are located at the splice boundary regions. In this context, Cali et al did not report any aberrant splicing for the R385 (1184 G → T) mutation.[10] Mutations that may lead to truncated proteins are shown *(below gene structure)*. Of these, mutations that lead to premature chain termination, or introduction of a stop translation codon are indicated *(large box)*. Mutations affecting splicing are also shown *(below box)*. These may lead to exon skipping, frame-shift and premature chain termination, or mRNA instability. For simplicity, large deletion mutations are not depicted.

CTX subjects where *CYP7A* is markedly up-regulated.[16,17] Further, side-chain hydroxylations and cleavage to form cholic acid via *CYP3A* are fivefold higher in $CYP27^{-/-}$ mice than in CTX subjects. Thus, fewer early bile acid precursors (7α-hydroxycholesterol) are formed in $CYP27^{-/-}$ mice (they have a much greater capacity to convert early bile acid precursors to cholic acid because *CYP3A* is markedly increased), so they are more resistant to loss of *CYP27* activity relative to humans. Variations in *CYP3A 4* (alternative side chain hydroxylation) in humans may thus account for the variability in the clinical phenotype. This is an enticing possibility that will need to be explored in future studies.

REFERENCES

1. van Bogaert L, Scherer HJ, Epstein E: Une Forme Cerebrale de la Cholesterinose Genezalisee. Paris, Masson et Cie, 1937.

2. Menkes JH, Schimschock JR, Swanson PD: Cerebrotendinous xanthomatosis: The storage of cholestanol within the nervous system. Arch Neurol 1968;19:47.

3. Salen G: Cholestanol deposition in cerebrotendinous xanthomatosis: A possible mechanism. Ann Intern Med 1971;75:843.

4. Salen G, Grundy SM: The metabolism of cholestanol, cholesterol and bile acids in cerebrotendinous xanthomatosis. J Clin Invest 1973;52:2822.

5. Setoguchi T, Salen G, Tint GS, et al: A biochemical abnormality in cerebrotendinous xanthomatosis: Impairment of bile acid biosynthesis associated with incomplete degradation of the cholesterol side chain. J Clin Invest 1974;531.

6. Hoshita T, Yasuhara M, Une M, et al: Occurrence of bile alcohol glucuronides in bile of patients with cerebrotendinous xanthomatosis. J Lipid Res 1980;21:1015.

7. Berginer VM, Salen G, Shefer S: Long-term treatment of cerebrotendinous xanthomatosis with chenodeoxycholic acid. N Engl J Med 1984;311:1649.

8. Batta AK, Shefer S, Batta M, et al: Effect of chenodeoxycholic acid on biliary and urinary bile acids and bile alcohols in cerebrotendinous xanthomatosis: Monitoring by high performance liquid chromatography. J Lipid Res 1985;26:690.

9. Batta AK, Salen G, Shefer S, et al: Increased plasma bile alcohol glucuronides in patients with cerebrotendinous xanthomatosis: Effect of chenodeoxycholic acid. J Lipid Res 1987;28:1006.

10. Cali JJ, Hsieh CL, Francke U, et al: Mutations in the bile acid biosynthetic enzyme sterol 27-hydroxylase underlie cerebrotendinous xanthomatosis. J Biol Chem 1991;266:7779.

11. Berginer VM, Shany S, Alkalay D, et al: Osteoporosis and increased bone fractures in cerebrotendinous xanthomatosis (CTX). Metabolism 1993;42:69.

12. Salen G, Berginer VM, Shore V, et al: Increased concentrations of cholestanol and apolipoprotein B in the

cerebrospinal fluid of patients with cerebrotendinous xanthomatosis: Effect of chenodeoxycholic acid. N Engl J Med 1987;315:1233.

13. Skrede S, Bjorkhem I, Buchmann MS, et al: A novel pathway for biosynthesis of cholestanol with 7α-hydroxylated C27-steroids as intermediates, and its importance for the accumulation of cholestanol in cerebrotendinous xanthomatosis. J Clin Invest 1985;75:448.

14. Salen G, Shefer S, Tint GS, et al: Biosynthesis of bile acids in cerebrotendinous xanthomatosis: Relationship of bile acid pool sizes and synthesis rates to hydroxylations at C-12, C-25 and C-26. J Clin Invest 1985;76:744.

15. Rosen HA, Reshef A, Maeda N, et al. Markedly reduced bile acid synthesis but maintained levels of cholesterol and vitamin D metabolites in mice with disrupted sterol 27-hydroxylase gene. J Biol Chem 1998;273: 14805.

16. Honda A, Salen G, Matsuzaki Y, et al: Differences in hepatic levels of intermediates in bile acid biosynthesis between Cyp27$^{-/-}$ and CTX. J Lipid Res 2001;42:291.

17. Honda A, Salen G, Matsuzaki Y, et al: Side chain hydroxylations are markedly up-regulated in Cyp27$^{-/-}$ mice but not in cerebrotendinous xanthomatosis. J Biol Chem 2001;276:34579.

18. Lee M-H, Hazzard S, Carpten JD, et al: Fine mapping mutation analyses, and structural mapping of cerebrotendinous xanthomatosis in U.S. pedigrees. J Lipid Res 2001;42:159.

19. Salen G, Batta AK, Tint GS, et al. Comparative effects of lovastatin and chenodeoxycholic acid on plasma cholestanol levels and abnormal bile acid metabolism in cerebrotendinous xanthomatosis. Metabolism 1994;43:1018.

20. Leiterdorf E, Reshef A, Meiner V, et al: Frameshift and splice-function mutations in the sterol 27-hydroxylase gene cause cerebrotendinous xanthomatosis in Jews of Moroccan origin. J Clin Invest 1993;91:2488.

21. Bjorkhem I, Diczfalusy U, Lutjohann D: Removal of cholesterol from extrahepatic sources by oxidative mechanisms. Curr Opin Lipid 1999;10:161.

22. Verrips A, Hoefsloot LH, Steenbergen GC, et al: Clinical and molecular genetic characteristics of patients with cerebrotendinous xanthomatosis. Brain 2000; 123:908.

CHAPTER

54

Glycogen Storage Diseases

Salvatore DiMauro

Serenella Servidei

Seiichi Tsujino

The concentration of glycogen in skeletal muscle (about 1 g/100 g fresh tissue) is second only to that in liver (up to 6 g/100 g tissue). Liver glycogen serves mainly to keep blood glucose constant, whereas muscle glycogen is exclusively for internal consumption and is one of the major fuels for muscle contraction.[1]

The immediate source of energy for contraction and relaxation derives from the hydrolysis of adenosine triphosphate (ATP), but ATP stores are meager, and ATP resynthesis depends on four metabolic processes: (1) oxidative phosphorylation; (2) anaerobic glycolysis; (3) the creatine kinase (CK) reaction, converting phosphocreatine (PCr) to ATP; and (4) the adenylate kinase reaction that catalyzes the conversion of two molecules of adenosine diphosphate (ADP) to one molecule of ATP and one of adenosine monophosphate (AMP); this is coupled to the adenylate deaminase reaction converting AMP to inosine monophosphate (IMP).

Quantitatively, oxidative phosphorylation is by far the most important source of energy. Anaerobic glycolysis plays a relatively minor role, essentially limited to conditions of sustained *isometric* contraction, when blood flow and oxygen delivery to exercising muscles are drastically reduced. Conversely, aerobic glycolysis is an important source of energy, especially during the more common, *dynamic* form of exercise, such as walking or running. Accordingly, the pathophysiology of glycogenoses due to defects of glycogenolysis or glycolysis relates more to the impairment of aerobic than anaerobic glycolysis.

There are 14 glycogen storage diseases (GSD) associated with specific defects of glycogen synthesis (GSD IV), glycogen breakdown (GSD I, II, III, V, VI, and VIII), or glycolysis (GSD VII to XIV) (Fig. 54–1). Two of these, GSD I and VI, affect mainly the liver, cause neurologic

symptoms only indirectly (e.g., hypoglycemic seizures), and will not be considered here. Of the remaining twelve entities, some affect muscle exclusively because the genetic defect involves a muscle-specific protein (e.g., myophosphorylase in GSD V) or, more often, the muscle-specific subunit of a multimeric enzyme (e.g., subunit M of phosphofructokinase in GSD VII). Others affect multiple tissues either because the enzyme is a single polypeptide (e.g., acid maltase in GSD II) or because the mutated muscle-specific subunit of a multimeric enzyme is shared with non-muscle isoforms, causing partial defects in other tissues (e.g., compensated hemolytic anemia in GSD VII).[2]

Clinical Features

Glycogen storage diseases cause two main clinical presentations (Tables 54-1 and 54-2; see also Fig. 54–1).

The first syndrome is characterized by acute, recurrent, reversible muscle dysfunction, manifesting as exercise intolerance or myalgia, with or without painful cramps (contractures), and often culminating in muscle breakdown (rhabdomyolysis) and myoglobinuria. This is the typical clinical picture of patients with defects in glycogen breakdown (phosphorylase b-kinase [PHK] deficiency [GSD-VIII] and phosphorylase deficiency [GSD V]) or defects in glycolysis (phosphofructokinase [PFK] deficiency [GSD VII], phosphoglycerate kinase [PGK] deficiency [GSD IX], phosphoglycerate mutase [PGAM] deficiency [GSD X], β enolase deficiency [GSD XIII], and lactate dehydrogenase [LDH] deficiency [GSD XI]).

Typically, patients experience myalgia, premature fatigue, and stiffness or weakness of exercising muscles, which is relieved by rest. The type and amount of exercise

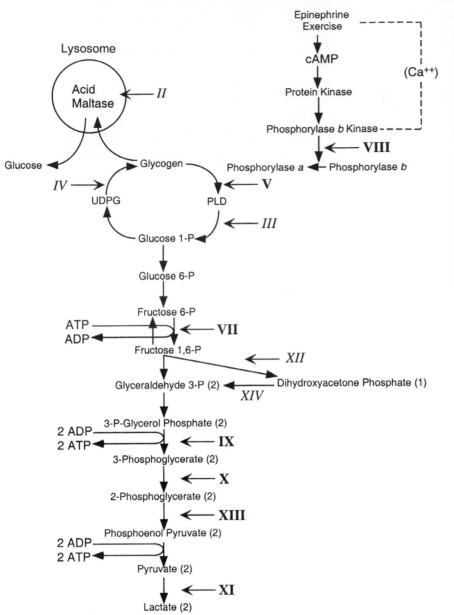

FIGURE 54–1. Scheme of glycogen metabolism and glycolysis. Roman numerals indicate enzymes whose deficiencies are associated with glycogen storage diseases (GSD): II, acid maltase; III, debrancher; IV, brancher; V, myophosphorylase; VII, muscle phosphofructokinase (PFK-M); VIII, phosphorylase b-kinase (PHK); IX, phosphoglycerate kinase (PGK); X, phosphoglycerate mutase (PGAM); XI, lactate dehydrogenase (LDH); XII, aldolase-A; XIII, β-enolase; XIV, triosephosphate isomerase (TPI). Bold numerals indicate GSD causing exercise intolerance, cramps, and myoglobinuria; italicized numerals indicate GSD causing weakness.

needed to precipitate symptoms vary from patient to patient, but two types of exertion are more likely to cause problems: brief intense isometric exercise, such as lifting heavy weights, or less intense but sustained dynamic exercise, such as walking uphill. Some patients learn to adjust their activities and lead relatively normal lives. However, when they exceed their limited exercise tolerance, they experience painful cramps and may develop myoglobinuria, with the attendant risk of renal shutdown. Myoglobinuria occurs in about 50% of patients with myophosphorylase deficiency (McArdle disease); it is less common in defects of glycolysis, and least common in PHK deficiency. Uncomplicated episodes of myoglobinuria are followed by complete clinical recovery.

The "second wind" phenomenon is characteristic of McArdle disease and much less common in PFK deficiency: when patients slow down or pause briefly at the

first appearance of symptoms, they can resume exercising with better endurance. This is related to increased muscle blood flow and increased availability of oxidizable blood-borne fuels (free fatty acids and glucose).

Onset is in childhood, and most patients describe their symptoms as lifelong, but severe cramps and myoglobinuria are rarely reported before adolescence. These disorders appear to be nonprogressive, but fixed weakness tends to set in with increasing age, especially in McArdle disease and in PFK deficiency. This is probably related to chronic muscle damage induced by everyday activities.

Extramuscular symptoms are rare. Jaundice and gouty arthritis may occur in PFK deficiency, reflecting hyperuricemia and hemolytic anemia. Hemolytic anemia and mental retardation may accompany myopathy in PGK deficiency. Dystocia and dermatological problems were reported in some patients with LDH deficiency.

TABLE 54–1. Glycogenoses Causing Exercise Intolerance, Cramps, and Myoglobinuria

Enzyme GSD no.	Non-muscle tissues affected	Isozyme or subunit	Chromosomal location	Common mutations
Phosphorylase b-kinase GSD VIII		$PHK\alpha_M$ PHKβ?	Xq12-13 16q12-13	
Phosphorylase GSD V		M	11q13	R49X (Whites)
PFK GSD VII	RBC	PFK-M	12q	Δ5 (Ashkenazi)
PGK GSD IX	RBC CNS	PGK-1	Xq13	
PGAM GSD X		PGAM-M	7p13-12.3	
LDH GSD XI	Smooth muscle skin	LDH-A	11p15.4	
β-enolase GSD XIII		β	17pter-q11	

CNS, central nervous system; RBC, red blood cells.

Rare, atypical phenotypes include fatal infantile myopathies in myophosphorylase or PFK deficiencies.

The second syndrome is characterized by progressive weakness involving limb and trunk muscles but usually sparing extraocular and facial muscles. This is the typical presentation of the single defect in glycogen synthesis (brancher deficiency, GSD IV), the single lysosomal glycogenosis (acid maltase deficiency, GSD II), debrancher deficiency (GSD III), and two glycolytic defects (aldolase A deficiency [GSD XII], and triosephosphate isomerase [TPI] deficiency [GSD XIV]).

The weakness is severe and generalized in infants with acid maltase deficiency (AMD). Some of these infants have isolated myopathy, whereas others have multisystem involvement, with massive cardiomegaly, less severe hepatomegaly, and, sometimes, macroglossia (Pompe disease). Patients with the childhood or adult-onset varieties of AMD have truncal and proximal limb myopathies often simulating muscular dystrophies or polymyositis. Early involvement of respiratory muscles is typical of AMD.

In debrancher deficiency (GSD III), weakness often becomes manifest in adult life and may be severe and generalized or milder and predominantly distal. Patients with distal weakness are often thought to have Charcot-Marie-Tooth disease or motor neuron disease.

Extramuscular involvement is extremely common in this group of glycogenoses and may contribute to the weakness. As previously mentioned, cardiomegaly dominates the clinical picture of infantile AMD (Pompe disease). Cardiomegaly can also be seen in infants with PHK

deficiency (GSD VIII) and in children with brancher deficiency (GSD IV). In debrancher deficiency (GSD III), cardiac involvement is common but cardiomegaly or overt cardiac symptoms are rare.

Hepatosplenomegaly, cirrhosis, and hepatic failure are common causes of death in children with brancher deficiency (GSD IV), but hepatomegaly may be associated with myopathy in less severely affected patients. In contrast, hepatomegaly and liver dysfunction often resolve spontaneously in patients with debrancher deficiency, some of whom develop myopathy later in life.

Both central and peripheral nervous systems are involved in infantile AMD (Pompe disease). Peripheral neuropathy is not uncommon in debrancher deficiency. An adult variant of brancher deficiency (adult polyglucosan body disease, APBD) is characterized by progressive upper and lower motor neuron disorder associated with sensory loss, sphincter problems, and, in about one half of the patients, dementia. Mental retardation has been reported in the single patient with TPI deficiency.

Diagnostic Evaluation

In patients with exercise intolerance, cramps, and myoglobinuria, GSD should be considered in the differential diagnosis, especially when the following clinical features are observed: (1) symptoms occur invariably in association with exercise and the muscles that ache or swell are those that had been exercised; (2) symptoms are triggered by sustained isometric exercise; (3) ischemic exercise causes visible cramps; (4) resting serum CK is elevated

TABLE 54–2. Glycogenoses Causing Fixed Weakness

Enzyme GSD no.	Non-muscle tissues affected	Isozyme or subunit	Chromosomal location	Common mutations
α-Glucosidase GSD, II	heart CNS liver		17q23-q25	IVS1-13t > g (Whites) Δ18 9 (Dutch) R854X (African-American)
Debrancher GSD III	liver heart		1p21	4455delT (North African Jews)
Brancher GSD IV	liver heart brain (APBD)		3p12	Y329S (APBD)
Aldolase GSD XII	RBC	Ald A	16q22-24	
TPI GSD XIV	RBC brain		12p13	
Lafora disease	brain nerve	laforin	6q	

APBD, adult polyglucosan body disease; CNS, central nervous system; RBC, red blood cells.

outside episodes of myoglobinuria. These features help distinguish GSD from the two other metabolic derangements causing similar symptoms, disorders of lipid metabolism, and defects of the mitochondrial respiratory chain. In disorders of lipid metabolism, there are no overt cramps, episodes of myoglobinuria are not triggered exclusively by exercise (prolonged fasting being a major precipitating factor), the offending exercise is prolonged rather than strenuous, and interictal CK is normal. In disorders of the respiratory chain, premature fatigue is the dominating feature, there is myalgia but no cramps, and myoglobinuria is often precipitated by repetitive exercise.[1]

The forearm ischemic exercise—which fails to increase venous lactate when there is a block anywhere in glycogenolysis or glycolysis (see Fig. 54–1)—is still useful, but is falling out of favor for two main reasons: (1) it depends on the ability and willingness of the patient to exercise vigorously; and (2) it is painful and may provoke local muscle damage with myoglobinuria.

Secure diagnosis of these disorders—of which all but one (PGK deficiency) are due to defects of muscle-specific enzymes—once required muscle biopsy for biochemical (or, less reliably, histochemical) documentation of the enzyme deficiency. Although muscle biopsy is still needed in most cases, it can be bypassed in some patients in whom a probable clinical diagnosis can be confirmed by molecular analysis of genomic DNA isolated from blood cells.[3] For this to happen, however, a few mutations associated with the disease in question must be especially frequent, at least in the ethnic group to which the patient belongs. Some of the most common mutations are listed in Tables 54–1 and 54–2.

In patients with weakness and without involvement of other tissues, the differential diagnosis from muscular dystrophies, neurogenic disorders, and inflammatory myopathies may be very difficult in the absence of a muscle biopsy, in part because serum CK levels can be very high in AMD and debrancher deficiency. The predominant involvement of respiratory muscles in AMD is a useful clue to the diagnosis.

Pathology

In GSD with exercise intolerance and myoglobinuria, muscle biopsy typically shows subsarcolemmal and less marked intermyofibrillar accumulations of glycogen, best revealed by the periodic acid-Schiff (PAS) reaction in semi-thin plastic-embedded sections. The glycogen storage may be mild enough to escape detection, especially in defects of terminal glycolysis (PGK, PGAM, and LDH deficiencies). Histochemical stains are available for myophosphorylase and PFK. Electron microscopy shows deposits of normal-looking glycogen beta particles in all forms except PFK deficiency.

In PFK deficiency, besides normal glycogen, there is accumulation of an abnormal polysaccharide, which stains intensely with PAS but is not digested by diastase.[4] Ultrastructurally, this polysaccharide is composed of finely granular and filamentous material, similar to the polyglucosan that accumulates in brancher deficiency and in Lafora disease (see later).

In some GSD with progressive weakness, muscle biopsies show massive accumulation of glycogen. This is especially true in both the myopathic and the generalized form of infantile AMD, in which muscle fibers take a "lacework" appearance, and ultrastructure shows both free and intralysosomal glycogen ("glycogenosomes") distorting the contractile system. Severe vacuolar myopathy, with large pools of free glycogen and some reactive glycogenosomes, is also characteristic of debrancher deficiency.[4] In contrast, glycogen storage in muscle was mild in the isolated patients with aldolase A deficiency and TPI deficiency. In brancher deficiency, the muscle biopsy shows pockets of polyglucosan, whose histochemical and ultrastructural features have been described earlier.

No histochemical reaction is available for AM, but the reaction for acid phosphatase, another lysosomal enzyme, is abnormally intense in patients with AMD.

Neuropathology has shown intralysosomal glycogen accumulation in Pompe disease, especially severe in anterior horn cells of the spinal cord (probably contributing to the flaccid weakness and explaining the tongue fasciculations often observed in these infants). Polyglucosan accumulates to various extent in all tissues of patients with brancher deficiency. In APBD, polyglucosan bodies are present in processes (but not in perikarya) of neurons and astrocytes in both gray and white matter. In sural nerve biopsies, often used for the diagnosis of APBD, polyglucosan bodies are abundant in the axoplasm of myelinated fibers and less abundant in unmyelinated fibers and Schwann cells.

Biochemical Findings

Glycogen storage diseases are defined by specific enzyme defects in muscle or other affected tissues. Residual activities are usually below 10% of normal in muscle, and are often explained by the presence of non-muscle isozymes. For example, in PGAM deficiency, the 5% residual muscle activity is due to the "heart" dimer, HH, and in LDH deficiency the same residual activity is due to the normal "heart" tetramer, H4. Immunochemical studies of muscle from patients with McArdle disease had shown lack of cross-reacting material (that is, enzyme protein) in most cases.[4] The explanation—we now know—is that the vast majority of white patients harbor a nonsense mutation in the first exon of the gene, which impedes protein synthesis.[4,5]

Why acid maltase deficiency—the defect of a single lysosomal polypeptide—should result in a generalized disorder (Pompe disease) and in a purely myopathic disorder (with onset in infancy, childhood, or adult life) remains unclear, because the enzyme defect is generalized in all forms. A small but crucially important difference in residual activity seems sufficient to protect non-muscle tissues in myopathic patients.

The differential tissue involvement in some patients with debrancher or brancher deficiency is difficult to explain because both enzymes are single polypeptides encoded by single genes. Accumulating evidence suggests that differential expression of a single gene may give rise to multiple isoforms, only some of which are affected by different mutations.

Molecular Genetic Findings

The genes encoding all proteins involved in GSD have been cloned, sequenced, and assigned to chromosomal loci (see Tables 54–1 and 54–2). Pathogenic mutations too numerous to be listed here have been identified for each disorder.[4] We will limit this discussion to a few general considerations.

There is striking genetic heterogeneity, often contrasting with relative clinical stereotypy. For example, at least 33 mutations have been identified in patients with McArdle disease, a clinically uniform disorder.[5] Conversely, the few patients with distinct phenotypes, such as fatal infantile myopathy or sudden infant death syndrome, harbored the most common mutation. Thus, genotype:phenotype correlations remain fuzzy, and not just for McArdle disease.

However, some interesting correlations are emerging. In AMD, for which about 50 mutations have been described, there is a reasonably good correspondence between severity of the mutation and severity of the clinical phenotype. Thus, deletions and nonsense mutations are usually associated with infantile AMD, whereas "leaky" mutations are associated with the adult-onset variant of the disease.[6] In brancher deficiency, a missense mutation (Y329S) that allows for substantial residual enzyme activity was found in patients with a mild form of hepatopathy, but also in seven patients with APBD, possibly explaining the late onset (although not the brain preference) of this disorder.[7]

As already mentioned, some mutations predominate in certain ethnic groups, presumably because of founder effects (see Tables 54–1 and 54–2), whereas others, presumably new mutations, are "private."

Animal Models

Spontaneously occurring animal models exist for several GSD. There are two forms of PHK deficiency in the mouse, an X-linked recessive "I" variant (resembling the human myopathic variant), and an X-linked dominant "V" variant.

Myophosphorylase deficiency has been documented in Charolais cattle and in Merino sheep and molecular defects have been identified in both species.[3] Clinical manifestations include exercise intolerance and myoglobinuria.

English springer spaniel dogs with PFK deficiency suffer from chronic hemolytic anemia and stress-related hemolytic crises, but do not show weakness, premature fatigue, or myoglobinuria. The different clinical phenotype is attributed to the relatively minor role of glycolysis in canine muscle and to the compensatory effect of the PFK-L subunit, which is partially expressed in muscle.

Among the GSD causing weakness, AMD is the only one for which a few animal models have been documented biochemically: these include Japanese quail, Lapland dog, and cattle.[6]

AMD is also the only GSD for which genetically engineered knockout mice have been obtained. Actually, in an attempt to boost glycogen accumulation in these mice, glycogen synthetase was upregulated, which altered the ratio of synthetase to branching enzyme and resulted in the deposition of polyglucosan[8] (as in human PFK deficiency).

Therapy

Patients with exercise intolerance and myoglobinuria should be warned about the risks of strenuous exercise, but encouraged to perform some aerobic exercise to avoid deconditioning.[9] A combination of high-protein diet and aerobic exercise has proved useful in patients with McArdle disease and may help in other GSD of this type. Vitamin B_6 supplementation and administration of creatine monohydrate showed some benefit in McArdle disease, but these results have to be confirmed. A first-generation adenovirus recombinant containing the full-length human myophosphorylase cDNA has been efficiently transduced into phosphorylase-deficient sheep and human myoblasts, where it restored enzyme activity.[10]

In AMD, enzyme replacement with recombinant human AM from rabbit milk resulted in marked improvement of cardiac and muscle function in four infants with Pompe disease.[11] High level production of recombinant human AM was obtained in Chinese hamster ovary cells. In a phase I/II clinical trial, the recombinant enzyme was administered intravenously to three infants with Pompe disease: cardiomegaly regressed and both cardiac and skeletal muscle functions improved. The infants had reached 16, 18, and 22 months of age at the time of the report.[12] Patients with childhood or adult AMD and respiratory insufficiency may need intermittent or permanent mechanically assisted ventilation.

In patients with debrancher or brancher deficiency and cirrhosis or liver failure, liver transplantation is an option: of 13 transplanted patients with brancher deficiency, nine had no cardiac or neuromuscular involvement in follow-ups varying from 0.7 to 13.2 years.[13]

Conclusion

Although human GSD were among the first inborn errors of metabolism to be described, the field is far from dormant.

Not only are new entities still being discovered, as exemplified by β-enolase deficiency,[14] but also previously unsuspected disorders are being unmasked as GSD. For example, the syndrome of hypertrophic cardiomyopathy and preexcitation due to mutations in *PRKAG2*, the gene for the γ2 regulatory subunit of AMP-activated protein kinase, is, in fact, a cardiac glycogenosis.[15]

More interesting to neurologists is the realization that Lafora disease is a bona fide GSD. Clinically, Lafora disease is characterized by seizures, myoclonus, and dementia (and, inconsistently, ataxia, dysarthria, spasticity, and rigidity). Onset is in adolescence and the course is rapidly progressive, with death before age 25 years in most cases. The pathologic hallmarks are the bodies described by Lafora: round, basophilic, strongly PAS-positive intracellular inclusions (3 nm to 30 nm in diameter) present only in neuronal perikarya and processes. Ultrastructurally, they are virtually identical to the polyglucosan bodies that accumulate in APBD. However, brancher activity is normal in Lafora disease. Linkage analysis in nine families localized the gene responsible for Lafora disease to chromosome 6q and mutations in the gene were identified.[16] The gene product, a tyrosine phosphatase named *laforin*, probably plays a role in the cascade of reactions controlling glycogen synthesis and degradation, and may result in an abnormally increased ratio of glycogen synthetase to brancher activity.

Acknowledgment

Part of the work described here was supported by a grant from the Muscular Dystrophy Association.

REFERENCES

1. DiMauro S, Haller RG: Metabolic myopathies: Substrate use defects. In: Schapira AHV, Griggs RC (eds): Muscles Diseases. Boston, Butterworth-Heinemann, 1999, pp 225–249.

2. DiMauro S, Lamperti C: Muscle glycogenoses. Muscle Nerve 2001;24:984–999.

3. El-Schahawi M, Tsujino S, Shanske S, DiMauro S: Diagnosis of McArdle's disease by molecular genetic analysis of blood. Neurology 1996;47:579–580.

4. Baynon RJ, Quinlivan RCM, Sewry CA: Selected disorders of carbohydrate metabolism. In Karpati G (ed): Structural and Molecular Basis of Skeletal Muscle Diseases. Basel, ISN Neuropath Press, 2002, pp 182–187.

5. DiMauro S, Andreu AL, Bruno C, Hadjigeorgiou GM: Myophosphorylase deficiency (Glycogenosis type V; McArdle disease). Curr Mol Med 2002;2:189–196.

6. Hirschhorn R: Glycogen storage disease type II: Acid alpha-glucosidase (acid maltase) deficiency. In Scriver CR, Beaudet AL, Sly WS, Valle D (eds): The

Metabolic and Molecular Bases of Inherited Disease. New York, McGraw-Hill, 1995, pp 2443–2464.

7. Lossos A, Meiner Z, Barash V, et al: Adult polyglucosan body disease in Ashkenazi Jewish patients carrying the Tyr329 Ser mutation in the glycogen-branching enzyme gene. Ann Neurol 1998;44:867–872.

8. Raben N, Danon MJ, Lu N, et al: Surprises of genetic engineering: A possible model of polyglucosan body disease. Neurology 2001;56:1739–1745.

9. Haller RG: Treatment of McArdle disease. Arch Neurol 2000;57:923–924.

10. Pari G, Crerar MM, Nalbantoglu J, et al: Myophosphorylase gene transfer in McArdle's disease myoblasts in vitro. Neurology 1999;53:1352–1354.

11. Van den Hout JMP, Reuser AJJ, de Klerk JBC, et al: Enzyme therapy for Pompe disease with recombinant human alpha-glucoside from rabbit milk. J Inher Metab Dis 2001;24:266–274

12. Amalfitano A, Bengur AR, Morse RP, et al: Recombinant human acid alpha-glucosidase enzyme therapy for infantile glycogen storage disease type II: Results of a phase I/II clinical trial. Genet Med 2001;3:132–138.

13. Matern D, Starzl TE, Arnaout W, et al: Liver transplantation for glycogen storage disease types I, III, and IV. Eur J Pediatr 1999;158:S43–S48.

14. Comi GP, Fortunato F, Lucchiari S, et al: β-enolase deficiency, a new metabolic myopathy of distal glycolysis. Ann Neurol 2001;50:202–207.

15. Arad M, Benson DW, Perez-Atayde AR, et al: Constitutively active AMP kinase mutations cause glycogen storage disease mimicking hypertrophic cardiomyopathy. J Clin Invest 2002;109:357–362.

16. Minassian BA, Ianzano L, Meloche M, et al: Mutation spectrum and predicted function of laforin in Lafora's progressive myoclonus epilepsy. Neurology 2000;55:341–346.

Disorders of Lipid Metabolism

Stefano Di Donato

Franco Taroni

Mitochondrial oxidative metabolism of fatty acids (FA) is a major source of energy, particularly at times of stress or fasting, and its contribution to energy homeostasis is especially important in heart, liver, and skeletal muscle.[1,2] Abnormalities of lipid catabolism as possible causes of human disease were first suggested in the late 1960s by morphologic observations of excessive accumulation of lipid droplets within muscle fibers of a young woman who had attacks of muscle weakness lasting from a few weeks to several years.[3] The lipid accumulation in muscle was associated with morphologic abnormality of mitochondria. In 1973, DiMauro and Melis-DiMauro discovered carnitine palmitoyltransferase (CPT) deficiency, the first enzyme defect of mitochondrial FA oxidation to be described.[4] The patient was a 29-year-old man who suffered from recurrent episodes of muscle pain and pigmenturia triggered by prolonged exercise, especially when the patient fasted. Since this description, 14 autosomal recessive defects have been identified, involving almost all enzyme steps in the pathway (Table 55–1).[2,5–7] With the exception of medium-chain acyl-CoA dehydrogenase (MCAD) deficiency, which has a high frequency (1:10,000 to 1:30,000 births) among Northern European Caucasians,[5] these disorders are uncommon and the prevalence rate is unknown for most of them.

PATHOPHYSIOLOGY

The immediate source of chemical energy for muscle contraction is the hydrolysis of ATP to ADP. ATP can be regenerated from ADP and the high-energy compound phosphocreatine, but during long-term exercise the rephosphorylation of ADP to ATP requires the utilization of other fuels, such as carbohydrate, FA, and ketones.

Skeletal muscle can use carbohydrate or lipid as fuel, depending on the degree of activity. The respiratory quotient or respiratory exchange ratio (RER) of resting muscle is close to 0.8, indicating an almost total dependence on the oxidation of FA.[1] During the early phase of exercise (up to approximately 45 minutes), energy is derived mainly from blood glucose and from muscle glycogen metabolism. During prolonged exercise, there is a gradual shift from glucose to FA utilization and, after a few hours, approximately 70 percent of the skeletal-muscle energy requirement is met by mitochondrial oxidation of long-chain FA (LCFA). Heart is also largely dependent on LCFA oxidation for its functional activity.[1]

Mitochondrial oxidation of lipids is a complex process that requires a series of enzymatic reactions (Fig. 55–1).[5,8] Schematically, plasma-free FA delivered into the cytosol are first activated to their corresponding acyl-coenzyme A (CoA) thioesters at the outer mitochondrial membrane by acyl-CoA synthetase(s). Unlike short-chain (C_4-C_6) and medium-chain (C_8-C_{12}) acyl-CoAs, long-chain (C_{14}-C_{20}) acyl-CoAs cannot enter mitochondria directly. The mitochondrial CPT enzyme system, in conjunction with a carnitine/acylcarnitine translocase (CACT), provides the active carnitine-dependent mechanism whereby long-chain acyl-CoAs are transported from the cytosolic compartment into the mitochondrion, where β-oxidation occurs. L-carnitine is supplied for this reaction by a plasma-membrane sodium-dependent carnitine transporter (CT). Once in the mitochondria, FA are oxidized by repeated cycles of four sequential reactions, acyl-CoA dehydrogenation, 2-enoyl-CoA hydration, L-3-hydroxy-acyl-CoA dehydrogenation, and 3-ketoacyl-CoA thiolysis. The final step of each cycle in the β-oxidation spiral is the release of two molecules of

TABLE 55-1. Molecular Genetics of Fatty-Acid β-Oxidation Disorders

Deficiency	MIM No.[1]	Gene Name	Chromosomal Localization	Gene Structure	cDNA, Coding Region	Mutations Identified	Prevalent Mutation
Long-chain fatty-acid oxidation							
Fatty-acid transport	–	nd	nd	nd	nd	–	nd
CT	212140	SLC22A5	5q33.1	10 exons	1674 bp	++	none
CPT1, liver	255120	CPT1A	11q13	partial	2322 bp	+	none
CACT	212138	SLC25A2	3p21.31	9 exons	903 bp	+	none
CPT2	255110	CPT2	1p32	5 exons	1974 bp	++	439C>T
	600650						Ser113Leu
	600649						
β-oxidation spiral							
VLCAD	201475	ACADVL	17p11.2-11.13	20 exons	1968 bp	+++	none
MTP, type 1 (LCHAD)	600890	HADHA	2p23	20 exons	2289 bp	+	1528G>C Glu474Gln
MTP, type 2 (LCEH/LCHAD/LCKT)	143450	HADHB	2p23	16 exons	1422 bp	+	none
Medium- and short-chain fatty-acid oxidation							
β-oxidation spiral							
MCAD	201450	ACADM	1p31	12 exons	1263 bp	+++	985A>G Lys304Glu
SCAD	201470	ACADS	12q22	10 exons	1239 bp	+	625G>A Gly185Ser 511C>T Arg147Trp
SCHAD	601609	HADHSC	4q22-q26	nd	nd	–	nd
MCKAT	602199	–	nd	nd	nd	–	nd
2,4-Dienoyl-CoA reductase	222745	DECR1	8q21.3	10 exons	nd	–	nd
Multiple acyl-CoA dehydrogenation defects							
ETF							
α-subunit	231680	ETFA	15q23-25	nd	999 bp	+	797C>T Thr266Met
β-subunit	130410	ETFB	19q13.3	nd	765 bp	+	none
ETF:QO	231675	ETFDH	4q33-qter	nd	1851 bp	+	none
Riboflavin responsive	–	–	–	–	nd	–	nd

nd, not determined. CT, carnitine transporter; CPT, carnitine palmitoyltransferase; CACT, carnitine/acylcarnitine translocase; VLCAD, very-long-chain acyl-CoA dehydrogenase; MTP, mitochondrial trifunctional protein; LCHAD, long-chain 3-hydroxyacyl-CoA dehydrogenase; LCEH, long-chain 2-enoyl-CoA hydratase; LCKT, long-chain 3-ketoacyl-CoA thiolase; MCAD and SCAD, medium- and short-chain acyl-CoA dehydrogenase, respectively; SCHAD, short-chain 3-hydroxyacyl-CoA dehydrogenase; MCKAT, medium-chain 3-oxoacyl-CoA thiolase; ETF, electron transfer flavoprotein; ETF:QO, coenzyme Q oxidoreductase.

[1]Mendelian Inheritance in Man [MIM]. Online MIM database (OMIM™): <http://www3.ncbi.nlm.nih.gov/Omim/searchomim.html>

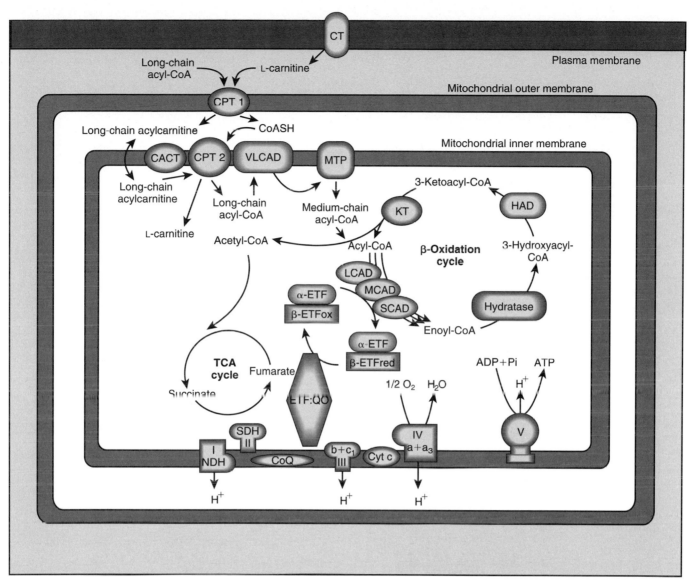

FIGURE 55–1. Schematic representation of the functional and physical organization of FA β oxidation enzymes in mitochondria. Enzymes that use FAD as a coenzyme are indicated in red. *CACT*, carnitine/acylcarnitine translocase; *CoQ*, coenzyme Q; *CPT1*, carnitine palmitoyltransferase 1; *CPT2*, carnitine palmitoyltransferase 2; *CT*, plasma membrane high-affinity sodium-dependent carnitine transporter (OCTN2); *Cyt c*, cytochrome *c*; *ETF*, electron transfer flavoprotein (*ox*, oxidized; reduced); *ETF:QO*, ETF:coenzyme Q oxidoreductase; *HAD*, L-3-hydroxyacyl-CoA dehydrogenase; *Hydratase*, 2-enoyl-CoA hydratase; *I*, respiratory chain complex I (*NDH*, NADH:coenzyme Q reductase); *II*, respiratory chain complex II (*SDH*, succinate dehydrogenase); *III*, respiratory chain complex III (*b*, cytochrome *b*; *c1*, cytochrome *c1*); *IV*, respiratory chain complex IV (cytochrome *c* oxidase—*a*, cytochrome *a*, and *a3*, cytochrome *a3*); *KT*, 3-ketoacyl-CoA thiolase; *MTP*, mitochondrial trifunctional protein; *V*, respiratory chain complex V (ATP synthase); *VLCAD, LCAD, MCAD, SCAD*, very-long-, long-, medium-, and short-chain acyl-CoA dehydrogenase, respectively. (From DiDonato S, Taroni F: Defects of fatty acid metabolism. In Karpati G [vol ed]: Structural and Molecular Basis of Skeletal Muscle Diseases. Switzerland, ISN Neuropath Press, 2002, p 191.)

acetyl-CoA and a fatty acyl-CoA that is two carbon atoms shorter. Multiple enzymes that exhibit partially overlapping chain-length specificity catalyze each reaction.[8] Thus, four distinct FAD-dependent acyl-CoA dehydrogenases have been identified. Similarly, there are two 2-enoyl-CoA hydratases, two NAD+-dependent L-3-hydroxy-acyl-CoA dehydrogenases, and two 3-ketoacyl-CoA thiolases with specificity for long- and short-chain acyl-CoAs. Evidence

for the presence of a medium-chain 3-ketoacyl-CoA thiolase has also been reported.[6] Complete catabolism of long-chain acyl-CoAs in mitochondria is accomplished by the action of two distinct, albeit coordinated, β-oxidation systems.[2] One is located on the mitochondrial inner membrane and is specifically involved in the oxidation of LCFA. The other system, composed of soluble enzymes located in the mitochondrial matrix, is responsible for the β-oxidation of medium-and short-chain acyl-CoAs (see Fig 55–1). Finally, mitochondrial FA β-oxidation is tightly coupled to both the tricarboxylic acid (TCA) and the respiratory chain. Thus, while acetyl-CoA released can enter the TCA cycle, the electrons of the FAD-dependent acyl-CoA dehydrogenases and the NAD+-dependent L-3-hydroxy-acyl-CoA dehydrogenases are transferred to the respiratory chain.

In skeletal muscle, impairment of LCFA transport across the mitochondrial membrane or defects in the β-oxidation pathway result in two main phenotypes,[1] a chronic myopathy or an acute muscle disorder characterized by rhabdomyolysis with paroxysmal myoglobinuria. When patients exercise for a prolonged period, glycogen store may be exhausted and rhabdomyolysis may occur. Fasting worsens the situation because it reduces the availability of both muscle glycogen and blood glucose, further increasing the dependence of muscle on FA metabolism. In some cases, reduced hepatic production of ketone bodies deprives muscle of another alternative fuel. Diversion of nonoxidized fatty acyl-CoA to triacylglycerol synthesis can explain the formation of lipid vacuoles observed in skeletal muscle of patients presenting with chronic myopathy.[1]

Possible pathogenic mechanisms for the development of cardiomyopathy in some patients with LCFA oxidation defects include both inadequate energy supply in the heart and myocardial damage and arrhythmogenesis due to the toxic effects of elevated intracellular concentration of long-chain acylcarnitines.[5]

CLINICAL FEATURES

Defects of fatty acid mitochondrial β-oxidation cause autosomal recessive disorders of infancy and childhood, though some patients present later in life. Overall, the clinical syndromes associated with FA oxidation disorders result from the failure of FA-oxidizing tissues to respond to increased energy demands. The main clinical features of FA oxidation disorders are illustrated in Table 55–2. Symptomatic hypoglycemia, characteristically associated with impaired ketogenesis, is often the earliest clinical manifestation and can be observed in nearly all these disorders.[2] Recurrent episodes of hypoketotic hypoglycemia, with or without concomitant brain involvement, are the most common presentation in the newborn or infant. Nausea and vomiting, hypotonia, drowsiness, and coma are also frequent. Sometimes attacks are triggered by fasting or minor viral infections. Infants and young children are at greater risk of having problems with fasting adaptation because, compared to adults, their basal metabolism is higher and some key enzymes involved in energy production and glucose homeostasis work at lower rates.

The acute and frequently life-threatening presentation in early infancy requires differential diagnosis from other encephalopathies of infancy, such as those caused

TABLE 55–2. Clinical Features Associated with Mitochondrial Fatty-Acid β-Oxidation Disorders*

Hepatic Signs

Hypoglycemia associated with low ketones (hypoketotic hypoglycemia)

Reye's-like syndrome

Steatosis

Acute hepatic failure

Sudden infant death syndrome (SIDS)

Muscle Signs

Hypotonia

Weakness and wasting

Proximal myopathy with lipid storage

Exercise intolerance and muscle pain with increased levels of creatine kinase

Episodic rhabdomyolysis (with occasional paroxysmal myoglobinuria)

Cardiac Signs

Hypertrophic and dilated cardiomyopathy

Progressive heart failure

Arrhythmias

Cardiac arrest

Sudden infant death syndrome (SIDS)

Nervous System Signs

Permanent brain damage due to hypoglycemia, arrhythmias, or cardiac arrest

Microgyria, cortical atrophy, and neuronal heterotopia

Pigmentary retinopathy

Peripheral sensorimotor neuropathy

Malformations

Renal dysplasia and nephromegaly*

Polycystic kidney

Facial dysmorphism

Brain malformations

*Proximal and distal tubulopathy is observed in CPT1 deficiency.

by hypoxia, space-occupying lesions, and drug or toxin ingestion. This is important because (1) a few defects of β-oxidation can be effectively cured, such as carnitine deficiency and riboflavin-responsive multiple acyl-CoA dehydrogenase deficiency, and (2) early diagnosis may help to prevent acute metabolic attacks, mental retardation, epilepsy, severe brain damage, and death.[9] Some infants with these diseases can also die abruptly without any obvious preceding symptoms, a picture reminiscent of two relatively common but pathogenetically ill-defined disorders of infancy: Reye's hepatic encephalopathy and sudden infant death syndrome (SIDS). Some infants survive the acute metabolic attacks but show poor growth, impaired psychomotor development, dystonia, spastic tetraplegia, and intractable seizures—the devastating effects of acidosis and acute energy shortage on the developing brain. Nervous system involvement is usually secondary to severe acidotic and hypoglycemic attacks, though patients with trifunctional protein deficiency may have retinitis pigmentosa and peripheral neuropathy.[2] Infants with severe defects of CPT2, ETF, or ETF:QO, however, can present congenital malformations of the brain (microgyria, neuronal heterotopia) and, sometimes, facial dysmorphism reminiscent of Zellweger syndrome. In addition to metabolic symptoms, patients often have cardiomyopathy. Primary carnitine deficiency, carnitine/acylcarnitine translocase deficiency, CPT2 deficiency, VLCAD deficiency, and MTP deficiency are all associated with various forms of heart disease.

Patients with onset in late infancy, childhood, or adulthood tend to have more chronic disorders characterized by progressive myopathy or cardiomyopathy, sometimes associated with mild metabolic symptoms such as nausea and drowsiness, or with altered laboratory tests such as hypoglycemia or poor rise of blood ketone concentrations in provocative tests. Disorders of lipid mitochondrial metabolism may cause two main clinical syndromes in muscle: (1) progressive weakness with hypotonia in approximately 35% of cases (e.g., carnitine transporter and carnitine/acylcarnitine translocase defects) or (2) acute, recurrent, reversible muscle dysfunction with exercise intolerance and acute muscle breakdown (rhabdomyolysis) with myoglobinuria in approximately 65% of cases (e.g., deficiencies of CPT2, very-long-chain acyl-CoA dehydrogenase, or trifunctional protein). Approximately 40% of patients affected with FA oxidation disorders, except CPT1 and MCAD deficiencies, present with significant muscular involvement.[9] Because of the dependence of heart and skeletal muscle on LCFA oxidation, cardiomyopathy (typically hypertrophic but sometimes dilated) and skeletal myopathy (chronic such as lipid storage myopathy or acute such as paroxysmal myoglobinuria) are commonly observed in LCFA oxidation defects. They are extremely rare in disorders of medium- and short-chain FA oxidation.

Because clinical presentation is of limited help in differential diagnosis, the only way to reach a definitive diagnosis is to analyze body fluids for accumulating metabolites and to study tissues for specific enzymes of fatty acid metabolism. Because most of the organic acids accumulating in β-oxidation defects are effectively cleared from the blood by the kidneys, gas chromatography-mass spectrometry (GC-MS) analysis of 24-hour urine specimens usually reveals a pattern of metabolites characteristic of a specific disease and is therefore the test of choice.[6] In addition, genetic testing is now available for almost all of these disorders, and prevalent mutations

have been identified in some (MCAD, LCHAD, and CPT2 deficiencies), which makes molecular screening feasible.[7]

DEFECTS OF MITOCHONDRIAL FATTY ACID OXIDATION

Carnitine Transporter Deficiency (Primary Carnitine Deficiency)

As discussed previously, L-carnitine (β-hydroxy-γ-N-trimethylamino-butyrate) has an essential role in the transport of LCFA into mitochondria for β-oxidation. Carnitine deficiency can be part of a number of inherited or acquired diseases (secondary carnitine deficiencies).[1,5] Primary carnitine deficiency (PCD) is an autosomal recessive disorder characterized by increased losses of carnitine in the urine and decreased carnitine concentration (usually less than 5% of normal) in plasma, heart, and skeletal muscle, caused by a defect of the high-affinity ($K_m = 5 \, \mu M$) plasma membrane sodium-dependent carnitine transporter (CT, OCTN2). Two major clinical presentations are associated with CT deficiency[5]: (1) a slowly progressive hypertrophic or dilated cardiomyopathy with lipid storage myopathy, occurring between 1 and 7 years of age; and (2) acute recurrent episodes of hypoglycemic hypoketotic encephalopathy usually occurring between 3 months and 2.5 years of age. These two phenotypes are not mutually exclusive, as in some families both metabolic and cardiomuscular presentations have been described.

CT deficiency (PCD) should be distinguished from secondary carnitine deficiency. In PCD, carnitine content is low in tissues (muscle, heart, liver) and in plasma (1% to 5% of the normal mean[10]). GC-MS analysis of urine does not show dicarboxylic aciduria, which is seen in patients with secondary carnitine deficiency due to fatty-acid oxidation defects.[1] Morphologic features include lipid storage in skeletal muscle, heart, and liver.[1] Once suspected, the defect of plasmalemmal CT should be ultimately confirmed by carnitine uptake investigations in cultured skin fibroblasts[10] or by molecular analyses.[11]

PCD patients respond well to high-dose oral L-carnitine supplementation (usually 100 to 200 mg/kg per day),[5,10] which restores plasma and liver carnitine levels to normal, whereas muscle carnitine levels remain low.[1] Nevertheless, patients gradually recover muscle strength, and heart function returns rapidly to normal, so that cardiokinetic therapy can be discontinued.[5] Also, attacks of hypoglycemia tend to disappear.[5,10]

In 1998, the gene encoding OCTN2, a novel organic cation transporter, was identified as a high-affinity sodium-dependent carnitine transporter in humans.[12] The OCTN2 cDNA codes for a 557 amino acid protein with 12 transmembrane domains. The corresponding gene, *SLC22A5* (solute carrier family 22, organic cation transporter, member 5), is composed of 10 exons and is located on chromosome 5q31.1. This locus is syntenic to the murine *jvs* (juvenile visceral steatosis) model locus on chromosome 11. *OCTN2* is strongly expressed in kidney, skeletal muscle, heart, and placenta.[12]

Nezu et al identified four mutations in the *SLC22A5* gene in three families with carnitine uptake defect.[13] A number of other mutations were reported soon thereafter, which abolish or severely impair carnitine transport when expressed in heterologous cells.[11] Most of the mutations were nonsense mutations associated with no residual carnitine transport activity. In a very few cases, "leaky" missense mutations have been identified, which retain residual carnitine transport activity.[11] However, there is a clear lack of genotype-phenotype correlation.[11]

Carnitine Palmitoyltransferase Deficiency

A number of biochemical and molecular studies have now firmly established that the carnitine palmitoyltransferase (CPT) system is composed of two distinct acyltransferases, CPT1, located on the inner side of the outer mitochondrial membrane, and CPT2, located on the inner side of the inner mitochondrial membrane.[14] Deficiencies of CPT1 and CPT2 have been extensively reviewed.[15,16]

CPT1 Deficiency

This disorder is commonly referred to as the "hepatic" form of CPT deficiency. It was first documented in an 8-month-old female who presented with encephalopathy, fasting hypoglycemia, hypoketonemia, and low plasma insulin concentrations without evidence of muscular disorder. Since then, about 15 more patients presenting with acute liver failure have been described.[16] In most cases, onset was before the second year of life.

Hypoglycemia may cause lethargy, coma, or partial or generalized seizures and may result in permanent motor deficit (hemiplegia), epilepsy (grand mal seizures), or psychomotor developmental delay. The characteristic lack of muscular or myocardial involvement can be explained by the existence of at least two tissue-specific isoforms of CPT1.[14,16] One is expressed in liver and fibroblasts (L-CPT1, CPT1A), which is mutated in patients,[16] and the other is expressed in skeletal muscle and heart (M-CPT1, CPT1B). Elevation of urinary dicarboxylic acids is never observed. Another distinctive feature of CPT1 deficiency is the increase in plasma carnitine levels, which are usually low in other fatty-acid oxidation disorders. In infants with disorders of mitochondrial fatty-acid oxidation, elevated plasma concentrations of total carnitine (usually approximately twice normal with a normal free-to-esterified ratio) may be a highly specific clue for CPT1 deficiency. The disease is ultimately diagnosed by documenting CPT1 deficiency in liver and fibroblasts with normal activity in muscle. Patients with isolated deficiency of muscle CPT1 have not yet been described.

CPT2 Deficiency

Three clinical phenotypes are associated with CPT2 deficiency: a myopathic form with juvenile-adult onset, an infantile form with hepatic, muscular, and cardiac involvement, and a lethal neonatal form with developmental abnormalities. In all cases, the enzyme defect can be demonstrated in every tissue examined (e.g., skeletal muscle, liver, fibroblasts, platelets, leukocytes). The most frequent clinical phenotype is commonly referred to as the "muscular" form of CPT deficiency. It is the most common disorder of lipid metabolism in muscle, one of the most common inherited disorders of mitochondrial FA oxidation,[9] and a major cause of hereditary recurrent myoglobinuria in both children and young adults.[17] Since the first description in 1973,[4] more than 150 patients suffering from recurrent attacks of aching muscle pain, stiffness, rhabdomyolysis, and myoglobinuria have been reported.[15,16] In approximately 80% of cases, age at onset is between 6 and 20 years. Among patients with the most typical presentation (i.e. exercise-induced myoglobinuria in adults), there is a 5.5:1 predominance of males over females. It seems that, in general, affected women or girls have milder symptoms, such as exercise- or fever-induced myalgia without pigmenturia.[15]

The clinical hallmark of the disease is paroxysmal myoglobinuria. Attacks of myoglobinuria are most often precipitated by prolonged exercise (exertional myoglobinuria).[17] Unlike patients with glycolytic defects, patients with CPT2 deficiency do not show reduced tolerance to brief strenuous exercise, do not experience a "second-wind" phenomenon (switch to utilization of fatty acids) and may not feel premonitory symptoms. In a smaller group of patients, mostly children, infection, usually of viral etiology, and/or fever and leukocytosis are the primary precipitating factors.[17]

The "muscular" form of CPT2 deficiency is usually a benign disease with a favorable outcome, provided that acute renal insufficiency, a potential complication of massive myoglobinuria, is adequately managed. In rare nonclassic cases, CPT2 deficiency can manifest as a severe life-threatening infantile hepatocardiomuscular form (CPT2 deficiency type 2) or a fatal neonatal-onset form (CPT2 deficiency type 3).[2,16] The infantile form (approximately 10 patients reported) is characterized by hypoketotic hypoglycemia, liver failure, cardiomyopathy, and mild signs of muscle involvement.[2,18] The disease is often fatal before 1 year of age. In addition to these symptoms, features of brain and kidney dysgenesis are frequently observed in the neonatal-onset variant.[2] This form is usually lethal during the first month of life.

This striking clinical heterogeneity of a single enzyme defect remains unexplained. However, some researchers[2] have suggested a correlation between residual

LCFA oxidation rates and phenotypic presentation. In the classic form, outside episodes of myoglobinuria and at-rest serum CK levels are normal. During acute episodes of rhabdomyolysis, there are massively increased levels of myoglobin ($\geq$200 ng/mL) in the urine and greatly increased levels of serum CK (20-fold to 400-fold) of muscle origin (CK-MM). Serum and muscle carnitine levels are usually normal. Urinary organic acid profile is also normal.

Diagnosis is ultimately made by demonstrating the enzyme defect in the patients' tissues. Widely different CPT2 levels have been reported, due to different assay conditions. Also, in most reported cases, the assays used did not discriminate between CPT1 and CPT2 activities. Optimal results are obtained with the "backward assay"[18] in the presence of 1% octyl glucoside, a strong detergent that fully releases active CP2 while inactivating CPT1 activity.[14] Despite the predominant muscular symptomatology, the enzyme defect is expressed in tissues other than skeletal muscle and can thus be detected in fibroblasts, leukocytes, platelets, and liver. Because the magnitude of CPT2 residual activity in peripheral blood leukocytes is similar to that observed in skeletal muscle (approximately 12% and 7%, respectively, when expressed as CPT2-to-citrate-synthase ratio), muscle biopsy is not required and the diagnosis can be confidently made by measuring CPT2 activity in either fresh or frozen isolated leukocytes.

Effective prevention of attacks may be accomplished by instituting a high-carbohydrate, low-fat diet with frequent and regularly scheduled meals, by avoiding the known precipitating factors (fasting, cold, prolonged exercise), and by increasing slow-release carbohydrate intake during intercurrent illness or sustained exercise.[15,16]

Two distinct genes for liver and muscle human CPT1 have been identified. The liver *CPT1* gene *(L-CPT1, CPT1A)* is located on chromosome 11q13.1, while the muscle *CPT1* gene *(M-CPT1, CPT1B)* is located on chromosome 22q13.33. Mutations in the liver-specific gene *CPT1A* have been reported in two patients.[16]

The human *CPT2* gene has been identified and characterized,[19,20] and approximately 20 mutations have been identified.[7,16] Most of the mutations are "private." However, a "common" mutation (Ser113Leu) can be identified in $\geq$50% of mutant alleles in patients of different ethnic origins with myopathic CPT2 deficiency.[21] Two other mutations were found to recur, albeit with a lesser frequency, a missense mutation Pro50His[20,22] and a frameshift mutation 413delAG.[22] This latter mutation was present in 20% of mutant alleles in the group of 59 patients investigated by Taggart et al,[22] and all carriers were of Ashkenazi Jewish ancestry, suggesting a defined ethnic origin. Currently, mutations can be detected in approximately 90% of patients with muscular CPT2 deficiency. Except for the

413delAG frameshift mutation, no other mutation abolishes enzyme activity completely. By contrast, null mutations have been found in patients with the lethal neonatal-onset form.[15] Mutation analysis suggested a certain genotype-phenotype correlation. For example, all mutations reported so far in the homozygous state are associated with either the muscular (Pro50His, Ser113Leu, Glu174Lys) or the generalized (Phe383Tyr, Tyr628Ser, Arg631Cys) phenotype.[2,18,20,21] However, compound heterozygotes harboring one adult-type mutation and one infantile-type mutation seem at risk for "crises" such as severe hepatic presentation or cardiac arrest.[16]

Carnitine/Acylcarnitine Translocase Deficiency

Carnitine/acylcarnitine translocase (CACT) deficiency belongs to the group of the defects of long-chain fatty-acid transport across the mitochondrial membrane, and may not be very rare, having been observed in more than 20 patients since the first description in 1992.[5] The disease is usually heralded by a life-threatening episode in the neonatal period, characterized by neonatal distress with hyperammonemia, variable hypoglycemia, heartbeat disorders, and muscle involvement with weakness and high serum CK.[5] The disease is often fatal within the first two years of life because of the deleterious consequences of long-chain acylcarnitine accumulation, which may cause untreatable episodes of arrhythmia. The human CACT gene has recently been cloned. The transcript is 1.2 kb in length and encodes a 301-amino acid protein composed of six transmembrane α-helices. The gene is located on chromosome 3p21.31. Molecular defects have been identified in several patients.[7]

Very-Long-Chain Acyl-CoA Dehydrogenase Deficiency

Very-long-chain acyl-CoA dehydrogenase deficiency (VLCAD) was first described in 1985 and attributed to a defect of the matrix enzyme long-chain acyl-CoA dehydrogenase (LCAD).[2] Following the discovery of VLCAD in 1992, it became clear that patients originally thought to suffer from LCAD deficiency had in fact VLCAD deficiency,[6] and more than 100 cases have been described.[7] The disease is clinically heterogeneous and can cause three major phenotypes: (1) a presentation resembling the muscular form of CPT2 deficiency with rhabdomyolysis and myoglobinuria, usually triggered by exercise or fasting; (2) a severe childhood form, with early onset of dilated or hypertrophic cardiomyopathy, recurrent episodes of hypoketotic hypoglycemia, and high mortality rate (50% to 75%); and (3) a milder childhood form, with later onset of hypoketotic hypoglycemia and dicarboxylic aciduria, low mortality, and rare cardiomyopathy. Most patients suffer from the severe cardiomyopathic form with early onset and poor outcome.[7] Isolated recurrent myoglobinuria has been reported in more than 10 patients,[23] with onset between 7 and 40 years of age. Fasting, exercise, or infections generally precipitated the episodes. Although the main complaints are reminiscent of CPT2 deficiency, the myalgia is more severe and the episodes more numerous. The diagnosis of VLCAD deficiency in an adult is difficult. Plasma LCFA profile by gas chromatography-mass spectrometry can be helpful for diagnosis because it may reveal an increase of tetradecaenoic ($C_{14:1}$) acid or $C_{14:1}$ and $C_{14:2}$ acylcarnitines, which persists even after the patient has fully recovered.[23] The diagnosis of VLCAD deficiency is ultimately based on the demonstration of reduced palmitoyl-CoA ($C_{16:0}$) dehydrogenation in skeletal muscle or cultured fibroblasts.

Patients have been treated with a dietary regimen consisting of avoidance of fasting and a high-carbohydrate, low-fat diet with or without supplementation with medium-chain triglyceride oil, riboflavin, or L-carnitine. This therapy has proved effective in reducing the recurrence of crises and in correcting both cardiac and muscle dysfunction.[23]

VLCAD is a mitochondrial membrane-bound homodimer with subunit size of approximately 66.5 kDa. The *ACADVL* gene spans approximately 5.4 kb of genomic DNA and has been mapped to chromosome 17p13.[7] More than 60 disease-causing mutations have been identified, none of which seemed to predominate.[7] In a molecular survey of 55 unrelated patients, Andresen et al identified 58 mutations and found some genotype-phenotype correlation.[7] Patients with the severe childhood phenotype had mutations that resulted in no residual enzyme activity, whereas patients with the milder childhood and adult phenotypes had mutations that resulted in some residual enzyme activity.

Mitochondrial Trifunctional Protein Deficiency

Mitochondrial trifunctional protein (MTP) deficiency is one of the latest additions to the list of mitochondrial FA oxidation disorders. The enzyme is a heterooctamer of four α-subunits, harboring long-chain 2-enoyl-CoA hydratase (LCEH) and long-chain L-3-hydroxyacyl-CoA dehydrogenase (LCHAD) activities, and 4 β-subunits harboring long-chain 3-ketoacyl-CoA thiolase (LCKT) activity. The disease is relatively frequent, with more than 60 patients reported thus far.[6,24] Clinical manifestations of the disease are characteristically associated with urinary excretion of C_6-C_{14} 3-hydroxydicarboxylic acids. Cases described before the discovery of MTP were reported as LCHAD deficiency. Patients can now be classified into two groups: those with long-chain 3-hydroxyacyl-CoA dehydrogenase (LCHAD) deficiency and those with MTP deficiency (combined enzyme deficiency).[6,24]

LCHAD Deficiency

The vast majority (≥85%) of MTP-deficient patients have an isolated deficiency of long-chain 3-hydroxyacyl-CoA dehydrogenase (LCHAD) activity with relative preservation of LCEH and LCKT activities and nearly normal amounts of both α- and β-subunits.[6] The disease is clinically heterogeneous.[24] In infancy and early childhood, hypoglycemic encephalopathy with or without severe hepatic involvement is the most common presentation. Other manifestations include chronic myopathy, paroxysmal myoglobinuria, and cardiomyopathy. Mortality is high (approximately 50%), the main cause of death being cardiac decompensation during a metabolic attack. However, cardiomyopathy in patients who survive acute episodes tends to resolve with dietary therapeutic measures (low-fat/high-carbohydrate diet associated with medium-chain triglyceride oil supplementation).[24] Later in childhood, predominant manifestations are episodes of rhabdomyolysis with muscle pain and weakness. Among the distinctive features of LCHAD deficiency are progressive pigmentary retinopathy and peripheral neuropathy. Also characteristic of this disorder is the occurrence of syndromes such as HELLP (hemolysis, elevated liver enzymes, and low platelets) and AFLP (acute fatty liver of pregnancy) in pregnant women with an affected fetus.[24]

MTP Deficiency (Combined Enzyme Deficiency)

In a smaller group of patients, all activities harbored by MTP are deficient, albeit to different extents, and both α- and β-subunits are barely detectable by immunoblot analysis.[6] In the relatively few patients with verified MTP deficiency, clinical manifestations are similar to those observed in patients with isolated LCHAD deficiency, although in general the clinical presentation is more severe and carries a higher mortality rate.[6] In very few cases, however, a benign late-onset neuromuscular phenotype was described, characterized by recurrent episodes of exercise-induced rhabdomyolysis.[24] This presentation closely resembled the adult form of CPT2 deficiency, except for the association of peripheral neuropathy. The occurrence of peripheral sensory-motor polyneuropathy appears to be a distinctive feature of both LCHAD and MTP deficiency and has been ascribed to a direct nerve toxicity of long-chain 3-hydroxy FA intermediates,[25] although this mechanism remains to be documented.

Both the gene for the α-subunit (*HADHA*) and that for the β-subunit (*HADHB*) map to the same region of chromosome 2p23. Because the distance between the two loci is quite short, the two genes are located side by side, as are the two (A and B subunit) genes of the bacterial fatty-acid β-oxidation multienzyme complex. Notably, both *HADHA* and *HADHB* genes share a common bidirectional promoter region, which would suggest a tight coupling between the synthesis of the two subunits.[26]

LCHAD deficiency appears to be a relatively common β-oxidation defect,[6,24] with an estimated frequency of at least 1:50,000 births in northern Europe.[24] Molecular studies have uncovered a prevalent missense mutation (1528G>C) that results in the Glu510Gln amino acid substitution in the LCHAD domain of α-subunit. This mutation fully inactivates the LCHAD component of MTP without affecting the hydratase or thiolase. The mutation can be detected in approximately 90% of LCHAD-deficient alleles,[6] thus making molecular screening for the disease quite feasible. However, the relative frequency of this mutation may be lower in Southern Europe (S DiDonato, F Taroni, unpublished observations). No apparent genotype-to-phenotype correlation has been observed, as patients homozygous for this mutation show widely different phenotypes.[6,24]

Unlike LCHAD deficiency, the molecular basis of MTP deficiency is heterogeneous. Mutations have been identified in both α- and β-subunits,[25] which result in severely but more evenly reduced activities of all three enzyme components of the MTP.[24] Formation of the $\alpha_4\beta_4$ enzyme complex is essential for MTP function, and the α- and β-subunit mutations in MTP-deficient patients apparently interfere with assembly of the enzyme complex.

Medium-Chain Acyl-Coa Dehydrogenase (MCAD) Deficiency

MCAD deficiency, together with CPT2 deficiency, is the most frequent disease of β-oxidation. Since the first report in 1982,[27] more than 400 patients have been identified worldwide, with a striking prevalence of Caucasians of Anglo-Saxon origin.[27] The frequency in the United States has been determined by newborn screening to be 1:15,000.[7] Typical symptoms include fasting intolerance, nausea, vomiting, hypoketotic hypoglycemia, lethargy, and coma beginning within the first 2 years of life. Clinical manifestations, however, are variable, and some patients may be asymptomatic, being recognized through family screening. On the other hand, some patients died suddenly, suggesting a correlation between MCAD deficiency and SIDS.[27] Patients have dicarboxylic aciduria. Adipic, suberic, and sebacic acids are detected in their urines, but C_{12}-C_{14} dicarboxylic acids, the hallmarks of VLCAD deficiency, are absent. Carnitine and β-hydroxybutyrate tend to be inappropriately low in plasma.[27] Unlike what happens in defects of LCFA oxidation, skeletal muscle and heart involvement is extremely rare in MCAD deficiency. However, Zierz and Engel found that 7 out of 15 patients with Reye's-like syndrome attacks initially diagnosed as having "systemic carnitine deficiency" had, in fact, MCAD deficiency. Later in childhood, the metabolic attacks ceased, but the patients developed a mild lipid storage myopathy.[1] Other researchers also described an MCAD-deficient patient carrying the common 985G mutation who presented late in life with rhabdomyolysis and acute encephalopathy after strenuous exercise.[2]

Early diagnosis and treatment of MCAD deficiency can result in good long-term outlook. Noninvasive diagnosis is greatly facilitated by fast-atom-bombardment (FAB)-MS analysis showing increased urinary excretion of hexanoylglycine, suberylglycine, and phenylpropionylglycine, in addition to the most common dicarboxylic acids.[27] Other FAB-MS studies indicate, however, that increased urinary octanoylcarnitine is probably the most useful diagnostic marker of MCAD deficiency, because it is detectable in high amounts in blood even between metabolic attacks.[27] Avoidance of fasting and maintenance of adequate caloric intake may prevent life-threatening metabolic attacks.

Deficiency of MCAD has been documented in most tissues, including cultured fibroblasts, lymphocytes, and liver.[27] The residual enzyme activity is 2% to 10% of normal.

The gene for MCAD is located on human chromosome 1p31 and is composed of 12 exons that span approximately 44 kb of genomic DNA.[7] In 1990, molecular genetic studies carried out by four research groups have simultaneously proven that most MCAD-deficient patients carry a point mutation in exon 11 at nucleotide 985 of the coding region.[7] This mutation is an A-to-G transition, which changes a highly conserved lysine at position 304 of the mature MCAD subunit into a glutamate. The mutation causes impairment of tetramer assembly and instability of the protein.[28] Most MCAD patients were shown to inherit this mutation in the homozygous configuration, suggesting a high frequency of the 985G mutation in the general population. In worldwide studies of Caucasian patients, the 985A → G transition was found in 90% of the mutant MCAD alleles.[7]

Riboflavin-Responsive Multiple Acyl-CoA Dehydrogenase Deficiency

Riboflavin (vitamin B_2) is the water-soluble precursor of two flavin coenzymes: flavin mononucleotide (FMN) and flavin adenine dinucleotide (FAD). Riboflavin cannot be synthesized in mammals, so they are entirely dependent on dietary supply. In mitochondria, several flavoproteins play a crucial role in the catabolism of fatty acids, carbohydrates (pyruvate), and amino acids. These include the straight-chain acyl-CoA dehydrogenases of the β-oxidation system (SCAD, MCAD, LCAD, and VLCAD), the electron transfer flavoprotein (ETF) and its dehydrogenase (ETF:QO), and a number of other dehydrogenases.[29]

Riboflavin-responsive multiple acyl-CoA dehydrogenase deficiency(RR-MADD),also known as riboflavin-responsive glutaric aciduria type 2, is a genetic metabolic disorder characterized by impaired oxidation of fatty acids due to multiple deficiencies of SCAD, MCAD, LCAD, and VLCAD. There are two major clinical phenotypes: (1) an infantile form with nonketotic hypoglycemia, hypotonia, failure to thrive, and acute metabolic episodes reminiscent of Reye's syndrome or MCAD deficiency; and (2) a juvenile form characterized by progressive proximal lipid storage myopathy.[1,30] There is usually an abnormal urinary excretion of organic acids that is compatible with glutaric aciduria type 2 or ethylmalonic-adipic aciduria.[1] Carnitine content in plasma and tissues is variably reduced. Culture in riboflavin-depleted medium is necessary to demonstrate the defect in fibroblasts.[29] Activities of SCAD, MCAD, and VLCAD are found to be reduced in isolated muscle mitochondria, with SCAD and MCAD activities being affected to a greater extent.[30] Not only are SCAD and MCAD activities severely impaired, but also their protein mass is markedly reduced, as demonstrated by Western blot analysis.[30] ETF and ETF:QO activities appear to be unaffected, while reductions of respiratory chain complexes I and II activities have been reported.[30]

The clinical, morphologic, biochemical, and physiologic responses to oral riboflavin supplementation (100 to 300 mg/day oral riboflavin) are usually dramatic,[30] with rapid improvement of muscle weakness and wasting and disappearance of signs of lipid accumulation at muscle biopsy. Riboflavin supplementation also normalizes the activities of SCAD and MCAD, and restores to normal the amount of protein mass.

No information is available on the molecular and genetic bases of this disorder. Reduced availability of intramitochondrial FAD, causing accelerated turnover of apoenzyme proteins, seems to be a likely explanation for RR-MAD. Cellular riboflavin uptake and FMN/FAD synthesis were normal in fibroblasts of two patients.[29,30] Potential sites of the defect may be FMN/FAD cellular uptake, mitochondrial transport of flavin cofactors, or their intramitochondrial synthesis.

Acknowledgments

Part of the original work cited was made possible by the valuable contribution of Drs. Silvia Baratta, Patrizia Cavadini, Barbara Garavaglia, Cinzia Gellera, Federica Invernizzi, Eleonora Lamantea, and Elisabetta Verderio and the generous support of Telethon-Italia to F.T.

REFERENCES

1. DiDonato S: Disorders of lipid metabolism affecting skeletal muscle: Carnitine deficiency syndromes, defects in the catabolic pathway, and Chanarin disease. In Engel AG, Franzini-Armstrong C (eds): Myology, 2nd ed. New York, McGraw-Hill, 1994, pp 1587–1609.

2. Taroni F, Uziel G: Fatty-acid mitochondrial b-oxidation and hypoglycaemia in children. Curr Opin Neurol 1996;9:477–485.

3. Bradley WG, Hudgson P, Gardner-Medwin D, Walton JN: Myopathy associated with abnormal lipid metabolism in skeletal muscle. Lancet 1969;1:495–498.

4. DiMauro S, Melis-DiMauro P: Muscle carnitine palmitoyltransferase deficiency and myoglobinuria. Science 1973;182:929–931.

5. Stanley CA: Carnitine disorders. Adv Pediatr 1995;42:209–242.

6. Wanders RJ, Vreken P, den Boer ME, et al: Disorders of mitochondrial fatty acyl-CoA beta-oxidation. J Inherit Metab Dis 1999;22:442–487.

7. Gregersen N, Andresen BS, Corydon MJ, et al: Mutation analysis in mitochondrial fatty acid oxidation defects: Exemplified by acyl-CoA dehydrogenase deficiencies, with special focus on genotype-phenotype relationship. Hum Mutat 2001;18:169–189.

8. Kunau WH, Dommes V, Schulz H: β-oxidation of fatty acids in mitochondria, peroxisomes and bacteria: A century of continued progress. Prog Lipid Res 1995; 34:267–342.

9. Saudubray JM, Martin D, de Lonlay P, et al: Recognition and management of fatty acid oxidation defects: A series of 107 patients. J Inherit Metab Dis 1999;22:488–502.

10. Garavaglia B, Uziel G, Dworzak F, et al: Primary carnitine deficiency: Heterozygote and intrafamilial phenotypic variation. Neurology 1991;41:1691–1693.

11. Wang Y, Taroni F, Garavaglia B, Longo N: Functional analysis of mutations in the OCTN2 transporter causing primary carnitine deficiency: Lack of genotype-phenotype correlation. Hum Mutat 2000;16: 401–407.

12. Tamai I, Ohashi R, Nezu J, et al: Molecular and functional identification of sodium ion-dependent, high affinity human carnitine transporter OCTN2. J Biol Chem 1998;273:20378–20382.

13. Nezu J, Tamai I, Oku A, et al: Primary systemic carnitine deficiency is caused by mutations in a gene encoding sodium ion-dependent carnitine transporter. Nat Genet 1999;21:91–94.

14. McGarry JD, Brown NF: The mitochondrial carnitine palmitoyl transferase system: From concept to molecular analysis. Eur J Biochem 1997;244:1–14.

15. Taroni F: Carnitine palmitoyltransferase deficiency. In Gilman S, Goldstein GW, Waxman SG (eds): Neurobase. La Jolla, CA, Arbor, 1995.

16. Bonnefont JP, Demaugre F, Prip-Buus C, et al: Carnitine palmitoyltransferase deficiencies. Mol Genet Metab 1999;68:424–440.

17. Tein I, DiMauro S, DeVivo DC. Recurrent childhood myoglobinuria. Adv Pediatr 1990;37: 77–117.

18. Taroni F, Verderio E, Fiorucci S, et al: Molecular characterization of inherited carnitine

palmitoyltransferase II deficiency. Proc Natl Acad Sci U S A 1992;89:8429–8433.

19. Finocchiaro G, Taroni F, Rocchi M, et al: cDNA cloning, sequence analysis and chromosomal localization of human carnitine palmitoyltransferase. Proc Natl Acad Sci U S A 1991;88:661–665.

20. Verderio E, Cavadini P, Montermini L, et al: Carnitine palmitoyltransferase II deficiency: Structure of the gene and characterization of two novel disease-causing mutations. Hum Mol Genet 1995;4:19–29.

21. Taroni F, Verderio E, Dworzak F, et al: Identification of a common mutation in the carnitine palmitoyltransferase II gene in familial recurrent myoglobinuria patients. Nat Genet 1993;4:314–320.

22. Taggart RT, Smail D, Apolito C, Vladutiu GD: Novel mutations associated with carnitine palmitoyltransferase II deficiency. Hum Mutat 1999;13:210–220.

23. Pons R, Cavadini P, Baratta S, et al: Clinical and molecular heterogeneity in very-long-chain acyl-coa dehydrogenase deficiency. Pediatr Neurol 2000;22:98–105.

24. Tyni T, Pihko H: Long-chain 3-hydroxyacyl-CoA dehydrogenase deficiency. Acta Paediatr 1999;88:237–245.

25. Ibdah JA, Tein I, Dionisi-Vici C, et al: Mild trifunctional protein deficiency is associated with progressive neuropathy and myopathy and suggests a novel genotype-phenotype correlation. J Clin Invest 1998;102:1193–1199.

26. Orii KE, Orii KO, Souri M, et al: Genes for the human mitochondrial trifunctional protein alpha- and beta-subunits are divergently transcribed from a common promoter region. J Biol Chem 1999;274:8077–8084.

27. Roe CR, Coates PM: Mitochondrial fatty acid oxidation disorders. In Scriver CR, Beaudet AL, Sly WS, Valle D (eds): The Metabolic and Molecular Bases of Inherited Disease, 7th ed. New York, McGraw-Hill, 1995, pp 1501–1533.

28. Yokota I, Saijo T, Vockley J, Tanaka K: Impaired tetramer assembly of variant medium-chain acyl-Coenzyme A dehydrogenase with a glutamate or aspartate substitution for lysine 304 causing instability of the protein. J Biol Chem 1992;267:26004–26010.

29. Rhead W, Roettger V, Marshall T, Amendt B. Multiple acyl-coenzyme A dehydrogenation disorder responsive to riboflavin: Substrate oxidation, flavin metabolism, and flavoenzyme activities in fibroblasts. Pediatr Res 1993;33:129–135.

30. Antozzi C, Garavaglia B, Mora M, et al: Late-onset riboflavin-responsive myopathy with combined multiple acyl coenzyme A dehydrogenase and respiratory chain deficiency. Neurology 1994;44:2153–2158.

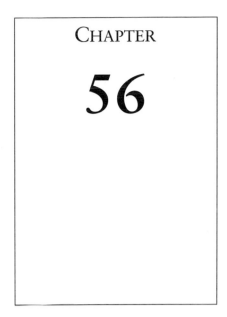

Disorders of Galactose Metabolism

Louis J. Elsas II

CLINICAL FEATURES

Classic galactosemia is a disease of newborns characterized by prolonged neonatal jaundice, bleeding diathesis, feeding intolerance, lethargy, *Escherichia coli* sepsis, hypotension, and, if untreated, death. This autosomal recessive trait is caused by absent function of galactose-1-phosphate uridyl transferase (GALT) (E.C. 2.7.7.12). If lactose ingestion continues, it results in accumulation of galactose, galactose-1-phosphate, and galactitol in cells, blood, and urine.[1,2] Severity of disease varies directly with the degree of GALT impairment and the load of ingested galactose.

Elevation of blood galactose occurs in this evolutionarily conserved galactose metabolic pathway from mutations impairing function of two other enzymes (Fig. 56–1). Deficiency of UDP galactose-4-epimerase (GALE) increases erythrocyte galactose-1-p and galactose in the presence of normally functioning GALT. Clinically, newborns are asymptomatic, but occasional families are described with later-onset, progressive neurologic dysfunction in GALE deficiency.[3,4] Galactosemia and excess urinary galactitol accumulation occurs in galactokinase (GALK) deficiency. Patients with GALK deficiency have neonatal and childhood cataracts without hepatocellular or neurologic dysfunction.[5] To prevent primary signs and symptoms for all of these enzyme-deficient, inherited disorders of galactose metabolism, lactose (galactose)-restricted diets are implemented during the first days of life.[6]

DISEASE INCIDENCE

The incidence of GALT deficiency is derived from many newborn, population-based screening programs. Severe mutations either in homozygous or compound heterozygous genotypes have an incidence of about 1:35,000 newborns. However, less severe mutations that impair erythrocyte GALT activity below 15% of normal and increase erythrocyte galactose-1-phosphate have an incidence of about 1:8,000 newborns.[2] The incidence of GALK deficiency is unknown in the general population, but it is probably less than 1:100,000. However, within inbred isolates such as the Romani Gypsy, the prevalence is 1:1600, and the carrier rate is as high as 5%.[7] GALE deficiency has an estimated prevalence of 1:23,000 in Japan, and 1:64,000 in white Americans. A benign but frequent form is found in African Americans with a frequency of 1:6200.[4,8]

DIAGNOSTIC EVALUATION

Diagnosis of all three disorders involves quantitation of analytes, enzyme analysis, and mutational analysis. In classic galactosemia (GALT deficiency), erythrocyte galactose-1-P and urinary galactitol are elevated, GALT enzyme is less than 5% of control, total body galactose oxidation to CO_2 is less than 5% recovery in two hours, and GALT mutations (Table 56–1) are defined.[2,9] In GALK deficiency, urinary galactitol is markedly elevated, erythrocyte Gal-1-P is normal, and the GALK enzyme is

TABLE 56–1. The Genetics of Three Enzymes of Galactose Metabolism and Their Mutations That Produce Human Disease

Deficient Enzyme	Chromosomal Location	Some Common Mutations	Ethnic Origin	Clinical Severity
GALT (galactose-1-P-uridyltransferase)	9p13	Q188R	Northern Europe	Severe
		S135L	Africa	Moderate
		K285N	S. Germany/Croatia	Severe
		L195P	Europe	Severe
		Y209C	Asia	Severe
		F161S	Europe	Severe
		N314D	Panethnic	Benign
		5Kbdel	Ashkenazim	Severe
		IVS2 nt2a→g (167 more)	Hispanic	Moderate
GALK (galactokinase)	17q24	P28T	Roma Gypsies	Cataracts
		R68C	Caucasian	Cataracts
		T288M	Caucasian	Cataracts
		R256W	Japan	Cataracts
		A384P	Caucasian	Cataracts
		T344M	Japan	Cataracts
		G349S	Japan	Cataracts
		410delg	Japan	Cataracts
		509-510delgt (12 more)	Japan	Cataracts
GALE (UDP galactose-4-epimerase)	1p36	L183P	Pakistani/Caucasian	Late childhood mental retardation
		N34S	Pakistani/Caucasian	Late childhood mental retardation
		G90E	Asia	Mental retardation
		D103G	Asia	Mental retardation
		K257R	Africa	Benign
		V94M	British	Pervasive delays Hepatomegaly
		L313M	Asia	Benign
		D103G	British	Benign

impaired. In GALE deficiency, erythrocyte galactose and Gal-1-P are elevated but the GALT enzyme is normal, and GALE is deficient in erythrocytes.[3,4] Some mutations that produce impaired enzyme function in these three genes are listed in Table 56–1.

PATHOPHYSIOLOGY: CLINICAL MANIFESTATIONS

GALT Deficiency

The galactose metabolic pathway shown in Figure 56–1 is evolutionarily conserved. This pathway produces energy and CO_2 from glucose-1-phosphate and maintains the pools of UDPglucose and UDPgalactose that are essential substrates for glycogen synthesis and the post-translational production of glycoproteins and glycolipids. This pathway is essential for glycobiology and the formation of cerebrosides, sphingomyelin, membrane receptors, and secreted hormones. These macromolecules are essential to the development of the nervous system. As can be seen in Figure 56–1, there are two pathways available to maintain homeostasis of UDPglucose and UDPgalactose concentrations even when GALT is impaired. These include production of UDPglucose from UGP and GALE activity to maintain UDPgalactose. Expression microarray experiments with GALT-deficient yeast and their revertants defined the toxic effects of galactose-1-phosphate.[10] Galactose-1-P inhibited glucose-1-phosphate pyrophosphorylase (UGP), thus decreasing the amount of both UDPglucose and UDPgalactose. In humans, the concentration of these compounds controls important

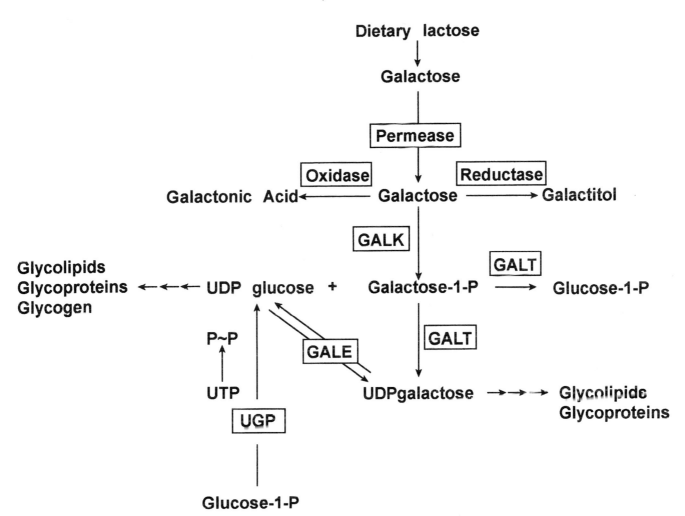

FIGURE 56–1. Metabolic pathway for conversion of human milk to galactose, glucose-1 P, UDPglucose, and UDPgalactose. Trivial names for enzymes are boxed in black. Three enzymes produce galactosemia when impaired in humans: GALT (galactose-1-phosphate uridyltransferase), GALE (UDP-galactose-4-epimerase), and GALK (galactokinase). Normally, end-products of galactose metabolism include CO_2 production from glucose-1-P and the synthesis of glycogen, glycolipid, and glycoproteins. The production of UDPglucose requires the UTP-dependent enzyme, glucose-1-phosphate pyrophosphorylase (UGP). Alternate pathways for accumulated galactose are indicated and include the increased production of galactitol and galactonic acid. Galactonic acid is metabolized through the pentose pathway, while galactitol accumulates in cells as an end product.

neonatal functions, including bilirubin conjugation; brain myelin formation; and post-translational processing of many secreted proteins, such as FSH, and membrane-attached receptors. The pathophysiologic effects of GALT deficiency in the newborn include rising direct bilirubin (and kernicterus), hepatocellular failure, growth failure, cataracts, and—if untreated—mental retardation, hearing loss, tremor, spasticity, and seizures. Approximately 10% of newborns with GALT deficiency have *E. coli* sepsis and die.[2] Lethal sepsis may result from reduced glycoprotein cell wall barriers to intestinal bacteria owing to reduced galactosyl and neuraminic acid residues on surface proteins.[10] If the infant with GALT deficiency is detected within a few days of life and galactose is removed from the diet, there is rapid remission of hepatocellular damage and normalization of health.

Public health newborn screening programs have reduced the lethality of classic galactosemia, but chronic effects of GALT deficiency were recognized as children grew older. This enigmatic set of chronic problems included verbal dyspraxia (56%); reduced IQ (46%); cataracts (10%); ovarian failure (up to 85% in females); ataxia and tremors (18%); and growth delay (before puberty).[2,11–13] The mechanisms producing these chronic conditions are not known. Some could be embryologic in origin and caused by severely impaired GALT with "toxic" effects of galactose-1-P, and reduced concentrations of UDPglucose and UDPgalactose available for glycoproteins and glycolipids in rapidly dividing fetal cells. Intracellular accumulation of galactitol is known to cause cataracts and seizures by its osmotic effects in lens epithelium and neurons, respectively.[5]

Galactokinase Deficiency

Cataracts without hepatic, ovarian, or central nervous system pathology are found in GALK (galactokinase) deficiency. As compared to GALT deficiency, galactitol but not galactose-1-P is accumulated through the alternate aldose reductase pathway (see Fig. 56–1). The accumulation of galactitol in lens fibers produces an osmotic gradient, swelling of cells, loss of permeability, cell death, and scarring. This process also occurs in GALT deficiency and is progressive if galactose intake continues.

Epimerase Deficiency

GALE (epimerase) deficiency is benign in newborns ascertained by screening.[3] There is a bias of ascertainment regarding clinical outcome where GALE deficiency is identified in families expressing pervasive mental delays. At a molecular level, some mutations such as V94M are found in more than one family, produce dysfunctional enzyme in vitro, and are presumed to cause disease in humans.[4] The accumulation of heterozygous mutations in GALK, GALT, or GALE may become "sensitivity" genes for more common adult disorders such as ovarian failure, presenile dementia, liver failure, and early cataract formation. Some mutations in GALT and GALE have a "dominant negative" effect on the normal allele and multiple heterozygous mutations in this important glycobiologic pathway may have additive effects producing organ pathology. Molecular studies in these disorders are of research interest.

DIAGNOSTIC EVALUATION

Population Screening

Because GALT (transferase) deficiency can be lethal yet preventable in the neonatal period, population-based newborn screening is used to identify and urgently treat affected newborns. The GALT enzyme is measured in erythrocytes from dried blood on filter paper using enzyme-linked, fluorometric methods. In classic galactosemia, there is no GALT activity (complete lack of fluorescence), and variant galactosemia is detected by partial impairment of fluorescence. In hot, humid months, prevalence of these variant forms is greater due to the instability of mutant GALT dimeric proteins.[14-16] State-based laboratories also use accumulation of galactose and galactose-1-P as part of the screening process.

FOLLOW-UP CONFIRMATION

A complete or partial positive screening test should immediately be followed by removal of lactose from the diet, retrieval of the newborn, and definition of the GALT biochemical phenotype and molecular genotype.[9,16] GALT enzyme is quantitated from erythrocytes and its isoforms identified by isoelectric focusing. Additional studies include quantitation of erythrocyte galactose-1-P, urinary galactitol, and molecular genotyping of the GALT gene. The nine mutations listed in Table 56–1 account for 75% of the mutant GALT alleles in America. All of the above are available through commercial laboratories on an emergency status.[14] An additional study, the "breath test" quantitates total body oxidation of ^{13}C-galactose to $^{13}CO_2$ expired in the infant's breath. Clinically significant impaired GALT is indicated by: GALT enzyme activity below 5% of control; erythrocyte galactose-1-phosphate above 2.5 mg/deciliter; urinary galactitol above 150 mmole per mole of creatinine; and cumulative percent dose of ^{13}C-galactose expired in 2 hours as $^{13}CO_2$ in breath below 5%.[2,9,11,13] This full set of diagnostic tests confirms the diagnosis of galactosemia and provides a basis for prognosis. For example, there is no GALT activity in erythrocytes from homozygotes harboring the S135L mutation common in African Americans with GALT-deficient galactosemia, but total body oxidation of ^{13}C-galactose to $^{13}CO_2$ is normal, and prognosis is good if patients are detected and treated in the newborn period.[17,18] In contrast, there is no erythrocyte GALT activity in the Q188R mutation common in Caucasians of Northern European descent, but patients who are homozygous for Q188R have less than 5% of ^{13}C-galactose recovered as $^{13}CO_2$ in their breath test. If the Q188R mutation is either homozygous or associated with another "severe" mutant allele listed in Table 56–1, outcome for dyspraxic speech and for ovarian failure is increased approximately tenfold.[11,15]

Differential Diagnosis

The diagnosis of galactosemia should be entertained in any infant with prolonged neonatal jaundice, bleeding diathesis, progressive hepatocellular dysfunction, congenital cataracts, or E. coli sepsis. Quantitation of erythrocyte galactose-1-P, urinary galactitol, GALT enzyme assay in erythrocytes, GALT molecular genotype, and galactose oxidation studies are available.[2] Differential diagnosis will include other causes for hepatocellular dysfunction such as hepatitis, biliary obstruction, and other rare inborn errors such as Niemann-Pick disease, hereditary fructose intolerance, tyrosinemia type 1, neonatal hemochromatosis, and infantile Wilson's disease.

The diagnosis of GALE (epimerase) deficiency is entertained when population-based newborn screening results indicate elevated RBC galactose-1-P and galactose but erythrocyte GALT activity is normal. Most newborns remain asymptomatic, but may develop cataracts or mental retardation later in life if untreated. The diagnosis is made by finding reduced GALE (epimerase) activity in erythrocytes, fibroblasts, or transformed lymphoblasts cultured from the patient. Molecular analysis of the GALE gene is available on a clinical basis.[2,4]

GALK deficiency will not be detected by most public health newborn screening programs and should be suspected in any patient with congenital or early-onset cataracts. Diagnosis is suspected on finding increased urinary galactitol and confirmed by finding reduced GALK (galactokinase) in peripheral erythrocytes. Molecular analysis of the GALK gene is available on a clinical basis.[2,5] Molecular analysis of GALK is important when considering whether heterozygosity for GALK deficiency may predispose to more common adult-onset cataracts. The erythrocyte enzyme analysis alone for GALK may not differentiate heterozygosity from homozygous normal. Further molecular analysis is recommended if there is concern about a mutation acting as a sensitivity gene in familial cataracts of adult onset.

THERAPY AND PREVENTION

Treatment of galactosemia is exclusion of galactose from the newborn's diet. This means essentially eliminating lactose-containing milk and substituting soy formulas before irreversible damage to the brain occurs.[6] Because endogenous galactose production continues, strict avoidance of all casein-derived proteins as well as lactose itself is necessary in young children. Some fruits and vegetables such as watermelons and tomatoes contain bioavailable galactosides and should be avoided. Education of parents and older children is important about the galactose content of foods. Lists of the galactose content of foods are available. Calcium supplements are necessary, and approximately 350 mg to 1000 mg ionized calcium per day should be prescribed for infants or older children on soy-based formulas. Lactose is often used as filler for medications by the pharmacy and should be avoided. Lactulose is used in managing the hyperammonemia of liver disease, but contains gram quantities of free lactose and must be avoided in newborns with liver disease in which GALT deficiency has not been ruled out.

LONG-TERM MANAGEMENT

During early childhood, it is necessary to evaluate neurologic status, speech, and ovarian and lens functions. Speech therapy can prevent later "learning disabilities" if diagnosis and intervention are provided before age 2 years.[12,13] In females, estrogen creams for dermatitis and replacement therapy may be indicated when ovarian failure is present. Ophthalmologic evaluation for cataracts may be required periodically if erythrocyte galactose-1-phosphate and urinary galactitol are not kept within therapeutic range by diet.

Determination of the galactose-1-phosphate content of erythrocytes and urinary galactitol is useful in monitoring adherence to and effectiveness of the diet. Erythrocyte galactose-1-phosphate should be kept below 3.5 mg/dL, but will remain in this above-normal range owing to endogenous galactose production. Concentrations above this level increase the odds ratio for developing dyspraxia and ovarian failure.[11–13] Urinary galactitol should be below 150 mmole per mole of creatinine.[13]

PRIMARY PREVENTION

Galactosemia is inherited as an autosomal recessive trait. Primary prevention of galactosemia involves heterozygote detection and preconceptual counseling of at-risk family members and parents of galactosemic children. Prenatal monitoring is available in the early second trimester by GALT enzyme analysis of cultured amniotic fluid cells or chorionic villus cells.[19] A cellular phenotype from the proband's cultured dermal cells is a prerequisite for prenatal monitoring of a fetus at risk. Mutational analysis of GALT DNA from fetal cells is the most sensitive and specific prenatal diagnostic method. To use mutational analysis, the genotype of the proband must be known. Late-trimester analysis of galactitol in amniotic fluid is useful. Using GC/MS or HPLC, galactitol from amniotic fluid in affected fetuses ranges from 5.9 μM to 10.6 μM (0.23 μM to 1.6 μM is normal). There is no evidence that restricting maternal lactose intake will influence the intracellular overproduction by affected fetal cells of either galactose-1-P or galactitol.[19]

PROGNOSIS

If a galactose-restricted diet is provided within the first week of life and continued throughout life, the presenting hepatotoxic symptoms resolve quickly and prognosis is good. If the diagnosis of GALT-deficient galactosemia is not established within days of life, the infant treated only with intravenous antibiotics and partially restricted lactose intake will demonstrate relapsing and episodic jaundice, and bleeding from altered hemostasis. With delayed treatment, complications such as mental and growth retardation are likely. Despite early and adequate therapy, the long-term outcome in older children and adults with "severe" galactosemia can include speech defects, poor growth, poor intellectual function, neurologic deficits (predominantly extrapyramidal findings with tremor and ataxia), and ovarian failure.[11–13,20] Localized galactitol accumulation may cause pseudo-tumor and seizures. Outcome and the "disease burden" can be predicted based on the GALT genotype, age at which successful therapeutic control was achieved, and compliance with galactose restrictions. Currently, the most sensitive prognostic test for treated infants is the galactose-oxidation breath test. If total body oxidation of ^{13}C-D-galactose to ^{13}CO$_2$ in the breath test is greater than 5% at 2 hours, outcome is good.[14] In contrast, a GALT genotype of Q188R/Q188R gives an odds ratio of 9.61 for dyspraxic speech and 8.33 for ovarian failure.[11,12]

FUTURE RESEARCH

The galactose metabolic pathway outlined in Figure 56–1 is evolutionarily conserved and required for production of energy through glucose-1-phosphate and for essential galactosylation and glycosylation of glycolipids and glycoproteins through UDPglucose and UDPgalactose. UDPglucose concentrations also requlate glycogen synthesis. It is imperative to better understand how multiple "mutations" affect regulation of flux from galactose as a substrate to these products. The biology of galactose metabolism and its link to energy production through mitochondrial OX/PHOS, and post-translational processing are important sets of basic research objectives to better understand neural and optic lens development as well as ovarian and hepatic function in humans.

MODEL SYSTEMS

The yeast *Saccharomyces cerevisiae* has been a good model system for these research objectives. However, the mouse with absent GALT has failed to reproduce the pathology of human galactosemia.[10,21] Perhaps understanding what alternate paths protect the mouse will clarify the pathophysiology of human galactosemia.

REFERENCES

1. Mason HH, Turner ME: Chronic galactosemia: Report of case with studies on carbohydrates. Am J Dis Child 1935;50:359–374.

2. Galactosemia. Gene Reviews 2002. http://www.geneclinics.org

3. Gitzelman R: Deficiency of uridine diphosphate galactose 4-epimerase in blood cells of an apparently normal infant. Helv Paediatr Acta 1972;27:125–130.

4. Quimby BB, Alano A, Almashaner S, et al: Characterization of two mutations associated with epimerase-deficiency galactosemia by use of a yeast expression system for human UDP-galactose-4-epimerase. Am J Hum Genet 1997;61:590–598.

5. Stambolia ND, Ai Y, Sidjamin D, et al: Cloning of the galactokinase cDNA and identification of mutations in two families with cataracts. Nat Genet 1995;10:307–312.

6. Elsas LJ, Acosta PB: Nutritional support of inherited metabolic disease. In Shils ME, Olson JA, Shike M, Ross (eds): Modern Nutrition in Health and Disease. Philadelphia, Williams & Wilkins, 1999, pp 1003–1057.

7. Kalaydjieva L, Perez-Lezaun A, Angelichera D, et al: A founder mutation in the GK1 gene is responsible for galactokinase deficiency in Roma Gypsies. Am J Hum Genet 1999;65:1299–1307.

8. Alano A, Almashaner S, Chinsky J, et al: Molecular characterization of a unique patient with epimerase deficiency galactosemia. J Inherit Metab Dis 1998;21:341–350.

9. Elsas LJ, Langley SD, Steele E, et al: Galactosemia: A strategy to identify new biochemical phenotypes and molecular genotypes. Am J Hum Genet 1995;56:630–639.

10. Lai K, Elsas LJ: Overexpression of human UDP-glucose pyrophosphorylase rescues galactose-1-phosphate uridyltransferase deficient yeast. Biochem Biophys Res Acta 2000;271:392–400.

11. Guerrero NV, Singh RH, Manatunga A, et al: Risk factors for premature ovarian failure in females with galactosemia. J Pediatr 2000;137:833–841.

12. Robertson A, Singh RH, Guerrero NV: Outcomes analysis of verbal dyspraxia in classic galactosemia. Genet Med 2000;2:142–148.

13. Webb A, Singh RH, Kennedy MJ, Elsas LJ: Predictors of verbal dyspraxia in galactosemia. Pediatr Res 2002 (in press).

14. Elsas LJ, Lai K: The molecular biology of galactosemia. Genet Med 1998;1:40–48.

15. Lai K, Willis AC, Elsas LJ: The biochemical role of glutamine-188 in human galactose-1-phosphate uridyltransferase. J Biol Chem 1999;274:6559–6566.

16. Elsas LJ: Newborn screening. In Rudolph AM, Hoffman JIE, Rudolph CD (eds): Rudolph's Pediatrics. New York, Appleton & Lange, 1996, pp 282–289.

17. Lai K, Langley SD, Singh RH, et al: A prevalent mutation for galactosemia among black Americans. J Pediatr 1996;128:89–95.

18. Lai K, Elsas LJ: Structure-function analysis of a common mutation in Blacks with transferase-deficiency galactosemia. Mol Genet Metab 2001;74:264–272.

19. Elsas LJ: Prenatal diagnosis of galactose-1-phosphate uridyltransferase (GALT)-deficient galactosemia. Prenat Diagn 2001;21:302–303.

20. Waggoner DD, Buist NR, Donnell GN: Longterm prognosis in galactosemia: Results of a survey of 350 cases. J Inherit Metab Dis 1990;13:802–818.

21. Leslie ND, Yager KL, McNamara PD, et al: A mouse model of galactose-1-phosphate uridyltransferase deficiency. Biochem Molec Med 1996;59:7–12.

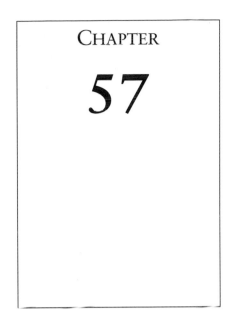

CHAPTER 57

Inborn Errors of Amino Acid Metabolism

William L. Nyhan

Richard Haas

Heritable disorders of amino acid metabolism affect the central nervous system in a variety of ways. The pathogenesis of clinical disease may reflect the accumulation of compounds, such as phenylalanine or leucine, which cause toxicity proximal to the defective enzyme. These compounds are essential nutrients but are highly toxic in large concentrations. Other compounds are natural neuropharmacologic agents or neurotransmitters, such as 4-hydroxybutyrate and glycine, respectively. Metabolic disease can also affect the brain by failing to make an essential product such as tetrahydrobiopterin (BH_4) in the hyperphenylalaninemias. It is characteristic of these disorders that there is a symptom-free period after birth during which toxic intermediates accumulate or deficiencies develop. Carnitine deficiency occurs secondarily in disorders in which CoA derivatives accumulate; the carnitine esters formed are preferentially excreted in the urine.[1] Supplementation with carnitine is therapeutically useful in amounts calculated to maximize the excretion of detoxifying carnitine esters, but not in amounts sufficient only to restore normal free carnitine concentrations. Because of the limited repertoire of response, especially in the very young infant, it is not necessary for the clinician to have intimate understanding of all of the pathways affected by genetic disease. Rather, there should be a logical approach to narrowing down the diagnosis. The initial laboratory tests are available in routine clinical laboratories. Among the most important is the test for ketonuria. Its presence in a neonate signifies an organic aciduria. A positive dinitrophenylhydrazine (DNPH) test is a screen for maple syrup urine disease. The blood should be examined for pH, electrolytes, glucose, and ammonia. Concentrations of lactic acid and uric acid are useful. Specific diagnostic biochemical genetic testing should be the next step, including quantitative assessment of amino acids in plasma, analysis of organic acids in urine, analysis of carnitine levels in blood and urine, and acylcarnitine profiles. These tests usually lead to the diagnosis. Enzymatic or molecular mutational diagnosis provides confirmation and is helpful in heterozygote detection and prenatal diagnosis.

CLASSIC ORGANIC ACIDEMIAS

The classic organic acidemias include propionic acidemia, methylmalonic acidemia, multiple carboxylase deficiency, isovaleric acidemia, and 3-oxothiolase deficiency.

Clinical Features and Diagnostic Evaluation

The classic clinical presentation of the organic acidemias[2] is vomiting, anorexia, and lethargy followed rapidly by life-threatening ketosis and acidosis, leading to dehydration, coma, apnea, and, in the absence of successful intensive care, death. Episodes of ketosis and acidosis are recurrent following infection or the dietary intake of the amounts of protein usual in infancy. Ketonuria is massive and, in infancy, complicated by hyperammonemia. Large quantities of glycine are often found. Effects of accumulated organic acids on the marrow are evidenced by neutropenia, thrombocytopenia, and anemia.

Specific findings in individual disorders include the alopecia and bright red, scaly dermal eruption of multiple carboxylase deficiency. Biotinidase deficiency displays ataxia, optic and auditory nerve degeneration, and spastic paraplegia. The acrid smell of isovaleric acidemia may be diagnostic. Renal tubular acidosis and chronic interstitial nephritis complicate methylmalonic acidemia.

Neurologic consequences of these disorders (seizures, hypotonia, spasticity, dystonia, chorea, and developmental delay) usually appear to be consequences of the acute episode and presence or absence of hypovolemic shock, hypoglycemia, or neonatal hyperammonemia more than consequences of the actual disease. Leigh encephalopathy has been seen in biotinidase deficiency. Stroke involving the basal ganglia, characteristic lesions on MRI and CT scan, clinical hemiplegia, or death can complicate methylmalonic and propionic acidemia.[3] The more general imaging picture of organic acidemia is that of hypomyelination, cerebral atrophy, or edema of the white matter in an acute episode.

Definitive diagnosis is by organic acid analysis of the urine. The hallmark metabolites of altered propionate metabolism, hydroxypropionate and methylcitrate, are seen in propionic acidemia, methylmalonic acidemia (MMA), and multiple carboxylase deficiency. In MMA, methylmalonate is also seen. In multiple carboxylase deficiency, 3-hydroxyisovalerate and 3-methylcrotonyl-glycine are also seen. The diagnostic metabolite for isovaleric acidemia is isovalerylglycine; the metabolites are tiglylglycine and 2-methyl-3-hydroxybutyrate for oxo-thiolase deficiency.

Pathology

Neuropathology reveals spongiform dysmyelination. A patient with infarction of the basal ganglia presented with endothelial cell swelling and vascular proliferation. Calcification of the basal ganglia occurs in biotinidase deficiency.

Biochemical Findings

The defect in propionic acidemia is in propionyl-CoA carboxylase, which catalyzes the conversion of propionyl-CoA to methylmalonyl-CoA. The defect in methylmalonic acidemia is in the methylmalonyl CoA mutase, which catalyzes the conversion of methylmalonyl CoA to succinyl CoA. Enzymes can be assayed in lymphocytes, cultured fibroblasts, or tissues. Activity in most patients is less than 2% of control. Prenatal diagnosis can be made by assay of enzyme in cultured amniocytes or chorionic villus cells. It is more reliable by direct gas chromatography mass spectrometry (GCMS) analysis of amniotic fluid for methylcitrate and/or methylmalonate.

In multiple carboxylase deficiency, primary defects are in holocarboxylase synthetase, which carries out the attachment of biotin to newly synthesized carboxylase proteins, and in biotinidase. Isovaleryl-CoA dehydrogenase, the site of the defect in isovaleric acidemia, has been assayed in fibroblasts.

Immunochemical Findings

Propionyl CoA carboxylase has an α and β subunit. In immunotitration, neither pccA nor pccBC contain cross-reacting material (CRM). Among patients in the Mut° group of methylmalonyl CoA mutase, immunotitration studies have revealed some to have some CRM, albeit reduced, whereas others have none. Immunochemical studies have detected mutation in the mutase that interferes with the transport of the enzyme into the mitochondria.

Molecular and Genetic Data

The mode of inheritance in each condition is autosomal recessive. Prevalence is unknown except for methylmalonic acidemia and biotinidase deficiency, in which neonatal screening indicated incidences of 1:48,000 to 1:60,000.

The gene for the α-chain of propionyl CoA carboxylase has been localized to chromosome 13; the gene for the ß-chain has been localized to chromosome 3, at 3q13.3-22. Mutations have been identified, such as a deletion in an intron in the ß gene that causes a frame shift and exon skipping, as well as a mutation in the ß gene responsible for 8 of 28 mutant alleles in Caucasian patients.[4] The gene for MMA mutase has been cloned, and its locus mapped to chromosome 6 p12-21.2. In the Mut° group, reduced amounts of mutase mRNA have been found. Mutations have been identified, clustering near the carboxy terminus, the site of cobalamin binding. The gene for isovaleryl-CoA dehydrogenase has been cloned and localized to chromosome 15q 12–15. A mutation has been identified that results in a truncated precursor protein that is inefficiently imported into mitochondria and bound to membrane. The gene for holocarboxylase synthetase has been cloned and located at chromosome 21q 22.1. The cDNA encodes 726 amino acids. A spectrum of mutations has been identified in 25 patients studied. A 1VS10+G>A was the most commonly found in European patients. Expression of mutant genes led to activities ranging from 0.2% to 22% of control, consistent with a spectrum of clinical severity.

Therapy

Treatment follows from a specific diagnosis. Multiple carboxylase deficiency is usually exquisitely sensitive to biotin, and usually 10 mg per day of oral biotin will reverse all manifestations of the disease. Ocular or auditory nerve damage in biotinidase deficiency may not be reversible. Methylmalonic acidemia that is responsive to vitamin B_{12} is much easier to manage than those that are not, but dietary therapy is always required, as it is in propionic acidemia and isovaleric acidemia. The principle of dietary therapy is in the restriction of protein containing the precursors to just those quantities required for anabolism and growth (and no more), along with adequate amounts of calories. Carnitine supplementation reverses the deficiency of free carnitine that regularly occurs in these conditions and forms carnitine esters of accumulated toxic organic acid CoA esters; these carnitine esters are readily excreted in the urine. In isovaleric acidemia, glycine supplementation accomplishes a further detoxification by the excretion of increased amounts of isovalerylglycine.

Propionic acidemia and methylmalonic acidemia have been treated with hepatic transplant, and there has been prompt cessation of acute episodes of metabolic imbalance.[5]

GLUTARIC ACIDURIA TYPE I

Clinical Features and Diagnostic Evaluation

Glutaric aciduria type I (GA I) is a degenerative neurologic disorder characterized by spasticity, dystonia, intellectual impairment, and choreoathetosis.[6] Encephalitis-like presentations tend to follow intercurrent illness and are followed by neurologic deterioration with dyskinesia and dystonic extensor and flexor spasms. Bilateral subdural collections of fluid have led to mistaken diagnoses of child abuse. Macrocephaly and particularly a head circumference curve that crosses normal development lines should suggest the diagnosis. CT or MRI classically reveals frontotemporal atrophy in a bat wing appearance.

Pathology

Neuropathology reveals striatal degeneration, extensive neuronal loss, and gliosis in the caudate and putamen. There may be severe spongiform changes in the white matter.

Biochemical Findings

Key diagnostic findings on organic acid analysis of the urine are large amounts of glutaric acid and 3-hydroxyglutaric acid, as well as glutaconic acid. Prenatal diagnosis may be made by direct GCMS assay of glutaric acid in the amniotic fluid.

The basic defect is in the glutaryl CoA dehydrogenase enzyme and is demonstrable in leukocytes and cultured fibroblasts as well as in liver. There is heterogeneity in amount of residual activity.

Molecular and Genetic Data

The gene is located on the short arm of chromosome 19. A number of mutations have been defined.[7] A splice site mutation has been identified in a population of Canadian Indians in whom the disease is common. Glutaric aciduria is also common among the Amish of Pennsylvania.

Therapy

Treatment with a diet low in protein to restrict the intake of lysine and tryptophan rapidly decreases the excretion of glutaric acid and other metabolites. Riboflavin and carnitine are also employed. Early diagnosis and—in acute crisis—prompt intravenous administration of large amounts of glucose and water appear to be useful in preventing neurodegeneration.

4-HYDROXYBUTYRIC ACIDURIA

Clinical Features and Diagnostic Evaluation

4-Hydroxybutyric aciduria is an unusual inborn error in the metabolic pathway for 4-aminobutyrate (GABA) in which the compound that accumulates has neuropharmacologic activity.[8,9]

Patients have all had neurologic abnormalities, including seizures, mental retardation, hyperactivity, somnolence, and spastic diplegia. 4-Hydroxybutyric acid produces seizures in animals. CT or MRI scans may be normal or show generalized cerebral atrophy. The detection of 4-hydroxybutyric acid by GCMS is diagnostic.

Biochemical Findings

The molecular defect is in the succinic semialdehyde dehydrogenase enzyme, which is predominantly active in brain. It can be assayed in lymphocytes and cultured human lymphoblasts. Accumulated succinic semialdehyde is promptly converted to 4-hydroxybutyrate.

Molecular and Genetic Data

Inheritance is autosomal recessive. Consanguinity has frequently been reported, and heterozygotes can be detected by assay of the enzyme in lymphocytes or lymphoblasts. Prenatal diagnosis is available by direct GCMS analysis of the amniotic fluid and enzyme assay on chorionic villus samples.

Therapy

The only available treatment is pharmacologic control of seizures.

PHENYLKETONURIA AND DISORDERS OF BIOPTERIN METABOLISM

Clinical Features and Diagnostic Evaluation

Phenylketonuria (PKU) is the classic error of amino acid metabolism. It serves as a model for the control of genetic disease because screening programs in every developed country detect infants with elevated blood concentrations of phenylalanine. This permits effective early intervention and therefore prevents mental retardation, the most important consequence of the disease. In untreated PKU, the intelligence quotient (IQ) is usually less than 30. Patients also have fair skin, blond hair, and blue eyes. Itching or an eczematoid rash may occur. Spastic paraplegia and seizures occur in some, and microcephaly in a few. Behavior is hyperkinetic. The EEG is abnormal. Neuroimaging studies in untreated PKU have revealed cerebral atrophy or calcification. Cranial calcification has also been reported in patients with abnormal biopterin metabolism. Each of these defects leads to a situation in which phenylalanine cannot be converted to tyrosine, although the phenylalanine hydroxylase apoenzyme is normal.

Diagnosis of PKU is by a positive screening test for phenylalanine on a drop of whole blood collected on filter paper. This must be confirmed by a quantitative test for phenylalanine and tyrosine in the blood. In classic PKU, the phenylalanine is more than 1200 mmol/L and the tyrosine is low. The urine gives a positive green color test for phenylpyruvic acid on the addition of 10% $FeCl_3$. Diagnosis in patients with defective hydroxylase cofactor metabolism is by administration of tetrahydrobiopterin. Tetrahydrobiopterin reduces phenylalanine levels in patients with cofactor defects, but it does not change phenylalanine levels in patients with PKU. Another diagnostic test is measurement of pterins in urine and dihydropteridine reductase in blood.

Pathology

Neuropathology reveals diminution in the size of the brain, gliosis, and delayed myelination. Spongy myelin changes correlate with decreased lipid content of white matter. Myelination ultimately takes place, but it is delayed.

Biochemical Findings

The defective enzyme in PKU is phenylalanine hydroxylase, which normally is expressed only in liver. It converts phenylalanine to tyrosine. In its absence, phenylalanine accumulates and is converted to phenylpyruvic acid, phenyllactic acid, phenylacetic acid, and phenylacetylglutamine. Phenylacetic acid accounts for the odor of the patient with untreated PKU.

Tetrahydrobiopterin is an essential cofactor for the phenylalanine hydroxylase enzyme. In the course of the reaction, tetrahydrobiopterin is oxidized to dihydrobiopterin, and it must be reduced with nicotinamide-adenine dinucleotide (NADH) in a reaction catalyzed by dihydropteridine reductase. Patients may have defects in this enzyme or in the synthesis of BH_4, catalyzed by GTP cyclohydrolase and dihydrobiopterin synthase.[10]

Each of these defects leads to a situation in which phenylalanine cannot be converted to tyrosine, although the phenylalanine hydroxylase apoenzyme is normal.

Immunochemical Findings

In classic PKU, the activity of phenylalanine hydroxylase is undetectable, and immunochemical studies have revealed no CRM.

Molecular and Genetic Data

PKU occurs in about 1:10,000 to 1:15,000 births. Biopterin abnormalities are found in 1% to 2% of hyperphenylalaninemic individuals. The gene for human phenylalanine hydroxylase has been cloned in man and mouse[11–13] and localized to chromosome 12q. At least 31 mutations in the human hydroxylase gene have been identified. Two mutations, expressed as zero activity and no CRM, accounted for almost half of the northern European patients studied: an arginine to tryptophan change in exon 12 and a splicing mutation in intron 12. Some 9 of 31 abnormal alleles involved cytosine-phosphate-guanine dinucleotides (CpG), which are known to be hot spots for mutation.

Therapy

Clinical manifestations may be successfully prevented by detection in neonatal screening and restriction of dietary intake of phenylalanine. We aim to maintain blood concentrations less than 300 µmol/L. Patients with biopterin abnormalities are treated with tetrahydrobiopterin.[14] In addition, therapy includes administration of dopamine, 5-hydroxytryptophan, and carbidopa. Carbidopa is necessary to inhibit peripheral decarboxylases that would prevent these compounds from entering the central nervous system.

NONKETOTIC HYPERGLYCINEMIA

Clinical Features and Diagnostic Evaluation

In nonketotic hyperglycinemia (NKH), the enzyme responsible is usually expressed only in brain and liver, and the diagnosis is made based on accumulation of glycine in the cerebrospinal fluid. Most patients present in the early days of life with life-threatening illness.[15] Hiccups are common and may occur prenatally. There is rapid progression to coma and respiratory arrest. Ventilatory assistance must be provided, or death ensues. A majority of patients die in the neonatal period, many without diagnosis. In those who survive the early crisis, there is little evidence of psychomotor development. Intractable seizures are the rule. Neonates are hypotonic or flaccid. Eventually they become spastic, hyperreflexic, and often opisthotonic. Most are microcephalic.

The classic abnormality of the EEG in NKH is a burst suppression pattern. Hypsarrhythmia has been encountered.

Neuroimaging on CT or MRI shows cerebral atrophy and white matter hypomyelination. The corpus callosum is abnormally thin.

NKH is phenotypically heterogeneous. A small number of patients have atypical milder clinical presentations. This disease may produce isolated mild mental retardation. It may also present as a neurodegenerative disease similar to Tay-Sachs or Krabbe disease. The corpus callosum is abnormally thin.

Pathology

Neuropathology reveals spongy change in the myelin. It is the characteristic finding, particularly in older patients. On electron microscopy, vacuoles are within the myelin sheaths.

Biochemical Findings

Concentrations of glycine in the plasma range from 6 to 12 mg/dL (mean concentration 7.5 mg/dL; concentration of control 1 mg/dL).

The excretion of glycine in the urine is enormous, often over 1 g/day. The ratio of glycine in the cerebrospinal fluid to that of the plasma is employed to make the diagnosis. In control individuals, the ratio is less than 0.04; in NKH, the ratio is greater than 0.10.

The fundamental defect in the glycine cleavage system has been demonstrated in liver and brain. Activity is demonstrable in chorionic villus samples, and this has been used for prenatal diagnosis.

The glycine cleavage system is composed of four proteins now designated P, H, T, and L. The P protein contains pyridoxal phosphate and catalyzes the decarboxylation of glycine. The H protein is a lipoic-acid–containing protein, which is the aminomethyl carrier protein. The T protein is a tetrahydrofolate requiring flavoprotein that transfers carbon 2 of glycine to tetrahydrofolate. The L protein is a dihydrolipoyl dehydrogenase that catalyzes the oxidation of the lipoic acid of the H protein to its disulfide. The overall reaction yields ammonia, carbon dioxide, and single carbon tetrahydrofolate, which in the presence of another molecule of glycine becomes the hydroxymethyl group of serine. The reaction is localized to the mitochondria.

Study of the specific components of the system that were abnormal in the glycine cleavage system revealed eight patients with defects in the P protein, four in the T protein, and one in the H protein. Phenotypically the classic neonatal type of NKH is usually associated with virtual absence of the P protein.

Molecular and Genetic Data

The gene for the P protein cDNA has been cloned, and a number of mutations have been identified.[16] In one patient with a large deletion, no immunoreactive protein could be found. Another classic patient had complete absence of P protein activity, but had immunoreactive P protein as well as mRNA. In this patient, a three base deletion was found leading to a deletion of the phenylalanine 756. The mutation in the classic disease found commonly in Finland has been identified as a G to T point

mutation of nucleotide 1691 leading to a serine to leucine change at amino acid 566 of the P protein.

Therapy

There is no satisfactory treatment for NKH. Administration of sodium benzoate in doses sufficient to decrease cerebrospinal fluid levels of glycine reduces intractable seizures.

MAPLE SYRUP URINE DISEASE

Clinical Features and Diagnostic Evaluation

In maple syrup urine disease (MSUD), the classic presentation is early neonatal hypertonicity and opisthotonus. Deep tendon reflexes are increased, and there may be clonus. Generalized seizures are common. Lethargy progresses rapidly to coma, apnea, and death, unless intubation and artificial ventilation are initiated promptly.

The EEG in MSUD may show generalized slowing or paroxysmal discharges. Neuroimaging on CT or MRI shows a generalized decrease in attenuation in the white matter, which resolves with treatment and time. There may be cerebral atrophy and, in acute coma, cerebral edema.

The clinical phenotype is variable. Intermediate, intermittent, and thiamine-responsive variants have been described. All of these variants have more residual enzyme than the classic form.[17] The disease is never intermittent; it is virtually always chemically recognizable. Only the acute symptoms are intermittent. Nevertheless, an acute episode in a variant patient may be fatal.

MSUD can be detected in newborn screening by the elevation of leucine in spots of blood. Confirmation of the diagnosis[18] is by quantitative analysis of plasma amino acids. Levels of leucine, valine, isoleucine, and alloisoleucine are elevated. The 2-ketoacid derivatives of these amino acids may be detected by organic acid analysis of the urine. A simple screening test is to add dinitrophenylhydrazine, which makes a yellow precipitate with these ketoacids.

Biochemical Findings

All forms of branched-chain ketoaciduria result from deficiency of branched-chain alpha-ketoacid dehydrogenase. The activity of the dehydrogenase enzyme is usually measured in lymphocytes, fibroblasts, or lymphoblasts by measuring the conversion of 14C-leucine to $14CO_2$. There is some correlation between clinical severity and amount of residual enzyme activity. Heterozygotes can be detected and prenatal diagnosis accomplished by assay of cultured amniocytes or chorionic villus samples.

MSUD is an autosomal recessive disorder. Incidence was 1:290,000 in the New England Newborn

Screening Program. It is 1:760 in the Pennsylvania Mennonites.

Molecular and Genetic Data

Branched-chain ketoacid dehydrogenase is an enzyme complex composed of three major subunits. Defects have been localized in a small number of patients to the E1, E2, or E3 proteins. E3 deficiency also causes lactic acidemia.

Northern and Western blotting studies have identified five different types of abnormality in components of the decarboxylase, and the cDNA of each component has been cloned. The $E1\alpha$ gene is located on chromosome 19q13.1–13.2, and the E1ß on 6p21–22. The E2 gene has been localized to chromosome 1. At least seven mutations in the E1a gene have been identified. In the Mennonite population, the common mutation is a T to A change that produces a missense Y393N.[19] The same mutation was found in a compound with an eight-base deletion causative of a downstream nonsense codon.[20] In an intermediate phenotype patient, there was a compound of a missense and one frame shift in $E1\alpha$. Other mutations have been found in $E1\alpha$, but only one in E1ß—a deletion in Japanese patients.[21] Eleven mutations have been reported in E2.[22] Two missense mutations have been found in E3.[23] A thiamine-responsive patient was found to have a 17-bp insertion and a Phe–215 to Cys missense mutation in the E2 mRNA.[24]

Therapy

A few patients have responded to treatment with large doses of thiamine. Therefore, newly diagnosed patients should be tested for thiamine responsiveness. Doses employed have ranged between 10 and 300 mg/day.

The treatment of MSUD consists of the provision of a diet low in branched-chain amino acids. Preparations of branched-chain amino acid-free amino acid mixtures are helpful. Neonatal screening is important. Optimal treatment before damaging ketoacidotic episodes occur can promote normal brain development.

Acute episodes of coma should be treated aggressively. An anabolic approach is to employ branched-chain amino acid-free parenteral or enteral nutrition to lay down branched chain amino acids into protein.[25] Once the acute episode is controlled, protein and branched-chain amino acid intake is limited to provide the minimum quantity of branched-chain amino acids necessary for growth. Patients must be carefully followed by monitoring plasma amino acid concentrations repeatedly.

Animal Models

Animal models have been described for a number of disorders of amino acid metabolism. There is a naturally occurring phenylketonuric mouse. Other models include hepatorenal tyrosinemia, histidinemia, sarcosinemia, and tyrosine hydroxylase deficiency. A bovine model of MSUD has been shown to have a single base pair substitution in the DNA for the $E1_\alpha$ subunit, which produces a stop codon.

Conclusion and Future Research Directions

Recognition of inborn errors of amino acid metabolism represented the beginning of molecular medicine and the first verification of the one-gene one-enzyme conceptualization. They continue to provide insights into the working of the body, and there is much to be learned. The variety of clinical expression is enormous. Many have effects on the nervous system.

The future can bring new knowledge about the nature of mutations and how they lead to the variety of enzyme defects and clinical phenotypes. When gene therapy can give stable expression, heritable disorders of amino acid metabolism should be prime targets.

REFERENCES

1. Wolff IA, Le TP, Haas R, et al: Carnitine reduces fasting ketogenesis in patients with disorders of propionate metabolism. Lancet 1986;1:289–291.

2. Nyhan WL, Ozand PT: Atlas of Metabolic Disease. London, Chapman and Hall, 1998.

3. Haas RH, Marsden DL, Capistrano-Estrada S, et al: Acute basal ganglia infarction in propionic acidemia. J Child Neurol 1995;10:18–22.

4. Tahara T, Kraus JP, Rosenberg LE: An unusual insertion/deletion in the gene encoding the beta-subunit of propionyl-CoA carboxylase is a frequent mutation in Caucasian propionic acidemia. Proc Natl Acad Sci U S A 1990;87:1372–1376.

5. Leonard JV, Walter JH, McKiernan PJ: The management of organic acidemias: The role of transplantation. J Inher Metab Dis 2001;24:309–311.

6. Hoffmann GF, Trefz FK, Barth PG, et al: Glutaryl-CoA dehydrogenase deficiency: A distinct encephalopathy. Pediatrics 1991;88:1194–1203.

7. Nyhan WL, Zschocke J, Hoffmann G, Stein DE, et al: Glutaryl-CoA dehydrogenase deficiency presenting as 3-hydroxyglutaric aciduria. Molec Genet Metab 1999;66:199–204.

8. Chambliss KL, Gray RGF, Rylance G, et al: Molecular characterization of methylmalonate semialdehyde dehydrogenase deficiency. J Inherit Metab Dis 2000;23:497.

9. Ishiguro Y, Kajita M, Aoshima T, et al: The first case of 4-hydroxybutyric aciduria in Japan. Brain Devel 2001;23:128–130.

10. Smith I, Leeming RJ, Cavanagh NP, et al: Neurological aspects of biopterin metabolism. Arch Dis Child 1986;61:130–137.

11. Okano Y, Eisensmith RC, Butler F, et al: Molecular basis of phenotypic heterogeneity in phenylketonuria. N Engl J Med 1991;324:1232.

12. Haefele JM, White G, McDonald JD. Characterization of the mouse phenylalanine hydroxylase mutation Pah (enu3). Mol Genet Metab 2001;72:27–30.

13. Waters PJ, Parniak MA, Hewson AS, Scriver CR: Alterations in protein aggregation and degradation due to mild and severe missense mutations (A104D, R157N) in the human phenylalanine hydroxylase gene (PAH). Human Mutat 1998;12:344–354.

14. Smith I, Hyland K, Kendall B, et al: Clinical role of pteridine therapy in tetrahydrobiopterin deficiency. J Inherit Metab Dis 1985;8:39–45.

15. Tada K: Nonketotic hyperglycinemia: Clinical and metabolic aspects. Enzyme 1987;38:27–35.

16. Tada K, Kure S: Non-ketotic hyperglycinaemia: Molecular lesion, diagnosis and pathophysiology. J Inherit Metab Dis 1993;16:691.

17. Goedde HW, Langelbeck V: Clinical and biochemical genetic aspects of intermittent branched-chain ketoaciduria. Acta Paediatr Scand 1970;59:83.

18. Fernhoff PM, Fitzmaurice N, Milner J, et al: Coordinated system for comprehensive newborn metabolic screening. South Med J 1982;75:529–532.

19. Matsuda I, Nobukuni Y, Mitsubuchi H, et al: AT-to-A substitution in the E1 alpha subunit gene of the branched-chain alpha-ketoacid dehydrogenase complex in two cell lines derived from Menonite maple syrup urine disease patients. Biochem Biophys Res Commun 1990;172:646.

20. Chuang JL, Fisher CR, Cox RP, Chuang DT: Molecular basis of maple syrup urine disease: Novel mutations at the E1 alpha locus that impair E1 (alpha 2 beta 2) assembly or decrease steady-state E1 alpha mRNA levels of branched-chain alpha-keto acid dehydrogenase complex. Am J Hum Genet 1994;55:297–304.

21. Nobukuni Y, Mitsubuchi H, Akaboshi I, et al: Maple syrup urine disease: Complete defect of the E1-beta subunit of the branched chain alpha-ketoacid dehydrogenase complex due to deletion of an 11-bp repeat sequence which encodes a mitochondrial targeting leader peptide in a family with the disease. J Clin Invest 1991;87:1862–1866.

22. Fisher CW, Fisher CR, Chuang JL, et al: Occurrence of a 2-bp (AT) deletion allele and a nonsense (G-to-T) mutant allele at the E2 (DBT) locus of six patients with maple syrup urine disease: Multiple-exon skipping as a secondary effect of the mutations. Am J Hum Genet 1993;52:414–424.

23. Liu T-C, Kim H, Arizmendi C, et al: Identification of two missense mutations in a dihydrolipoamide dehydrogenase-deficient patient. Proc Natl Acad Sci U S A 1993;90:235.

24. Fisher CW, Lau KS, Fisher CR, et al: A 17-bp insertion and a Phe215-Cys missense mutation in the dihydrolipoyl transacylase (E2) mRNA from a thiamine-responsive maple syrup urine disease patient WG–34. Biochem Biophys Res Commun 1991;174:804–809.

25. Nyhan WL, Rice-Kelts M, Klein J, Barshop BA: Treatment of the acute crisis in maple syrup urine disease. Arch Pediatr Adolesc Med 1998;152:593–598.

Disorders of the Urea Cycle

Lewis J. Waber

The reactions of the urea cycle provide the main mechanism for the disposition of waste nitrogen in humans and most other mammals. The cycle accomplishes the net conversion of the nitrogen atoms in one molecule each of ammonium and aspartate to urea. Whereas ammonium is toxic, urea is relatively inert, soluble in water, and readily excreted in the urine. The cycle requires the sequential action of five enzymes: mitochondrial carbamoylphosphate synthetase I (CPS), mitochondrial ornithine transcarbamylase (OTC), cytosolic argininosuccinate synthetase (AS), cytosolic argininosuccinate lyase (AL), and cytosolic arginase (AR).

The function of the cycle also requires a transport system to shuttle intermediates across the mitochondrial membranes. Activity of the first enzyme of ureagenesis, carbamoylphosphate synthetase, requires an activator, N-acetylglutamate which is synthesized in the mitochondrial matrix by N-acetylglutamate synthetase. Deficiency of the transporter causes the hyperammonemia, hyperornithinemia, homocitrullinemia (HHH) syndrome. Deficiency of N-acetylglutamate synthetase causes a phenotype similar to CPS deficiency. This chapter will not review those defects further.

Defects in any of the enzymes of ureagenesis result in hyperammonemia and accumulation of other nitrogenous products, notably glutamine and alanine. The hyperammonemia causes cerebral dysfunction, cerebral edema, and death. Early diagnosis and treatment may avert premature death and severe cerebral damage. All the enzyme deficiencies are inherited as autosomal recessive traits except for OTC deficiency, which is X-linked.

This chapter is based on a chapter from the previous edition of this volume by Mize and Waber.[1] A comprehensive review of the urea cycle enzymes was published in 2001.[2]

Clinical Features and Diagnostic Evaluation

Neonatal Presentation

Children are normal at birth and remain so for at least 24 hours. They become tachypneic and develop respiratory alkalosis caused by stimulation of the respiratory center by ammonia. They develop poor feeding, vomiting, lethargy, seizures, and coma. Ammonia levels may rise above 1000 μmol/L. Without treatment, death occurs as a result of irreversible cerebral edema. Severe neonatal hyperammonemic coma nearly invariably leads to permanent neurologic damage. Later, affected children are at risk for episodes of hyperammonemia brought on by viral infections, otitis media, or inadvertent feeding of a high-protein meal.

Late-Onset Presentations

Partial deficiencies of urea cycle enzymes cause varying degrees of protein intolerance, vomiting, failure to thrive, and developmental delay. Episodes of hyperammonemia causing transient ataxia and confusion are common. The hyperammonemia may resolve rapidly with intravenous glucose infusions and go unrecognized if ammonia is not measured.

Female carriers of OTC deficiency, which is X-linked, can be completely asymptomatic or have a variety of symptoms, including (1) hyperammonemic coma indistinguishable from that of affected males; (2) severe hyperactivity, mental retardation, and ataxia; and (3) protein intolerance and avoidance.[3] About 20% of female heterozygotes manifest at the least protein intolerance. Menstruation or childbirth may increase the risk for hyperammonemic episodes. Patients with episodic unexplained confusion or ataxia often self-select a low-protein diet.

Arginase Deficiency

Patients with arginase deficiency do not present with hyperammonemic coma. They have milder hyperammonemia, typically in the 200 to 300 μmol/L range. The most prominent features are progressive spasticity, particularly in the legs, and mild mental retardation. Some patients have protein intolerance and avoidance, similar to patients with late-onset presentations of the other urea cycle defects.

Diagnostic Evaluation

Symptomatic individuals with urea cycle defects have ammonia levels above 300 μmol/L at the time of diagnosis. Levels in neonates are often well above 1000 μmol/L at the time of presentation. Symptomatic individuals with lesser elevations of ammonia are unlikely to have a defect in the urea cycle.

Plasma amino acid quantitation may establish the diagnosis. Typical amino acid patterns are given in Table 58–1. In summary, amino acid patterns in CPS and OTC deficiencies are identical: elevated glutamine (above 1000 μmol/L in symptomatic individuals) and decreased citrulline (<5 μmol/L). Patients with OTC deficiency have orotic aciduria when they are hyperammonemic. Patients with AS deficiency (citrullinemia) have hyperglutaminemia and citrulline levels typically above 1000 μmol/L. Arginine levels may be low (<40 μmol/L). Patients with AL deficiency (argininosuccinic aciduria) have hyperglutaminemia, moderately elevated citrulline levels (200 to 300 μmol/L), and hypoargininemia, and show the presence of argininosuccinic acid and its anhydrides. Patients with AR deficiency (argininemia) have elevated arginine levels (>400 μmol/L) and milder hyperglutaminemia.

Diagnostic suspicions can be confirmed by enzyme assays. Arginase can be assayed in red cells or cultured fibroblasts. AS and AL can be assayed in fibroblasts, although plasma amino acid patterns are usually diagnostic for those disorders. Assaying CPS and OTC requires liver tissue. Enzymatic diagnosis of OTC heterozygotes is particularly problematic since the distribution of enzyme in the liver is patchy, reflecting patterns of X-chromosome inactivation. Allopurinol loading may induce orotic aciduria or

TABLE 58–1. Biochemical and Molecular Properties of Urea Cycle Enzymes

Enzyme	Chromosomal location	Cellular location	Tissue expression	Biochemical phenotype of deficiency	
				Plasma amino acids	Urine organic acids
Carbamoyl phosphate synthetase I EC 6.3.4.16 MIM 237300*	2q35	Mitochondrial matrix	Liver	Decreased citrulline, Increased glutamine, alanine Decreased arginine	Unremarkable
Ornithine transcarbamylase EC 2.1.3.3 MIM 311250*	Xp21.1	Mitochondrial matrix	Liver, intestine	Decreased citrulline, Increased glutamine, alanine Decreased arginine	Increased orotic acid
Argininosuccinate synthetase EC 6.3.4.5 MIM 215700*	9q34	Cytosol	Liver, fibroblasts	Increased citrulline, Increased glutamine, alanine Decreased arginine	Unremarkable
Argininosuccinate lyase EC 4.3.2.1 MIM 207900*	7cen-q11.2	Cytosol	Liver, fibroblasts	Moderately increased citrulline, increased argininosuccinate and anhydrides, increased glutamine, alanine Decreased arginine	Unremarkable
Arginase EC 3.5.3.1 MIM 207800*	6q23	Cytosol	Liver, erythrocytes	Increased arginine	Unremarkable

orotidinuria in heterozygotes,[4] but the predictive value of the test is low in individuals without a family history. Direct sequencing of the OTC gene may be the best diagnostic test for females suspected of being OTC heterozygotes.

Pathology

Although there is heterogeneity among these disorders, neuropathologic observations have been remarkably uniform across the enzyme deficiencies. Postmortem studies have demonstrated global derangements of neural development, if not degeneration.[5] In mild OTC deficiency in girls, there has been severe cerebral shrinkage and brain collapse, resembling acquired hepatocerebral degeneration. Terminal events due to neonatal hyperammonemia are associated with brain edema and mitochondrial changes in Alzheimer type II astrocytes. Cystic necrosis at the cortical gray-white matter junction has been rarely noted with mild neuron changes. Computed tomographic (CT) scans and pathologic examination have shown other changes such as brain stem encephalitis and cerebral atrophy. In several patients without preceding coma, seizure, or cardiopulmonary arrest, lesions resembling infarcts have been reported, namely mild ventriculomegaly and bifrontal lesions on CT scans and high signal lesions on MRI scans that are evident in a watershed zone between anterior and middle cerebral areas. These changes are difficult to interpret in light of varying extent of injury and metabolic control in these patients. Myelination defects or neuron loss in the basal nuclei and occasional cerebellar heterotopias have been reported in patients with AL and OTC deficiencies; myelination delay and astrocytic nuclear swelling have occurred without neuronal damage in AL deficiency. Some patients with AL deficiency may develop portal fibrosis.

Biochemical (Enzymatic) Findings

Figure 58–1 shows that the mature forms of the first two enzymes in the pathway (CPS and OTC) are mitochondrial, and the last three (AS, AL, and AR) are cytoplasmic. The complete urea cycle is expressed functionally in parenchymal cells of the liver and, to a much lesser extent, in the kidney; intestinal mucosa expresses activities for the mitochondrial enzymes. Biochemical properties of the six enzymes are shown in Table 58–1.

Two human arginase isozymes (AI and AII) exist. Arginase I, abundant in the cytosol of hepatocytes, is primarily responsible for the urea generated in the urea cycle. Arginase II in the mitochondrial matrix appears to be involved primarily in ornithine production.

Expression of Urea Cycle Enzymes

The entire cycle is expressed in hepatocytes. Within the liver, expression is highest in cells near the portal triads. CPS constitutes as much as 30% of mitochondrial protein

in liver. Glutamine synthetase is expressed in hepatocytes surrounding the hepatic veins. Conversely, glutaminase is expressed in cells in the portal triads. It thus appears that systemic ammonium is converted to glutamine, a high-affinity, low-capacity process. The glutamine is hydrolyzed and the ammonium converted to urea in the portal cells, a high-capacity, low-affinity process. Conversely, ammonium produced by glutamine degradation or digestive absorption in the intestine reaches the portal triads and is converted into urea. Only a small amount of portal vein-derived ammonia appears to be metabolized to glutamine directly.

Part of the urea cycle is also present in the kidney (the cytosolic enzymes) and in the intestine (the mitochondrial enzymes). Intestine contains CPS and OTC and is capable of producing citrulline from ammonium and ornithine. The gut also contains ornithine aminotransferase (OAT) and is capable of synthesizing ornithine from glutamate. The kidney uses glutamine as the source of ammonium ions as a means of excretion of excess acid into the tubular fluid. Glutamine carbon is converted to glucose. The kidney also takes up citrulline and releases arginine. The source of the citrulline is the intestine. This reaction is a major source of arginine synthesis and explains why arginine is not an essential amino acid in normal humans.

The net result is an active shuttle of glutamine within the liver and between gut, liver, and kidney. The intestine uses glutamine as a fuel, producing ammonium, citrulline, and alanine. The ammonium reaches the liver and is converted either to urea or glutamine. The gut-produced citrulline is not removed by the hepatocytes. Instead, it serves as a source for arginine synthesis in the kidney. Systemically produced ammonia would be preferentially converted to glutamine near the hepatic veins. The glutamine can serve as a source of urinary ammonium (acid excretion) or of urea, depending on whether it was broken down in the kidney or in the liver.

In the absence of effective urea cycle activity, only the glutamine-producing reactions would be active in the liver, hence the extreme hyperglutaminemia characteristic of urea cycle disorders. Similarly, a defect in any of the urea cycle enzymes will vitiate the intestinal-renal pathway for arginine synthesis, making arginine an essential amino acid.

Molecular-Genetic Data (Including Mutations)

Single genes encode each enzyme of the urea cycle. A variety of mutations responsible for deficiencies of OTC, AS, AL, and AR have been described. Some of the basic information is summarized in Table 58–1.

Carbamylphosphate Synthetase I

CPS comprises two large subunits of 160,000 daltons. It has been mapped to chromosome 2q35.[6] The gene produces a 5 kb mRNA. Like other mitochondrial enzymes,

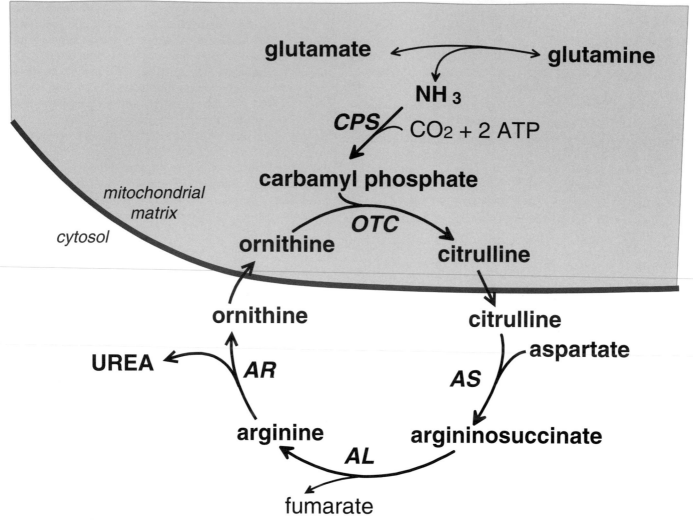

FIGURE 58–1. The urea cycle. Substrates in the pathway of nitrogen removal are indicated in boldface type. Enzymes of the cycle are indicated in boldface italic type. Other molecules are indicated in regular type. AL, argininosuccinate lyase; AR, arginase; AS, argininosuccinate synthetase; CPS, carbamoylphosphate synthetase; OTC, ornithine transcarbamylase.

CPS is synthesized in the cytosol as a prepeptide, imported into the mitochondria via a specific transport system, cleaved by a peptidase to remove the leader sequence, and assembled into the active protein. Summar[7] has reported several mutations causing CPS deficiency.

Ornithine Transcarbamylase

Much is known about the human *OTC* gene and its mutations. The gene was mapped to band Xp2i.1 by in situ hybridization.[8] This places the gene in the region of the loci for Duchenne muscular dystrophy and glycerol kinase. An OTC cDNA was first isolated from rats, then from humans. The human, rat, and mouse mRNAs are all of similar lengths, about 1600 bases. The coding portion contains a leader sequence for 32 amino acids followed by 322 amino acids for the mature enzyme. The OTC leader peptide has been used as a model for the study of mitochondrial import processes. Residues 8 through 22 of the human OTC leader peptide contain the informa-tion necessary to direct import into the mitochondria. The leader peptide is basic, containing four arginine residues and no acidic residues. Genomic analysis has revealed that the *OTC* gene covers over 85 kb of DNA.

Many mutations in the *OTC* gene have been described.[9] Some patients have deletions detectable by Southern blotting. This is not the case in most families. Some mutations, however, affect restriction cleavage sites. Nucleotide 245 may be a "hot spot" for mutation (ARG-to-GLN) associated with late-onset OTC deficiency. Some families with OTC deficiency have the same mutation found in the *spf-ash* mouse model of mild OTC deficiency, with 1% to 4% of residual enzyme activity; despite this rel-atively low activity, patients developed normally.

Argininosuccinate Synthetase

The *AS* gene is located at 9q34,[10] close to the ABO blood group locus. A cDNA clone for the gene was isolated in 1981. In addition to this expressed gene, there are 14 pseudogenes scattered over the genome. The expressed gene is 64 kb in size and has 14 exons. It codes for an RNA 1600 bases long. Analysis of a full-length cDNA predicted 412 amino acids, with a subunit molecular weight of 46,400. Because the enzyme is cytoplasmic, no leader sequences or processing is necessary for activity.

Because the enzyme is expressed in fibroblasts, analysis of gene expression in mutants is much easier than in CPS or OTC deficiencies, in which hepatocytes must be studied. Kobayashi and coworkers[11] identified 20 mutations in patients with citrullinemia. One (IVS-6AS) was common in Japanese patients, but no common mutation was found in patients of other ethnic backgrounds.

Argininosuccinate Lyase

A cDNA clone for *AL* was isolated in 1986. The predicted enzyme would contain 463 amino acids and have a molecular weight of approximately 52,000. *AL* has been mapped to the long arm of chromosome 7 (7cen-ql.2) by in situ hybridization.[12] The gene has 16 exons and is 35 kb long.

Arginase

A cDNA clone for human arginase was isolated in 1985. Using somatic cell hybrids and in situ hybridization techniques, the gene was mapped to 6q23 the next year.[13] The gene is 11.5 kb long and contains eight exons. The predicted protein has 322 amino acids and a molecular weight of 35,000. Molecular and immunologic studies have shown that the genes for arginase I and arginase II are not homologous. Nine mutations associated with arginase deficiency have been described.[14]

Animal Models

A few models for urea cycle defects are known. These include a Holstein-Friesian calf model of citrullinemia, and two sparse-fur mouse models for OTC deficiency. One, *spf*, has a mutation that appears to affect mRNA processing. The other, *spf-ash* (associated with abnormal skin and hair), has a missense mutation in the gene that causes aberrant mRNA splicing.

In the *spf* mouse, hepatic OTC activity of affected males approximates 10% of that found in unaffected male litter mates and is associated with urinary bladder stones composed mostly of orotic acid.

In the *spf-ash* mutation, male mice have 5% to 10% of normal OTC, yet develop only slight hyperammonemia and otherwise grow quite well. OTC reduction is less pronounced in the intestine than in the liver compared with the *spf* mouse, and CPS I activity is also significantly modified.

Chronic or Subacute Hyperammonemia

Chronic or subacute hyperammonemia has been induced in rats independent of genetic defects of the urea cycle.

Rats have been injected with urease, which causes isolated hyperammonemia. In another ammonium acetate mouse model, nuclear magnetic resonance spectroscopy suggested a fall in cerebral tricarboxylic acid–cycle activity. In this model, further inhibition of glutamine accumulation by inhibition of glutamine synthetase (by L-methionine sulfoximine) prevented cerebral edema (as indicated by increased brain water), suggesting that a common mechanism, for example, idiogenic osmoles, may cause brain swelling. A similar rabbit model of acute ammonium acetate hyperammonemia has been developed.

Therapy

Acute Hyperammonemic Coma

Dialysis is the most effective method of removing waste nitrogen, reducing hyperammonemia, and restoring a normal metabolic balance. Hemodialysis is most effective, although peritoneal dialysis is more accessible in many centers. Exchange transfusion is ineffective for the removal of significant quantities of waste nitrogen.

Adjunctive measures are to provide at least 60% of the recommended daily allowance for calories parenterally. Intravenous sodium benzoate (250 mg/kg per day) and sodium phenylacetate (250 to 500 mg/kg per day) have been useful but not sufficient for treating acute hyperammonemic coma. At this time, these medications are not approved for intravenous use in the United States and are available only as investigational new drugs. Extreme care must be used in administering these drugs as deaths from inadvertent overdoses have been reported.[15] Intravenous arginine at 200 mg/kg per day is beneficial in treating hypoargininemia in all the disorders. In AS deficiency (citrullinemia) and AL deficiency (argininosuccinic aciduria), larger doses up to 800 mg/kg per day are useful in promoting ammonia excretion.[16]

Long-Term Management

The objective is to reduce the body load of waste nitrogen while allowing for normal growth and development with as normal a diet as possible.[17] Goals should be to maintain ammonia concentrations in the normal range and glutamine concentrations below 500 μM without essential amino acid or arginine deficiency.[18]

Diet Management

The diet must be adjusted to provide adequate calories and protein for growth. Some patients may require only a low protein diet (1.2 to 2.0 g/kg per day), sometimes with a protein-free caloric supplement. When a satisfactory nitrogen balance cannot be maintained by diet alone, drug therapy should be added (discussed later). Drugs are nearly always required for patients with neonatal presentations. If adequate protein cannot be provided from natural sources without causing nitrogen accumulation and hyperammonemia, some or all of the natural protein can be replaced by products providing "protein" as a mixture of essential amino acids.

Drug Therapy

The development of alternative pathway therapy,[19] the use of drugs that are conjugated with nitrogen-containing substances and excreted in the urine has allowed long-term survival. Arginine and sodium phenylbutyrate[20] are the most useful drugs to promote urinary nitrogen excretion. Sodium phenylbutyrate has replaced sodium benzoate and sodium phenylacetate in oral drug therapy regimens.

CPS and OTC Deficiencies. Oral sodium phenylbutyrate 500 to 800 mg/kg per day, plus oral L-citrulline (up to 200 mg/kg per day) is used to maintain normal serum arginine.

AS Deficiency (Citrullinemia). Oral L-arginine at 400 to 800 mg/kg per day; sodium phenylbutyrate (500 to 800 mg/kg per day) is usually necessary.

AL Deficiency (Argininosuccinic Aciduria). Oral L-arginine at 400 to 800 mg/kg per day is used.

Arginase Deficiency. Sodium phenylbutyrate at 500 mg/kg per day is used.

Transplantation

Medical therapy is usually sufficient for patients with AS and AL deficiencies, although the patients have episodic hyperammonemia. Given the difficulties of treatment of the most severe cases of OTC and CPS deficiencies, liver transplantation may be the best therapeutic modality. Liver transplantation corrects the major metabolic defects but exposes the patients to the risks of long-term immunosuppression.[21]

Conclusion and Future Directions

Urea cycle disorders cause severe neurologic impairment if not diagnosed and treated rapidly. Knowledge of the underlying biochemistry has allowed effective treatments to be designed. Medical therapy must be started before hyperammonemia causes permanent neurologic damage, making rapid diagnosis imperative. Although it is effective, medical therapy does not eliminate episodic hyperammonemia.

One promising new modality for early diagnosis is newborn screening using tandem mass spectrometry.[22] AS, AL, and AR deficiencies can be diagnosed using the amino acid profile generated by this screening procedure. CPS and OTC deficiencies do not create unique amino acid profiles detectable by the screen, although suspicion may be increased if hyperglutaminemia is found. In any case, given the rapidity of onset of hyperammonemia in the neonatal onset disorders, there may not be sufficient time for the screen to be completed before damage is done.

Gene therapy offers the possibility of more definitive treatment. Successful gene therapy will most likely require targeting the hepatocytes because the complete cycle is expressed in those cells. A gene therapy trial for OTC deficiency was terminated after the death of one of the research subjects, apparently due to an adverse reaction to the adenovirus vector.[23] Improved vectors and new techniques to improve expression levels may make gene therapy a viable therapeutic modality in the future.

REFERENCES

1. Mize CM, Waber LJ: Urea cycle disorders. In Rosenberg RN, Prusiner SB, DiMauro S, et al (eds): The Molecular and Genetic Basis of Neurological Disease. Boston, Butterworth-Heinmann, 1997, pp 1151–1174.
2. Brusilow SW, Horwich AL: Urea cycle enzymes. In Scriver CR, Beaudet AL, Sly WS, Valle D (eds): The Metabolic and Molecular Basis of Inherited Disease. New York, McGraw-Hill, 2001, pp 1909–1963.
3. Batshaw ML, Msall M, Beaudet AL, Trojak J: Risk of serious illness in heterozygotes for ornithine transcarbamylase deficiency. J Pediatr 1986;108:236–241.
4. Sebesta I, Fairbanks LD, Davies PM, et al: The allopurinol loading test for the identification of carriers for ornithine carbamoyltransferase deficiency: Studies in a healthy control population and females at risk. Clin Chim Acta 1994;224:45–54.
5. Harding BN, Leonard JV, Erdohazi M: Ornithine carbamoyl transferase deficiency: A neuropathological study. Eur J Pediatr 1984;141:215–220.
6. Summar ML, Dasouki MJ, Schofield PJ, et al: Physical and linkage mapping of human carbamyl phosphate synthetase I and reassignment from 2p to 2q35. Cytogenet Cell Genet 1995;71:266–267.
7. Summar ML: Molecular genetic research into carbamoyl-phosphate synthase I: Molecular defects and linkage markers. J Inherited Metabolic Disease 1998;21:30–39.
8. Lindgren V, de Martinville B, Horwich AL, et al: Human ornithine transcarbamylase locus mapped to band Xp21.1 near Duchenne muscular dystrophy locus. Science 1984;226:698–700.
9. Tuchman M, Matsuda I, Munnich A, et al: Proportions of spontaneous mutations in males and females with ornithine transcarbamylase deficiency. Am J Med Genet 1995;55:67–70.
10. Northrup H, Lathrop M, Lu S-Y, et al: Multilocus linkage analysis with the human argininosuccinate synthetase gene. Genomics 1989;5:442–444.
11. Kobayashi K, Kakinoki H, Fukushige T, et al: Nature and frequency of mutations in the argininosuccinate synthetase gene that cause classical citrullinemia. Hum Genet 1995;96:454–463.

12. Todd S, McGill JR, McCombs JL, et al: cDNA sequence, interspecies comparison and gene mapping analysis of argininosuccinate lyase. Genomics 1989;4: 53–59.

13. Sparkes RS, Dizikes GJ, Klisak I, et al: The gene for human liver arginase (ARG1) is assigned to chromosome band 6q23. Am J Hum Genet 1986;39:186–193.

14. Uchino T, Snyderman SE, Lambert M, et al: Molecular basis of phenotypic variation in patients with argininemia. Hum Genet 1995;96:255–260.

15. Praphanphoj V, Boydjiev SA, Waber LJ, et al: Three cases of intravenous sodium benzoate and sodium phenylacetate toxicity occurring in the treatment of acute hyperammonemia. J Inherit Metab Dis 2000;23: 129–136.

16. Brusilow SW, Danney M, Waber L, et al: Treatment of episodic hyperammonemia in children with inborn errors of urea synthesis. N Engl J Med 1984; 310:1630–1634.

17. Feillet F, Leonard JV: Alternative pathway therapy for urea cycle disorders. J Inherit Metab Dis 1998;21:101–111.

18. Maestri NE, McGowan KD, Brusilow SW: Plasma glutamine concentration: A guide to the management of urea cycle disorders. J Pediatr 1992;121: 259–261.

19. Brusilow SW, Valle DL, Batshaw ML: New pathways of nitrogen excretion in inborn errors of urea synthesis. Lancet 1979;452–454.

20. Brusilow SW: Phenylacetylglutamine may replace urea as a vehicle for waste nitrogen excretion. Pediatr Res 1991;29:147–150.

21. Whitington PF, Alonso EM, Boyle JT, et al: Liver transplantation for the treatment of urea cycle disorders. J Inherit Metab Dis 1998;21:112–118.

22. Anonymous: Serving the family from birth to the medical home. A report from the Newborn Screening Task Force convened in Washington DC, May 10–11, 1999. Pediatrics 2000;106:383–427.

23. Raper SE, Yudkoff M, Chirmule N, et al: A pilot study of in vivo liver-directed gene transfer with an adenoviral vector in partial ornithine transcarbamylase deficiency. Hum Gene Ther 2002;12:163–175.

Disorders of Glucose Transport

Darryl C. De Vivo

Dong Wang

Juan M. Pascual

Transport of water-soluble molecules across tissue barriers has been a subject of increasing interest since 1952.[1] Widdas proposed that the transport of glucose across the erythrocyte membrane required a carrier mechanism to facilitate diffusion. In hindsight, these observations were prescient. Two major families of glucose transporters have been discovered.[2,3] These discoveries have provided important insights into three genetically determined human diseases.

One major family includes the concentrative Na+/glucose transporters (SGLT) otherwise known as active co-transporters or symporters. These symporters are energized by H+ or Na+ gradients. These gradients are generated and maintained by ATP-dependent ion pumps. Three types of concentrative Sglts have been identified: Sglt1, Sglt2, and Sglt3. Secondary structure analysis suggests 14 transmembrane α-helices. Sglt1 is responsible for glucose absorption from the intestinal tract. Sglt2, together with Sglt1, is responsible for glucose absorption in the renal tubules. The peptide sequence of mammalian Sglt1 was determined in 1987 by expression cloning of its cDNA.[4] The deduced peptide chain contains 664 amino acids arranged in 14 transmembrane domains and exposing both amino and carboxyl termini to the extracellular space. The *SGLT1* (locus SLC5A1) gene is localized to chromosome 22q12.3 (UCSC Human Genome Project Working Draft, June 2002 Assembly; http://genome.cse.ucsc.edu) and spans 72 kb. The gene contains 15 exons. Two other *SGLT* genes are now known to exist (*SGLT2* and *SGLT3*) in addition to several homologous genes of uncertain functionality.[5] *SGLT2* (locus SLC5A2) is localized to chromosome 16p11.2, and the protein is expressed in kidney and, to a lesser degree, in ileum. *SGLT3* gene (locus SLC5A4) is localized to chromosome

22p12.3 near the *SGLT1* gene locus (UCSC Human Genome Project Working Draft, June 2002 Assembly; http://genome.cse.ucsc.edu). The Sglt3 protein may represent a duplication of the Sglt1 protein.

Mutations in the *SGLT1* gene cause the glucose-galactose malabsorption syndrome (OMIM 182380).[6] The glucose-galactose malabsorption syndrome was described in 1962.[7,8] Both reports, one from Sweden and the other from France, described a familial entity of early onset characterized by watery acid diarrhea and life-threatening dehydration. The symptoms typically begin before the fourth day of life and respond to the elimination of glucose and galactose in the feedings. This syndrome has no direct neurologic symptomatology, and is only mentioned here for the sake of completeness.

The other major family of glucose transporters is the GLUT gene family. These transporters facilitate passive diffusion of glucose across tissue barriers by energy-independent stereo-specific mechanisms.

In the mid-1980s, Mueckler and colleagues discovered a protein that facilitated the diffusion of glucose across the epidermis cell membrane.[9] Later, Birnbaum et al made similar observations in the rat brain and the two groups proceeded to clone and sequence the gene encoding the Glut1 protein.[10] The gene was assigned to human chromosome 1 and localized further to the short arm (1p34.2) (UCSC Human Genome Project Working Draft, April 2002 Assembly; http://genome.cse.ucsc.edu). Since 1985, additional proteins have been identified that are responsible for the facilitated diffusion of hexoses across tissue barriers.[11] These *GLUT* genes are a subset of genes within a large superfamily of transport facilitators. This superfamily of transport facilitators is designated SLC2A for solute carrier 2A according to the HUGO Gene

Nomenclature Committee.[12–14] *GLUT6* was identified as a pseudogene, and *GLUT7*, initially reported to encode a microsomal transporter, later was shown to be a cloning artifact.[15] These earlier missteps have been corrected as new information has emerged. The current understanding of this *GLUT* gene family has been reviewed.[2,11,16] The *GLUT* family includes 12 *SLC2A* genes, numbered 1–12, encoding 12 Glut proteins. A thirteenth member of the GLUT family is the myoinositol transporter, HMIT1. Joost and Thorens in their concluding remarks stated that "it appears reasonable to assume that (essentially) all members of the family are now identified."[11] The genes encoding three GLUT proteins (1, 5, and 7) are localized to the short arm of chromosome 1: *GLUT1* to 1p34.2, and *GLUT5* and *GLUT7* to 1p36.2. These three gene loci are separated by approximately 40 Mbp. *GLUT1* is highly expressed in erythrocytes and brain, *GLUT5* is highly expressed in intestine, testis and kidney; and *GLUT7* expression currently is unknown. The *GLUT7* gene is contiguous to the *GLUT5* gene on chromosome 1p36.2 and the GLUT7 protein has a high degree of similarity (58% identical amino acids) compared with the fructose-specific GLUT5 protein. The GLUT5 protein is known to be present in brain microglia although its function in these cells remains unclear.

Human Glut1 has a molecular mass of 54,117 Da, has a single N-linked oligosaccharide and 12 transmembrane segments. (Fig. 59–1). Mueckler et al visualized the Glut1 transporter as an aqueous sugar translocation pathway through the lipid bilayer via the clustering of several transmembrane helices.[9,17] Cloherty and colleagues have proposed that the Glut1 transporter is a cooperative homotetramer, each protein presenting a translocation pathway that alternates between uptake and export states.[18,19] The model also predicts that at any instant two subunits represent uptake and two subunits represent exit states. We have been able to examine the bidirectional flux of glucose, dehydroascorbic acid and water in the wild-type and mutant Glut1 proteins using mutations that we have discovered in patients with the Glut1 deficiency syndrome (Glut1DS). Our studies with a T310I pathogenic missense mutation provide experimental results strongly suggesting the presence of two channels per Glut1 monomer, one of which can be blocked by the mutation T310I.[20]

Two human diseases result from mutations of Glut family proteins. The first is the Fanconi-Bickel syndrome (OMIM 227810) and the second is the Glut1 deficiency syndrome (OMIM 606777).

The Fanconi-Bickel syndrome was first described in 1949[21] and originally named hepatorenal glycogenosis

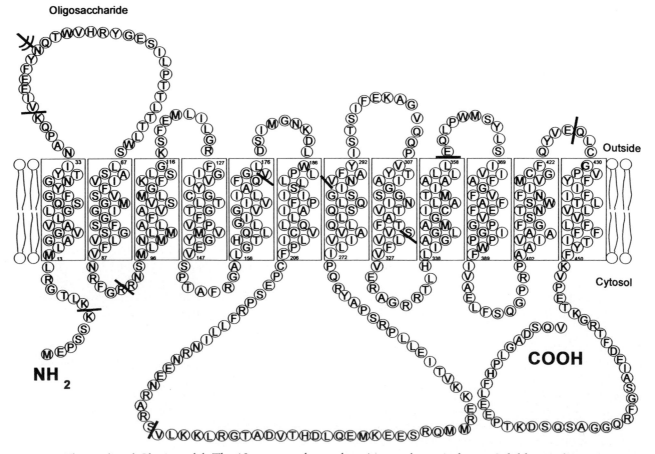

FIGURE 59–1. The predicted Glut1 model. The 12 transmembrane domains are shown in *boxes*. *Solid bars* indicate the location of introns in the GLUT1 gene.

with renal Fanconi syndrome. This first patient presented at age 6 months with failure to thrive, polydipsia, and constipation. Later in childhood, he developed osteopenia, short stature, hepatomegaly, and tubular nephropathy. The nephropathy was associated with glycosuria, phosphaturia, aminoaciduria, and intermittent proteinuria. These urinary metabolites were accompanied by hypophosphatemia and hyperuricemia. The liver was filled with glycogen and fat. Distinctively, ketotic hypoglycemia was evident preprandially and hyperglycemia was evident postprandially. This distinctive feature is the result of the multi-functional role of Glut2 in the pancreas and the liver. These patients may exhibit intestinal malabsorption and diarrhea, but they do not have any primary neurologic complaints.

The *GLUT2* gene was cloned in 1988[22] and localized to chromosome 3q26.2 (UCSC Human Genome Project Working Draft, June 2002 assembly; http://genome.cse.ucsc.edu/). The gene contains eleven exons and ten introns spanning about 30 kb. A mutation in the *GLUT2* gene was identified in the original case by Santer et al (1997).[23] Most patients with the Fanconi-Bickel syndrome are homozygous for the disease-related mutations consistent with an autosomal recessive pattern of inheritance. Some patients have been shown to be compound heterozygotes.[24]

Glut1DS was first described in 1991.[25] Since that time, approximately 100 patients have been identified in the United States and elsewhere throughout the world.[2,26] Mueckler et al had cloned the gene encoding the protein that catalyses the uptake of glucose into red blood cells.[9] Later, this protein was shown to be immunochemically identical to the Glut1 protein in brain microvessels and in brain astrocytes.[27,28] The clinical syndrome, in and of itself, argues forcefully for the concept that glucose transport across the blood-brain-barrier (BBB) is an important rate-limiting event and contributes, in ways not yet fully understood, to impaired early brain growth and functional development. The clinical signature of Glut1DS is the presence of hypoglycorrhachia and low CSF lactate concentration in the absence of hypoglycemia. Other conditions causing hypoglycorrhachia commonly cause elevated CSF lactate. Examples include mitochondrial diseases, intracranial infection, and subarachnoid hemorrhage. Several treatment strategies have been pursued, none optimal, as it relates to the developmental encephalopathy associated with this clinical syndrome. The ketogenic diet has been effective in controlling seizures but has had little measurable effect on the associated cognitive impairment and behavioral disturbances. As the number of cases increases worldwide, it becomes more important to expand our understanding of the clinical phenotypes and to explore alternative treatment strategies designed to mitigate the brain injury associated with impaired glucose transport across the BBB during early neurologic development.

Glut1 is highly expressed in brain tissues, including the endothelial cells of the brain microvessels and the astrocytes. The neurologic symptoms can be traced directly to a metabolic disturbance of the glial-endothelial complex that is fundamental to the integrity of the BBB. As a result, the remainder of this chapter focuses exclusively on the clinical and molecular features of the Glut1DS.

CLINICAL FEATURES

The phenotypic spectrum of Glut1DS is becoming broader as more patients are being diagnosed. The clinical signature of the classical phenotype is an infantile-onset epileptic encephalopathy associated with delayed neurologic development, deceleration of head growth, acquired microcephaly, incoordination, and spasticity. The two children described by De Vivo and colleagues in 1991 exhibited these neurologic signs. The presence of hypoglycorrhachia led the investigators to speculate that there was a defect in the transport of glucose across the BBB. Seven years later, these speculations were substantiated. The first patient had a large-scale deletion involving one *GLUT1* allele causing hemizygosity, and the second patient had a heterozygous nonsense mutation (Y449X).[29] Three clinical phenotypes have been defined with the acquisition of more patients. The first phenotype (classical) is a developmental encephalopathy with seizures. Seizures typically begin within the first 4 months of life. The prenatal and perinatal histories, birth weights, and Apgar scores are normal. The earliest epileptic events include apneic episodes and episodic eye movements simulating opsoclonus. The infantile seizures are clinically fragmented and the electro-encephalographic correlate is that of multifocal spike-wave discharges.[30] Seizures become more synchronized with brain maturation and present clinically as generalized events associated with classical 2.5- to 4-Hz spike and wave discharges electrically. Five seizure types have been described in these patients, including generalized tonic or clonic seizures, myoclonic seizures, atypical absence, atonic, and unclassified seizures. The frequency of clinical seizures varies considerably from one patient to another. Some have daily seizures, whereas others have only occasional seizures separated by days, weeks, or months. As a rule, the clinical seizures respond poorly to anti-epileptic drugs, and disappear rapidly after beginning a ketogenic diet.

These patients suffer other paroxysmal events and it remains unclear whether these events are epileptic or non-epileptic nosologically. Paroxysmal events include intermittent ataxia, confusion, lethargy or somnolence, alternating hemiparesis, abnormalities of movement or posture, total body paralysis, sleep disturbances, and recurrent headaches. The frequency of the neurologic symptoms fluctuates unpredictably and may be influenced by environmental factors such as fasting or fatigue.[31] The patients have degrees of speech and language impairment. Dysarthria is common. Both receptive and expressive language skills are affected, but expressive language skills are disproportionately affected. Varying degrees of cognitive impairment have been described ranging from learning disabilities to severe mental retardation. Social adaptive behavior is a strength in these children. They are remarkably comfortable in the group setting and interact comfortably with their peer group and with adults.

Acquired microcephaly occurs in 50% of patients and deceleration of head growth is more common. However, a small number of patients continue to experience normal head growth.

Non-classic phenotypes also have been identified. One patient has mental retardation and intermittent ataxia without any clinical seizures[32] and one patient has a movement disorder characterized by choreoathetosis and dystonia. The movement disorder responded to a ketogenic diet.[33] These non-classic phenotypes, thus far observed in about 5% to 10% of the Glut1DS patient population, indicate that diagnostic studies should be performed on all infants and children with unexplained neurologic symptoms, including epilepsy, mental retardation, and movement disorders.

The physical findings relate to the pyramidal, extrapyramidal, and cerebellar systems predominantly and consist of varying degrees of spasticity, dystonia, and ataxia. The limb tone generally is increased, tendon reflexes are brisk, and Babinski signs are present. The gait abnormality is best described as a spastic ataxia. No consistent abnormalities of ocular fundi, cranial nerves, or sensation have been described, and the general physical examination is normal. These children have a tendency to be slightly smaller than their peers.

The differential diagnosis has continued to expand as the Glut1DS phenotypic spectrum has broadened. Several patients have been investigated for an occult neuroblastoma because of the opsoclonus-like eye movement abnormalities in early infancy. Other infantile-onset metabolic encephalopathies may be associated with infantile-onset seizures, developmental delay, and deceleration of head growth, including chronic hypoglycemic syndromes and disorders of amino acid and organic acid metabolism. Rett syndrome and Angelman syndrome have been considered occasionally, and many patients have been diagnosed initially with cerebral palsy.

LABORATORY FEATURES

Examination of the cerebrospinal fluid is essentially diagnostic in the correct clinical setting. All patients have hypoglycorrhachia and low-normal or low lactate concentrations. This profile is specific for Glut1DS in the absence of hypoglycemia. The CSF-glucose concentrations generally are in the mid-30s (mg/dl) and seldom, if ever, exceed 40 mg/dl. The CSF lactate values are always lower than 1.4 mM.

Brain MRI and CT imaging generally are normal. Minor, nonspecific abnormalities have been described in some patients with slight degrees of brain hypotrophy. The PET scan is distinctively abnormal.[34] The abnormalities include a global reduction of glucose uptake with more severe hypometabolism in the medial temporal lobes and the thalami. The thalamic hypo-metabolism is accentuated by the relatively increased uptake of glucose in the basal ganglia.

The electroencephalographic abnormalities, described earlier, include generalized spike or poly-spike wave discharges in approximately 50% of patients, mild diffuse slowing in 33%, focal epileptiform discharges in 10% to 15%, and focal slowing in 5% to 10%. In infancy, the EEG abnormality is focal with temporal and posterior spike discharges. Later in childhood, the EEG pattern is generalized with spike-wave epileptiform discharges.

The erythrocyte glucose uptake study is a valuable screening test and should be carried out in all patients with an appropriate clinical syndrome and associated hypoglycorrhachia. The Glut1 protein in the erythrocyte membrane is immunologically and chemically identical to the Glut1 isoform in cerebral microvessels.[27] The rate of 3-o-methyl-D-glucose uptake by freshly isolated, washed erythrocytes in vitro is decreased in patients compared to controls. The assay is relatively specific and sensitive for Glut1DS, but false negatives have been observed.[35] Chronic hyperglycemic conditions including diabetes mellitus also may produce false positives by causing downregulation of Glut1 receptors in tissue membranes.[2]

Fluorescence in situ hybridization (FISH) studies are available and can be performed on blood lymphocytes or cultured skin fibroblasts.[29] Three patients with Glut1DS have been determined to be hemizygous by FISH analysis (Fig. 59–2). This number represents approximately 10% of patients who have been confirmed at the molecular level.

GLUT1 genomic analysis is indicated in patients who are negative by FISH assay. Genomic DNA can be extracted from the patient's blood or cultured skin fibroblasts or other available tissues. We have identified 30 heterozygous mutations including 18 missense mutations, 3 nonsense mutations, 3 insertions, 3 microdeletions 9 and 3 splice site mutations (Fig. 59–3).

PATHOLOGY

Currently, there is nothing known regarding neuropathology in Glut1DS. One patient died from hemorrhagic pancreatitis while being treated with a ketogenic diet.[36] Neuropathology was not described. Microcephaly is known to occur, and thalamic hypometabolism is distinctive on PET scanning. Animal models, when developed, likely will provide important information regarding neuropathology in Glut1DS.

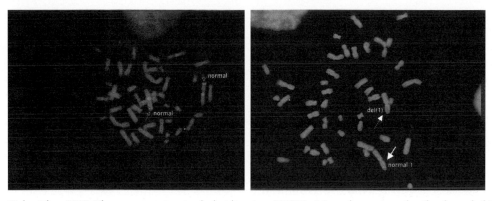

FIGURE 59–2. (See Color Plate VIII) Fluorescence in situ hybridization (FISH). Metaphase spreads of cultured skin fibroblasts from the Glut1DS patients were probed with a fluorescence labeled DNA probe specific for GLUT1. *A*, Patient #12 carried a heterozygous deletion (1086delG); the two alleles of GLUT1 were indicated by *arrows* with "normal." *B*, Patient #24 was hemizygous for GLUT1 in the short arm of chromosome 1 indicated by *arrows* with "normal 1" and "del(1)."

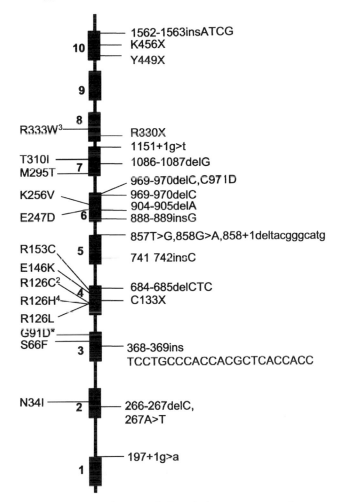

FIGURE 59–3. Distribution of identified mutations in Glut1DS on the GLUT1 gene. The 30 identified mutations currently reported (29, 45, 59, 60) are shown in the diagram. The three hemizygous mutations are not represented. The ten exons are shown in filled boxes. The line represents the 9 introns, 5′ and 3′ untranslated regions on the GLUT1 gene. The number on the top right corner of the mutation indicates the number of patients carrying the same mutation. (From Klepper J, Willemsen M, Verrips A, et al: Autosomal dominant transmission of GLUT1 deficiency. Hum Mol Genet 2001;10:63–68.)

BIOCHEMISTRY

Study of Glut1DS patients has provided clinical proof of principle that glucose transport across the BBB can be a rate-limiting step for brain metabolism.[37] Historically, glucose was considered the obligate fuel for brain metabolism under any and all circumstances. In 1967, ketone bodies were shown to substitute partially for glucose during conditions that favor chronic ketosis.[38] Glucose, after entering the brain, is phosphorylated irreversibly to glucose-6-phosphate and metabolized in the pentose phosphate shunt, Embden-Meyerhoff pathway, or converted to glycogen. The pentose phosphate shunt is important for nucleic acid synthesis. The Embden-Meyerhoff pathway permits glycolytic conversion of glucose to pyruvate. Glycogen synthesis provides a source of fuel during periods of metabolic stress. Decreased entry of glucose into the brain limits these three pathways and potentially contributes to the pathophysiology of Glut1DS.

Ketone bodies enter the brain by a monocarboxylic transport (MCT) system and are metabolized exclusively within the mitochondrial matrix to acetyl-CoA.[39] Ketone bodies provide an alternative source of acetyl-CoA in conditions that affect pyruvate synthesis from glucose. These conditions include the Glut1DS, pyruvate dehydrogenase deficiency, and other rare defects of cerebral glycolysis.[40]

Magistretti has proposed a bold new theory of brain metabolism by suggesting that lactate, derived from glucose in the astrocyte, is metabolized by the neuron as its principal energy source.[41] The Magistretti theory is thought-provoking, but not without its critics.[42] Others had shown GLUT3 on the neuronal membrane.[43] These issues and interpretations are directly relevant to an understanding of brain metabolism and Glut1DS pathophysiology. The Magistretti theory would suggest that the limitation of glucose transport across the BBB and the astrocyte membrane would limit glycogen storage and synthesis of lactate in the astrocyte. This suggestion is consistent with our observations that the CSF lactate is low-normal or low in patients with Glut1DS. Decreased lactate production by the astrocyte would limit uptake into the neuron, possibly causing secondary energy failure in this brain cell. The development of an animal model will allow these speculations to be investigated directly.

GENETICS

Glut1DS generally presents as a new mutation and behaves as a cellular co-dominant trait with haploinsufficiency. Most patients have private mutations distributed throughout the 12 transmembrane domains of the *GLUT1* gene (see Fig. 59–3). Several families have been recognized documenting an autosomal dominant pattern of inheritance over two or more generations (Fig. 59–4).

The first family (see Fig. 59–4A) was reported in 1999 and in complete detail in 2001.[44–46] Five patients in three generations were affected in the first family. The affected family members manifested mild to severe seizures, developmental delay, ataxia, hypoglycorrhachia in the three patients undergoing lumbar puncture, and decreased erythrocyte uptake studies. Several interesting caveats were identified in this family. The affected grandfather lived until age 78 years. He had been gainfully employed and fathered four children. He had learned of a home remedy that would mitigate his neurologic symptoms. He would take a dose of honey when anticipating the onset of symptoms. Minutes later he would feel better. This home remedy was passed on to his two affected children, one man and one woman. Each had similar symptoms. The daughter recognized a peculiar sensitivity to coffee and to caffeine-containing beverages. As a result, she avoided such beverages since childhood. She also benefited from carbohydrates when symptomatic. She had three children, as shown in Figure 59–4A. Her daughter is healthy and her two sons are neurologically impaired and unable to carry on daily living activities independently. The two boys and their mother had hypoglycorrhachia, decreased red blood cell glucose uptake, and a heterozygous Glut1 R126H missense mutation.

The second familial case was reported by Klepper et al.[47] The father had two daughters by separate marriages (see Fig. 59–4B). Each affected family member suffered seizures, mild to moderate mental retardation, hypoglycorrhachia, and decreased red blood cell uptake studies. The two daughters also had ataxia. Their condition was associated with a heterozygous G91D missense mutation in exon 3.

A third family involving a mother and her son has been identified (see Fig. 59–4C).[48] The son suffered apnea, seizures, hypoglycorrhachia, and nystagmus in infancy. Glucose uptake studies were decreased in the red blood cells of both of them and a heterozygous R126C missense mutation was identified by analysis of their genomic DNA.

Other patterns of inheritance also have been identified including paternal mosaicism[49] and compound heterozygosity.[50] In this case, the patient inherited a K256V missense mutation from his asymptomatic mother, and an R126L missense mutation occurred spontaneously in the paternal allele. The R126L and the K256V missense mutations were present in trans, producing the state of compound heterozygosity.

ANIMAL MODELS

Several animal models have been developed to assess the pathophysiology of glucose transporter mutations. Homozygous *GLUT2* gene disruption causes hyperglycemia and hypoinsulinemia in mice. These animals demonstrate an abnormal glucose tolerance and a loss of insulin control by glucose on gene expression.[51] GLUT2 is necessary for maintaining normal glucose homeostasis and normal development and function of the endocrine pancreas. The clinical counterpart for the mouse GLUT2 knockout model is the Fanconi-Bickel syndrome.

A GLUT4 mouse knockout model also has been developed. The female mice exhibit normal blood glucose concentrations, both in the fed and the fasted states, and normal glucose tolerance. The male mice show elevated postprandial blood glucose concentrations compared to control mice. Other glucose transporter isoforms were unchanged in the setting of *GLUT4* haploinsufficiency in this gene-targeted knockout mouse model. The fed blood insulin levels in the male and female mice were elevated 5- to 6-fold, indicating that the *GLUT4* knockout mice were insulin resistant. The male mice with heterozygous GLUT4 knockout genotype resemble humans with non-insulin dependent diabetes mellitus. Both the mutant mice and the humans with non-insulin dependent diabetes mellitus have reduced muscle glucose uptake, hypertension, and histopathologic abnormalities in the heart and liver.[52] GLUT4 knockout mice also had shown reduction in growth rates and shortened life span, possibly resulting from the reported cardiac hypertrophy.

Creation of a GLUT1 mouse model was unsuccessful until relatively recently. Heilig has succeeded in

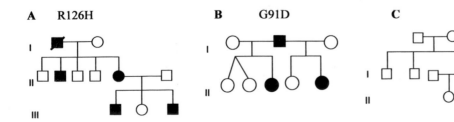

A R126H **B** G91D **C**   FIGURE 59–4. Pedigrees of the three families with Glut1DS.

creating a transgenic antisense mouse model for GLUT1 haploinsufficiency. His studies indicate that the homozygous mutant mice develop a significant embryopathy with various neurologic malformations, including microcephaly, anencephaly, anophthalmia, and caudal regression. These neurologic malformations simulate abnormalities in infants of diabetic mothers. A gene-targeted homologous knockout mouse model currently is being produced in our laboratory and the phenotypic manifestations in the heterozygous and homozygous states have yet to be evaluated (Wang, Pascual, De Vivo, unpublished data). These models, in development, will permit investigators to examine the neurochemical, neuropathologic, and neurobehavioral consequences of GLUT1 loss of function during fetal and postnatal developments.

THERAPY

The ketogenic diet was introduced in 1991 as a possible treatment for Glut1DS before it was confirmed that there was a decrease in glucose transport across tissue barriers.[25] Ketone bodies are transported across tissue barriers by monocarboxylic transporters. As a result, ketone bodies are available as an alternative brain fuel source and can be taken up directly into brain cells. The regional distribution of ketone body utilization in the brain is incompletely understood, and the clinical circumstances suggest that the diet is highly effective in controlling the epileptic complications, but it has no clear benefit on the behavioral disturbances. Additional studies are necessary to answer this question directly. Most patients suffer deceleration of head growth during infancy and 50% develop microcephaly with measurements falling below the third percentile. It remains uncertain what brain elements are primarily at risk. Astroglial proliferation continues postnatally. Other postnatal events include myelinization, dendritic arborization, and synaptogenesis. Any or all of these structural developments could be vulnerable in the postnatal period because of cerebral energy failure, and these vulnerabilities seemingly are only partially protected by the state of chronic ketosis.[53] Transport of glucose across tissue barriers is influenced by other factors. Chronic hyperglycemia causes downregulation of glucose transporters, whereas chronic hypoglycemia or acute hypoxia causes upregulation of Glut1 transporters. Alpha lipoic acid (thioctic acid) has been shown to facilitate glucose transport in cultured skeletal muscle cells that are Glut4 dependent.[54] Similar, although less convincing studies, have been carried out in Glut1 transport systems. We recommend, without convincing clinical evidence, that patients take α-lipoic acid supplements.[55] The patient response has been modest but the dose taken by mouth may be inadequate to approximate the in vitro corrective effects.[56]

Barbiturates are known to inhibit transport of glucose. Most patients with infantile-onset seizures are treated with phenobarbital, the most commonly used anti-epileptic drug. Parents have reported anecdotally that phenobarbital not only fails to improve seizure control, but also may worsen their child's neurobehavioral state. We have shown that in vitro barbiturates aggravate the Glut1 transport defect in erythrocytes from patients with Glut1DS.[57] We have made similar observations with methylxanthines, also known to inhibit transport of glucose by Glut1.[58] One patient, described earlier (see Fig. 59–4A), reported that she was unduly sensitive to coffee and had avoided this beverage since childhood.[45] We therefore advise patients to avoid barbiturates, coffee, and other caffeine-containing beverages.

All infants and young children are placed on a ketogenic diet as soon as Glut1DS is suspected. The more definitive laboratory studies can be carried out after the ketogenic diet is started without obscuring the results. Older children and adults become increasingly noncompliant and some have chosen to resume a regular diet even though their symptoms relapse and seizures recur.

FUTURE RESEARCH

Additional studies will need to focus on several aspects of the clinical syndrome as one attempts to develop more effective treatments for Glut1DS. The phenotypes are broader than originally expected and include examples of developmental encephalopathy with seizures, developmental encephalopathy without seizures, mental retardation with or without intermittent ataxia, and disorders of movement, including choreoathetosis and dystonia. The single most important clinical laboratory observation is a low CSF glucose concentration. This finding, coupled with a low normal or low CSF lactate value in the absence of hypoglycemia, is essentially diagnostic of the condition. Greater use of a lumbar puncture as a diagnostic tool or the development of an alternative diagnostic procedure that provides equivalent information is necessary to identify more patients with nonclassic phenotypes. Also, there is significant phenotypic variability within this patient population and there is no clear correlation between phenotype and genotype. Two gene hot spots have been suggested by studies and correlations of phenotype and genotype at these molecular loci will be informative. The Glut1 transporter is multifunctional and is known to transport other molecules including galactose, dehydroascorbic acid, and water. Whether the multifunctional role of Glut1 contributes to the phenotypic variability remains to be determined.

Alternative dietary regimens also need to be explored, including a high carbohydrate diet fortified with uncooked cornstarch to maintain the blood glucose concentrations in a higher range. Pharmacologic agents also may be helpful in achieving this goal. For example, diazoxide is a known inhibitor of pancreatic beta cell insulin release. Diazoxide opens the sulfonylurea receptor-potassium channel complex, resulting in islet cell hyperpolarization and inhibition of insulin release. Glucagon also raises blood glucose by stimulating gluconeogenesis and glycogenolysis, and by inhibiting glucose uptake by hepatic and muscle tissues. Diazoxide may prove helpful as a daily treatment to raise the interprandial blood glucose concentrations and glucagon may prove helpful in treating acute paroxysmal events.

The availability of mouse models will facilitate studies of neurobehavior, neuropathology, neurochemistry, and neurophysiology.

CONCLUSION

Glut1DS has emerged as the prototype for disorders that affect BBB function. This is the first example of a genetically determined disorder that interferes with the orderly transfer of important brain nutrients across the BBB and into brain cells. This condition is the result of haploinsufficiency and it is transmitted as an autosomal dominant trait. It is one of several examples of genetically determined metabolic diseases that produce familial epilepsy.

Our continuing studies now show that Glut1DS also may cause other neurologic disturbances, including mental retardation and intermittent movement disorders. Seizures, when present, appear in infancy, and we encourage physicians to perform a lumbar puncture as part of the diagnostic assessment. However, it is less likely that physicians will perform a lumbar puncture in patients with mental retardation or movement disorders. As a result, the critical diagnostic observation will be overlooked, namely hypoglycorrhachia and low normal or low CSF lactate concentration.

One of the consequences is misdiagnosing a treatable condition. These patients respond to a ketogenic diet. The diet appears most effective in managing the paroxysmal aspects of the syndrome, including the seizures, intermittent loss of function, and disorders of movement. There is insufficient evidence, thus far, to determine whether early treatment with a ketogenic diet will mitigate the neurobehavioral elements of the syndrome. Intuitively, one would expect that early treatment would be beneficial in these neurologic domains as well.

The condition is evident in the developing brain but the functional consequences appear to develop postnatally. Certain brain regions appear to be more vulnerable than others, typical of most metabolic diseases that affect the developing nervous system. PET scan studies have shown that there is a global reduction in glucose uptake and metabolism, and a rather selective hypometabolism of the thalami. In contrast, there appears to be a relative hypermetabolism of the basal ganglia. The clinical findings parallel these observations to some degree. Patients principally have abnormalities referable to pyramidal, extra-pyramidal, and cerebellar systems with a global disturbance of cognition.

Much work needs to be done to explain the regional insults during early neurologic growth and development, and other studies are necessary to determine whether the patient needs to be treated with a ketogenic diet throughout life or only during the critical period of brain development, when the brain metabolic rate for glucose is at its highest.

Similar studies also need to be developed to investigate other glucose transporters that are expressed in brain tissue. GLUT3 is expressed on neuronal membranes and one can only speculate as to the phenotype associated with mutations in this gene. Similarly, there are now a family of genes dedicated to the transport of monocarboxylic acids (MCTs). Egress of lactic acid from the brain and entry of ketone bodies into the brain are dependent on MCTs. Also, lactate entry into the neuron requires the presence of an MCT on this cell membrane particularly if the Magistretti hypothesis is correct.

The development of animal models with mutations of the GLUT genes and the MCT genes will accelerate our observations and improve our speculations regarding human conditions with expected neurologic phenotypes.

REFERENCES

1. Widdas WF: Inability of diffusion to account for placental glucose transfer in the sheep and consideration of kinetics of a possible carrier transfer. J Physiol 1952;118:23–29.

2. De Vivo DC, Wang D, Pascual JM, Ho YY: Glucose transporter protein deficiency syndromes. Int Rev Neurobiol 2002;51:259–288.

3. Joost HG, Bell GI, Best JD, et al: Nomenclature of the GLUT/SLC2A family of sugar/polyol transport facilitators. Am J Physiol Endocrinol Metab 2002;282:974–976.

4. Hediger MA, Ikeda T, Coady M, et al: Expression of size-selected mRNA encoding the intestinal Na/glucose cotransporter in *Xenopus laevis* oocytes. Proc Natl Acad Sci U S A 1987;84:2634–2637.

5. Wright EM: Renal Na$^{(+)}$-glucose cotransporters. Am J Physiol Renal Physiol 2001;280:F10–F18.

6. Turk E, Zabel B, Mundlos S, et al: Glucose/galactose malabsorption caused by a defect in the Na$^+$/glucose cotransporter. Nature 1991;350: 354–356.

7. Lindquist B, Meeuwisse G: Chronic diarrhoea caused by monosaccharide malabsorption. Acta Paediatr 1962;674–685.

8. Laplane R, Polonovski C, Etienne M, et al: L'inttolerance aux sucres a transfert intestinal actif. Arch Fr Pediatr 1962;895–944.

9. Mueckler M, Caruso C, Baldwin SA, et al: Sequence and structure of a human glucose transporter. Science 1985;229:941–945.

10. Birnbaum MJ, Haspel HC, Rosen OM: Cloning and characterization of a cDNA encoding the rat brain

glucose-transporter protein. Proc Natl Acad Sci U S A 1986;83:5784–5788.

11. Joost HG, Thorens B. The extended GLUT-family of sugar/polyol transport facilitators: Nomenclature, sequence characteristics, and potential function of its novel members (review). Mol Membr Biol 2001;18:247–256.

12. Marger MD, Saier MH Jr: A major superfamily of transmembrane facilitators that catalyse uniport, symport and antiport. Trends Biochem Sci 1993;18:13–20.

13. Saier MH, Jr., Beatty JT, Goffeau A, et al: The major facilitator superfamily. J Mol Microbiol Biotechnol 1999;1:257–279.

14. Sauer N, Stadler R:. A sink specific H+/monosaccharide co-transporter from *Nicotiana tabacum*: Cloning and heterologous expression in baker's yeast. Plant J 1993;4:601–610.

15. Burchell A: A re-evaluation of GLUT 7. Biochem J 1998;331(pt 3):973.

16. Ho Y-Y, Wang D, De Vivo D: Glucose transporters. Wiley Encyclopedia Molecular Med 2001;5: 1441–1446.

17. Mueckler M, Makepeace C: Analysis of transmembrane segment 10 of the Glut1 glucose transporter by cysteine-scanning mutagenesis and substituted cysteine accessibility. J Biol Chem 2002;277: 3498–3503.

18. Cloherty EK, Diamond DL, Heard KS, Carruthers A: Regulation of GLUT1-mediated sugar transport by an antiport/uniport switch mechanism. Biochemistry 1996;35:13231–13239.

19. Cloherty EK, Levine KB, Carruthers A: The red blood cell glucose transporter presents multiple, nucleotide-sensitive sugar exit sites. Biochemistry 2001;40:15549–15561.

20. Iserovich P, Wang D, Ma L, et al: Changes in glucose transport and water permeability resulting from the T310I pathogenic mutation in Glut1 are consistent with two transport channels per monomer. J Biol Chem 2002;277:30991–30997.

21. Fanconi G, Bickel H:. Die chronische Aminoacidurie (Aminosaeurediabetes oder nephrotisch-glukosurisscher Zwergwuchs) bei der Glykogenose und Cystinkrankheit. Helv Paediat Acta 1949; 359–396.

22. Fukumoto H, Seino S, Imura H, et al: Sequence, tissue distribution, and chromosomal localization of mRNA encoding a human glucose transporter-like protein. Proc Natl Acad Sci U S A 1988;85: 5434–5438.

23. Santer R, Schneppenheim R, Dombrowski A, et al: Mutations in GLUT2, the gene for the liver-type glucose transporter, in patients with Fanconi-Bickel syndrome. Nat Genet 1997;17:324–326.

24. Santer R, Groth S, Kinner M, et al: The mutation spectrum of the facilitative glucose transporter gene SLC2A2 (GLUT2) in patients with Fanconi-Bickel syndrome. Hum Genet 2002;110:21–29.

25. De Vivo DC, Trifiletti RR, Jacobson RI, et al: Defective glucose transport across the blood-brain barrier as a cause of persistent hypoglycorrhachia, seizures,

and developmental delay. N Engl J Med 1991;325:703–709.

26. Klepper J, Voit T: Facilitated glucose transporter protein type 1 (GLUT1) deficiency syndrome: Impaired glucose transport into brain—a review. Eur J Pediatr 2002;161:295–304.

27. Kalaria RN, Gravina SA, Schmidley JW, et al: The glucose transporter of the human brain and blood-brain barrier. Ann Neurol 1988;24:757–764.

28. Harik SI, Kalaria RN, Andersson L, et al: Immunocytochemical localization of the erythroid glucose transporter: Abundance in tissues with barrier functions. J Neurosci 1990;10:3862–3872.

29. Seidner G, Alvarez MG, Yeh JI, et al: GLUT-1 deficiency syndrome caused by haploinsufficiency of the blood-brain barrier hexose carrier. Nat Genet 1998;18:188–191.

30. Leary L, Wang D, Nordli D, et al: Seizure characterization and electrographic features in Glut-1 deficiency syndrome. Epilepsia 2002 (in press).

31. von Moers A, Brockmann K, Wang D, et al: EEG features of Glut-1 deficiency syndrome. Epilepsia 2002;43:941–945.

32. Overweg-Plandsoen W, Groener JEM, Brouwer O, et al: GLUT 1 deficiency without epilepsy, an unusual cause for developmental delay. Brain Dev 2002;24 (in press).

33. Friedman JR, Thiele EA, Wang D, et al: Early onset dystonia/choreoathetosis/ataxia secondary to GLUT-1 deficiency, responsible to ketogenic diet. Movement Disorders 2002 (in press).

34. Pascual JM, van Heertum RL, Wang D, et al: Imaging the metabolic footprint of Glut1 deficiency on the brain. Ann Neurol 2002;52:458–464.

35. Klepper J, Garcia-Alvarez M, O'Driscoll KR, et al: Erythrocyte 3-o-methyl-D-glucose uptake assay for diagnosis of glucose-transporter-protein syndrome. J Clin Lab Anal 1999;13:116–121.

36. Stewart WA, Gordon K, Camfield P: Acute pancreatitis causing death in a child on the ketogenic diet. J Child Neurol 2001;16:682.

37. Lund-Andersen H, Kjeldsen CS: Uptake of glucose analogues by rat brain cortex slices: Membrane transport versus metabolism of 2-deoxy-D-glucose. J Neurochem 1977;29:205–211.

38. Owen OE, Morgan AP, Kemp HG, et al: Brain metabolism during fasting. J Clin Invest 1967;46:1589–1595.

39. De Vivo DC: The effects of ketone bodies on glucose utilization. In FA Welsh (ed): Cerebral Metabolism and Neural Function, Baltimore, Williams & Wilkins, 1980, pp 243–254.

40. De Vivo DC, Leary L, Wang D: Glut-1 deficiency syndrome and other glycolytic defects. J Child Neurol 2002 (in press).

41. Magistretti PJ: Cellular bases of functional brain imaging: Insights from neuron glia metabolic coupling. Brain Res 2000;886:108–112.

42. Chih CP, Lipton P, Roberts EL, Jr: Do active cerebral neurons really use lactate rather than glucose? Trends Neurosci 2001;24:573–578.

43. Vannucci SJ, Maher F, Simpson IA: Glucose transporter proteins in brain: Delivery of glucose to neurons and glia. Glia 1997;21:2–21.

44. Brockmann K, Korenke G, Moers A, et al: Epilepsy with seizures after fasting and retardation—The first familial cases of glucose transporter protein (GLUT1) deficiency. Europ J Paed Neurol 1999;3:90–91.

45. Brockmann K, Wang D, Korenke CG, et al: Autosomal dominant glut-1 deficiency syndrome and familial epilepsy. Ann Neurol 2001;50:476–485.

46. Wang D, Brockmann K, Korenke CG, et al: Glut-1 deficiency syndrome (Glut-1DS): Autosomal dominant transmission of the R126H missense mutation. Ann Neurol 2001;50:S125.

47. Klepper J, Willemsen M, Verrips A, et al: Autosomal dominant transmission of GLUT1 deficiency. Hum Mol Genet 2001;10:63–68.

48. Ho Y-Y, Wang D, Hinton V, et al: Glut-1 deficiency syndrome: Autosomal dominant transmission of the R126C missense mutation. Ann Neurol 2001;50: 125.

49. Wang D, Ho YY, Pascual JM, et al: Glut-1 deficiency syndrome (Glut-1 DS): R333W genotype and paternal mosaicism. Ann Neurol 2001;50:124.

50. Wang D, Pascual JM, Ho YY, et al: Glut-1 deficiency syndrome (Glut-1 DS): A severe phenotype associated with compound heterozygosity in *trans*. Ann Neurol 2001;50:S125.

51. Guillam MT, Hummler E, Schaerer E, et al: Early diabetes and abnormal postnatal pancreatic islet development in mice lacking Glut-2. Nat Genet 1997;17: 327–330.

52. Stenbit AE, Tsao TS, Li J, et al: GLUT4 heterozygous knockout mice develop muscle insulin resistance and diabetes. Nat Med 1997;3:1096–1101.

53. De Vivo DC, Garcia-Alvarez, M, Ronen, GM, et al: Glucose transport protein deficiency: An emerging syndrome with therapeutic implications. Int Pediatr 1995;10:51–56.

54. Klip A, Tsakiridis T, Marette A, Ortiz PA: Regulation of expression of glucose transporters by glucose: A review of studies in vivo and in cell cultures. Faseb J 1994;8:43–53.

55. De Vivo DC, Garcia AM, Tristschler HJ: Deficiency of glucose transporter protein type 1: Possible therapeutic role for alpha-lipoic acid (thioctic acid). Diabetes und Stoffwechsel 1996;5:36–40.

56. Kulikova-Schupak R, Ho YY, Kranz-Eble P, et al: Stimulation of GLUT-1 gene transcription by thioctic acid and its potential therapeutic value in Glut-1 deficiency syndrome (GLUT-1DS). J Inherit Metab Dis 2001;S106.

57. Klepper J, Fischbarg J, Vera JC, et al: GLUT1-deficiency: Barbiturates potentiate haploinsufficiency in vitro. Pediatr Res 1999;46:677–683.

58. Ho YY, Yang H, Klepper J, et al: Glucose transporter type 1 deficiency syndrome (Glut1DS): Methylxanthines potentiate GLUT1 haploinsufficiency in vitro. Pediatr Res 2001;50:254–260.

59. Klepper J, Wang D, Fischbarg J, et al: Defective glucose transport across brain tissue barriers: A newly recognized neurological syndrome. Neurochem Res 1999;24:587–594.

60. Wang D, Kranz-Eble P, De Vivo DC: Mutational analysis of GLUT1 (SLC2A1) in Glut-1 deficiency syndrome. Hum Mutat 2000;16:224–231.

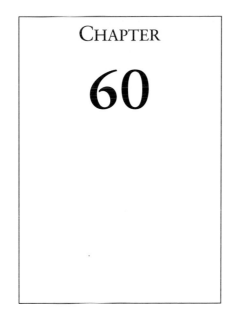

CHAPTER

60

Maple Syrup Urine Disease: Clinical and Biochemical Perspectives

David T. Chuang

Rody P. Cox

Jacinta L. Chuang

The oxidative degradation of branched-chain amino acids (BCAAs) leucine, isoleucine, and valine begins with reversible transamination by coupling with α-ketoglutarate to give rise to the corresponding branched-chain α-ketoacids (BCKAs)—α-ketoisocaproate (KIC), α-keto-β-methylvalrate (KMV) and α-ketoisovalerate (KIV).[1] These ketoacids are translocated into mitochondria where they are irreversibly decarboxylated by a single branched-chain α-ketoacid dehydrogenase (BCKD) complex. The resultant branched-chain acyl-CoAs are further degraded through separate remaining reactions in the BCAA flux. Acetoacetate and succinyl-CoA from leucine and valine, respectively, serve as fuels, whereas acetyl-CoA produced from leucine or isoleucine is a precursor for fatty acids and cholesterol synthesis. The oxidation of BCKAs takes place in liver, kidney, muscle, heart, brain, and adipose tissue.

Maple syrup urine disease (MSUD) or branched-chain ketoaciduria is an autosomal recessive disorder caused by deficiency in the BCKD complex.[2] This mitochondrial enzyme complex is composed of three catalytic and two regulatory components,[3] and its activity is regulated through reversible phosphorylation-dephosphorylation.[4] MSUD is a complex disorder because a mutation in any one component of the BCKD complex may produce the disease. There are currently five distinct clinical phenotypes (classic, intermediate, intermittent, thiamine-responsive, and E3-deficient), based on severity of symptoms, age of onset, and protein component affected.[1]

presentation is the most common (occurring in approximately 75% of patients) and the most severe form of the disease.[1] The first symptoms are difficulty in feeding, with vomiting. The levels of BCAAs are markedly increased in blood, CSF, and urine. In classic MSUD, the bulk of the BCKAs is derived from leucine. The presence of alloisoleucine derived from L-isoleucine is diagnostic for MSUD. Progressive weight loss and neurologic signs of alternating hypertonic and hypotonic posturing occur. Dystonic extension of the arms resembling decerebrate rigidity is often observed. A maple syrup or burnt sugar odor is present in the diapers.[5] Seizures and coma may occur leading to death if not treated. Untreated classic MSUD patients usually die within the first few months of life from metabolic crisis and neurologic deterioration, which are often precipitated by infection or other stresses. Surviving patients, who initiate dietary therapy late by restricting BCAA levels,[6] generally suffer from severe neurologic damage including mental retardation, spasticity, or hypotonia and occasionally cortical blindness. However, there is wide variation in the age of onset and rapidity of neurologic damage even among siblings.[7] Physical examination usually shows a bulging frontal bone, generalized hyperreflexia with spasticity, a Babinski sign, dystonic posturing, and severe psychomotor retardation.[1,5,7] Cranial nerve palsy with bilateral ptosis, ophthalmoplegia, and bilateral facial nerve paralysis has been described in some patients.[8]

CLINICAL PRESENTATION OF CLASSIC MSUD

Children with classic MSUD appear normal at birth, but within 4 to 7 days they develop encephalopathy. This

NEUROPATHOLOGY OF MSUD

Edema of the brain was noted in the initial description of the disease, with the brain weighing 650 g rather than the 410 g expected in a normal infant of similar age.[5] The

635

major findings in the brain of MSUD patients occur in the white matter. There was failure of myelination with no signs of demyelination, glial reaction, or neuronal degeneration.[5] Defective myelination also was accompanied by a striking spongy degeneration of the white matter, with decreased number of oligodendroglial cells. The pyramidal tracts of the spinal cord, the myelin around the dentate nuclei, the corpus callosum, and the cerebral hemispheres are most affected. A moderate degree of astrocytic hypertrophy is present in the white matter of most patients. Impressive alterations are also noted in the cerebellum with necrosis of the granular cell layer, but the molecular and Purkinje cell layers are preserved.[1] In patients treated with restricted diets,[6] the neuropathologic findings are similar but less pronounced. Chemical analysis of the brain shows reduction in the lipid content. Proteolipids and cerebrosides are particularly affected, indicating reduced amounts of myelin.

VARIANT TYPES OF MSUD

Milder forms of MSUD have been reported.[1] An intermittent form of the disease presents with episodic ketoacidosis precipitated by infections or excess protein intake. Between episodes, the subjects are asymptomatic with normal psychomotor development. The BCAA and BCKA levels are also normal between exacerbations but rise dramatically during ketoacidotic episodes. An intermediate form of MSUD was described, in which BCAAs and BCKAs are moderately elevated but there is no obvious ketoacidosis. Mental retardation and psychomotor delay is present. The diagnosis of MSUD in these patients is usually delayed until the first or second year of life. Institution of dietary therapy often results in some improvement. Fibroblasts from patients with the intermittent and intermediate forms of MSUD have residual decarboxylation activity that is greater than 2% and as high as 25% to 40% of normal.[1] The residual decarboxylation activity in cells from variant MSUD patients could not be directly related to the phenotype, although it correlated with tolerance for dietary proteins.[9]

A thiamine-responsive type of MSUD was convincingly documented by Scriver and associates.[10] An 11-month old female infant had excessive BCAAs and BCKAs in the urine and exhibited developmental retardation. The patient was placed on a low protein diet and 10 mg of thiamine hydrochloride per day was administered. The BCAAs in plasma fell within several days. Withdrawal of thiamine resulted in a prompt rise of plasma BCAAs to prethiamine treatment levels. Reinstituting thiamine again resulted in a dramatic response. Thiamine responsiveness has been reported in other MSUD subjects but biochemical improvement required several weeks to months of therapy.[1]

Dihydrolipoyl dehydrogenase (E3) deficiency is a rare disorder.[1] The phenotype is dominated by severe lactic acidosis with relatively modest elevations of BCKAs and BCAAs.[11] Because E3 is a common component of the pyruvate, α-ketoglutarate, and branched-chain α-ketoacid dehydrogenase complexes (see later), its deficiency causes impairment of all three mitochondrial α-ketoacid dehydrogenase complexes. Infants develop persistent lactic acidosis between 8 weeks and 6 months of age. The clinical course is marked by progressive neurologic deterioration that includes movement disorders, hypotonia, and seizures. Death usually ensues within the first year of life. The neuropathology shows demyelination and cavitation primarily in the basal ganglia, thalamus, and brain stem.

GENETICS AND PREVALENCE

MSUD is clearly a mendelian recessive disorder as documented by family studies, and more recently by molecular genetic detection of recessive mutations in families.[1] Prevalence depends on the population studied. In Mennonites, 1 in 176 live births is afflicted with classic type MSUD.[12] A large collaborative study of 2.8 million newborns showed an incidence of MSUD at 1:180,000 live births.[13]

MACROMOLECULAR ORGANIZATION AND COMPONENT REACTIONS

The mammalian BCKD complex is one member of the highly conserved mitochondrial α-ketoacid dehydrogenase complexes, comprising pyruvate dehydrogenase complex (PDC), α-ketoglutarate dehydrogenase complex (α-KGDC), and the BCKD complex, all with similar structures and functions.[3] The mammalian BCKD complex consists of three catalytic components: a heterotetrameric ($\alpha_2\beta_2$) branched-chain α-ketoacid decarboxylase or E1, a homo-24-meric dihydrolipoyl transacylase or E2, and a homodimeric dihydrolipoamide dehydrogenase or E3. The E1 and E2 components are specific for the BCKD complex, whereas the E3 component is common to all three α-ketoacid dehydrogenase complexes.[3] In addition, the mammalian BCKD complex contains two regulatory enzymes: a specific kinase and a specific phosphatase, which regulate activity of the BCKD complex through phosphorylation (inactivation)/dephosphorylation (activation) cycles.[4] The six distinct subunits, whose multiple copies with cofactors and prosthetic groups make up the mammalian BCKD complex, are shown in Table 60–1. The BCKD complex is organized around a cubic E2 core to which 12 copies of E1, 6 copies of E3, and unknown numbers of the kinase and the phosphatase molecules are attached through ionic interactions (Fig. 60–1). The molecular mass of the BCKD multienzyme complex is estimated to be 4×10^6 daltons.

The reaction steps catalyzed by the three enzyme components are also shown in Figure 60–1. The E1 component catalyzes a thiamine pyrophosphate (TPP)-

TABLE 60–1. Component Enzymes and Subunit Composition of the Mammalian Branched-Chain α-Ketoacid Dehydrogenase (BCKD) Complex

Component	Molecular Mass (daltons)	Prosthetic Group (P) and Cofactor (C)
BCKA decarboxylase (E1)	1.7×10^5 ($\alpha_2 \beta_2$)	TPP (C)
α Subunit	46,500	Mg^{2+} (C)
β Subunit	37,200	K^+
Dihydrolipoyl transacylase (E2)	1.1×10^6 (α_{24})	Lipoic acid (P)
subunit	46,518*	
Dihydrolipoyl dehydrogenase (E3)	1.1×10^5 (α_2)	FAD (C)
subunit	55,000	
BCKD kinase	1.8×10^5 (α_4)	Mg^{2+} (C)
subunit	43,000	
BCKD phosphatase	4.6×10^5 (?)	None
subunit	33,000	

*Calculated from the amino acid composition deduced from a bovine E2 cDNA. The E2 subunit migrates anomalously as a 52-kDa species in SDS-PAGE.
BCKA, branched-chain α-ketoacid; TPP, thiamine pyrophosphate.

mediated decarboxylation of the α-ketoacids and the subsequent reduction of the lipoyl moiety, which is covalently bound to E2. The reduced lipoyl moiety and the lipoyl domain serve as a "swinging arm" to transfer the acyl group from E1 to CoA, giving rise to acyl-CoA. The E3-component, with tightly bound flavin adenine dinucleotide (FAD), reoxidizes the dihydrolipoyl residue of E2 with NAD+ as the ultimate electron acceptor. The net or overall reaction is the production of branched-chain acyl-CoA, CO_2, and NADH from the α-ketoacids (reaction 1).

$$R\text{-}CO\text{-}COOH + CoA\text{-}SH + NAD^+ \rightarrow R\text{-}CO\text{-}S\text{-}CoA + CO_2\uparrow + NADH + H^+$$

CRYSTAL STRUCTURE OF THE E1 COMPONENT

The mammalian E1 component contains two α and two β subunits with $M_r = 45,500$ and 37,800, respectively, as deduced from amino acid composition (see Table 60–1). The E1 component has a size of $M_r = 166,600$, and requires K+ ions, $MgCl_2$, and TPP for activity. The crystal structure of the human E1 component has recently been determined at 2.7-Å resolution.[14] The overall $\alpha_2\beta_2$ heterotetrameric structure of human E1 is shown in Figure 60–2A. The tetrahedral arrangement dictates that each subunit is in contact with the other three subunits. Subunits α, α', β, and β' are designated such that the α and the β subunits, when combined, correspond to one polypeptide of the related dimeric yeast transketolase. The assembly of human E1 proceeds through the αβ heterodimeric intermediate, and the assembly of equivalent αβ and α'β' heterodimers produce the native heterotetramer.[15] Prominent features in the structure of human heterotetramer include the crossover of the N-terminal tails of the two α-subunits and the C-terminal extensions of the same subunits that provide interactions with the β subunits. The small C-terminal extension of the α subunit is critical for the $\alpha_2\beta_2$ assembly of human E1 and is the site of the prevalent Mennonite mutation (Y393N-α) (see Fig. 60–2B).

The binding pocket for cofactor TPP is located at the interface between α and β' or α' and β subunits (see Fig. 60–2A). The TPP-binding motif, Gly-Asp-Gly(X)$_{28-30}$NN in the α subunit forms an integral part of the cofactor-binding fold. Residues Glu76-β' and Ser162-α are bound to N1' and the C4' amino group of the aminopyrimidine ring, respectively. These two conserved active-site residues directly participate in the TPP-mediated decarboxylation reaction. The coordination of the Mg^{2+} ion and the interactions of TPP with amino acid residues from α and β subunits are also conserved in TPP-dependent enzymes. It is noteworthy that K+-ion binding sites are found in both α and β subunits. These novel K+ ion coordinations play important roles in stabilizing the TPP-binding fold, as well as maintaining the integrity of the E1 heterotetramer. The two phosphorylation sites Ser292-α and Ser302-α are located close to the active site. The conserved His291-α binds to a phosphate group in cofactor TPP, and may have a direct role in catalysis, as suggested by the *Pseudomonas* E1 structure.[16] The C-terminal end of the β subunit binds to the E2 component, confirming the topology previously deduced from sedimentation studies and dark-field electron microscopy.

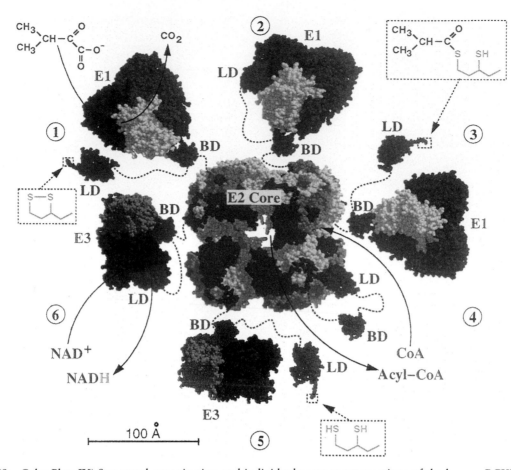

FIGURE 60–1. (See Color Plate IX) Structural organization and individual component reactions of the human BCKD complex. The macromolecular structure (4×10^6 Da in size) is organized about a cubic transacylase (E2) core (based on the structure of *Azotobacter* pyruvate dehydrogenase E2), to which a decarboxylase (E1) (based on the *Pseudomonas* BCKD E1 structure), a dehydrogenase (E3) (according to the structure of *Azotobacter* pyruvate dehydrogenase E3) are attached through ionic interactions. E2 of the BCKD complex contains 24 identical subunits with each polypeptide made up of three folded domains: lipoyl (LD), E1/E3-binding (BD), and the E2 core domains that are linked by flexible regions (represented by *dotted lines*). E1 $\alpha_2\beta_2$ heterotetramers or E3 homodimers are attached to BD. The mammalian BCKD kinase and BCKD phosphatase (not shown) presumably bind to LD. E1 catalyzes the TPP-mediated oxidative decarboxylation of α-ketoacids. The TPP-hydroxyacylidene moiety is transferred to a reduced lipoyl prosthetic group *(in the box)* on LD. The flexible LD carries S-acyldihydrolipoamide to the active site in the E2 core to generate acyl-CoA. The reduced lipoyl moiety on LD is oxidized by E3 on BD with a concomitant reduction of NAD$^+$. (From Ævarsson A, Seger K, Turley S, et al: Crystal structure of 2-oxoisovalerate dehydrogenase and the architecture of 2-oxo acid dehydrogenase multienzyme complexes. Nat Struct Biol 1999;6:785–792.)

STRUCTURAL BASIS FOR MSUD MUTATIONS

There are 19 known MSUD missense mutations that result in amino acid substitutions in the E1α and E1β subunits of the human E1 heterotetramer.[1] Based on the newly determined human E1 structure, these mutations can now be classified into three groups.[14] Group 1 consists of mutations affecting cofactor TPP-binding. The most notable mutation in this group (N222S-α) is involved in coordination to the Mg^{2+} ion. Asn-222 provides a ligand to the metal ion through the side-chain carbonyl group, which cannot be replaced by the hydroxyl group of the Ser side chain. R114W-α and R220W-α are two similar mutations in that each wild-type residue binds to

phosphate oxygen atoms of TPP through ionic interactions. Replacement of either residue with an aromatic Trp residue disrupts the charge interaction required for tight TPP binding. An intriguing mutation is the T166M-α, which is involved in the ligation to K$^+$ in one of the novel metal ion-binding sites. Because K$^+$ binding stabilizes the TPP-binding pocket, a disruption of the metal ion coordination by the T166M-α mutation interferes with cofactor binding.

Group 2 encompasses mutations that impair subunit interactions. The most notable mutations in this group are Y393N-α, F364C-α, and Y368C-α. These wild-type aromatic residues are located in the so-called "Mennonite region" or C-terminal portion of the α subunit (see Fig. 60–2B). The human E1 structure discloses that Tyr-393

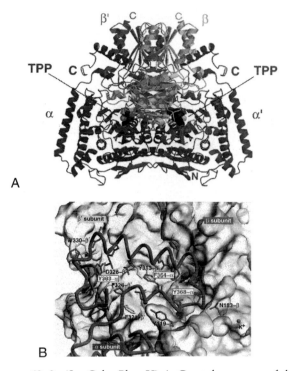

A

B

FIGURE 60–2. (See Color Plate X) *A*, Crystal structure of the human E1 heterotetramer at 2.7-Å resolution. Each of the two identical 400-residue α subunits is composed of a large domain containing mostly α helices. The α subunit also shows an extended *N*-terminal tail and a small helical *C*-terminal domain. Each of the two identical β subunits of 346 residues is divided into two domains of similar size. They correspond to the *N*-terminal and *C*-terminal halves of the polypeptide. Each domain of the β subunit comprises four parallel central β strands with several helices packed in variable orientations against the β strands. Interactions between the equivalent αβ and α′β′ heterodimeric intermediates result in the assembly of the 167-kDa E1 heterotetramer. Each human E1 binds two TPP molecules, two Mg^{2+} and four K^+ ions. *B*, E1α MSUD mutations in the "Mennonite" region impede interactions of the α subunit with the β or β′ subunit. The *C*-terminal domain of E1α subunit shown as a coil backbone is packed against semi-transparent surfaces of the β and β′ subunits. Selected side chains are marked and the three aromatic residues Tyr-393-α, Phe-364-α, and Tyr-368-α that are affected in MSUD are boxed. This segment of the E1α chain is called the "Mennonite" region due to the presence of the prevalent Y393N-α mutation in this population. Tyr-393-α is hydrogen-bonded to Asp-328-β′, in the β′ subunit. Phe-364-α is packed against Tyr-313-β′, also in the β′ subunit. Tyr-368-α is packed against the β subunit at the α/β subunit interface. (From Ævarsson A, Chuang JL, Wynn RM, et al: Crystal structure of human branched-chain α-ketoacid dehydrogenase and molecular basis of multienzyme complex deficiency in maple syrup urine disease. Structure 2000;8:277–291.)

and Phe-364 in the α subunit are hydrogen-bonded to residues in the β′ subunit (see Fig. 60–2*B*). Mutations in these aromatic residues abolish the α | β′ or α′ | β interactions that are necessary for dimerization of the αβ het-

erodimeric intermediates. This defect produces permanently locked inactive heterodimers as shown in an earlier study.[14] The Y368C-α mutation is related to the interactions between α | β and α′ | β′ subunits. The substitution of a Tyr residue with a Cys is likely to impede the formation of the heterodimeric intermediate during E1 assembly. Other mutations in the E1α subunit in this group are A209D-α, A240P-α, G245R-α and R252H-α. The two missense mutations in the β subunit H156R-β and N126Y-β also alter E1 subunit interactions. His156-β is critical for homologous β | β′ interactions. The side chain of His156-β in one β subunit is, like a knob, embedded into a pocket formed by residues from the other β subunit. Substitution of His156-β with an Arg residue disrupts the normal hydrogen bonding between H156-β and residues on the β′ subunit. These adverse effects prevent association between the two β subunits during the $\alpha_2\beta_2$ assembly of human E1.

Group 3 comprises mutations affecting the hydrophobic core of E1. The T265R-α and I281T-α mutations in the E1α subunit are adjacent to each other and are in the hydrophobic core of the human E1. Introduction of a large and charged Arg-side chain in T265R-α or a polar Thr-side chain in I281T-α apparently disrupts the packing of the hydrophobic core, resulting in a dysfunctional E1. Other mutations in this group are G204S-α, A208T-α and M64T-α. The occurrence of missense mutations affecting the hydrophobic core of the E1α subunits raises the possibility for the development of chemical therapeutics to mitigate the MSUD phenotype.

TRIMETHYLAMINE N-OXIDE CORRECTS E1 ASSEMBLY DEFECTS IN VITRO

The naturally occurring osmolyte trimethylamine N-oxide (TMAO) is present in high concentrations in coelacanth (sharks) and marine elasmobranchs (rays). It counteracts the damaging effects of concentrated urea on protein folding and stability in these organisms. The possible effect of TMAO on the activity of MSUD mutant E1 carrying amino acid substitutions in the Mennonite region (see Fig. 60–2*B*) was studied in vitro.[17] Figure 60–3 shows that E1 activity of the three E1α MSUD mutants Y368C-α, F364C-α and Y393N-α is insignificant below 0.4 M TMAO. Rapid rises in residual E1 activity were obtained at 0.5 M or higher TMAO concentrations. The highest degree of activation occurs at 1 M TMAO concentration for all three MSUD mutants, with Y368C-α at 50%, F364C-α at 39%, and Y393N-α at 17% of the wild-type specific activity. At higher than 1 M TMAO concentrations, elevated residual E1 activities decline precipitously. The TMAO-rescued Y368C-α mutant E1 activity is stable, particularly in the presence of cofactor TPP and E2, even after the removal of the osmolyte.

The effect of TMAO on mutant E1 assembly was also investigated. As described above, the Y393N-α Mennonite mutation leads to trapped inactive

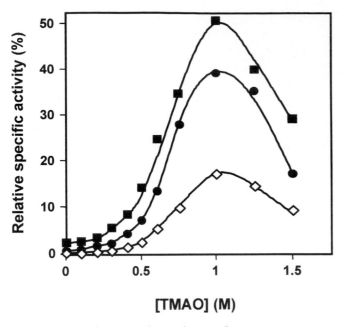

FIGURE 60–3. The optimal stimulation of MSUD mutant E1 occurs at 1 M TMAO concentration. Y368C-α (solid square), F364C-α (solid circle), and Y393N-α (open diamond) mutant E1 at 0.2 mg/ml were incubated with different concentrations of TMAO at 23°C for 16 hours. After centrifugation at 12,000 rpm at 4°C for 10 minutes, aliquots were taken from the supernatant for radiochemical E1 activity assay and protein concentration determination. Specific activity was calculated for each sample and expressed as a percentage of the specific activity of wild-type E1. TMAO, trimethylamine N-oxide. (From Song JL, Chuang DT : Natural osmolyte trimethylamine N-oxide corrects assembly defects of mutant branched-chain α-ketoacid dehydrogenase in maple syrup urine disease. J Biol Chem 2001;276:40241–40246.)

heterodimers, which were separated on a sucrose density gradient. After 16 hours of incubation with 0.75 M TMAO at 23°C, the Y393N-α mutant E1 sedimented as a heterotetramer on the same sucrose density gradient, similar to wild-type E1 without TMAO treatment. Fractions that contained Y393N-α heterodimers before TMAO incubation did not exhibit E1 activity. The conversion of the mutant αβ heterodimers to mutant $\alpha_2\beta_2$ heterotetramers after TMAO treatment coincided with the presence of E1 activity. Similar results were obtained with F364C-α and Y368C-α mutant E1. The data provide direct evidence that TMAO corrects assembly defects in MSUD by promoting the conversion of trapped inactive mutant heterodimers into active heterotetramers. Moreover, during chaperonins GroEL/GroES-mediated refolding, the recovered activity of Y368C mutant E1 is 17-fold higher in the presence of TMAO than in its absence. In contrast, TMAO has no effect on the renatured wild type E1 activity under similar conditions. Delayed addition of TMAO during refolding of Y368C-α mutant E1 does not affect the activation of E1 activity

by the osmolyte. These findings suggest that the TMAO exerts its effects after the mutant E1 is folded and trapped in the heterodimeric conformation. Therefore, chaperonins and TMAO work in tandem to enhance the recovery of enzyme activity during refolding of mutant E1.

The beneficial effects of TMAO on the phenotypes of certain genetic diseases have been demonstrated at the cell culture level. For example, TMAO at 100 mM has been shown to reverse defective trafficking of ΔF508 cystic fibrosis transmembrane conductance regulator in A1-5 cells and enhance antigen presentation in antigen-presenting cells. A serum concentration of 50 mM TMAO with a long half-life of 18 to 21 hours has been achieved in a mouse model. These findings offer an auspicious prospect for the use of "chemical chaperones" such as TMAO as an approach to eradicate human diseases caused by protein misfolding. The results presented in this study demonstrate for the first time that the TMAO is capable of correcting assembly defects associated with MSUD after folding and at the step of the trapped heterodimeric ensemble. Whether these in vitro results have direct application in the treatment of MSUD patients needs to be addressed by cell culture and animal studies.

STRONG CORRELATION BETWEEN THIAMINE-RESPONSIVE MSUD AND E2 MUTATIONS

Since the first description of a thiamine-responsive MSUD patient (WG-34) by Scriver and associates,[10] the biochemical mechanism for this clinical phenotype has been a subject of intense interest. It was speculated that the E1 component was defective as it utilizes TPP, a derivative of thiamine for decarboxylation of BCKAs. Therefore, the first report by Fisher et al, that the E2 component is deficient in Scriver's thiamine-responsive patient (WG-34), was entirely unexpected.[18] This finding was later confirmed by nucleotide sequencing, which showed that the WG-34 thiamine-responsive patient carried F215C and IVSdel[–3.2kd:–14] mutations in the E2 subunit.[19] Another thiamine-responsive patient was later studied by whole-body [1-^{3}C] leucine oxidation while on a BCAA restricted diet; thiamine supplements at 200 mg/d increased her rate of $^{13}CO_2$ release from undetectable to 14.2% of normal levels.[20] This patient is compound-heterozygous for the K278K and the 15- to 20-kb deletion alleles.

Two additional documented thiamine-responsive patients have also been studied.[21] Both patients were found to carry E2 mutations; one is compound-heterozygous for the P73R and G292R substitutions and the other carries an R223G substitution and the IVSdel[–3.2kb:–14] deletion. A survey of the known MSUD mutations shows that 10 of the 27 E2 MSUD alleles, including the aforementioned, are associated with the thiamine-responsive phenotype.[1] These data establish a good correlation between the thiamine-responsive phenotype and the E2 MSUD mutations. Equally important, thus far none of the E1α-deficient MSUD patients have exhibited a thiamine-responsive phenotype. It should also be noted that 10 other E2 mutations are related to the milder intermediate or intermittent phenotype.[1] These patients are not reported to be thiamine-responsive. Nevertheless, the recommendation is that these E2-deficient MSUD patients with milder symptoms should receive thiamine supplements in their diets, which on a long-term basis may prove beneficial. The biochemical mechanism for thiamine response in E2-deficient MSUD patients remains unknown. Because a normal E1 component is present in these patients, TPP may exert its residual effects by augmenting residual E1 activity. The requirement for high doses of thiamine may be explained by a reduced affinity of E1 for TPP in the absence of a normal E2 component. Additional biochemical studies are needed to substantiate or differentiate these possibilities.

STABLE CORRECTION OF MSUD BY RETROVIRAL GENE TRANSFER

As the first step for somatic gene therapy for MSUD, Koyata et al[22] have carried out a retroviral gene transfer of a normal E1α cDNA into cultured lymphoblasts from a Mennonite patient carrying the homozygous Y393N-α mutation. To facilitate gene transfer, a full-length normal E1α cDNA containing the complete mitochondrial targeting sequence was inserted into a replication-incompetent LN vector. The recombinant retroviral vector was packaged in ectropic Gp+E86 cells, followed by replication in amphotropic PA317cells. High titers of the recombinant retroviruses were used to transduce Mennonite MSUD lymphoblasts. Transduced G418-resistant cells showed normal rates of decarboxylation with [1-¹⁴C] KIV as the substrate. The corrected phenotype was stable for up to 14 weeks without the antibiotic selection, which was the duration of the study. Western blotting of the lysates from transduced cells showed that the expression of normal E1α subunits was partially restored, similar to that observed in the transient correction with the EBO vector. Integration of the normal cDNA into the chromosome of the host MSUD cells was established by the restriction fragment patterns in Southern blotting. This study demonstrates the feasibility of correcting assembly-defective E1α mutation by retroviral gene transfer.

Mueller et al[23] described stable correction of E2-deficient MSUD by introduction of a normal E2 cDNA into skin fibroblasts from a patient with MSUD. The retroviral gene transfer was mediated by the MFG vector packaged in CRIP producer cells. Transduction of the E2-deficient MSUD cells with the recombinant viruses restored [1-¹⁴C] leucine decarboxylation to 93% of the normal level. Stable expression of BCKD activity lasted for at least 7 weeks. Immunofluorescent patterns showed that the expressed normal E2 was correctly targeted to mitochondria.

Because MSUD is a hepatic disease and the liver is a non-growing organ, integration of the normal gene into hepatocyte chromosomes may be difficult because retroviral gene integration requires cell replication. However, MSUD has an advantage in that the BCAAs are transaminated in muscle followed by the circulation of BCKAs to the liver for degradation. Retroviral gene transfer into various cell types such as T cells, endothelial cells, myoblasts, or others by the methods established in the above two studies may be effective in ameliorating the disease phenotype.

CONCLUSION

MSUD is arguably an under-appreciated metabolic disorder because of its rare occurrence in the general population. However, the disease has severe neurologic and metabolic consequences caused by the toxicity of the accumulated BCKAs. These manifestations often prove fatal or lead to mental retardation in surviving patients. MSUD is therefore a dreadful disease to individual patients and their families, as well as to certain kindred such as Mennonites, where the incidence of the disease is high as a result of consanguinity. Currently, the only effective, although less than perfect, therapy (other than liver transplantation) is special diets that contain reduced levels of BCAAs.

The six genetic loci associated with MSUD confer the large variations in clinical phenotypes, and complicate the identification and mutational analysis of the affected gene. The mitochondrial BCKD complex, which is deficient in MSUD, has been, and continues to be, a fertile ground for studying how human mutations impede catalysis, assembly, and protein-to-protein interactions of the macromolecular multi-enzyme complex. The strong correlation between E2 mutations and the thiamine-responsive MSUD phenotype suggests a potential role of the vitamin in mitigating mild variants of the disease. The recent determination of three-dimensional structures for components of the human BCKD complex has provided a powerful further impetus to these efforts. The biochemical approach may ultimately prove fruitful in developing more effective therapies for MSUD. The recent use of a natural osmolyte trimethylamine N-oxide to correct, in part, the E1 assembly defect resulting from the prevalent Y393N-α mutation in Mennonite patients constitutes a step in this direction.

Acknowledgments

This work was supported by grants DK-26758 from the National Institutes of Health and I-1286 from the Welch Foundation.

REFERENCES

1. Chuang DT, Shih VE: Maple syrup urine disease (branched-chain ketoaciduria). In Scriver CR, Beaudet AL, Sly WS, et al: The Metabolic and Molecular Basis of Inherited Disease, 8th ed. New York, McGraw-Hill, 2001, pp 1971–2006.

2. Dancis J, Hutzler J, Levitz M: Metabolism of the white blood cells in maple syrup urine disease. Biochim Biophys Acta 1960;43:342–345.

3. Chuang DT, Chuang JL, Wynn RM, Song JL: The branched-chain α-ketoacid dehydrogenase complex, human. In Creighton TE (ed): Encyclopedia of Molecular Medicine, vol 5. John Wiley & Sons, New York, 2001, pp 393–396.

4. Harris RA, Hawes JW, Popov KM, et al: Studies on the regulation of the mitochondrial alpha-ketoacid dehydrogenase complexes and their kinases. Adv Enzyme Regul 1997;37:271–293.

5. Menkes JH, Hurst PL, Craig JM: New syndrome: Progressive familial infantile cerebral dysfunction associated with an unusual urinary substance. Pediatrics 1954;14:462–467.

6. Snyderman SE, Norton PM, Roitman E, Holt LE: Maple syrup urine disease, with particular reference to dietotherapy. Pediatrics 1964;34:454–472.

7. Dancis J, Leviz M, Miller S, Westall RG: Maple syrup urine disease. Br Med J 1959;1:91–93.

8. Chhabria S, Tomasi LG, Wong PWK: Ophthalmoplegia and bulbar palsy in variant forms of MSUD. Ann Neurol 1979;6:71–72.

9. Dancis J, Hutzler J, Snyderman SE, Cox RP: Enzyme activity in classical and variant forms of maple syrup urine disease. Pediatrics 1972;81:312–320.

10. Scriver CR, MacKenzie S, Clow CL, Delvin E: Thiamine responsive maple syrup urine disease. Lancet 1971;1:310–312.

11. Munnich A, Saudubray JM, Taylor J, Charpentier C, et al: Congenital lactic acidosis, alpha-ketoglutaric aciduria and variant form of maple syrup urine disease due to a single enzyme defect: Dihydrolipoyl dehydrogenase deficiency. Acta Paediatr Scand 1982;71: 167–171.

12. Marshall L, DiGeorge A: Maple syrup urine disease in the old order Mennonites. Am J Hum Genet 1981;33:139.

13. Naylor GW, Guthrie R: Newborn screening for maple syrup urine disease (branched-chain ketoaciduria). Pediatrics 1978;61:262–266.

14. Ævarsson A, Chuang JL, Wynn RM, et al: Crystal structure of human branched-chain α-ketoacid dehydrogenase and molecular basis of multienzyme com-plex deficiency in maple syrup urine disease. Structure 2000;8:277–291.

15. Wynn RM, Davie JR, Chuang JL, et al: Impaired assembly of E1 decarboxylase of the branched-chain α-ketoacid dehydrogenase complex in type IA maple syrup urine disease. J Biol Chem 1998;273:13110–13118.

16. Ævarsson A, Seger K, Turley S, et al: Crystal structure of 2-oxoisovalerate dehydrogenase and the architecture of 2-oxo acid dehydrogenase multienzyme complexes. Nat Struct Biol 1999;6:785–792.

17. Song J-L, Chuang DT: Natural osmolyte trimethylamine N-oxide corrects assembly defects of mutant branched-chain α-ketoacid dehydrogenase in maple syrup urine disease. J Biol Chem 2001;276: 40241–40246.

18. Fisher CW, Chuang JL, Griffin TA, et al: Molecular phenotypes in cultured maple syrup urine disease cells. Complete $E_1\alpha$ cDNA sequence and mRNA and subunit contents of the human branched-chain α-keto acid dehydrogenase complex. J Biol Chem 1989;264: 3448–3453.

19. Fisher CW, Lau KS, Fisher CR, et al: A 17-bp insertion and a Phe215Cys missense mutation in the dihydrolipoyl transacylase (E2) mRNA from a thiamine-responsive maple syrup urine disease patient WG-34. Biochem Biophys Res Commun 1991;174:804–809.

20. Ellerine NP, Herring WJ, Elsas LJ, et al: Thiamin-responsive maple syrup urine disease in a patient antigenically missing dihydrolipoamide acyl-transferase. Biochem Med Metab Biol 1993;49:363–374.

21. Chuang JL, Cox RP, Chuang DT: E2 transacy-lase-deficient (type II) maple syrup urine disease. Aberrant splicing of E2 mRNA caused by internal intronic deletions and association with thiamine-responsive phenotype. J Clin Invest 1997;100:736–744.

22. Koyata H, Cox RP, Chuang DT: Stable correction of maple syrup urine disease in cells from a Mennonite patient by retroviral-mediated gene transfer. Biochem J 1993;295:635–639.

23. Mueller GM, McKenzie LR, Homanics GE, et al: Complementation of defective leucine decarboxyla-tion in fibroblasts from a maple syrup urine disease patient by retrovirus-mediated gene transfer. Gene Ther 1995;2:461–468.

CHAPTER 61

Metabolic Disorders— Congenital Disorders of Glycosylation

Marc C. Patterson

The congenital disorders of glycosylation (CDG) are a family of anabolic diseases with variable multisystem manifestations. All result from defective activity of enzymes that participate in the modification of proteins and other macromolecules by the addition and processing of oligosaccharide side chains (glycosylation). Disorders of N-linked and O-linked glycosylation have been described.[1] Strictly speaking, the galactosemias and mucolipidoses II and III fall into this group. They will not be further discussed here because they have traditionally been separately categorized. The catabolism of glycoproteins largely occurs in lysosomes, catalyzed by specific hydrolases. The glycoproteinoses result from deficiencies in these enzymes.

N-glycosylation is localized to the endoplasmic reticulum (ER) and Golgi apparatus in eukaryocytes, and is essential to survival.[2] The process occurs in three distinct phases.[3] In the first phase, oligosaccharides are synthesized in a series of reactions catalyzed by enzymes located on the cytoplasmic surface of the ER membrane. Glucose (Glc), fucose (Fuc), and mannose (Man) derived from the diet are activated through linkage to nucleotide bases, and are then sequentially attached to dolichol pyrophosphate (Dol-PP) anchored in the ER membrane to yield a branched-chain structure containing two N-acetylglucosamine (GlcNAc) molecules and eight mannose molecules ($GlcNAc_2Man_8$). This complex is then *flipped* from the cytoplasmic to the luminal face of the ER membrane, where additional saccharides are added to form $Dol-PP-GlcNAc_2Man_9Glc_3$ (the lipid-linked oligosaccharide [LLO] precursor). The LLO interacts with the oligosaccharyltransferase complex (OST), and attaches to growing polypeptide chains through amide bonds with asparagine (Asn) residues that are associated with serine (Ser) residues in an Asn-X-Ser motif.

In the second phase, the external glucose residues of the oligosaccharide chains are trimmed by alpha-glucosidases to yield a $GlcNAc_2Man_9Glc_1$ side chain that enters the calnexin-calreticulin deglycosylation-reglycosylation cycle. Proteins that are appropriately folded are deglycosylated and are able to proceed along the ER-Golgi pathway. Those that are not folded correctly remain in the cycle until they are either appropriately folded or degraded.

In the third phase of N-glycosylation, the nascent glycoprotein passes from the ER through the Golgi apparatus, where it is exposed to gradually increasing pH and a series of enzymes that first trim the N-glycans to a core of mannose residues and then add more saccharides to produce complex, tissue-specific glycoforms. For any given protein, a family of glycoforms is produced, such that the net function of the protein represents the mean activity of the population of glycoforms.

Observations from animal studies suggest that optimal function is achieved when there is a balance between hypoglycosylation and excessive glycosylation.[4] For example, the (hypoglycosylated) *MGATV* –/– mouse is relatively protected from tumor growth and metastasis,[5] but is more susceptible to autoimmune diseases than controls[6] (discussed later).

Two phases of N-glycosylation may be conceptualized: a tightly controlled early phase (in the ER) leading to the production of a limited number of glycoproteins of high and consistent quality, followed by the Golgi phase, in which modifiable structural and functional diversity is conferred on glycoproteins through tissue-specific processing of glycans.

Clinical Features and Diagnostic Evaluation

The CDG syndromes are summarized in Table 61–1. The current nomenclature recognizes three groups.[7] Group I includes those disorders characterized by impaired syn-thesis of the lipid-linked oligosaccharide and its attachment to the growing polypeptide chain. All members of this group have a type 1 pattern of transferrin glycoforms. Group II includes defects in the processing of N-glycans. Group X was established for those patients with evidence of abnormal glycosylation in whom the underlying enzy-

TABLE 61–1. Congenital Disorders of Glycosylation—Classification

N-*glycosylation*
Group I: *Defects in assembly of* N-*glycans*

Type	Enzyme	Gene	Key features	Less common features
Ia	Phosphomannomutase 2	PMM2	Mental retardation (MR), hypotonia, esotropia, lipodystrophy, cerebellar hypoplasia, strokelike episodes, seizures	Cardiomyopathy, pericardial effusions, coagulopathy
Ib	Phosphomannose isomerase	PMI	Hepatic fibrosis, protein-losing enteropathy, coagulopathy, hypoglycemia	
Ic	α, 1-3 Glucosyltransferase	ALG6	Moderate MR, hypotonia, esotropia, epilepsy	Ataxia, pigmentary retinopathy
Id	α, 1-3 Mannosyltransferase (mannosyltransferase VI)	ALG3	Profound psychomotor delay, optic atrophy, acquired microcephaly, iris colobomas; hypsarrhythmia	
Ie	Dolicholphosphate mannose synthase	DPM1	Severe MR, epilepsy, hypotonia, mild dysmorphism	
If	Mannose-P-dolichol utilization defect 1	MPDU1	Short stature, ichthyosis, psychomotor retardation, pigmentary retinopathy	
Ig	Dolichol-P-mannose: dolichol mannosyltransferase	ALG12	Hypotonia, facial dysmorphism, psychomotor retardation, acquired microcephaly, frequent infections	

Group II: *defects in* N-*glycan processing*

IIa	β, 1-2 N-acetylglucos-aminyltransferase	MGAT2	MR, dysmorphism, stereotypies, seizures	
IIb	α, 1-2 glucosidase	GLS1	Dysmorphism, hypotonia, seizures (death at 2½ months)	
IIc	GDP fucose transporter defect	FUCT1	Recurrent infections, persistent neutrophilia, MR, microcephaly, hypotonia (normal transferrin IEF)	
IId	β-1,4-galactosyltransferase	βGalT1	Hypotonia (myopathy), spontaneous hemorrhage, Dandy-Walker malformation	

Group X: *Unknown genetic basis*

?		?	Includes former type III	Hemolytic anemia, thrombo-cytopenia, Budd-Chiari syndrome, corneal dystrophy

O-*Glycosylation*

	(Xylose β, 1-4) galactosyltransferase I	XGPT	Progeroid Ehlers-Danlos syndrome; macrocephaly, joint hyperextensibility	
	Glucuronyltransferase N-acetyl-D-glucosaminyl-transferase	EXT1 EXT2	Multiple exostoses (diaphyseal, juxtaepiphyseal)	Long bone sarcomas in 3% (associated with loss of heterozygosity)

matic and genetic basis has not yet been determined. This classification superseded previous designations of these disorders as the "diasialotransferrin developmental deficiency" (DDD) syndrome and the "carbohydrate deficient glycoprotein syndrome" (CDGS), reflecting growing appreciation of the biochemical and clinical spectrum of this family of diseases. All of these disorders are autosomal recessive, and, except for CDG-1b (PMI deficiency), all produce primary dysfunction of the nervous system.

The most frequently recognized phenotype is CDG-1a (phosphomannomutase [PMM2] deficiency). The clinical progression of the typical (severe) phenotype has been classified into four phases. The first is the infantile phase, with varying combinations of dysmorphism, abnormal fat distribution (supragluteal and vulval fat pads, focal lipoatrophy), inverted nipples, cryptorchidism, esotropia, recurrent infections, cardiomyopathy or pericardial effusions, coagulopathies, nephrotic syndrome, hypothyroidism, life-threatening episodes of hepatic failure, and unexplained coma. Mortality may be up to 20% in this phase. In the second phase (the remainder of the first decade), children experience seizures and stroke-like episodes, often precipitated by intercurrent infections. The third phase (second decade) is marked by slowly progressive cerebellar ataxia and wasting of the legs, accompanied by progressive visual loss secondary to pigmentary retinopathy. In the fourth phase, the adult phase, the picture is one of moderate mental retardation with severe ataxia and hypogonadism, with or without skeletal deformities. As is the case for most inborn errors of metabolism, the availability and application of biochemical tests has led to the identification of milder and partial phenotypes of CDG. For example, early reports stressed the ubiquity of cerebellar hypoplasia in CDG-Ia. One girl with CDG Ia had normal computed tomography (CT) of the head at 9 months, with progressive atrophy on CT at 2 years, and magnetic resonance imaging (MRI) at 9 years. The authors concluded that the (olivoponto) cerebellar hypoplasia reported in infancy in most children with CDG-Ia likely results from atrophy of antenatal onset,[8] rather than hypoplasia proper.

Phosphomannose isomerase deficiency (CDG-Ib) is the only form of CDG for which effective therapy is available (discussed later). It has no primary neurologic manifestations, the burden of disease falling on the liver, gastrointestinal tract, kidney, and coagulation system. Published cases on CDG-Ib are summarized by Babovic-Vuksanovic and colleagues.[9] Two further cases with essentially similar features have been reported in abstract form.

CDG-Ic results from glucosyltransferase I deficiency. Thirty patients, about half of whose studies are unpublished, have been recognized.[1] CDG-Ic has a milder phenotype than CDG-Ia, characterized by moderate psychomotor retardation, hypotonia, esotropia,

seizures, and ataxia. Abnormalities of glycoproteins are also less consistent and less severe.

A boy with microcephaly, optic atrophy, iris colobomas, epilepsy, spastic quadriparesis, and profound psychomotor delay was initially classified as type IV CDGS. Subsequently, he was found to have deficient mannosyltransferase VI activity, and is now categorized as having CDG-Id.[7,10]

CDG-Ie is a severe phenotype, in which findings include marked psychomotor delay, profound hypotonia, microcephaly, cortical blindness, and intractable seizures associated with elevated creatine kinase (CK), depressed antithrombin III (AT III) and a type 1 pattern of transferrin glycoforms.[11] Some children have dysmorphic features, including down slanting palpebral fissures, flat occiput and nasal bridge, hemangiomas of the occiput and sacrum, a high narrow palate, and mild limb shortening. Dolichol phosphate mannose synthase activity is markedly diminished in all cases.

Three children have been described with severe psychomotor retardation and variable features, including growth retardation, optic atrophy, ichthyosis, dysmorphism (parietal bossing and thin lips), hypo- or hypertonia, enlarged subarachnoid spaces, thrombocytopenia, transient deficiency of growth hormone and insulin-like growth factor I, and mild elevations of creatine kinase (CK). All have mutations in *MPUD1/Lec35*, leading to deficient function of the Lec35 protein (discussed later).[12] Schenk and colleagues hypothesize that Lec35 protein acts as a chaperone for dolichol phosphate in the endoplasmic reticulum (ER) membrane, ensuring appropriate lateral spacing of Dol-P-Man and Dol-P-Glc. In the absence of such spacing, these compounds may form rafts that alter local concentration gradients, impairing synthesis of the LLO and its accessibility to the oligosaccharyltransferase complex.

The index patient with CDG-Ig was born to consanguineous parents, and had congenital hypotonia and facial dysmorphism. Her development was markedly delayed and she had progressive microcephaly, feeding difficulties, and poor growth. She had frequent upper respiratory tract infections that are associated with IgA deficiency. The activity of Dolichol-P-mannose:dolichol mannosyltransferase, was severely deficient.[13]

Three children have been reported with CDG-IIa.[14] They were of Belgian, Iranian, and French descent, and all had severe psychomotor delay, acquired microcephaly and growth retardation, and variable combinations of hypotonia, ventricular septal defects, craniofacial dysmorphism (thin lips, hooked nose, large ears, hypertrophied gums, and short neck), stereotypies, and coagulation defects. All have impaired activity of the Golgi enzyme, N-acetylglucosaminyl transferase II (GlcNAc II, GnT II), and an increase in tri- and mono-sialotransferrin (type II pattern).

The index case of CDG-IIb was a girl born with marked hypotonia and craniofacial dysmorphism (prominent occiput, scalp alopecia, short palpebral fissures, long eyelashes, broad nose, retrognathia, and a high arched palate).[15] She also had generalized edema, thoracic scoliosis, hypoplastic genitalia, and overlapping fingers. Subsequently she developed progressive hepatomegaly, respiratory failure, and seizures. The child died at 74 days of age despite supportive care. Transferrin glycoforms were normal, but urine contained an abnormal tetrasaccharide whose analysis led to the recognition of glucosidase I deficiency.

CDG-IIc was first described as leukocyte adhesion deficiency, type 2 (LAD II). Affected individuals have persistent marked neutrophilia, recurrent nonpurulent skin infections and periodontitis, short stature, microcephaly and delayed psychomotor development.[16] Fucosylation of glycoproteins is impaired by GDP fucose transporter deficiency. This includes sialyl-Lewis X (sLeX), a key ligand for selectins that act as endothelial adhesion molecules. Transferrin glycoforms are normal in this form of CDG.

The first case of CDG-IId[17] was a boy with macrocephaly secondary to a Dandy-Walker malformation with hydrocephalus, transient cholestasis, hypotonia and progressive elevation of CK secondary to myopathy, coagulation abnormalities, and a unique pattern of transferrin glycoforms, with elevation of tri-, di-, mono- and a-sialo transferrin. Analysis of the glycosylation pathway led to the finding of β-1, 4-galactosyltransferase deficiency.

CDG should be considered in any child (or adult) with otherwise unexplained hypotonia, seizures, mental retardation or delayed development, as well as the additional features described earlier. Indeed, any child with unexplained multisystem disease and apparently disparate findings could have CDG. The likelihood of CDG is strongest when the neurologic signs are combined with systemic abnormalities, particularly coagulopathies, hepatocellular dysfunction, gastrointestinal disturbances (protein-losing enteropathy and cyclic vomiting), endocrinopathy (hypogonadism, hyperinsulinemic hypoglycemia, and hypothyroidism), and cardiac disease (hypertrophic cardiomyopathy and pericardial effusion).

Pathology

Biopsy and postmortem studies have been performed in CDG-Ia, and are summarized in a review by Jaeken and coworkers.[18] Findings have included olivopontocerebellar atrophy, with neuronal dropout and gliosis throughout the neuraxis. Dandy-Walker malformations have been reported in both CDG-Ia and CDG-IId.[17] Myelin loss and Schwann cell inclusions have been reported in peripheral nerves. The liver may be enlarged, and shows microvesicular steatosis, fibrosis, and inclusions in hepatocytes. Renal cysts, testicular fibrosis, and aging changes in epidermal collagen have also been observed. Dysostosis and gross skeletal deformities (pectus carinatum and kyphoscoliosis) are found in some cases.

Liver biopsy in CDG-Ib has shown fibrosis in some cases and ductal plate hypoplasia in at least one other case.[9]

Postmortem examination of the child with CDG-IIb found hepatic cholangiofibrosis, macrovesicular steatosis, and enlarged lysosomes. Parenchymal cells contained inclusions with concentric lamellae; similar structures were observed in macrophages. The brain showed increased weight, slightly delayed myelination, and widespread ballooning of neurons that contained empty, membrane-bound vacuoles on electron microscopy.[15]

Biochemical (Enzymatic) Findings

Characterization of transferrin glycoforms is the most widely used screening test for CDG. Group I CDG is associated with shift in transferrin isoforms from a predominance of tetra- and tri-sialo species to variable increases in a-, mono-, and di-sialo-species. The pattern in group II is more variable, with an increase in tri- and monosialotransferrin in CDG-IIa, a unique pattern in CDG-IId (as described earlier), and normal patterns in CDG-IIb and CDG-IIc. False positives occur in genetic variants of transferrin, actively imbibing alcoholics, galactosemia, and hereditary fructose intolerance. False negatives have been observed in preterm babies and some patients with CDG-Ia, whose transferrin IEF was initially abnormal.[19] Intensification of the classic type 1 pattern has been described in CDG-Ia patients treated with mannose.

Assessment of transferrin glycoforms was originally performed using slab gel immunoelectrophoresis, and later by ion-exchange chromatography linked with immunoassay or high performance liquid chromatography. These methods require substantial time (from hours to days), and the exact nature of the glycoforms measured is uncertain. A single-step technique combining online immunoaffinity-postconcentration-mass spectrometry can determine the relative abundance of transferrin isoforms using less than 5 microliters of blood in less than 30 minutes.[20] This technique could be used for large-scale population screening for CDG.

AT III, other coagulation factors, thyroxine-binding globulin, alpha-1-antitrypsin, glycoprotein hormones, and serum lysosomal enzymes may be assayed to complement the screening for transferrin isoforms.

When a patient has a typical phenotype, direct enzyme measurement or genotyping may be considered. In some patients with CDG-Ia, the activity of PMM2 has overlapped with that of heterozygotes, mandating genotyping. Common mutations (R141H, F119L) should be screened for first, followed by a search for other mutations if these are not present, or are present on only one allele. Genomic sequencing may be necessary in some cases, where the pathogenic mutations involve splice site donors (discussed later).

Assays of PMM and PMI activity are readily available in most western countries. Patients with a type I transferrin glycoform pattern should have PMM and PMI activity assayed first. If these are negative, and genotyping is either not indicated or is negative, direct collaboration with a research glycobiologist is necessary.

Molecular-Genetic Data

Molecular and genetic data are summarized in Table 61–2, and current data may be accessed online at http://www.kuleuven.ac.be/med/cdg/. As in many other uncommon recessive disorders, patients with CDG are either homozygous for mutations associated with a founder effect (particularly in geographically or genetically restricted populations), or are compound heterozygotes for private mutations. Genomic sequencing has been necessary in some forms of CDG where the mutations occurred in splicing donor sites (PMI and ALG6).

Most genotyping information is available for CDG-1a. Phosphomannomutase 2 is the 246 amino acid product of the *PMM2* gene, localized to chromosome 16p13. Mutations have been described throughout the gene. The most frequent mutation overall is R141H. In Scandinavian populations, R141H and F119L together account for 72% of cases, and R141H/F119L is the most frequent genotype. Statistical analysis suggests that homozygosity for R141H should be observed with a frequency of 1 in 20,000, but no such cases have been found. R141H recombinant protein lacks useful activity, and Jaeken and Matthijs[1] have concluded that the R141H/R141H genotype is lethal. The same authors have estimated a frequency of CDG-1a as high as 1 in 20,000 based on a frequency of other mutations between 1 in 300 and 1 in 400.

Genotype-phenotype correlation is not always consistent. For example, G691A has been associated with severe manifestations in several cases, but a child who was a compound heterozygote for A647T/G691A had a relatively benign course.[8] The steps in N-glycosylation are tightly interlinked, so that mutations in genes other than that giving rise to the primary syndrome might act as modifiers. Data from one group support this hypothesis. Studies in yeast mutants and humans with CDG-Ia found that the presence of the T911C mutation in one allele *ALG 6* was associated with a more severe phenotype in both cell lines and patients with mutations in both *PMM2* alleles.[21]

Most cases of CDG-1b are associated with missense mutations of the *PMI* gene, involving highly conserved amino acids. Patients homozygous for three of these mutations (M51T, D131N, and R152Q) have been described.

CDG-1c was the first of the congenital disorders of glycosylation in which the human biochemistry was deduced from studies in yeast. The human ortholog of yeast *ALG6* lies in 1p22.3 and contains 14 exons stretching over 55 kb. The most frequent mutations are listed in Table 61–2.

Animal Models

Murine models of MGAT 1, 2, 3, and 5 deficiency have been described.[22] The *MGATI*–/– mouse dies at embryonic day 9.5 with failure of neural tube closure and abnormal vascular development and body symmetry. An *MGATI* –/– chimera has emphasized the role of *MGATI* gene products in the normal embryonic development of epithelial tissues. The *MGATII* –/– mouse is born with multiple anomalies and dies in the neonatal period. Hypoglycosylation reduces the rate of tumor growth by impairing signaling pathways in *MGATIII* –/– and *MGATV*–/– mice.[5] This protection comes at the expense of an increased risk of autoimmune disease in the *MGATV*–/– model.[6] These animals show enhanced T-cell receptor (TCR) clustering, perhaps secondary to reduced spatial separation of TCRs by hypoglycosylated galectins. The functional consequence is activation of cell-mediated immunity by what would otherwise be subthreshold stimuli.

The experience with these models has emphasized the specificity of discrete stages in the pathway of glycosylation commensurate with the variable phenotypes observed in human CDG.

Therapy

Mannose supplementation partially or completely corrects the hypoglycosylation of multiple conjugates in fibroblast cultures from patients with CDG 1a and 1b, where cellular GDP-mannose levels are low, but not in cells from patients with CDG 1e, where GDP mannose levels are normal.[23] Plasma mannose concentrations are lower in CDG 1a patients than in controls, and oral mannose supplementation in healthy volunteers and patients boosts plasma concentrations. Despite these encouraging preliminary data, neither oral nor intravenous mannose supplementation produces clinical or biochemical improvement in patients with CDG1a. In some cases, mannose supplementation has been associated with exaggeration of the abnormal pattern of transferrin glycoforms.

CDG1b (phosphomannose isomerase deficiency) has shown variable response to oral mannose supplementation.[9,24] In some cases, there was virtually complete resolution of clinical manifestations with return of laboratory markers to normal or near normal. Older individuals with irreversible tissue damage are less likely to respond in this fashion.

Oral fucose therapy for CDG-IIc (leukocyte adherence deficiency II) has proved effective in bringing about clinical and laboratory improvement in the single patient treated.[25] The patient's episodes of febrile illness abated, persistent neutrophilia resolved, and psychomotor development improved. In this case, the use of pharmacologic doses of the substrate presumably activated the otherwise minor fucose salvage pathway, allowing sidestepping of

TABLE 61–2. Genotype-Phenotype Data

Type and Gene	Chromosome	Size	Mutations
1a/PMM2	16p13	~8 exons	R141H and F119L: >70% in Scandanavia, >50% overall. R141H homozygous assumed lethal. Most mutations missense
1b/PMI	15	5 kb/8 exons	13 mutations; 11/13 missense M51T, D131N, R152Q homozygotes described. Others: c 166-167ins C, S102L, M138T, I140T, IVS4-1G >C, R219Q, G250S, Y255C, I398T, R418H
1c/ALG6	1p22.3	55 kb/ 14 exons	A333V – four homozygotes, 13/20 alleles; IVS3+5G > A; S170I, G227E, del 1299, F304S (polymorphism), del L444, S478P
1d/ALG3		>5kb/9 exons	G118D; W71R homozygotes
1e/DPM1	20q13	24 kb/–	R92G (homozygous), 331-343 del, 628 del C
1f/MPDU1	–	–	M1T, G73E, L74S, L119P, 511 del C
Ig/ALG12		2.5 kb transcript	T571G (homozygous)
IIa/MGAT2	14q21	1.3 kb/1 exon	Q31X, S290F, H262R (homozygous); D267H, N318D/C339X
IIb/GCS1	2p12-13	2.8 kb/–	R486T/F652L
IIc/FUCT1	–	–	R147T, T308R
IId/BGALT1	9	–	1031–1032 ins C
EDS/XGALT1	–	–	A186D/L206P
MHE/EXT1,2,3	8q23-24	250kb/11 exons	50 mutations in EXT1; >70% cause premature termination of transcript
	11p11-12	100kb/16 exons	25 mutations
	19p		

the genetic defect and adequate fucosylation of glycoconjugates.

There are no data on the role of mannose supplementation in the rare phenotypes of CDG, although the experience with CDG-1a suggests that this is unlikely to be a fruitful approach to therapy.

Conclusion

The CDG are a diverse and growing family of diseases whose study promises to yield insights into many fundamental processes that involve the participation of glycoproteins, including fetal development, regulation of immunity, and tumor genesis. Continued progress in the field is predicated on the education and alertness of clinicians, who must consider CDG in patients with a wide range of presentations, and partnering with glycobiologists to pursue characterization of novel glycosylation defects.

Mannose and fucose therapy are beneficial to a small number of patients at present. Understanding the discrepancy between the in vitro and in vivo effects of mannose in CDG-Ia may lead to better therapy for these patients. It is also likely that knowledge gained from studies of CDG will translate into therapies for other disorders in which glycoproteins play a role, including developmental disorders, cancer, and immune disorders.

REFERENCES

1. Jaeken J, Matthijs G: Congenital disorders of glycosylation. Annu Rev Genomics Hum Genet 2001;2:129–151.

2. Aebi M, Hennet T: Congenital disorders of glycosylation: Genetic model systems lead the way. Trends Cell Biol 2001;11:136–141.

3. Helenius A, Aebi M: Intracellular functions of N-linked glycans. Science 2001;291:2364–2369.

4. Freeze HH, Westphal V: Balancing N-linked glycosylation to avoid disease. Biochimie 2001;83: 791–799.

5. Granovsky M, Fata J, Pawling J, et al: Suppression of tumor growth and metastasis in Mgat5-deficient mice. Nat Med 2000;6:306–312.

6. Demetriou M, Granovsky M, Quaggin S, Dennis JW: Negative regulation of T-cell activation and autoimmunity by Mgat5 N-glycosylation. Nature 2001; 409:733–739.

7. Aebi M, Helenius A, Schenk B, et al: Carbohydrate-deficient glycoprotein syndromes become congenital disorders of glycosylation: An updated nomenclature for CDG. First International Workshop on CDGS. Glycoconj J 1999;16:669–671.

8. Mader I, Dobler-Neumann M, Kuker W, et al: Congenital disorder of glycosylation type Ia: Benign clin-

ical course in a new genetic variant. Childs Nerv Syst 2002;18:77–80.

9. Babovic-Vuksanovic D, Patterson MC, Schwenk WF, et al: Severe hypoglycemia as a presenting symptom of carbohydrate-deficient glycoprotein syndrome. J Pediatr 1999;135:775–781.

10. Korner C, Knauer R, Stephani U, et al: Carbohydrate deficient glycoprotein syndrome type IV: Deficiency of dolichol-P-Man:Man(5)GlcNAc(2)-PP-dolichol mannosyltransferase. Embo J 1999;18:6816–6822.

11. Kim S, Westphal V, Srikrishna G, et al: Dolichol phosphate mannose synthase (DPM1) mutations define congenital disorder of glycosylation Ie (CDG-Ie). J Clin Invest 2000;105:191–198.

12. Schenk B, Imbach T, Frank CG, et al: MPDU1 mutations underlie a novel human congenital disorder of glycosylation, designated type If. J Clin Invest 2001;108:1687–1695.

13. Chantret I, Dupre T, Delenda C, et al: Congenital disorders of glycosylation type Ig as defined by a deficiency in dolichol-P-mannose: Man7GlcNAc2-PP-dolichol mannosyltransferase. J Biol Chem 2002;30:30.

14. Cormier-Daire V, Amiel J, Vuillaumier-Barrot S, et al: Congenital disorders of glycosylation IIa cause growth retardation, mental retardation, and facial dysmorphism. J Med Genet 2000;37:866–884.

15. De Praeter CM, Gerwig GJ, Bause E, et al: A novel disorder caused by defective biosynthesis of N-linked oligosaccharides due to glucosidase I deficiency. Am J Hum Genet 2000;66:1744–1756.

16. Anderson DC, Smith CW: Leukocyte adhesion deficiencies. In Beaudet AL, Valle D, Sly WS (eds): The Metabolic and Molecular Bases of Inherited Disease. New York, McGraw-Hill, 2001, pp 4829–4856.

17. Peters V, Penzien JM, Reiter G, et al: Congenital disorder of glycosylation IId (CDG-IId)—a new entity. Clinical presentation with Dandy-Walker malformation and myopathy. Neuropediatrics 2002;33:27–32.

18. Jacken J, Matthijs G, Carchon H, Van Schaftingen E: Defects of N-glycan synthesis. In Beaudet AL, Sly WS, Valle D (eds): The Molecular and Metabolic Bases of Inherited Disease. New York, McGraw-Hill, 2001, pp 1601–1622.

19. Patterson MC: Screening for "prelysosomal disorders": Carbohydrate-deficient glycoprotein syndromes. J Child Neurol 1999;14:16–22.

20. Bergen HR, Lacey JM, O'Brien JF, Naylor S: Online single-step analysis of blood proteins: The transferrin story. Anal Biochem 2001;296:122–129.

21. Westphal V, Kjaergaard S, Schollen E, et al: A frequent mild mutation in ALG6 may exacerbate the clinical severity of patients with congenital disorder of glycosylation Ia (CDG-Ia) caused by phosphomannomutase deficiency. Hum Mol Genet 2002;11:599–604.

22. Dennis JW, Warren CE, Granovsky M, Demetriou M: Genetic defects in N-glycosylation and cellular diversity in mammals. Curr Opin Struct Biol 2001;11:601–607.

23. Rush JS, Panneerselvam K, Waechter CJ, Freeze HH: Mannose supplementation corrects GDP-mannose deficiency in cultured fibroblasts from some patients with congenital disorders of glycosylation (CDG). Glycobiology 2000;10:829–835.

24. Niehues R, Hasilik M, Alton G, et al: Carbohydrate-deficient glycoprotein syndrome type Ib. Phosphomannose isomerase deficiency and mannose therapy. J Clin Invest 1998;101:1414–1420.

25. Marquardt T, Luhn K, Srikrishna G, et al: Correction of leukocyte adhesion deficiency type II with oral fucose. Blood 1999;94:3976–3985.

CHAPTER

62

Disorders of Glutathione Metabolism

Ellinor Ristoff

Agne Larsson

Glutathione (γ-glutamyl-cysteinyl-glycine, GSH) is found in most living cells in high concentration (up to 10 mM).[1] For instance, the mammalian brain contains 1 to 3 mM GSH in all regions.[2] Glutathione takes part in several fundamental biologic functions, including handling of reactive oxygen species, detoxification of xenobiotics and carcinogens, redox reactions, biosynthesis of DNA and leukotrienes, and neurotransmission or neuromodulation (Fig. 62–1).

Most of the GSH is intracellular and less than 1% is usually present in an oxidized or disulfide form (GSSG). Up to 20% of total GSH is found in the mitochondria, which do not contain the enzymes needed for GSH synthesis. Glutathione, therefore, seems to be imported to the mitochondria from the cytosol. Glutathione has been thought to be a storage form of cysteine because the concentrations of intracellular cysteine are usually one or two orders of magnitude lower than those of GSH.

Hardly any GSH seems to be transported across the blood-brain barrier. All the enzymes of the γ-glutamyl cycle, as well as GSH disulfide reductase, GSH peroxidase, thiol transferases, GSH-S-transferases, superoxide dismutase, and catalase are present in the brain. Astrocytes contain substantially higher levels of GSH than neurons, and it has been suggested that they protect the brain against reactive oxygen species and provide cysteine to restore GSH pools in the neurons. In addition to GSH, ascorbate is an important antioxidant in the brain, and both antioxidants may act synergistically. Astrocytes and the spinal cord contain high-affinity binding sites for GSH and it has been postulated that GSH may be an endogenous agonist of N-methyl-D-aspartate (NMDA) glutamate receptors.[3] Low cellular levels of GSH in neuronal cultures are associated with increased fragility and

susceptibility to toxic agents. A decreased concentration of GSH may also trigger apoptosis.[2]

The turnover of GSH is catalyzed by enzymes of the γ-glutamyl cycle (Fig. 62–2). In this review we concentrate on inborn errors of the γ-glutamyl cycle, with special emphasis on neurologic features, diagnostic evaluation, and molecular genetics. We do not discuss other disorders of GSH metabolism, such as GSH peroxidase deficiency, GSH reductase deficiency, and glucose-6-phosphate dehydrogenase deficiency.

Because GSH participates in so many important functions, it might be expected that humans with severe GSH deficiency would not survive. Nevertheless, patients with mutations in the γ-glutamyl cycle do exist. The γ-glutamyl cycle involves six enzymes (see Fig. 62–2). The biosynthesis of the tripeptide GSH is catalyzed by the consecutive action of γ-glutamylcysteine synthetase and GSH synthetase. Glutathione acts as a feedback inhibitor of γ-glutamylcysteine synthetase. The initial degradative step is catalyzed by γ-glutamyl transpeptidase, which transfers the γ-glutamyl group to an acceptor—for example, an amino acid—to form γ-glutamyl amino acids. The latter dipeptides are substrates of γ-glutamyl cyclotransferase, which catalyzes release of the γ-glutamyl residue as 5-oxoproline (pyroglutamic acid), which is then converted to glutamate by 5-oxoprolinase. In humans, hereditary deficiencies have been described in four of the six enzymes, namely, γ-glutamylcysteine synthetase, GSH synthetase, γ-glutamyl transpeptidase, and 5-oxoprolinase.[1] Mutants are still to be found in γ-glutamyl cyclotransferase and in the dipeptidase. Most of the mutations are leaky, which means that the patients have considerable residual enzyme activity. Knockout mice of γ-glutamylcysteine synthetase and γ-glutamyl transpeptidase[4,5]

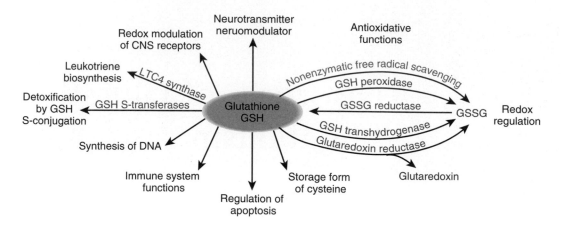

FIGURE 62–1. Examples of postulated biologic functions of glutathione.

are used as a model to study the biologic roles of GSH. Cultured cells from patients with inborn errors in the metabolism of GSH also provide unique experimental models.

For further information about disorders of GSH metabolism and the role of GSH in the nervous system, the reader is referred to other reviews.[1,2]

CLINICAL FEATURES AND DIAGNOSTIC EVALUATION

Patients with genetic defects in the γ-glutamyl cycle are rare. All four verified defects are inherited as autosomal recessive traits.

γ-Glutamylcysteine synthetase deficiency (OMIM 230450) has been described in more than 10 patients from 7 families. All patients had well-compensated hemolytic anemia. Two siblings also had generalized aminoaciduria and developed spinocerebellar degeneration and a neuromuscular disorder with peripheral neuropathy and myopathy in their thirties.[6] One of them became psychotic after being treated with sulfonamide for a urinary tract infection. Another patient, reported to have a learning disability with dyslexia, was regarded as mentally retarded,[7] but physical and neurologic examinations were normal. The diagnosis of γ-glutamylcysteine synthetase is established by finding a low activity of the enzyme together with low levels of γ-glutamylcysteine and GSH. Mutation analysis can be done.

Glutathione synthetase deficiency (OMIM #266130) has been confirmed in more than 60 patients in approximately 50 families. About 25% of all patients with this condition died in childhood—often in the neonatal period—because of acidosis, electrolyte imbalance,

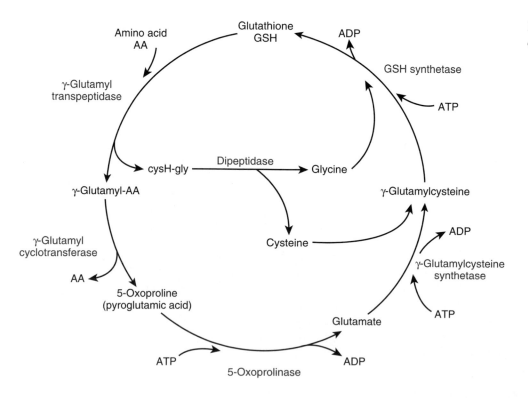

FIGURE 62–2. The γ-glutamyl cycle.

infections, and convulsions. Among the surviving patients, three clinical phenotypes can be distinguished: mild, moderate, or severe.[8] Patients with mild GSH synthetase deficiency have hemolytic anemia as the only clinical symptom. Patients with moderate GSH synthetase deficiency usually present in the neonatal period with metabolic acidosis, 5-oxoprolinuria, and hemolytic anemia. Those with severe GSH synthetase deficiency develop progressive neurologic symptoms (e.g., mental retardation, seizures, spasticity, ataxia), and may suffer from recurrent bacterial infections due to defective granulocyte function. The acidosis in this condition is due to overproduction of 5-oxoproline (pyroglutamic acid) as a consequence of defective feedback regulation of γ-glutamylcysteine synthetase by subnormal levels of GSH. γ-Glutamylcysteine thus accumulates in excessive amounts and is then converted by γ-glutamyl cyclotransferase into 5-oxoproline and cysteine. The excessive formation of 5-oxoproline exceeds the capacity of 5-oxoprolinase and accumulates in body fluids, causing metabolic acidosis and 5-oxoprolinuria. Patients with moderate or severe GSH synthetase deficiency usually excrete gram quantities (up to 30 g/d) of 5-oxoproline in the urine, whereas those with mild GSH synthetase deficiency maintain cellular levels of GSH that are usually sufficient to prevent accumulation of 5-oxoproline.

Eye involvement can occur in patients with the severe form, including retinal pigmentation, crystalline opacity of the lenses, reduced adaptation to darkness, and abnormal electroretinograms.[9] Because the retina is part of the CNS, these changes indicate brain involvement. In these patients, the dipeptide γ-glutamylcysteine is synthesized and may, in part, substitute for GSH.

The diagnosis is based on low activity of GSH synthetase and low levels of GSH, and can be confirmed by mutation analysis. In families with severe GSH synthetase deficiency, prenatal diagnosis has been performed by analysis of enzyme activity in samples of chorionic villi or cultured amniocytes, and by determining 5-oxoproline levels in amniotic fluid. If the mutant alleles in the family have been identified, prenatal diagnosis can also be made by mutation analysis.[1]

γ-Glutamyl transpeptidase deficiency (OMIM 231950) has been reported in five patients in four families.[1] Three of these had involvement of the central nervous system with psychomotor retardation, mental retardation, and absence epilepsy. It is uncertain whether these symptoms are directly related to the enzyme deficiency. All patients had glutathionuria (up to 1 g/d; controls <10 mg/d). The diagnosis is based on finding glutathionuria, elevated levels of GSH in plasma, and decreased activity of γ-glutamyl transpeptidase in nucleated cells, serum/plasma and/or urine (<10%). Patients also have increased urinary levels of γ-glutamylcysteine and cysteine.

In most tissues, including the brain, 5-oxoprolinase is the enzyme in the γ-glutamyl cycle with the lowest cat-alytic capacity. *5-Oxoprolinase deficiency* (OMIM 260005) has been reported in eight patients in six families. 5-Oxoprolinase deficiency is clinically heterogeneous. Patients have a variety of clinical symptoms, including mental retardation, microcephaly, neonatal hypoglycemia, microcytic anemia, renal stone formation, and enterocolitis. All patients with 5-oxoprolinase deficiency have had 5-oxoprolinuria (4 to 10 g/d).[1] The decreased activity of 5-oxoprolinase in nucleated cells reduces the conversion of 5-oxoproline to glutamate. 5-Oxoproline accumulates in body fluids and is excreted in the urine. Because the amounts are less than those found in patients with GSH synthetase deficiency, metabolic acidosis is usually not present. The diagnosis is based on finding 5-oxoprolinuria and low activity of 5-oxoprolinase.

Other causes of 5-oxoprolinuria, apart from GSH synthetase deficiency and 5-oxoprolinase deficiency, should be considered in the diagnostic work-up.[1] These include diet (certain infant formulas and tomato juice); severe burns; Stevens-Johnson syndrome; inborn errors of metabolism outside the γ-glutamyl cycle (e.g., X-linked ornithine transcarbamylase deficiency, urea cycle defects, tyrosinemia, homocystinuria); certain drugs, such as paracetamol, vigabatrin, and antibiotics (flucloxacillin and netilmicin); malnutrition, pregnancy, and prematurity.

PATHOLOGY

Several patients with GSH synthetase deficiency have died, but only a few have been autopsied. Only one of these patients survived the first year of life, and died at age 28 years. An autopsy of the CNS revealed selective atrophy of the granule cell layer of the cerebellum, focal lesions in the frontoparietal cortex, and bilateral lesions in the visual cortex and thalamus.[10] The lesions in the brain resemble those seen after intoxication with mercury—that is, Minamata disease—and it was suggested that treatment of severe GSH synthetase deficiency with antioxidants might be beneficial.[10] Autopsies in other patients with GSH synthetase deficiency, who died in the neonatal period, showed lesions related to intrauterine hypoxia, hemorrhages, infections, generalized cerebral atrophy with asymmetric and partly large gyri, and cerebral necrosis.

BIOCHEMICAL FINDINGS

In the diagnostic work-up, it is important to remember that erythrocytes contain an incomplete γ-glutamyl cycle; they lack both γ-glutamyl transpeptidase and 5-oxoprolinase. Both of these enzymes must be analyzed in nucleated cells, such as leukocytes or cultured fibroblasts. In most tissues, 5-oxoproline is the rate-limiting degradative enzyme.

Patients with *γ-glutamylcysteine synthetase* or *GSH synthetase deficiency* have low activity of the corresponding enzymes in erythrocytes and nucleated cells. The enzymes can be measured as described elsewhere.[1,11] Glutathione synthetase can also be measured in cultured amniocytes or chorionic villi (authors' unpublished results). Patients usually have a residual enzyme activity of 1% to 30% of the normal mean, and heterozygous carriers about 50% of the normal mean. Patients with γ-glutamylcysteine synthetase deficiency have 1% to 20% of the normal mean of GSH and γ-glutamylcysteine in erythrocytes, whereas patients with GSH synthetase deficiency have low levels of GSH in erythrocytes and fibroblasts, and accumulate γ-glutamylcysteine.[12] *Glutathione* can be measured with the 5,5′-dithiobis(2-nitrobenzoic acid) GSH recycling assay,[13] or HPLC.[14] Patients with GSH synthetase deficiency also have 5-oxoprolinuria (up to 1 g/kg/d). *5-Oxoproline* can be determined by gas chromatography-mass spectrometry. 5-Oxoprolinuria is usually detected when a patient suspected of having a metabolic disease is screened for organic acids in the urine. The diagnosis of γ-glutamylcysteine synthetase and GSH synthetase deficiency can be confirmed with mutation analysis.

Patients with *γ-glutamyl transpeptidase deficiency* have low enzyme activity in nucleated cells, serum/plasma and urine (<10% of the normal mean) and high levels of GSH in plasma and urine (the excretion in urine may be as high as 1 g/d; controls <10 mg/d). The cellular levels of GSH are normal. γ-Glutamyl transpeptidase in nucleated cells can be determined with the method described by Wright and colleagues.[15]

Patients with *5-oxoprolinase deficiency* have low activity of 5-oxoprolinase in nucleated cells, elevated levels of 5-oxoproline in body fluids and increased urinary excretion of 5-oxoproline (4 to 10 g/d, controls <50 mg/d). 5-Oxoprolinase in nucleated cells can be measured as described elsewhere.[1]

MOLECULAR-GENETIC DATA

Human *γ-glutamylcysteine synthetase* is a heterodimer consisting of a heavy (catalytic) and a light (regulatory) subunit. The gene for the heavy subunit has been localized to chromosome 6p12 and the gene for the light subunit to chromosome 1p21.[16,17] The heavy subunit (molecular weight 73 kDa) has catalytic activity and is responsible for the feedback inhibition by GSH. The light subunit (molecular weight 28 kDa) is catalytically inactive, but plays an important regulatory role by lowering the K_m of γ-glutamylcysteine synthetase for glutamate and raising the K_i for GSH.[18] Two different mutations in the heavy subunit have been identified in two families with γ-glutamylcysteine synthetase deficiency.[7,11]

Human *GSH synthetase* is a homodimer with a subunit size of 52 kDa. The three dimensional structure of the GSH synthetase enzyme has been determined.[19] The gene has been localized to chromosome 20q11.2, and it consists of 13 exons.[20,21] Because the human genome

appears to contain only one GSH synthetase gene, the various clinical forms of GSH synthetase deficiency must reflect different mutations in this single gene. So far, 21 different mutations have been identified. Most are missense mutations and they are located in all exons except exons 2 and 3. In seven patients, no mutation has yet been found in the coding exons, and it is therefore important to study the introns and the promoter region. No simple correlation has been found between genotype and phenotype. The manifestations of many diseases, previously regarded as monogenic and inherited in a strict mendelian fashion, have now been shown to be modified by several genes and by environmental factors.

The human *γ-glutamyl transpeptidase* gene family is composed of at least seven different gene loci and several of them are located on the long arm of chromosome 22.[1] γ-Glutamyltranspeptidase is a heterodimer with subunits of 21 kDa and 38 kDa that result from the processing of a single precursor polypeptide. The enzyme is membrane-bound with its active site facing the external side of the cell. No mutations have been identified in patients with γ-glutamyl transpeptidase deficiency.

The mammalian *5-oxoprolinase* enzyme has not yet been studied extensively. It seems to be composed of two identical subunits of 140 kDa.

ANIMAL MODELS

A number of experimental methods have been used to study the roles of the individual enzymes in the γ-glutamyl cycle by inducing an experimental deficiency. For this purpose, cultured cells, tissue slices, rodent models, and knockout mice have been used.[1]

A selective inhibitor of *γ-glutamylcysteine synthetase*, L-buthionine-S, R-sulfoximine (BSO), is transported into many tissues, but not across the blood-brain barrier. The levels of GSH decrease in rodent tissues after a few doses of BSO to about 10% to 20% of controls.[1] A knockout mouse for γ-glutamylcysteine synthetase (the heavy subunit) has been made and it shows that homozygous embryos fail to gastrulate and die before day 8.5 of gestation.[4] This mouse model involves complete GSH deficiency and lethality results from apoptotic cell death. However, cell lines from homozygous mutant blastocysts grow indefinitely in GSH-free medium supplemented with N-acetylcysteine. The authors concluded that GSH is essential for mammalian development, but dispensable in cell culture, and the functions of GSH, rather than GSH itself, are essential for cell growth.

No selective inhibitor of mammalian *GSH synthetase* has been identified, and so far no knockout mouse is available.

Several inhibitors of *γ-glutamyl transpeptidase* exist. The administration of such inhibitors to mice causes glutathionuria and glutathionemia. After acivicin treatment, there is an increase of urinary thiols, including GSH, γ-glutamylcysteine, and cysteine. A knockout mouse for γ-glutamyl transpeptidase has been developed: these animals suffer from glutathionuria, postnatal growth failure, lethargy, reduced life span, and infertility.[5]

In mice, the administration of competitive inhibitors of *5-oxoprolinase*, such as L-2-imidazolidone-4-carboxylate or D,L-3-methyl-5-oxoproline, significantly reduces the metabolism of 5-oxoproline and the concentration of 5-oxoproline in the urine.[1]

THERAPY

Patients with γ-glutamylcysteine synthetase and GSH synthetase deficiency should avoid drugs known to precipitate hemolytic crises in patients with glucose-6-phosphate dehydrogenase deficiency, for example, phenobarbital, acetylsalicylic acid, and sulfonamides.

In patients with GSH synthetase deficiency, the most important prognostic parameters for survival and long-term favorable outcome are early diagnosis, correction of acidosis, and early supplementation with vitamins C and E.[8] The acidosis is corrected with bicarbonate, citrate, or tris-hydroxymethyl aminomethane (THAM). The recommended dose of vitamin C (ascorbic acid) is 100 mg/kg/d and of vitamin E (α-tocopherol) 10 mg/kg/d. Because N-acetylcysteine (NAC) protects cells in vitro from oxidative stress, NAC supplementation (15 mg/kg/d) has been suggested for GSH-deficient patients. However, 2002 findings question the treatment with NAC.[22]

No specific treatment has been proposed or tried in patients with 5-oxoprolinase deficiency or γ-glutamyl transpeptidase deficiency.

CONCLUSION

Patients with genetic defects in the metabolism of GSH are rare. The mode of inheritance is autosomal recessive, which means that such patients are often the result of consanguineous marriages and, therefore, may be homozygous for other recessive genes. The phenotype may thus be the result of several genetic defects. Furthermore, patients with various symptoms, such as mental retardation, are more likely to be investigated for metabolic defects. The association between genotype (GSH metabolic defect) and phenotype must therefore be interpreted with caution. Additional studies of more patients with inborn errors in the metabolism of GSH are necessary to clarify the biologic functions of GSH.

Glutathione is involved in several fundamental biologic functions, including free radical scavenging. Living organisms are constantly exposed to toxic compounds, some of which are produced by the organism itself. Oxygen radical stress occurs in all aerobic organisms as a result of aerobic metabolism. It is postulated that some patients with GSH synthetase deficiency develop neurologic symptoms because GSH deficiency causes oxidative damage to DNA and other macromolecules that accumulate in tissues, including the brain, where certain regions may be more vulnerable than others. The brain is particularly sensitive to oxidative injury because of its high energy requirement and high rate of oxygen consumption. The presence of high levels of polyunsaturated fatty acids, the essentially nonregenerative nature of neurons, and the relatively low activities of the enzymatic antioxidants, superoxide dismutase, catalase, and GSH peroxidase in the CNS are additional factors that contribute to vulnerability.

The finding, in one patient with GSH synthetase deficiency, that postmortem lesions were confined to certain regions of the brain supports the hypothesis that GSH is an important scavenger of reactive oxygen species. It is postulated that low levels of GSH trigger apoptosis and the neurologic symptoms in some of the patients may be due to excessive apoptosis. Some data also suggest that GSH is a neuromodulator and neurotransmitter in the CNS, where specific high-affinity binding sites for GSH may exist.[3] Glutathione plays an important role in maintaining the redox balance in the cells. Moreover, human brain tissue can synthesize significant amounts of leukotrienes that, in addition to mediators of inflammation and host defense, may have neuromodulatory functions in the brain.[23] The synthesis of cysteinyl leukotrienes requires GSH and is decreased in patients with GSH deficiency.

Premature infants have less oxidative stress defense than term infants and they are at risk of exposure to high concentrations of oxygen in inhaled air as well as increased oxidative stress as a result of infections and inflammation.[24] Oxidative stress seems to play an important role in the pathogenesis of several conditions in the newborn infant, such as bronchopulmonary dysplasia, retinopathy of prematurity, necrotizing enterocolitis, and periventricular leukomalacia. These conditions are far more common than inborn errors in the metabolism of GSH. It is important to clarify the biologic functions of GSH and the pathophysiologic mechanisms by studying patients with inborn errors of GSH metabolism. This is essential for greater understanding, better genetic counseling of affected families, and more effective treatment to prevent damage of the CNS and other tissues.

Acknowledgments

This study was supported by grants from the Swedish Medical Research Council (4792), Frimurarebarnhuset in Stockholm Foundation, the Swedish Society of Medicine, the Linnéa and Josef Carlsson Foundation, the Ronald McDonald Foundation, and the Sven Jerring Foundation.

REFERENCES

1. Larsson A, Anderson M: Glutathione synthetase deficiency and other disorders of the gamma-glutamyl cycle. In CF Scriver, AL Beaudet, WS Sly, D Valle (eds): The Metabolic and Molecular Bases of Inherited Disease, 8th ed. New York, McGraw Hill, 2001, pp 2205–2216.

2. Shaw C: Glutathione in the Nervous System. Bristol, Taylor & Francis, 1998.

3. Janaky R, Ogita K, Pasqualotto BA, et al: Glutathione and signal transduction in the mammalian CNS. J Neurochem 1999;73:889–902.

4. Shi ZZ, Osei-Frimpong J, Kala G, et al: Glutathione synthesis is essential for mouse development but not for cell growth in culture. Proc Natl Acad Sci U S A 2000;97:5101–5106.

5. Harding CO, Williams P, Wagner E, et al: Mice with genetic gamma-glutamyl transpeptidase deficiency exhibit glutathionuria, severe growth failure, reduced life spans, and infertility. J Biol Chem 1997;272:12560–12567.

6. Richards FD, Cooper MR, Pearce LA, et al: Familial spinocerebellar degeneration, hemolytic anemia, and glutathione deficiency. Arch Intern Med 1974;134:534–537.

7. Beutler E, Gelbart T, Kondo T, Matsunaga AT: The molecular basis of a case of gamma-glutamylcysteine synthetase deficiency. Blood 1999;94: 2890–2894.

8. Ristoff E, Mayatepek E, Larsson A: Long-term clinical outcome in patients with glutathione synthetase deficiency. J Pediatr 2001;139:79–84.

9. Larsson A, Wachtmeister L, von Wendt L, et al: Ophthalmological, psychometric and therapeutic investigation in two sisters with hereditary glutathione synthetase deficiency (5-oxoprolinuria). Neuropediatrics 1985;16:131–136.

10. Skullerud K, Marstein S, Schrader H, et al: The cerebral lesions in a patient with generalized glutathione deficiency and pyroglutamic aciduria (5-oxoprolinuria). Acta Neuropathol 1980;52: 235–238.

11. Ristoff E, Augustson C, Geissler J, et al: A missense mutation in the heavy subunit of gamma-glutamylcysteine synthetase gene causes hemolytic anemia. Blood 2000;95:2193–2196.

12. Larsson A, Mattsson B, Hagenfeldt L, Moldeus P: Glutathione synthetase deficient human fibroblasts in culture. Clin Chim Acta 1983;135:57–64.

13. Anderson ME: Determination of glutathione and glutathione disulfide in biological samples. Methods Enzymol 1985;113:548–555.

14. Luo JL, Hammarqvist F, Andersson K, Wernerman J: Surgical trauma decreases glutathione synthetic capacity in human skeletal muscle tissue. Am J Physiol 1998;275(2 pt 1):E359–E365.

15. Wright EC, Stern J, Ersser R, Patrick AD: Glutathionuria: Gamma-glutamyl transpeptidase deficiency. J Inherit Metab Dis 1980;2:3–7.

16. Sierra-Rivera E, Summar ML, Dasouki M, et al: Assignment of the gene (GLCLC) that encodes the heavy subunit of gamma-glutamylcysteine synthetase to human chromosome 6. Cytogenet Cell Genet 1995;70:278–279.

17. Sierra-Rivera E, Dasouki M, Summar ML, et al: Assignment of the human gene (GLCLR) that encodes the regulatory subunit of gamma-glutamylcysteine synthetase to chromosome 1p21. Cytogenet Cell Genet 1996;72:252–254.

18. Huang CS, Anderson ME, Meister A: Amino acid sequence and function of the light subunit of rat kidney gamma-glutamylcysteine synthetase. J Biol Chem 1993;268:20578–20583.

19. Polekhina G, Board PG, Gali RR: Molecular basis of glutathione synthetase deficiency and a rare gene permutation event. EMBO J 1999;18:3204–3213.

20. Whitbread L, Gali RR, Board PG: The structure of the human glutathione synthetase gene. Chem Biol Interact 1998;111:35–40.

21. Gali RR, Board PG: Sequencing and expression of a cDNA for human glutathione synthetase. Biochem J 1995;310:353–358.

22. Ristoff E, Hebert C, Njalsson R, et al: Glutathione synthetase deficiency. J Inherit Metab Dis 2002 (in press).

23. Mayatepek E: Leukotriene C4 synthesis deficiency: A member of a probably underdiagnosed new group of neurometabolic diseases. Eur J Pediatr 2000;159:811–818.

24. Saugstad OD: Update on oxygen radical disease in neonatology. Curr Opin Obstet Gynecol 2001;13: 147–153.

Purines

William L. Nyhan

Inherited defects of purine and pyrimidine metabolism have been well documented in 11 different syndromes, many of which are associated with neurologic abnormalities.[1] Lesch-Nyhan disease is the most common and best studied disorder in this group.[2–5] It was first described as a syndrome in 1964 in two brothers aged 4 and 8 years, respectively.[6] The defect is a lack of the activity of the enzyme hypoxanthine guanine phosphoribosyltransferase (HPRT) (Fig. 63–1).[7] HPRT catalyzes the reaction in which the purines hypoxanthine and guanine are reutilized to form their respective nucleotides, inosinic acid (IMP) and guanylic acid (GMP). The gene for HPRT is located on the X chromosome, and the disorder occurs almost exclusively in males. Phenotypic heterogeneity in the expression of symptoms is seen and correlates with varying degrees of residual HPRT activity.[8]

CLINICAL FEATURES AND DIAGNOSTIC EVALUATION

Affected infants typically develop normally for the first 4 to 6 months and have no positive findings on the neurologic examination. The first sign of the disease is usually a manifestation of crystalluria, often described as "orange sand" in the diapers. Delayed neurologic development is apparent within the first year, and the affected child does not learn to sit alone or loses this ability if sitting has been achieved. The child never learns to stand unassisted or walk. If securely fastened around the chest, the child is able to sit in a chair. During the first year, extrapyramidal signs develop. Involuntary movements are choreic and athetoid as well as dystonic. Opisthotonic spasms are regularly present. Signs of pyramidal tract involvement develop during the first years of life, and the accompanying spasticity is severe and may lead to dislocation of the hips. Patients have hyperreflexia, and ankle clonus and a positive Babinski response are present in most. Scissoring of the legs is common. Dysarthria and dysphagia are other features of the disease, and the dysarthria can combine with the motor defect to make proper assessment of the patient's mental capabilities difficult. Most patients eat poorly, and most of them vomit. The vomiting becomes incorporated into their abnormal behavior, so at least some of it appears semivoluntary.

Mental development may be retarded; the IQ, as measured, is usually in the range of 40 to 70. However, the behavior and the motor defect make testing difficult. Some patients have had normal cognitive function, and a few have been successful mainstream students. Aggressive, self-injurious behavior is one of the most distinctive features of Lesch-Nyhan disease and in our experience has always been present in patients with the fully developed syndrome. However, there are probably exceptions to every rule. Among 22 patients from Spain,[5] one patient whose relatives displayed the full syndrome including self injurious behavior was observed until age 21 years without displaying this behavior, and another with two typical Lesch-Nyhan uncles had reached 6 years of age without self-injurious behavior. Patients bite their lips and fingers with resulting loss of tissue, sometimes including phalanges of the fingers or the tongue. Patients are not insensitive to pain, and they scream in pain when they bite and are usually relieved when restrained to prevent self-injury. Physical restraint and extraction of teeth are the only effective methods of preventing the behavior. Aggressive behavior is also directed to others; they bite, hit, or kick, and verbal aggression becomes common. The abnormal behavior appears to be compulsive and beyond the control of the patient, who is often remorseful about the behavior.

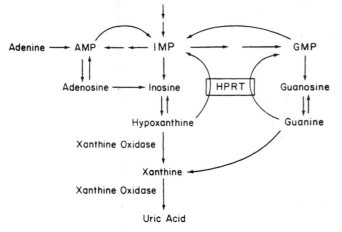

FIGURE 63–1. Reactions catalyzed by HPRT. PRPP = 5-phosphoribosyl-1-pyrophosphate.

Hyperuricemia is characteristic; serum uric acid levels are usually between 5 and 10 mg/dL. The excretion of uric acid is 3 to 4 mg of uric acid per 1 mg creatinine (1.9 +/– 0.9 mmol/mole creatinine). Normal children excrete less than 1 mg uric acid/mg creatinine. A mean of 0.2 mmol/mole creatinine was reported[5] for 20 controls. The consistent finding of this elevated uric acid to creatinine ratio and its relative ease of measurement usually make it a useful initial screening test for the disease,[9] but patients may have normal serum levels if they are efficient excreters and particularly if adult male standards are used for normal values. Urinary data for uric acid can be spuriously low as a result of bacterial contamination. The clinical consequences of hyperuricemia are manifestations shared with gout: arthritis, tophi, painful crystalluria, hematuria, nephrolithiasis, urinary tract infection, and in untreated patients renal failure. Patients have also manifested megaloblastic anemia, in some severe enough to require regular blood transfusions. Macrocytosis or megaloblastic changes in the marrow have also been found in the absence of clinical anemia.

A preliminary diagnosis of classic Lesch-Nyhan syndrome can be made based on the phenotype. A serum concentration in a child of more than 4 to 5 mg uric acid/dL and a urine uric acid to creatinine ratio of 3 to 4 are supportive. However, a definitive diagnosis requires analysis of HPRT enzyme activity, which is most consistently assayed in erythrocyte lysate.

PATHOLOGY

The most significant pathologic feature is the normality of the central nervous system. The accumulation of uric acid in soft tissue tophi yields an amorphous powdery histologic picture. In joints, an inflammatory response surrounds crystallized needles of sodium urate engulfed by leukocytes. In the renal parenchyma, the inflammatory response results in fibrosis and renal failure.

BIOCHEMICAL FINDINGS

HPRT (EC 2.4.2.8.) catalyzes the reaction of hypoxanthine and guanine with PRPP to form their nucleotides (see Fig. 63–1). HPRT is ubiquitously expressed in cells of the human body, with highest levels found in the basal ganglia. The subcellular localization is cytoplasmic. IMP and GMP are produced from the de novo pathway as well as from the HPRT-catalyzed salvage pathway. In HPRT deficiency, the underutilization of hypoxanthine and guanine leads to increased excretion of the degradation product uric acid, and the accompanying underutilization of PRPP gives rise to increased activity in the de novo pathway, increasing uric acid production. Plasma levels of hypoxanthine and xanthine are only slightly elevated because of the efficiency of hepatic xanthine oxidase, but this enzyme is not active in brain and high levels of hypoxanthine are found in the cerebrospinal fluid. The other consequence of increased de novo pathway activity is the elevation in levels of 5-aminoimidazole-4-carboxamide (AICA) and its corresponding ribonucleoside (AICAR).

In Lesch-Nyhan disease, the activity of HPRT in erythrocytes approximates zero. A number of patients have been described in whom HPRT activity is low, but they do not have the full clinical phenotype displayed by the classic Lesch-Nyhan patient. Patients with HPRT deficiency generally belong to one of three groups: those with all features of Lesch-Nyhan disease, those with the neurologic manifestations and hyperuricemia, and those with hyperuricemia only. In some patients with partial HPRT deficiency, the abnormal enzyme is readily distinguished as different from both control and Lesch-Nyhan HPRT activity. However, no consistent correlation between enzyme activity as measured in the red cell lysate and clinical phenotype has emerged. However, a rough inverse correlation between HPRT activity and the severity of the clinical symptoms was found when enzyme activity was measured in intact cultured fibroblasts.[8] Classic Lesch-Nyhan patients exhibited HPRT activities below 1.4% of normal. Patients with neurologic symptoms and hyperuricemia had HPRT activities ranging from 1.6% to 8% of normal. In the hyperuricemic group, the lowest reported activity was 8% of normal and the highest around 60%.

In partial variants with neurologic disease, hyperuricemia is present together with the typical extrapyramidal and pyramidal symptoms found in the classic

Lesch-Nyhan patient. Intelligence is normal or near normal and behavior is normal. The neurologic examination of these patients is indistinguishable from that of the patient with classic Lesch-Nyhan disease.

A distinct clinical phenotype with partial HPRT deficiency (7.5% of normal enzyme activity) has been reported in a family with four affected members. Each member displayed a phenotype of atypical neurologic disease characterized by spasticity, increased deep tendon reflexes, and a positive Babinski response but no dystonia or choreoathetosis; mental retardation was mild.

IMMUNOCHEMICAL FINDINGS

Biochemical analysis of structural variants of the enzyme, purified from cells of HPRT-deficient patients, has been reported in a limited number of cases. Many mutant forms of the enzyme could be biochemically distinguished from the normal enzyme based on altered electrophoretic mobility, thermolability, altered kinetics, or decreased affinity for HPRT antibodies. This was, however, seldom possible for the enzyme of classic Lesch-Nyhan patients. The enzyme is unstable when purified, and antibodies seldom give standard precipitations with antigen.

MOLECULAR AND GENETIC DATA

The gene for HPRT is coded on the X chromosome and mapped to the distal part of the long arm at position Xq2.6-Xq2.7.

The disease is transmitted in an X-linked recessive fashion. It is almost exclusively a disease of the male, but six affected females have been observed.[10] The human gene spans approximately 44 Kb of DNA over nine exons, and the sequence of the entire 57 Kb gene has been determined.[11] The sequences determined for the cDNA matched completely the 218 amino acid sequence that had previously been determined for the enzyme protein.[12] The transcriptional promoter region is like that of other housekeeping genes with many copies of the GGGCGG sequence, but lacking CAAT-like and TATA-like sequences characteristic of most mRNA-coding genes.

In the majority of patients with HPRT deficiency, there is no gross alteration of the gene, and approximately 85% of Lesch-Nyhan patients produce detectable amounts of normal-sized HPRT mRNA in their cells.[13–15] These findings were obtained through studies of a large number of HPRT-deficient individuals, by Southern and Northern analyses, using an HPRT cDNA probe and several different restriction endonucleases. Southern analysis is of limited value in detecting mutant forms of HPRT. As can be expected, major alteration of the HPRT gene usually results in the classic Lesch-Nyhan phenotype. Sometimes a point mutation results in the loss or the gain of a specific endonuclease restriction site and gives a different Southern blot pattern as compared with normal. HPRT Toronto was one of the first HPRT

mutants to be examined in this fashion. Amino acid sequence analysis had revealed a glycine for arginine substitution.[16] The nucleotide substitution in HPRT Toronto could be predicted, and it was shown that this would result in the loss of a Taq I restriction site. This information could then be applied in restriction fragment length polymorphism (RFLP) analysis of DNA from affected and carrier members of this particular family.[17] In most instances of HPRT deficiency, however, RFLP analysis is not informative.

The introduction of the polymerase chain reaction (PCR) and the continued refinement of DNA sequence analysis have revolutionized the field of inherited diseases and the characterization of specific mutations. These approaches have led to the identification of 236 different HPRT mutations.[15] The spectrum is heterogeneous, but most variants represent point mutations. Most families studied have displayed a unique mutation; the same mutation has only rarely been found in unrelated pedigrees. About 85% of patients produce detectable amounts of HPRT mRNA of normal sizes. Classic Lesch-Nyhan patients have had a major mutation often leading to essentially no activity of the enzyme, as well as deletions detectable by Southern analysis. Large alterations include duplications such as one resulting from recombination of Alu sequences in introns 6 and 8.[18] In other Lesch-Nyhan patients, a single gene substitution produced a nonsense mutation that led to a stop mutation and coded for a markedly truncated protein. In some instances a point mutation has led to the removal of a splice site creating an aberrant mRNA and protein. Missense mutations in Lesch-Nyhan patients have generally been nonconservative; for instance, an aspartic acid for a glycine at position 16; a leucine for phenylalanine at position 74; and a tyrosine for an aspartic acid at position 201.[15] A CpG mutational hot spot was identified at arginine 51 of the HPRT protein.[19] This may represent deamination of 5-methylcytosine to thymine. This position has been mutated 11 times among reported patients.[15]

In the neurologic variant group of patients, point mutations have been the rule, and the types of change observed have been relatively conservative. For instance, changing a valine to a glycine[19] would not be expected to make a major difference in protein structure. Others had changes such as an isoleucine to a threonine. In these patients and in the partial or hyperuricemic variants, no deletions, stop codons, or major rearrangements were observed. In HPRT$_{Salamanca}$, there were two mutations: a T-to-G change at position 128 and a G-to-A change at 130.[19] These changes resulted in the substitution of two adjacent amino acids at position 43 and 44: methionine to arginine and aspartic acid to asparagine. These would not appear to be particularly nonconservative, but the phenotype was probably the mildest of the neurologic variants observed. They may have reflected another observation—that the milder mutations have tended to cluster at the amino terminal end of the enzyme. Point mutations in Lesch-Nyhan patients have been more likely sited in areas important to substrate binding and catalytic activity. Patients with the Lesch-Nyhan syndrome often had mutations that altered predicted protein size, while in one series[5] no partial variant had such a mutation changing protein size.

Four female patients with typical Lesch-Nyhan phenotypes including self-injurious behavior have all been the result of nonrandom inactivation of the X-chromosome carrying the normal HPRT gene.[10] In one patient, there was an affected brother and the mother and a sister were carriers of the same C→T transition at position 508 that changed arginine 169 to stop. In the other three patients, the mothers were not carriers, and the mutation in the HPRT gene was a de novo genetic event. In one amino deletion occurred on the maternal X, in the second a nonsense mutation in exon 3, and in the third a point mutation in the paternal X, each followed by nonrandom inactivation of the nonmutant X. A fifth girl represented an X chromosomal translocation. The sixth was one of the identical twins, the twin of the patient being normal; the affected twin was an example of extremely skewed inactivation. The phenotypically normal twin and the mother were extremely skewed in the opposite direction, the normal situation in carriers of mutations that lead to the Lesch-Nyhan disease.

Heterozygote detection is complicated in this disease. Random inactivation of the X chromosome leads to a mosaic pattern of activity of X-linked enzymes in two populations of cells in accordance with the Lyon hypothesis. However, carriers of the gene for the classic Lesch-Nyhan disease always have normal HPRT activity in erythrocytes and leukocytes, probably reflecting selection against the HPRT negative cells very early in embryonic development. The most widely employed enzymatic method of heterozygote detection takes advantage of the fact that hair follicles are largely clonal, containing either HPRT-positive or HPRT-negative cells only. Enzyme assay is carried out on each individual hair root of the sample of sufficient size, usually 30 hairs, to provide statistical reliability.

When mutation has been defined in a family, assay of the DNA for its presence or absence can be done conveniently on peripheral blood. This is facilitated in case of those mutations that interfere with or create a restriction site, permitting the development of a simplified method. Otherwise, oligonucleotides specific for recognizing the mutation can be employed for detection. Heterozygotes are detected by hybridization of the allele-specific oligonucleotide to the DNA. Alternatively, oligonucleotides specific for regions surrounding the known mutation are manufactured and used to PCR-amplify genomic DNA, which is subsequently analyzed for presence of the mutation by nucleotide sequence analysis.[20] Because the spectrum of mutations in HPRT deficiency has turned out to be very heterogeneous, molecular-based diagnosis requires individually tailored analysis in most families.

Prenatal diagnosis can be performed by assay of the enzyme in amniocytes[21] and chorionic villus cells.[22] Amniocytes are assayed either by cell lysis as for the red blood cell or by the intact cell method. A sizable number of affected and nonaffected fetuses have been detected in this way. When analyzing chorionic villus cells, care must be taken to control the activity of 5′-nucleotidase, which is high enough in this tissue to catabolize all the IMP produced by HPRT, thus making normal cells appear to be HPRT deficient.[22] Any molecular method described here for carrier detection can also be used for prenatal diagnosis, if the particular mutation in the family is known. Definition of the mutation in a family makes molecular prenatal diagnosis the method of choice. It can be applied to amniocytes or chorionic villus cells.

ANIMAL MODELS OF HPRT DEFICIENCY

Animal models for self-injurious behavior resembling that seen in the Lesch-Nyhan patient have been created by the administration of high doses of caffeine or theophylline. The underlying mechanism is not clear in either case, but a role for endogenous adenosine has been proposed in view of the pharmacologic actions of caffeine and theophylline as antagonists at the adenosine receptor. High doses of clonidine have been reported to induce self-injurious behavior in mice, and the mechanism might operate through blocking of adenosine receptors. Amphetamine and amphetamine-related drugs, when given repeatedly or in high doses, also induce self-injurious behavior in mice and rats, and this is probably an effect of increased dopamine release. One of the most well-characterized models for self injurious behavior was described in rats treated neonatally with 6-hydroxydopamine (6-OHDA). 6-OHDA administered intracisternally in the neonatal brain leads to destruction of dopaminergic nerve fibers. When these animals later are given dopamine or a D1 agonist, self-injurious behavior is induced. This dopamine triggered behavior is not seen after treatment of adult rats with 6-OHDA. Similar response to dopamine challenge was displayed by monkeys, in which nigrostriatal dopamine neurons were denervated in the neonatal period through surgical lesion of the brain stem. These observations have led to the hypothesis that even late manifesting self-injurious behavior may be the result of neonatal depletion of dopamine.

Self-injurious behavior similar to that exhibited by the Lesch-Nyhan patient can be induced in these different animal models, and the underlying mechanism in some of them appears to be related to abnormalities in the dopaminergic system. However, it is obvious that the basic biochemical defect, that is, HPRT deficiency, is not present. This renders them of little value in studies of the relationship between the absence of HPRT activity and the occurrence of cerebral manifestations of disease.

The first HPRT-deficient animal model was created in the mouse. Similar but slightly different approaches produced an animal model of HPRT deficiency. Embryonic stem cells were used for the selection of HPRT-deficient cells, which either arose spontaneously or were produced by retroviral insertional mutagenesis. HPRT-negative embryonic stem cells were introduced into mouse blastocysts to produce chimeric mice, which were screened for HPRT deficiency. Heterozygous females were then mated to produce HPRT-deficient males.

It has been interesting but somewhat disconcerting to learn that in spite of the total absence of HPRT activity in these animals, they seem to develop normally and do not exhibit any of the neurologic symptoms associated with Lesch-Nyhan disease. Excess uric acid does not accumulate in mice, because unlike humans, mice express the uricase enzyme that metabolizes uric acid to allantoin, which is readily excreted.

However, measurements of dopamine levels in the forebrains of these HPRT-negative mice have yielded values of 20% to 30% depletion compared with normal. A 70% to 90% depletion of dopamine has been found in the basal ganglia of three Lesch-Nyhan patients studied postmortem. It has been speculated that the mouse might be less dependent than humans on the purine salvage pathway for maintaining adequate intracellular levels of purine nucleotides and that this might be particularly true for cells of the basal ganglia. Nevertheless, the mouse model may be useful in the development of therapy for Lesch-Nyhan disease.

THERAPY

The excessive uric acid production in these patients is best treated with daily administration of allopurinol. A dose of 20 mg/kg/day promptly leads to normal plasma concentrations of uric acid and prevention of symptoms related to hyperuricemia. The reduction of uric acid is paralleled by increases in urinary levels of hypoxanthine and xanthine. Because these patients cannot reutilize hypoxanthine, the levels of these oxypurines can become quite high. The solubility of hypoxanthine is much higher than uric acid, so this purine will not cause calculi. On the other hand, xanthine is even less soluble than uric acid, so xanthine calculi can be a problem. For some patients, it becomes necessary to measure the concentration of oxypurines to arrive at the optimal dose of allopurinol. However, the potential complication of xanthine stone formation should not deter treatment with allopurinol. A high fluid intake is recommended. Alkalinization of the urine is not useful.

Allopurinol administration does not affect the neurologic or behavioral manifestations of the disease. Effective management of the self injurious behavior is physical restraint and in some cases extraction of teeth. Numerous trials with different drugs have been tested in the past, and no effective therapy is available for these manifestations.

Allogeneic bone marrow transplant was successfully accomplished in a 22-year-old Lesch-Nyhan patient.[23] Because there is no gross neuropathologic abnormality in Lesch-Nyhan disease, it cannot be ruled out that a circulating toxin causes the central nervous system damage. If so, it may be of benefit to restore HPRT activity in the hematopoietic system. However, in this patient, no improvement of neurologic or behavioral symptoms was observed, although the HPRT activity in the patient's blood was normal. Hyperuricemia was also not improved. It might not be possible, however, to reverse the cerebral symptoms in an adult, and it would be of interest to know how a presymptomatic Lesch-Nyhan patient would respond to bone marrow transplant. However, at least five other bone marrow or cord blood stem cell transplants have been carried out in Lesch-Nyhan patients, and all have died of complications of the procedure. Future attempts at therapy will undoubtedly include gene therapy. In several studies, introduction of retroviral-based vectors containing HPRT cDNA into HPRT-negative cultured cells have resulted in complete or partial correction of the metabolic defect in these cells.[24] Mouse bone marrow cells expressing human HPRT after retroviral transfer were transplanted into murine hosts, and the recipient animals expressed the human protein in spleen and bone marrow for up to 4 months.[25] In one study, HPRT-negative rat fibroblasts that expressed human HPRT after retroviral gene transfer were injected into the brains of adult rats. Human HPRT was detected in the brains of these animals for up to 2 months following the treatment. Because previous studies on bone-marrow transplant and enzyme transfer in Lesch-Nyhan patients have not been successful in improving neurologic symptoms, it may be argued that the HPRT gene has to be targeted to cells in the central nervous system to produce effective gene replacement. To this end, a recombinant herpes simplex type 1 virus vector containing the human HPRT gene was constructed and used to infect mice in vivo by direct intrathecal injection. Human HPRT mRNA was subsequently detected in the brains of these animals, but not in tissues outside the central nervous system. It was not resolved in this study, however, whether the herpes simplex type I virus vector directed synthesis of human HPRT protein in these animals.

CONCLUSION AND FUTURE RESEARCH DIRECTIONS

Lesch-Nyhan disease remains the best model for the effects of mutation in a gene on the biochemistry of the body in the causation of abnormal behavior. Its effects on the neurologic phenotype of these patients are also distinct and provocative. Much progress has been made. The enzymatic defect is known and readily tested for in clinical situations. The gene has been cloned and its chromosomal position identified. An enormous number of mutations have been identified.

This molecular work will continue, and it is likely that further insights into the relations between mutation and enzyme structure and function and between genotype and phenotype will develop.

A major goal for research is understanding the pathogenesis of the neurologic and behavioral features of the disease, and how they result from the enzyme defect. It appears likely that these understandings will lead to treatment. Gene therapy is more problematic. It appears clear that the peripheral correction will not be enough. The enzyme will have to function in the central nervous system. This too is a realizable goal.

REFERENCES

1. Sege-Peterson K, Nyhan WL: Clinical disorders of purine and pyrimidine metabolism. In Berg BO (ed): Principles of Child Neurology. New York, McGraw Hill, 1996, pp 1177–1199.

2. Nyhan WL, Ozand PT: Atlas of Metabolic Diseases. London, Chapman and Hall, 1998, pp 376–388.

3. Christie R, Bay C, Kaufman IA, et al: Lesch-Nyhan disease: Clinical experience with nineteen patients. Dev Med Child Neurol 1982;24:293.

4. Nicklas JA, O'Neill JP, Jinnah HA, et al: Lesch-Nyhan Syndrome. GeneClinics: Available at http://www.genetics.org/profiles/ins/details.html 2000.

5. Puig JG, Torres RJ, Mateos FA, et al: The spectrum of hypoxanthine-guanine phosphoribosyltransferase (HPRT) deficiency. Clinical experience based on 22 patients from 18 Spanish families. Medicine 2001;80:1.

6. Lesch M, Nyhan WL: A familial disorder of uric acid metabolism and central nervous system function. Am J Med 1964;36:561.

7. Seegmiller JE, Rosenbloom FM, Kelley WN: Enzyme defect associated with a sex-linked human neurological disorder and excessive purine synthesis. Science 1967;155:1682.

8. Page T, Bakay B, Nissinen E, Nyhan WL: Hypoxanthine guanine phosphoribosyl transferase variants: Correlation of clinical phenotype with enzyme activity. J Inherit Metab Dis 1981;4:203.

9. Kaufman JM, Greene ML, Seegmiller JE: Urine uric acid to creatinine ratio: Screening test for disorders of purine metabolism. J Pediatr 1968;73:583.

10. De Gregorio L, Nyhan WL, Serafin E, Chamoles NA: An unexpected affected female patient in a classical Lesch-Nyhan family. Mol Genet Metab 2000;69:263.

11. Edwards A, Voss H, Rice P, et al: Automated DNA sequencing of the human HPRT locus. Genomics 1990;6:593.

12. Wilson JM, Tarr GE, Mahoney WC, Kelley WN: Human hypoxanthine-guanine phosphoribosyl-transferase. Complete amino acid sequence of the erythrocytes enzyme. J Biol Chem 1982;257:10978.

13. Yang TP, Patel PI, Chinault AC, et al: Molecular evidence for new mutation at the HPRT locus in Lesch-Nyhan patients. Nature 1984;310:412.

14. Gordon RB, Emmerson BI, Stout JT, Caskey CT: Molecular studies of hypoxanthine-guanine phosphoribosyltransferase mutations in six Australian families. Aust N Z J Med 1987;17:424.

15. Jinnah HA, De Gregorio L, Harris JC, et al: The spectrum of inherited mutations causing HPRT deficiency: 75 new cases and a review of 196 previously reported cases. Mutat Res 2000;463:309.

16. Wilson JM, Kelley WN: Molecular basis of hypoxanthineguanine phosphoribosyltransferase deficiency in a patient with the Lesch-Nyhan syndrome. J Clin Invest 1983;71:1331.

17. Wilson JM, Frossard P, Nussbaum RL, et al: Hyman hypoxanthine phospho-ribosyltransferase: Detection of a mutant allele by restriction endonuclease analysis. J Clin Invest 1983;72:767.

18. Marcus S, Steen AM, Andersson B, et al: Mutation analysis and prenatal diagnosis in a Lesch-Nyhan family showing non-random X-inactivation interfering with carrier detection tests. Hum Genet 1992;89:395.

19. Sege-Peterson K, Chambers J, Page T, et al: Characterization of mutations in phenotypic variants of hypoxanthine phosphoribosyltransferase deficiency. Hum Mol Genet 1992;1:427.

20. Gibbs RA, Nguyen P, Edwards A, et al: Multiplex DNA deletion detection and exon sequencing of the hypoxanthine phosphoribosyltransferase gene in Lesch-Nyhan families. Genomics 1990;7:235.

21. Gibbs DA, McFadyen IR, Crawford MA, et al: First trimester prenatal diagnosis of Lesch-Nyhan syndrome. Lancet 1984;2:1180.

22. Page T, Broock RL: A pitfall in the prenatal diagnosis of Lesch-Nyhan syndrome by chorionic villus sampling. Prenat Diagn 1990;10:153.

23. Nyhan WL, Page T, Gruber HE, Parkman R: Bone marrow transplantation in Lesch-Nyhan disease. Birth Defects Original Articles Series 1986;22:113.

24. Willis R, Jolly DJ, Miller AD, et al: Partial phenotypic correction of human Lesch-Nyhan (hypoxanthine-guanine phosphoribosyltransferase deficient) lymphoblasts with a transmissible retroviral vector. J Biol Chem 1984;259:7842.

25. Miller AD, Eckner RJ, Jolly DJ, et al: Expression of a retrovirus encoding human HPRT in mice. Science 1984;23:795.

CHAPTER

64

The Porphyrias

D. Montgomery Bissell

The acute hepatic porphyrias compose a group of genetically and biochemically distinct diseases, all with a neuropsychiatric presentation consisting of mental changes, neurovisceral pain, and generalized seizures. The challenge to the neurologist is to recognize the condition before instituting therapy with drugs such as anticonvulsants, which can intensify or prolong the attack. Although the clinical presentation can be highly suggestive of porphyria, none of the symptoms is unique to these diseases. Therefore, a high index of suspicion generally is required. Quantitative analysis of porphyrins and porphyrin precursors in urine and feces provides a definitive diagnosis. Therapy centers on the administration of heme (as hematin or heme arginate), which compensates for the principal metabolic deficiency of these diseases. Prevention involves screening of potential genetic carriers and education as to the conditions that increase the risk of an acute attack. Animal studies and limited human data suggest that genetic carriers can experience progressive, albeit subclinical, neurologic damage in the absence of acute symptoms. In general, however, when properly managed, porphyria is not a cause of long-term disability.

HEME AND PORPHYRIN METABOLISM

The porphyrias represent a group of disturbances in which intermediates or by-products in the pathway of heme synthesis are produced in excess. Early clinical observations established the existence of more than one type of porphyria, the most prominent of which were recognized as hereditary.[1,2] With elucidation of the pathway of heme synthesis, the biochemical relationship of these diseases to one another was defined. Moreover, the pat-

tern of overproduction associated with an individual type pointed to a block at a specific step in the pathway of heme synthesis. In the 1960s and 1970s, assays of the enzymes of the pathway were developed, confirming that each type of porphyria represented an inherited deficiency of one of these proteins. The genes encoding these enzymes have all been cloned and analyzed for mutations.

PATHWAY OF HEME SYNTHESIS

The building blocks of heme are succinyl CoA and glycine, which combine to form δ-aminolevulinic acid (ALA), the first committed intermediate of the pathway. In subsequent reactions, two molecules of ALA combine to form porphobilinogen (PBG), the pyrrole subunit of the heme ring. Four PBGs are linked, yielding an intermediate linear tetrapyrrole, hydroxymethylbilane, which is cyclized to the initial porphyrin of the pathway, uroporphyrinogen-I. Because PBG is asymmetric, having one acetyl and one propionyl substituent, four porphyrin isomers are theoretically possible: a regular head-to-tail linkage of the four PBG units (type I), reversal of two adjacent units (type II), reversal of one unit (type III), and reversal of two opposite units (type IV). The only isomers found in nature are types I and III, with type III representing the physiologic intermediate in heme synthesis (Fig. 64–1). The conversion of uroporphyrinogen to coproporphyrinogen and protoporphyrinogen involves decarboxylation of the side-chains, with conversion of acetyl substituents to methyl groups and (in protoporphyrinogen) two of the propionyls to vinyls (see Fig. 64–1). Decarboxylation produces intermediates of progressively decreasing water solubility,

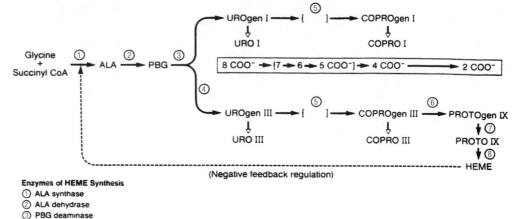

FIGURE 64–1. The pathway of heme synthesis. Between two arms of the pathway that depict the isomer I and isomer III porphyrin, the number of carboxyl substituents for each porphyrin is shown *(box)*. ALA, δ-aminolevulinic acid; COPRO, coproporphyrin; PBG, porphobilinogen; PROTO, protoporphyrin; URO, uroporphyrin.

which is reflected in the excretory route of these compounds in vivo: ALA, PBG, and uroporphyrin appear in urine, coproporphyrin in both urine and feces, and protoporphyrin only in feces.

    The true porphyrin intermediates in heme synthesis are the porphyrinogens together with protoporphyrin. The conversion of uroporphyrinogen and coproporphyrinogen to the corresponding porphyrins represents an irreversible oxidation. Uroporphyrin and coproporphyrin have no biologic role and are destined for excretion. Normally, they represent a minute fraction of the total flow of intermediates through the pathway.

REGULATION OF HEME AND PORPHYRIN SYNTHESIS

The pattern of heme precursors in urine or feces for each of the porphyrias is shown in Figure 64–1. Each porphyria can be viewed as resulting from a partial block to the flow of precursors along the pathway, with excess excretion of the intermediates that precede the enzyme deficiency. The pathway as a whole is regulated by its end product, heme. ALA synthase, the enzyme mediating the initial step of the pathway (see Fig. 64–1), governs the flow of precursors into the pathway, and its activity is subject to feedback inhibition by heme. With induction of heme-requiring proteins (such as hepatic cytochrome P-450 after the administration of barbiturates), heme use is increased. This lifts the feedback inhibition of ALA synthase, allowing increased flow of precursors along the pathway. If the pathway is compromised by a defective enzyme (as in the hereditary porphyrias), a prolonged, exaggerated increase in ALA synthase results, with marked overproduction of intermediates prior to the block, which gives rise to the excretion patterns shown in Figure 64–1.

PORPHYRIA: CLINICAL ASPECTS

Classification of Porphyrias

The porphyrias are grouped according to their predominant manifestation (neurologic or cutaneous) and the tissue in which porphyrin overproduction is most evident (liver or bone marrow) (Table 64–1).[1,2] Liver and bone marrow are sites of relatively high production of heme for synthesis of microsomal cytochromes and hemoglobin. Given this, it is unclear why some porphyrias are expressed predominantly in liver and others largely or exclusively in bone marrow. Another question concerns the relationship between the manifestations of porphyria and overproduction of heme precursors. Cutaneous disease in porphyria correlates with overproduction of porphyrins, which is expected because porphyrins are photosensitizers. However, the same correlation does not exist between neurologic symptoms and levels of heme precursors (ALA, PBG, or both) for the acute porphyrias. Although all the acute (neurologic) porphyrias involve a major disturbance in hepatic heme synthesis, alterations in nonhepatic cells may underlie some disease manifestations. Heme synthesis presumably occurs in all nucleated cells because it is required for the production of heme proteins (e.g., mitochondrial cytochromes); thus, cellular heme deficiency rather than overproduction of pathway intermediates may be the underlying metabolic lesion, as discussed in the Pathogenesis of Neurologic Symptoms section.

Clinical Manifestations

Descriptions of the clinical presentation of the various porphyrias are available in reviews.[1,2] This chapter focuses on neurologic manifestations of the acute attack porphyrias, a group comprising acute intermittent por-

TABLE 64–1. Classification of Hereditary Porphyrias

	*Acute (Neurologic)**	*Cutaneous**
Hepatic		
Acute intermittent	+++	0
Coproporphyria	++	+
Variegate	++	++
Cutanea tarda	0	++
ALA uria*	+	0
Erythropoietic		
Congenital (Gunther's)	0	+++
Protoporphyria	0	++

*0, symptom complex absent; +, mild when symptomatic; ++, moderate when symptomatic; +++, severe when symptomatic; ALA, δ-aminolevulinic acid

phyria, hereditary coproporphyria, variegate porphyria, and (most likely) δ-aminolevulinic aciduria. Although these types are genetically and biochemically distinct, their presentation as acute diseases is essentially identical. Patients typically seek medical attention for abdominal or back pain, which is aching more often than colicky but can suggest inflammation of a hollow viscus. An important differentiating point in porphyric pain is the lack of fever, leukocytosis, or rebound tenderness. Constipation is often present. It may be chronic, worsening at the time of an attack. Characteristically, abdominal x-ray discloses a gas pattern pointing to ileus rather than mechanical obstruction.

Psychosis or seizures can be part of the initial presentation of a porphyric attack. If present, a history of abdominal pain, nausea, or vomiting during the preceding days suggests porphyria rather than a primary neuropsychiatric disorder. Mental abnormalities accompany acute attacks in 50% to 75% of cases and range from depression to delusions; frank psychosis is unusual.[3] King George III of the English House of Stuart suffered from a psychosis that has been attributed to porphyria. If he had porphyria, which is doubtful,[4,5] it was atypical. Most commonly, patients are judged "hysterical" or drug seeking, because their need for pain relief is not supported by the physical findings. So striking is this aspect of the acute illness that some patients unfortunately have progressed to flaccid paralysis or commitment for psychiatric care without a correct diagnosis. Electroencephalograms are diffusely abnormal, as in metabolic encephalopathies. The Klüver-Bucy syndrome, consisting of aggressive oral and hypersexual behavior attributed to a temporal lobe lesion, has also been described.[6] In all instances, electrolyte abnormalities should be excluded. Hyponatremia may accompany acute attacks or result from initial treatment of an attack with intravenous dextrose and water. It can be severe enough to affect mental status.

Seizures may be the presenting manifestation of porphyria and represent a particular challenge to the neurologist in that many of the widely used long-acting anticonvulsants are contraindicated in porphyria. The seizures most often are generalized and thus per se do not point to porphyria. However, a history of preceding abdominal pain or of chronic complaints (such as constipation) may suggest the diagnosis. A history of dark urine is helpful but not always present. When the diagnosis is suspected, treatment (other than measures to suppress the seizures) should be withheld pending the results of a rapid test for urine PBG (see diagnosis section).

Neuropathy occurs in approximately 40% of acute attacks,[7] generally 1 to 4 weeks after onset but in rare cases as late as 11 weeks.[7] Weakness is the predominant manifestation and is usually proximal and symmetric. It can involve the upper extremities, the lower extremities, or both (Table 64–2). The rate of neurologic progression is highly variable among individual patients but can be

TABLE 64–2. Symptoms and Signs in Acute Hepatic Porphyria at Presentation

Symptom	*Frequency (%)*	*Sign*	*Frequency (%)*
Abdominal pain	95	Tachycardia	80
Extremity pain	50	Dark urine	74
Back pain	29	Motor deficit	60
Chest pain	12	Proximal limbs	48
Nausea, vomiting	43	Distal limbs	10
Constipation	48	Generalized	42
Diarrhea	43	Altered mentation	40
		Hypertension	36
		Sensory deficit	26
		Seizure	20

Note. Data from Ridley [7] and Stein and Tschudy [90]: studies of acute intermittent porphyria. The findings in hereditary coproporphyria and variegate porphyria are similar [1,2].

rapid, with flaccid tetraplegia and respiratory paralysis appearing within a few days. Cranial nerve involvement, when present, involves nerves X and VII most frequently.[7] Monocular or total blindness can occur and has been attributed to vasospasm[8-10]; it is usually transient but can be permanent.[9] In patients with altered mental function, magnetic resonance imaging (MRI) has suggested the posterior leukoencephalopathy syndrome, with improvement following hematin administration.[10] Sensory disturbances occur in as many as 50% of patients in some series and may precede the motor neuropathy.[7] These consist of paresthesias and numbness (usually distal) and are unimpressive in relation to the motor signs.

Neuropathologic Findings

In early autopsy studies, demyelination was more prominent than axonal degeneration, suggesting a primary disorder of Schwann cells.[8,11] The patchy nature of the process also was emphasized, with damage only at intervals along a nerve or affecting some nerves but not others within a bundle and no relationship to blood vessels or the perineurium.[11] Subsequent reports, however, with one describing a sural nerve biopsy during the early phase of an attack,[12] provided evidence for primary axonal degeneration.[7] Nerve conduction studies support this, being typically in the normal or low-normal range,[13,14] and the time course and pattern of recovery of motor function (proximal to distal) are more consistent with axonal regeneration than with Schwann cell repair.[7]

DIAGNOSIS

In a first presentation of acute porphyria, the diagnosis is seldom obvious. The principal complaints of abdominal or back pain are not specific, and many of the associated manifestations are helpful more for excluding a surgical emergency than for directing attention to porphyria. Thus, specific laboratory tests are always required for establishing the diagnosis and for characterizing the type of porphyria in an individual case (Table 64–3).

A hallmark of the acute porphyrias (other than δ-aminolevulinic aciduria, which manifests increased ALA

rather than PBG) is marked elevation of PBG in urine. This can be established rapidly, if only qualitatively, with the two-step Watson-Schwartz test. In the first step, urine is mixed with Ehrlich's aldehyde reagent (p-dimethylaminobenzaldehyde in hydrochloric acid), which forms a pink complex with PBG. Although lack of an initial pink reaction product constitutes a negative result, a red complex is not by itself specific for PBG. Urobilinogen, among other substances present in normal urine, reacts with Ehrlich's reagent. For a correct interpretation of the test, the pink complex must be tested for solubility in water. In the second step, the solution is adjusted to pH 4 (with a saturated solution of sodium acetate) and then extracted with n-butanol. The PBG complex remains in the aqueous (lower) layer, whereas that due to urobilinogen and most other chromogens partitions into butanol. When performed in this manner, the Watson-Schwartz test yields few false positives.[15] The test is insensitive to concentrations of PBG below 10 mg/liter, which is of no consequence for emergent evaluation of symptomatic patients because PBG concentrations in urine during acute attacks invariably exceed this level.[15] Given its relative insensitivity, however, the Watson-Schwartz test is not used to identify asymptomatic genetic carriers of acute porphyria. In practice, all positive Watson-Schwartz test results should be confirmed and quantified with a column assay,[16] which is widely available.

The Watson-Schwartz test is distinct from a porphyrin screen, which is offered by many laboratories. The latter is a qualitative test for porphyrins (not ALA or PBG) and is of value mainly in dermatologic diagnosis. It does not differentiate acute (neurologic) from chronic (cutaneous) porphyria.

Identifying the type of porphyria requires quantitative assay of ALA, PBG, and porphyrins in urine and feces. As presented in Table 64–4 and Figure 64–1, a specific pattern of excretion is associated with each type of acute porphyria. This information can be supplemented by assay in cell lysates of specific enzyme deficiencies. This is particularly important in acute intermittent porphyria (AIP) for the reason that a sizable fraction of carriers have normal urine analyses when asymptomatic. A study from Sweden found that in carriers confirmed by

TABLE 64–3. Normal Values for Porphyrins and Porphyrin Precursors*

	Urine (24 hours)	Feces (Dry Weight)	Erythrocytes
ALA	<57 pmol (<7.5 mg)	—	—
PBG	<9 pmol (<2 mg)	—	—
URO	12–60 nmol (0.01–0.05 mg)	trace	—
COPRO	76–382 nmol (0.05–0.25 mg)	<76 nmol/g (<50 pg/g)	<23 nmol/liter (<1.5 pg/dl)
PROTO	—	<215 nmol/g (<120 pg/g)	<1.3 pmol/liter (<75 pg/dl)

*Column chromatographic and solvent extraction methods are used to quantify ALA and PBG [16] and the porphyrins [130]. ALA, δ-aminolevulinic acid; PBG, porphobilinogen; URO, uroporphyrin; COPRO, coproporphyrin; PROTO, protoporphyrin.

TABLE 64–4. Profile of Heme Precursors in the Porphyrias

Type of Porphyria	Enzyme Defect	Precursors Present in Increased Amount*			
		Urine	Feces	Plasma	Red Blood Cells
Acute intermittent	3[†]	ALA, **PBG**, URO		ALA, PBG	
Hereditary coproporphyria	5	PBG, URO, COPRO	**COPRO**	COPRO	
Variegate porphyria	7	PBG, URO, COPRO	COPRO < **PROTO**	COPRO, PROTO	
δ-Aminolevulinic aciduria	2	**ALA**, COPRO			PROTO
Cutanea tarda	5	**URO** > COPRO	URO	URO	
Congenital erythropoietic	4	URO >> COPRO	URO, COPRO	URO	**URO**
Protoporphyria	8		PROTO	PROTO	**PROTO**
Secondary porphyrinuria	?	(URO) **COPRO**			

*Bold type denotes the precursor that is characteristically increased. ALA, δ-aminolevulinic acid; PBG, porphobilinogen; URO, uroporphyrin; COPRO, coproporphyrin; PROTO, protoporphyrin.

[†]For a key to the enzymes of heme synthesis, see Figure 64–1.

DNA analysis, 44% had a normal urine PBG.[17] The defective enzyme in AIP, PBG deaminase (PBG-D, also known as uroporphyrinogen-I synthase), is present in erythrocytes, making its assay convenient. Because PBG-D does not fluctuate with disease activity, it is a useful adjunct to urine studies in screening for genetic carriers among family members of an index case. On average, affected individuals have 50% of normal activity. Problems include the fact that the porphyric and normal ranges overlap by about 20%; in addition, in some families PBG-D activity is reduced in nonerythroid tissues but is normal in erythrocytes. The basis for the latter finding has been determined and is described later in the Molecular Genetics section. Patients with subclinical hemolysis also may have false negative tests. PBG-D

activity is highest in young erythrocytes and may reach the normal range in states of increased red cell turnover. These various circumstances account for a falsely normal PBG D determination in about 25% of known carriers. Nonetheless, by combining urine studies, PBG-D activity, and pedigree analysis, 80% to 90% of carriers of AIP can be identified.[17,18]

The enzymes that are defective in hereditary coproporphyria and variegate porphyria, respectively, are coproporphyrinogen oxidase and protoporphyrinogen oxidase. Although assays for both exist, they require extracts of nucleated cells and are research procedures. Carriers are identified by fecal porphyrin analysis (Fig. 64–2), which in the case of variegate porphyria, has a sensitivity of approximately 75%.[19]

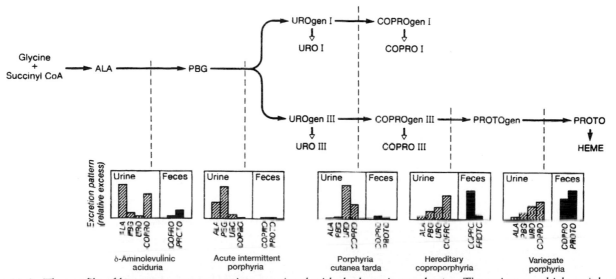

FIGURE 64–2. The profile of heme precursor excretion associated with the hepatic porphyrias. The points at which an inherited enzyme deficiency compromises the flow of precursors are shown (dashed vertical lines). For specific enzymes affected and key to abbreviations, see Figure 64–1.

A fourth type of acute porphyria is δ-aminolevulinic aciduria, which may be the rarest of the acute porphyrias. It is clinically silent except in individuals who are homozygous for defective PBG synthase.[20] Its diagnostic feature is marked elevation of urinary ALA and coproporphyrin as well as very low activity (<5% of normal) of erythrocyte PBG synthase. The urine pattern resembles that seen in heavy metal intoxication, which should be excluded.

Differential Diagnosis

In patients with progressive weakness due to acute porphyria, the entity most likely to be considered is acute ascending polyneuropathy, the Guillain-Barré syndrome. Several differential points are worth noting. An ascending paralysis (classic in Guillain-Barré, albeit not always present) is rare in acute porphyria.[22] Abdominal pain, constipation, and tachycardia precede the acute neurologic illness in porphyria but either are not present or are coincidental in Guillain-Barré. Also, beyond the first few days of the illness, the protein concentration of the cerebrospinal fluid in Guillain-Barré reaches abnormal levels and mononuclear cells may be present, whereas cerebrospinal fluid is usually normal throughout an attack of porphyria.[22] The most important differential point is the presence of PBG in urine.

In some respects, the symptoms of lead intoxication and hereditary tyrosinemia mimic those of acute porphyria. In both, urinary ALA is increased, which is due to inhibition of ALA dehydrase. In lead intoxication, the peripheral neuropathy is predominantly (if not exclusively) motor, as in porphyria, and central nervous system function may be depressed as well. The urine porphyrin pattern (isolated elevation of urine ALA and coproporphyrin) points to the correct diagnosis, which is established with a blood lead determination.

Hereditary tyrosinemia is a disease of tyrosine catabolism[23] involving a mutation in the gene for fumarylacetoacetate hydrolase (FAH). Its inheritance is autosomal recessive. Defective FAH leads to buildup in the liver of toxic fumarylacetoacetate and succinyl acetone, an inhibitor of ALA dehydrase. Thus, a biochemical hallmark of the disease is high levels of ALA (but not PBG) in blood and urine. Most interestingly, many of the symptoms, including abdominal pain and neurologic crises, resemble acute porphyria,[23,24] suggesting that ALA causes the neurologic component of acute porphyria (discussed later). The differentiation of hereditary tyrosinemia from acute porphyria on clinical grounds is straightforward. Tyrosinemia manifests in infancy or early childhood. Acute porphyria, by contrast, is rare before puberty.[25] Even in the homozygous form of hereditary coproporphyria or variegate porphyria, photocutaneous disease is the predominant manifestation in childhood; neuropsychiatric manifestations are minimal or absent.[26,27] Additionally, hereditary tyrosinemia is

associated with vitamin D-resistant rickets, aminoaciduria, and clinically evident liver disease, none of which occurs in acute porphyria.

Secondary Coproporphyrinuria

The evaluation of acute porphyria generally requires quantitative measurement of heme precursors in urine and feces. A frequent finding from screening studies is an isolated increase in urine coproporphyrin. This result is nonspecific, occurring in a wide range of conditions,[28] and is termed *secondary coproporphyrinuria* (see Table 64–4). It should not be construed as evidence of hereditary porphyria.

PATHOGENESIS OF NEUROLOGIC SYMPTOMS

The relationship between altered heme metabolism and the neuropsychiatric symptoms of acute porphyria is a conundrum despite investigation spanning many years; several hypotheses remain active (Table 64–5). Although the genetic lesion varies for the three acute porphyrias, overproduction of ALA and PBG is common to all. Attention has focused on ALA, in large part because both lead intoxication and hereditary tyrosinemia share clinical features with acute porphyria and both involve overproduction of ALA.

ALA as a Neurotoxin

ALA has two postulated mechanisms of toxicity. One hypothesis, which has received fairly detailed study, is based on the resemblance of ALA to the inhibitory neurotransmitter, γ-aminobutyric acid (GABA).[29,30] GABA is

TABLE 64–5. Neuropathogenesis of Acute Porphyria

Hypotheses

Neurotoxicity of ALA

　? Pro-oxidant

　? Reduces melatonin production by the pineal gland

ALA as a false neurotransmitter

　? GABA analogue

Neural heme deficiency

　? failure of endogenous synthesis

　? failure of exogenous supply (e.g., from liver)

Altered tryptophan metabolism

　(→ increased CNS serotonin)

Effects of hematin

　Consistent with any of the above

ALA, δ-aminolevulinic acid; GABA, γ-aminobutyric acid; CNS, central nervous system.

present in the myenteric plexus of the guinea pig intestine, where it may inhibit peristalsis.[31] Thus ALA, acting as a GABA agonist, could produce the ileus associated with acute porphyria. Several in vitro studies exist on the mechanism of GABAergic actions of ALA, although in most cases effects were seen only at supra-physiologic concentrations of ALA (Table 64–6). Although the concentration of ALA at the synapse is unknown, its level in neural tissue appears to be about 10% of that in plasma. In brain, this may be due to both the blood-brain barrier and limited activity of the heme synthetic pathway, which is low at baseline in neural tissue and noninducible by drugs such as barbiturates.[33]

The second hypothesis focuses on ALA as a neurotoxin. In the presence of a cuprous or ferrous ion, ALA undergoes oxidation to 4,5-dioxovaleric acid, releasing oxygen radicals,[34–36] which may be directly damaging.[37–41] Experimentally, ALA has been shown to alter mitochondrial permeability and to cause thiol oxidation, actions that are blocked by radical scavengers.[37] The clinical relevance of these observations remains to be established. In two patients with AIP, antioxidant therapy for 8 weeks produced no detectable benefit.[42]

A problem for either hypothesis is the fairly poor correlation between the level of blood ALA, which can range widely in genetic carriers, and neurologic symptoms.[29,43] It has been shown only that patients with a history of acute porphyria have more pronounced chronic deficits (motor and sensory) than do asymptomatic carriers,[44] possibly because patients with attacks have experienced higher average blood ALA than have asymptomatic carriers.

Heme Deficiency and Altered Tryptophan Metabolism

Increased production of ALA (and PBG) is an indirect result of a partial block of the heme synthetic pathway. A direct consequence of this defect is heme deficiency, which may be present in neural tissues as well as the liver.[1] It remains unclear whether neural cells meet their need for heme through endogenous production or by importing exogenous heme. The latter possibility at least exists with hepatocytes as the possible source.[45] The proteins that more rapidly turn over heme would be most affected by an acute shortage of heme. Tryptophan pyrrolase, which catalyzes the conversion of tryptophan to kynurenine, is one of these proteins. This enzyme has heme as its prosthetic group but binds it with a relatively low affinity such that even in the normal state, it is only half-saturated with heme. Therefore, it is particularly susceptible to inactivation during heme deficiency. Such inactivation in theory shunts tryptophan from the kynurenine pathway to the tryptophan hydroxylase pathway, which yields 5-OH-tryptamine (serotonin). The predicted result is a serotonergic state, and this is consistent with studies in animals[46] and conceivably accounts for some porphyric manifestations, such as a heightened sensitivity to sedatives. Blood tryptophan is increased in some patients with AIP, with serotonin and its urinary metabolite, 5-hydroxyindole acetic acid, both increasing during acute attacks.[47,48] These changes are reversed by administration of heme.[48,49] Further work is needed to relate tryptophan metabolism to symptoms in acute porphyria.

Plasma melatonin also decreases in patients with acute porphyria.[48,50] This is a surprise, given that serotonin, the substrate for melatonin production, is increased. However, unlike the changes in serotonin and other metabolites of tryptophan, the drop in melatonin is unaffected by heme administration[48] and thus does not appear to reflect a state of heme deficiency in the pineal, which produces melatonin. The defect in melatonin production occurs also in rats with high circulating ALA.[51] Given that the pineal is outside the blood-brain barrier, it is likely to be more affected by systemic ALA than are other parts of the brain. Whether the loss of melatonin production represents a direct toxicity of ALA or a GABAergic effect is uncertain. The fact that administered GABA has a similar effect supports the latter possibility.[51] Deficient melatonin (and loss of circadian variation) may account for some of the prodrome of acute porphyria (mood disturbances, insomnia), although this remains to be proven. It is interesting that melatonin is an antioxidant and, in experimental systems, counters the pro-oxidant effects of ALA.[39–41,52] This opens the possibility that a primary loss of melatonin sensitizes the

TABLE 64–6. Effects of ALA on GABA Metabolism in Vitro[*]

Observation	Effective (ALA)	Reference
Inhibition of high-affinity uptake of GABA by cortical synaptosomes	10^{-3} to 10^{-4} M	131
Inhibition of potassium-stimulated release of GABA from preloaded synaptosomes	10^{-4} to 10^{-6} M	135
Inhibition of GABA uptake into neurons	10^{-3} M	137
CSF (ALA) in acute porphyria	2×10^{-5} to 2×10^{-7} M	132
Plasma (ALA) in acute porphyria	10^{-4} to 10^{-6} M	138
Inhibition of muscimol binding to synaptic membranes	10^{-3} M	139

[*]ALA = δ-aminolevulinic acid; GABA = γ-aminobutyric acid; CSF = cerebrospinal fluid.

patient to the neurotoxic effects of ALA. Alternatively, loss of melatonin may be secondary to the high levels of ALA associated with acute attacks. Longitudinal studies of patients between and during attacks will be necessary to address this question.

The postulated mechanisms of neural dysfunction described here are not mutually exclusive. On the contrary, they could be additive because they involve different aspects of heme regulation and neuronal physiology. Perhaps this is why no single hypothesis has yet provided a complete explanation of the neurologic syndrome in acute porphyria. The fact that administered heme fails to restore melatonin to normal levels may lend insight into facets of the acute attack that are due to altered melatonin and to elevated ALA and heme deficiency.

CHEMICAL AND PHYSIOLOGIC INDUCERS OF ACUTE PORPHYRIA

Most acute attacks of porphyria involve a known precipitating factor, although some are apparently spontaneous. Most often, the precipitating factor is a pharmaceutical, and lists of offending drugs have been compiled. The length of some lists creates the impression that no drug is safe. A preferred approach is to group drugs according to their estimated hazard level and to include apparently safe drugs.[1,2,22,53] The most hazardous pharmaceuticals are those that stimulate hepatic heme synthesis. By inducing synthesis of apocytochrome P-450, they indirectly create a demand for new heme. The most important class of inducers includes the barbiturates and related compounds. Clinical experience confirms the risk of these agents to carriers of acute porphyria (Table 64–7). While this presents a problem for the treatment of seizure disorders, for virtually all other clinical indications, less risky and effective agents are available.

Test systems exist to prospectively judge the risk of therapeutic agents to carriers of porphyria. These consist of the rat liver in vivo, chick embryo liver in ovo, and chick embryo hepatocytes in culture. Each system provides a quantitative estimate of the ability of a pharmaceutical to induce porphyrin or heme synthesis. The correlation between experimental data and clinical experience is less than perfect. Compounds such as diazepam, which are inducers in chick embryo hepatocytes (probably the most sensitive of the test systems), have been used with impunity in porphyria. Conversely, relatively poor inducers in experimental systems, such as clonazepam, have not been entirely benign in patients.[54] Discordant findings, however, are the exception rather than the rule, even though interspecies differences in the response to xenobiotics may be expected. Anecdotal reports of drugs that have been used without adverse consequences in individual patients have little value. Similar reports exist for even the most dangerous drugs, when patients have received them inadvertently.[55] A reasonable approach is

to categorize all medications that have been linked to at least one well-documented attack of acute porphyria as "hazardous" and to label any chemicals that are active in a test system but not yet implicated as a cause of acute porphyria in humans as "possibly hazardous."[53,56] A third and important category comprises drugs that are not inducers of cytochrome P-450 and have never precipitated acute porphyria; this includes some extremely useful agents.

TABLE 64–7. Use of Medications in Porphyria

Unsafe	Believed to Be Safe
Anticonvulsants	
Barbiturates	Bromides
Carbamazepine	Diazepam
Clonazepam	Gabapentin
Ethosuximide	Magnesium sulfate
Felbamate	
Phenytoin	
Primidone	
Tiagabine	
Valproic acid	
Hypnotics/Sedatives	
Barbiturates	Chloral hydrate
Chlordiazepoxide	Chlorpromazine
Ethchlorvynol	Diphenhydramine
Glutethimide	Lithium
Meprobamate	Lorazepam
Methyprylon	Meclizine
	Trifluoperazine
Other	
α-Methyldopa	Adrenocorticotropic hormone
Danazol	Allopurinol
Ergot preparations	Aminoglycosides
Estrogens	Aspirin
Griseofulvin	Codeine
Imipramine	Colchicine
Pentazocine	Furosemide
Pyrazinamide	Ibuprofen
Sulfonamides	Insulin
	Meperidine
	Morphine
	Naproxen
	Warfarin

A physiologic condition that predisposes humans to acute porphyria is fasting. Based on studies in experimental animals, fasting appears to sensitize the heme synthetic pathway to the effects of an inducing drug. It has been suggested that the previously discussed changes in tryptophan metabolism contribute to the carbohydrate-sensitive state by inhibiting hepatic gluconeogenesis.[57]

Female sex steroids also are involved in acute exacerbations. This inference is based on the fact that attacks are more common in women than in men (despite an even distribution of the genetic defect) and have a peak incidence in the third and fourth decades of life; attacks before puberty are rare. Exacerbations in some women are cyclic, occurring just before menstruation, although it can be difficult to distinguish the early symptoms of acute porphyria from premenstrual complaints.

MOLECULAR GENETICS

The inherited enzymatic defect for each of the acute porphyrias has been identified (see Fig. 64–2). Each protein has been purified, all of the corresponding genes cloned, and mutational analysis performed.[63-70] The most extensively studied of these enzymes is PBG deaminase, which is mutated in AIP. According to a study of 3350 Western European individuals, the prevalence of the defective gene is around 1:1650.[71] A single copy, located on chromosome 11,[72] gives rise to two transcripts that encode proteins of 44 and 42 kDa, respectively.[73] The smaller of the two is expressed solely in erythroid cells, whereas the larger is ubiquitous. The gene has two transcriptional start sites (Fig. 64–3), and each promoter has been examined by DNase-I hypersensitivity mapping and by functional studies of deletion mutants in transgenic mice or erythroleukemia cells. The promoter for the erythroid form, which drives the smaller transcript, is tissue specific, sharing motifs with other erythroid-specific genes such as globins.[74,75] Erythroid cells also have a mecha-

nism for premature termination of transcription from the upstream promoter, to exclude interference with the tissue-specific promoter.[75] The complete genomic sequence for PBG deaminase has been published,[76] and analysis of defects in individual families with AIP has revealed more than 150 mutations.[77] Studies of PBG deaminase from *Escherichia coli* indicate that key functional domains are conserved in the human enzyme. Several mutations that are clustered in exons 10 and 12, giving rise to inactive protein, affect residues in the active site.[78,79]

Variation in Tissue Expression of Porphobilinogen Deaminase

Before DNA analysis, the first indication of genetic heterogeneity among carriers of AIP came with the observation that in rare families, the expected deficiency of PBG-D was present only in nucleated cells, contrary to usual findings of reduced activity in erythrocytes as well as nucleated cells.[80] Analysis of the genetic transcriptional unit for PBG-D in erythroid and nonerythroid tissues has provided an explanation for this finding. The mutation in families with AIP but normal erythroid PBG-D appears to involve nucleotide changes at the first exon-intron junction.[80,81] Because these lie upstream of the second start site, the erythroid transcript is unaffected. Most mutations are distal and therefore affect both forms of the enzyme.

Variation in the Production of Mutant Porphobilinogen Deaminase

A different form of heterogeneity has been inferred by comparison of active PBG-D and total immunoprecipitable enzyme protein in various families with AIP. While in most cases there is a similar decrease in enzyme activity and total enzyme protein, in approximately 15%, the ratio of enzyme activity to total enzyme protein is less than 1, indicating a mutation that results in enzymatically inactive but stable PBG-D.[82]

Mutation analysis has not proved to be useful for predicting the likelihood or frequency of acute porphyric attacks, except in the case of one Swedish study.[83] This is consistent with an important role for medications and other environmental factors in the pathogenesis of acute attacks. The multiplicity of defects also means that molecular genetic methods have not been applied to diagnosis except for identifying carriers in individual large kindreds. Denaturing gradient gel electrophoresis has the necessary sensitivity for genetic screening[86] but is not a technique that lends itself to routine laboratory use. Substantial genetic heterogeneity has been documented also in hereditary coproporphyria[84] and variegate porphyria.[85]

ANIMAL MODELS

The traditional models of acute porphyria involve the administration of chemicals that cause rapid degradation

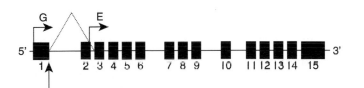

FIGURE 64–3. Structure of the PBG deaminase gene (not to scale). The respective start sites for transcription of the general (G) and erythroid (E) forms are shown (right-angle arrows). The splicing event that excludes exon 2 in the normal G transcript is also shown (dotted-line caret between exons 1 and 3). The inferior arrow (*) shows the location of a splice-junction mutation that results in deficiency of the ubiquitous form of PBG-D, but it is upstream of the start site for the erythroid form. This type of mutation is responsible for AIP cases with deficient PBG-D in the liver but normal activity in erythrocytes.

of hepatic microsomal heme and thus induce a disturbance in heme homeostasis that biochemically resembles the human disease. The prototype inducer is allyl isopropylacetamide[58]; its mechanism of action has been studied in detail. It undergoes activation on cytochrome P-450 to a radical species, which forms a covalent adduct with one of the pyrrole nitrogens of the enzyme's heme constituent. The modified heme is unstable and undergoes degradation.[59] This sequence of events, in which cytochrome P-450 participates in its own destruction, has been termed *suicide inactivation*. The most potent inducing agents block a step in heme synthesis as well as accelerate the turnover of cytochrome P-450 heme, thus rapidly creating a heme-deficient state in the liver.[60]

While these models have illuminated several important aspects of hepatic heme regulation, none has reproduced the neurologic abnormalities of human porphyria. To address this problem, researchers developed a mouse with a null mutation in PBG deaminase.[61] Homozygous mutant mice died in utero, as expected. Although heterozygotes had 50% of normal hepatic enzyme activity (as in AIP), they exhibited no biochemical or behavioral abnormalities. Even after challenge with phenobarbital, urinary excretion of ALA was normal. Reasoning that the mouse might require more than a 50% deficiency in PBG deaminase for disease manifestations, the investigators created a second mouse line with a partial defect in one allele and crossed it with the mouse line bearing the null allele. PBG deaminase in the compound mutant heterozygote was 30% of normal. Although baseline ALA excretion remained low (less than twofold increase above normal), phenobarbital administration elicited a marked increase in hepatic ALA synthase activity and urinary ALA.[61] Most importantly, over a period of 6 to 16 months, the animals developed neurologic deficits characterized as muscle weakness and loss of motor function; histology showed axonal degeneration. Nerve conduction was essentially unaltered. Because the neurologic syndrome proceeds in mice with normal or minimally elevated ALA, the authors concluded that it reflects an underlying neural heme deficiency rather than ALA toxicity. While the model mimics certain aspects of AIP in humans, phenobarbital administration failed to produce acute symptoms such as seizures or rapidly progressive paralysis. Additionally, the neuropathology that developed chronically in the mutant mice appears to be much more severe than that reported for asymptomatic human carriers of AIP.[44,62] Nevertheless, this model should lend itself to dissecting the mechanisms of neurologic damage in porphyria.

THERAPY

Acute Attacks

The initial management is directed at pain relief, support for complications such as hyponatremia, and elimination of factors that may have precipitated the attack. The use of chlorpromazine for pain relief has been advocated, although excessive sedation can be troublesome. Anecdotal reports support the use of propranolol, which counters the tachycardia present in most patients and may also relieve pain.[87] If used, propranolol should be introduced at a low dose, as hypotensive reactions have occurred in some patients.[88] In many cases, adequate analgesia requires meperidine or morphine. For patients with a clear-cut acute attack, the risk of addiction is minimal. A remission, either spontaneous or with hematin administration, can be expected within a few days, at which point analgesic medication is terminated.

Hyponatremia often accompanies acute attacks of porphyria and may contribute to neurologic abnormalities. Although not always present on admission, hyponatremia nonetheless can emerge rapidly with administration of intravenous fluids (e.g., dextrose in water). Its basis is debated. In some patients, high urine osmolarity suggests the syndrome of inappropriate secretion of antidiuretic hormone (SIADH), whereas in others, hypovolemia may be the underlying problem.[89] Because the presence of SIADH cannot be assumed, water restriction should be avoided in favor of saline administration, with diuretics as needed.

All nonessential medications, in addition to those implicated as a cause of acute attacks, should be discontinued. For reversing a fasting state (present in most patients because of pain and nausea), carbohydrate is given with the goal of providing approximately 400 g dextrose daily. Although this therapy has not been tested in controlled trials, it is supported by clinical experience.[90]

Administration of heme, as hematin, constitutes definitive therapy, on the premise that heme deficiency is the principal metabolic abnormality in acute porphyria. The initial studies of hematin were carried out in gravely ill patients but established that the intravenously administered material was effective in suppressing overproduction of ALA and PBG.[91] Subsequent work from several groups demonstrated the clinical efficacy of this treatment,[92–94] leading to the current recommendation that hematin be used early in the course of an acute attack if not as first-line therapy.[1,2] In patients without neurologic signs, conservative care involving the measures outlined earlier may be pursued for 2 to 3 days, supplemented by hematin after this period if the clinical picture is unchanged or deteriorating. In patients presenting with neurologic signs, hematin is started as early as possible, together with carbohydrates and supportive care.

Heme itself (ferriprotoporphyrin IX) is essentially insoluble in aqueous media but dissolves readily in alkaline solutions (e.g., 0.1 M sodium carbonate, pH 8.0). In this form, it is termed *hydroxyheme*, or *hematin*. Hematin is unstable in solution[95,96] and thus has been formulated in dry form for reconstitution immediately prior to infusion (Panhematin, Abbott Laboratories, Chicago,

Illinois). Heme may be rendered soluble also by complexing it with the amino acid arginine to form heme arginate, which is stable in solution and essentially identical to hematin with respect to its metabolic and clinical effects.[97] It is marketed in 40% 1,2-propanediol and 10% ethanol (Normosang, Clinica, Helsinki, Finland; available in Europe but not in the United States). A third preparation is heme-albumin (methemalbumin). It has received relatively little use, and data on its stability are limited.[49]

Freshly prepared hematin (or heme-arginate) is given at a dose of 1.5 to 2.0 mg/kg body weight by slow intravenous infusion (over 10 minutes). Initially, it was recommended that a dose be given every 12 hours,[98] but a single daily administration appears to be equally effective.[94] Urinary PBG and symptoms are monitored. With effective levels of administered heme, PBG drops after 24 to 48 hours, reaching less than 20% of the preinfusion level after 48 to 72 hours. A symptomatic response is apparent 72 to 96 hours after the initiation of therapy[94] and is typically dramatic, as judged by markedly reduced pain, improved mental status, and a diminishing need for analgesia. Objective neurologic signs, however, respond variably depending on the underlying pathology. Neurodegeneration is unaffected by hematin, although its progression may be halted.[99]

Despite the efficacy of intravenous hematin, resistance to this treatment and failure have been reported.[100,101] In at least some cases, this represents mishandling of the compound. Hematin decays in solution, even when refrigerated, and thus must be given directly after its preparation; the decayed form is ineffective.[95] Another problem is accuracy of diagnosis. In genetic carriers who are acutely ill, it can be difficult to establish with certainty whether symptoms are due to porphyria or to an unrelated problem. The level of urinary PBG provides a rough guide. If urinary PBG is less than 25 mg per 24 hours, an acute flare of porphyria is unlikely,[94] regardless of the severity of the symptoms. In two patients with *subacute* porphyria-like symptoms and urinary PBG that was elevated but less than 25 mg per 24 hours, hematin infusion was ineffective.[94] In short, true hematin resistance or failure appears to be rare. Indeed, if the material has been correctly prepared and infused, the lack of a response should call the diagnosis into question.

Adverse effects of hematin are minor and infrequent, provided that the recommended dose is not exceeded. Hematin in large amounts is known to be nephrotoxic; one patient receiving an unusually large dose exhibited renal failure, which was transient.[102] Chemical phlebitis occurs in approximately 4% of infusions, presumably owing to the alkalinity of the solution. Using as large a vein as possible and applying a slow infusion rate minimizes this. Anticoagulant effects of hematin were noted in early reports, manifested as prolonged prothrombin time and reduced platelets.[103,104] The abnormalities were transient, and clinically significant bleeding was unusual. Anticoagulant effects appear to be attributable to decayed hematin[95,96] and should be minimal with freshly reconstituted material. Heme arginate reportedly does not affect coagulation parameters.[97] Nonetheless, caution is recommended in administering any of these preparations to patients with impaired coagulation or a bleeding tendency.

Premenstrual Exacerbations

Changes in reproductive hormones occurring during menstruation may exacerbate acute porphyria. The initial approach is symptomatic therapy along with elimination of medications that may be hazardous in porphyria (see Table 64–7). If these measures are ineffective, or if the patient develops objective signs of porphyria during periods of symptoms, ovulatory suppression with analogues of gonadotropin-releasing hormone may be helpful.[105,106] The latter are peptides that have no demonstrable porphyria-inducing activity, in contrast to the synthetic gonadal steroids in oral contraceptives, which have been linked to attacks in some patients.[107] In anecdotal reports, administration of hematin, given weekly or timed to the expected onset of symptoms, also has been effective.[108] Danazol appears to induce porphyria and should be avoided.[109]

Seizures

If seizures are present, they generally occur at the onset of an acute attack. They can be suppressed with intravenous diazepam. The use of magnesium sulfate also has been recommended, based on its efficacy in eclamptic seizures,[110] but experience with this agent in acute porphyria is very limited.[111] Hematin or heme arginate should be administered but, as noted, acts only after a lag period of 3 to 4 days.

Treatment of chronic seizures in genetic carriers of acute porphyria is singularly difficult because many of the first-line agents have been implicated in acute attacks.[54,112–114] Barbiturates and related compounds (e.g., phenytoin) are absolutely contraindicated (see Table 64–7). Individual patients may tolerate carbamazepine or valproic acid, although the risk of a porphyric exacerbation is substantial.[54,112,115] Gabapentin has been effective in a few reported cases and without complications.[116,117] Studies of porphyrin induction in cultured liver cells also support the use of gabapentin but suggest that felbamate, lamotrigine, and tiagabine should be avoided.[118]

Bromides have fallen out of favor as an anticonvulsant but are safe in porphyria and apparently effective.[54,113] Despite their narrow therapeutic index and the necessity for close monitoring, they have been used in the modern era for childhood epilepsy that is resistant to standard therapy, with good effect.[119–122] A conservative approach is to initiate therapy with 10 mg/kg per day, taken in divided doses with food to minimize gastric irritation.[120] A serum level of 80 to 100 mg/dl is targeted, but this may need to be adjusted to achieve the desired clinical effect or to reduce side effects. Serum bromide is assayed by a colorimetric procedure[123] that is simple but may not be available in clinical laboratories. Bromide ion interferes with the serum chloride determination by ion-specific electrode, resulting in an apparent hyperchloremia. Side effects, occurring in all patients who achieve anticonvulsant levels of bromide, consist primarily of sedation, an acneiform skin eruption, and gastrointestinal symptoms. Toxic effects ("bromism") include psychosis and ataxia. Bromide is eliminated through the kidneys. Although its half-life is long (approximately 12 days), excretion can be accelerated by the administration of sodium chloride and diuretics.

Hematin is impractical as chronic therapy because it must be given intravenously; also, iron accumulation is at least a theoretical concern. Orally administered heme is ineffective, because it is degraded by intestinal heme oxygenase.[93]

Genetic Therapy

With cloning of the relevant genes and the development of methods for targeting DNA to erythroid cells[124] or hepatocytes,[125,126] the tools for gene therapy are available. Their application to severe forms of erythropoietic porphyria is attractive, because these diseases lack effective treatment and can cause disfiguring skin damage. In the case of the acute hepatic porphyrias, however, two considerations reduce enthusiasm for gene therapy. The first is the fact that the vast majority of genetic carriers have no symptoms if the circumstances associated with acute attacks can be avoided. Second, it is unclear whether correction of the defect in the liver would necessarily alter the neurologic manifestations (see Pathogenesis of Neurologic Symptoms section). In short, with proper identification and education of carriers, the risks of genetic therapy outweigh the benefits.

PROGNOSIS

In a series reported in 1969,[7] 10 of 29 acute porphyric attacks with neuropathy were fatal. The current mortality rate is substantially lower than this, most likely as a result of heightened awareness of the disease and tests for the genetic trait, with screening of possible carriers and early diagnosis. Undoubtedly, hematin treatment and improved intensive care also have had a positive effect.

Given that most acute attacks are precipitated by an identifiable factor, repeat episodes are avoidable with appropriate education of the patient and occur in fewer than 20% of those who have had an acute attack. Neurologic deficits, when present, resolve slowly, proceeding from proximal to distal muscles, consistent with axonal regrowth. Although permanent sequelae have

been described,[127] complete recovery is the rule over an average time of 10.6 months after the acute episode.[7]

Acute porphyria may manifest as an altered mental state. Given the difficulty of the diagnosis, the question of whether mental institutions have a disproportionate number of people with unrecognized porphyria has been raised. Patients hospitalized for mental illness have been surveyed for reduced activity of PBG-D and elevated urinary PBG. The results are mixed. One study found an unexpectedly high prevalence of abnormal tests,[128] although few if any of the patients with positive results had a history suggestive of past episodes of acute porphyria. In another study, the prevalence of positive tests did not differ from that in the control population.[129] For patients with a recognized acute attack who are under appropriate therapy, mental disturbances resolve promptly; there is no association of these diseases with a chronic major psychosis.[3] Also, in the absence of specific treatment, spontaneous remission is frequent. For these reasons, porphyria is unlikely to be an underlying problem in patients with chronic mental illness.

REFERENCES

1. Bissell DM: Haem metabolism and the porphyrias. In Millward-Sadler GH, Wright R, Arthur MJP (eds): Wright's Liver and Biliary Disease, 3rd ed. London, WB Saunders, 1992, p 397.

2. Anderson KE: The porphyrias. In Zakim D, Boyer TD (eds): Hepatology: A Textbook of Liver Disease, 3rd ed. Philadelphia, Saunders, 1996, p 417.

3. Patience DA, Blackwood DHR, McColl KEL, Moore MR: Acute intermittent porphyria and mental illness—a family study. Acta Psychiatr Scand 1994;89:262.

4. Brownstein S: George III: A revised view of the royal malady. J Hist Neurosci 1997;6:38.

5. McDonagh AF, Bissell DM: Porphyria and porphyrinology—the past 15 years. Semin Liver Dis 1998; 18:3.

6. Guidotti TL, Charness ME, Lamon JM: Acute intermittent porphyria and the Klüver-Bucy syndrome. Johns Hopkins Med J 1979;145:233.

7. Ridley A: The neuropathy of acute intermittent porphyria. Quart J Med 1969;8:307.

8. Gibson JB, Goldberg A: The neuropathology of acute porphyria. J Pathol Bacteriol 1956;71:495.

9. Lai CW, Hung T, Lin WSJ: Blindness of cerebral origin in acute intermittent porphyria. Arch Neurol 1977;34:310.

10. Utz N, Kinkel B, Hedde JP, Bewermeyer H: MR imaging of acute intermittent porphyria mimicking reversible posterior leukoencephalopathy syndrome. Neuroradiology 2001;43:1059.

11. Naef RW, Berry RG, Schlesinger MS: Neurologic aspects of porphyria. Neurology 1958;9:313.

12. Thorner PS, Bilbao JM, Sima AA, Briggs S: Porphyric neuropathy: An ultrastructural and quantitative case study. Can J Neurol Sci 1981;8:281.

13. Albers JW, Robertson WC, Daube JR: Electrodiagnostic findings in acute porphyric neuropathy. Muscle Nerve 1978;1:292.

14. Flugel KA, Druschky KF: Electromyogram and nerve conduction in patients with acute intermittent porphyria. J Neurol 1977;214:267.

15. Pierach CA, Cardinal R, Bossenmaier I, Watson CJ: Comparison of the Hoesch and the Watson-Schwartz tests for urinary porphobilinogen. Clin Chem 1977;23:1666.

16. Davis JR, Andelman SL: Urinary delta-aminolevulinic acid (ALA) levels in lead poisoning. 1. A modified method for the rapid determination of urinary delta-aminolevulinic acid using disposable ion exchange chromatography columns. Arch Environ Health 1967;15:53.

17. Andersson C, Thomell S, Floderus Y, et al: Diagnosis of acute intermittent porphyria in northern Sweden: An evaluation of mutation analysis and biochemical methods. J Intern Med 1995;237:301.

18. Lamon JM, Frykholm BC, Tschudy DP: Family evaluations in acute intermittent porphyria using red cell uroporphyrinogen I synthetase. J Med Genet 1979;16:134.

19. von und zu Fraunberg M, Kauppinen R: Diagnosis of variegate porphyria—hard to get? Scand J Clin Lab Invest 2000;60:605.

20. Bird TD, Hamernyik P, Nutter JY, Labbe RE: Inherited deficiency of delta-aminolevulinic acid dehydratase. Am J Hum Genet 1979;31:662.

21. de Verneuil H, Doss M, Brusco N, et al: Hereditary hepatic porphyria with delta aminolevulinate dehydrase deficiency: Immunologic characterization of the non-catalytic enzyme. Hum Genet 1985;69:174.

22. Sergay SM: Management of neurologic exacerbations of hepatic porphyria. Med Clin North Am 1979;63:453.

23. Gentz J, Johansson S, Lindblad B, et al: Excretion of delta aminolevulinic acid in hereditary tyrosinemia. Clin Chim Acta 1969;23:257.

24. Strife CF, Zuroweste EL, Emmett EA, et al: Tyrosinemia with acute intermittent porphyria: Aminolevulinic acid dehydratase deficiency related to elevated urinary aminolevulinic acid levels. J Pediatr 1977;90:400.

25. Badcock NR, O'Reilly DA, Zoanetti GD, et al: Childhood porphyrias: Implications and treatments. Clin Chem 1993;39:1334.

26. Murphy GM, Hawk JLM, Magnus IA, et al: Homozygous variegate porphyria: Two similar cases in unrelated families. J Roy Soc Med 1986;79:361.

27. Mustajoki P, Tenhunen R, Niemi KM, et al: Homozygous variegate porphyria: A severe skin disease of infancy. Clin Genet 1987;32:300.

28. Doss MO: Porphyrinurias and occupational disease. Ann N Y Acad Sci 1987;514:204.

29. Becker DM, Kramer S: The neurological manifestations of porphyria: A review. Medicine 1977;56:411.

30. Silbergeld EK: Role of altered heme synthesis in chemical injury to the nervous system. Ann N Y Acad Sci 1987;514:297.

31. Brennan MJW, Cantrill RC: Delta-aminolevulinic acid is a potent agonist for GABA autoreceptors. Nature 1979;280:514.

32. Paterniti JR, Simone JJ, Beattie DS: Detection and regulation of delta-aminolevulinic acid synthetase activity in the rat brain. Arch Biochem Biophys 1978;189:86.

33. Percy VA, Shanley BC: Studies on haem biosynthesis in rat brain. J Neurochemistry 1979;33:1267.

34. Hiraku Y, Kawanishi S: Mechanism of oxidative DNA damage induced by delta-aminolevulinic acid in the presence of copper ion. Cancer Res 1996;56:1786.

35. Douki T, Onuki J, Medeiros MH, et al: DNA alkylation by 4,5-dioxovaleric acid, the final oxidation product of 5-aminolevulinic acid. Chem Res Toxicol 1998;11:150.

36. Di Mascio P, Teixeira PC, Onuki J, et al: DNA damage by 5-aminolevulinic and 4,5-dioxovaleric acids in the presence of ferritin. Arch Biochem Biophys 2000;373:368.

37. Hermes-Lima M: How do Ca2+ and 5-aminolevulinic acid-derived oxyradicals promote injury to isolated mitochondria? Free Radic Biol Med 1995;19:381.

38. Costa CA, Trivelato GC, Pinto AM, Bechara EJ: Correlation between plasma 5-aminolevulinic acid concentrations and indicators of oxidative stress in lead-exposed workers. Clin Chem 1997;43:1196.

39. Carneiro RC, Reiter RJ: Melatonin protects against lipid peroxidation induced by delta-aminolevulinic acid in rat cerebellum, cortex and hippocampus. Neuroscience 1998;82:293.

40. Princ FG, Maxit AG, Cardalda C, et al: In vivo protection by melatonin against delta-aminolevulinic acid-induced oxidative damage and its antioxidant effect on the activity of haem enzymes. J Pineal Res 1998;24:1.

41. Karbownik M, Tan D, Manchester LC, Reiter RJ: Renal toxicity of the carcinogen delta-aminolevulinic acid: Antioxidant effects of melatonin. Cancer Lett 2000;161:1.

42. Thunell S, Andersson D, Harper P, et al: Effects of administration of antioxidants in acute intermittent porphyria. Eur J Clin Chem Clin Biochem 1997;35:427.

43. Ackner B, Cooper JE, Gray CH, et al: Excretion of porphobilinogen and delta-aminolevulinic acid in acute porphyria. Lancet 1961;1:1256.

44. Wikberg A, Andersson C, Lithner FL: Signs of neuropathy in the lower legs and feet of patients with acute intermittent porphyria. J Intern Med 2000;248:27.

45. Bissell DM, Liem HH, Muller-Eberhard U: Secretion of haem by hepatic parenchymal cells. Biochem J 1979;184:689.

46. Litman DA, Correia MA: Elevated brain tryptophan and enhanced 5-hydroxytryptamine turnover in acute hepatic heme deficiency: Clinical implications. J Pharmacol Exp Therap 1985;232:337.

47. Correia MA, Litman DA, Lunetta JM: Drug-induced modulations of hepatic heme metabolism. Ann N Y Acad Sci 1987;514:248.

48. Puy H, Deybach JC, Baudry P, et al: Decreased nocturnal plasma melatonin levels in patients with recurrent acute intermittent porphyria attacks. Life Sci 1993;53:621.

49. Bonkovsky HE, Healey JE Lourie AN, Gerron GG: Intravenous heme-albumin in acute intermittent porphyria: Evidence for repletion of hepatic hemoproteins and regulatory heme pools. Am J Gastroenterol 1991;86:1050.

50. Bylesjo I, Forsgren L, Wetterberg L: Melatonin and epileptic seizures in patients with acute intermittent porphyria. Epileptic Disord 2000;2:203.

51. Puy H, Deybach JC, Bogdan A, et al: Increased delta aminolevulinic acid and decreased pineal melatonin production. A common event in acute porphyria studies in the rat. J Clin Invest 1996;97:104.

52. Qi W, Reiter RJ, Tan DX, et al: Melatonin prevents delta-aminolevulinic acid-induced oxidative DNA damage in the presence of Fe2+. Mol Cell Biochem 2001;218:87.

53. Disler PB, Blekkenhorst GH, Eales L, et al: Guidelines for drug prescription in patients with the acute porphyrias. S Afr Med J 1982;64:656.

54. Bonkowsky HE, Sinclair PR, Emery S, Sinclair JE: Seizure management in acute hepatic porphyria: Risks of valproate and clonazepam. Neurology 1980;30:588.

55. Slavin SA, Christoforides C: Thiopental administration in acute intermittent porphyria without adverse effect. Anesthesiology 1976;44:77.

56. Moore MR: International review of drugs in acute porphyria. Internat J Biochem 1980;12:1089.

57. Correia MA, Lunetta JM: Acute hepatic heme depletion: Impaired gluconeogenesis in rats. Semin Hematol 1989;26:120.

58. Meyer UA, Marver HS. Chemically induced porphyria: Increased microsomal heme turnover after treatment with allylisopropylacetamide. Science 1971;171:64.

59. Correia MA, Farrell GC, Olson S, et al: Cytochrome P-450 heme moiety: The specific target in drug-induced heme alkylation. J Biol Chem 1981;256:5466.

60. De Matteis F, Stonard M: Experimental porphyrias as models for human hepatic porphyrias. Semin Hematol 1977;14:187.

61. Lindberg RL, Porcher C, Grandchamp B, et al: Porphobilinogen deaminase deficiency in mice causes a neuropathy resembling that of human hepatic porphyria. Nat Genet 1996;12:195.

62. Kochar DK, Poonia A, Kumawat BL, et al: Study of motor and sensory nerve conduction velocities, late responses (F-wave and H-reflex) and somatosensory evoked potential in latent phase of intermittent acute porphyria. Electromyogr Clin Neurophysiol 2000;40:73.

63. Ishida N, Fujita H, Fukuda Y, et al: Cloning and expression of the defective genes from a patient with δ-aminolevulinate dehydratase porphyria. J Clin Invest 1992;89:1431.

64. Deybach J-C, Puy HK: Porphobilinogen deaminase gene structure and molecular defects. J Bioenerg Biomembr 1995;27:197.

65. Astrin KH, Desnick RJ: Molecular basis of acute intermittent porphyria: Mutations and polymorphisms in the human hydroxymethylbilane synthase gene. Hum Mutat 1994;4:243.

66. Warner CA, Yoo H, Roberts AG, Desnick RJ: Congenital erythropoietic porphyria: Identification and expression of exonic mutations in the uroporphyrinogen III synthase gene. J Clin Invest 1992;89:693.

67. Martasek P, Camadro JM, Delfau-Larue M, et al: Molecular cloning, sequencing, and functional expression of a cDNA encoding human coproporphyrinogen oxidase. Proc Natl Acad Sci U S A 1994;91:3024.

68. Fujita H, Kondo M, Taketani S, et al: Characterization and expression of cDNA encoding coproporphyrinogen oxidase from a patient with hereditary coproporphyria. Hum Mol Genet 1994;3:1807.

69. Martasek P, Nordmann Y, Grandchamp B: Homozygous hereditary coproporphyria caused by an arginine to tryptophan substitution in coproporphyrinogen oxidase and common intragenic polymorphisms. Hum Mol Genet 1994;3:477.

70. Nishimura K, Taketani S, Inokuchi H: Cloning of a human cDNA for protoporphyrinogen oxidase by complementation in vivo of a hemG mutant of Escherichia coli. J Biol Chem 1995;270:8076.

71. Nordmann Y, Puy H, Da Silva V, et al: Acute intermittent porphyria: Prevalence of mutations in the porphobilinogen deaminase gene in blood donors in France. J Intern Med 1997;242:213.

72. Namba H, Narahara R, Tsuji K, et al: Assignment of human porphobilinogen deaminase to 1 Iq24. Iq24.2 by in situ hybridization and gene dosage studies. Cytogenet Cell Genet 1991;57:105.

73. Chretien S, Dubart A, Beaupain D, et al: Alternative transcription and splicing of the human porphobilinogen deaminase gene result either in tissue-specific or in housekeeping expression. Proc Natl Acad Sci U S A 1988;85:6.

74. Porcher C, Pitiot G, Plumb M, et al: Characterization of hypersensitive sites, protein-binding motifs, and regulatory elements in both promoters of the mouse porphobilinogen deaminase gene. J Biol Chem 1991;266:10562.

75. Porcher C, Picat C, Daegelen D, et al: Functional analysis of DNase-I hypersensitive sites at the mouse porphobilinogen deaminase gene locus. J Biol Chem 1995;270:17368.

76. Yoo HW, Warner CA, Chen CH, Desnick RJ: Hydroxymethylbilane synthase: Complete genomic sequence and amplifiable polymorphisms in the human gene. Genomics 1993;15:21.

77. Whatley SD, Woolf JR, Elder GH: Comparison of complementary and genomic DNA sequencing for the detection of mutations in the HMBS gene in British patients with acute intermittent porphyria: Identification of 25 novel mutations. Hum Genet 1999;104:505.

78. Brownlie PD, Lambert R, Louie GV, et al: The three-dimensional structures of mutants of porphobilinogen deaminase: Toward an understanding of the structural basis of acute intermittent porphyria. Protein Sci 1994;3:1644.

79. Shoolingin-Jordan PM: Porphobilinogen deaminase and uroporphyrinogen III synthase: Structure, molecular biology, and mechanism. J Bioenerg Biomembr 1995;27:181.

80. Grandchamp B, Picat C, Kauppinen R, et al: Molecular analysis of acute intermittent porphyria in a Finnish family with normal erythrocyte porphobilinogen deaminase. Eur J Clin Invest 1989;19:415.

81. Grandchamp B, Picat C, Mignotte V, et al: Tissue-specific splicing mutation in acute intermittent porphyria. Proc Natl Acad Sci U S A 1989;86:661.

82. Desnick RJ, Ostasiewicz LT, Tishler PA, Mustajoki P: Acute intermittent porphyria: Characterization of a novel mutation in the structural gene for porphobilinogen deaminase. J Clin Invest 1985;76:865.

83. Andersson C, Floderus Y, Wikberg A, Lithner F: The W198X and R173W mutations in the porphobilinogen deaminase gene in acute intermittent porphyria have higher clinical penetrance than R167W. A population-based study. Scand J Clin Lab Invest 2000;60:643.

84. Lamoril J, Puy H, Whatley SD, Martin C, et al: Characterization of mutations in the CPO gene in British patients demonstrates absence of genotype-phenotype correlation and identifies relationship between hereditary coproporphyria and harderoporphyria. Am J Hum Genet 2001;68:1130.

85. Whatley SD, Puy H, Morgan RR, et al: Variegate porphyria in Western Europe: Identification of PPOX gene mutations in 104 families, extent of allelic heterogeneity, and absence of correlation between phenotype and type of mutation. Am J Hum Genet 1999;65:984.

86. Tchernitchko D, Lamoril J, Puy H, et al: Evaluation of mutation screening by heteroduplex analysis in acute intermittent porphyria: Comparison with denaturing gradient gel electrophoresis. Clin Chim Acta 1999;279:133.

87. Beattie AD, Moore MR, Goldberg A, Ward RL: Acute intermittent porphyria: Response of tachycardia and hypertension to propranolol. Br Med J 1973;3:257.

88. Bonkowsky HL, Tschudy DP: Hazard of propranolol in treatment of acute porphyria. Br Med J 1974;4:47.

89. Bloomer JR, Berk PD, Bonkowsky HL, et al: Blood volume and bilirubin production in acute intermittent porphyria. N Engl J Med 1971;284:17.

90. Stein JA, Tschudy DP: Acute intermittent porphyria: A clinical and biochemical study of 46 patients. Medicine 1970;49:1.

91. Bonkowsky HL, Tschudy DP, Collins A, et al: Repression of the overproduction of porphyrin precursors in acute intermittent porphyria by intravenous infusions of hematin. Proc Natl Acad Sci U S A 1971;68:2725.

92. Watson CJ, Pierach CA, Bossenmaier I, Cardinal R: Postulated deficiency of hepatic heme and repair by hematin infusions in the "inducible" hepatic porphyrias. Proc Natl Acad Sci U S A 1977;74:2118.

93. Lamon JM, Frykholm BC, Hess RA, Tschudy DP: Hematin therapy for acute porphyria. Medicine 1979;58:252.

94. Bissell DM: Treatment of acute hepatic porphyria with hematin. J Hepatol 1988;6:1.

95. Goetsch CA, Bissell DM: Instability of hematin used in the treatment of acute hepatic porphyria. N Engl J Med 1986;315:235.

96. Jones RL: Hematin-derived anticoagulant: Generation in vitro and in vivo. J Exp Med 1986;163:724.

97. Tenhunen R, Tokola O, Linden IB: Haem arginate: A new stable haem compound. J Pharm Pharmacol 1987;39:780.

98. Dhar GJ, Bossenmaier I, Petryka ZJ: Effects of hematin in hepatic porphyria. Further studies. Ann Intern Med 1975;83:20.

99. Bosch EP, Pierach CA, Bossenmaier I, et al: Effect of hematin in porphyric neuropathy. Neurology 1977;27:1053.

100. McColl KE, Moore MR, Thompson GG, Goldberg A: Treatment with haematin in acute hepatic porphyria. Q J Med 1981;198:161.

101. Herrick AL, Moore MR, McColl KEL, et al: Controlled trial of haem arginate in acute hepatic porphyria. Lancet 1989;1:1295.

102. Dhar GJ, Bossenmaier I, Cardinal R: Transitory renal failure following rapid administration of a relatively large amount of hematin in a patient with acute intermittent porphyria in clinical remission. Acta Med Scand 1978;203:437.

103. Morris DL, Dudley MD, Pearson RD: Coagulopathy associated with hematin treatment for acute intermittent porphyria. Ann Intern Med 1981;95:700.

104. Glueck R, Green D, Cohen I, Ts'ao C: Hematin: Unique effects on hemostasis. Blood 1983;61:243.

105. Anderson KE, Spitz IM, Bardin CW, Kappas A: A gonadotropin releasing hormone analogue prevents cyclical attacks of porphyria. Arch Intern Med 1990;150:1469.

106. Herrick AL, McColl KE, Wallace AM, et al: LHRH analogue treatment for the prevention of premenstrual attacks of acute porphyria. Q J Med 1990;75:355.

107. Perlroth MG, Marver HS, Tschudy DP: Oral contraceptive agents and the management of acute intermittent porphyria. JAMA 1965;94:1037.

108. Lamon JM, Bennett M, Frykholm BC, Tschudy DP: Prevention of acute porphyric attack by intravenous hematin. Lancet 1978;2:492.

109. Hughes MJ, Rifkind AB: Danazol, a new steroidal inducer of δ-aminolevulinic acid synthetase. J Clin Endocrinol Metab 1981;52:549.

110. Lucas MJ, Leveno KJ, Cunningham FG: A comparison of magnesium sulfate with phenytoin for the prevention of eclampsia. New Engl J Med 1995;333:201.

111. Taylor RL: Magnesium sulfate for AIP seizures. Neurology 1981;31:1371.

112. Larson AW, Wasserstrom WR, Felsher BF, Shih JC: Posttraumatic epilepsy and acute intermittent porphyria: Effects of phenytoin, carbamazepine, and clonazepam. Neurology 1978;28:824.

113. Magnussen CR, Doherty JM, Hess RA, Tschudy DP: Grand mal seizures and acute intermittent porphyria: The problem of differential diagnosis and treatment. Neurology 1975;25:1121.

114. Schoenfeld N, Greenblat Y, Epstein O, Atsmon A: The influence of carbamazepine on the heme biosynthetic pathway. Biochem Med 1985;34:280.

115. Morgan CJ, Badawy AA: Effects of acute carbamazepine administration on haem metabolism in rat liver. Biochem Pharmacol 1992;43:1473.

116. Tatum WO, Zachariah SB: Gabapentin treatment of seizures in acute intermittent porphyria. Neurology 1995;45:1216.

117. Zadra M, Grandi R, Erli LC, et al: Treatment of seizures in acute intermittent porphyria: Safety and efficacy of gabapentin. Seizure 1998;7:415.

118. Hahn M, Gildemeister OS, Krauss GL, et al: Effects of new anticonvulsant medications on porphyrin synthesis in cultured liver cells: Potential implications for patients with acute porphyria. Neurology 1997;49:97.

119. Livingston S, Pearson PH: Bromides in the treatment of epilepsy in children. J Dis Child 1953;86:717.

120. Woody RC: Bromide therapy for pediatric seizure disorder intractable to other antiepileptic drugs. J Child Neurol 1990;5:65.

121. Okuda K, Yasuhara A, Kamei A, et al: Successful control with bromide of two patients with malignant migrating partial seizures in infancy. Brain Dev 2000;22:56.

122. Ryan M, Baumann RJ: Use and monitoring of bromides in epilepsy treatment. Pediatr Neurol 1999;21:523.

123. Wuth O: Rational bromide treatment. JAMA 1927;88:2013.

124. Kasahara N, Dozy AM, Kan YW: Tissue-specific targeting of retroviral vectors through ligand-receptor interactions. Science 1994;266:1373.

125. Gupta S, Aragona E, Vemuru RP, et al: Permanent engraftment and function of hepatocytes delivered to the liver: Implications for gene therapy and liver repopulation. Hepatology 1991;14:144.

126. Pages JC, Andreoletti M, Bennoun M, et al: Efficient retroviral-mediated gene transfer into primary culture of murine and human hepatocytes: Expression of the LDL receptor. Hum Gene Ther 1995;6:21.

127. Sorenson AW, With TK: Persistent pareses after porphyric attacks. Acta Med Scand 1971;190:219.

128. Tishler PV, Woodward B, O'Connor J, et al: High prevalence of intermittent acute porphyria in a psychiatric patient population. Am J Psych 1985;142:1430.

129. Jara-Prado A, Yescas P, Sanchez FJ, et al: Prevalence of acute intermittent porphyria in a Mexican psychiatric population. Arch Med Res 2000;31:404.

130. Schwartz S, Berg MH, Bossenmaier I, Dinsmore H: Determination of porphyrins in biological materials. Methods Biochem Anal 1960;8:221.

131. Muller WE, Snyder SH: δ-Aminolevulinic acid: Influences on synaptic GABA receptor binding may explain CNS symptoms of porphyria. Ann Neurol 1977;2:340.

132. Gorchein A, Webber R: Delta-aminolevulinic acid in plasma, cerebrospinal fluid, saliva and erythrocytes: Studies in normal, uraemic and porphyric subjects. Clin Sci 1987;72:103.

133. Russell VA, Lamm MCL, Taljaard JJF: Effects of δ-aminolaevulinic acid, porphobilinogen and structurally related amino acids on 2-deoxy-glucose uptake in cultured neurons. Neurochem Res 1982;7:1009.

134. Helson L, Braverman S, Mangiardi J: δ-Aminolevulinic acid effects on neuronal and glial tumor cell lines. Neurochem Res 1993;18:1255.

135. Brennan MJW, Cantrill RC: Delta-Aminolaevulinic acid and amino acid neurotransmitters. Mol Cell Biochem 1981;38:49.

136. Bornstein JC, Pickett JB, Diamond I: Inhibition of the evoked release of acetylcholine by the porphyrin precursor delta-aminolevulinic acid. Neurology 1979;5:94.

137. Percy VA, Lamm MC, Taljaard JJ: Delta-aminolaevulinic acid uptake, toxicity, and effect on (14C) gamma-aminobutyric acid uptake into neurons and glia in culture. J Neurochem 1981;36:69.

138. Shanley BC, Percy VA, Neethling AC: Pathogenesis of neural manifestations in acute porphyria. S Afr Med J 1977;51:458.

139. Emanuelli T, Pagel FW, Alves LB, et al: 5-Aminolevulinic acid inhibits (3H)muscimol binding to human and rat brain synaptic membranes. Neurochem Res 2001;26:101.

CHAPTER

65

Friedreich's Ataxia and Iron Metabolism

Massimo Pandolfo

Friedreich's ataxia (FA) is an autosomal recessive disease characterized by progressive neurologic and cardiac abnormalities. It has a prevalence of around 2×10^{-5} in Caucasians, accounting for one half of the overall hereditary ataxia cases and three fourths of those with onset before age 25 years in this ethnic group. There are local clusters of FA owing to a founder effect, such as those observed in Rimouski, Québec, and in Kathikas-Arodhes, Cyprus. FA may not exist in nonwhite populations.

The first symptoms usually appear in childhood, but age of onset may vary from infancy to adulthood. Atrophy of sensory and cerebellar pathways causes ataxia, dysarthria, fixation instability, deep sensory loss, and loss of tendon reflexes. Corticospinal degeneration leads to muscular weakness and extensor plantar responses. Hypertrophic cardiomyopathy may contribute to disability and cause premature death. Other common problems include kyphoscoliosis, pes cavus, and, in 10% of patients, diabetes mellitus.

The FA gene *(FRDA)* encodes a small mitochondrial protein, frataxin, which is produced in insufficient amounts in the disease as a consequence of a GAA triplet repeat expansion in the first intron of the gene. Frataxin deficiency leads to excessive free radical production in mitochondria, progressive iron accumulation in these organelles, and dysfunction of Fe-S center containing enzymes (in particular, respiratory complexes I, II, and III, and aconitase).

CLINICAL FEATURES

Rigorous diagnostic criteria were established in the late 1970s and early 1980 by the Québec Collaborative group and by Anita Harding. After the gene discovery in 1996,

the phenotype has been extended beyond the limits fixed by these criteria (Table 65–1).

The typical age of onset of FA is around puberty, but it may be earlier or later, even in late adult life (late-onset Friedreich's ataxia, LOFA). Age of onset may dramatically vary within a sibship, a phenomenon now in part explained by the dynamic nature of the underlying mutation.

Gait instability and generalized clumsiness are the most frequent symptoms at onset. Typically, the patient is a child who starts to sway when walking and falls easily. The child may be active in sports and have shown no clues of the impending neurologic illness. More commonly, the child is considered "clumsy" for some time before the overt appearance of symptoms. Scoliosis, often considered to be idiopathic, may precede the onset of ataxia. Rare patients (5%) are diagnosed with idiopathic hypertrophic cardiomyopathy and treated as such for up to 3 years before the appearance of neurologic symptoms.

Mixed cerebellar and sensory ataxia is the hallmark of the disease. It begins as truncal ataxia causing swaying, imbalance, and falls. At the very beginning, balance and gait abnormalities are subtle and may be revealed only as a difficulty in tandem gait and in standing on one foot. Subsequently, gait becomes frankly ataxic, with irregular steps, veering, and difficulty in turning. Loss of upright stability becomes evident when standing with feet close together and is worsened by eye closure (positive Romberg sign). With further progression, gait becomes broad-based, with frequent losses of balance, at first requiring intermittent support (furniture, walls, an accompanying person's arm), then a cane, then a walker. Patients become completely unable to stand with feet together, then need support even with their feet apart. Eventually, on average 10 to 15 years after onset, patients

TABLE 65–1.

Diagnostic Criteria for FRDA		*Frequency of Signs and Symptoms Observed in 59 Consecutive Patients with a Positive Molecular Test for Friedreich's Ataxia*	
Autosomal recessive inheritance			
Onset before age 25			
Within five years of onset		Ataxia	100%
Limb and truncal ataxia showing evolution in a two-year period		Deep sensory loss in lower limbs	89%
Absent tendon reflexes in legs		Dysarthria	83%
Extensor plantar responses		Cardiomyopathy	79%
Motor NCV >40 m/sec in upper limbs with small or absent SAPs		Lower limb areflexia	75%
Five years after onset		Square-wave jerks	75%
Above criteria, plus dysarthria		Upper-limb areflexia	72%
Additional criteria, not essential for diagnosis, present in >two thirds of cases		Scoliosis	68%
Scoliosis		Babinski sign	62%
Pyramidal weakness in legs		Pes cavus	58%
Absent reflexes in upper limbs		Weakness in lower limbs	46%
Distal loss of joint position and vibration sense in lower limbs		Distal amyotrophy	26%
Abnormal EKG		Decreased muscle tone in lower limbs	22%
Other criteria, present in <50% of cases		Carbohydrate intolerance	18%
Nystagmus		Optic atrophy	13%
Optic atrophy		Cerebellar atrophy at MRI	11%
Deafness		Increased muscle tone in lower limbs	7%
Distal weakness and wasting		Hearing loss	6%
Pes cavus			
Diabetes			

lose the ability to walk, stand, and sit without support. Evolution is variable, however, and some patients with mild cases are still ambulatory decades after onset.

Limb ataxia appears after truncal ataxia. Fine-motor skills become impaired, with increasing difficulty in activities such as writing, dressing, and handling utensils. Dysmetria and intention tremor are evident. Ataxia is progressive and unremitting, though periods of relative stability are frequent at the beginning of the illness.

With rare exceptions, dysarthria appears within 5 years from clinical onset. It consists of slow, jerky speech with sudden utterances, and progresses until speech becomes almost unintelligible. Dysphagia, particularly for liquids, appears only with advanced disease. Modified foods, then a nasogastric tube or gastrostomy feedings are eventually required.

Loss of position and vibration sense is invariable, but may not be evident at onset. Perception of light touch, pain, and temperature, initially normal, tends to decrease with advancing disease. Loss of tendon reflexes in the lower limbs was considered essential for the diagnosis. However, a minority of patients with a positive molecular test for FA (FA with retained reflexes, FARR), have elicitable, sometimes even exaggerated reflexes with spasticity. Extensor plantar responses are found in most patients. Muscular weakness becomes severe only with advanced disease. Ataxia and not weakness is the primary cause for loss of ambulation. Even when patients become wheelchair-bound, they still maintain, on average, 70% of their normal strength in lower limbs. In general, the combination of sensory neuropathy and pyramidal tract degeneration results most often in the typical picture of areflexia associated with extensor plantar responses. However, sometimes one component prevails. Such partial pictures are usually observed in milder cases. Muscle tone is often normal at onset. However, with advancing pyramidal involvement and particularly when deambulation becomes severely impaired, many patients complain of spasms in the lower limbs, mostly nocturnal. Despite limited involvement of lower motor neurons, distal amyotrophy in the lower limbs and in the hands is frequent even early in the course of the disease. When patients are wheelchair-bound, disuse atrophy occurs.

The typical oculomotor abnormality of FA is fixation instability with square-wave jerks. Various combinations of cerebellar, vestibular, and brain stem oculomotor signs may be observed, but gaze-evoked nystagmus is uncommon and ophthalmoparesis does not occur. About 30% of patients develop optic atrophy, with or without visual impairment. Sensorineural hearing loss affects about 20% of patients. Optic atrophy and sensorineural hearing loss tend to be associated with each other.

Cognitive functions are well preserved, though there are reports of slowed information processing speed not accompanied by major prefrontal cortex and mood disorders. Accordingly, mental retardation and learning disabilities do not seem to be more prevalent in patients with FA than in the general population. On the other hand, FA, as any disease causing substantial physical disability, may have a substantial impact on academic, professional, and personal development if not properly managed.

Shortness of breath (40%) and palpitations (11%) are the most common symptoms of heart involvement. The electrocardiogram (EKG) shows inverted T-waves in essentially all patients, ventricular hypertrophy in most, conduction disturbances in about 10%, and supraventricular ectopic beats and atrial fibrillation on occasion. Repeated EKG recordings are the most sensitive test to detect FA cardiomyopathy. Echocardiography and Doppler-echocardiography demonstrate concentric hypertrophy of the ventricles (62%) or asymmetric septal hypertrophy (29%), with diastolic function abnormalities.

About 10% of FA patients develop diabetes mellitus, and 20% have carbohydrate intolerance. The mechanisms are complex, involving beta cell, atrophy, and peripheral insulin resistance. Oral hypoglycemic drugs may initially control some cases, but insulin is eventually necessary. Diabetes may increase the burden of disease, complicate the neurologic picture, and promote potentially fatal complications. Kyphoscoliosis may cause pain and cardiorespiratory problems. Pes cavus and pes equinovarus may further affect ambulation. Autonomic disturbances, most commonly cold and cyanotic legs and feet, become increasingly frequent as the disease advances. Parasympathetic abnormalities such as decreased heart rate variability parameters have been reported. Urgency of micturition is rare.

Variant Phenotypes

A positive molecular test for FA is found in up to 10% of patients with recessive or sporadic ataxia who do not fulfill the classical clinical diagnostic criteria for the disease. A reanalysis of these cases revealed that no clinical finding or combination of findings characterizes FA exclusively or is necessarily present in positive cases. Even

neurophysiologic evidence of axonal sensory neuropathy is very rarely absent in patients with a proven molecular diagnosis. Overall, however, the classic features of FA, including cardiomyopathy, are highly predictive of a positive test. Absence of cardiomyopathy and moderate to severe cerebellar cortical atrophy, demonstrated by MRI, appear to be the best predictors of a negative test. In the author's opinion, a molecular test for FA, along with MRI and neurophysiologic investigations, is indicated in the initial workup of all cases of sporadic or recessive degenerative ataxia, regardless of whether they fulfill the diagnostic criteria.

Neurophysiologic Investigations

Sensory nerve action potentials (SNAPs) are severely reduced or, most often, lost. Motor and sensory (when measurable) nerve conduction velocities (NCVs) are instead within or just below the normal range. These findings clearly distinguish an early case of FA from a case of hereditary demyelinating sensorimotor neuropathy. Degeneration of both peripheral and central sensory fibers also results in dispersion and delay of somatosensory evoked potentials (SEPs). Brain stem auditory evoked potentials (BAEPs), beginning from the most rostral component, wave V, progressively deteriorate in all patients. Visual evoked potentials (VEPs) are commonly (50% to 90%) reduced in amplitude with a normal P 100 latency. Central motor conduction velocity, determined by cortical magnetic stimulation, is slower than normal, and, contrary to sensory involvement, this slowing becomes more severe with increasing disease duration.

Biochemical Investigations

Attention is currently focused on iron metabolism and oxidative stress. Blood iron, iron-binding capacity, and ferritin are normal, but there is an increase in circulating transferrin receptors. In addition, several markers of oxidative stress are increased, including urinary 8-hydroxy-2'-deoxyguanosine (8OH2'dG), a marker of oxidative DNA damage, and plasma malondialdehyde, a marker of lipid peroxidation.

Neuroimaging

The characteristic neuroimaging finding in FA is the thinning of the cervical spinal cord. It can be detected on sagittal and axial magnetic resonance (MRI) images, along with signal abnormalities in the posterior and lateral columns. Brain stem, cerebellum, and cerebrum are apparently normal, but quantitative studies showed that these structures are smaller in FA patients compared with healthy controls. The extent of this diffuse atrophy correlates with clinical severity. Vermian and lobar cerebellar atrophy only occurs in more severe and more advanced cases and is usually mild. In fact, marked cerebellar atrophy early in the course of the disease is a strong predictor of a negative molecular test for FA. However, TC-HMPAO single-photon emission computed tomography (SPECT) reveals a decrease in cerebellar blood flow, more than expected for the limited degree of atrophy. Positron emission tomography (PET) scans with fluorodeoxyglucose (FDG) as tracer reveal an increased glucose uptake in the brain of FA patients who are still ambulatory. As the disease progresses, glucose consumption decreases and patients lose their ability to walk, eventually becoming subnormal. Although not yet fully explained, this abnormality may relate to mitochondrial dysfunction.

Proton magnetic resonance spectroscopy (^{1}H-MRS) is now used in FA. It is a noninvasive technique that does not require the use of radioactive tracers, and it is able to quantify in vivo metabolites present in millimolar concentrations with a spatial resolution down to a few cubic centimeters. The neuronal marker N-acetyl-aspartate (NAA), lactate, choline (Cho), and creatine-phosphocreatine (Cr) are metabolites that can be measured by this technique. In FA, MRS analysis of skeletal muscle and heart showed a reduced rate of ATP synthesis after exercise, which is inversely correlated to GAA expansion sizes, and is improved by coenzyme Q10 treatment. There are no published data for the brain.

Prognosis

On average, typical FA patients become wheelchair-bound 15 years after onset. Milder cases may remain ambulatory much longer; severe cases may lose deambulation in childhood. Early onset and left ventricular hypertrophy predict a faster rate of progression. The burden of neurologic impairment, cardiomyopathy, and diabetes if present, shortens life expectancy. Despite older studies indicating that most patients die in their thirties, survival may be significantly prolonged with appropriate treatment of diabetes and cardiac symptoms (particularly arrhythmias) and prevention and management of complications resulting from prolonged neurologic disability. Carefully assisted patients may live several more decades.

DIAGNOSIS

Nonhereditary diseases may cause early-onset, progressive ataxia with a chronic course. MRI will reveal posterior fossa tumors and malformations, including platybasia and basilar impression, as well as the lesions of multiple sclerosis. Detection of antigliadin and antiendomysial antibodies points to a diagnosis of gluten sensitivity, which may cause a progressive and treatable cerebellar syndrome even in the absence of gastrointestinal symptoms and signs of malabsorption.

Rare metabolic disorders may resemble FA. In particular, a FA-like clinical picture occurs in some cases of isolated vitamin E deficiency, an autosomal recessive disease due to defective conjugation of the vitamin to lipoproteins. Differentiating features of isolated vitamin E deficiency include a less severe peripheral neuropathy, the common occurrence of nodding head tremor and pigmentary retinopathy, and lack of cardiomyopathy. A similar neurologic picture may occur when vitamin E deficiency is secondary to a genetic disorder of lipoproteins (e.g., abetalipoproteinemia) or to malabsorption.

Early-onset cerebellar ataxia (EOCA) with retained reflexes constitutes a heterogeneous category of disorders that even includes atypical FA cases. Again, early prominent cerebellar atrophy is found only in non-FA cases. The recent mapping of two ataxia-oculomotor apraxia loci and the cloning of one of them now provide a molecular basis for more EOCA cases.

DNA testing is the gold standard to confirm a clinical diagnosis of FA, for carrier detection and for prenatal diagnosis. It is discussed in the clinical and molecular genetics section.

PATHOLOGY

Central Nervous System

Degeneration of the posterior columns of the spinal cord is the hallmark of the disease. Atrophy is more severe in the Goll than in the Burdach tract, therefore the longest fibers originating more caudally are most affected. The spinocerebellar tracts, the dorsal more than the ventral, and their neurons of origin, Clarke's column, also become atrophic. In the brain stem, atrophy involves the gracilis and cuneate nuclei and the medial lemnisci, particularly in their ventral portion deriving from the gracile nuclei, as well as the cranial nerve sensory nuclei and entering roots of the V, IX and X nerves, the descending trigeminal tracts, the solitary tracts, and the accessory cuneate nuclei, corresponding to Clarke's column in the spinal cord. Overall, FA severely affects the sensory systems providing information to the brain and cerebellum about the position and speed of body segments. The motor system is directly affected as well: the long crossed and uncrossed corticospinal motor tracts are atrophic, more so distally, suggesting a "dying back." There is a variable loss of pyramidal neurons in the motor cortex, while motor neurons in the brain stem and in the ventral horns of the spinal cord are less affected. In the cerebellum, cortical atrophy occurs late and is mild, while atrophy of the dentate nuclei and of superior cerebellar pedunculi is prominent. Quantitative analysis of synaptic terminals indicates a loss of contacts over Purkinje cell bodies and proximal dendrites. The auditory system and the optic nerves and tracts are variably affected. The external pallidus and subthalamic nuclei may show a moderate cell loss. Finally, since many patients with FA die as a consequence of heart disease, widespread hypoxic changes and focal infarcts are often found in the central nervous system (CNS).

In the peripheral nervous system, the major abnormalities occur in the dorsal root ganglia (DRG), where a loss of large primary sensory neurons is observed, accompanied by proliferation of capsule cells that form clumps called "Residualknötchen" of Nageotte. Loss of large myelinated sensory fibers is prominent in peripheral nerves, while the fine, unmyelinated fibers are well preserved. Interstitial connective tissue is increased. This sensory axonal neuropathy is an early event in the course of the disease and, according to some authors, is scarcely progressive.

Heart

Ventricular walls and interventricular septum are thickened. Hypertrophic cardiomyocytes are found early in the disease and are intermingled with normal-appearing ones. Then, atrophic, degenerating, even necrotic fibers progressively appear; there is diffuse and focal inflammatory cell infiltration; and connective tissue increases. In the late stage of the disease, with extensive fibrosis, the cardiomyopathy becomes dilatative. A variable number of cardiomyocytes, from less than 1% to more than 10%, show intracellular iron deposits. This is a specific finding in FA and a direct consequence of the basic biochemical defect.

Other Organs

More than three fourths of FA patients have kyphoscoliosis, mostly as a double thoracolumbar curve resembling the idiopathic form. Pes cavus, pes equinovarus, and clawing of the toes are found in about one half of the cases. Patients with diabetes (about 10%) often show a loss of islet cells in the pancreas, which is not accompanied by the autoimmune inflammatory reaction found in type I diabetes.

CLINICAL AND MOLECULAR GENETICS

Gene Structure and Expression

The FA gene *(FRDA)* is localized in the proximal long arm of chromosome 9 and is composed of 7 exons spread over 95 kb of genomic DNA. The major (and probably only functionally relevant mRNA) is 1.3 kb and corresponds to the first 5 exons, numbered 1 to 5a. The encoded protein, predicted to contain 210 amino acids, is called frataxin. In adult humans, frataxin mRNA is most abundant in the heart and spinal cord, followed by liver, skeletal muscle, and pancreas. In mouse embryos, expression starts in the neuroepithelium at embryonic day 10.5 (E10.5), then reaches its highest level at E14.5. Into the postnatal period, the highest levels are found in the spinal cord, particularly at the thoracolumbar level, and in the dorsal root ganglia. The developing brain is also very rich in frataxin mRNA, which is abundant in the proliferating neural cells in the periventricular zone, in the cortical plates, and in the ganglionic eminence.

The Intronic GAA Triplet Repeat Expansion

FA is the consequence of frataxin deficiency. Most patients are homozygous for the expansion of a GAA triplet repeat sequence (TRS) in the first intron; 5% are heterozygous for a GAA expansion and a point mutation in the frataxin gene. Repeats in normal chromosomes contain up to about 40 triplets; there are 90 to more than 1000 triplets in FA chromosomes. Expanded alleles show meiotic and mitotic instability. Lengths of the GAA TRS corresponding to pathologic FRDA alleles can adopt a triple helical structure in physiologic conditions and inhibit transcription in vivo. Two triplexes may associate to form a novel DNA structure called sticky DNA that has been shown to inhibit transcription in vitro by sequestering RNA polymerase.

As expected by the fact that smaller expansions allow a higher residual expression of the frataxin gene, the severity and age of onset of the disease are in part determined by the size of the expanded GAA repeat, in particular of the smaller allele. A number of studies have shown a direct correlation between the size of GAA repeats and earlier age of onset, earlier age when confined to a wheelchair, more rapid rate of disease progression, and presence of nonobligatory disease manifestations indicative of more widespread degeneration. However, differences in GAA expansions account for only about 50% of the variability in age of onset. Other factors that influence the phenotype may include somatic mosaicism for expansion sizes, variations in the frataxin gene, modifier genes, and environmental factors.

Frataxin Point Mutations

About 2% of FA chromosomes carry GAA repeat of normal length, but have missense, nonsense, or splice site mutations ultimately affecting the frataxin coding sequence. FA patients carrying a frataxin point mutation are in all cases compound heterozygotes for a GAA repeat expansion. Therefore, as GAA expansion homozygotes, they express a small amount of normal frataxin that is thought to be essential for survival (see Animal Models section). About 2% of the FA chromosomes have a normal GAA repeat but carry missense, nonsense, or splice site mutations ultimately affecting the frataxin coding sequence. All affected individuals with a point mutation so far identified are heterozygous for an expanded GAA repeat on the other homologue of chromosome 9. Missense mutations have so far been identified only in the C-terminal portion of the protein corresponding to the mature intramitochondrial form of frataxin. Nonsense and most missense mutations result in a typical FA phenotype, while a few missense mutations are associated with milder atypical phenotypes with slow progression, suggesting that the mutated proteins preserve some residual function. The G130V mutation in particular is associated with early onset but slow progression, no dysarthria, mild limb ataxia, and retained reflexes. For unclear reasons, optic atrophy is more frequent in patients with point mutations of any kind (50%).

DNA Testing

Polymerase chain reaction (PCR) or Southern blot can be used to directly detect the intronic GAA expansion. PCR requires only a small amount of DNA, but high-quality DNA is extremely important. Ambiguous results, particularly in heterozygote detection, can be resolved by subsequent hybridization of PCR products with an oligonucleotide probe containing a GAA or CTT repeat. Southern blot requires more DNA and is less accurate for determining the number of repeats, but it will not miss a heterozygote when heterozygosity detection is crucial.

The question of the lower limit for an expansion to be pathologic, so far reported to be 66 triplets, is not so critical in FA as in dominant unstable repeat diseases. The diagnosis is anyway strongly supported when the other chromosome carries a fully expanded GAA repeat or a frataxin point mutation. In vitro data indicate that repeats exceeding about 50 triplets start to adopt a triplex structure and may form sticky DNA, suggesting that they may be pathologic. Length and sequence of the repeat must both be taken into account in uncertain cases. Interruptions of the GAA triplet repeat sequence prevent the formation of a triplex structure and sticky DNA in vitro. In vivo, interrupted or variant repeats are occasionally found and may be nonpathologic up to the equivalent of 130 triplets.

Testing for point mutation is done in research laboratories. No mutation in the coding sequence could be identified in up to 40% of compound heterozygous patients in some series. Some of them may actually have a different disease and carry a GAA expansion by chance, given its high frequency (1:90) in Caucasians. One such case has been documented.

Individuals with an FA-like phenotype but no GAA expansion most likely have mutations at a different locus. Homozygosity for frataxin point mutations has never been reported. If such cases exist, they should have consanguineous parents, but biologic reasons argue against their existence; mouse models demonstrated that complete absence of frataxin or the presence of only abnormal frataxin is incompatible with life.

Frataxin Function

Frataxin does not resemble any protein of known function. It is highly conserved during evolution, with homologues in mammals, invertebrates, yeast, and plants. The

protein is targeted to the mitochondrial matrix. Most of our knowledge about the functional role of frataxin comes from the investigation of yeast cells in which the frataxin homologue gene (YFH1) has been deleted. $\Delta yfh1$ strains progressively lose respiratory competence and mitochondrial DNA (rho°). Iron accumulates in mitochondria, more then tenfold in excess of wild type, at the expense of cytosolic iron. These cells become hypersensitive to H_2O_2, indicating the occurrence of Fenton chemistry. Loss of respiratory competence requires the presence of iron in the culture medium, and occurs more rapidly as iron concentration is increased, suggesting that permanent mitochondrial damage is the consequence of iron toxicity. Normal human frataxin is able to complement the defect in $\Delta yfh1$ cells, while mutated human frataxin is unable to do so, indicating that the function of yfh1p is conserved in human frataxin. It is interesting that the expression of yeast and human frataxin is not regulated by iron levels, and its mRNA does not contain an iron-responsive element. A series of publications described the ternary structure of its bacterial homologue, CyaY. All studies agree that mature frataxin is a compact, globular protein containing an N-terminal α helix, a middle β sheet region composed of seven β strands, a second α helix, and a C-terminal coil. The α helices are folded upon the β sheet, with the C-terminal coil filling a groove between the two α helices. On the outside, a ridge of negatively charged residues and a patch of hydrophobic residues are highly conserved suggesting that they interact with a large ligand, probably a protein. However, experiments aimed at identifying a protein partner of frataxin, mostly by using the yeast two-hybrid method, have so far failed. Frataxin does not have any feature resembling known iron-binding sites, and the NMR study failed to identify any structural change after iron addition. This is in contrast with biochemical data that suggested that frataxin binds iron in a high molecular weight complex, possibly protecting it from free radicals. This issue needs to be resolved if the function of frataxin is to be understood.

Hypotheses on the Pathogenesis of Friedreich's Ataxia

Altered iron metabolism, oxidative stress, and mitochondrial dysfunction all occur in FA. Iron accumulation has been detected in myocardial cells and in the dentate nucleus. There is a moderate but significant increase of mitochondrial iron in fibroblasts. A high level of circulating transferrin receptor suggests a relative cytosolic iron deficit, as observed in the yeast model. Oxidative stress is demonstrated by lipid peroxidation and oxidative DNA damage products in plasma and urine and by the sensitivity of FA fibroblasts to low doses of H_2O_2. As for mitochondrial dysfunction, the same Fe-S enzyme defects found in $\Delta yfh1$ yeast (deficit of respiratory complexes I, II, and III, and of aconitase) are found in affected tissues from FA patients. In vivo, MRS analysis of skeletal muscle shows a reduced rate of ATP synthesis, which is inversely correlated to GAA expansion sizes, and may be improved by coenzyme Q10. Increased free radical production was directly shown in P19 cells engineered to produce reduced levels of frataxin. Furthermore, these cells as well as in fibroblasts from FA patients show abnormal antioxidant responses. In particular, an increase in mitochondrial SOD triggered by iron in normal cells is blunted in FA cells. Finally, abnormal free radical production during differentiation of multipotent frataxin-deficient cells adversely affects neuronal differentiation and increases apoptosis, an observation that may have implications for the human disease.

ANIMAL MODELS

The early embryonic lethality of frataxin KO mice has complicated the effort to generate a vertebrate animal model of the disease. A viable mouse model was eventually obtained through a conditional gene-targeting approach. A heart and striated muscle frataxin-deficient line and a line with more generalized, including neural, frataxin deficiency were recently generated. These mice reproduce important progressive pathophysiologic and biochemical features of the human disease. These features are cardiac hypertrophy without skeletal muscle involvement in the heart and striated muscle frataxin-deficient line; large sensory neuron dysfunction without alteration of the small sensory and motor neurons in the more generalized frataxin-deficient line; and deficient activities of complexes I to III of the respiratory chain and of the aconitases in both lines. Time-dependent intramitochondrial iron accumulation occurs in the heart of the heart and striated muscle frataxin-deficient line. These animals provide an important resource for pathophysiologic studies and for testing of new treatments. However, they still do not mimic the situation occurring in the human disease because conditional gene targeting leads to complete loss of frataxin in some cells at a specific time in development, while FA is characterized by partial frataxin deficiency in all cells and throughout life. Therefore, there is still a need to develop new animal models of the disease. An attempt was made to create a model by generating GAA expansion knock-in mice, but animals carrying a GAA expansion in heterozygosity with a KO allele still make enough frataxin (20% of normal) to present a normal phenotype.

THERAPY

There is no established treatment to stop or slow down the degenerative process, but new knowledge derived from the characterization of the FA gene product is starting to change this picture. Based on the hypothesis that iron-mediated oxidative damage plays a major role in the pathogenesis of FA, removal of excess mitochondrial iron

and/or antioxidant treatment may in principle be attempted. Removal of excess mitochondrial iron is problematic with currently available drugs. Desferrioxamine (DFO) is effective in chelating iron in the extracellular fluid and cytosol, not directly in mitochondria. Furthermore, DFO toxicity may be higher when there is no overall iron overload. Thus, chelation therapy has a number of unknowns: It is probably better tested in pilot trials involving a small number of closely monitored patients. Iron depletion by phlebotomy, though less risky, presents the same uncertainties concerning possible efficacy. As far as antioxidants are concerned, these include a long list of molecules with specific mechanisms of action and pharmacokinetic properties. To have the potential to be effective in FA, an antioxidant must protect against damage caused by the free radicals involved in the disease (in particular OH); act in the mitochondrial compartment; and cross the blood-brain barrier. At this time, CoQ derivatives, like its short-chain analog idebenone, appear to be interesting molecules and are the object of pilot studies. These molecules seem to be particularly effective in treating FA cardiomyopathy because they reduce heart size and activate ATP production, as shown by MRS.

Attempts at symptomatic treatment utilize drugs affecting neurotransmitters acting in the cerebellar circuitry. Tested compounds include cholinergic agonists (physostigmine and choline), neuropeptides (TRH), serotoninergic agonists (5-OH tryptophan and buspirone), and the dopaminergic drug amantadine. Overall, results have not been encouraging.

Rehabilitation programs should include exercises aimed at maximizing the residual capacity of motor control. Orthopedic interventions are sometimes necessary, including surgical correction of severe scoliosis and correction of foot deformity in patients who can walk.

FUTURE RESEARCH

New knowledge on frataxin function and FA pathogenesis is needed to progress toward an effective treatment of the disease. The biochemistry of frataxin needs to be elucidated and its still elusive primary function identified. The functional role of frataxin at the cell biology level needs to be better defined, in particular its role in iron metabolism, antioxidant defenses, and mitochondrial function. The effects of frataxin deficiency also have to be better investigated. Attention must be focused on subtle consequences, such as perturbed intracellular signaling, as well as physical consequences of abnormal iron distribution and free radical production. Pharmacologic agents that counteract specific effects of frataxin deficiency need to be identified. In the long term, gene replacement, protein replacement, or reactivation of the expression of endogenous frataxin may be cures and are worth exploring. Regarding the last possibility, studies on the structure and properties of the GAA repeat expansion may also be essential.

REFERENCES

1. Adamec J, Rusnak F, Owen WG, et al: Iron-dependent self-assembly of recombinant yeast frataxin: Implications for Friedreich ataxia. Am J Hum Genet 2000;67:549–562.

2. Babcock M, de Silva D, Oaks R, et al: Regulation of mitochondrial iron accumulation by Yfh1, a putative homolog of frataxin. Science 1997;276: 1709–1712.

3. Campuzano V, Montermini L, Moltó MD, et al: Friedreich ataxia: Autosomal recessive disease caused by an intronic GAA triplet repeat expansion. Science 1996;271:1423–1427.

4. Chamberlain S, Shaw J, Rowland A, et al: Mapping of mutation causing Friedreich ataxia to human chromosome 9. Nature 1988;334:248–250.

5. Cossée M, Dürr A, Schmitt M, et al: Frataxin point mutations and clinical presentation of compound heterozygous FA patients. Ann Neurol 1999;45: 200–206.

6. Cossée M, Puccio H, Gansmuller A, et al: Inactivation of the FA mouse gene leads to early embryonic lethality without iron accumulation. Hum Mol Genet 2000;9:1219–1226.

7. Dhe-Paganon S, Shigeta R, Chi YI, et al: Crystal structure of human frataxin. J Biol Chem 2000;275: 30753–30756.

8. Geoffroy G, Barbeau A, Breton G, et al: Clinical description and roentgenologic evaluation of patients with Friedreich ataxia. Can J Neurol Sci 1976;3: 279–286.

9. Harding AE: Friedreich ataxia: A clinical and genetic study of 90 families with an analysis of early diagnosis criteria and intrafamilial clustering of clinical features. Brain 1981;104:589–620.

10. Jiralerspong S, Ge B, Hudson TJ, Pandolfo M: Manganese superoxide dismutase induction by iron is impaired in FA cells. FEBS Lett 2001;509:101–105.

11. Lodi R, Hart PE, Rajagopalan B, et al: Antioxidant treatment improves in vivo cardiac and skeletal muscle bioenergetics in patients with Friedreich's ataxia. Ann Neurol 2001;49:590–596.

12. Miranda C, Santos MM, Ohshima K, et al: Frataxin knock-in mice. FEBS Lett 2002;512:291–297.

13. Musco G, Stier G, Kolmerer B, et al: Towards a structural understanding of Friedreich ataxia: The solution structure of frataxin. Structure Fold Des 2000;8:695–707.

14. Puccio H, Simon D, Cossée M, et al: Mouse models for FA exhibit cardiomyopathy, sensory nerve defect and Fe-S enzyme deficiency followed by intramitochondrial iron deposits. Nat Genet 2001;27:181–186.

15. Rötig A, deLonlay P, Chretien D, et al: Frataxin gene expansion causes aconitase and mitochondrial iron-sulfur protein deficiency in Friedreich ataxia. Nat Genet 1997;17: 215–217.

16. Rustin P, von Kleist-Retzow JC, Chantrel-Groussard K, et al: Effect of idebenone on cardiomyopathy in Friedreich ataxia: A preliminary study. Lancet 1999; 354:477–479.

17. Sakamoto N, Chastain PD, Parniewski P, et al: Sticky DNA: Self-association properties of long GAA• TTC repeats in R• R• Y triplex structures from Friedreich ataxia. Mol Cell 1999;3:465–475.

18. Sakamoto NK, Ohshima KL, Montermini LM, et al: Sticky DNA, a self-associated complex formed at long GAA• TTC repeats in intron 1 of the Frataxin gene, inhibits transcription. J Biol Chem 2001;276: 27171–27177.

19. Santos M, Ohshima K, Pandolfo M: Frataxin deficiency enhances apoptosis in cells differentiating into neuroectoderm. Hum Mol Genet 2001;10:1935–1944.

Disorders of Copper Metabolism: Wilson Disease and Menkes Disease

John H. Menkes

WILSON DISEASE

Wilson disease (WD) is an autosomal recessive disorder of copper metabolism associated with cirrhosis of the liver and degenerative changes in the basal ganglia. The first description of the disease and its pathologic anatomy was provided by Wilson in 1912.[1] For many years it was believed that WD was due to ceruloplasmin deficiency. It has now become evident that absence of ceruloplasmin causes aceruloplasminemia, which results in a severe disorder of iron metabolism presenting during the fourth decade of life with dysarthria, dystonia, and dementia.[2]

Molecular and Biochemical Pathology

Copper homeostasis is an important biologic process. By balancing intake and excretion, the body avoids copper toxicity on the one hand, and on the other hand ensures the availability of adequate amounts of it for a variety of vital enzymes. Cellular copper transport consists of three processes: copper uptake, intracellular distribution and utilization, and copper excretion.[3] The WD gene, *ATP7B*, codes for a P-type ATPase (WND) that is expressed in a variety of tissues, most highly in liver. It is required for the transport of copper into the hepatocyte secretory pathway, its incorporation into ceruloplasmin, and its excretion into bile.[3] Details of normal copper metabolism are presented in Culotta and Gitlin.[4]

More than 200 mutations of the *ATP7B* gene have been described.[5] Some mutations are population-specific, and others are common in many nationalities. Most patients are compound heterozygotes.[6] The genetic mutations are responsible for a reduced biliary transport and excretion of copper, and an impaired formation of ceruloplasmin (Fig. 66–1).[4]

Pathology

Abnormalities in copper metabolism result in a deposition of the metal in several tissues. The liver shows a focal necrosis that leads to a coarsely nodular, postnecrotic cirrhosis. The nodules vary in size and are separated by bands of fibrous tissues of different widths. Some hepatic cells are enlarged and contain fat droplets, intranuclear glycogen, and clumped pigment granules; other cells are necrotic with regenerative changes in the surrounding parenchyma. Electron microscopic studies indicate that copper is initially spread diffusely within cytoplasm. As the disease progresses, the metal is sequestered within lysosomes, which become increasingly sensitive to rupture. Copper probably initiates and catalyzes oxidation of the lysosomal membrane lipids, resulting in lipofuscin accumulation. Copper also induces mitochondrial dysfunction in liver, probably mediated via mitochondrial copper accumulation.

In brain, the basal ganglia show the most striking alterations. They have a brick-red pigmentation; spongy degeneration of the putamen frequently leads to the formation of small cavities.[1] Microscopic studies reveal a loss of neurons, axonal degeneration, and large numbers of protoplasmic astrocytes, including giant forms termed Alzheimer cells. Opalski cells, also seen in WD, are generally found in gray matter. They are large cells with a rounded contour and finely granular cytoplasm. They probably represent degenerating astrocytes. Copper is deposited in the pericapillary area and within astrocytes, but it is uniformly absent from neurons and ground substance. Lesser degenerative changes are seen in the brainstem, dentate nucleus, substantia nigra, and convolutional white matter. Copper is also found throughout the cornea, particularly the substantia propria.

Normal hepatocyte copper metabolism

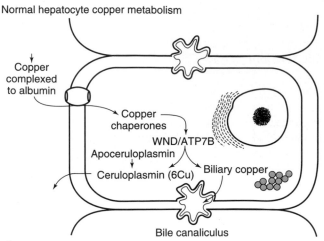

A

Wilson disease hepatocyte copper metabolism

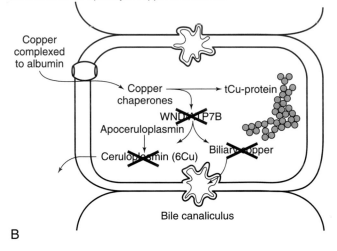

B

FIGURE 66–1. Normal hepatocyte copper metabolism and effects of Wilson disease mutation. *A,* Copper complexed to albumin is transported into hepatocytes, then escorted to sites of incorporation into copper-containing enzymes and proteins. The WND/*ATP7B* copper transporter is necessary for incorporation of copper into ceruloplasmin and for excretion of copper into bile. *B,* In Wilson disease, excess copper accumulates. Reactive species generated by copper ions damage hepatocytes. The hepatocytes release copper, causing damage to other tissues and organs. (From Dr. Jennifer A. Cuthbert, Department of Internal Medicine, Southwestern Medical School, the University of Texas Southwestern Medical Center, Dallas, Texas.)

Clinical Manifestations

If left untreated, WD is a progressive condition with a tendency toward temporary clinical improvement and arrest.[7] The condition occurs in all races, with a particularly high incidence in Eastern European Jews, Italians from southern Italy and Sicily, and people from some small islands in Japan (groups with a high rate of inbreeding). Approximately 40% of patients present with overt or subclinical evidence of liver disease. In a fair number of cases, primarily in young

children, initial symptoms can be hepatic, such as jaundice or portal hypertension, and the disease can assume a rapidly fatal course without any detectable neurologic abnormalities.[8] Less frequently, WD presents as an acute or intermittent Coombs-negative, nonspherocytic anemia accompanied by leukopenia and thrombocytopenia.

In 40% of patients, the first clinical manifestation is neurologic (Table 66–1). The first signs are usually bulbar; these can include indistinct speech and difficulty in swallowing. A rapidly progressive dystonic syndrome is not unusual. In essence, WD is a disorder of motor function; there are no sensory symptoms or reflex alterations. In a large proportion of patients, behavioral and psychiatric manifestations predominate, and almost every patient suffers from a psychiatric disorder some time in the course of the disease.[9]

The intracorneal, ring-shaped pigmentation, first noted by Kayser and Fleischer, might be evident to the naked eye or might appear only with slit-lamp examination. It can antedate overt symptoms of the disease and has been detected even in the presence of normal liver functions.

Generally, MRI correlates better with clinical symptoms than CT. It demonstrates abnormal signals (hypointense on T1-weighted images, and hyperintense on T2-weighted images) most commonly in the putamen, thalami, and the head of the caudate nucleus. The midbrain is also abnormal, as are the pons and cerebellum.

Diagnosis

When WD presents with neurologic manifestations, some diagnostic features are the progressive extrapyramidal

TABLE 66–1. Initial Neurologic Signs in 31 Patients with Wilson Disease

Sign	Percentage of Patients
Dysarthria	97
Dystonia	65
Dysdiadochokinesia	58
Rigidity	52
Abnormal posture	42
Abnormal gait	42
Abnormal facial expression	39
Tremor	32
Abnormal eye movements	32
Drooling	23
Bradykinesia	19
Motor impersistence	19
Frontal release signs	19
Athetosis	10

Data adapted from Brewer GJ, Yuzbasiayan-Gurkan V. Wilson disease. Medicine 1992;71:139.

symptoms commencing after the first decade of life, such as abnormal liver function, aminoaciduria, cupriuria, and absent or decreased ceruloplasmin. The concentration of ceruloplasmin in plasma is normally between 20 and 40 mg/dL. It is reduced in Menkes disease, iron and copper deficiency, nephrotic syndrome, and in normal infants. Some 5% to 20% of patients with WD have normal levels of the copper protein. The presence of a Kayser-Fleischer ring is the single most important diagnostic feature; its absence in a patient with neurologic symptoms rules out the diagnosis of WD. The ring is not seen in the majority of presymptomatic patients, nor in some patients in whom WD presents with hepatic symptoms.[10] In affected families, the differential diagnosis between heterozygotes and presymptomatic homozygotes is of utmost importance, inasmuch as it is generally accepted that presymptomatic homozygotes should be treated preventively. Low ceruloplasmin levels in an asymptomatic family member only suggest the presymptomatic stage of the disease; some 10% to 20% of heterozygotes have ceruloplasmin levels below 15 mg/dl. Since gene carriers comprise about 1% of the population, gene carriers with low ceruloplasmin values are seen forty times more frequently than patients with WD and low ceruloplasmin values. Whenever the diagnosis is in doubt, an assay of liver copper is indicated. In all confirmed cases of WD, hepatic copper is greater than 3.9 µmol/g dry weight (237.6 µg/g) as compared to a normal range of 0.2 to 0.6 µmol/g.

Linkage analysis can identify the presymptomatic patient in families with one or more informative family members. Because of the large number of mutations causing the disease, polymerase chain reaction-based screening of mutations can be laborious. About one third of North American WD subjects have a point mutation (His 1069Glu), and screening for this mutation can be performed rapidly.[11] A combination of mutation and linkage analysis is required for prenatal diagnosis.

Therapy

Whether symptomatic or asymptomatic, all WD patients require treatment. Treatment aims to initially remove the toxic amounts of copper and to secondarily prevent tissue reaccumulation of the metal.[12] Treatment can be divided into two phases. First, toxic copper levels are brought under control; then maintenance therapy is initiated. There is no currently agreed-upon regimen for treatment of the new patient with neurologic or psychiatric symptoms. In the past, most centers recommended starting patients on D-penicillamine. This drug is effective in promoting urinary excretion of copper. However, a significant number of patients have adverse reactions such as worsening of neurologic symptoms. Because of these side effects, many institutions now advocate initial therapy with ammonium tetrathiomolybdate or triethylene tetramine dihydrochloride (trientine). Zinc acetate is the optimum drug for maintenance therapy, and for the treat-

ment of the presymptomatic patient. It acts by inducing intestinal metallothionein (MT) by as much as 15-fold.[13] MT has a high affinity for copper and prevents its entrance into blood. Zinc is far less toxic than penicillamine but is much slower acting. Trientine in combination with zinc acetate has been suggested for patients who present in hepatic failure. Orthotopic liver transplant can be helpful for the patient who presents with end-stage hepatic disease. The procedure appears to correct the metabolic defect and can reverse neurologic symptoms.[14] Diet does not play an important role in the management of WD, although Brewer recommends restriction of liver and shellfish during the first year of treatment.[12]

On the previously mentioned regimens, neurologic symptoms start to improve 5 to 6 months after therapy has begun and is generally complete in 24 months. As shown by serial neuroimaging studies, there is a significant regression of lesions within thalamus and basal ganglia. As a rule, patients remain normal if they are started on therapy prior to the evolution of symptoms. Patients who have had hepatic disease exclusively do well, and in 80%, hepatic functions return to normal. About 40% of patients who present with neurologic symptoms become completely asymptomatic and remain so. Patients with the mixed hepatocerebral picture do poorly. Less than 25% recover completely, and about 25% continue to deteriorate, often with the appearance of seizures.[8]

MENKES DISEASE

Menkes disease (MD), also known as kinky hair disease, is a multifocal degenerative disease of gray matter first described in 1962 by Menkes et al.[15] Some 10 years later, Danks et al[16] found serum copper and ceruloplasmin levels to be reduced and suggested that the primary defect in MD involved copper metabolism. In 1993, three groups of workers isolated the gene *(ATP7A)* whose defect is responsible for the disease, and found that it encoded a transmembrane copper-transporting P-type ATPase (MNK), and that the disease results from a widespread defect in intracellular copper transport, and consequent copper maldistribution

Molecular and Biochemical Pathology

ATP7A, the gene for MD, is located at Xq13. It encodes for an energy-dependent, copper-transporting P-type membrane ATPase (MNK).[17] The structural homology between the two genes is extremely high in the 3' two thirds of the genes, but there is considerable divergence between them in the 5' one third.[17] *ATP7A* is expressed in all tissue with the exception of liver. It consists of six metal-binding domains, eight transmembrane domains, and domains for phosphatase, phosphorylation, and ATP binding (Fig. 66–2).[17] At basal copper levels, the protein is located in the trans-Golgi network, the sorting station for proteins exiting from the Golgi apparatus, where it is

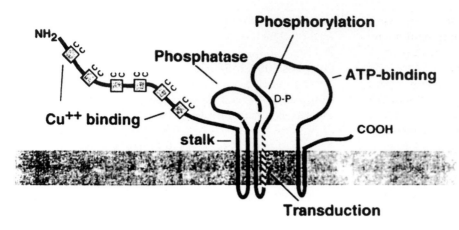

FIGURE 66–2. Model for the proposed gene product of the MNK gene. Boxes with paired cysteines (C) represent putative copper-binding protein motifs. D-P represents the phosphorylation site. Exon 10 of the MNK gene is skipped at a low level in several normal tissues. This does not alter the reading frame, but results in the loss of two of the eight transmembrane domains. (From Dr. S. Packman, Division of Genetics, Department of Pediatrics, University of California–San Francisco School of Medicine, San Francisco, California.)

involved in copper uptake into its lumen.[18] At increased intracellular and extracellular copper concentrations, the MNK protein shifts toward the plasma membrane, presumably to enhance removal of excess copper from the cell.[18]

The characteristic abnormality in copper metabolism as expressed in the human infant is a maldistribution of body copper, a result of defective copper transport across the placenta, the gastrointestinal tract, and the blood-brain barrier.[3] The consequence is a failure of copper incorporation into a variety of essential enzymes.[17,19] Patients absorb little or no orally administered copper; when the metal is given intravenously, they experience a prompt rise in serum copper and ceruloplasmin. As a result of impaired copper efflux, the copper content of cultured fibroblasts, myotubes, and lymphocytes derived from patients with MD is several times greater than that of control cells.[20]

Pathology

Because of defective activity of the metalloenzymes, a variety of pathologic changes are set into motion. In skin, the elastin fibers are reduced in number, and consist of thin strands of amorphous elastin associated with numerous microfibrils.[21] Cerebral and systemic arteries are tortuous with irregular lumens and frayed and split intimal linings. These abnormalities reflect the failure in elastin and collagen cross-linking caused by a decrease in functional activity of copper-dependent lysyl oxidase.

Anatomical changes within the brain are believed to result from reduced activity of the various copper-containing enzymes, in particular, from mitochondrial dysfunction, from vascular lesions, or from a combination of the two factors. Gross examination of the brain discloses diffuse atrophy; unilateral or bilateral subdural hematomas are commonly present. There is extensive focal degeneration of gray matter with neuronal loss and gliosis and an associated axonal degeneration in white matter.[15] Cellular loss is prominent in the cerebellum. Purkinje cells are most affected; many are lost, and others show abnormal dendritic arborization ("weeping willow") and periso-

matic processes. Focal axonal swellings ("torpedoes") are also observed.[15] On electron microscopy, there are a variety of mitochondrial abnormalities.[22]

Clinical Features

MD is an X-linked disorder; its frequency has been estimated at 0.8 to 2:100,000 live male births. Most of the clinical manifestations can be explained by the low activities of the various copper-containing enzymes. These include cytochrome c oxidase, lysyl oxidase, superoxide dismutase, peptidylglycine α-amidating monooxygenase, tyrosinase, dopamine-β-hydroxylase, and ascorbic acid oxidase.

The clinical manifestations of MD are quite variable. In part, the variability can be explained by a large number of mutations. These include mutations that lead to splicing abnormalities, small duplications, nonsense mutations, and missense mutations. To date, all mutations detected have been unique for each given family, and almost all have been associated with a decreased level of the mRNA for the copper-transporting ATPase. There is no good genotype-phenotype correlation. In the allelic variant of MD, occipital horn syndrome, the full length MNK protein is absent, but the truncated MND protein is expressed and is localized to the endoplasmic reticulum.[23]

Baerlocher and Nadal,[24] and Kaler[25] have provided a comprehensive review of the clinical features. In the classic form, symptoms appear during the neonatal period. Most commonly, there is hypothermia, hypoglycemia, poor feeding, and impaired weight gain. Less often there is a fatal hemorrhagic diathesis and multiple congenital fractures. Cephalhematomas can be prominent in infants born vaginally. The appearance of hair is often unremarkable at birth; newborns can have little or no hair, or normally pigmented hair.[25] Other patients present with seizures, delayed development, or failure to thrive. The most striking finding is the abnormal hair. It is colorless and friable. On examination under the microscope, a variety of abnormalities are evident, most commonly pili torti (a hair shaft which is flattened and twisted 180 degrees on its own axis). Monilethrix (an elliptical swelling of the hair shafts with intervening tapered constrictions), and trichorrhexis nodosa (small beaded swelling of the hair shaft with fractures at regular intervals) are also seen.[15]

Other organs can also be involved. Optic discs are pale, and there are microcysts of the pigment epithelium and iris. Hydronephrosis, hydroureter, and diverticula or rupture of the bladder has been reported. Radiographs of long bones show a variety of abnormalities. They include osteoporosis, metaphyseal spurring, a diaphyseal periosteal reaction, and scalloping of the posterior aspects of the vertebral bodies. Skull radiographs can reveal the presence of wormian bones in the lambdoidal and posterior sagittal sutures.

Neuroimaging studies frequently disclose cerebral atrophy, areas of low density within the cortex, impaired myelination and tortuous and enlarged intracranial vessels. Asymptomatic subdural hematomas are almost invariable.

The course is inexorably downhill, but the rate of neurologic deterioration varies from one patient to the next. There are recurrent infections of the respiratory and urinary tracts. Sepsis and meningitis are fairly common, and there is evidence for dysfunction of the cellular immune responses.

Diagnosis

The clinical history of developmental arrest or regression, hypotonia, and seizures, and the appearance of the infant, in particular the unusual hair, should suggest the diagnosis. Reduced levels of serum ceruloplasmin and copper levels are diagnostic of MD. Urinary copper is variable; normal, reduced, and even elevated levels have been reported. This assay is therefore of no value for the diagnosis of MD.

Heterozygotes are mostly asymptomatic, and do not show any biochemical abnormalities. However areas of pili torti constitute between 30% and 50% of the hair. Prenatal diagnosis has been based on the increased copper content of cultured amniocytes and chorionic villus samples.

Therapy

Because symptoms of MD are the consequence of impaired activity of the various copper-containing enzymes, copper supplementation would seem to be a rational means of treating this condition. However, neither oral nor parenteral administration of copper has been effective, even though the latter induces a rapid rise of both ceruloplasmin and copper. Copper histidinate has been suggested, but due to the considerable clinical heterogeneity of patients with MD the effectiveness of this therapy is difficult to evaluate.

REFERENCES

1. Wilson SAK: Progressive lenticular degeneration: A familial nervous disease associated with cirrhosis of the liver. Brain 1912;34:295–509.

2. Gitlin JD. Aceruloplasminemia. Pediatr Res 1998; 44:271–276.

3. Loudianos G, Gitlin JD. Wilson's disease. Sem Liver Dis 2000;353–364.

4. Culotta VC, Gitlin JD: Disorders of copper transport. In Scriver CR, Beaudet AL, Sly WS, et al (eds): The Metabolic and Molecular Bases of Inherited Disease, 8th ed. New York, McGraw-Hill, 2000, pp 3105–3126.

5. Wu ZY, Wang N, Lin MT, et al: Mutation analysis and the correlation between genotype and phenotype of Arg778Leu mutation in Chinese patients with Wilson disease. Arch Neurol 2001;58:971–976.

6. Thomas GR, Forbes JR, Roberts EA, et al: The Wilson disease gene: Spectrum of mutations and their consequence. Nat Genet 1995;9:210–217.

7. Scheinberg IH, Sternlieb I: Wilson's Disease, 2nd ed. Philadelphia, WB Saunders, 1999.

8. Arima M, Takeshita K, Yoshino K, et al: Prognosis of Wilson's disease in childhood. Eur J Pediatr 1977;126: 147–154.

9. Portala K, Westermark K, Ekselius L, von Knorring L: Personality traits in treated Wilson's disease determined by means of the Karolinska Scales of Personality (KSP). Eur Psychiatry 2001;16:362–371.

10. Scott J, Golan JL, Samourian S, Sherlock S: Wilson's disease, presenting as chronic active hepatitis. Gastroenterology 1978;74:645–651.

11. Shah AB, Chernov I, Zhang HT, et al: Identification and analysis of mutation in the Wilson disease gene *(ATP7B)*: Population frequencies, genotype-phenotype correlation, and functional analyses. Am J Hum Genet 1997;61:317–328.

12. Brewer GJ: Practical recommendations and new therapies for Wilson's disease. Drugs 1995;50:240–249.

13. Sturniolo GC, Mestriner C, Irato P, et al: Zinc therapy increases duodenal concentrations of metallothionein and iron in Wilson's disease patients. Am J Gastroenterol 1999;94:334–338.

14. Emre S. Atillasoy EO, Ozdemir S, et al: Orthotopic liver transplantation for Wilson's disease: A single-center experience. Transplantation 2001;72: 1232–1236.

15. Menkes JH, Alter M, Weakley D, et al: A sex-linked recessive disorder with growth retardation, peculiar hair, and focal cerebral and cerebellar degeneration. Pediatrics 1962;29:764–779.

16. Danks DM, Campbell PE, Stevens BJ, et al: Menkes' kinky hair syndrome: An inherited defect in copper absorption with widespread effects. Pediatrics 1972;50:188–201.

17. Harrison MD, Dameron CT: Molecular mechanisms of copper metabolism and the role of the Menkes disease protein. J Biochem Mol Toxicol 1999;13:93–106.

18. Andrews NC: Mining copper transport genes. Proc Nat Acad Sci U S A 2001;98:6543–6545.

19. Vulpe CD, Packman S: Cellular copper transport. Ann Rev Nutr 1990;15:293–322.

20. Tümer Z, Horn N:w Menkes disease: Recent advances and new aspects. J Med Genet 1997;34: 265–274.

21. Pasquali-Ronchetti I, Baccarani-Contri M, Young RD, et al: Ultrastructural analysis of skin and aorta from a patient with Menkes disease. Exp Mol Pathol 1994;61:36–57.

22. Yoshimura N, Kudo H. Mitochondrial abnormalities in Menkes' kinky hair disease (MKHD). Acta Neuropathol (Berl) 1983;9:296–303.

23. Francis MJ, Jones EE, Ponnambalam S, et al: A Golgi localization signal identified in the Menkes recombinant protein. Hum Mol Gent 1998;7:1245–1252.

24. Baerlocher K, Nadal D: Das Menkes-syndrom. Ergeb Inn Med Kinderheilkd 1988;57:77–144.

25. Kaler SG. Menkes disease. Adv Pediatr 1994; 41:263–304.

CHAPTER

67

The Influence of α-Tocopherol, Caloric Restriction, and Genes on Life Span

Richard Mayeux

Longevity in any population is the result of a decrease in the cumulative mortality across all ages. However, over the last few decades the trend toward increasing survival into old age for developed countries has been a result of decreasing mortality rates among the older segment of the population. Between 1950 and 1995, the mortality rates for women between age 80 and 90 years declined by 50%.[1] Men have also made substantial gains in life span but at a much slower pace. Improvements in environmental hygiene, social welfare, health care systems, and advances in medicine worldwide have contributed to the current trends in longer life span. Research has also shown that life style and socioeconomic status have important influences. Dietary factors, particularly the consumption of antioxidants and caloric restriction, may have profound effects on longevity in laboratory animals, but their effect on human aging has not been fully explored. Genes that influence longevity and life span are also poorly understood, but are considered important based on studies of aging in model systems, and to some degree in humans.

For nearly 3 decades, it has been known that biologic aging occurs as a result of influences at the genetic and epigenetic level. The finding that normal human and animal cells in culture undergo a finite number of population doublings in vitro offered the first clues that aging begins at the cellular level. Specific pathways involving metabolism have been implicated in longevity.[2] Studies show that a large number of genes may control cell destiny by regulating replication or senescence.[3] For example, variations in genes involved in metabolic control mechanisms in yeast and in insulin-signaling pathways in nematodes (*Caenorhabditis elegans*) and fruit flies (*Drosophila melanogaster*) significantly extend life span.

Mutations in genes resulting in dwarfism can extend life span in rodents by the effect of these variants on growth hormone, which in turn, affects insulin signaling and metabolism. As might be expected, mammals are more complex than lower organisms because mutations in genes that modulate apoptosis have also been found to affect life span. Some of these pathways have been investigated in relation to human aging, but the complexity of human aging and longevity show only minimal parallels.

PATHOPHYSIOLOGY OF LONGEVITY AND SENESCENCE

Aging is physiologically complex. Theories for the biologic bases of aging have been developed covering a wide range of molecular systems. The mitochondrial theory of aging implicates oxidative stress within the cell leading to the accumulation of mtDNA mutations and oxygen-free radicals. The rate of oxidative damage within the mitochondria may represent the biologic clock of aging. Genes that affect life span in model systems include those that encode signal transduction proteins and participate in the regulation of mitochondrial metabolism.[4] The telomere-telomerase hypothesis of aging proposes that telomere loss results in replicative senescence within the cell and that telomerase activation results in immortalization.[5] The telomere is a complex structure composed of both DNA and other proteins, and may serve as another type of molecular clock that tallies the number of cell divisions and limits further divisions at a predetermined point. The precise role of telomeres in predicting and limiting cellular life span nonetheless remains unclear.[6] It is hypothesized that longevity in humans depends on optimal functioning of the immune system. Certain changes in the major histocompatibility complex (MHC), known to control a variety of immune functions, can be associated with the altered life span in strains of mice. Human studies have shown contradictory results regarding the association between longevity and some HLA-DR alleles or HLA-B8, DR3 haplotype, known to be involved in the antigen nonspecific control of immune response.[7]

The accumulation of somatic mutations during life has also been proposed as a cause of aging. There is an invariant relationship between life span and number of random somatic mutations. Studies at a number of gene loci have shown that somatic mutations of a variety of types accumulate with age. Dietary restriction, which prolongs life span, results in slowed accumulation of some somatic mutations in mice. Conversely, senescence-accelerated mice that have been bred to have a shortened life span show accelerated accumulation of somatic mutations.[8]

Brain function during senescence may also provide a key to understanding longevity. The brains of elderly individuals without dementia show an overall reduction in brain volume and weight, and enlargement of brain ventricles. These changes are, in part, due to nerve cell loss, but accurate estimates of neuronal loss are difficult to make. There are losses of synapses and dendritic pruning in the aged brain, but these occur in selected areas, rather than globally. The neuropathologic features of Alzheimer's disease are not marked among genuinely intact elderly people. It is hypothesized that Alzheimer's disease is an example of accelerated brain aging. However, since there is a strong genetic contribution to developing this disease, it may not be the inevitable consequence of old age, even if quite frequent.[9]

Depending on the strain, studies in aged mice also show age-related changes in the sensorimotor performance, spontaneous behavior, and in learning and memory tasks. Complex learning, such as in the Morris water maze task of spatial learning, can be dramatically affected, whereas simple discrimination learning is only impaired in the oldest animals. Changes in sensorimotor ability and locomotor activity do not account for the learning impairments.[10]

CALORIC INTAKE AND α-TOCOPHEROL

Caloric intake decreases about 20% to 30% among the elderly because of decline in physical activity and resting metabolic rate for most people.[11] Other factors such as depression and alterations in taste and odor perception also contribute. Except for genetic manipulation, caloric restriction has been found to be the only reproducible method shown to slow aging and increase longevity in laboratory animals. Clarification of the underlying biologic mechanisms remains intensively investigated. The beneficial effect of caloric restriction on longevity has been investigated in a controlled study of nonhuman pri-

mates. In humans, caloric reduction lowers body weight, which in turn lowers blood pressure, and may reduce blood levels of lipoproteins, glucose, and insulin. Combined with exercise, reduced calories can also improve coronary artery disease and extend life span. There are other effects such as lower body temperatures and a slower age-related decline in circulating levels of androgenic hormones.

Caloric restriction increases resistance of neurons to dysfunction and degeneration, and improves behavioral outcome in animal models of Alzheimer's disease.[12] However, a significant benefit of caloric restriction may be a decreased risk of age-related disorders such as diabetes, cardiovascular disease, cancer, and dementia.

Alternative mechanisms have been proposed to explain the effects of caloric restriction. For example, caloric restriction in mice may retard aging by inducing a metabolic shift in protein turnover that decreases macromolecular damage. Lee et al[13] observed an increase in transcriptional activity for genes related to the up-regulation of gluconeogenesis, fatty acid synthesis, and increased synthesis and turnover of proteins. During caloric restriction in young and old rodents, this pathway involves increase in mRNA expression of genes involved in hepatic gluconeogenesis, glucose 6-phosphatase, and phosphoenolpyruvate carboxykinase. There is also an increase in peripheral protein turnover, which augments gluconeogenesis. Spindler[14] has proposed that caloric restriction both enhances and maintains protein turnover and renewal, which in turn, contributes to the extension of life in laboratory animals. However, each species may have specific effects related to caloric restriction. In a comparison of young and old rhesus monkeys, gene expression analysis revealed selective up-regulation of genes involved in inflammation and oxidative stress, and down-regulation of genes involved in mitochondrial electron transport and oxidative phosphorylation.[15]

Drugs that mimic the beneficial effect of caloric restriction, such as 2-deoxyglucose, have also been shown to lower plasma insulin levels and body temperature in rats and nonhuman primates.[16] Caloric restriction or the use of medications that have the same effect in humans will need careful investigation before implementing treatment or recommendations.

While there may be advantages to caloric restriction, there may also be disadvantages. For example, with the decrement in caloric intake there is also a decrease in micronutrient consumption, most notably α-tocopherol, which declines approximately 30%.[17] α-Tocopherol is one of the most biologically active antioxidants in vivo. α-Tocopherol is a fat-soluble vitamin that is abundant in foods in some forms. As a nutrient, α-tocopherol is the most effective lipid-soluble antioxidant in the biologic membrane preventing free radical damage, and it is important for both normal brain development and maintenance during late life. In model systems such as cell culture, α-tocopherol acts as an oxygen-free radical scavenger and limits lipid peroxidation. In aged rats, for example, the unusual decline in long-term potentiation (LTP) in the dentate gyrus of the hippocampus is prevented by dietary supplementation of α-tocopherol.[18] In laboratory animals, Bondy et al[19] reported that dietary manipulation with antioxidants can also alter the changes during senescence that result in oxidative damage to macromolecules, increasing the production of nitric oxide synthase and reactive oxygen species. Whether α-tocopherol supplementation can impede the progression of age-related degenerative disorders associated with oxidative damage remains uncertain. However, Sano et al[20] found that α-tocopherol at doses of 2000 IU/day delayed progression to the more advanced stages of Alzheimer's disease over a 10-month period.

The generation of reactive oxygen species in mitochondria (also an important mechanism for aging) and the subsequent effect of oxidative damage to cellular macromolecules is well established. It is unclear whether caloric restriction or use of supplemental dietary antioxidants such as α-tocopherol can be used to slow or prevent this effect in humans. Support for antioxidant use is mainly limited to the extension of average life span in laboratory animals. Investigations to date have been observational rather than rigorous clinical trials. Clearly, there is a need for further work to examine preventative interventions.

GENETICS OF AGING AND LIFE SPAN IN HUMANS

Compared to the average person, family members of centenarians are four times as likely to live past 85 years.[21] Human monozygotic twins are more likely to be concordant for life span than dizygotic twins, particularly among the oldest twins. However, it is predicted that only one third or less of the variance in longevity in humans is attributed to genetic factors. Investigating the correlation of age at death between parents and their offspring has proven difficult because secular trends in environmental conditions impede meaningful comparisons. Though a large number of studies imply that genetic variation influences longevity in humans, the extent to which this occurs directly or indirectly is unclear. Heritability of longevity, defined as the degree to which total years of life or age at death is shared among family members has been estimated from investigations of human twins, isolated and founder populations. Mitchell et al[22] provided estimates of the heritability of human longevity from several recently published studies of twins and geographically isolated populations. Estimates of the heritability of life span among twins are highly variable, ranging from 10% among twins reared apart, to as high as 50% among same-sex twin pairs. Among 2,872 Danish twins, variance was attributed to genetic and environmental factors. The authors modeled both genetic and environmental factors, not shared and shared within the family, and they

estimated heritability of longevity to be 25%. A small sex-difference was caused by a greater impact of non-shared environmental factors among women. Heritability was constant over the three 10-year birth cohorts included. There was little evidence for effect of shared environmental factors.[23] Among Swedish twins, intra-pair correlation for life span was similar to that among Danish twins, but lower for men than for women. The age at death did not influence the outcome. The authors also compared twins reared apart to twins reared together and concluded that most of the variance in longevity was explained by environmental factors. Over the total age range, 30% of the variance in longevity was attributable to genetic factors, and almost all of the remaining variance was due to unshared individual specific environmental factors.[24] As summarized by Mitchell et al,[22] the methods used to estimate heritability across studies varied considerably, possibly contributing to the variation.

Mitchell et al[22] also reviewed three large cohort studies involving large multigenerational families. Heritability estimates varied from 0% to 32%. The highest percentages were found among genealogies of six large New England families. Heritability of life span in the older-order Amish also indicates that 25% of the variation may be due to genetic factors. Parent and offspring ages at death were highly correlated, as were ages of death among siblings.[22] The strongest effects were for parents and siblings surviving past the age of 75 years. The authors concluded that genetic influences on life span might vary at different ages. As noted by these authors, premature death in a parent is a strong risk factor for premature death among offspring. Because susceptibility to disease also increases with age, "mortality determinants" among older individuals may be very different from those among younger persons.

Studies of centenarians imply much stronger genetic effects. Compared with siblings of individuals who did not survive past age 73 years, siblings of centenarians were four times more likely to live to age 85 years or older.[21] Centenarians are also more healthy and generally more active than individuals 10 to 20 years younger.[21,25]

It may be argued that absence of disease-causing genetic variants throughout life must certainly promote longevity. Alternatively, extreme longevity can be mediated by variations in genes that provide protection against diseases during middle and late life. To that end, a genetic linkage study among families of centenarians has identified a locus on chromosome 4.[26]

Using a series of 137 families characterized by extreme longevity defined as survival past the age of 98 years for at least one member of the family, Puca et al[26] found statistically significant evidence favoring linkage to a region on chromosome 4. Male siblings were 91 years or older and female siblings were 95 years or older. Although a specific variant in a gene has not been identified, the finding of excess allele sharing among elderly family members offers the opportunity to identify a genetic explanation. Other regions on different chromosomes showed smaller peaks, suggesting the possibility of other genetic mutations or variants. This work will need to be confirmed by others, and fine mapping of this region will be required to isolate the gene.

Finch and Ruvkun[2] have also proposed a significant role for the nervous system in aging and longevity. Genes that affect life span affect neural mechanisms involved in hormones that regulate vitality and growth throughout life. The nervous system is particularly implicated in the control of life span via the effects of insulin signaling in the brain on metabolism and reproduction. Mutations in these same pathways in model organisms alter the normal protective mechanisms for neurons. The accumulation of oxygen-free radicals, protein conformational changes, decline in chaperone functions, and secondary loss of energy production in mitochondria can also result in neuronal degeneration and subsequent mortality.

KNOWN GENETIC VARIANTS AND LONGEVITY

Variant alleles in genes such as apolipoprotein-E *APOE* have also been shown to promote life span, though inconsistently.[3] Because of their associations with diseases of aging, variations in genes encoding the angiotensin-converting enzyme methylenetetrahydrofolate reductase and in MHC haplotypes have also been associated with longevity (but less consistently).[2] Several genetic variants, particularly those associated with cardiovascular disorders, have been investigated for their potential association with longevity (Table 67–1). While some variants have been confirmed, most have not. Nonetheless, there is a remarkable consistency in the functions of these genes and their disease relationships.

Mutations in a gene encoding a helicase and exonuclease have been identified as the etiology of Werner's syndrome, a rare autosomal disorder causing progeria.[27] Severe atherosclerosis and a higher frequency of cancer as well as rapid aging during young adulthood are the main features of this disorder. However, variant alleles or polymorphisms at the Werner locus have not been found to affect aging in humans. Mice without *Klotho*, a gene that encodes a type I membrane protein and shares homology with glycosides, age prematurely. *Klotho*-deficient mice develop normally during the first month of life, but then rapidly develop growth retardation, become inactive, and die by the second month.[28] Investigators have indentifed a polymorphism in the human gene on chromosome 13q12 that has been associated with longevity (defined as survival to age 75 years or older). Although intriguing, investigations of progeria-like syndromes are limited because they do not always characterize the extent and diverse nature of aging.

APOE has been extensively investigated because of its role in lipid metabolism, ischemic cardiovascular disease, and Alzheimer's disease. There are three common alleles of *APOE*: ε2, ε3, and ε4. While the ε3 allele is the most common allele and generally present in two copies in about 60% to 80% of humans, ε4 is considered to be the ancestral allele. The frequency of *APOE*-ε4 varies worldwide from 40.7% among Pygmies to 2% to 3% among some Asian populations. Variation at the APOE locus has also been related to longevity. The ε4 allele is associated with a shorter life span compared to the other alleles, while the ε2 allele has been associated with extreme longevity.[29,30] Although the mechanism by which the ε2 allele extends life is unknown, Reich et al[31] have proposed an interaction between *APOE* and oxidative stress. They showed that compared to mice fed a normal diet, those fed an α-tocopherol–deficient diet had higher levels of isoprostanes and neuroprostanes, mark-

TABLE 67–1. Genes in which at least one variant allele has been associated with longevity in humans

Gene	Function	Disease Association
APOE	Lipoprotein metabolism	Alzheimer's disease, cardiovascular disease
APOB	Cholesterol homeostasis	Coronary artery disease
APOA-IV	Lipoprotein metabolism	None
ACE	Rennin-angiotensin system	Hypertension, cardiovascular disease
HLA class I	Immune response	Immune disorders
Factor V	Blood coagulation	Myocardial infarction, thromboembolism
Fibrinogen	Plasma coagulation factor	Coronary artery disease
MTHFR (methylene-tetrahydrofolate reductase)	Homocysteine methylation	Cardiovascular disease, cancer susceptibility
MtDNA	Oxidative phosphorylation	Mitochondrial diseases
Klotho	Microvascular activity	None

Data adapted from De Benedictis G, Tan Q, Jeune B, et al: Recent advances in human gene-longevity association studies. Mech Ageing Dev 2001; 122:909–920.

ers of free-radical–mediated damage. Moreover, *APOE*-null mice showed an even greater elevation. α-tocopherol supplementation markedly limited this effect in both normal and *APOE*-null mice on normal or α-tocopherol–deficient diets. Thus, the lack of *APOE* may increase susceptibility to oxidative damage. At least in animal models, this can be prevented by α-tocopherol supplementation.

CONCLUSION

Longevity is influenced by a complex interaction between genetic, social, and environmental factors.[2] Among the environmental factors, dietary factors may be of greatest interest because of the potential ability to intervene if a rational means become available. The ability of α-tocopherol supplementation to limit the progression of oxidative stress in aged laboratory animals and to slow the progress to more advanced stages of Alzheimer's disease in some individuals illustrates the therapeutic potential of this compound. Genes that influence life span are still being investigated. However, when they are discovered, new pathways will be identified that may also prove to be important targets for intervention. Environmental and behavioral factors such as diet may play a role throughout life in the maintenance of good health and longevity. However, much more work is required to fully understand the way in which dietary factors such as α-tocopherol interact with genes to influence longevity.

Acknowledgments

This work is from the Taub Institute on Alzheimer's Disease and the Aging Brain, the Gertrude H. Sergievsky Center, and the Departments of Neurology and Psychiatry in the College of Physicians and Surgeons.

Support was provided by Federal Grants AG/ES18732, AG07232, AG08702, the Charles S. Robertson Memorial Gift for Alzheimer's Disease Research from the Banbury Fund, and the Blanchette Hooker Rockefeller Foundation.

REFERENCES

1. Vaupel JW, Carey JR, Christensen K, et al: Biodemographic trajectories of longevity. Science 1998;280:855–860.

2. Finch CE, Ruvkun G: The genetics of aging. Annu Rev Genomics Hum Genet 2001;2:435–462.

3. Barzilai N, Shuldiner AR: Searching for human longevity genes: The future history of gerontology in the post-genomic era. J Gerontol A Biol Sci Med Sci 2001; 56:83–87.

4. Camougrand N, Rigoulet M: Aging and oxidative stress: Studies of some genes involved both in aging and in response to oxidative stress. Respir Physiol 2001;128:393–401.

5. Harley CB: Telomerase is not an oncogene. Oncogene 2002;21:494–502.

6. Stewart SA, Weinberg RA: Senescence: Does it all happen at the ends? Oncogene 2002;21:627–630.

7. Caruso C, Candore G, Romano GC, et al: Immunogenetics of longevity. Is major histocompatibility complex polymorphism relevant to the control of human longevity? A review of literature data. Mech Aging Dev 2001;122:445–462.

8. Morley A: Somatic mutation and aging. Ann N Y Acad Sci 1998;854:20–22.

9. Anderton BH: Aging of the brain. Mech Ageing Dev 2002;123:811–817.

10. Gower AJ, Lamberty Y: The aged mouse as a model of cognitive decline with special emphasis on studies in NMRI mice. Behav Brain Res 1993;57:163–173.

11. Morley JE: Anorexia, sarcopenia, and aging. Nutrition 2001;17:660–663.

12. Mattson MP: Emerging neuroprotective strategies for Alzheimer's disease: Dietary restriction, telomerase activation, and stem cell therapy. Exp Gerontol 2000;35:489–502.

13. Lee CK, Klopp RG, Weindruch R, Prolla TA: Gene expression profile of aging and its retardation by caloric restriction. Science 1999;285:1390–1393.

14. Spindler SR: Calorie restriction enhances the expression of key metabolic enzymes associated with protein renewal during aging. Ann N Y Acad Sci 2001; 928:296–304.

15. Kayo T, Allison DB, Weindruch R, Prolla TA. Influences of aging and caloric restriction on the transcriptional profile of skeletal muscle from rhesus monkeys. Proc Natl Acad Sci U S A 2001;98:5093–5098.

16. Roth GS, Ingram DK, Lane MA. Caloric restriction in primates and relevance to humans. Ann N Y Acad Sci 2001;928:305–315.

17. Wakimoto P, Block G: Dietary intake, dietary patterns, and changes with age: An epidemiological perspective. J Gerontol A Biol Sci Med Sci 2001;56 Spec No 2:65–80.

18. Murray CA, Lynch MA: Dietary supplementation with vitamin E reverses the age-related deficit in long term potentiation in dentate gyrus. J Biol Chem 1998; 273:12161–12168.

19. Bondy SC, Yang YE, Walsh TJ, et al: Dietary modulation of age-related changes in cerebral prooxidant status. Neurochem Int 2002;40:123–130.

20. Sano M, Ernesto C, Thomas RG, et al: A controlled trial of selegiline, alpha-tocopherol, or both as treatment for Alzheimer's disease. The Alzheimer's Disease Cooperative Study. N Engl J Med 1997;336: 1216–1222.

21. Perls TT, Bubrick E, Wager CG, et al: Siblings of centenarians live longer. Lancet 1998;351:1560.

22. Mitchell BD, Hsueh WC, King TM, et al: Heritability of life span in the old order Amish. Am J Med Genet 2001;102:346–352.

23. Herskind AM, McGue M, Holm NV, et al: The heritability of human longevity: A population-based study of 2872 Danish twin pairs born 1870–1900. Hum Genet 1996;97:319–323.

24. Ljungquist B, Berg S, Lanke J, et al: The effect of genetic factors for longevity: A comparison of identical and fraternal twins in the Swedish Twin Registry. J Gerontol A Biol Sci Med Sci 1998;53:441–446.

25. Perls T, Levenson R, Regan M, Puca A. What does it take to live to 100? Mech Aging Dev 2002;123:231–242.

26. Puca AA, Daly MJ, Brewster SJ, et al: A genome-wide scan for linkage to human exceptional longevity identifies a locus on chromosome 4. Proc Natl Acad Sci U S A 2001;98:10505–10508.

27. Martin GM, Oshima J: Lessons from human progeroid syndromes. Nature 2000;408:263–266.

28. Arking DE, Krebsova A, Macek M, et al: Association of human aging with a functional variant of klotho. Proc Natl Acad Sci U S A 2002;99:856–861.

29. Schachter F, Faure-Delanef L, Guenot F, et al: Genetic associations with human longevity at the APOE and ACE loci. Nat Genet 1994;6:29–32.

30. Frisoni GB, Louhija J, Geroldi C, Trabucchi M: Longevity and the epsilon2 allele of apolipoprotein E: The Finnish Centenarians Study. J Gerontol A Biol Sci Med Sci 2001;56:M75–M78.

31. Reich EE, Montine KS, Gross MD, et al: Interactions between apolipoprotein E gene and dietary alpha-tocopherol influence cerebral oxidative damage in aged mice. J Neurosci 2001;21:5993–5999.

32. De Benedictis G, Tan Q, Jeune B, et al: Recent advances in human gene-longevity association studies. Mech Aging Dev 2001;122:909–920.

CHAPTER

68

Vitamins: Cobalamin and Folate

Michael Shevell

David S. Rosenblatt

COBALAMIN

Absorption, Transport, and Metabolism

Cobalamin (Cbl, vitamin B_{12}) is an essential cofactor for two intracellular reactions: (1) mitochondrial methylmalonyl CoA mutase, which converts methylmalonyl CoA to succinylCoA and (2) cytosolic methionine synthase, which generates methionine from homocysteine. Inherited disorders of either transport or metabolism of cobalamin results in deficient activity in either one or both of these enzymes.[1]

Dietary cobalamin is obtained almost exclusively from animal sources. Free dietary cobalamin is initially bound to salivary glycoprotein R binders (haptocorrin, transcobalamin I). Proteolytic hydrolysis of R binders occurs in the acidic milieu of the stomach, subsequent to which Cbl binds to parietal cell secreted intrinsic factor (IF) in the proximal ileum. The resulting Cbl-IF complex then binds to specific enterocyte brush border localized receptors (likely cubilin) in the distal ileum. The Cbl-IF surface receptor complex is then internalized through endocytosis and undergoes lysosomal degradation that releases the bound cobalamin. This intracellular cobalamin is then bound to transcobalamin II (TCII) and released into the portal circulation.[2]

Circulating systemic cobalamin is bound to both TCI and TCII, but TCII is the physiologically active form. Through pinocytosis of this bound complex, cobalamin enters the cells and is initially processed in the lysosome where the TCII undergoes proteolytic degradation. Upon release from the lysosome, the central cobalt atom of cobalamin is in the trivalent state and undergoes a series of reduction reactions to the monovalent state. Monovalent cobalamin is either converted to methylcobalamin

(MeCbl) or is taken up by the mitochondria and converted to adenosylcobalamin (AdoCbl). MeCbl is the cofactor and a methyl donor for methionine synthase, while AdoCbl is the cofactor for methylmalonyl CoA mutase.[3]

Inherited disorders of cobalamin are traditionally separated into those resulting from defects in absorption, transport, and cellular uptake of the vitamin and those resulting from defects in intracellular processing.[4]

Disorders of Absorption, Transport, and Cellular Uptake

These disorders are characterized clinically by the core findings of megaloblastic anemia. Developmental delay and myelopathy may also be seen. These disorders may result from: (1) absent or deficient intrinsic factor,[5] (2) deficient enterocyte uptake and transport of Cbl-IF (Imerslund-Gräsbeck syndrome),[6] or (3) deficiency of TCII.[7] Failure to thrive may also be a feature of both Imerslund-Gräsbeck syndrome and TCII deficiency. Extended duration of illness and delayed or inadequate treatment is associated with the prominence of neurologic symptoms in the setting of TCII deficiency.[3] This is particularly true if the anemia is treated with folate alone in the absence of cobalamin.

In IF deficiency and Imerslund-Gräsbeck syndrome, there is low-serum Cbl, normal gastric function and morphology, and absence of autoantobodies to IF. In TCII deficiency, serum Cbl may be normal because TCI levels are normally much higher than TCII levels. Megaloblastic anemia is an almost constant feature. Homocystinuria and methylmalonic aciduria may be present, but at levels below that encountered for the disorders of intracellular Cbl metabolism. The Schilling test is abnormal in both deficient IF and defective enterocyte transport. It is correctable in the former by a source of human IF and not correctable in the latter. The Schilling test may or may not be abnormal in the setting of TCII deficiency as TCII may also be involved in the transcytosis of Cbl through the enterocyte. For most patients with TCII deficiency, serum TCII is not detectable by electrophoresis; however, some patients will have immunoreactive TCII, which has abnormal Cbl-binding properties.[3]

Inheritance for these disorders is autosomal recessive. The gene for hereditary IF deficiency has been localized to chromosome 11q13, and the cDNA has been cloned.[8] No mutations in affected patients have been identified. For Imerslund-Gräsbeck syndrome, interest has focused on cubilin, which has been identified as the probable Cbl-IF receptor. Linkage studies in multiplex Scandinavian families with this syndrome have localized the gene to 10p12.[9] This is the same region to which cubilin maps. Disease-specific mutations in cubilin have been found in some Finnish families.[10] The TCII gene is on chromosome 22, and both deletion and nonsense mutations have been identified in affected individuals.[11]

Treatment of these disorders requires systemic Cbl given IM initially to replete body stores then on an ongoing maintenance basis. A spectrum of outcomes is possible, and reversal of neurologic symptoms has been reported; however this largely depends on the duration of symptoms before the initiation of treatment. Folate supplementation will assist in the reversal of hematologic abnormalities but should not be given without concurrent adequate Cbl treatment.[3]

Disorders of Intracellular Metabolism

Eight inherited defects in intracellular Cbl metabolism have been identified by somatic cell complementation analysis (cblA to cblH).[1,4] These disorders typically feature more severe metabolic disturbances than those encountered in disorders of Cbl absorption, transport, and uptake. Furthermore, these disorders have elucidated distinct steps in the normal pathway of intracellular Cbl utilization (Fig. 68–1).

Three defects (cblC, cblD, cblF) result in both homocystinuria and methylmalonic aciduria. There is a deficiency in the synthesis of both AdoCbl and MeCbl in cultured fibroblasts. cblC is the most common of these diseases, with more than 150 patients. cblC typically presents in the first year of life with megaloblastic anemia, feeding difficulties, hypotonia, and lethargy progressing to significant neurologic impairment in which

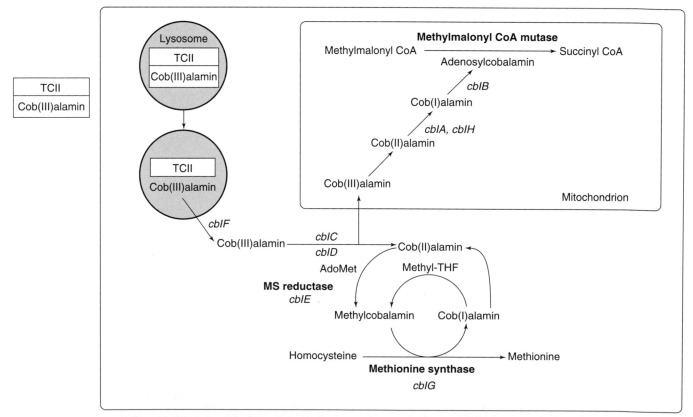

FIGURE 68–1. Intracellular cobalamin metabolism showing lysosomal, cytoplasmic, and mitochondrial compartments. AdoMet = S-adenosylmethionine; cblA, cblH = location of complementation groups cblA–cblH; Cob(III)alamin = B_{12a} = Cbl^{3+}; Cob(II)alamin = B12r = Cbl^{2+}; Cob(I)alamin = B_{12s} = Cbl^{1+}; MS = methionine synthase; Methyl-THF = methyltetrahydrofolate; TCII = transcobalamin II.

seizures and a pigmentary retinopathy are frequent.[12] Late-onset cblC occurs less frequently and is characterized by mental status changes (delirium, psychosis) and long tract findings. A similar biochemical profile is apparent in cblD, which has been described in only two brothers.[13] Clinical manifestations were milder, with cognitive disability and behavioral changes apparent. However, cells from these brothers complemented with those from cblC patients. Both cblC and cblD feature a defect in the process of reduction of the central cobalt atom from the trivalent to divalent state following the efflux of Cbl from the lysosome. The genes for these disorders have not been identified. Autosomal recessive inheritance is presumed; however, X-linked inheritance cannot be ruled out for cblD. The cblF disorder has been identified in 6 patients; the defect involves the failure of Cbl to exit the lysosome.[14] Clinical presentation has been quite variable with feeding difficulties, skin changes, hypotonia, and developmental delay. The gene for this disorder has not been identified.

Disorders with impaired MeCbl synthesis alone include two distinct complementation classes: cblE and cblG. These patients have both megaloblastic anemia and neurologic symptoms.[2-4] Most patients present early on with significant feeding difficulties and failure to thrive. Developmental delay, nystagmus, tonic changes, and visual impairment often occur. Late-onset cases from both complementation classes have been reported, frequently manifesting neuropsychiatric symptoms and/or myelopathy. Cerebral atrophy and white matter changes have been apparent on neuroimaging studies. These patients have megaloblastic anemia and homocystinuria in the absence of methylmalonic aciduria. Cultured fibroblasts reveal reduced MeCbl synthesis, whereas AdoCbl synthesis is normal. Complementation analysis provides the definitive diagnosis. The defect in cblE is in methionine synthase reductase required by methionine synthase, and the defect in cblG is in the methionine synthase enzyme itself.[15] The methionine synthase gene has been localized to chromosome 1q43, and mutations have been identified in cblG patients.[16] The methionine synthase reductase gene has been localized to chromosome 5p15, and mutations have been reported in most cblE patients.[17]

Three complementation classes (cblA, cblB, and cblH) have been identified in isolated AdoCbl deficiency.[2-4] Early-onset and late-onset presentations have been described in cblA and cblB. The early-onset form featured acutely ill infants with recurrent vomiting, lethargy, and hypotonia; the later onset presented either indolently with developmental delay or acutely with metabolic decompensation. These patients have methylmalonic aciduria (Cbl responsive) without homocystinuria or megaloblastic anemia. AdoCbl synthesis is reduced in cultured fibroblasts, and complementation of cells with the other classes of intracellular Cbl defects and methylmalonyl CoA mutase deficiency is demonstrated.

In cblA and cblH, the defect appears to be in intramitochondrial reduction of the central cobalt atom of Cbl from the divalent to monovalent state.[18] In cblB, the defect is in the adenosyltransferase enzyme, which is the final stage in the synthesis of AdoCbl.[19] These disorders are autosomal recessive in inheritance; however, the gene for each has not yet been identified.

For all disorders of intracellular Cbl utilization, treatment consists of systemic pharmacologic Cbl supplementation.[15] Hydroxy-Cbl (OHCbl) is the preferred form of Cbl. For the cblC disorder, cyano-Cbl (CNCbl) has been shown to be ineffective. Betaine supplementation has been demonstrated to be helpful in cblC, cblE, and cblG. Protein restriction is useful in cblA, cblB, and cblH patients. Outcome is variable, depending largely on age of onset and delay in initiating treatment.

While not strictly a defect in intracellular Cbl utilization, owing to its clinical and biochemical similarity, methylmalonyl-CoA mutase (mutase) deficiency is best considered within the context of these disorders.[3] A nuclear coded intramitochondrial homodimer, mutase catalyzes the isomerization of methylmalonyl-CoA to succinyl-CoA, a key step in propionate catabolism that uses AdoCbl as an essential cofactor. Clinical variability in presentation ranges from acute neonatal ketoacidosis to subacute indolent courses characterized by developmental delay to asymptomatic cases detected on routine newborn screening.[20] Two biochemical phenotypes also exist relating to the amount of detectable mutase enzyme activity in cultured fibroblasts; mut^0 and mut^-.[21] Residual activity in the enzyme apparent upon stimulation with high concentrations of hydroxycobalamin in the culture medium characterizes the mut^- subclass. The mut^0 patients have an early and often fatal neonatal presentation, whereas the mut^- patients present typically in later infancy or childhood. Survival is usual for the mut^- patients; however there may be significant eventual morbidity, which need not be preceded by episodic acidosis and clinically apparent metabolic imbalance.[20] Inheritance is autosomal recessive, with the *MUT* gene localized to chromosome 6p12. Clinical and enzymatic correlations with documented mutations in the *MUT* locus have been demonstrated.[21] Many mutations have been identified, including three common mutations: G717V, E117X, N219Y. Treatment consists of dietary protein restriction, pharmacologic Cbl supplementation, and antimicrobial agents to reduce enteric anaerobic production of propionate. Carnitine supplementation in this setting may also be beneficial. In patients with absent mutase activity, Cbl supplementation is usually not effective.

FOLATE

Absorption, Transport, and Metabolism

Folates are essential cofactors for a variety of 1-carbon transfer reactions involved in the synthesis of purines, pyrimidines, and methionine as well as the catabolism of serine, glycine, and histidine. Dietary folates are predominantly polyglutamates that undergo intestinal hydrolysis to monoglutamates before absorption. Intestinal absorption is by a specific transport system, which also appears to mediate folate transport across the choroid plexus. Released into the portal circulation, folates are methylated in the liver and released into the systemic circulation. Cellular uptake is also mediated by specific transport systems.[2]

Folate metabolism is complex and linked to glycine and serine interconversion, pyrimidine nucleotide synthesis, purine biosynthesis, histidine catabolism (glutamate formiminotransferase), and methionine production from homocysteine (Fig. 68–2) Methylenetetrahydrofolate reductase (MTHFR) is necessary to generate methyltetrahydrofolate, a methyl donor for methionine synthase.[3]

Disorders of Absorption, Transport, and Cellular Uptake

Hereditary folate malabsorption (congenital malabsorption of folate) involves a defect in the common transport system for folate at the intestine and choroid plexus levels.[22] Clinical symptoms typically begin in the first few months of life and include megaloblastic anemia, failure to thrive, diarrhea, seizures (frequently intractable), and progressive neurologic deterioration. Intracranial calcifi-

cations have been observed in some patients. Serum, red blood cell, and cerebrospinal fluid folate levels are low. A severe abnormality in the intestinal absorption of orally administered folate is apparent. Inheritance is autosomal recessive. Although a putative cDNA for the intestinal folate transporter has been identified,[23] no mutations in affected patients have been reported. Treatment is the administration of pharmacologic amounts of folic acid, folinic acid, or MTHFR, usually by parenteral means.

Disorders of Intracellular Metabolism

Two disorders in intracellular folate metabolism have been described. Glutamate formiminotransferase deficiency has been reported in more than twelve patients. Clinical features have included cognitive disability ranging from mild to severe, with associated seizures and cortical atrophy observed in more severely affected individuals.[22] Speech delay may be a feature. The enzymatic defect affects histidine metabolism and results in excessive formiminoglutamate (FIGLU) excretion. However, the level of observed FIGLU excretion does not actually correlate with disease severity.[15] Other findings have included megaloblastic anemia, elevated histidine, and normal folate levels. Inheritance is autosomal recessive. The gene for human formiminoglutamate transferase is on chromosome 21.[15] It is not clear that

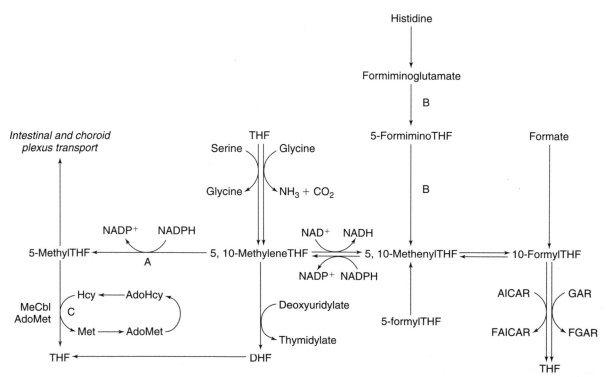

FIGURE 68–2. Folate metabolism showing sites (A, B, and C) of the confirmed enzymatic block involved in inborn errors of folate metabolism. A = methylenetetrahydrofolate reductase; B = glutamate formiminotransferase; formiminotetrahydrofolate cyclodeaminase; C = methionine synthase; AdoHcy = S-adenosylhomocysteine; AdoMet = S-adenosylmethionine; AICAR = 5-phosphoribosyl-5-aminoimidazole-4-carboxamide; DHF = dihydrofolate; GAR = 5-phosphoribosylglycinamide; Hcy = homocysteine; Met = methionine; THF = tetrahydrofolate.

treatment with folate in order to normalize FIGLU levels is necessary.[15]

More than 50 patients with MTHFR deficiency are known.[1] Phenotypic expression for this disorder is variable and includes (1) acute neurologic deterioration in early infancy; (2) developmental delay, seizures, and progressive neurologic impairment in childhood; and (3) myelopathy, psychiatric disease, and cerebrovascular events in adolescence and adulthood. The enzymatic defect results in deficient formation of MTHF, which results in reduced methylation of homocysteine to yield methionine. Thus, homocystinuria is apparent, although less than that observed in cystathionine synthase deficiency. Serum homocysteine is elevated, and serum methionine is low. There is no megaloblastic anemia. It is unclear if the neurologic features of MTHFR deficiency are the result of elevated homocysteine, low methionine, or interference in critical methylation reactions. Inheritance is autosomal recessive, and the gene is located on chromosome 1p36 with the cDNA well characterized.[24] Multiple mutations responsible for MTHFR deficiency have been identified.[25] Early treatment with betaine (which functions as a substrate for an alternative means of methyl transfer between homocysteine and methionine) is recommended. Folic acid, pyridoxine, methionine, and Cbl supplementation has also been used.[15]

A common polymorphism in MTHFR (677C→T) confers enzyme thermolability, and also causes a mild reduction in enzymatic deficiency.[26] Hyperhomocysteinemia has emerged recently as an important independent risk factor for vascular disease including stroke.[27] There is some suggestion, albeit still controversial, that the 677C→T polymorphism may also function as an independent risk factor for vascular disease.[26] Furthermore, it is known that periconceptional folate supplementation reduces the risk of offspring with neural tube defects in both low and high-risk groups. There is good evidence to suggest that the 677C→T polymorphism is a risk factor for neural tube defects.[28]

REFERENCES

1. Rosenblatt DS, Fenton WA: Inborn errors of cobalamin metabolism. In Banerjee R (ed): Chemistry and Biochemistry of Vitamin B_{12}. Baltimore, John Wiley & Sons, 1999, pp 367–384.

2. Fowler B: Genetic defects of folate and cobalamin metabolism. Eur J Pediatr 1998;157:60–66.

3. Shevell MI, Cooper BA, Rosenblatt DS: Inherited disorders of cobalamin and folate transport and metabolism. In Rosenberg RN, Prosiner SB, DiMauro E, Sardi RL (eds): The Molecular and Genetic Basis of Neurological Disease, 2nd ed. Boston, Butterworth-Heinemann, 1997, pp 1301–1322.

4. Rosenblatt DS: Inborn errors of folate and cobalamin metabolism. In Carmel R, Jacobsen DW (eds):

Homocysteine in Health and Disease. Cambridge, Cambridge University Press, 2001, pp 244–258.

5. Yang YM, Ducos R, Rosenberg AJ, et al: Cobalamin malabsorption in three siblings due to abnormal intrinsic factor that is markedly susceptible to acid and proteolysis. J Clin Invest 1985;76:2057–2065.

6. Gräsbeck R: Familial selective vitamin B_{12} malabsorption. N Engl J Med 1972;287:358.

7. Hall CA: The neurologic aspects of transcobalamin II deficiency. Br J Haematol 1992;80:117–120.

8. Hewitt JE, Gordon MM, Taggart RT, et al: Human gastric intrinsic factor: Characterization of cDNA and genomic clones and localization to human chromosome 11. Genomics 1991;10:432–440.

9. Kozyraki R, Kristiansen MM, Silahtaroglu A, et al: The human intrinsic factor-vitamin B_{12} receptor, cubilin: Molecular characterization and chromosomal mapping of the gene to 10p within the autosomal recessive megaloblastic anemia (MGA1) region. Blood 1998;91:3593–3600.

10. Aminoff M, Carter JE, Chadwick RB, et al: Mutations in CUBN, encoding the intrinsic factor-vitamin B_{12} receptor, cubilin, cause hereditary megaloblastic anaemia 1. Nat Genet 1999;21:309–13.

11. Li N, Rosenblatt DS, Kamen BA, et al: Identification of two mutant alleles of transcobalamin II in an affected family. Hum Mol Genet 1994;3:1835–1840.

12. Rosenblatt DS, Aspler AL, Shevell MI, et al: Clinical heterogeneity and prognosis in combined methylmalonic aciduria and homocystinuria (cblC). J Inherit Metab Dis 1997;20:528–538.

13. Goodman SI, Moe PG, Hammond KB, et al: Homocystinuria with methylmalonic aciduria: Two cases in a sibship. Biochem Med 1970;4:500–515.

14. Rosenblatt DS, Hosack A, Matiaszuk NV, et al: Defect in vitamin B_{12} release from lysosomes: Newly described inborn error of vitamin B_{12} metabolism. Science 1985;228:1319–1321.

15. Rosenblatt DS: Disorders of cobalamin and folate transport and metabolism. In Fernandez J, Saudubray JM, van den Berghe G (eds): Inborn Metabolic Disease: Diagnosis and Treatment, 3rd ed. New York, Springer-Verlag, 2000, pp 284–304.

16. Leclerc D, Campeu E, Goyette P, et al: Human methionine synthase: cDNA cloning and identification of mutations in patients of the cblG complementation group of folate/cobalamin disorders. Hum Mol Genet 1996;5:1867–1874.

17. Leclerc D, Wilson A, Dumas R, et al: Cloning and mapping of a cDNA for methionine synthase reductase, a flavoprotein defective in patients with homocystinuria. Proc Natl Acad Sci U S A 1998;95:3059–3064.

18. Cooper BA, Rosenblatt DS, Watkins D: Methylmalonic aciduria due to a new defect in adenosylcobalamin accumulation by cells. Am J Hematol 1990;34:115–120.

19. Fenton WA, Rosenberg LE: The defect in the cbl B class of human methylmalonic acidemia: Deficiency of cob(I)alamin adenosyltransferase activity in extracts of cultured fibroblasts. Biochem Biophys Res Commun 1981;98:283–289.

20. Shevell MI, Matiaszuk N, Ledley FD, Rosenblatt DS: Varying neurological phenotypes among mut^0 and mut$^-$ patients with methylmalonyl CoA mutase deficiency. Am J Med Genet 1993;45:619–624.

21. Ledley FD, Rosenblatt DS: Mutations in MUT methylmalonic acidemia: Clinical and enzymatic correlations. Hum Mutat 1997;9:1–6.

22. Rosenblatt DS, Fenton WA: Inherited disorders of folate and cobalamin transport and metabolism. In Scriver CR, Beaudet Al, Sy WS, Valle D (eds): The Metabolic and Molecular Bases of Inherited Disease (8th ed). New York, McGraw-Hill, 2001, pp 3897–3933.

23. Rosenblatt S, Whitehead VM: Cobalamin and folate deficiency: Acquired and hereditary disorders in children. Sem Hematol 1999;36:19–34.

24. Goyette P, Sumner JS, Milos R, et al: Human methylenetetrahydrofolate reductase: Isolation of cDNA, mapping and mutation identification. Nat Genet 1994;7:195–200.

25. Goyette P, Frosst P, Rosenblatt DS, Rozen R: Seven novel mutations in the methylenetetrahydrofolate reductase gene and genotype/phenotype correlations in severe methylenetetrahydrofolate reductase deficiency. Am J Hum Genet 1995;56:1052–1059.

26. Frosst P, Blom HJ, Milos R, et al: A candidate genetic risk factor for vascular disease: A common methylenetetrahydrofolate reductase mutation causes thermoinstability. Nat Genet 1995;10:111–113.

27. Diaz-Arrastia R: Homocysteine and neurologic disease. Arch Neurol 2000;57:1422–1428.

28. Christensen B, Arbour L, Tran P, et al: Genetic polymorphisms in methylenetetrahydrofolate reductase and methionine synthase folate levels in red blood cells and risk of neural tube defects. Am J Med Genet 1999;84:151–157.

Disorders of Biotin Metabolism: Treatable Neurologic Syndromes

Barry Wolf

Biotin is a water-soluble B-complex vitamin that consists of a heterocyclic ring with an aliphatic carbon side chain that ends in a carboxyl group (Fig. 69–1).[1] The latter group is covalently attached to the various carboxylases that use it as a coenzyme. One of the nitrogens (N–1) of the ureide portion of the ring is involved with transferring carbon dioxide from various substrates to their respective products. Biotin is the coenzyme for four carboxylases in humans that have important roles in gluconeogenesis, fatty acid synthesis, and the catabolism of several branch-chain amino acids. Three carboxylases are mitochondrial. Pyruvate carboxylase converts pyruvate to oxaloacetate, the initial step in gluconeogenesis. Propionyl CoA carboxylase catabolizes several branch-chain amino acids and odd-chain fatty acids. β-methyl-crotonyl CoA carboxylase is involved in the catabolism of leucine. The fourth carboxylase, acetyl CoA carboxylase, is mainly a cytosolic enzyme that converts malonyl CoA to acetyl CoA, the first step in the biosynthesis of fatty acids (although recent studies indicate a form of the enzyme in mitochondria).

Biotin is covalently attached to the various apocarboxylases by the enzyme biotin holocarboxylase synthetase. The carboxyl group of biotin is attached through an amide bond to an α-amino group of a specific lysine residue of the apoenzyme. This reaction occurs through two partial reactions. The first is the ATP-requiring phosphorylation of biotin resulting in biotinyl 5-AMP. In the second partial reaction, this intermediate reacts with apocarboxylases, resulting in biotinylated holoenzymes. After the carboxylases are degraded proteolytically to biocytin (biotinyl-lysine) or biotinyl peptides, the enzyme biotinidase (EC 3.5.1.12) cleaves the amide bond, releasing lysine or lysyl-peptides and free biotin, which can then be recycled.[2] Biotinidase also plays a role in the

processing of protein-bound biotin, thereby making the vitamin available to the free biotin pool. Recently, it has been shown that biotinidase transfers biotin from the cleavage of biocytin to histones.[3]

There are inherited isolated deficiencies in the three mitochondrial carboxylases. Each deficiency is due to a structural abnormality in one of them, whereas the activities of the other carboxylases are normal. Each disorder is inherited as an autosomal recessive trait. Affected children usually develop neurologic symptoms and metabolic compromise. All three isolated deficiencies are treated by dietary restriction and fail to respond to pharmacologic doses of biotin.

In addition to isolated carboxylase deficiencies, there are two other disorders characterized by deficient activities of at least the three mitochondrial biotin-dependent carboxylases. Initially, these disorders were designated early-onset or neonatal multiple carboxylase deficiency and late-onset or juvenile multiple carboxylase deficiency based on when symptoms appeared. It has now been shown that the first of these disorders is due to deficient activity of biotin holocarboxylase synthetase and the second is due to deficient activity of biotinidase. Both disorders have some symptoms in common. Most importantly, both can be treated effectively with pharmacologic doses of biotin. This chapter will discuss these two readily treatable biotin-responsive disorders.

BIOTIN HOLOCARBOXYLASE SYNTHETASE DEFICIENCY

Clinical and Neurologic Features

Children with biotin holocarboxylase synthetase deficiency usually exhibit breathing abnormalities such as

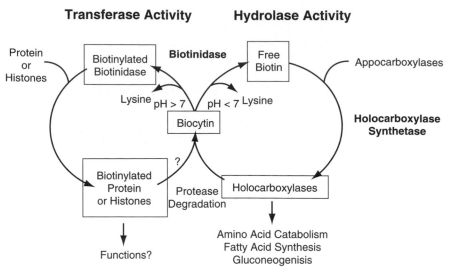

FIGURE 69–1. The biotin bi-cycle pathway. Holocarboxylase synthetase attaches biotin to various apocarboxylases and forms holocarboxylases. The holocarboxylases are then proteolytically degraded, forming biocytin. The biocytin is either cleaved by biotinidase at pH<7 recycling free biotin (biotinyl-hydrolase activity), or it is cleaved and the biotinidase is biotinylated at pH>7. The biotinylated biotinidase can then readily transfer the biotin to other proteins, such as histones (biotinyl-transferase activity). (From Hymes J, Wolf B: Biotinidase and its role in biotin metabolism. Clin Chim Acta 1996;255:1–11.)

tachypnea, hyperventilation, or apnea; feeding difficulties; hypotonia or hypertonia; seizures; lethargy; and irritability, which can result in developmental delay and coma.[1,4] Many children developed skin rash, and several had alopecia. All affected children have had metabolic ketoacidosis and organic aciduria. Abnormal urine odor was noted in several patients. Most of those evaluated had hyperammonemia. These children usually develop symptoms in the newborn period, but some have become symptomatic at several months of age, and one presented at 8 years. The findings on CT scan of the head are variable, ranging from normal to low-density changes scattered throughout the white matter of both cerebral hemispheres, with loss of demarcation between gray and white matter.[5] The EEG abnormalities are also variable, ranging from normal to diffusely abnormal with burst-suppression patterns.[5] These aberrant patterns may normalize with biotin treatment. Siblings of several of the children who had the same disorder have become comatose and died before a diagnosis was made or appropriate treatment was instituted. This disorder is inherited as an autosomal recessive trait. Because only a small number of patients have been reported, the gene frequency of the disorder cannot be estimated accurately.

Biochemical Findings and Laboratory Analysis

Holocarboxylase synthetase deficiency is usually suspected when high concentrations of the metabolites, α-hydroxyisovalerate, α-methylcrotonylglycine, α-hydroxypropionate, methylcitrate, and/or lactate are found in the urine of a child exhibiting some or all of the above clinical findings.[1,6] Prior to biotin treatment, the activities of the various mitochondrial carboxylases are deficient in extracts of the peripheral blood leukocytes. Within days after starting biotin therapy, the carboxylase activities increase to normal or near normal in these cells. Skin fibroblasts from these patients are deficient in the three mito-

chondrial carboxylase activities when cells are cultured in a medium containing low concentrations of biotin. Upon incubation of these cells in high concentrations of biotin, the carboxylase activities increase to normal or near normal. Definitive diagnosis requires the demonstration of deficient activity of holocarboxylase synthetase in peripheral blood leukocytes or skin fibroblasts. A simple assay of the first partial reaction in the holocarboxylase synthetase reaction was developed, and this activity was deficient in all children previously shown to have holocarboxylase synthetase deficiency. This assay allows a more rapid confirmation of the diagnosis of this disorder.

The Enzyme and the Enzyme Deficiency

Holocarboxylase synthetase has been studied in both bacterial and animal systems and is highly specific for biotin. The enzyme requires ATP and magnesium for activity. In rat, 70% of the holocarboxylase synthetase activity is located in the cytosol and the remaining 30% is in the mitochondria. Bovine holocarboxylase synthetase has been purified to homogeneity.[7] Using the protein sequence data, the cDNA for the enzyme was cloned and sequenced.[8] Simultaneously, a second group isolated the gene for the enzyme.[9] The gene for the holocarboxylase synthetase has been localized to chromosome 21q22.1.

The primary enzyme deficiency was demonstrated by several laboratories at about the same time.[10,11] Studies of the enzymes of many known patients with holocarboxylase synthetase deficiency have revealed elevated K_m values of biotin, ranging from 3 to 70 times that of normal, and the age of onset of symptoms in these children correlated negatively with the K_m values of biotin. Recently a child with the highest K_m of biotin had a very mild clinical course. Differences were noted in the stability of the mutant enzymes, suggesting biochemical heterogeneity for the disorder.

Multiple mutations have been identified in the gene that cause holocarboxylase synthetase deficiency.[12] Mutations within the biotin-binding region of the enzyme result in a protein with increased K_m values of biotin, whereas those outside of this region result in enzymes with normal K_m values, but reduced V_{max} values. Children with altered K_m values readily respond to biotin therapy, whereas those with normal K_m values respond to biotin, but usually not as well. One child who did not develop symptoms until 8 years of age has been reported with an abnormal gene-splicing mutation that results in decreased amounts of normal synthetase mRNA. Mutation analyses of children with this disorder may be useful in predicting phenotype.

Therapy

Most patients with holocarboxylase synthetase deficiency have improved markedly following oral administration of 10 mg of biotin per day. Biochemical abnormalities correct quickly with improvement of many, if not all, of the clinical symptoms. However, a child with one of the highest K_m values of biotin continued to excrete abnormal organic acids even when treated with 60 to 80 mg of biotin per day. Based on the differences in the K_m values of biotin for the synthetase in these patients, the necessity of administering higher concentrations of biotin must be determined on an individual basis. If treatment is delayed, many of the neurologic abnormalities will not be reversible with biotin therapy.

Prenatal Diagnosis and Prenatal Treatment

Prenatal diagnosis of holocarboxylase synthetase deficiency has been performed by demonstrating deficient activities of the mitochondrial carboxylases in cultured amniocytes. When these cells were cultured in medium supplemented with biotin, the carboxylase activities increased toward normal. In addition, affected fetuses have had elevations of α-hydroxyisovalerate and/or methylcitrate in their amniotic fluid, using stable isotope dilution techniques. Although the latter method is a simpler and more rapid method for prenatal diagnosis, both diagnostic procedures should be performed to confirm the diagnosis, using the same sample of amniotic fluid.

Prenatal treatment of holocarboxylase synthetase deficiency has been performed in two separate at-risk pregnancies. The mothers were treated with 10 mg of biotin orally, one from the 34th week of gestation and the other from the 23rd week of gestation. In both cases, the children were asymptomatic at birth, although in the second pregnancy the child became symptomatic after biotin was withheld for a short time. Once biotin treatment was reinstituted, the child's condition returned to normal. The diagnosis was confirmed in both children. Both have remained asymptomatic on biotin therapy. Because biotin treatment initiated at birth apparently prevents development of symptoms in affected newborns, it is unclear if prenatal treatment of affected children is necessary.

BIOTINIDASE DEFICIENCY

Clinical and Neurologic Features

In addition to the children with biotin holocarboxylase synthetase deficiency, there are patients who have been reported with seizure, skin rash, and/or hypotonia that first appears at several months of age.[1,13] Their urinary organic acids are consistent with those of children with multiple carboxylase deficiency. Similarly, the carboxylase activities in extracts of their peripheral blood leukocytes were deficient, and they increased following biotin administration. However, unlike the patients with holocarboxylase synthetase deficiency, these patients had normal carboxylase activities in extracts of their fibroblasts cultured in biotin-replete medium. It was initially proposed that these children have a defect in the intestinal or renal transport of biotin. However, in 1983 it was shown that these patients and other children with the late-onset form of multiple carboxylase deficiency actually have a deficiency of serum biotinidase activity.[14]

The most common neurologic features of this disorder are seizures and hypotonia. The most common types of seizures are generalized and tonic/clonic, but some children have exhibited partial, infantile spasms, or myoclonic seizures.[15] Several patients exhibited breathing abnormalities, such as hyperventilation, stridor, and apnea. Frequently they have cutaneous symptoms, including skin rash and varying degrees of alopecia. Sensorineural hearing loss[16,17] and eye problems, such as optic atrophy,[18] have been described in a large number of untreated children. Several patients have had cellular immunologic abnormalities, manifested by fungal infection. These immunologic aberrations are varied and may represent the effects of abnormal organic acid metabolites or biotin deficiency on normal function. Biotin therapy rapidly corrects the immunologic dysfunction. Some patients with biotinidase deficiency have manifested only one or two of these features, whereas others have exhibited a full spectrum of neurologic and cutaneous findings. The age of onset of symptoms varies from 1 week to 10 years, with a mean age from 3 to 6 months. As untreated children get older, they may exhibit ataxia and developmental delay. Several children have not developed symptoms until late childhood or adolescence.[19] They exhibited symptoms that were different from those of the younger affected children: spastic paraparesis often with rapid loss of vision with progressive optic neuropathy. The paraparesis markedly improved over months to years, whereas the scotomata resolved within weeks to months. Biotinidase deficiency is inherited as an autosomal recessive trait with parents exhibiting serum enzyme activities intermediate between that of the deficient and normal individuals.

Computerized axial tomography of the head has been performed in several affected children at different ages, but fails to reveal consistent findings.[5] The findings are usually normal but may reveal diffuse cerebral atrophy with or without low attenuation of the white matter, basal ganglia calcifications, enlargement of the ventricles, and even cysts. EEG findings range from normal to diffuse slow-wave activity that usually resolves with biotin treatment.

Biochemical Findings and Laboratory Analysis

The majority of patients exhibit metabolic ketolactic acidosis and organic aciduria similar to that seen in holocarboxylase synthetase deficiency. The most commonly elevated urinary organic acid is α-hydroxyisovalerate. These patients may have mild hyperammonemia. There was considerable variability in expression of this disorder even within a family. The absence of organic aciduria or metabolic ketoacidosis in a symptomatic child does not exclude this disorder.

The Enzyme and the Enzyme Deficiency

Biotinidase is found in many procaryotes and eukaryotes and in most mammalian tissues, particularly serum, liver, and kidney. Human biotinidase has been purified to homogeneity from serum and plasma by several groups.[20–22] The enzyme is a monomeric glycoprotein with a molecular weight of between 67,000 and 74,000 daltons. Using the protein sequence, the cDNA encoding the biotinidase gene was cloned and isolated[23] and the organization of the entire gene elucidated.[24]

Serum biotinidase is produced mainly in the liver. Biotinidase is localized intracellularly to the rough endoplasmic reticulum. Although the major function of biotinidase is to recycle biotin by cleaving biocytin and biotinyl-peptides, the enzyme has also been shown to biotinylate histones following the cleavage of biocytin. One study suggested that biotinidase functions as a biotin-binding protein in serum, whereas another study failed to support this. The exact site of biocytin cleavage or the metabolism of the enzyme in serum and tissues remains to be determined.

Biotinidase activity is determined by measuring the release of biotin from biocytin or a biocytin analogue, such as N-biotinyl p-aminobenzoate.[14] Other end-point and kinetic assays for biotinidase activity in serum and tissues are available. To our knowledge, all patients who have been tested using the natural and the artificial substrate have been shown to be deficient in both.

Patients with profound biotinidase activity have less than 10% mean normal activity. The parents of these children usually have serum enzyme activities intermediate between those of the patients and normal individuals. Deficient biotinidase activity has also been demonstrated

in extracts of leukocytes and fibroblasts from some of these patients. At least one patient has also been shown to have deficient biotinidase activity in his liver extract.

In addition to patients with profound biotinidase deficiency, a group of patients with partial deficiency, 10% to 30% of mean normal activity, have been identified by newborn screening. Clinical consequences of partial deficiency were not known until one child, who was identified by newborn screening but was not treated with biotin, developed hypotonia, skin rash, and hair loss at six months of age during a bout of gastroenteritis. The child's symptoms rapidly resolved with biotin treatment. It is possible that partial biotinidase deficiency is a problem only when affected individuals are exposed to certain stresses, such as starvation or infection. The full clinical spectrum of partial deficiency remains to be elucidated.

Multiple mutations have been described in symptomatic children with profound biotinidase deficiency.[25] Two mutations are common in children with profound biotinidase deficiency who were identified by newborn screening. When the mutations among children identified by newborn screening were compared with those of children ascertained by exhibiting symptoms, four mutations comprise about 60% of the abnormal alleles. Two mutations occurred in both populations but occurred in the symptomatic population at a significantly greater frequency. The other two common mutations occurred only in the newborn screening group. There is no clear genotype-phenotype correlation. In addition, almost all children with partial biotinidase deficiency have a single missense mutation on one allele in combination with a mutation for profound biotinidase deficiency on the other.

Pathophysiology

Serum biotinidase activity is not altered by biotin deficiency. This was demonstrated by the fact that several patients who became biotin deficient while being treated with parenteral hyperalimentation that lacked biotin had normal serum biotinidase activity. Biotinidase appears to play an important role in the processing of protein-bound biotin. This may occur either by secretion into the intestinal tract, where it can release biotin that can subsequently be absorbed, or by cleaving biocytin or biotinyl-peptides in the intestinal mucosa or in the blood.

Biotinidase activity in cerebrospinal fluid and in the brain is very low. This suggests that the brain may not be able to recycle biotin and, therefore, must depend on biotin that is transported across the blood-brain barrier. Several symptomatic children who failed to exhibit peripheral lactic acidosis or organic aciduria have had elevations of lactate and/or organic acids in their cerebrospinal fluid. This compartmentalization of the biochemical abnormalities may explain why neurologic symptoms usually appear before the other symptoms.

Most patients with biotinidase activity who have hearing loss have had this problem prior to biotin therapy. Hearing loss is usually irreversible, although several young affected children have shown some improvement with therapy. The mechanism causing the hearing loss remains to be determined.

Neuropathology

The brains of several children with biotinidase deficiency have been studied. They have revealed a variety of abnormalities. One patient was found to have cerebral degeneration and atrophy with an absence of the Purkinje cell layer with rarification of the granular layer and proliferation of the Bergmann layer. There was gliosis of the white matter and dentate nucleus, but the brainstem and cerebral peduncles were normal. There was focal necrosis with vascular proliferation and infiltration by macrophages, suggesting a subacute necrotizing myelopathy. There was acute meningoencephalitis of the entire central nervous system. In the second child, who died at 3 months of age, the brain revealed defective myelination, focal areas of vacuolization, and gliosis in the white matter of the cerebrum and cerebellum. There was also a mild gliosis in the pyramidal cellular layer of the hippocampus, and there were characteristic changes of viral encephalopathy in the putamen and caudate nucleus.

Therapy

All symptomatic children with biotinidase deficiency have improved after treatment with 5 to 10 mg of biotin per day. Biotin must be administered in the free form, as opposed to the bound form. The biochemical abnormalities and seizures rapidly resolve after biotin treatment, followed by improvement of the cutaneous manifestations. Hair growth returns over a period of weeks to months in the children with alopecia. Optic atrophy and hearing loss seem to be the most resistant to therapy, especially if a long period has elapsed between the time symptoms appeared and the time of diagnosis and initiation of treatment. Some treated children have rapidly achieved developmental milestones, whereas others have continued to show deficits.

Most patients with biotinidase deficiency excrete large quantities of biocytin in their urine, but there is no evidence of accumulation of this metabolite in the tissues. It remains to be determined whether biotin therapy is harmful, because it may increase the concentration of biocytin in these children.

Prenatal Diagnosis

Biotinidase activity is measurable in cultured amniotic fluid cells and in amniotic fluid. Therefore, the potential for prenatal diagnosis of biotinidase deficiency exists. Prenatal diagnosis has been performed in several at-risk pregnancies in which amniocentesis was performed because of advanced maternal age. The fetuses were unaffected, and this was confirmed after birth.

Neonatal Screening

Since biotinidase deficiency met many of the criteria for considering inclusion into a neonatal screening program, a colorimetric test for biotinidase activity was developed for determining biotinidase activity in the same blood spots currently used for other newborn screening tests.[26] About 25 states in the United States and 25 countries screen their newborns for biotinidase deficiency. The incidence of biotinidase deficiency is about 1:137,000 for profound biotinidase deficiency, 1:110,000 for partial biotinidase deficiency, and 1:61,000 for the combined incidence of profound and partial biotinidase deficiency. Most children with biotinidase deficiency have been Caucasian, and only several were African American or Asian.

CONCLUSION

Although deficient activities of biotin holocarboxylase synthetase and biotinidase have been shown to cause two biotin-responsive disorders, there is a small group of patients with biotin-responsive conditions who have neither holocarboxylase synthetase or biotinidase deficiency. A group of biotin-responsive children in Saudi Arabia with basal ganglia disease characterized by encephalopathy, dystonia, and quadriparesis have been shown to have a defect in a biotin transporter gene.[27] Therefore, there may be other disorders in biotin metabolism that need to be elucidated. In the process, we will surely better understand the normal intermediary metabolism of this vitamin and obtain clues about the etiology of other vitamin-responsive syndromes.

REFERENCES

1. Wolf B: Disorders of Biotin Metabolism. In Scriver CR, Beaudet AL, Sly WS, Valle D (eds): The Metabolic and Molecular Bases of Inherited Disease. New York, McGraw-Hill, 2001, 3935–3962.

2. Hymes J, Wolf B: Biotinidase and its role in biotin metabolism. Clin Chim Acta 1996;255:1–11.

3. Hymes J, Fleischhauer K, Wolf B: Biotinylation of histones by human serum biotinidase: Assessment of biotinyl-transferase activity in sera from normal individuals and children with biotinidase deficiency. Biochem Molecul Med 1995;56:76–83.

4. Coskun T, Tokatli A, Ozalp I: Inborn errors of biotin metabolism. Clinical and laboratory features of eight cases. Turk J Pediatr 1994;36:267–278.

5. Wolf B. Disorders of biotin metabolism: Treatable neurological syndromes. In Rosenberg R, Prusiner SB, Di Mauro S, et al (eds): The Molecular and Genetic Basis of Neurological Disease. Boston, Butterworth-Heinemann, 1992, pp 569–581.

6. Suormala T, Fowler B, Duran M, et al: Five patients with a biotin-responsive defect in holocarboxylase function: Evaluation of responsiveness to biotin therapy in vivo and comparative biochemical studies in vitro. Pediatr Res 1997;41:666–673.

7. Chiba Y, Suzuki Y, Aoki Y, et al: Purification and properties of bovine liver holocarboxylase synthetase. Arch Biochem Biophys 1995;313:8–14.

8. Suzuki Y, Aoki Y, Ishida Y, et al: Isolation and characterization of mutations in the human holocarboxylase synthetase cDNA. Nat Genet 1994;8:122–128.

9. Leon-Del-Rio A, Leclerc D, Akerman B, et al: Isolation of a cDNA encoding human holocarboxylase synthetase by functional complementation of a biotin auxotroph of *Escherichia coli*. Proc Natl Acad Sci U S A 1995;92:4626–4630.

10. Burri BJ, Sweetman L, Nyhan WL: Mutant holocarboxylase synthetase: Evidence for the enzyme defect in early infantile biotin-responsive multiple carboxylase deficiency. J Clin Invest 1981;68:1491–1495.

11. Saunders ME, Sherwood WG, Dutchie M, et al: Evidence for a defect of holocarboxylase synthetase activity in cultured lymphoblasts from a patient with biotin-responsive multiple carboxylase deficiency. Am J Hum Genet 1982;34:590–601.

12. Yang XB, Aoki YB, Li XB, et al: Structure of human holocarboxylase synthetase gene and mutation spectrum of holocarboxylase synthetase deficiency. Hum Genet 2001;109:526–534.

13. Wolf B, Heard GS, Weissbecker KA, et al: Biotinidase deficiency: Initial clinical features and rapid diagnosis. Ann Neurol 1985;18:614–617.

14. Wolf B, Grier RE, Secor-McVoy JR, Heard GS: Biotinidase deficiency: A novel vitamin recycling defect. J Inherit Metab Dis 1985;8:53–58.

15. Salbert BA, Pellock JM, Wolf B: Characterization of seizures associated with biotinidase deficiency. Neurology 1993;43:1351–1354.

16. Wolf B, Grier RE, Heard GS: Hearing loss in biotinidase deficiency. Lancet 1983;2:1365.

17. Wolf B, Spencer RF, Gleason AT: Hearing loss in common in symptomatic children with profound biotinidase deficiency. J Pediatr 2002;140:242–246.

18. Salbert BA, Astruc J, Wolf B: Ophthalmological findings in biotinidase deficiency. Ophthalmologica 1993;206:177–181.

19. Wolf B, Pomponio RJ, Norrgard KJ, et al: Delayed-onset profound biotinidase deficiency. J Pediatr 1998;132:362–365.

20. Craft DV, Goss NH, Chandramouli N, Wood HG: Purification of biotinidase from human plasma and its activity on biotinyl peptides. Biochemistry 1985;24:2471–2476.

21. Chauhan J, Dakshinamurti J: Purification and characterization of human serum biotinidase. J Biol Chem 1986;261:4268–4274.

22. Wolf B, Miller JB, Hymes J, et al: Immunological comparison of biotinidase in serum from normal and biotinidase-deficient individuals. Clin Chim Acta 1987;164:27–32.

23. Cole H, Reynolds TR, Buck GB, et al: Human serum biotinidase: cDNA cloning, sequence and characterization. J Biol Chem 1994;269:6566–6570.

24. Knight HC, Reynolds TR, Meyers GA, et al: Structure of the human biotinidase gene. Mamm Genome 1998;9:327–330.

25. Hymes J, Stanley CM, Wolf B: Mutations in BTD causing biotinidase deficiency. Hum Mutat 2001;200:375–381.

26. Wolf B: Worldwide survey of neonatal screening for biotinidase deficiency. J Inherit Metab Dis 1991;14:923–927.

27. Zang W, Al-Yamani E, Acierno JS, et al: Mutations in SCL19A3 encoding a novel transporter cause biotin-responsive basal ganglia disease. Am J Hum Genet 2001;69:195.

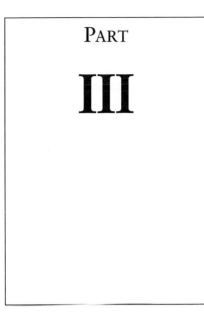

PART

III

PSYCHIATRIC DISEASE

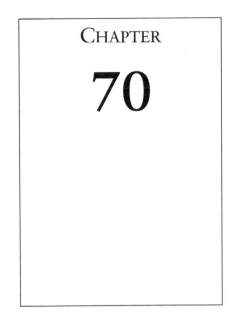

CHAPTER

70

Psychiatric Diseases: Challenges in Psychiatric Genetics

Maja Bucan

Edward S. Brodkin

Susceptibility to many severe neuropsychiatric disorders appears to have a genetic basis. Clustering of psychiatric disorders—such as schizophrenia, major depression, bipolar disorder, or autism—in families provides a first indication that the family members may share a common set of disease-causing genes. However, an exposure to similar environmental or cultural factors may also lead to such familial clustering. *Family, twin,* and *adoption studies* are commonly used to determine the degree of heritability of a disease or a trait, to determine the mode of inheritance and penetrance, and to estimate the number of genes that affect the disease or trait.[1] Data on the concordance rates of disease in monozygotic and dizygotic twins raised in the same family or raised apart provide a more direct way to assess heritability. Higher concordance rates in monozygotic versus dizygotic twins indicates a genetic component to disease susceptibility. Adoption studies have shown that, in general, an adoptee's risk of having a psychiatric disorder depends more on the affection status of the biologic parent than on that of the adoptive parent. Figure 70–1 illustrates heritability rates for several severe psychiatric disorders.

Although twin studies have provided strong evidence for the heritable nature of vulnerability to schizophrenia, major depression, bipolar disorder, and particularly autism, these studies have also revealed the genetic complexity of these disorders. For example, although the monozygotic concordance rate in autism is substantial (81%), it is not complete (less than 100%), indicating that the disease-susceptibility genes are not completely penetrant.[2-4] The more than twofold difference (25-fold in autism) in the concordance rate between monozygotic and dizygotic twins is an indication that the number of genes that contributes to this illness is large.

Great interest in the genetics of psychiatric disorders comes from the potential power of a genetic approach for the identification of disease genes and the elucidation of the molecular basis of pathophysiology. Biologic research in psychiatry has historically focused on the initial targets of psychiatric medications, such as neurotransmitter receptors and transporters; however, these studies have not unequivocally determined that abnormalities in these pathways represent the primary defects leading to disease pathophysiology. Positional or map-based cloning has the potential to identify disease-causing genes without previous knowledge about biochemical abnormalities or pathophysiology. For example, the Huntington disease locus was mapped, and subsequently the gene was identified in the absence of knowledge regarding the pathophysiologic basis for selective loss of neurons that is most severe in the caudate and putamen.[5,6]

In the next sections, we will summarize the current methodology in psychiatric genetics, and touch on the difficulties of psychiatric genetics, as well as some strategies that are being employed to try to overcome these difficulties. In particular, we will focus on the use of endophenotypes for psychiatric disorders and the use of animal models for the dissection of genetic pathways that may be related to psychiatric disease pathophysiology.

APPROACHES AND CHALLENGES IN PSYCHIATRIC GENETICS

A genetic approach toward the identification of a disease gene(s) starts with a collection of well-ascertained families or large cohorts of affected individuals. In the *linkage analysis* of preferably large pedigrees, one looks for segregation

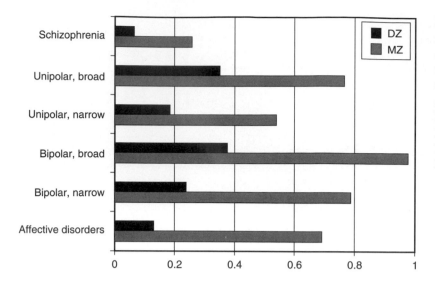

FIGURE 70–1. Concordance rates for psychiatric traits. DZ, dizygotic twin; MZ, monozygotic twin. (From Ott J: Statistical methods to discover susceptibility genes for nervous system diseases. In Chin HR, Moldin SO [eds]: Methods in Genomic Neuroscience. New York, CRC Press, pp 287–296.)

of the disease phenotype with molecular markers that are evenly distributed throughout the genome, with the goal of identifying a marker that is closely linked with the disease phenotype. A marker locus will appear linked to (or coinherited with) the disease phenotype owing to the physical proximity (and lower recombination rate) between the marker and the disease-causing locus in the genome. Currently available data on the chromosomal position of "linked" markers will reveal an approximate map location for a disease locus and provide a starting point for the positional cloning, that is, the molecular identification of a disease gene within that genomic region. This approach has been successfully employed for mapping and positional cloning of a large number of mendelian disease genes. In these single-gene disorders, a collection and closer examination of large multigenerational pedigrees segregating the disease gene reveals a mode of inheritance (dominant, recessive, or other) and provides initial material for the genetic linkage analysis. In the absence of large families, statistical analysis has to be conducted using pooled data from a number of families to evaluate the likelihood of linkage between a set of markers and a disease locus. The LOD (log of the odds) score method calculates and compares the likelihood ratio between linkage under the test hypothesis (that the marker and the disease locus are linked) and the neutral— "null"—hypothesis (that there is no linkage between the two loci).[7] The null hypothesis is that the recombination fraction between the two loci is one half (i.e., no linkage), whereas the test hypothesis allows all values of theta less one half. Thus there is no unique value of the likelihood under the test hypothesis. The LOD score is the logarithm (to base 10) of the ratio of the largest possible value of the likelihood under the test hypothesis to the (unique) value under the null hypothesis. By convention, a LOD score equal to or greater than 3 (equivalent to greater than 1000:1 odds in factor of linkage) indicates that evidence for linkage between the marker and the disease locus is significant. LOD score analysis of pedigrees with psychiatric disorders is complicated by the difficulty in determining the mode of

inheritance, as well as by the risk of pooling data from genetically heterogeneous families in which different genes, or sets of genes, may cause a similar clinical syndrome.

In addition to methods of linkage analysis that require large, phenotypically ascertained pedigrees, other powerful methods for identification of susceptibility genes are family-based methods that involve analysis of only affected family members or affected siblings (affected sib-pair method).[8] This nonparametric method does not require a specific model regarding mode of inheritance, nor does it require that assumptions be made about the number of loci involved. In general, if both siblings inherit the same allele from a parent, they are said to share this allele identical by descent (IBD), and if they inherit different alleles there is no IBD sharing. If both siblings share the same allele, but each sibling inherited that allele from a different parent, this allele sharing is not IBD, but only identical by state (IBS). If the disease locus and the marker locus are not linked, there is equal probability (the probability is exactly 0.5) that the same allele will be shared IBD by two affected siblings. Independent of mode of inheritance, when marker and disease loci are linked, there is an increased tendency for the two affected sibs or two affected family members to share the same marker allele IBD (the probability will be higher than 0.5).

Whereas linkage analysis requires access to families, *case-control association studies* require collection of a population-based sample composed of affected and unaffected individuals. The case-control association study involves statistical analysis of allele frequency for a marker locus in the unaffected control population, compared with that in the affected individuals. A significant association is assumed when one or more alleles occur significantly more often in affected than in unaffected individuals. Although it has been proposed that association studies have greater statistical power than linkage analysis to detect multiple loci of small effect,[9] the major problem with case-control association studies is the presence of highly variable allele frequencies in different ethnic groups, which makes the choice of an appropriate control group particularly difficult when there is population stratification.

The *transmission disequilibrium test* (TDT) combines aspects of the affected sib-pair sharing method and the case-control test of association method.[10,11] This method uses population-based tests for linkage disequilibrium (LD) or skewed transmission of one of the alleles from a heterozygous parent (A1A2) to their affected offspring. In the case of an unlinked marker, we expect equal (50% : 50%) transmission of alleles A1 and A2. In the case of a marker that is linked to the predisposing allele for a disease, one allele (let's say A1) will be inherited with the disease phenotype more often than expected by chance. In TDT, the same individuals, parents and affected offspring, provide both subjects and controls for linkage based on the concept of association. The TDT analysis is particularly useful as a follow-up of genome-wide linkage or LD analyses, because a large number of so called "trios" (both parents and an affected child) can be used in the TDT analysis for fine mapping of the candidate region(s).

Association studies on affected sibs can be performed using markers evenly spaced throughout the genome. However, dense genetic and physical maps and the currently available draft sequence of the human genome allow selection of polymorphic markers (simple sequence repeats or single-nucleotide polymorphisms—SNPs) close by or within *candidate genes*—known genes selected for study based on hypotheses regarding the pathophysiology or neurobiology of the disease. The association between the disease phenotype and a genetic variant of a candidate gene is particularly compelling when the variant is a functional polymorphism (e.g., a polymorphism in an exon coding region causing an amino acid change), which increases the likelihood that the polymorphism could be a disease-causing mutation. The candidate gene approach will continue to represent an important way to search for the susceptibility genes for psychiatric disorders,[12,13] particularly as the molecular neurobiologic underpinnings of behavioral anomalies are better understood through animal models.[14,15] Furthermore, the availability of databases with information on genetic variants in coding and noncoding conserved sequences surrounding every gene in the genome (SNP databases), together with data from systematic expression profiling, will allow for each of the 40,000 to 50,000 genes in the human genome to be considered or used as a candidate gene in linkage and association studies.

For many mendelian disorders, including neurologic disorders, diagnosis does not represent a major challenge. For example, in the case of Huntington chorea, the autosomal-dominant pattern of inheritance, together with the pronounced movement disorder that characterizes the disease, makes the classification of family members into "affected" and "unaffected," relatively straightforward. In many mendelian disorders, there are laboratory tests (biochemical, electrophysiologic, x-ray or MRI) that help greatly with diagnosis. However, in psychiatric disorders this classification is usually more difficult.

Currently, the *Diagnostic and Statistical Manual of Mental Disorders*, Fourth Edition (DSM-IV) is the standard source of *diagnostic criteria for psychiatric disorders*; however, there are several problems with the use of standard DSM psychiatric diagnoses as phenotypes for genetic studies. DSM definitions of "disorders" are based primarily on the fulfillment of a certain number of behavioral symptom criteria, but not on an understanding of the underlying biology of the disorders, which is still largely obscure, nor on specific biochemical or neuroimaging tests.

Each disorder that DSM-IV defines as a discrete entity, such as bipolar I disorder, is more likely to be a genetically heterogeneous group of diseases, each of which is caused by interactions among various sets of multiple genes and environmental factors. Moreover, as is usually the case in complex genetics, family members who share some susceptibility genes for bipolar I disorder do not necessarily manifest the same phenotype; conversely, individuals with the same phenotype do not necessarily share the same set of susceptibility genes. Thus, a proband with bipolar I disorder may share susceptibility genes in common with another family member, but this other family member may exhibit any one of a number of other phenotypes, including DSM-IV bipolar II disorder, single-episode or recurrent major depressive disorder, or schizoaffective disorder, due to the effect of environmental factors, modifier genes, or random developmental events on the expression of the susceptibility genes (variable expressivity) (Fig. 70–2). Alternatively, this other family member may have no DSM-IV diagnosis at all (reduced penetrance). Even those relatives who do not meet criteria for any DSM-IV diagnosis may nevertheless have milder, subthreshold forms of the phenotype, or may have more subtle neuropsychological, neurophysiologic, or neuroanatomic abnormalities that will not be detected without specialized testing. Thus, probands' relatives, who, in the past, may have been classified as unaffected in genetic studies using only DSM-IV criteria, may in fact show a subtle phenotype—an endophenotype—that is biologically related to the disease and that could contribute important information and statistical power to genetic studies. Genetic linkage studies of complex disease will benefit from dissection of these endophenotypes, in addition to dissection of the full clinical manifestations of the illness (discussed later).

There may be individuals who appear to have the same phenotype as affected individuals, but this phenotype may be caused by the effects of a completely different set of genes or environmental factors (phenocopies), or both. This *heterogeneity* of genes that may lead to the same or similar clinical manifestations in different families

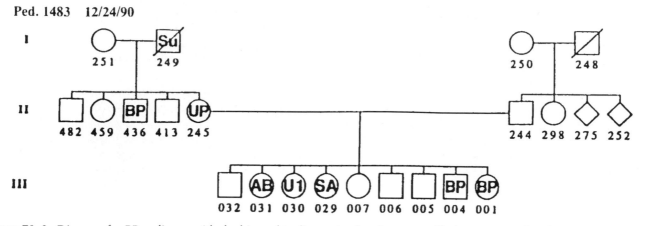

FIGURE 70–2. Diagram for BP pedigree, with the hierarchic diagnosis of each person. Circles represent females, squares are males, diamonds indicate sex unknown; a slash through the symbol indicates that the person is deceased. AB, anorexia and bulimia; BP, bipolar I and bipolar II w/major depression; SA, schizo-affective; SU, suicide; UI, single-episode unipolar; UP, unipolar (not excluded). (From Berrettini WH, Goldin LR, Martinez MM, et al: A bipolar pedigree series for genomic mapping of disease genes: Diagnostic and analytic considerations. Psychiatr Genet 1991;2:125–160.)

or populations is another confounding factor in the genetic analysis of psychiatric disorders. In the analysis of mendelian traits, a linkage analysis on an initial set of large families usually provides sufficient information on the genetic heterogeneity of the disease. Specifically, these initial studies may demonstrate whether the determined disease map location is consistent when additional families with the same clinical manifestation are tested for linkage. In psychiatric disorders, in the absence of large families in which it is likely that the same set of genes causes a clinical syndrome, linkage analysis has to be conducted by combining data from a large set of smaller families with potentially different susceptibility loci. Because of the high frequency of psychiatric disorders in the general population, the possibility that a different set of predisposing genes may be inherited from both parents is high. Several strategies have been employed to minimize the genetic heterogeneity of families studied in linkage analyses. A promising and commonly used approach is a pedigree analysis in geographically isolated populations.[16] Such populations can usually be traced to a limited number of founders (e.g., 50 to 500); therefore, it is likely that a smaller subset of disease susceptibility loci will be present in this isolated population relative to the number of susceptibility loci that might be present in the general population. More importantly, isolated populations have had fewer generations of genetic recombination (i.e., large chromosomal regions are in linkage disequilibrium), and, therefore, it should be easier to detect association between a disease and alleles or haplotypes at mapped marker loci. In several cases, genetic findings in population isolates, used to search for susceptibility genes for bipolar disorder (Old Order Amish and the Central Valley of Costa Rica) and for schizophrenia (Iceland and Finland), have been confirmed in studies on heterogeneous populations.[17–21] For a review, see Peltonen et al.[16]

Although heterogeneity is frequently mentioned as a major obstacle in the identification of genetic variants underlying neuropsychiatric traits, it is important to keep in mind that heterogeneity per se does not represent an insurmountable problem. In the case of dementia, heterogeneity and variable age-of-onset once seemed to represent an overwhelming obstacle in the understanding of the genetic underpinnings of this growing economic and social problem. However, research progress on Alzheimer's disease, for example, the most common form of dementia, has revealed that four genes account for 30% of the genetic variance. (For a review, see Tanzi and Bertram.[22]) Two critical factors that allowed for advances in the genetic understanding of Alzheimer's disease were the use of a narrow phenotype (early onset) and the identification of rare multigenerational families in which the disease segregates as an autosomal-dominant, fully penetrant form. The discovery of multigenerational pedigrees that exhibit simple genetic transmission of a particular behavioral disorder or syndrome might similarly advance psychiatric genetics. The research community has been making strong efforts to identify such families, but, to date, such families have been extremely rare.[23]

The *nature and frequency of mutations underlying psychiatric disorders* may represent additional reasons for difficulties in the genetic mapping of susceptibility loci. Many rare mendelian diseases are caused by missense mutations leading to loss-of-function or dominant negative phenotypes that may be more severe, robust, less variable, and more likely to be fully penetrant. In the case of complex disorders, and specifically psychiatric disorders, variations are likely to be more subtle, less penetrant, and perhaps more susceptible to gene-gene interaction effects or environmental effects.[24,25] It is possible that genetic variants that underlie complex traits will not be found within protein coding regions of genes (will not alter amino acids), but, rather, will occur in noncoding regulatory regions that will be difficult to identify in the absence of information on the nature of these regulatory regions. Currently, efforts are underway to use comparative sequence analysis to select regions that are evolutionarily conserved between mouse and human, as candidates for these regulatory elements and to include them, along with coding sequences, in the analysis of genetic variants in complex diseases.[24,25] In contrast to most mendelian diseases that are caused by rare genetic variants, common psychiatric disorders may be caused by genetic variants that are common in the general population and, therefore, these variants will be more difficult to distinguish as "disease-causing." This problem potentially could be overcome by the use of large sample sizes, which would provide greater statistical power than many previous studies have had.

Linkage to defined chromosomal regions has been reported for a number of common psychiatric disorders (see later chapters). However, difficulties in replicating the original linkages or associations in larger sets of families, as well as a failure to identify a small number of loci with a major effect, provide unequivocal evidence that these disorders are genetically complex; they are oligogenic (affected by a large number of loci with a small effect) and probably susceptible to epistatic effects (gene-gene interactions) and interaction with the environment. Given this oligogenic epistatic model, most linkage studies of psychiatric phenotypes are severely underpowered from a statistical standpoint. Based on the observed overlap of susceptibility loci for both bipolar disorder and schizophrenia in several chromosomal regions,[26] it has been suggested that certain chromosomal regions may be implicated in severe psychiatric disorders rather than causing susceptibility to specific clinical syndromes.[19] Moreover, despite tremendous efforts, the molecular identification of the relevant alleles within these loci has not been accomplished. Therefore, instead of relying solely on human genetic studies, we may need to elucidate the nature of disrupted pathways and patterns of gene interactions from studies of model organisms. These considerations have led psychiatric geneticists to revisit the issue of phenotypes. Rather than focusing only on the full clinical manifestations of the disease, which may represent the most extreme phenotype, psychiatric geneticists are now attempting to genetically dissect additional phenotypes that may be related to disease pathophysiology.

DIAGNOSIS AND GENETIC DISSECTION OF PSYCHIATRIC PHENOTYPES

Problems with the definition of phenotype will hinder any genetic study, regardless of the study design or the sophistication of the genotyping technology employed. Psychiatric geneticists have questioned whether their extremely slow progress in identifying susceptibility genes has been due, in part, to the use of inadequate phenotype definitions, specifically due to the exclusive use of DSM-III, DSM-IIIR, or DSM-IV diagnoses as phenotypes.

These considerations have led psychiatric geneticists to begin to identify and use endophenotypes (including neuropsychological, neurophysiologic, or neuroanatomic traits, or a combination of these) in genetic studies of psychiatric disorders.[27–30] *Endophenotypes* are thought to be indicators of pathophysiologic processes that mediate between susceptibility genes and full expression of the disease,[31] and these traits may be biologically and genetically simpler (influenced by a smaller number of genes and environmental factors) than the full DSM-IV diagnosis; therefore, endophenotypes are thought to provide a more sensitive measure of genetic susceptibility to disease than does diagnosis, and their genetic dissection is thought to be more tractable.[30–33] The use of endophenotypes in psychiatric genetics may be compared with the use of risk factors for atherosclerosis (e.g., blood pressure, cholesterol level) in genetic studies, rather than the exclusive use of myocardial infarction as a phenotype.[32]

Before a trait is accepted as a suitable endophenotype for psychiatric genetic studies, it should, ideally, have certain characteristics: It must be heritable, correlated with disease or disease severity, or both, (but not due to the effects of medication or disease sequelae), and present (but perhaps at lower levels) in unaffected relatives of an affected individual.[30,32] In the absence of an understanding of pathophysiology, it is difficult to prove definitively that a putative endophenotype is related to pathophysiology, but the characteristics just mentioned provide support that there is likely to be such a relationship. Great care should be taken in validating particular traits as endophenotypes, that is, in establishing and replicating the correlation between the endophenotype and the disorder, and in attempting to demonstrate that the trait is related to the pathophsyiology and is not simply an epiphenomenon. It is also quite helpful if the endophenotype remains stable across most of the human lifespan (developmentally stable), so that it can be measured in multiple generations of affected pedigrees.[30]

The use of endophenotypes may increase the power of psychiatric genetics studies in several ways. First, endophenotypes may enable investigators to begin to define biologic subtypes of psychiatric disorders, which would allow for studies of more genetically homogeneous populations.[30] Second, endophenotypes can be measured in all members of a pedigree, not just the members affected by DSM diagnoses, and the inclusion of all members of a pedigree in genetic analysis will increase the statistical power to detect genetic linkage. Third, in contrast to DSM categorical diagnoses (affected vs. unaffected), endophenotypes are often measured as quantitative variables, which provide genetic studies with greater statistical power to measure susceptibility genes of small effect on the phenotype.[33a] Fourth, genetic studies of endophenotypes can be carried out in the general population to identify genes that affect the traits, and thus identify genes that may lie in the biologic pathway of the disease. It is easier to recruit large numbers of subjects in the general population, rather than trying to recruit large numbers of families affected by a particular disease. These larger numbers will provide greater statistical power to detect genes. Through these studies, genetic loci can be identified that affect endophenotypes and thus that affect disease risk and biologic pathways involved in disease.[32]

Much of the early work on endophenotypes has been related to schizophrenia, although, increasingly, endophenotypes for other psychiatric disorders have been proposed. Ming Tsuang and coworkers have developed a concept called "schizotaxia" that consists of endophenotypes for schizophrenia, including negative symptoms (e.g., social withdrawal), neuropsychological deficits (e.g., attention impairments), and structural brain abnormalities (e.g., abnormal temporal lobe sulcal-gyral patterns), even in the absence of psychosis. This constellation of relatively subtle phenotypes affects 20% to 50% of nonpsychotic relatives of schizophrenic patients.[34,35] Neuroanatomic endophenotypes have been proposed for schizophrenia, including reductions in frontal and temporal gray matter volumes and increases in frontal and temporal sulcal cerebrospinal fluid (CSF) volume, compared with controls.[31]

Freedman and coworkers have used failure to inhibit the P50 auditory evoked response to repeated stimuli ("prepulses") as an endophenotype for schizophrenia.[36] These investigators reported a genome-wide linkage analysis that revealed significant linkage of this endophenotype to a polymorphism at the site of the alpha 7-nicotinic receptor.[36] Significant linkage was not found between this polymorphism and the full schizophrenia phenotype in this study, which may have been due to the low statistical power of the families to detect linkage to schizophrenia.[30] If this polymorphism is, in fact, related to the full schizophrenia phenotype, one would expect to find linkage with a sufficiently large sample size and, in fact, this has been reported.[37,37a] P50 and prepulse inhibition have also been suggested as separate endophenotypes for schizotypal personality disorder.[38]

Cornblatt and Malhotra argue that abnormalities in sustained attention, as measured by the Continuous Performance Test, Identical Pairs (CPT-IP), may be a useful endophenotype that reflects biologic susceptibility to schizophrenia.[39] Deficits in performance on this test have been reported in patients with various schizophrenia spectrum disorders (including schizotypal personality), as well as in non-psychotic relatives of patients. This attentional deficit may adversely affect the processing of social information and may contribute to deficits in social problem solving in schizophrenic patients.[39]

Event related potential P300 has been proposed as an endophenotype for schizophrenia, as well as alcoholism. Alcoholic individuals show a characteristic alteration in the amplitude of the P300 evoked brain potential, as do their unaffected sons who are at risk for alcoholism.[40,41] P300 amplitude in response to a variety of test stimuli has been shown to be heritable and has been successfully used in genetic linkage studies.[42,43] The study of other psychiatric disorders may benefit from this research and strategy as well. Lowering of mood induced by acute tryptophan depletion, which is thought to acutely lower brain serotonin levels, has been suggested as an endophenotype for vulnerability to major depression or bipolar disorder because this trait tends to be found in unaffected relatives of probands but not in controls.[44] In family studies of autism, there are often relatives (e.g., parents of autistic children) who do not meet criteria for autism, but rather exhibit milder abnormalities in social behavior, language, or other behaviors. These other individuals are now considered to show the "broad autism phenotype," an endophenotype that may increase the power of genetic studies of autism.[45]

Efforts have been made to find biologic subtypes and endophenotypes for obsessive-compulsive disorder (OCD) in order to study more genetically homogeneous groups of patients and to increase the power of genetic studies. For example, OCD has been subtyped based on the presence or absence of tics, and factor analyses of OCD have revealed four factors that may be studied separately in population studies: (1) obsessions and checking, (2) concerns with symmetry and ordering, (3) concerns with contamination and cleaning, and (4) hoarding behaviors.[46] Efforts have also been made to find biologic subtypes of attention deficit hyperactivity disorder (ADHD), to improve the power of genetic studies. For example, Smalley and coworkers assessed neurocognitive task performance and the occurrence of comorbid conditions (e.g., learning disability, conduct disorder) in order to try to refine the ADHD phenotype and identify more biologically homogenous subtypes of ADHD for genetic studies.[47]

An additional benefit of the study of endophenotypes is that they can be studied in animal models, particularly mice, for which there are powerful resources and methodologies for genetic analysis. Although it is extremely difficult to model the full clinical manifestations of psychiatric disorders in animals (because animals do not have humans' capacity for language and other higher cognitive functions that are disrupted in many psychiatric disorders), certain endophenotypes for psychiatric disorders can often be studied directly in both humans and animals. Therefore, it is important to consider the use of animal models as an additional research strategy that may advance psychiatric genetics.

ANIMAL MODELS

The study of endophenotypes in animal models provides opportunities to discover genetic and neurobiologic pathways that underlie these traits and that may be related to the pathophysiology of human psychiatric disorders. Many of the endophenotypes that have been studied in humans can be modeled accurately in animals. Once a behavioral paradigm has been established, there are several well-established methodologies for the genetic dissection of the traits in animals (especially mice), including (1) quantitative trait locus (QTL) analysis to identify genetic loci that account for differences between inbred mouse strains[48]; (2) the analysis of point mutations in mice that are induced by a mutagen, such as N-ethyl-nitrosourea (ENU), and cause a change in a phenotype of interest[49]; and (3) the analysis of knockout (null-mutant) or transgenic mice that have an induced change in a known gene.[14] A great advantage in the use of animal models is that both genetic and environmental factors can be carefully controlled, which is extremely helpful in the dissection of complex traits.

As an example of this approach, sensorimotor gating abnormalities in schizophrenia have been modeled well in animals.[50] Sensory gating is measured in both humans and animals as the level of prepulse inhibition (PPI) of startle response, that is, the level of attenuation of a startle response (acoustic or tactile) on presentation of a non–startle-inducing prepulse stimulus (Fig. 70–3). In humans, the startle response is measured as an eyeblink response or P50 auditory evoked response to repeated stimuli[36]; in animals PPI can be measured as a whole body response using a startle chamber. There is a substantial genetic influence on PPI in animals, as demonstrated by the differences between inbred mouse strains in this phenotype. There are several examples of single-gene mutant mice that show changes in PPI. Particularly interesting is the example of proline dehydrogenase (*Prodh-/-*) knockout mice, which show lower levels of PPI and elevated levels of brain proline relative to wild-type controls.[51] The homologous human gene, *PRODH2*, lies on chromosome 22q11 in a region that has been associated with schizophrenia and schizoaffective disorder. Approximately 20% to 30% of patients with microdeletions in chromosome 22q11 meet diagnostic criteria for schizophrenia or schizoaffective disorder and there is accumulating evidence that the *PRODH2/DGCR6* locus may be at least one of the loci within 22q11 that affects schizophrenia predisposition.[52-56] Thus, although certain human studies have found linkage of P50 abnormalities to the chromosomal region containing alpha 7-nicotinic receptor, lines of evidence from other human studies and animal models point to the involvement of the proline dehydrogenase gene in both schizophrenia and its endophenotype, PPI.[36,51,55] Certainly, multiple genetic and neurobiologic pathways affect the attentional abnormalities associated with schizophrenia, and these studies provide an example of the way that human and animal studies can work well together to elucidate these pathways. The convergence of human and mouse studies of schizophrenia and PPI is also demonstrated by a report that found evidence for the association of *Neuregulin 1* on chromosome 8p with schizophrenia in an isolated population.[20] These investigators also tested mice that were heterozygous for a mutation of *Nrg1* (the homozygous null mutation was lethal) and found that these mice showed increased levels of activity and impairments in PPI.

In addition to endophenotypes, there are certain types of behavioral disorders (e.g., use of addictive substances) that can be fairly well modeled in animals. Animal behavioral paradigms, such as place preference conditioning and drug self-administration, are thought to be very useful models of drug-seeking and drug abuse or dependence behaviors, or both, in humans. In these paradigms, animals will seek or self-administer many of the same drugs that are addictive in humans, including opiates and cocaine.[57] Neurobiologic and genetic studies of animals have led to the identification of particular genes (e.g., deltaFosB, CREB, corticotrophin releasing factor) and pathways that may be involved in mammalian responses to drugs of abuse.[58-60] Genes in these pathways will then provide useful candidate genes for human genetic association studies of drug addiction.

In summary, the genetic analysis of psychiatric disorders and human endophenotypes, on the one hand, and the genetic analysis of animal models of behavior and endophenotypes, on the other hand, are complementary; in fact, they are synergistic approaches that should be pursued simultaneously in order to maximize research progress in psychiatric genetics. Linkage studies of human psychiatric disorders, in both isolated and heterogeneous populations, have begun to converge on certain large chromosomal regions that are likely to harbor susceptibility genes, such as the region on chromosome 8p that has been found repeatedly in linkage studies of schizophrenia.[20,61-63,65] Candidate genes within these large chromosomal regions, such as *Neuregulin 1* in 8p, are being closely analyzed in humans.[20] Then, a series of alleles with mutations in these candidate genes in the mouse (loss-of-function, hypomorph, hypermorph, dominant-negative mutations, including those in coding and noncoding regions) can be studied for their function and their effect on behavior and endophenotypes.[20] Simultaneously, studies of animal models of behavior and endophenotypes (e.g., studies of single-gene mutants) have begun to reveal additional genes and genetic/neurobiologic pathways that affect these phenotypes. Animal studies allow for a great deal of experimental control over genes and environmental factors and access to brain tissue that is not possible in human studies. Thus animal models provide investigators with an invaluable opportunity to study gene and brain function, as well as gene–gene and gene–environment interactions. Genes found originally in animal studies can lead investigators to study the homologous human genes in association studies. Although some of the findings in animals may not hold true in humans, there are a growing number of cases in which the original discovery of a gene in animals reveals *a new functional role of a human gene* (e.g., the story with mutant mice and leptin/leptin receptor in obesity and mutant mice and dogs and narcolepsy),

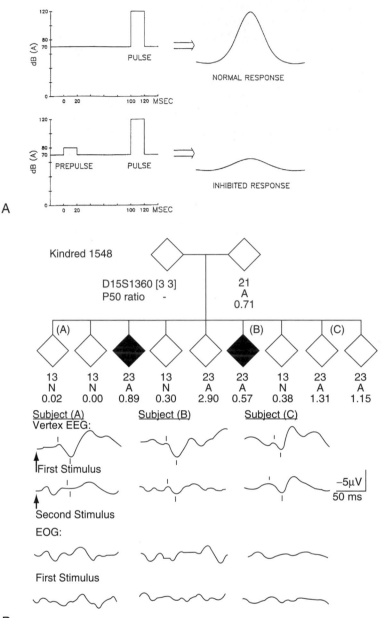

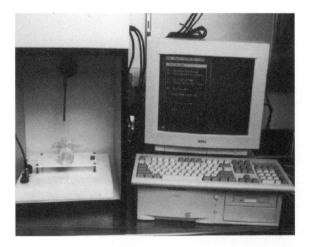

FIGURE 70–3. *A*, Diagrammatic representation of prepulse inhibition. The top figure *(A)* illustrates the pulse-alone trial in which startle is elicited by a 120-dB noise burst presented for 20 to 40 msec. The startle response is measured for 100 (animals) or 250 (humans) msec after the onset of the pulse. The lower figure illustrates the prepulse + pulse trial in which startle is inhibited by a weak prepulse given 30 to 1000 msec (in this case, 100 msec) before the same startle-eliciting pulse used in the pulse-alone trial. In experiments examining tactile rather than acoustic startle, the pulse is an air-puff to the neck (humans) or back (rats). *B*, Segregation of alleles of D15S1360 and P50 ratio in a portion of a family affected with schizophrenia. A indicates abnormal and N, normal, based on previously determined distributions of the P50 ratio for schizophrenic and normal subjects. Filled symbols represent schizophrenic subjects. The pedigree has been altered in several ways to protect subject confidentiality. Auditory-evoked responses to paired stimuli (arrows) demonstrate normal and abnormal P50 ratios in clinically unaffected siblings (A, C) and an abnormal P50 ratio in a schizophrenic sibling (B). A computer alogorithm identified the P50 waves in the vertex electroencephalogram (EEG) (marks below the tracings) and measured their amplitudes relative to the preceding negative peaks (marks above the tracings). Simultaneous electro-oculographic (EOG) recordings illustrate that the P50 wave was not generated by eye movement artifact. *C*, Acoustic startle response (ASR) and prepulse inhibition of startle (PPI) are measured in mice using a sound-attenuating chamber. The acoustic startle test consists of startle intensities at every 10 dB from 90 to 120 dB. The percent prepulse inhibition (PPI) protocol consists of a standard 120-dB startle stimulus preceded by a prepulse stimulus of 70 dB, 90 dB, or 95 dB. Acoustic startle and PPI are tested in the same session. (*A*, From Braff DL, Geyer MA: Sensorimotor gating and schizophrenia. Human and animal model studies. Arch Gen Psychiatry 1990;47:181–188. *B*, From Freedman R, Coon H, Myles-Worsley M, et al: Linkage of a neurophysiologic deficit in schizophrenia to a chromosome 15 locus. Proc Natl Acad Sci U S A 1997;94:587–592.)

regardless of whether disease-causing mutations in these genes have been found in humans.[66-69] Working simultaneously on human and animal studies, while paying close attention to the nature of the phenotypes studied, and taking advantage of the great advances in genome sequencing and genotyping technologies, should allow investigators to further unravel the complexities of psychiatric genetics.

Acknowledgments

The research of M.B. is supported by the National Institutes of Health, and the research of E.S.B. is supported by a Career Award in the Biomedical Sciences from the Burroughs Wellcome Fund. We thank W. Ewens, W. Berrettini, M. Burmeister, and members of our laboratories for helpful discussions and comments on the manuscript.

REFERENCES

1. Nussbaum RL, McInnes RR, Willard HS, et al: Genetics in Medicine, 6th ed. Philadelphia, WB Saunders, 2002.

2. Folstein S, Rutter M: Infantile autism: A genetic study of 21 twin pairs. J Child Psychol Psychiatry 1977; 18:297–321.

3. Steffenburg S, Gillberg C, Hellgren L, et al: A twin study of autism in Denmark, Finland, Iceland, Norway, and Sweden. J Child Psychol Psychiatry 1989; 30:405–416.

4. Bailey A, LeCouteur A, Gottesman I, et al: Autism as a strongly genetic disorder: Evidence from a British twin study. Psychol Med 1995;25:63–77.

5. Gusella JF, Wexler NS, Conneally PM, et al: A polymorphic DNA marker genetically linked to Huntington's disease. Nature 1983;306:234–238.

6. The Huntington's Disease Collaborative Research Group: A novel gene containing a trinucleotide repeat that is expanded and unstable on Huntington's disease chromosomes. Cell 1993;72(6):971–983.

7. Morton NE: Sequential tests for the detection of linkage. Am J Hum Genet 1955;7:277–318.

8. Weeks DE, Lange K: The affected-pedigree-member method of linkage analysis. Am J Hum Genet 1988;42:315–326.

9. Risch N, Merikangas K: The future of genetic studies of complex human diseases. Science 1996;273: 1516–1517.

10. Spielman RS, Ewens WJ: The TDT and other family-based tests for linkage disequilibrium and association. Am J Hum Genet 1996;59(5):983–989.

11. Ewens WJ, Spielman RS: Locating genes by linkage and association. Theor Popul Biol 2001;60(3): 135–139.

12. Tabor HK, Risch NJ, Myers RM: Opinion: Candidate-gene approaches for studying complex genetic traits: Practical considerations. Nature Rev Genetics 2002;3(5):391–397.

13. Glatt CE, Freimer NB: Association analysis of candidate genes for neuropsychiatric disease: The perpetual campaign. Trends Genet 2002;18(6):307–312.

14. Bucan M, Abel T: The mouse: Genetics meets behaviour. Nature Reviews Genetics 2002;3(2):114–123.

15. Seong E, Seasholtz AF, Burmeister M: Mouse models for psychiatric disorders: What is the benefit, where are the limits? (in press).

16. Peltonen L, Palotie A, Lange K: Use of population isolates for mapping complex traits. Nature Reviews Genetics 2000;1(3):182–190.

17. Ginns EI, Ott J, Egeland JA, et al: A genome-wide search for chromosomal loci linked to bipolar affective disorder in the Old Order Amish. Nat Genet 1996;12: 431–435.

18. McInnes LA, Escamilla MA, Service SK, et al: A complete genome screen for genes predisposing to severe bipolar disorder in two Costa Rican pedigrees. Proc Nat Acad Sci U S A 1996;93(23):13060–13065.

19. Ophoff RA, Escamilla MA, Service SK, et al: Genomewide linkage disequilibrium mapping of severe bipolar disorder in a population isolate. Am J Hum Genet 2002;71:656–574.

20. Stefansson H, Sigurdsson E, Steinhorsdottir V, et al: Neuregulin 1 and susceptibility to schizophrenia. Am J Hum Genet 2002;71:877–892.

21. Hovatta I, Varilo T, Suvisaari J, et al: A genome-wide screen for schizophrenia genes in an isolated Finnish subpopuation suggesting multiple susceptibility loci. Am J Hum Genet 1999;65:1114–1124.

22. Tanzi RE, Bertram L: New frontiers in Alzheimer's disease genetics. Neuron 2001;32(2):181–184.

23. Brunner HG, Nelen M, Breakefield XO, et al: Abnormal behavior associated with a point mutation in the structural gene for monoamine oxidase A. Science 1993;262:578–580.

24. Zwick ME, Cutler DJ, Aravinda C: Patterns of genetic variance in mendelian and complex traits. Annu Rev Genomics Hum Genet 2000;1:387–407.

25. Zwick ME, Cutler DJ, Chakraverti A, et al: Genetic variation analysis of neuropsychiatric traits. In Chin HR, Moldin SO (eds): Methods in Genomic Neuroscience. New York, CRC Press, 2001, pp 297–310.

26. Berrettini WH: Susceptibility loci for bipolar disorder: Overlap with inherited vulnerability to schizophrenia. Biol Psychiatry 2000;47:245–251.

27. Gershon ES, Goldin LR: Clinical methods in psychiatric genetics. I. Robustness of genetic marker investigative strategies. Acta Psychiatr Scand 1986;74: 113–118.

28. Lander ES: Splitting schizophrenia. Nature 1988;336:105–106.

29. Leboyer M, Bellivier F, Nosten-Bertrand M, et al: Psychiatric genetics: Search for phenotypes. Trends Neurosci 1998;21:102–105.

30. Freedman R, Adler LE, Leonard S: Alternative phenotypes for the complex genetics of schzophrenia. Biol Psychiatry 1999;45:551–558.

31. Cannon TD, Gasperoni TL, van Erp TGM, Rosso IM: Quantitative neural indicators of liability to schizophrenia: Implications for molecular genetic studies. Am J Med Genet 2001;105:16–19.

32. Almasy L, Blangero J: Endophenotypes as quantitative risk factors for psychiatric disease: Rationale and study design. Am J Med Genet 2001;105:42–44.

33. Moldin SO: Indicators of liability to schizophrenia: Perspectives from genetic epidemiology. Schizophrenia Bull 1994;20:169–184.

33a. Wijsman, EM, Amos CI: Genetic analysis of simulated oligogenic traits in nuclear and extended pedigrees: Summary of GAW10 contributions. Genetic Epidemiol 1997;14:719–735.

34. Tsuang MT: Defining alternative phenotypes for genetic studies: What can we learn from studies of schizophrenia? Am J Med Genet 2001;105:8–10.

35. Tsuang MT, Stone WS, Tarbox SI, Faraone SV: An integration of schizophrenia with schizotypy: Identification of schizotaxia and implications for research on treatment and prevention. Schizophr Res 2002;54:169–175.

36. Freedman R, Coon H, Myles-Worsley M, et al: Linkage of a neurophysiological deficit in schizophrenia to a chromosome 15 locus. Proc Natl Acad Sci U S A 1997;94:587–592.

37. Gershon ES, Badner JA, Goldin LR, et al: Closing in on genes for manic-depressive illness and schizophrenia. Neuropsychopharmacology 1998;18: 233–242.

37a. Freedman R, Leonard S: Editorial: Genetic linkage to schizophrenia at chromosome 15q14. Am J Med Genet 2001;105:655–657.

38. Cadenhead KS, Light GA, Geyer MA, et al: Neurobiological measures of schizotypal personality disorder: Defining an inhibitory endophenotype? Am J Psychiat 2002;159:869–871.

39. Cornblatt BA, Malhotra AK: Impaired attention as an endophenotype for molecular genetic studies of schiozophrenia. Am J Med Genet 2001;105:11–15.

40. Porjesz B, Begleiter H: Visual evoked potentials and brain dysfunction in chronic alcoholics. In Begleiter H (ed): Evoked Brain Potentials and Behavior. New York, Plenum, 1979, pp 277–302.

41. Begleiter H, Porjesz B, Bihari B, Kissin B: Event-related brain potentials in boys at risk for alcoholism. Science 1984;225:1493–1496.

42. Almasy L, Porjesz B, Blangero J, et al: Heritability of event-related brain potentials in families with a history of alcoholism. Am J Med Genet 1999; 88:383–390.

43. Williams JT, Begleiter H, Porjesz B, et al: Joint multipoint linkage analysis of multivariate qualitative and quantitative traits. II. Alcoholism and event-related potentials. Am J Hum Genet 1999;65:1148–1160.

44. Quintin P, Benkelfat C, Launay JM, et al:. Clinical and neurochemical effect of acute tryptophan depletion in unaffected relatives of patients with bipolar affective disorder. Biol Psychiatry 2001;50:184–190.

45. Piven J: The broad autism phenotype: A complementary strategy for molecular genetic studies of autism. Am J Med Genet 2001;105:34–35.

46. Leckman JF, Zhang H, Alsobrook JP, Pauls DL: Symptom dimensions in obsessive-compulsive disorder: Toward quantitative phenotypes. Am J Med Genet 2001;105:28–30.

47. Smalley SL, McCracken J, McGough J: Refining the ADHD phenotype using affected sibling pairs. Am J Med Genet 2001;105:31–33.

48. Brodkin ES, Nestler EJ: Quantitative trait locus analysis: A new tool for psychiatric genetics. Neuroscientist 1998;4:317–323.

49. Pinto LH, Takahashi JS: Functional identification of neural genes. In Chin HR, Moldin SO (eds): Methods in Genomic Neuroscience. New York, CRC Press, pp 65–90.

50. Braff DL, Geyer MA: Sensorimotor gating and schizophrenia. Human and animal model studies. Arch Gen Psychiatry 1990;47:181–188.

51. Gogos JA, Santha M, Takacs Z, et al: The gene encoding proline dehydrogenase modulates sensorimotor gating in mice. Nat Genet 1999;21:434–439.

52. Pulver AE, Nestadt G, Goldberg R, et al: Psychotic illness in patients diagnosed with velo-cardio-facial syndrome and their relatives. J Nerv Mental Dis 1994;182:476–478.

53. Bassett AS, Chow EWC: 22q11 deletion syndrome: A genetic subtype of schizophrenia. Biol Psychiatry 1999;46:882–891.

54. Murphy KC: Schizophrenia and velo-cardio-facial syndrome. Lancet 2002;359:426–430.

55. Liu H, Heath SC, Sobin C, et al: Genetic variation at the 22q11 PRODH2/DGCR6 locus presents an unusual pattern and increases susceptibility to schizophrenia. Proc Natl Acad Sci U S A 2002;99:3717–3722.

56. Chakravarti A: A compelling genetic hypothesis for a complex disease: PRODH2/DGCR6 variation leads to schizophrenia susceptibility. Proc Natl Acad Sci U S A 2002;99:4755–4756.

57. Koob GF, Nestler EJ: The neurobiology of drug addiction. J Neuropsychiatry Clin Neurosci 1997;9: 482–497.

58. Carlezon WA, Thome J, Olson VG, et al: Regulation of cocaine reward by CREB. Science 1998; 282:2272–2275.

59. Kelz MB, Chen J, Carlezon WA Jr, et al: Expression of the transcription factor deltaFosB in the brain controls sensitivity to cocaine. Nature 1999;401: 272–276.

60. Koob GF: Stress, corticotrophin-releasing factor, and drug addiction. Ann N Y Acad Sci 1999;897: 27–45.

61. Pulver AE, Lasseter VK, Kasch L, et al: Schizophrenia: A genome scan targets chromosomes 3p and 8p as potential sites of susceptibility genes. Am J Med Genet 1995;60:252–260.

62. Kendler KS., MacLean CJ, O'Neill FA, et al: Evidence for a schizophrenia vulnerability locus on chromosome 8p in the Irish study of high-density schizophrenia families. Am J Psychiatry 1996;153:1534–1540.

63. Levinson DF, Wildenauer DB, Schwab SG, et al: Additional support for schizophrenia linkage on chromosomes 6 and 8: A multicenter study. Am J Med Genet 1996;67:580–594.

64. Blouin JL, Dombroski BA, Nath SK, et al: Schizophrenia susceptibility loci on chromosomes 13q32 and 8p21. Nat Genet 1998;20:70–73.

65. Gurling HM, Kalsi G., Brynjolfson J, et al: Genomewide genetic linkage analysis confirms the presence of susceptibility loci for schizophrenia, on chromosomes 1q32.2, 5q33.2, and 8p21-22 and provides support for linkage to schizophrenia, on chromosomes 11q23.3-24 and 20q12.1-11.23. Am J Hum Genet 2001;68:661–673.

66. Zhang Y, Proenca R, Maffei M, et al: Positional cloning of the mouse obese gene and its human homologue. Nature 1994;372:425–432.

67. Tartaglia LA, Dembski M, Wang X, et al: Identification and expression cloning of a leptin receptor, OB-R. Cell 1995;83:1263–1271.

68. Chemelli RM, Willie JT, Sinton CM, et al: Narcolepsy in orexin knockout mice: Molecular genetics of sleep regulation. Cell 1999;98:437–451.

69. Lin L, Faraco J, Li R, Kadotani H, et al: The sleep disorder canine narcolepsy is caused by a mutation in the hypocretin (orexin) receptor 2 gene. Cell 1999;98:365–376.

SUGGESTED READINGS

American Psychiatric Association: Diagnostic and Statistical Manual of Mental Disorders, 4th ed. American Psychiatric Association, Washington, DC, 1994.

Berrettini WH: A bipolar pedigree series for genomic mapping of disease genes: Diagnostic and analytic considerations. Psychiatr Genet 1991;2:125–160.

Geyer MA, Swerdlow NR, Mansbach RS, Braff DL. Startle response models of sensorimotor gating and habituation deficits in schizophrenia. Brain Res Bull 1990;25:485–498.

Ott J: Statistical methods to discover susceptibility genes for nervous system diseases. In Chin HR, Moldin SO (cds): Methods in Genomic Neuroscience. New York, CRC Press, pp 287–296.

Tecott LH, Wehner JM: Mouse molecular genetic technologies: Promise for psychiatric research. Arch Gen Psychiatry 2001;58(11):995–1004.

Depression

Kerry J. Ressler
Charles B. Nemeroff

Unipolar major depression is a very common syndromal disorder that carries with it extreme morbidity and mortality. Epidemiologic and family studies consistently place the lifetime prevalence of the disorder at 5% to 12% in men and 10% to 22% in women.[1] It is a disorder with considerable morbidity, and current estimates suggest that it will soon rank second only to ischemic heart disease as a source of disability worldwide.[2] It is a source of significant mortality, with suicide occurring in 8% to 15% of patients who previously had been hospitalized for depression. Furthermore, depression is an independent risk factor for the development of coronary artery disease and stroke, and patients with comorbid depression have worse outcomes following myocardial infarction. In general, medically ill patients with depression suffer significantly more morbidity and mortality than do those without depression.

CLINICAL FEATURES

Diagnosis of Depressive Disorders

Because psychiatric disorders do not yet have biochemical or genetic markers of high specificity and sensitivity, psychiatric diagnosis in practice remains a purely clinical endeavor based on observation, interview, history, and collateral information. The *Diagnostic and Statistical Manual of Mental Disorders,* 4th edition (DSM-IV), provides a precise and consistent diagnostic framework for psychiatric disorders including information on prevalence, identification of risk factors, determination of optimal treatment modalities, and creation of preventative measures. The DSM-IV Mood Disorders section is composed of three major parts. The first describes the symptom clusters of

mood episodes, including major depressive, manic, hypomanic, and mixed episodes. The second part describes the criteria for the syndromes that are defined as mood disorders, including major depression and bipolar disorder, mood disorder owing to a general medical condition, and substance-induced mood disorder. The third part includes the specifiers that describe either the most recent mood episode or the course of recurrent episodes.

This chapter focuses on the neurobiology and genetics of the syndrome of unipolar depression, also called major depression, as contrasted with bipolar depression, the depressive phase of manic-depressive bipolar disorder. Major depressive disorder is defined by at least one major depressive episode, which is a two-week period of decreased functioning in which the patient has either depressed mood and/or anhedonia, in addition to at least four of the following symptoms: (1) significant weight change (loss or gain of 5% body weight), (2) insomnia or hypersomnia, (3) psychomotor agitation or retardation, (4) fatigue, (5) feelings of worthlessness or guilt, (6) decreased concentration/attention, (7) recurrent thoughts of death or suicidal behaviors.

Major depressive disorder is classified according to severity, presence of psychosis, and level of remission. Subtypes of major depression, based on symptom clustering or course, include catatonic, psychotic, melancholic, atypical, seasonal pattern, postpartum onset, chronic without remission, and early-onset, though the latter is not yet recognized as a separate subtype by the DSM. The subtypes that appear to have the most genetic or heritable validity as distinctly separate disorders appear to be early-onset, melancholic, atypical, seasonal, and psychotic. Early-onset is typically defined as having the first episode before age 25 years. Melancholic type indicates a symptom cluster of extreme anhedonia, lack of reactivity to any pleasurable stimuli, worsening morning symptoms, early morning awakening, marked psychomotor agitation or retardation, and significant anorexia or weight loss. Atypical depression refers to a subtype that is almost opposite of melancholic, with significant mood reactivity, appetite increase and weight gain, hypersomnia, leaden paralysis, and significant interpersonal rejection sensitivity. Major depression with seasonal onset, also known as seasonal affective disorder, describes depression with onset generally in winter months (during decreased light exposure) that tends to naturally remit during summer months. Its prevalence is increased in northern climates, and there is some evidence that it is responsive to artificial light therapy. Psychotic depression is characterized by the presence of psychosis, usually delusions.

Course

The course of major depression is variable. Symptoms generally develop over a period of days to weeks. A prodromal period including anxiety and mild depressive symptoms may predate the full episode by weeks to months. An untreated episode can last for 6 months or longer, regardless of age of onset. There is generally a complete remission of symptoms over time, but 20% to 30% of patients do not recover completely for months to years. The majority of patients who experience one major depressive episode, despite attaining a complete remission, will experience subsequent recurrences. The recurrence rate among individuals who have had three or more episodes of major depression is greater than 90%. There is also evidence that two factors place the patient at risk for more severe and refractory episodes in the future with less likelihood of achieving complete remission. They are (1) increased length of time before treatment and (2) increased number of previous episodes. The chronic subtype of major depression occurs in 5% to 10% of cases and is defined as continuously meeting criteria for major depressive episode for 2 or more years without remission.

Syndromes Secondary to Medical and Neurologic Disease

It is important that the clinician be aware that depressive symptoms from moderate to severe can occur in conjunction with numerous systemic medical illnesses (diagnosed as mood disorder with depressive features owing to a general medical condition).[3] For example, patients with Cushing's disease have up to a 67% lifetime prevalence of depression and high rates of anxiety disorders as well. Furthermore, these symptoms often precede hirsutism, stria, and other physical signs of the disease. Diabetes, both types I and II, are associated with up to a 33% lifetime prevalence. Coronary artery disease (CAD) and congestive heart failure patients have up to a 26% lifetime risk of depression. Also, there is a marked increased in cardiac morbidity and mortality in patients who have depression compared to matched cardiac patients without depression. Multiple cancers, most notably pancreatic carcinoma, are associated with depression, often preceding the diagnosis of the cancer.

Many neurologic diseases are especially prone to creating secondary depressive disorders. Patients with Parkinson's disease have been found to have a 40% to 50% lifetime prevalence of depression, with a significant portion having diminished serotonin metabolites in their CSF, and major depressive episode often predates the neurologic symptoms. Huntington's disease patients exhibit a lifetime prevalence of depression of ~40% and may show depressive symptoms prior to neurologic symptoms. Cerebrovascular disease is a very common cause of late-life depression, with a 30% to 50% lifetime prevalence of depression. Patients with multiple sclerosis frequently exhibit depression, with the prevalence rates as high as 50%, but they may also experience manic or hypomanic symptoms. Patients with Alzheimer's disease also have unusually high rates of depression.

Although it is common for clinicians to believe that depression is simply a sequelae of the inability to cope with a debilitating disease in these patients, both biologic and epidemiologic data suggest that this is not the primary factor. Instead, it appears that many of the biologic mechanisms leading to these systemic and neurologic diseases are also antecedents to the neurobiologic mechanisms of depression (e.g., loss of monoamine neurons in degenerative disorders, impairment to limbic regions of the brain secondary to cerebrovascular accidents, paraneoplastic syndromes, iatrogenic causes such as glucocorticoid therapy for rheumatoid arthritis or multiple sclerosis).

It is important for the clinician to look for and recognize depression in the medically ill patient, as well as to treat it aggressively. It has been shown repeatedly that depression in the neurologic or medically ill patient is quite responsive to antidepressant medication, and there is increasing evidence that morbidity and mortality are significantly reduced when depression is adequately treated in these patients.

PATHOLOGY: BIOCHEMICAL ALTERATIONS

Neurotransmitter Abnormalities

There are multiple lines of evidence that the brain stem monoamine systems are dysregulated in depression and anxiety disorders.[3–5] A vast literature has documented abnormalities in the norepinephrine (NE) and serotonin (5HT) systems, though there is also burgeoning evidence that dopamine (DA) may have a role in the disorder. The preponderance of evidence suggests that increased NE transmission or receptor supersensitivity occurs in combination with decreased 5HT transmission or receptor hyposensitivity.

It is unlikely, however, that the primary biologic "lesion" occurs directly within the NE and 5HT systems. Rather, these neurotransmitters have a role in the modulation of multiple neural systems including those mediating cognition, attention, affect regulation, memory, stress response, endocrine function, and sleep regulation. There is normally precise control of activity within the brain stem nuclei: the locus coeruleus (NE), raphe nucleus (5HT), and ventral tegmental area (DA). Depression appears to be a state in which these systems are dysregulated, resulting in abnormal modulation of the neural circuits that mediate many of the functions outlined above. This dysregulation likely occurs as a common end state of multiple factors thus creating the heterogeneous syndrome of major depression. Antidepressant treatment appears to bring these modulatory systems back to a state of homeostasis, allowing for a return to normal neurotransmitter regulation.

Norepinephrine Alterations

The initial catecholamine hypothesis by Schildkraut in 1965 proposed that abnormally low states of NE lead to depressive symptoms, whereas elevated NE states lead to euphoric or manic symptoms. Years of research to explore these relationships further have refuted this simple dichotomy (reviewed in references 3–5). Rather, there appears to be a complex dysregulation of NE levels and locus coeruleus (LC) firing in states of depression and anxiety. This may lead to increases or decreases in NE release coupled with altered sensitivities of presynaptic and postsynaptic receptors.

The principal findings that implicate dysregulation of the noradrenergic system have been comprehensively reviewed.[4–7] The most consistent data for patients with depression is as follows: (1) increased concentrations of plasma and CSF NE metabolites; (2) greater variability in the concentration of NE and NE metabolites compared to controls; (3) altered α_2 receptor binding in postmortem brains; (4) increased β-adrenergic receptors in postmortem tissue; (5) blunted growth hormone (GH) response to clonidine (an α_2 receptor agonist), especially in suicidal patients; and (6) consistent increase in tyrosine hydroxylase activity (the rate-limiting enzyme in NE production) in postmortem locus coeruleus.

In summary, although there is a range of variability regarding findings of NE and its metabolites and presynaptic and postsynaptic receptor dynamics, the findings consistently show abnormal NE turnover coupled with increased receptor sensitivity. This data suggest that at basal firing conditions, NE levels may indeed be lower than normal, but that more rapid LC firing in response to stress may lead to greater than normal NE transmission in conjunction with supersensitive postsynaptic receptors.

Serotonin Alterations

The serotonin hypothesis of depression posits a relative deficiency of brain serotonergic activity in depression. As with NE, indirect measures of precursor (tryptophan) availability and metabolite concentrations provided initial evidence for abnormalities in the system. As with the NE system in depression and anxiety, there are also alterations in 5HT receptor populations. Although there has been variability in this data, it has provided a consistent picture of decrease in serotonergic neural activity during depression.

This data has been reviewed in detail.[4,5] The principal consistent findings are (1) increased $5HT_2$ and decreased $5HT_{1a}$ receptor binding in postmortem brain tissue; (2) reduced serotonin transporter (SERT) binding in postmortem cerebral cortex and hippocampus; (3) reduced SERT binding in platelets and in the raphe nucleus, as assessed with functional brain imaging; (4) diminished prolactin release after fenfluramine and other 5HT secretagogues, suggesting a decreased serotonergic responsiveness; and (5) decreased serotonin metabolites (5HIAA) in cerebrospinal fluid (CSF), especially in suicidal patients. Finally, selective serotonin reuptake inhibitors (SSRIs) that increase the extracellular fluid concentration of 5HT are effective antidepressants. Overall, these data suggest that impaired serotonergic function is a biochemical trait that underlies the vulnerability for recurrent episodes of depression.

Dopamine Alterations

An increasingly impressive body of evidence supports a role for a relative DA neuronal deficiency in depression. These findings include (1) reduced concentrations of DOPAC, a major DA metabolite, in postmortem tissue of depressed suicide victims; (2) evidence from functional brain imaging studies using single proton emission tomography (SPECT) and positron emission tomography (PET) that have measured DA neuronal activity; (3) markedly blunted GH response to apomorphine, a DA receptor agonist, in depressed patients with a history of suicide attempts; (4) unusually high rates of depression in patients with Parkinson's disease, a disorder associated with DA neuronal cell death; (5) the overwhelming evidence for a critical role for DA in mediating reward and pleasure, the absence of which is generally acknowledged as the cardinal symptom of depression; and (6) the efficacy of DA reuptake blockers and DA agonists in the treatment of depression.

Corticotropin Releasing Factor and HPA Axis Alterations

Hyperactivity of the hypothalamic-pituitary-adrenal (HPA) axis in depressed patients is one of the most consistent findings in the literature on mood disorders (reviewed in references 4 and 8–10). These data support a preeminent role of hyperactivity of the corticotropin-releasing factor (CRF) neural circuits in depression. The most consistent findings are (1) elevated CSF CRF concentrations in depressed patients; (2) increased hypothalamic CRF immunoreactivity and CRF mRNA expression and decreased CRF receptor binding in postmortem frontal cortex of suicide victims; (3) increased adrenocorticotropic hormone (ACTH) and cortisol during depression; (4) blunted ACTH (and β-endorphin) response to intravenously administered CRF; (5) glucocorticoid and ACTH nonsuppression after dexamethasone administration or the combined dexamethasone/CRF test; and (6) administration of CRF directly into the CNS of laboratory animals mimics many cardinal features of depression, including decreased appetite, disrupted sleep, decreased libido, and anhedonia.

CRF hypersecretion is thought to occur in conjunction with monoamine abnormalities and limbic dysregulation. Activation of the fear-stress response circuitry leads to activation of the central nucleus of the amygdala (CeA) or the bed nucleus of the stria terminalis (BNST), a similar region of the "extended amygdala" involved in anxiety. Neurons from these regions release CRF in numerous brain areas in response to stress.[11] In addition, direct activation of the paraventricular nucleus (PVN) of the hypothalamus leads to CRF release that stimulates the secretion of ACTH from the anterior pituitary gland. It has been shown in several studies that CRF is elevated in CSF of patients with depression, neurologic disorders, and comorbid depression. As many as 75% of patients with major depression have overactivity of the HPA axis as characterized by hypercortisolemia. Evidence of significant alterations in CRF neuronal density and increased production suggest that depression involves a state of significantly altered neural circuitry mediating the stress response pathways. Consistent with data discussed below, neuroimaging studies have revealed a correlation between increased amygdala activation and plasma cortisol levels in depression.[12] Furthermore, dysregulation of NE and CRF systems occurring in conjunction with stress early in life may contribute to depression and anxiety symptoms in adulthood.[10]

Thyrotropin-Releasing Hormone and HPT Axis Alterations

There have also been consistent findings of abnormalities within the hypothalamic-pituitary-thyroid (HPT) axis in depression[4]: (1) increased CSF thyrotropin-releasing hormone (TRH) concentrations, (2) decreased nocturnal thyroid-stimulating hormone (TSH) concentrations, (3) blunted TSH response to intravenously administered TRH administration, and (4) unusually high rate of autoimmune thyroiditis in depressed patients. Clinically, it is recognized that augmentation of antidepressants with one of the thyroid hormones, T_3, is an effective means of converting antidepressant nonresponders to responders. Recently a new TRH receptor, TRH-R2, has been discovered that is distributed in thalamic, limbic,

and cortical brain regions. This is in marked contrast to the TRH-R1 that is limited in distribution to the hypothalamus and anterior pituitary. Additionally, little notice has been paid to the fact that the reticular nucleus of the thalamus expresses as much TRH peptide as the hypothalamus. Growing evidence suggests that this system may play a significant role in the sleep and attentional abnormalities found in depression. Indeed, two thirds of TRH in the central nervous system is extrahypothalamic. Further understanding of this system will surely prove fascinating, as it may be possible to incorporate the role of this neuropeptide regulatory system with the neurocircuitry information described above.

PATHOLOGY: FUNCTIONAL NEUROBIOLOGY

Brain Regions

Functional imaging experiments with positron emission tomography (PET) and functional magnetic resonance imaging (fMRI) have provided new insights into the brain regions and circuits involved in depression. Numerous studies have found changes in frontal cortical activity in depressed states.[12,13] In these studies, there appear to be differential activations of cortex. Dorsal prefrontal cortex (PFC) is generally suppressed in contrast to ventral PFC and orbital cortex which have been found to be more activated in depressed patients compared with controls.[12] Antidepressant treatment normalizes these alterations, increasing dorsal PFC activity and decreasing ventral and orbital PFC activity. The amygdala has been found to be consistently activated in depressed patients more than in nondepressed controls, with its imaged neural activity correlated with depression severity.[12] As with cortical abnormalities, the altered amygdala activity normalizes with antidepressant response and remission.

Some groups have examined the relationship of normal sadness to depression using emotion provocation paradigms.[13] The dorsal prefrontal areas (Brodmann area 9) are temporarily decreased in activity with transient sadness in healthy controls but remain decreased in activity in depressed patients. Furthermore, they found that ventral prefrontal areas similar to those discussed previously (subgenual cingulate, Brodmann area 25) are temporarily increased in normal sadness in healthy volunteers but remain increased in depressed patients. Although it also has been found that other cortical areas are altered in depression and sadness, these two regions (dorsal and ventral prefrontal cortex) show the most consistent results. These data suggest that a limbic circuit involving activation of ventral prefrontal areas and amygdala in combination with inhibition of dorsal prefrontal areas may mediate normal sadness as well as the abnormal mood states of depression. It appears that in major depression, the neural circuits that normally mediate the transient emotions of sadness, dysphoria, and anxiety are unable to return to baseline.

Neural Circuits Mediating Stress and Fear

The limbic circuitry mediating stress, fear, anger, and other emotions is thought to be critically involved in both depression and anxiety disorders (Fig. 71–1). In normal functioning, the amygdala serves to continuously compare sensory stimuli to previously learned aversive (fear/stress/pain mediating) or appetitive (approach/motivational/hedonic mediating) stimuli.[14] Recognition of previously associated stimuli activates the appropriate conditioned response pathway. The neural circuits mediating some of the amygdala-dependent behaviors have been clearly demonstrated. For example, the CeA as well as the BNST project extensively to the hypothalamic and brain stem circuitry that mediate the stress and fear response (e.g., hypothalamic paraventricular nucleus→HPA axis activation, central gray→freezing behavior, parabrachial nucleus→respiratory distress).[11] When the amygdala registers a comparison between current incoming stimuli that have previously been associated with fear or stress, the CeA and BNST are able to rapidly activate a distributed neural system engaging the fight-flight response.[15] Prefrontal cortex, with its highly

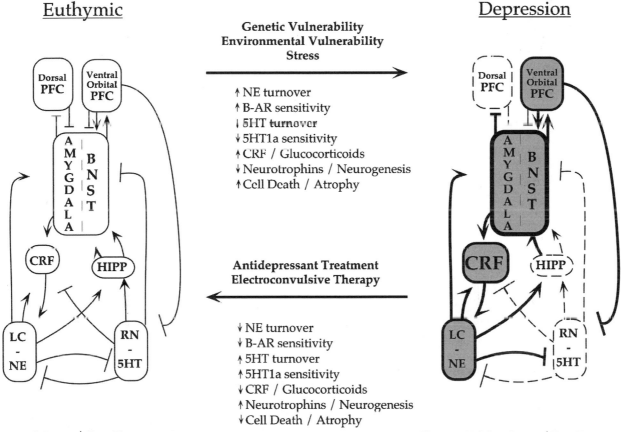

FIGURE 71–1. Neurotransmitter modulation of affective circuitry involved in depression. Brain stem modulatory nuclei, locus coeruleus with norepinephrine (LC-NE), and raphe nuclei with serotonin (RN-5HT) are shown with their primary excitatory (→) and inhibitory (–|) effects on limbic circuitry. During the euthymic state, stressful or fearful stimuli initially activate the LC-NE system via CRF release from the amygdala and the paraventricular nucleus of the hypothalamus. This is opposed by 5HT release that promotes aversion tolerance and decreases the stress response mediated by the amygdala/bed nucleus of the stria terminalis (BNST). There are reciprocal connections between amygdala and prefrontal cortical (PFC) areas. These areas are critical for extinction of fearful memories and aversion tolerance, however ventral prefrontal areas may also serve to activate amygdala and inhibit RN activity. Multiple genetic and environmental determinants lead to alterations in these systems resulting in a dysregulated state of functioning in depression. Increased activity *(thick lines)* and decreased activity *(hash lines)* are shown. In this state, the LC-NE system is hyperresponsive to stress or fear stimuli, and the RN-5HT system is hyporesponsive with decreased inhibition of stress reactivity. The cortical modulation of limbic reactivity is dysregulated and likely contributes to altered NE/5HT functioning.

refined information, has significant interconnectivity with the amygdala, and it may be required for extinction of aversive memories. This is consistent with the idea that cortical representations are able to modulate limbic associations—that rational thought should prevail over irrational fear or worry. It has been proposed that the dorsal prefrontal cortex is involved via these connections in regulating affect, providing cognitive control over emotions such as stress, fear, anger, anxiety, and frustration.[14,15] However, ventral prefrontal cortex appears to subserve emotional functions, and its interconnections with the amygdala may be mutually excitatory.

The physiology of the locus coeruleus (LC) is consistent with a nucleus critically involved in attention, vigilance, and orientation.[5,10,16] In awake behaving animals, the LC is most active when orienting to a novel, aversive, or stressful stimulus. NE stimulates potentially stressful memories and fear-stress responses in the amygdala. NE also increases long-term potentiation and contextual conditioning to aversive stimuli in hippocampus. This is consistent with the role of the LC-NE system in vigilance via activation of the fight-flight response. The CeA and BNST pathways release CRF onto the LC, which activates LC firing and NE release.

NE activation of cortex is complex, with decreased activation at too low or too high levels of release and optimal activation with midrange firing. Thus at high rates of activity, NE may lead to an overactivation of limbic pathways over cortical pathways, as presumably would promote survival if a rapid fight-flight response is needed. Finally, NE activation appears to have an inhibitory role on raphe firing.

In contrast to the LC, the raphe nuclei (RN) show highest firing during internally directed rhythmic movements and behaviors, with diminished firing when orienting to external stimuli.[17] 5HT from the RN mediates tolerance to aversive experience in the amygdala, potentially decreasing likelihood of a fight-flight response. 5HT appears to decrease context conditioning in hippocampus with aversive stimuli. These data are consistent with a role of the raphe-5HT system in homeostasis, decreased aggression, and tolerance to aversion. Raphe firing is inhibited both by NE from the LC and by orbital cortex activation. These regions of cortex are activated in correlation with sad or anxious emotion, and are thought to be important in control over amygdala activation.[12]

Normal Response to Stress

A working model for the role of this neural circuit in normal and pathologic responses to stress is as follows[5]: The brain stem monoamine circuits are modulatory systems that exhibit baseline levels of tonic firing and are exquisitely controlled by other neural pathways and complex regulatory loops. During normal functioning, in the presence of a safe environment with internally directed behaviors such as feeding or grooming, the RN are relatively active. Released 5HT acts to inhibit the LC and limbic pathways, leading to decreased sensitivity to arousal or stressful/aversive stimuli. During such states, executive cortical areas (dorsal PFC) prevail over limbic control of affect.

When the animal is exposed to stress, however, the balance shifts. Recognition of potentially stressful/aversive stimuli by amygdala pathways activates LC firing, and the RN is inhibited. LC activation of amygdala-hippocampal pathways increases the sensitivity to aversive/stressful stimuli further increasing hypothalamic CRF release and subsequently plasma cortisol levels. These combined shifts lead limbic pathways to prevail over prefrontal cortical pathways in the control of affect. The organism is primed in a state of arousal and prepared for initiation of the fight-flight stress response. In the healthy or euthymic condition, the individual returns to a baseline affective state when the stressful/aversive stimulus is gone.

Abnormal Regulation during Depressed and Anxiety States

In depressed states and in some anxiety states, the aforementioned neural systems are dysregulated. NE transmission is overactive via LC firing, receptor sensitivity, or both. In contrast, 5HT transmission is underactive via inhibited RN firing, decreased receptor sensitivity, or both. These neurotransmitter alterations contribute to overactivation of amygdala, BNST, and hippocampal areas activating the stress/fear response. Ventral cortical areas primarily associated with affect and strongly interconnected with the amygdala are also overactivated and may contribute to inhibition of RN firing. Resultant increases in CRF will further activate the LC-NE system promoting vigilance and stress/fear responsiveness, while increases in adrenal glucocorticoids and increased activity of autonomic, visceral, and neural pathways also occur. In this depressed or anxious state, the stimulus-response is shifted. A stimulus that might only lead to minimal arousal in the healthy "euthymic" state may now activate significant arousal and continual activation of the fight-flight pathways.

Depression as a Disorder of Decreased Neural Plasticity

There is considerable data that supports the hypothesis that stress, depression, and anxiety disorders induce degeneration of target neurons, perhaps mediated by cortisol.[18,19] Hippocampal atrophy has been reported in several studies of depression,[20] although discordant results have also appeared.[21] Glial cell loss and neuronal abnormalities have been observed in the prefrontal cortex in major depression. Noradrenergic axons have been found with decreased axonal arborization and density in stress models. Serotonergic axon sprouting appears to be dependent on BDNF, which appears to decrease after stress exposure. Thus, it appears that stress and disorders associated with chronic stress may increase neuronal atrophy and perhaps frank neuronal degeneration. Furthermore, hippocampal neurons undergo continuous proliferation well into adulthood. This continued neurogenesis is dependent on the presence of serotonin and inhibited by adrenal steroids,[19] both of which are altered in depression. Accumulating evidence shows that antidepressant treatment may reverse the atrophy of hippocampal neurons, increase cell survival, and increase monoamine axonal sprouting in both rodent and human.[18]

These changes in neuronal populations in the depressed state likely contribute to the dysregulated affective neural circuitry, and may lead to worsening symptoms and resistance to treatment. Decreased neuronal density and atrophy in the hippocampus and prefrontal cortex presumably contribute to decreased activity and responsiveness. These processes likely serve to maintain a state of imbalance in depression by decreasing the ability of cortical and hippocampal areas to inhibit or modulate the stress-fear pathways of the amygdala and interconnected circuitry. The depressed or anxious state is one in which these stress-fear pathways cannot be easily "shut off" or returned to normal, which leaves the individual in a chronic state of abnormal affective responsiveness.

Interaction between Neurobiology and Genetics

Current working models of depression at a neurobiologic level are heavily dependent on the concept of stress as a causal mediator of the depressed state. In fact, the data are most consistent with the hypothesis that depression is a quintessential disorder of gene-environment interaction. As discussed later, numerous family, adoption, and twin studies place the genetic loading at approximately 35% to 50% for the likelihood of developing depression with an environmental loading of 50% to 65%. Figure 71–2 shows genetic and environmental roles acting through development to influence the phenotype of trait vulnerability, which in combination with ongoing environmental stress may result in depression.

It is increasingly evident that the brain exhibits neural plasticity even into adulthood, and gene products act on neuronal processes to influence initial development as well as ongoing learning and homeostatic responsiveness in adulthood. However, the brain evolved to integrate environmental information, and it is biochemically and physically shaped by environment continuously. Therefore, the fact that depression is partially environmentally determined should be no more self-evident than the fact that congestive heart failure, lung cancer, or type II diabetes are complex genetic disorders that are also partially environmentally determined.

GENETICS: UNIPOLAR DEPRESSION AS A HERITABLE DISEASE

Family Association Studies

Numerous studies have been performed addressing the question, "Are family members of depressed patients more likely to be depressed than family members of nondepressed patients?" Familial aggregation studies take as the independent variables subjects with major depression and case controls without depression (controlling for relatively simple variables such as age, sex, and medical history). The dependent variables are the presence of depressive symptomatology in biologic relatives (usually first-degree). A meta-analysis[22] analyzed the extant literature on genetic epidemiologic studies of depression and found only five familial association studies that were well designed by the criteria of appropriate controls, diagnostic criteria, systematic recruitment, and direct determination of major depression versus bipolar diagnosis.

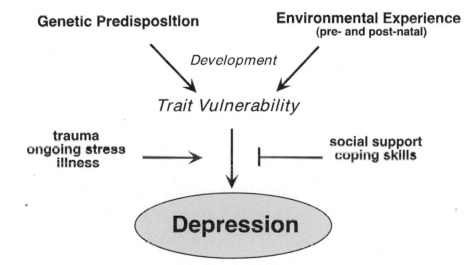

FIGURE 71–2. Genetic and environmental interactions mediating onset of depression, showing combined roles of genes and environment (contributing 35% to 50% of variance) in the development of major depression. It is thought that early environmental experience during development (including prenatal and perinatal insults and early familial interactions) interact with different genes leading to distinct traits or temperaments. Combinations of personality traits likely provide both protection and vulnerability to environmental insults (life events) during adolescence and adulthood.

TABLE 71–1. Risk of Major Depression in First-Degree Relatives from Family Association Studies

Study	Risk: Subject's Relatives	Risk: Control's Relatives	Odds Ratio
Tsuang, et al: Br J Psych 1980;37:497	15.2	7.5	2.2
Gershon, et al: Arch Gen Psych 1982;39:1157	16.6	5.8	3.2
Weissman, et al: Arch Gen Psych 1984;41:13	17.6	5.9	3.4
Maier, et al: Arch Gen Psych 1993;50:871	21.6	10.6	2.3
Weissman, et al: Arch Gen Psych 1993;50:767	21.0	5.5	4.6

Data from Sullivan PF, Neale MC, Kendler KS: Genetic epidemiology of major depression: Review and meta-analysis. Am J Psychiatry 2000; 157:1552–1562.

Studies from this meta-analysis are shown in Table 71–1. When all studies were analyzed together, there was a very strong association between major depression in the identified patient and first-degree relatives (p < .00005). Taken together, these studies indicate that major depression is familial. However, these studies are unable to differentiate genetic influences from familial environmental influences. As discussed above, considerable evidence suggests that the syndrome of depression results from a genetic-environmental interaction.

Adoption Studies

When compared with other psychiatric disorders, there are far fewer studies of adoption involving probands with unipolar depression compared to bipolar disorder or schizophrenia. Table 71–2 shows the three studies considered as well controlled. They clearly have their pitfalls, primarily in that the ability to gain diagnostic data on the biologic parent is very limited. Nonetheless, two of the studies provide suggestive evidence that the risk of developing major depression is significantly higher if the biologic parent suffered depression, regardless of the adoptive environment. This strongly suggests that a significant component of the relative risk for depression must be genetic. Nonetheless, these studies have limited statistical power and remain of relatively limited utility for determining heritable risk.

Twin Studies

As with other disorders, twin studies[23] have proved to be the most powerful tool to determine the relative contribution of heritability. Furthermore, the comparison of monozygotic twins to dizygotic twins allows for the critical variables of genes versus environment to be finely separated. This analysis and interpretation is based on the assumption that monozygotic and dizygotic twins receive similar environmental inputs. There is evidence that monozygotic twins are treated much more similarly than are dizygotic twins by their family members, especially early in development. Therefore, some differences between these two groups that were assumed to be genetic may be due to environmental factors. This argument and the data supporting this assumption are discussed in detail in reference 23. This same group performed a meta-analysis of the extant twin studies (Table 71–3) and determined that the best model to fit the entirety of the data was one in which genetic liability accounted for 37% of the risk of major depression.

This concatenation of data suggests that unipolar or major depression is clearly genetically heritable. These studies likely underestimate the genetic liability, because measurement error in terms of underdiagnosis or misdiagnosis lead to higher specific environment predictions and lower genetic variance predictions. Another recent study by Kendler and colleagues examined a longitudinal sample of twins in which repeated clinical assessments decreased measurement error. Indeed, this longitudinal study found genetic liability of major depression to be 66%.[27] This level approaches the heritability estimates found in bipolar disorder and schizophrenia.

GENETIC STUDIES: THE SEARCH FOR QUANTITATIVE TRAITS

Although the available data are incontrovertible concerning a genetic contribution to major depression, it appears

TABLE 71–2. Relative Risk of Major Depression in Adopted Offspring

Study	Population	Relative Risk if Biological Parents had Depression	
Von Knorring, et al: Arch Gen Psych 1983;40:943	56 adoptees, 115 controls	0.71	NS
Cadoret, et al: J Affective Disord 1985;9:155	48 depressed, 395 nondepressed	2.54	p=.05*
Wender, et al: Arch Gen Psych 1986;43:923	71 adoptees, 75 controls	7.24	p=.03

*Study initially did not meet p=.05 level when gender was separately examined. When Sullivan et al, 2000 reanalyzed data combining gender, significance was found.[22]

TABLE 71–3. Summary of Twin Studies and Hereditary Liability Estimates

Study (Patient Population)	Patient Population	Country	Sex	Concordance MZ	Concordance DZ	Genetic Liability	Shared Environment Liability	Specific Environment Liability
Kendler, et al: Behav Genet 1995;25:217	Clinical	Sweden	M	.50	.33	49%	21%	30%
			F	.32	.20	17%	0%	83%
McGuffin, et al: Arch Gen Psych 1996;53:129	Clinical	UK	M	.46	.15	58%	0%	42%
			F	.46	.22	38%	0%	62%
Lyons, et al: Arch Gen Psych 1998;55:468	Community	US	M	.23	.14	36%	0%	64%
Bierut, et al: Arch Gen Psych 1999;56:557	Community	Australia	M	.34	.30	24%	0%	76%
			F	.50	.37	44%	0%	56%
Kendler and Prescott: Arch Gen Psych 1999;56:39	Community	US	M	.41	.34	31%	0%	69%
			F	.47	.43	38%	0%	62%

Data from Sullivan PF, Neale MC, Kendler KS: Genetic epidemiology of major depression: Review and meta-analysis. Am J Psychiatry 2000; 157: 1552–1562.

likely that this syndrome arises from numerous genetic and environmental insults and may comprise a heterogeneous set of diseases. Given this heterogeneity, how can susceptibility genes for depression be identified? An increasingly important approach to this problem is the search for quantitative traits that may underlie depression (reviewed in reference 24). This approach is derived from an increasing recognition that the heritable component of depression does not arise from single genes that are necessary and sufficient to cause a disorder. Rather, such quantitatively inheritable traits likely arise from the interactions of multiple genes with the environment. A number of studies have now approached the problem of identifying the quantitative traits that underlie the heritable component of depression.

Kendler and colleagues examined the clinical characteristics of major depression as predictive variables of risk of depression in relatives.[25] Using the Virginia Twin Registry, they examined 3786 twin pairs, 1765 of whom had a lifetime history of the disorder, of whom 639 (36.2%) had affected co-twins. Their best-fit model suggested that number of episodes, duration of longest episode, and recurrent suicidal thoughts were the clinical features most predictive of risk for major depression in the co-twin. Surprisingly, age of onset and number of depressive symptoms did not predict twin relative risk. In fact, the only 2 symptoms of the 14 criteria from DSM-IV significantly correlated with increased co-twin risk: (1) suicidal thoughts (risk 1.4, p < .001) provided additional evidence for the genetic contribution to suicidality and (2) feelings of guilt had some predictive validity (risk 1.21, p = .03). These findings are consistent with the view that

depression is a syndromal definition and cannot be broken down into symptoms as quantitative markers for determining genetic causality. Nevertheless, it is quite likely that subtypes of depression characterized by greater severity (e.g., psychotic depression) may be more heritable.

In fact, an attempt has been undertaken to focus on defining subtypes of major depression that may be more heritable for association or linkage studies. One study examined a subtype of depression based on age of onset, early-onset recurrent major depressive disorder (RE-MDD),[26] which some evidence suggest is the most familial form of the disorder. The population was defined as having a first episode before age 25 years, and having had at least two episodes of nonpsychotic, unipolar major depression. Eighty-one families having probands with RE-MDD were ascertained, and familial association studies were performed. The associations in these families were compared to population prevalence rates for RE-MDD. This study supported a sex-independent, mendelian dominant mode of inheritance for RE-MDD. This and other similar evidence suggest that a major locus contributes to the expression of RE-MDD, and possibly other mood disorders. However, the methods used do not allow the determination of whether the same major locus is segregating across families or whether multiple major loci are involved (genetic heterogeneity).

DSM-IV described subtypes of major depression (melancholic, atypical, postpartum, and seasonal) based on symptomatic clustering from validated epidemiologic prevalence studies. Unfortunately, there is little evidence that these subtypes delineate separate qualitative diseases that can be genetically separable. Melancholic depression is the oldest recognized variant of depression, and well-controlled twin studies have examined its heritability.[27] In this study, there was increased risk of the co-twin having major depression if the proband had major depression, melancholic subtype. However, the genetic contribution of melancholic and nonmelancholic depression seemed largely to reflect depression severity per se and not melancholia.

A different approach to understanding the genetic basis of depression takes the view that the 50% to 60% variance of depression accounted for by stressful life events may be mainly due to an interaction with genetic traits. For example, different personality traits may lead a person to engage in more risk-taking behavior, while other traits may lead to poorer coping skills. These traits might be primarily genetically determined, thus placing the person at an increased likelihood of depression in response to environmental stressors.

To examine these questions, McGuffin and colleagues examined sibling pairs of depressed probands and healthy controls in the Cardiff Depression Study.[28] They sought to determine whether there might be a common familial factor influencing vulnerability to depression and the experiencing of life events. They used a sib-pair design of familial association with 108 probands with major depression and their siblings compared with 105 healthy controls and siblings. Outcomes were based on diagnostic interviews, and data were collected concerning adverse life events. Lifetime relative risk of unipolar depression in siblings of depressed subjects compared to control siblings was 9.74. However, there was no significant difference in life event measures in proband siblings compared to controls. Thus, there appeared to be no evidence for a common factor contributing to both depression and life events in this study. Therefore, they conclude that the >60% variance in depression accounted for by life events/environment was not likely genetically determined. A similar study by the same group looked specifically at risk-taking or sensation-seeking

behavior. Surprisingly, they found that sensation seeking correlated negatively with depression, though sensation seeking itself seemed to be an independent familial trait. It appeared that although sensation seeking correlated positively with life events, these were not the more severe events that are typically associated with precipitating depressive episodes. Thus, it does not appear that sensation seeking is a risk factor for depression and may in fact even be slightly protective.

Another aspect of personality that has been extensively studied as a vulnerability factor to depression is the trait of neuroticism. Although *neurosis*, a term last used in DSMII, is an imprecise term that encompasses many aspects of personality, neuroticism, per se, has been objectively measured. In the last decade, a five-factor model of personality has emerged, with personality being considered a result of five dimensions: extroversion, agreeableness, conscientiousness, neuroticism, and openness.[29,30] These factors have been found to have considerable heritability and may be akin to genetically determined temperaments (discussed later). Neuroticism, defined by a collection of anxiety traits and negative emotionality, has been repeatedly shown as an independent risk factor for depression (Table 71–4). Although a rigorous understanding of personality is far from complete and other approaches define neuroticism as made up of temperamental traits such as high harm avoidance and character traits such as low self-directedness,[31] it remains a useful measure of trait vulnerability.

Similarly, it is thought that behavioral temperament is largely genetically inherited. Such temperamental differences in individuals likely then lead to differential responses to environmental experience. In a well-designed series of studies, Kagan and colleagues have shown that about 20% of healthy children are born with a temperament that predisposes them to be highly reactive to novel events and fearful of unfamiliar people and environments.[32] They termed this trait behavioral inhibition. Furthermore, this trait appears to be heritable and is pres-

TABLE 71–4. Neuroticism as a Contributing Trait for Major Depression

Study	Measure	Results of Neuroticism Traits
Weissman, et al: Am J Psych 1978;135:797	Neuroticism Scale (Maudsley Personality Inventory) 8- to 48-month prospective study	Most important predictor of long-term outcome after treatment
Charney, et al: Am J Psych 1981;138:1601	DSM-III diagnosis of personality disorder inpatient chart review	Related to earlier onset and worse outcome ($p <.001$)
Black, et al: J Affect Disord 1988;14:115	DSM-III diagnosis of personality disorder case-controlled study	Poorer response to medication and poorer recovery ($p <.025$)
Duggan, et al: J Affect Disord 1995;35:139	Neuroticism score of Eysenck Personality Inventory family association study	Increased risk of depression in probands and relatives
O'Leary and Costello: J Affect Disord 2001;63:67	Neuroticism Scale (Maudsley Personality Inventory) 18-month prospective study	Higher neuroticism scores correlate with longer time to remission ($p<.01$)

ent in infancy. Through prospective studies, these temperamental influences have been shown to place "reactive" infants and behaviorally inhibited children at higher risk for anxiety and affective disorders as adolescents.

Both the neuroticism trait in adults and the behavioral inhibition temperament in children seem to depend more on symptomatology that is associated with anxiety than depression, per se. However, it is clear that anxiety and depression are likely quantitative spectrum disorders with remarkable comorbidity of both syndromes and symptoms, and are not, in fact, easily separable. There is now evidence that anxiety and depression have common genetic origins. Furthermore, the phenotypic differences between anxiety and depression appear to be dependent upon the environment. Thus vulnerability, as indexed by the personality scale of neuroticism, overlaps genetically to a substantial extent with both anxiety and depression.[33]

Kendler's group has scrutinized the role of genetic-environmental interaction by evaluating the role of stressful life events in depression in women from twin pairs. Their data suggest that a genetic vulnerability to major depression may be expressed only if an individual is exposed to stressful life events. Thus, major depression is a disorder in which vulnerability may occur through multiple genetic pathways. It is clear that the interaction between genetic vulnerability and environmental experience determines the vulnerability to major depression.

MOLECULAR GENETICS

Although there are linkage studies underway using genome-wide screens that may well be informative in bipolar disorder and schizophrenia, there are no published data available from such studies examining major depression. However, numerous candidate gene linkage studies have been conducted using polymorphisms of genes that encode proteins thought to be involved in the biochemical pathways underlying depression or in the treatment of depression. The majority of these studies have revealed either no significant linkage or have shown statistically that the polymorphism shows no linkage (LOD < −2) to depression (Table 71–5).

TABLE 71–5. Candidate Gene Linkage Studies in Unipolar Depressive Disorders: Negative Findings

Gene or Loci	Illness	Study	Size	Result	Reference
NET	Major Depression (MD)	Association	329	NS	Zill, et al: Neuropsychopharm 2002;26:489
Golf	MD	Association	321	NS	Zill, et al: Psychiatr Genet 2002;12:17
Alpha2 adr	MD	Linkage	17 families	LOD< −2	Wang, et al: J Affect Disord 1992;25:191
Esterase-D 13q14	MD	Linkage	8 families	NS	Wesner, et al: J Stud Alcohol 1991;52:609
DopaBH 9q34	MD + BP	Linkage	5 families	NS	Sherringto, et al: Biol Psych 1994;36:434
HLA	MD + BP	Linkage	10 families	NS	Suarez and Croughan: Psychiatr Res 1982;7:19
HLA linkage Chr 6	MD + BP	Linkage	19 families	NS	Suarez and Reich: Arch Gen Psych 1984;41:22
MAOA	MD + BP	Association	403	NS	Syagailo, et al: Am J Med Genet 2001;105:168
Tryp Hyd, 5HT2A, 5HT2C, 5HTTLR, DRD4, DAT1, COMT	MDD	Association	274	NS	Frisch, et al: Mol Psychiatry 1999;4:389
D2, D3, TH	MD + BP	Linkage	23 families	NS	Serretti, et al: J Affect Disord 2000;58:51
38 SSTRPs (linked to 12 candidate genes)	MD, recurrent	Linkage	34 families	NS	Neiswanger, et al: Am J Med Genet 1998;81:443
Chromosomes 16, 18, 21, 4	MD, recurrent	Linkage	5 families	NS	Balciuniene, et al: Mol Psychiatry 1998;3:162
30 markers (linked to multiple candidate genes)	Depressive spectrum	Linkage	27 families	NS, (except 9q LOD=1.7)	Wilson, et al: Biol Psychiatry 1989;26:163

TABLE 71–6. Candidate Gene Linkage Studies in Unipolar Depressive Disorders: Positive Findings

Gene (Polymorphism)	Population	Study	Size	OR or LOD	Reference
SERT (5HTTLPR short allele)	Neuroticism	Association	397	p <.01 association with Neuroticism	Greenberg, et al: Am J Med Gen 2000;96:202
SERT (5HTTLPR short allele)	Neuroticism and Anxiety	Association	505	7%–9% inheritance of anxiety p <.01	Lesch, et al: Science 1996;274:1527
SERT (VNTR)	Major Depression	Association	276	OR = 6.95	Ogilvie, et al: Lancet 1996; 347:731
SERT (5HTTLPR)	MD (Melancholia)	Association	158	p = .007 small positive association	Gutierrez, et al: Human Gen 1998;103:319
SERT pro (5HTTLPR)	MD or BP	Association	1024	p = .02, OR = 1.53	Collier, et al: Mol Psychiatry 1996;1:453
5HT2C (c23s)	Major Depression	Association	2063	p = .006 small positive association	Lerer, et al: Mol Psychiatry 2001;6:579
5HT2A	Fibromyalgia	Association	283	p = .008 positive association	Bondy, et al: Neurobiol Dis 1999;6:433
5HT2A (102 T/C polym)	MD (SAD)	Association	323	OR = 7.57, p = .002	Arias, et al: Mol Psychiatry 2001;6:239
TH (HUMTH01)	Insulin-Resistance Depression	Association	465	p <.0001 Insulin resistant association with TH	Chiba, et al: Metabolism 2000;49:145

In contrast, studies of the serotonin reuptake transporter *(SERT)* and, to a lesser extent, 5HT receptors have been recently fruitful (Table 71–6). In multiple studies by different groups, a polymorphism within the promoter of the serotonin transporter (5HT transporter linked promoter region—*5HTTLPR*) has been repeatedly linked to depression, anxiety, and neuroticism traits. This polymorphism exists about 1000 base pairs upstream of the transcription initiation site for *SERT* within the promoter region. It has been shown that the short allele variant is associated with reduced *SERT* gene expression, reduced *SERT* binding, and reduced 5HT uptake.[34] These data suggest that decreased expression of the *SERT* gene is associated with increased neuroticism traits and increased risk for depressive or anxiety disorders. These studies are consistent with the biochemical data that serotonin-containing neurons in the brain may contribute to personality traits and play a role in the risk for depression. Another polymorphism within the *SERT* gene with a variable number of tandem repeats (VNTR) has been reported to be associated with major depression, although other studies have not replicated this finding. While it does not explain all of the genetic variance contributing to major depression, *SERT* appears to be a gene that, when not optimally expressed, places the individual at increased risk for neuroticism and depression.

Recently, an unexpected and exciting finding has appeared in a related area. Gratacos and colleagues have identified a duplication on human chromosome 15 as a significant susceptibility factor for panic and phobic disorders.[35] One of the candidate genes in this region is a neurotrophic factor receptor (NTK3) that is abundantly expressed in the locus coeruleus, the primary site for norepinephrine production. Given the high degree of comorbidity and shared symptomatology of anxiety disorders and depression, it will be interesting to see if this duplication increases the risk for some types of depression. This finding will likely rejuvenate the cytogenetic approach to examining familial forms of depression.

ANIMAL MODELS

There have been a number of animal models developed to study depression. Virtually all of these have focused on either developmental or environmental stress to produce a depressed phenotype.[3,4] More recent genetic animal models have been created through the use of mice with transgenic DNA insertion or homologous recombination (knockouts). One of the most impressive models to date is arguably the $5HT_{1A}$ receptor knockout.[36] Mice lacking this receptor have been shown to exhibit anxiety and fear behavior in several behavioral paradigms. The same group has recently used elegant molecular biology techniques to "rescue" the phenotype of these knockout animals by replacing the $5HT_{1A}$ receptor with transgenesis. Using a tissue-specific promoter that has limited expression, the $5HT_{1A}$ gene is replaced within neurons of the hippocampus, amygdala, and forebrain, but specifically not the raphe nuclei.[37] This limited expression is sufficient to rescue the behavioral phenotype of $5HT_{1A}$ knockout mice, suggesting that it is the $5HT_{1A}$ gene in these target areas that contributes to anxiety-like behavior, and not its role in autofeedback within the raphe. Finally, using a conditional gene that can be replaced for limited periods of time, they showed that the replacement is only necessary during development. If the $5HT_{1A}$ gene is replaced only during the first months of life, but is absent again in adulthood, the animal shows normal levels of anxiety-like behavior as an adult. However, if it is replaced only in adulthood and not earlier during development, the behavioral phenotype is not restored. These data elegantly reveal how a specific interaction between a gene, environment, and development can lead to establishing normal and abnormal adult anxiety-like behavior.

Although other 5HT receptors and the 5HT transporter have also been studied by this knockout method, such manipulations have not resulted in specific increases in anxiety-like or depressive behavior. A different approach has been taken to create a neuron-specific knockout of the glucocorticoid (GR) and mineralocorticoid (MR) receptors.[38] It appears that in the GR knockout, feedback inhibition of hypothalamic CRF secretion is blocked, but amygdala expression of CRF is unaltered. These GR-deficient animals have diminished anxiety responses in the dark/light box and elevated O-maze, spending more time in open, lighted regions than controls. In contrast, MR knockout animals have greatly increased CRF levels and exhibit an increase in HPA-axis activity. These MR-deficient animals also exhibit significant increases in anxiety-like behavior. These studies are in their early phases and need to be considered in the context of the complexity (including possible memory loss) of these animals. Nonetheless, they are consistent with the hypothesis that corticosteroid responsiveness in the brain is a critical mediator of stress and likely contributes to the environmental stress—gene interaction.

Interestingly, CRF knockout mice displayed no significant alterations in anxiety or depression. This may be due to redundant functions of CRF with the recently discovered CRF homologue urocortin. Nonetheless, when CRF is overproduced via a transgenic approach, animals show increased anxiety-like behavior. Additionally, the $CRFR_1$ and $CRFR_2$ receptor knockouts both show significant alterations in anxiety-like behavior.[39] $CRFR_1$ mutant mice have impaired stress responses and display decreased anxiety-like behavior. In contrast, $CRFR_2$ mutant animals are hypersensitive to stress and display increased anxiety-like behavior. When a double mutant animal is made, both sexes display increased anxiety-like behavior, though the males show significantly more. Furthermore the $CRFR_2$ genotype of the mother affects the anxiety-like behavior of the male pups, such that a pup born to a heterozygous or homozygous mutant mother displays more anxiety-like behavior, regardless of pup genotype. This seems to be due to the anxiety/stress state of the mother during pup development. These results implicate the known CRF receptors as well as the role of environment—gene interaction in the development of anxiety or depressive behavior.

In summary, animal models using targeted mutagenesis of candidate genes have been used with success to model anxiety-like and some depression-like phenotypes. As more candidate genes are discovered via genome screens for quantitative trait markers, molecular biology will allow the scrutiny of the function of those genes within relevant neural circuits.

THERAPY

In experimental studies, there are rapid effects of antidepressants on the firing rate of certain neurons and associated increase in the release of neurotransmitter. However, there is often a 3- to 5-week lag between the initiation of antidepressant action and clinical efficacy in both depression and anxiety disorders. Thus the alterations in these systems after chronic, not acute, antidepressant treatment is key to understanding their mechanism(s) of action. The selective serotonin reuptake inhibitors (SSRIs), the combined serotonin/norepinephrine reuptake inhibitors (SNRIs), and the tricyclic antidepressants (TCAs) all appear to act, at least in part, by inhibiting the reuptake of 5HT and/or NE neurotransmitters at the synaptic cleft. Thereby they create an initial increase in neurotransmitter availability (Table 71–7). The changes that occur after chronic antidepressant treatment are quite complicated, however, and likely result from the homeostatic mechanisms of autoreceptors and feedback projections that regulate this neural circuitry.

The data for changes in NE neurotransmission following chronic antidepressant treatment have been relatively consistent. They are (1) decrease in concentrations of NE and its metabolites in CSF occurs after chronic administration of noradrenergic and serotonergic antidepressants, (2) decrease in locus coeruleus firing rate occurs with chronic antidepressant treatment, (3) down regulation of β-adrenergic receptors occurs after chronic antidepressant treatment and electroconvulsive therapy (ECT), and (4) decrease in tyrosine hydroxylase activity within the locus coeruleus occurs after chronic antidepressant treatment and ECT. Thus, it has become increasingly accepted that long-term antidepressant treatment is associated with, and may depend on, decreasing transmission of the locus coeruleus–NE system.[4,5,7,10]

As opposed to NE, the raphe 5HT system appears to exhibit increased activity with chronic antidepressant treatment.[4–6] Evidence for this includes (1) increased 5HT concentrations in forebrain and raphe occur after chronic antidepressant treatment, which is demonstrated by microdialysis; (2) increased prolactin responsiveness to tryptophan or fenfluramine challenge occurs with chronic antidepressant treatment, suggesting enhanced 5HT responsiveness; (3) increased density and sensitivity of postsynaptic $5HT_{1A}$ receptors occurs with antidepressant treatment and ECT; and (4) decreased serotonin transporter density has been reported with chronic antidepressant treatment, suggesting increased synaptic concentrations of 5HT. Together, these data convincingly demonstrate that long-term antidepressant treatment is

TABLE 71–7. Mechanism of Action of Currently Available Antidepressants

Mechanism	Antidepressant	
Primarily serotonin reuptake inhibitor	Clomipramine	Fluoxetine
	Citalopram	
Primarily norepinephrine reuptake inhibitor	Nortriptyline	
	Reboxetine	
Mixed norepinephrine/serotonin reuptake inhibitor	Amitriptyline	Paroxetine
	Imipramine	Duloxetine
	Venlafaxine	Milnacipran
Mixed serotonin/dopamine reuptake inhibitor	Sertraline	
Serotonin reuptake inhibitor + 5HT2 receptor antagonist	Nefazodone	
	Trazodone	
Serotonin 5HT2R and 5HT3R antagonist + norepinephrine α 2 R antagonist	Mirtazapine	
Monoamine oxidase inhibitors (inhibit breakdown of 5HT/NE/DA)	Phenylzine	Isocarboxazid
	Tranylcypromine	

associated with, and may depend upon, increasing transmission of the raphe nuclei serotonin system.[4–7,10]

Mechanism of Antidepressant Drug Action

It may be counterintuitive that the alterations in overall NE and 5HT activity would shift in opposite directions with antidepressant treatment. These changes appear to occur in both systems whether the treatment is 5HT reuptake specific, NE reuptake specific, or ECT. This suggests that there are systemic changes that occur in the treatment of depression that serve to alter both NE and 5HT neuromodulatory systems. It appears that the combination of $5HT_{1A}$ autoreceptor desensitization, $\alpha2$ autoreceptor sensitization, and βAR desensitization all result in an increase in $5HT_{1A}$ postsynaptic transmission and a decrease in βAR transmission.[6] Through such alterations in receptor regulation and interactions between the excitatory NE and inhibitory 5HT system, antidepressants appear to work through correcting dysregulated NE transmission and increasing 5HT transmission.

Despite the apparent similarity of NE-acting or 5HT-acting antidepressants on the NE and 5HT systems, it has been reproducibly shown that serotonergic-specific or noradrenergic-specific antidepressants depend on the availability of 5HT and NE, respectively, for their antidepressant efficacy.[7] Rapid depletion of 5HT, but not NE, induces rapid relapse in depressed patients during SSRI-induced remission. Similarly, rapid depletion of NE, but not 5HT, induces rapid relapse in depressed patients who have achieved remission with noradrenergic antidepressants. However, healthy volunteers and patients in remission no longer on antidepressants do not appear to be sensitive to monoamine depletion. These results suggest

that monoamines play a critical role in modulating other neurobiologic systems involved in recovery from depression, rather than representing the primary pathophysiologic cause of depression.

Through these mechanisms, serotonergic, noradrenergic, and dual-acting antidepressants appear to reset the dysregulated neural systems, perhaps in similar ways. In general, 5HT and NE neurotransmission is increased and decreased, respectively. It is thought that these changes decrease amygdala and ventral prefrontal hyperactivity, thus increasing tolerance to aversion and increasing dorsal prefrontal control over affective response. ECT appears to exert similar chronic effects on these symptoms. Although the mechanism(s) of action of ECT remain obscure, one hypothesized mechanism is via strengthening of prefrontal cortex connectivity with limbic structures secondary to seizure activity. Psychotherapy may produce similar effects on these systems, via increasing cognitive and cortical control over limbic pathways. Shifting the balance of NE and 5HT activity would also result in decreased adrenal glucocorticoid levels and increased neurotrophic factor activity, slowly increasing neuronal density and axonal growth.[18] The slow time course of antidepressant response may reflect the combined time courses of the relatively early adaptation of monoamine transmission and receptor sensitivity, the later increases in strength of cortical modulation of limbic circuitry, and the delayed increases in neurotrophic factor–mediated neuronal growth and arborization.

CONCLUSION AND FUTURE DIRECTIONS

Unipolar major depressive disorder is a disorder of significant prevalence and morbidity. It is clearly a heritable disorder, and genetic influences appear to account for 30% to 50% of vulnerability to it. Despite this evident genetic role, the underlying pathophysiology is clearly heterogeneous. It appears that abnormalities in multiple gene pathways may lead to a similar endpoint. The interaction between neural development, genes, and environment render major depression one of the quintessential disorders of shared interaction between gene and environment. A combination of genetic predisposition and environmental stress appear to lead to similar alterations in the CNS systems that underlie affective responsiveness. Candidate gene studies to date suggest a potentially preeminent role of polymorphisms within the serotonin reuptake transporter. These polymorphisms may increase the risk of personality traits that increase vulnerability to depression following environmental insults. Animal models support a role for abnormalities of both the 5HT system and the CRF system in increasing risk of anxiety and depressive symptomatology. Through animal and human imaging, the neural circuitry involving dorsal and ventral prefrontal cortical interactions with limbic subcortical structures is being elucidated. Furthermore, a model of how brain stem monoamine neuronal circuitry may modulate these systems is being clarified.

The only linkage and association studies that have been published investigating genetic loci for major depression have used a relatively small number of candidate genes. Future hypothesis-neutral linkage studies performed with genomewide scans will allow for identification of novel genetic loci that underlie the genetic variance of depression. A better understanding of the quantitative traits that increase vulnerability to depression will be critical for progress in such linkage studies. More advanced imaging techniques are currently being undertaken that utilize specific positron emission tomography (PET) ligands in humans with depression. Additionally, advancing micro-PET applications in transgenic rodents will soon allow gene circuit interactions to be visualized. Thus, it will soon be possible to approach the genetic mechanisms of vulnerability to depression, the role of these genes in transgenic models, and the role of these genes in the neural circuits that underly affective response. These types of studies will further the understanding of depressive symptomatology and the pathophysiology of major depression, as well as enhance treatment options for these debilitating disorders.

REFERENCES

1. Kessler RC, Zhao S, Blazer DG, Swartz M: Prevalence, correlates, and course of minor depression and major depression in the National Comorbidity Survey. J Affect Disord 1997;45:19–30.

2. Murray CJ, Lopez AD: Global mortality, disability, and the contribution of risk factors: Global burden of disease study. Lancet 1997;349:1436–1442.

3. Kaplan H, Sadock B (eds): Comprehensive Textbook of Psychiatry, 6th ed. Baltimore, Williams and Wilkins, 1995.

4. Schatzberg A, Nemeroff C (eds): Textbook of Psychopharmacology. Washington, DC, American Psychiatric Press, 1998.

5. Ressler KJ, Nemeroff CB: Role of serotonergic and noradrenergic systems in the pathophysiology of depression and anxiety disorders. Depress Anxiety 2000;12:2–19.

6. Blier P: Crosstalk between the norepinephrine and serotonin systems and its role in the antidepressant response. J Psychiatry Neurosci 2001;26:3–10.

7. Delgado PL: Depression: The case for a monoamine deficiency. J Clin Psychiatry 2000;61:7–11.

8. Ladd CO, Huot RL, Thrivikraman KV, et al: Long-term behavioral and neuroendocrine adaptations to adverse early experience. Prog Brain Res 2000;122: 81–103.

9. Holsboer F: Stress, hypercortisolism and corticosteroid receptors in depression: Implications for therapy. J Affect Disord 2001;62:77–91.

10. Koob GF: Corticotropin-releasing factor, norepinephrine, and stress. Biol Psychiatry 1999;46: 1167–1180.

11. Davis M: The role of the amygdala in conditioned and unconditioned fear and anxiety. In Aggleton J (ed): The Amygdala: A Functional Analysis, 2nd ed. New York, Oxford University Press, 2000, pp 213–288.

12. Drevets WC: Neuroimaging studies of mood disorders. Biol Psychiatry 2000;48:813–829.

13. Mayberg HS, Liotti M, Brannan SK, et al: Reciprocal limbic-cortical function and negative mood: Converging PET findings in depression and normal sadness. Am J Psychiatry 1999;156:675–682.

14. Lang PJ, Davis M, Ohman A: Fear and anxiety: Animal models and human cognitive psychophysiology. J Affect Disord 2000;61:137–159.

15. LeDoux J: The Emotional Brain: The Mysterious Underpinnings of Emotional Life. New York, Simon and Schuster, 1996.

16. Robbins T, Everitt B: Central norepinephrine neurons and behavior. In Bloom F, Kupfer D (eds): Psychopharmacology: The Fourth Generation of Progress. New York, Raven Press, 1995, pp 363–372.

17. Jacobs B, Fornal C: Activity of serotonergic neurons in behaving animals. Neuropsychopharmacology 1999;21:9–15.

18. Duman R, Malberg J, Thome J: Neural plasticity to stress and antidepressant treatment. Biol Psychiatry 1999;46:1181–1191.

19. Gould E: Serotonin and hippocampal neurogenesis. Neuropsychopharmacology 1999;21:46–51.

20. Bremner J, Narayan M, Andersen E, et al: Hippocampal volume reduction in major depression. Am J Psychiatry 2000;157:115–118.

21. Muller M, Lucassen P, Tassouridis A: Neither major depression nor glucocorticoid treatment affects the cellular integrity of the human hippocampus. Eur J Neurosci 2001;14:1603–1612.

22. Sullivan PF, Neale MC, Kendler KS: Genetic epidemiology of major depression: Review and meta-analysis. Am J Psychiatry 2000;157:1552–1562.

23. Kendler KS: Twin studies of psychiatric illness: Current status and future directions. Arch Gen Psychiatry 1993;50:905–915.

24. Eley TC, Plomin R: Genetic analyses of emotionality. Curr Opin Neurobiol 1997;7:279–284.

25. Kendler, KS, Gardner CO, Prescott CA: Clinical characteristics of major depression that predict risk of depression in relatives. Arch Gen Psychiatry 1999;56:322–327.

26. Maher BS, Marazita ML, Zubenko WN, et al: Genetic segregation analysis of recurrent, early-onset major depression: Evidence for single major locus transmission. Am J Med Genet 2002;114:214–221.

27. Kendler KS: The diagnostic validity of melancholic major depression in a population-based sample of female twins. Arch Gen Psychiatry 1997;54:299–304.

28. Farmer A, Harris T, Redman K, et al: Cardiff depression study: A sib-pair study of life events and familiality in major depression. Br J Psychiatry 2000;176:150–155.

29. Briggs S, Assessing the five-factor model of personality description. J Personality 1992;60:253–293.

30. Petersen T, Bottanari K, Alpert J, et al: Use of the five-factor inventory in characterizing patients with major depressive disorder. Compr Psychiatry 2001;42:488–493.

31. Cloninger R: Temperament and personality. Curr Opin Neurobiol 1994;4:266–273.

32. Kagan J, Snidman N: Early childhood predictors of adult anxiety disorders. Biol Psychiatry 1999;46:1536–1541.

33. Kendler KS, Walters EE, Neale MC, et al: The structure of the genetic and environmental risk factors for six major psychiatric disorders in women: Phobia, generalized anxiety disorder, panic disorder, bulimia, major depression, and alcoholism. Arch Gen Psychiatry 1995;52:374–383.

34. Lesch KP, Bengel D, Heils A, et al: Association of anxiety-related traits with a polymorphism in the serotonin transporter gene regulatory region. Science 1996;274:1527–1531.

35. Gratacos M, Nadal M, Nartin-Santos R, et al: A polymorphic genomic duplication on human chromosome 15 is a susceptibility factor for panic and phobic disorders. Cell 2001;106:367–379.

36. Gingrich JA, Hen R: Dissecting the role of the serotonin system in neuropsychiatric disorders using knockout mice. Psychopharmacology (Berl) 2001;155:1–10.

37. Gross C, Zhuang X, Stark K, et al: Serotonin1A receptor acts during development to establish normal anxiety-like behaviour in the adult. Nature 2002;416:396–400.

38. Gass P, Reichardt HM, Strekalova T, et al: Mice with targeted mutations of glucocorticoid and mineralocorticoid receptors: Models for depression and anxiety? Physiol Behav 2001;73:811–825.

39. Bale, TL, Picetti R, Contarino A, et al: Mice deficient for both corticotropin-releasing factor receptor 1 (CRFR1) and CRFR2 have an impaired stress response and display sexually dichotomous anxiety-like behavior. J Neurosci 2002;22:193–199.

CHAPTER

72

Bipolar Disorder

Carol A. Mathews

Victor I. Reus

Nelson B. Freimer

Bipolar disorder (BP), also known as manic-depressive illness, is an episodic mood disorder characterized by recurrent episodes of mania and depression alternating with periods of normal mood. BP has an important societal impact, and if untreated, can be a significant cause of morbidity and mortality. Individuals with BP have high levels of impairment in social, marital, and occupational functioning, and up to 50% abuse alcohol or other substances.[1] In 1990, BP was the sixth leading cause of disability worldwide.[2] At least 25% of individuals with BP attempt suicide, and up to 15% will die from suicide.[3] In addition, untreated mood disorders can worsen the prognosis of medical disorders; individuals with mood disorders not only become medically ill more often than the general population, they are also more likely to die from cardiovascular disease.[4]

CLINICAL FEATURES AND DIAGNOSTIC EVALUATION

BP is characterized by cyclical changes in mood, cognition, and behavior.[5] Manic, depressed, and mixed states all occur in BP, and psychotic symptoms are also common. Mania, which is required for a diagnosis of BP, consists of an abnormally elevated mood, characterized by euphoria, expansiveness, and/or irritability. Other classic features include inflated self-esteem, grandiosity, low frustration tolerance, increased need for immediate gratification, decreased impulse control, an increase in provocative behaviors, and an increase in goal-directed activity (social, work-related, or creative). In addition, increased energy, decreased need for sleep, sexual or religious preoccupation, and racing thoughts are often noted.

Depression consists of a pervasive or consistently low mood in conjunction with neurovegetative and cognitive features such as difficulty sleeping, low energy, anhedonia, social isolation, and changes in appetite.[5] Depressive episodes in BP are similar to those in unipolar depression, although atypical depressions and psychotic depressions occur more often in BP than in unipolar depression. Depression is a characteristic part of BP, but it is not a necessary component; approximately 10% of patients with BP never have a clear depressive episode.[1]

Mixed states, also called dysphoric mania, are defined as the simultaneous co-occurrence of the full symptoms of mania and depression although a broader definition (some, but not necessarily all, symptoms of mania and depression co-occurring) is also common.[1] Depending on the definition used, between 15% and 70% of BP patients will experience a mixed episode, and about 50% of inpatient hospitalizations for BP are for mixed states.[1] It is unknown whether mixed states represent a more severe form of BP or whether they represent an etiologically distinct form of the illness.

BP is generally thought of as being part of a group of affective illnesses that also includes BP type II (BP II), cyclothymia, recurrent unipolar depressive disorder, and schizoaffective disorder, manic type (Fig. 72–1), although the etiologic relationship between these disorders is not known.[1] BP II is perhaps the most closely related clinically to BP I, and is characterized by episodes of depression and hypomania, a period of persistently elevated mood associated with a clear change in functioning, but not severe enough to cause marked impairment.[5] Hypomania can in certain cases even be associated with an improvement in functioning. Cyclothymia is defined

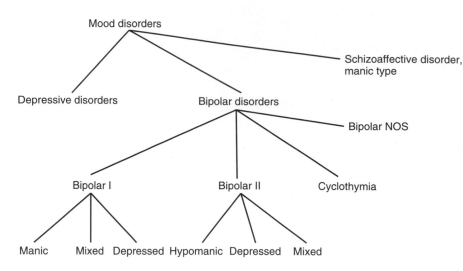

FIGURE 72–1. The spectrum of mood disorders. (From Goodwin FK, Jamison KR: Manic-Depressive Illness. Oxford University Press, New York, 1990.)

by episodes of hypomania that alternate with periods of depressive symptoms not meeting severity or duration criteria for a full depressive episode.[5] Schizoaffective disorder incorporates episodes of clear mania and/or depression, but also chronic psychotic symptoms that persist in the absence of mood symptoms.[5]

Like all psychiatric disorders, BP is an empirical diagnosis; there are no laboratory or imaging studies that can be used to make or confirm the diagnosis. Therefore, diagnostic schemas are required. The most commonly used diagnostic schema in clinical practice and in research is the *Diagnostic and Statistical Manual of Mental Disorders,* 4th edition (DSM IV). To make a

DSM IV diagnosis of BP, several conditions must be met. The fundamental requirement is a distinct period of abnormal mood (expansive, elevated, or irritable) along with at least three of the associated cognitive and behavioral symptoms discussed above. Because of the similarities between the mood spectrum disorders, objective evidence of impairment such as hospitalization or disruption of function is also required. Similarly, DSM IV criteria specifically exclude individuals whose symptoms can be attributed to the direct effects of a medication, substance, or medical condition. Table 72–1 shows DSM IV criteria for a manic episode, the fundamental component of BP.

TABLE 72–1. DSM IV Criteria for Manic Episode

A distinct period of abnormally and persistently elevated, expansive, or irritable mood, lasting at least 1 week (or any duration if hospitalization is necessary)

During the period of mood disturbance, three or more of the following symptoms persist (four if the mood is only irritable) and are present to a significant degree:

Inflated self-esteem or grandiosity

Decreased need for sleep (e.g., feels rested after only 3 hours of sleep)

More talkative than usual or pressure to keep talking

Flight of ideas or subjective experience that thoughts are racing

Distractibility (i.e., attention too easily drawn to unimportant or irrelevant external stimuli)

Increase in goal-directed activity (at work, at school, or sexually) or psychomotor agitation

Excessive involvement in pleasurable activities that have a high potential for painful consequences (e.g., engaging in unrestrained buying sprees, sexual indiscretions, or foolish business investments)

The symptoms do not meet criteria for a Mixed Episode

The mood disturbance is sufficiently severe to cause marked impairment in occupational functioning or in usual social activities or relationships with others, or to necessitate hospitalization to prevent harm to self or others, or there are psychotic features.

The symptoms are not due to the direct physiological effects of a substance (e.g., a drug of abuse, a medication or other treatment) or a general medical condition (e.g., hyperthyroidism).

Note: Manic-like episodes that are clearly caused by somatic antidepressant treatment (e.g., medication, electroconvulsive therapy, light therapy) should not count toward a diagnosis of Bipolar I disorder.
From Diagnostic and Statistical Manual of Mental Disorders, 4th Edition, American Psychiatric Press, Inc. Used with Permission.

EPIDEMIOLOGY

BP occurs worldwide and affects 1% to 2% of the population. The lifetime prevalence of BP I is between 0.5% and 1.5%, and the lifetime prevalence of BP II is estimated at 0.5%, although more recent genetic studies have suggested that it may actually be more common than BP I.[3] BP affects all races equally and occurs with equal frequency in men and women, although the age of onset (usually late teens or early twenties) is somewhat earlier for men than women.[1] Childhood onset, although rare, does occur, and it is often difficult to recognize because behavioral disturbances tend to predominate over emotional symptomatology.[3]

THERAPY

Treatment of BP is directed at mood stabilization and involves different categories of psychopharmacologic agents, depending on the phase of illness. Traditional mood stabilizers, which include lithium carbonate and a variety of anticonvulsant drugs, such as carbamazepine, valproate, and lamotrigine, appear to have prophylactic as well as acute antimanic efficacy; lithium and lamotrigine have demonstrable antidepressant benefit as well. Other anticonvulsants, such as gabapentin, topiramate, tiagabine, and zonisamide also may possess some efficacy in the treatment of BP, although well-controlled trials are still few.[6-7]

In addition to traditional mood stabilizers, atypical antipsychotic drugs have now been shown to possess specific antimanic effects, and possibly acute antidepressant efficacy as well.[6] Olanzapine is the only atypical antipsychotic approved by the U.S. Food and Drug Administration for acute mania, but clinical usage and a few preliminary studies indicate that olanzapine's therapeutic effects in acute mania are likely shared by clozapine, risperidone, quetiapine, and ziprasidone.[6] Benzodiazepines are frequently utilized in the acute management of mania. However, their effects seem limited to control of psychomotor agitation and sleep disturbance, and evidence for prophylactic efficacy is lacking.[8] Antidepressant drugs are judiciously used to treat depressive episodes in the course of BP, but may accelerate cycle frequency and precipitate progression into mania.[8]

The proven prophylactic effects of lithium and several of the anticonvulsant drugs have stimulated investigation of possible common mechanisms of action. One early hypothesis that proposed that lithium's beneficial effects are dependent on inositol depletion has recently received additional support.[9] Using a model system that focused on neuronal growth, an independent group of investigators has recently shown that valproate, carbamazepine, and lithium each act on the inositol trisphosphate (IP_3) pathway and that a novel oligopeptidase inhibitor can inhibit the action of all three drugs.[9] Other investigators, focusing on lithium's inhibition of PKC,

have begun to explore the possible efficacy of other PKC inhibitors, such as tamoxifen, in BP.[10] Inhibition of glycogen synthase kinase-3 (GSK-3) by lithium and valproate represents another target effect of exploration, as do similar drug effects on neurotrophic signaling cascades, such as the mitogen activated protein kinase (MAP) pathway.[10] Validation of the conclusion that the correlated biochemical effects are responsible for the mechanisms of action remains problematic. Ideally, such changes should occur at therapeutic concentrations of the drug, involve known pathways in the circuitry of emotional response, and be relevant to existing animal models of predictive drug efficacy.

The growing evidence that mood disorders may be associated with neuronal loss and atrophy, and that lithium, other mood stabilizers, and antidepressant drugs all have neuroprotective effects suggests that drug treatment may have optimal effects on the course of illness if instituted at an early stage and continued long term. At this point, however, clinical empirical data in support of this hypothesis are lacking.

PATHOLOGY

Postmortem studies of BP disorder have documented changes in brain volume and neuronal or glial cell count, as well as changes in neuropeptide level and function. A reduction of glial cell number and density has been reported in patients with BP and major depressive disorder (MDD), as has a change in signal activity, particularly in the prefrontal cortex.[11] An increase in the number of large pigmented neurons in the locus caeruleus has also been observed.[11]

An increased number of vasopressin, oxytocin, and corticotropin releasing hormone expressing neurons have been found in the paraventricular nucleus of the hypothalamus in brains of patients with BP and MDD, and a decrease in neuropeptide Y mRNA levels in the prefrontal cortex in individuals with BP.[11] Increased signal transduction via adenyl cyclase activity and decreased inositol levels were also noted in the prefrontal cortex of BP brains.[11] Together, these findings suggest that abnormalities in signal transduction pathways, particularly in the prefrontal cortex, may be involved in the pathophysiology of BP.

Post-mortem studies of BP must, however, be interpreted with caution. Comparison of BP tissue to control tissue is confounded by the effects of acute and chronic medication treatment, and it is unclear which changes represent state or trait phenomena (i.e., whether enduring neuroanatomical changes are to be expected in a cyclical disorder with periods of normality or remission). Owing to these difficulties and the relative scarcity of appropriate brain tissue, advances in technology have served to shift the focus away from neuropathology toward structural and functional neuroimaging, which can incorporate a significantly greater number of subjects and can be done at all phases of illness, allowing examination of state and trait changes.

NEUROIMAGING

Structural neuroimaging studies, which include computed tomography (CT), magnetic resonance imaging (MRI), and magnetic resonance spectroscopy (MRS), have focused primarily on volumetric or area measures of particular brain structures. The most replicated finding in CT and MRI studies has been of a greater number of signal hyperintensities in white matter regions of BP subjects compared with healthy age-matched controls and with other psychiatric comparison groups. Although these hyperintensities occur more commonly in frontal or parietal/frontal areas, there is no consistent localization. Prefrontal cortical areas of bipolar patients are smaller in volume compared to healthy subjects, while subcortical regions, specifically the amygdala and the striatum/basal ganglia, show evidence of enlargement.[12] Cerebellar vermal atrophy and lateral ventriculomegaly have also been reported in BP subjects, although the evidence for this is more equivocal.[12]

Functional neuroimaging studies (positron emission tomography or PET, single-photon emission computed tomography or SPECT, and, more recently, functional magnetic resonance imaging or fMRI) have measured both changes in brain metabolism and changes in blood flow. In general, studies of glucose metabolism suggest that changes related to affective state occur primarily in the frontal cortical regions, where metabolism decreases during depression and normalizes or increases during mania.[12] These findings are not specific to BP, however, and may be more indicative of state-related changes than they are illness-specific. Cerebral blood flow studies show essentially the same patterns.[12] During depression, frontal and temporal cortical regions show decreased blood flow, especially in the left hemisphere.[12] Studies of blood flow during mania are more inconsistent. Functional changes in glucose and phospholipid metabolism in the prefrontal cortex and the subcortical regions, specifically in the amygdala and the striatum/basal ganglia, appear to be state rather than trait-related and more prominent in depression than in mania. Dopamine-binding studies suggest that there may also be lower frontal dopamine D_1-receptor binding in bipolar patients, as well as higher caudate dopamine D_2-receptor density in bipolar patients with psychosis.[12]

Overall, neuroimaging studies indicate abnormalities in the cortical and subcortical regions of the brains of bipolar patients, particularly in the prefrontal cortex. White matter atrophy or underdevelopment may also be present, leading to ventriculomegaly. Integration of these findings suggests dysfunction in one or more of the frontal-subcortical pathways, particularly in the orbitofrontal-subcortical circuit (thought to modulate empathic and socially-appropriate behaviors). Loss of activity in these pathways may lead to a loss of modulatory input to the prefrontal cortex, causing hypo- or hyperactivated states.[12]

BIOCHEMISTRY

Most of what is known about the biochemistry and cellular neurobiology of BP comes from our understanding of the mechanism of action of effective treatments for BP, in particular, the use of lithium and the anticonvulsants. As with the neuroimaging studies, understanding the pathophysiology of BP is complicated by the fact that it is a cyclical disorder, and that the biochemical underpinnings for the states of mania and depression may be very different than those for BP itself. Several biochemical pathways have been examined or implicated in BP, including the monoaminergic system, cellular signaling pathways involving protein kinase C, and systems involving adenylate cyclase.

Studies of the biogenic amines originated with the observation that antidepressants (which block monoamine reuptake) can trigger manias, shorten cycle length in individuals with BP, or worsen long-term outcome of BP.[13] In addition, receptors for the biogenic amines are concentrated in the limbic system, an anatomic region implicated in the regulation of sleep, appetite, arousal, and sexual function.[13] Alterations in the noradrenergic, dopaminergic, serotonergic, and cholinergic systems have been reported in patients with BP,[13] but likely represent secondary rather than primary pathophysiologic effects.

Accordingly, signal transduction pathways, which can affect the functional balance between multiple neurotransmitter systems, have been examined intensively. In particular, long-term changes in excitability in the protein kinase C (PKC) and the adenylyl cyclase (AC) systems have been hypothesized to regulate mood cycling in BP disorder.[13,14]

Lithium, an effective mood stabilizer, has been shown to exert complex effects on the activity of adenylyl cyclase (AC), primarily increasing basal AC activity and attenuating receptor-mediated responses to AC (Fig. 72–2).[13–17] In vitro, lithium administration inhibits the stimulation of AC by directly inhibiting the catalytic subunit. In acute treatment, Mg^{2+} can reverse these effects, suggesting that lithium directly competes with magnesium for binding. In chronic treatment, lithium increases basal AC levels and attenuates the β-adrenergic mediated effects. Mg^{2+} does not reverse the chronic effects of lithium.[13] Lithium has also been shown to act on the receptor-mediated second messenger system by affecting G protein function directly. Lithium attenuates the inhibitory G protein (G_i) by stabilizing it in its inactive conformation, but does not have any direct effect on G protein levels.[13] This removal of the inhibition by G_i may result in the elevations in basal AC levels discussed above

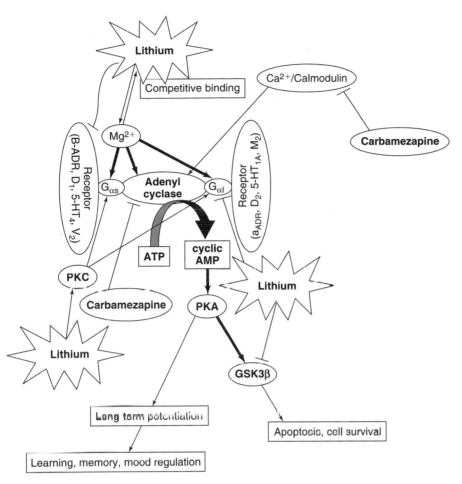

FIGURE 72–2. The adenylyl cyclase system. (Courtesy of Angela Eastvold.)

and cause a relative change in the equilibrium of the active and inactive protein conformations, stabilizing the system and preventing the development of supersensitive adrenergic, dopaminergic, or serotonergic receptors.[10] Carbamazepine, an anticonvulsant that has proven efficacy in BP, also causes an overall "dampening" of the AC system, in this case acting directly on AC to decrease cyclic AMP as well.[13]

Lithium, at therapeutic levels, also exerts effects on the PKC signaling cascade (Fig. 72–3). As with the AC system, acute and chronic lithium exposure each produces responses in different PKC isoenzymes. Acute lithium exposure alters several PKC-mediated responses, and chronic lithium exposure causes a decrease in phorbol ester mediated responses, and a subsequent downregulation of specific PKC isoenzymes.[10] An acidic protein, myristoylated alanine-rich C kinase substrate (MARCKS), which has been implicated in regulating long-term neuroplastic events, is the primary substrate for PKC.[13] Chronic lithium administration dramatically reduces MARCKS expression in the hippocampus, an effect that is not immediately reversed upon lithium discontinuation.[10,13] The action of lithium on MARCKS is dependent upon both the inositol concentration and the level of receptor-mediated activation of PI hydrolysis in the hippocampus. Valproic acid, another anticonvulsant that is effective in treating mania, produces similar effects on the PKC isozymes and on expression of MARCKS in the hippocampus, suggesting that this system is indeed important in BP.[13] PKC may also be involved in phosphorylating the G proteins of the AC system.[13]

In addition to pharmacologic data, more direct evidence of involvement of signaling pathways in BP exists. BP patients have higher levels of $G\alpha_s$ in the frontal, temporal, and occipital cortices, as well as evidence of increased $G\alpha_s$ activity. In addition, increased PKC activity and isozyme levels have been reported in the brains of BP subjects.[17] Both antidepressants and lithium also affect other cell-signaling pathways that are involved in regulating cell survival and cell death, including cAMP-responsive element-binding protein (CREB), brain-derived neurotrophic growth factor (BDNF), and the bcl-2 and mitogen-activated protein (MAP) kinases.[10] Lithium increases levels of bcl 2, a cytoprotective protein, in human neuronal cells, and inhibits the activity of glycogen synthase kinase 3β (GSK 3β), which has a role in regulating neuronal survival via numerous transcription factors, including CREB.[10] GSK 3β in turn is regulated by PKC. Chronic lithium treatment has also been shown to increase total gray matter content in the human brain, a possible consequence of its neuroprotective effects.

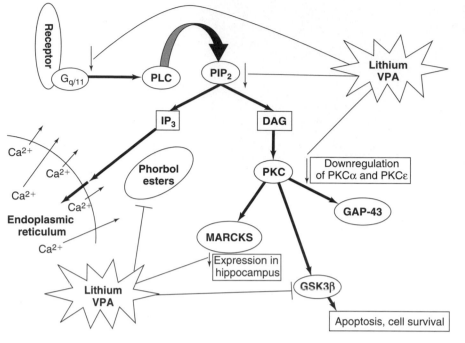

FIGURE 72–3. The protein kinase C system. (Courtesy of Angela Eastvold.)

GENETIC APPROACHES TO THE STUDY OF COMPLEX DISORDERS

Genetic mapping studies have been highly successful in elucidating the molecular basis of disorders with simple mendelian inheritance, but have so far contributed relatively little new knowledge about traits that are etiologically complex. Unfortunately, such complexity characterizes most neuropsychiatric disorders, including BP. Mapping a complex disorder requires addressing factors such as incomplete penetrance (expression of the phenotype in only some of the individuals carrying the disease genotype), the presence of phenocopies (forms of the disease that are not caused by genetic factors), locus heterogeneity (different genes causing the same disease in different families or populations), polygenic inheritance (multiple genes acting together to cause disease), or multifactorial inheritance (gene and environment interacting to cause a trait or disease). Several complementary strategies may mitigate the effect of various sources of complexity on genetic mapping. These strategies include the use of information from multiple types of genetic epidemiologic studies, careful delineation of phenotypes for genetic investigation, and choosing an advantageous study population.

EPIDEMIOLOGIC APPROACHES

Genetic investigations are dependent on demonstration that the disorder in question is familial, and on knowledge of the degree of genetic contribution and the mode of inheritance. These steps are undertaken using epidemiologic approaches such as twin studies, relative risk determinations, and segregation analyses.

Twin studies compare the concordance rates of a disorder in monozygotic and dizygotic twins. For a disorder that is strictly determined by genetic factors, the concordance rate should be 100% in monozygotic twin pairs and 25% or 50% in dizygotic twin pairs, depending on whether the disease is recessive or dominant, respectively. For a disorder in which genetic factors are important but not exclusive, the concordance rates should be greater for monozygotic than for dizygotic twins, assuming that the influence of environment is the same for both types of twin pairs; when genetic factors do not play a role, the concordance rates should not differ between the twin pairs.[15]

Relative risk is defined as the rate of occurrence of a trait for the relatives of an affected individual divided by the rate of occurrence for the general population.[15] A relative risk of >1 suggests a genetic etiology, and the magnitude of the measure gives an estimate of the genetic contribution to the disease. Relative risks can be calculated for sibling pairs, parent-offspring pairs, and various other types of family relationships. Likely mode of transmission can be determined by comparing the degree of relative risk for each type of relationship.

Segregation analysis compares the observed number of individuals with a particular trait to the expected number within a given family, assuming a particular mode of inheritance, and then compares the likelihood of observing these data under a specified genetic model to the likelihood of observing the data under other genetic models. Segregation analyses are useful for establishing whether there is a genetic component to the disorder in question, and for estimating the likely mode of inheritance within a particular family or group of families.[15]

Despite the fact that little is known about the pathophysiology of BP, evidence for a genetic component is strong. The relative risk of BP for first-degree relatives of individuals with BP I is seven times that of the general population, and the risk of BP II is also increased. Twin studies have indicated that the concordance rate for BP among monozygotic twins is between 60% and 90%, while the concordance rate among dizygotic twins is closer to that for first-degree relatives (around 8%). Finally, the biologic relatives of adopted individuals with BP are at greater risk for BP than are the adoptive relatives.[3,16]

Although the genetic epidemiology studies strongly support a genetic contribution to BP, the mode of transmission is less clear. It is currently believed that BP is genetically heterogeneous, with multiple genes playing at least some role in its development. What role they play and how they interact with one another has yet to be elucidated, however. Some, but not all, segregation analyses have provided support for a locus of major effect. Other studies have suggested that several genes acting in a multiplicative way may be a more realistic model. In addition, phenomena such as anticipation (where successive generations of affected individuals suffer from an earlier onset or a more severe form of the disorder because of instability in the genetic mutation) and differential maternal and paternal inheritance have also been hypothesized. Anticipation is seen in other neuropsychiatric disorders such as Huntington's disease and fragile X syndrome, and in these disorders is secondary to a trinucleotide repeat sequence that expands in successive generations.[16]

Once genetic epidemiology has provided as much information as possible about the genetic basis of a trait and the phenotype has been defined, the next step is to search for specific sequence variants that contribute to susceptibility to the disorder, using candidate gene studies or genome screens. A candidate gene is one whose location and protein product are known, and that is hypothesized to play a role in the pathophysiology of the disorder, although sometimes genes with unknown functions that are located in a particular chromosomal region of interest are also considered via this approach. Because the pathophysiology of most neuropsychiatric disorders is not well-understood, candidate genes have traditionally been derived from pharmacologic response data or from cytogenetic data (including translocations and deletions) indicating a candidate region. A number of candidate genes for BP have been examined, principally involving serotonergic, dopaminergic, and adrenergic receptor, transporter, and enzymatic or metabolic genes.

Candidate gene studies have principally been based on association analyses. Whereas linkage studies attempt to find cosegregation of a genetic marker and a disease gene within a family or families, association studies examine whether a particular allele occurs more frequently in affected individuals within a population. Association studies of candidate genes look for an association between a specific variant allele within or near a gene of interest and the disease, with the assumption that the variant is actually the mutation that is causing the disease.

Of the 20 or more genes that have been examined, none have provided strong evidence for a role in BP susceptibility.[16] The most widely studied has been the serotonin transporter gene (chromosome 17q). The promoter region of the serotonin transporter gene has an insertion/deletion polymorphism that shows differential gene expression, leading to speculation that it may be a functional polymorphism for BP. Although positive associations have been reported, numerous negative studies also exist.[16] These mixed results may mean that the serotonin transporter gene is a risk factor for some individuals with BP, and that the variation between studies is due to genetic heterogeneity among affected individuals. However, it is more likely that these findings are false positives. Most of the positive findings have occurred in case-control studies, which are subject to high false-positive rates due to underlying differences in allele frequency between cases and controls for reasons unrelated to disease status. Family-based studies, which control for the problems of differential allele frequencies by using parental chromosomes as controls, have been negative or equivocal for linkage to the serotonin transporter.[16]

Similar problems exist for all other candidate genes as well, with both positive and negative studies reported. Because of the problems in interpreting such results, several investigators have turned to meta-analysis as a way to assess the association data for a particular candidate gene in its entirety. This approach has the advantage of increased power by combining a number of small studies, although problems leading to false positive results in the original studies may be compounded in a meta-analysis. Meta-analyses have been done for multiple candidate genes, including the 5-HTT gene, the monoamine oxidase A (MAOA) gene, the dopamine D3 receptor gene (DRD3), and the tyrosine hydroxylase gene.[19-22] Neither the DRD3 gene nor the tyrosine hydroxylase gene showed any evidence of association with BP. The meta-analyses for the MAOA gene and the 5-HTT gene, each of which examined two separate polymorphisms within the gene or in the promoter region, gave positive results for one polymorphism but not the other ($p = 0.02$ for MAOA, $p = 0.049$ for 5-HTT). The significance of these results is unclear, as the p values, although nominally significant, are no longer statistically significant when corrected for multiple testing. In addition, these studies did not report tests for homogeneity across studies, a crucial factor in the interpretation of meta-analyses. Also, in the case of the MAOA gene, the association studies were done with silent polymorphisms; so far no functional variants in the MAOA gene have been identified that are associated with BP.

The other approach to identifying BP susceptibility loci is through a search for linkage.

Several strategies have been developed to map disease genes through linkage analysis, all based on identifying genetic marker alleles that are shared by affected individuals identical by descent (IBD), i.e., inherited from a common ancestor along with a linked disease gene. Alleles or haplotypes that are shared IBD must be differentiated from those that are shared identical by state (IBS). Alleles that are shared IBS, rather than IBD, are shared by affected individuals for a variety of other reasons, such as the same mutation in an allele occurring twice in a population. Dense, closely spaced marker maps are critical for determining whether an allele is shared IBD or IBS. Markers closely surrounding an allele shared IBD will also be shared IBD, whereas markers closely surrounding an allele shared IBS will not show sharing among affected individuals.[16]

Searching for areas of linkage to the disorder of interest has traditionally been done using pedigree (lod score) analysis. A pedigree analysis consists of scanning the genome or a portion of the genome in one or more affected pedigrees, calculating a lod score at each marker position, and identifying the chromosomal regions that show a significant deviation from what would be expected under the conditions of independent assortment (chance). Pedigree analysis is best done in families of three or four generations, where affected individuals are separated by two to six meiotic steps. For simple mendelian disorders where the mode of inheritance is known, a lod score of 3 has been considered to be significant evidence for linkage.[17] In complex disorders in which the mode of inheritance is unknown (and it is common practice to use hundreds of genetic markers and multiple genetic models), one can expect to find false positives (regions that are significant at $p < 0.05$, corresponding to a lod score of >1), by chance alone, approximately 24 times (once per chromosome). The frequent use of multiple markers and multiple genetic models, as well as uncertainties in estimates of penetrance level and allele frequencies for many disorders, increases the likelihood of a false-positive result, and creates a problem as to what represents acceptable evidence for linkage. In instances in which multiple genetic markers are tested, a lod score of 3.4 has been suggested as sufficient evidence for linkage. When multiple genetic models are used, the formula $3 + \log(t)$, where t is the number of tests performed, has been suggested. Under these parameters, a lod score of 3.4 or higher would be required to provide significant evidence of linkage if more than one model is used, and a lod score of 4 would be required if ten models are used.[17] Many investigators argue that these criteria are in fact too stringent, as they assume that each model is independent of the others, which is not the case in mapping studies. Some investigators have argued that for complex traits, where genetic heterogeneity is likely to be prominent, a lod score of >1 is significant. For this reason, a classification system for reporting linkage based on dense genome scans has been proposed. This system suggests four levels of statistical significance for evaluating the results of a genome screen. These include suggestive evidence ($p = 0.001$), significant linkage ($p = 0.0001$), highly significant linkage ($p = 0.00002$), and confirmed linkage (significant linkage from one or more initial studies that has subsequently been confirmed in a follow-up or additional sample).[17]

Although the criteria listed above suggest that replication of the finding in a separate sample is necessary to confirm linkage, it is important to note that failure to replicate a linkage finding in another population does not necessarily mean that there is no linkage at that locus. Failure to replicate the finding may be due to genetic heterogeneity, diagnostic differences between the study populations, or statistical fluctuation. In such cases, extension studies in the original population or a meta-analysis of all studies may help to confirm or refute the initial finding.

NONPARAMETRIC APPROACHES

In addition to traditional parametric approaches such as the pedigree method, multiple nonparametric approaches have been developed to address the problem of searching for linkage in the presence of genetic heterogeneity, incomplete penetrance, and unknown modes of transmission. These approaches do not require the specification of a model or the attendant parameters such as allele frequencies, mutation and recombination rates, etc. They are less powerful in their ability to detect linkage than a correctly specified linkage model, but are often more robust in the face of genetic complexity. Another advantage of nonparametric methods is that lod score analysis of a small number of large families can be very sensitive to small changes in a few data points (for example, a change from unaffected status to affected status), whereas nonparametric analyses (usually done on a large number of small families) tend to normal distributions and are thus less affected by such changes. The most commonly used nonparametric methods are based on sib pair analysis. Sib pair analysis examines the frequency with which sib pairs concordant for a trait share a particular region of the genome compared with the frequency that is expected under random segregation. The analysis is based on the concept that siblings share approximately 50% of their genomes IBD. In this method, siblings are genotyped, and population frequencies and parental genotypes are used to estimate the proportion of genes shared IBD at each site for each sib pair. If a group of unrelated sib pairs with a certain trait shares a particular area of the genome significantly more than 50% of the time (the proportion of sharing expected under conditions of random segregation), that area of the genome is considered likely to be linked to the trait in question. Those pairs concordant (or discordant) for each genetic locus can then be compared via statistical tests. Although it is possible to do sib pair analyses using both affected and unaffected siblings, usually only affected-affected sib pairs are evaluated because little information is gained by including unaffected sib pairs and because excluding these individuals alleviates the problem of incomplete penetrance.[15]

Linkage searches can be done either through investigation of selected candidate regions or through a whole genome screen. This approach assumes that there are no known specific areas of interest within the genome and involves screening the entire genome with evenly spaced markers in an attempt to find an area or areas of linkage. Genome screens are becoming increasingly more common for genetic studies of psychiatric disorders, because of limited success with the candidate gene method, as well as a relative lack of candidate areas.

The earliest genetic studies of BP used information about the clinical presentation of the disorder to identify likely areas of interest in the genome. In one of the first to report positive linkage findings, investigators noted that in several families BP and other affective disorders appeared to be inherited in an X-linked fashion, and, further, that they appeared to co-segregate with colorblindness and G6PD deficiency, which map to the X chromosome. Initial linkage studies of the X chromosome gave lod scores between 4 and 9.[16] Early studies of chromosome 11 were similar to those for the X chromosome. These studies, which were done in large Amish pedigrees heavily loaded for BP, and based on previous suggestions of linkage to this region, reported lod scores of around 4.[16] Not surprisingly, these findings generated a great deal of interest. However, replication studies in other populations failed to produce positive results for either the X chromosome or for chromosome 11, and extension and reanalysis of the original data also failed to support the findings. The most likely explanation for this is that the initial linkage studies on the X chromosome used variations in phenotype (colorblindness and G6PD deficiency) as markers rather than DNA polymorphisms. Such markers are less informative, and recombinations are frequently missed. Also, errors in G6PD status of some individuals were identified, and some previously unaffected individuals later developed BP. These changes in phenotype also affected the linkage results.[16] For chromosome 11, the most significant change between the original study and the follow up was a change in affection status (from unaffected to affected) in two members of the original pedigree. These two individuals did not share the alleles of interest in the original two markers, and this single change lowered the lod scores to below 2. Attempts to extend the study by adding a new branch of the pedigree also showed no significant evidence for linkage.[16]

The failure to replicate and/or extend these early linkage findings, which initially appeared to be so promising, illustrates the sensitivity of genetic findings of complex traits to phenotype definition, and the importance of considering the entire genome in linkage studies. Genomewide screens have now become the approach of choice for BP, given the relative lack of information about pathophysiology, and the lack of success with candidate gene approaches. These studies have an important advantage in that they do not require a priori knowledge of the biologic underpinnings of BP.

Most of the genome screens done to date for BP support the idea that the disorder is heterogeneous, and suggest that many, if not all, genes for BP confer a modest susceptibility risk rather than being genes of major effect. So far, there are at least four chromosomal areas that show some evidence for linkage—chromosomes 18, 4p, 21q, and 12q, as well as a number of other areas that may also play a role.

Chromosome 18 Pericentromeric

The evidence that there is at least one susceptibility gene for BP on chromosome 18 is mounting, although the precise location remains unclear, and there may in fact be more than one important region. The first report of linkage to chromosome 18 came from a partial genome screen, which identified a region of interest near the centromere. Because this was a linkage analysis using pedigree data, model specification was required, and the results were analyzed using both recessive and dominant models. Of the positive lod scores reported, no clear pattern was observed; some markers were positive under a recessive model in some families, some were positive under a dominant model, and some were positive under both models. Nonparametric tests, which do not require a mode of inheritance to be specified, provided somewhat stronger evidence for linkage, but again, there were no clear patterns. Additional genotyping in the area of interest supported the linkage finding and subsequently narrowed the region to about 11 to 15 Mb from the p telomere, with a maximum lod score of 2.32.[16]

Attempts to replicate this finding in other populations have been mixed. Although at least two groups have found no evidence for linkage to the pericentromeric region of chromosome 18 in their samples, one group found evidence to support linkage to this region. Hypothesizing that a parent-of-origin effect might play a role in the inheritance of BP, they divided their sample into those families in which the disorder appeared to be inherited from the paternal side and those in which the disorder appeared to be inherited from the maternal side, and analyzed these groups both together and separately. Using nonparametric methods, they found evidence for excess allele sharing in several markers in the pericentromeric area of chromosome 18 (18p11) using a broad diagnostic category, which included BP I and II and recurrent major depression. Since this finding, two other groups have also reported evidence of a parent-of-origin effect in this area of chromosome 18.[16]

18q and 18p

The same group that initially reported support for a parent-of-origin effect near the centromere also analyzed markers all along chromosome 18 in their families, and found excess allele sharing in the area of 18q as well. Although the supporting evidence for linkage in the 18p area previously described was obtained under a broad diagnostic category, the evidence for linkage in the 18q region was found under a relatively narrow diagnostic category, which included only BP I and BP II disorder. The results for 18q were somewhat strengthened when the pedigrees were divided into paternal and maternal samples. Two point lod scores in the area of 18q were between 2.6 and 3.5 in the paternal pedigrees, the peak multipoint lod score in this area was 3.11, and there was evidence of excess allele sharing for several markers in the area. When this group attempted to replicate their findings in a new sample of BP pedigrees using the same diagnostic criteria as the original study, they found evidence for excess allele sharing among affected sib pairs in two markers in the region of interest on 18q (18q21), but little evidence for linkage on 18p. Support for the parent-of-origin effect was also reduced in this new sample. Analysis of these BP families combined with the original study set strengthened the evidence for linkage in this region, although most of the linkage was shown to come from allele sharing between sibling pairs with BP II and not from those with BP I.[16]

Another genome screen was conducted for BP I only, in two large Costa Rican pedigrees, and also gave evidence for linkage on 18q, although in a region somewhat below the area previously reported, as well as in an area on 18p. When the 18q region was further examined, shared haplotypes were found in most affected individuals; 23 of the 26 affected individuals in the two families shared some portion of a core haplotype in this area.

Because of the continued suggestion of one or more susceptibility loci located on chromosome 18, other groups have also examined this area for evidence of linkage. Several of these groups have found some evidence for linkage, although weak, at or near 18q23, as well as near 18q12. In an attempt to consolidate the various results, a meta-analysis of some of the chromosome 18 linkage data was conducted.[23] This study did not include data from all of the chromosome 18 studies, but did include approximately 700 families, and attempted to standardize the data for pooling and comparison. This study found evidence of excess allele sharing at the tip of 18p, as well as in the pericentromeric region of 18 when a broad phenotype was used. There was less evidence for association on the long arm of chromosome 18 from this study, although there were some isolated markers that showed evidence of excess sharing under one model or another. Results of the meta-analysis under a narrow phenotypic model were not reported.

The combined evidence of these studies, although somewhat contradictory and confusing, points to at least two different susceptibility loci on chromosome 18, one on 18p and one on 18q. These loci, if they represent true areas of linkage, are different in intriguing ways. The 18p finding is perhaps the most difficult to explain, as for most studies a single marker explains the majority of the positive findings, and each study points to a different marker. In addition, the evidence for a locus in this area appears to be strongest in individual families; the evidence actually diminishes when families are combined; and it is strongest under a broad phenotype definition that includes not only BP but also major depression. This suggests that this area may harbor a susceptibility locus for affective disorder in general rather than for BP specifically.

In contrast, the 18q finding extends over several markers, and is robust to the addition of new families. Although different markers were tested in the different studies, they all lie within the area of the larger haplotype noted in the Costa Rican families. Finally, this finding is dependent on a narrow phenotypic definition—the evidence weakens or disappears when the phenotype is expanded to include major depression, suggesting that this locus may be more specific for BP.

Chromosome 4p

Another possible susceptibility locus for BP is on chromosome 4, suggested from a genome screen of 12 Scottish families with affected individuals diagnosed as BP I and BP II. One of these families showed a peak multipoint lod score of 4.8 under an autosomal dominant model. Haplotype analysis identified seven markers that were shared by all 11 affected individuals and by 14 of 16 of those affected with recurrent major depression.[16] When the other 11 families were added, the maximum lod score dropped to between 2.9 and 3.3. There was, however, evidence for locus heterogeneity in these families, with only approximately 30% to 35% of the families likely to be linked to this locus. Under the assumption of genetic heterogeneity, the maximum lod score for the combined families increased to 4.1.

At least two other studies have also provided supporting evidence of a potential susceptibility locus at 4p. A lod score of 2 was found at the original marker of interest in a subsequent study of Danish families, and a study of German families showed evidence of allele sharing at the same marker. The group that performed the original study has now reportedly narrowed the area of interest on chromosome 4p to approximately 9 cM using haplotype analysis.[16]

Chromosome 21

The initial report of linkage on chromosome 21 came from a partial genome screen of 47 multigenerational BP families completed in 1994. This study initially gave high lod scores for ten markers on 21q22.3 in one family (the maximum lod score was 3.41) under an autosomal dominant model, as well as significant results in this region using an affected-pedigree-member approach. A recent replication study by the same group in an additional 40 families reported a peak heterogeneity lod score of 3.35, with 50% of the families studied contributing to the linkage results. However, other studies examining this region have been equivocal. Although there have been two reports of excess allele sharing among individuals with BP, there have also been studies that have found no evidence for linkage to BP in this region.[16] Interpretation of the linkage results on chromosome 21q is therefore difficult.

Other Regions of Interest

Interest in the X chromosome as a potential region of linkage for BP continues, despite the revision of findings of the early studies. At least two groups have reported linkage to Xq24-27, with one group reporting a lod score of 3.9 in one BP family. However, these reports have not been replicated, and X-linked inheritance does not appear to be a major mode of transmission in the majority of bipolar families.[16]

At least one group has also reported linkage to chromosome 22q11-3 (lod scores of between 2 and 3.5).[16] This region may be of particular interest because it has also been linked to schizophrenia, and has been reported to harbor genes that are induced in microarray studies of methamphetamine-treated rats, which have been used as a model of psychosis. Although the linkage findings to BP have not been replicated, it is possible that 22q11 may harbor a gene that confers risk for psychosis, rather than being specific for BP.

Results of a complete genome screen in a kindred of old-order Amish that subsumed the pedigrees from the earlier studies also showed promising potential areas of linkage, including the areas of 6pter-p24, 13q13, and 15q11-qter.[16] One marker in each area gave p values of 0.001 or less in these families using nonparametric methods. Using lod score analysis, however, none of the markers had a lod score greater than 3, and none of the flanking markers were strongly positive. In addition, there was no evidence of shared haplotypes. Although it is possible, and perhaps very likely, that these findings represent false positives, these areas should be more closely examined using additional markers and additional families in order to further explore the possibility that they contain susceptibility loci.

GENOME-WIDE ASSOCIATION STUDIES

Candidate gene studies focused on a few genes are unlikely to succeed in disorders where the pathophysiology is incompletely understood, as is the case with neuropsychiatric disorders. However, it may soon be possible to conduct genomewide candidate gene studies; there will be sequence variants identified in virtually all brain-expressed genes, and these variants can be tested for association to BP. There is also increasing interest in applying association methods to genomewide screens based on genotyping of densely spaced sequence variants. These variants would not have to be candidate alleles themselves, but would be expected to be in close proximity to candidate alleles. They would be detected based on detection of linkage disequilibrium (LD) with disease susceptibility alleles; that is, these alleles will be inherited IBD by affected individuals and therefore will be presenting such individuals more frequently than expected by random segregation.[16] LD studies have traditionally been used to complement traditional pedigree analyses, either to further narrow a region of interest that has already been identified or to confirm a previous finding. However, these methods are now being used for whole genome screens, particularly for diseases in which traditional linkage studies have been unsuccessful. These studies have one great advantage over a traditional pedigree analysis. Because affected individuals are chosen from an entire population rather than from one or a few pedigrees, only the population size and the frequency of the disease limit the number of potential subjects. For disorders in which genetic heterogeneity or incomplete penetrance are likely to be factors, maximizing the number of affected individuals that can be included in the analysis is extremely important. In addition, expanding the potential sample pool allows investigators to more rigidly define the disease phenotype, thereby increasing the likelihood that the phenotype under investigation is due to a major gene effect.

THE USE OF ISOLATED POPULATIONS

Genomewide LD studies are not yet feasible in heterogeneous populations; affected individuals in such populations are so distantly related to one another that the regions of LD around disease susceptibility variants is very small and cannot be detected using currently available polymorphic markers. However, LD mapping may currently be feasible in some population isolates that have been recently founded. In such isolates, the population descends from a small number of original founders.[18] Over time, recombination across the generations will gradually diminish the length of the chromosomal regions that are shared IBD, and most individuals will share very little of the genome with one another. However, individuals who share a common trait or disease in such a population may have inherited the same susceptibility allele and are therefore more likely than random individuals in the population to share marker alleles that are in LD with the susceptibility allele. In recently founded isolates, these affected individuals may be less than 20 generations removed from their common ancestors, and therefore may demonstrate LD for sizable genomic segments around disease susceptibility genes. Available markers are sufficiently densely spaced to detect such LD in a genomewide screen.

LD based genome screening studies of BP have already been initiated using samples from the recently founded isolate of the Central Valley of Costa Rica. These studies have used particularly narrow diagnostic classifications (BP I with at least two psychiatric hospitalizations). The most interesting localization to emerge so far from these studies is on 8p12-21.[24] As with the region on 22q11, this region has also been identified as a potential area of linkage in schizophrenia, and may represent a more general susceptibility locus for psychotic disorders.

ANIMAL MODELS

Although animal models have historically been used to further our understanding of the etiology and pathophysiology of complex disorders, designing an appropriate animal model for BP is complicated by the fact that the majority of symptoms are changes in emotional or cognitive state that are difficult to represent in model systems. For this reason, most animal models of mania have focused on easily quantifiable behavioral traits that are often associated with the condition, primarily hyperactivity and arousal.[1] One way of inducing hyperactivity is via administration of amphetamine, which acts as a dopamine agonist and increases locomotion and aggression, and causes stereotyped behaviors such as sniffing and an increased startle response in rats. Other methods have included morphine administration, serotonin depletion using parachlorophenylalanine, and brain lesions in various anatomical structures, including the hippocampus, frontal cortex, globus pallidus, ventral tegmentum, and a number of others.[1] The drug-induced hyperactivity states have been shown to respond to treatment with lithium, neuroleptics, or cholinergic agonists.[1] Taken together, these models in general indicate that activation of the dopaminergic and serotonergic systems results in an increase in locomotor activity and arousal, both fundamental characteristics of mania. All of these models produce chronic changes rather than cyclical changes, however, making their relevance to BP somewhat limited.

Other animal models that have been proposed for BP focus more on the cyclic nature of the disorder. These include changes in circadian rhythm, including the rhythms of activity and rest that occur in all mammals, as well as the cyclical rhythm of rest and hyperactivity that occur when an animal is placed in a novel environment. Although animal models of these paradigms are scarce, the cyclicity seen when an animal is placed in a novel environment has been studied, and both the amplitude and frequency of the cycles have been shown to be reduced by administration of lithium.[1]

ENDOPHENOTYPES

The genetic studies of BP in the Amish illustrate many of the inherent difficulties of doing genetic analysis in complex disorders. The Amish appear to be a perfect population for such investigations; they are an isolated population with known genealogies, clean phenotypes with little comorbidity, and large extended families. However, the linkage findings for BP in this group have so far been inconsistent and/or contradictory, and even in this ideal population no evidence for linkage has withstood attempts at confirmation or replication. For this reason, some investigators have suggested the use of endophenotypes to further inform their genetic studies of BP. Endophenotypes are defined as alternative phenotypes that are related to a disease phenotype, but are likely to be more simple genetically than the diseases themselves.[25] Endophenotypes traditionally include biochemical or pathologic disease changes, such as the presence of neurofibrillary tangles in Alzheimer's disease; serum or cerebrospinal fluid levels of metabolites, hormones, or trophic factors such as insulin levels in diabetes; and biophysical markers such as abnormalities in responses to evoked potentials in schizophrenia. Analyzing endophenotypes has been a useful strategy in identifying susceptibility genes for other complex disorders, most notably the long Q-T syndrome. In this syndrome, a specific electrocardiogram finding that appeared to have a more straightforward inheritance pattern was used as the phenotype of interest because the inheritance patterns of the syndrome were complex.[25] A variety of approaches for endophenotyping BP have been suggested, including the use of abnormal biochemical, neuroanatomical, neurophysiologic, or neurocognitive changes associated with BP or identified from animal models of BP. Other options include subgrouping by genetic epidemiology (family history, maternal or paternal inheritance), treatment response, symptom severity, or the presence of comorbid disorders such as panic disorder.[25] Some of these approaches have been attempted, with little success to date, while others are still being explored. Some of the more promising endophenotype studies include linkage analysis of clinical response to lithium treatment, sensitivity to cholinergic activity (cholinergic agents can cause depression, while anticholinergic agents can trigger mania), sensitivity to psychostimulants, REM sleep latency, and the presence of white matter hyperintensities, all of which are correlated with BP and are thought or known to segregate within families.[25] However, the extent to which these factors are familial remains unclear, and the utility of the approaches remains more theoretical than practical at the present time.

CONCLUSION

The study of BP is entering an exciting phase. With the development of new technologies, our understanding of the neuroanatomy, biochemistry, and pathophysiology of BP is rapidly increasing. Advances in approaches to the genetic study of complex disorders have led to a number of possible chromosomal locations for BP. The identification of susceptibility genes, while so far elusive, is clearly possible. Perhaps most importantly, it is now possible to combine the various avenues of research into more concerted approaches, allowing for a more in-depth understanding of the pathology of BP as well as the functioning of the normal brain.

REFERENCES

1. Goodwin FK, Jamison KR: Manic Depressive Illness. New York, Oxford University Press, 1990.

2. Murray CJL, Lopez AD (eds): The Global Burden of Disease and Injury Series, Volume 1: A Comprehensive Assessment of Mortality and Disability from Diseases, Injuries, and Risk Factors in 1990 and Projected to 2020. Cambridge, Harvard University Press, 1996.

3. Keck PE, McElroy SL, Arnold LM: Advances in the pathophysiology and treatment of psychiatric disorders: implications for internal medicine. Bipolar disorder. Med Clin North Am 2001;85:645–661.

4. Connerny I, Shapiro PA, McLaughlin JS, et al: Relation between depression after coronary artery bypass surgery and 12-month outcome: A prospective study. Lancet 2001;358:1766–1771.

5. American Psychiatric Association: Mood disorders. In Diagnostic and Statistical Manual of Mental Disorders, 4th ed. Washington, DC, American Psychiatric Press, 1994, 317–391.

6. McElroy SL, Keck PE: Pharmacologic agents for the treatment of acute bipolar mania. Biol Psych 2000;48:539–557.

7. Sachs GS, Thase ME: Bipolar disorder therapeutics: Maintenance treatment. Biol Psych 2000;48: 573–581.

8. Bowden CL, Gitlin MJ, Keck PE, et al: Practice guideline for the treatment of patients with bipolar disorder, revision. Am J Psych 2002;159:1–50.

9. Williams RSB, Cheng L, Mudge AW, Harwood AJ. A common mechanism of action for three mood-stabilizing drugs. Nature 2002:417:292–295.

10. Manji HK, Chen G, Hsiao JK, et al: Regulation of signal transduction pathways by mood stabilizing agents: Implications for the pathophysiology and treatment of bipolar affective disorder. In Manji HK, Bowden CL, Belmaker RH (eds): Bipolar Medications: Mechanisms of Action. Washington, DC, American Psychiatric Press, 2000, 129–177.

11. Vawter MP, Freed WJ, Kleinman JE: Neuropathology of bipolar disorder. Biol Psych 2000; 48:486–504.

12. Strakowski SM, BelBello MP, Adler C, et al: Neuroimaging in bipolar disorder. Bipolar Disorders 2000;2:148–161.

13. Manji HK, Lenox RH: Signaling: Cellular insights into the pathophysiology of bipolar disorder. Biol Psych 2000;48:518–530.

14. Mork A, Jensen JB: Effects of lithium and other mood-stabilizing agents on the cyclic adenosine monophosphate signaling system in the brain. In Manji HK, Bowden CL, Belmaker RH (eds): Bipolar Medications: Mechanisms of Action. Washington, DC, American Psychiatric Press, 2000, 109–128.

15. Lander ES, Schork NJ: Genetic dissection of complex traits. Science 1994;265:2037–2047.

16. Potash JB, DePaulo JR Jr: Searching high and low: A review of the genetics of bipolar disorder. Bipolar disorders 2000;2:8–26.

17. Lander E, Kruglyak L: Genetic dissection of complex traits: Guidelines for interpreting and reporting linkage results. Nat Genet 1995;11:241–247.

18. Escamilla MA. Population isolates: Their special value for locating genes for bipolar disorder. Bipolar Disorders 2001;3:299–317.

19. Furlong RA, Ho L, Rubinsztein JS, et al: Analysis of the monoamine oxidase A (MAOA) gene in bipolar affective disorder by association studies, meta-analyses, and sequencing of the promoter. Am J Med Genet 1999;88:398–406.

20. Furlong RA, Ho L, Walsh C, et al: Analysis and meta-analysis of two serotonin transporter gene polymorphisms in bipolar and unipolar affective disorders. Am J Med Genet 1998;81:58–63.

21. Elvidge G, Jones I, McCandless F, et al: Allelic variation of a BalI polymorphism in the DRD3 gene does not influence susceptibility to bipolar disorder: Results of analysis and meta-analysis. Am J Med Genet 2001; 105:307–311.

22. Furlong RA, Rubinsztein JS, Ho L, et al: Analysis and metaanalysis of two polymorphisms within the tyrosine hydroxylase gene in bipolar and unipolar affective disorders. Am J Med Genet 1999;88:88–94.

23. Dorr DA, Rice JP, Armstrong C, et al: A meta-analysis of chromosome 18 linkage data for bipolar illness. Genet Epidemiol 1997;14:617–622.

24. Ophoff RA, Escamilla MA, Service SK, et al: Genome-wide linkage disequilibrium mapping of severe bipolar disorder in a population isolate. Am J Hum Genet 2002;71:565–574.

25. Lenox RH, Gould TG, Manji HK. Endophenotypes in bipolar disorder. Am J Med Genet 2002;114:391–406.

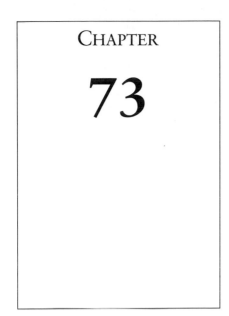

CHAPTER 73

Schizophrenia

David W. Volk

David A. Lewis

Individuals afflicted with schizophrenia usually experience a lifetime of disability and emotional distress.[1] Schizophrenia is manifest as a wide range of signs and symptoms indicative of disturbances in cognitive, emotional, perceptual, and motor processes. The initial formal descriptions of schizophrenia more than a century ago highlighted the substantial differences across affected individuals in the specific constellation of clinical features and the severity and course of the illness exhibited. This clinical heterogeneity, in concert with the identification of differences across individuals in the presence and magnitude of various brain abnormalities, supports the idea that what we recognize clinically as schizophrenia is likely to encompass a set of disorders that differ with respect to their underlying causes and pathophysiologic mechanisms.

This complexity has made the identification of specific etiologic factors in schizophrenia a great challenge. Available data indicate that genetic, environmental, and developmental factors all contribute to the risk of developing schizophrenia, although the specific combinations of factors that may give rise to the illness remain elusive. The apparent discrepancies in the literature, in terms of positive findings and failures to replicate particular genetic linkage or environmental risk factors, may to some degree reflect the complex nature of schizophrenia. Thus, as is the case for many human disease states, the clinical syndrome termed *schizophrenia* may represent the endpoint of many different pathogenetic paths.

CLINICAL FEATURES AND DIAGNOSTIC EVALUATION

The clinical presentation of schizophrenia involves a diverse range of signs and symptoms classified into three groups: (1) distortions in normal brain functions (positive symptoms), (2) reductions in normal brain functions (negative symptoms), and (3) cognitive deficits.[1,2] Positive symptoms include: (1) disturbances in sensory processes such as hallucinations, usually auditory in nature, but can be visual, olfactory, or haptic; (2) disturbances in thought content, such as delusions, frequently with persecutory or nihilistic themes; and (3) disorganization of thought processes, which results in speech or other forms of language that are illogical and lack meaningful associations. Negative symptoms typically include the reduced or inappropriate expression of emotions, reduced initiative and drive, poverty of speech, disinterest in normal pleasurable activities, and social withdrawal. Cognitive deficits in schizophrenia include a reduction in general intellectual functioning, deficits in working memory, poor executive function with deficient processing of complex information, and reduced attention. Positive symptoms are the clinical features most responsive to currently available antipsychotic medications, and it is now recognized that the relatively treatment-resistant negative and cognitive symptoms may be the most chronic and debilitating aspects of the illness. Indeed, cognitive deficits appear to be the best predictor of long-term prognosis.

These diagnostic clinical features of schizophrenia frequently become apparent in the late second to third decade of life, with the average age of onset generally about five years earlier in males than females. Prior to the clinical onset of the illness, premorbid features, including subtle deficits in motor, cognitive, and social abilities, may be evident in childhood. Later, the prodromal phase, which typically occurs in adolescence, includes attenuated positive symptoms, such as ideas of reference and magic thinking, mood symptoms such as anxiety and dysphoria, and cognitive symptoms such as distractibility and social withdrawal. Distinguishing these prodromal signs from normal behavioral changes during adolescence may be very difficult. The gradual transition from the prodromal phase to the acute phase of schizophrenia may be associated with the introduction of new stressors in life that typically occur in late adolescence such as college, military, and exposure to drugs and alcohol.

The life course of schizophrenia is variable, ranging from a single episode with no relapses to a more serious course of repeated episodes throughout life with increasing impairment. While the majority of patients recover from the initial episode, most patients (>80%) also relapse during the subsequent 5 years. Factors associated with a more positive outcome include absence of prominent premorbid signs, acute onset of the illness with a shorter duration of the initial episode, and prompt and continued use of antipsychotic medications.

ETIOLOGIC FACTORS

Genetic Liability

Several convergent lines of evidence support a critical role of inheritance in the etiology of schizophrenia.[3] For example, family, twin, and adoption studies have demonstrated that the morbid risk of schizophrenia in the relatives of affected individuals increases with the percentage of shared genes. In contrast to the 1% incidence of schizophrenia in the general population, schizophrenia occurs in approximately 2% of the third-degree relatives (e.g., first cousins) of an individual with schizophrenia, 2% to 6% of second-degree relatives (e.g., nieces, nephews), and 6% to 17% of first-degree relatives (e.g., parents, siblings, or children). In addition, if one member of a twin pair has the illness, the risk of schizophrenia in the other twin is approximately 17% for fraternal twins and approaches 50% for identical twins. Other lines of evidence indicate that the familial nature of schizophrenia is not due to shared environmental factors. For example, when the biologic children of individuals with schizophrenia are adopted away, their risk of developing schizophrenia is elevated, as expected for first-degree relatives, and is much higher than the general population rates of schizophrenia present in their adoptive families. Furthermore, the offspring of identical twins discordant for schizophrenia have elevated rates of the disorder, regardless of whether the parent was affected or unaffected.

Thus, the etiology of schizophrenia clearly involves genetic factors, with the heritability of the disorder estimated at approximately 80%. However, about 60% of all persons with schizophrenia have neither a first- or second-degree relative with the disorder. In addition, given that the degree of concordance for schizophrenia among monozygotic twins is only about 50%, genetic liability alone is not sufficient for the clinical *appearance* of the disorder. These observations suggest both that the genetic predisposition to schizophrenia is complex and that additional, nongenetic factors are required for the inherited risk to become manifest.

Environmental Risk

Because inheritance alone cannot account for schizophrenia, substantial effort has been expended to identify the potential etiologic role of a variety of environmental factors. The importance of these factors is demonstrated by the fact that in twin studies, the nonshared environment accounts for almost all of the liability for schizophrenia attributable to environmental effects. A wide variety of adverse events, especially during early development, have been associated with an increase in the relative risk of schizophrenia.[4] For example, a history of in utero events, such as severe maternal malnutrition during the first trimester or maternal influenza during the second trimester of pregnancy, and a variety of complications during labor or delivery, has been found with increased frequency in individuals with schizophrenia. In addition, factors associated with place of birth appear to increase the later risk of schizophrenia. For example, urban births are associated with approximately twice the risk of schizophrenia as rural births, and may account for a much greater percentage of the affected population than genetic liability. However, it is important to note that most individuals with these life events do not develop schizophrenia.

Developmental Processes

Based on these findings, most models of the etiology of schizophrenia propose additive and/or interactive effects between multiple susceptibility genes and environmental factors. Furthermore, the temporal delay between environmental events of possible etiologic significance and the appearance of clinical illness has played a major role in the idea that schizophrenia may be a disorder of neural development. In addition, numerous observations of subtle disturbances in motor, cognitive, and social functions during childhood and adolescence of individuals who later manifest schizophrenia have been viewed as evidence of disturbances in neurodevelopmental processes.[4]

The view of schizophrenia as a developmental disorder has also been inferred from postmortem studies that generally have failed to find evidence of gliosis, whether examined by Nissl staining or immunoreactivity for GFAP, in the brains of individuals with schizophrenia. Furthermore, glial membrane turnover, as assessed by magnetic resonance spectroscopy, does not appear to be increased at illness onset or in subjects with chronic schizophrenia. This apparent absence of gliosis has been interpreted to exclude typical neurodegenerative processes as operative in schizophrenia. Given the epidemiologic data for perinatal brain damage as a precursor of the illness, the absence of gliosis seems surprising from a neurodevelopmental perspective given that the brain may be able to mount a gliotic response as early as the second trimester of gestation. On the other hand, loss of neurons and other types of disturbances may transpire in either the developing or adult brain without a sustained glial reaction. Consequently, the absence of gliosis may only be informative regarding the possible mechanisms of brain abnormalities in schizophrenia, and not their timing.

Interactive Mechanism

Thus, the available data suggest that schizophrenia may encompass a heterogeneous group of disorders whose etiopathogenesis involves the interplay of polygenetic influences and environmental risk factors operating on brain maturational processes. The complexity of these potential interactions clearly complicates the study of the molecular mechanisms of illness. On the one hand, schizophrenia may be a single disease process with a range of severity and clinical manifestations across individuals, determined by the extent to which different brain regions or circuits are affected. Alternatively, the clinical heterogeneity may indicate that what we recognize as schizophrenia represents, in fact, a constellation of different disease processes that share some phenotypic features. Differentiating among these possibilities awaits the definitive identification of specific etiologic factors.

Together, these findings contribute to the current state of exciting, but not fully substantiated, hypotheses regarding the etiopathogenesis of schizophrenia. In terms of revealing the molecular basis of this illness, the existing literature is limited by the fact that any particular finding (1) may be restricted to the specific subset of subjects studied, (2) may represent a secondary process that is associated with the illness but that does not reflect the primary causal mechanisms, or (3) may represent a false positive observation, given the number of different molecules that have been studied. For these and other reasons, it is not possible at this time to present a comprehensive, definitive review of the molecular basis of schizophrenia. Thus, we have chosen to highlight studies illustrating different and complementary approaches that have yielded interesting data regarding altered molecular systems and candidate genetic liabilities in schizophrenia.

MOLECULAR SYSTEMS

Molecular Alterations in the Context of Neural Circuitry

In order to understand how disease-related alterations at the molecular level produce disturbed brain function, the actions of the molecules of interest must be considered within the constraints provided by the neural circuits that produce or utilize them. Clues regarding the affected neural circuits come from reports of structural brain abnormalities in individuals with schizophrenia, such as enlargement of the lateral and third ventricles, and reduced volume of the cortical gray matter.[4] The latter changes do not appear to represent a uniform abnormality. They appear to affect preferentially certain association cortices including those located in the dorsal prefrontal cortex (PFC), the superior temporal gyrus, and limbic areas such as the hippocampal formation and anterior cingulate cortex. These structural abnormalities have been observed in first-episode, never-medicated subjects with schizophrenia, and may be present prior to the clinical onset of illness, suggesting that they reflect the primary disease process and are not a secondary consequence of the illness or of its treatment.

Of these brain regions, the PFC is of particular interest. Subjects with schizophrenia consistently perform poorly on certain cognitive tasks that are subserved by circuitry involving the dorsal PFC, such as those requiring working memory.[5,6] In addition, these subjects fail to show normal activation of this brain region when attempting to perform such tasks. Disturbances in working memory and related cognitive functions may be the most persistent and, over the long-term, the most debilitating symptoms of schizophrenia. In addition, the long-term prognosis for individuals with schizophrenia appears to be best predicted by the degree of cognitive impairment. Thus, understanding the molecular basis for abnormalities in PFC circuitry may be particularly important for improving clinical outcome.

Many postmortem studies have reported a 5% to 10% reduction in cortical thickness (with a corresponding increase in cell-packing density but no change in total neuron number) in the dorsal PFC of subjects with schizophrenia. Although the size of some PFC neuronal populations, particularly pyramidal neurons in deep layer 3, is smaller in schizophrenic subjects, the increase in cell-packing density is also likely to reflect a decrease in the number of axon terminals, distal dendrites, and dendritic spines that represent the principal components of cortical synapses.[7] Indeed, it has been reported that the density of basilar dendritic spines on PFC layer 3 pyramidal neurons is decreased in subjects with schizophrenia. Furthermore, it has been found that levels of synaptophysin, a presynaptic terminal protein, is decreased in the PFC of subjects with schizophrenia in multiple studies. Finally, levels of N-acetyl aspartate, a marker of axonal and/or neuronal integrity, are reduced in the PFC of subjects with schizophrenia. Thus, convergent lines of evidence from neuroimaging and postmortem studies suggest that schizophrenia is associated with synaptic alterations in the PFC.[1] Consequently, in the following subsections, we review findings that address the molecular bases and consequences of synaptic-related abnormalities in the PFC in schizophrenia.

Presynaptic Machinery

Gene chips or microarrays provide a powerful approach for examining the mRNA expression levels of thousands of genes simultaneously. A postmortem study of gene expression profiling in the dorsal PFC (area 9) of subjects with schizophrenia revealed that, of over 250 gene groups examined, the most consistently altered group of genes included those whose protein products are involved in the machinery of presynaptic function.[8] That is, decreased tissue mRNA levels were found for proteins located on or associated with synaptic vesicles or the presynaptic membrane, and proteins known or hypothesized to play a role in the release of neurotransmitters, such as N-ethylmaleimide sensitive factor, synapsin II, synaptotagmin 5, and synaptogyrin 1. Although the extent to which the reported transcript changes are converted into alterations at the protein level remains to be determined, other studies of individual synapse-associated proteins (e.g., synaptophysin, SNAP-25) have generally found reductions in the PFC of subjects with schizophrenia.

Interestingly, although subjects with schizophrenia appear to share a common abnormality in the control of synaptic transmission, they also differ according to the specific combination of presynaptic genes that showed reduced expression. These differences suggest at least two tentative conclusions. First, the observation that only a subset of the transcripts within this gene group were reduced in a given subject tends to argue against the finding representing simply a consequence of an overall reduction in the number of PFC synapses in schizophrenia. Second, the pattern of different genes showing altered expression in different subjects may be consistent with a polygenic mode of inheritance for schizophrenia. Perhaps consistent with this view, a number of the chromosomal loci that have been implicated in schizophrenia (discussed later) contain genes encoding proteins related to presynaptic function.

Metabolic Processes

The disturbances in DLPFC function in schizophrenia also appear to be associated with altered metabolism in this brain region.[5] For example, the normal increases in glucose utilization and blood flow present in the dorsal PFC when subjects are asked to perform certain cognitive tasks are markedly blunted in subjects with schizophrenia, compared to the large activations and blood flow increases seen in normal subjects. Considerable efforts have been made to determine the cellular mechanisms that may underlie these apparent alterations in brain metabolism in schizophrenia. Observations by magnetic resonance spectroscopy, in both chronically ill and never-medicated, first-episode subjects with schizophrenia, suggest that changes in the concentration of high-energy phosphate molecules (including ATP, phosphocreatine, and phospholipid metabolites) may reflect the cellular mechanisms underlying these metabolic disturbances. In addition, it has been reported that the expression levels of various metabolic genes, or the tissue concentrations of

proteins encoded by these genes, are reduced in postmortem brain tissue from subjects with schizophrenia.

Middleton and colleagues recently used cDNA microarrays to examine the expression profile of genes composing major metabolic pathways in postmortem samples of PFC area 9 from matched pairs of subjects with schizophrenia and controls.[9] Of the 71 metabolic pathways assessed, only 5 showed consistent changes in expression in schizophrenia. Specifically, reduced expression levels were identified for the transcripts of genes whose protein products are involved in the regulation of ornithine and polyamine metabolism, the mitochondrial malate shuttle system, the transcarboxylic acid (TCA) cycle, aspartate and alanine metabolism, and ubiquitin metabolism. Parallel in situ hybridization studies were also conducted in macaque monkeys treated chronically with haloperidol in a manner that mimicked the clinical use of this antipsychotic medication. Interestingly, although most of the metabolic genes that showed decreased expression in the subjects with schizophrenia were not similarly altered in the monkeys, the transcript encoding the cytosolic form of malate dehydrogenase displayed a marked treatment-associated increase in expression. These findings suggest that metabolic alterations in the PFC of subjects with schizophrenia reflect highly specific abnormalities, at least at the level of gene expression, and that the therapeutic effect of antipsychotic medications may, in part, be mediated by the normalization of some of these alterations in gene expression.

Although the cause of altered levels of these transcripts remains to be determined, the high metabolic demands placed on neurons by the processes involved in synaptic communication suggest that these changes are related to the synaptic abnormalities present in the PFC in schizophrenia.

GABA Neurotransmission

Recent studies also suggest that certain neuronal populations and circuits may be most compromised by these alterations in synaptic machinery and metabolism. For example, disturbances in inhibitory (GABA) neurons appear to play a prominent role in the dysfunction of PFC circuitry in schizophrenia.[10,11] Presynaptic markers of the synthesis, release, and reuptake of GABA have been reported to be decreased in postmortem samples from schizophrenia subjects. Furthermore, these alterations have been consistently reported to occur at the level of gene expression in the PFC. For example, the expression of mRNAs encoding glutamate decarboxylase (GAD$_{67}$, a synthesizing enzyme for GABA) and the GABA membrane transporter (GAT-1, responsible for reuptake of GABA into the nerve terminal) is also reduced. Some of these alterations have been reported in both hemispheres of the PFC and also in the temporal cortex, suggesting that dysfunction of inhibitory circuitry in cortical association regions may be a common feature of schizophrenia. Studies have also reported that several markers of inhibitory neurotransmission are unchanged in subjects with major depressive disorder, with or without psychotic features, suggesting that alterations in GABA neurotransmission may be relatively specific to the diagnosis of schizophrenia, or at least not associated primarily with either depression or psychosis. Finally, treatment with haloperidol does not appear to account for the reduction in presynaptic GABA markers in schizophrenia, since monkeys treated with haloperidol for a year in a manner that mimicked clinical use did not show differences in several inhibitory markers in the PFC.

Inhibitory neurons in the cerebral cortex contain heterogeneous subpopulations of neurons that exhibit unique anatomical, biochemical, and electrophysiologic properties reflecting specialized functional roles in the regulation of neuronal activity and working memory. For example, chandelier neurons provide a linear array of axon terminals (cartridges) that exclusively synapse along the axon initial segment of pyramidal neurons, which is the site of action potential generation. Chandelier neurons are also among the minority of GABA neurons that express the calcium-binding protein parvalbumin and exhibit a fast-spiking, nonadapting firing pattern. These characteristics suggest that chandelier neurons are anatomically positioned and functionally adapted to powerfully regulate the output of pyramidal neurons. In contrast, double-bouquet neurons, which express the calcium-binding proteins calbindin or calretinin and exhibit a regular-spiking, adaptive firing pattern, provide axon terminals that target more distal dendritic sites on pyramidal cells or other GABA neurons. Thus, knowledge of whether disturbances in GABA neurotransmission are predominantly localized to individual subpopulations of inhibitory neurons may provide insight into dysfunction of the PFC in schizophrenia.

Interestingly, recent studies have indeed found that alterations in inhibitory neurotransmission in schizophrenia appear to be most prominent in a subset of PFC GABA neurons that includes chandelier cells.[12] For example, the protein level of GAT-1 appears to be selectively reduced in the axon terminals of chandelier cells. In addition, in PFC area 9, the relative cellular levels of expression of GAD_{67} and GAT-1 mRNAs are actually normal in the majority of inhibitory neurons, but are undetectable in a subset of neurons in the same cortical layers where chandelier cells are located. These findings do not appear to reflect a reduction in the number of GABA neurons since most studies have not found a decrease in PFC neuron number or density in schizophrenia. Furthermore, the protein and mRNA expression levels of parvalbumin, but not calretinin, are reduced in subjects with schizophrenia, suggesting that the affected subset of neurons probably includes chandelier cells but not double-bouquet cells. Interestingly, chandelier neurons may play a critical role in working memory

processes suggesting that alterations in chandelier cells may be particularly relevant to the working memory dysfunction present in schizophrenia.[10]

The consequences of alterations in presynaptic GABA markers on inhibitory signaling can be further understood through studies of postsynaptic $GABA_A$ receptors, since changes in extracellular GABA levels appear to result in compensatory changes in $GABA_A$ receptors. Earlier studies of postsynaptic $GABA_A$ receptors in the PFC of subjects with schizophrenia found increases in radiolabeled muscimol binding that are most prominent at the pyramidal cell body, but no change or a decrease in benzodiazepine binding. However, $GABA_A$ receptors are composed of pentamers of subunits, most commonly including at least one of each of the α, β, and γ subunit classes, and ligand-binding studies are not able to detect selective differences in individual $GABA_A$ receptor subunits. Genetic studies have failed to find evidence of a linkage between polymorphisms of major $GABA_A$ receptor subunit genes and schizophrenia. Analyses of the mRNA expression of the major $GABA_A$ receptor subunits in the PFC in subjects with schizophrenia have also failed to find differences in schizophrenia, although some studies have reported increases in the $α_1$ subunit mRNA expression and a reduction in the short isoform of the $γ_2$ subunit. However, studies of mRNA expression, which is confined to the cell soma, do not allow an analysis of differences in the distinctive subcellular distributions of different $GABA_A$ receptor subunits present in individual neurons.

To understand the consequences of disturbances in GABA neurotransmission in chandelier neurons in schizophrenia, it is critical to determine whether $GABA_A$ receptors located at the principal postsynaptic targets of chandelier cells (axon initial segments or AIS of pyramidal cells) are affected.[12] Interestingly, in the superficial layers of human cerebral cortex, the $α_2$ subunit of the $GABA_A$ receptor is prominently localized to pyramidal neuron AIS. A recent study found an increase in the density of pyramidal neuron AIS immunoreactive for the $α_2$ subunit in the PFC of subjects with schizophrenia. There was no increase in subjects with major depression. The density of $α_2$-labeled AIS was inversely correlated to the density of GAT-1-labeled cartridges in subjects with schizophrenia. Thus, in schizophrenia, $GABA_A$ receptors appear to be upregulated at pyramidal neuron AIS in response to deficient GABA neurotransmission at chandelier axon terminals. These data further demonstrate that disturbances in inhibition at the chandelier neuron–pyramidal neuron synapse may be a critical component of prefrontal cortical dysfunction in schizophrenia.

The pathophysiologic mechanism that results in selective disturbances in chandelier neurons, but not in the majority of cortical inhibitory neurons, is not understood. For example, it is possible that chandelier neurons have an intrinsic abnormality related to the unique gene products or electrophysiologic properties that distinguish them from the other subtypes of inhibitory neurons that appear to be unaffected in schizophrenia. For example, while calretinin is expressed in human frontal cortex before birth, parvalbumin does not appear until age 3 to 6 months. Reynolds and Beasley hypothesize that the absence of this neuroprotective calcium-binding protein may create a neonatal window of vulnerability to neurotoxic events selectively in the cells that normally would eventually express parvalbumin.[13] However, the nature of such neurotoxic events is unknown, and the mechanism in which these insults could alter the functional properties of these neurons without resulting in cell death remains unclear. Alternatively, inhibitory neurotransmission may be reduced in chandelier neurons in response to a reduction in their excitatory inputs. For example, morphologic changes in PFC layer 3 pyramidal neurons, and reduced neuronal number in the mediodorsal nucleus of the thalamus, have been reported in subjects with schizophrenia. Interestingly, in monkey PFC area 46, the dendrites of parvalbumin-containing cells are preferentially targeted by axon terminals from local pyramidal neurons and receive inputs from the mediodorsal nucleus of the thalamus. However, experimental models of the effects of reduced excitatory input to chandelier neurons have not been published.

Costa and colleagues have proposed a novel hypothesis that a deficiency of reelin, an extracellular matrix protein, may contribute to alterations in inhibitory neurotransmission in the PFC in schizophrenia.[14] Their studies have revealed decreases in reelin protein and mRNA expression in multiple brain regions, including prefrontal and temporal cortex, hippocampus, caudate, and cerebellum. However, with the exception of the hippocampus, these findings await independent replication. Studies of the reelin haploinsufficient mouse, which expresses approximately half of the normal levels of reelin protein and mRNA, have demonstrated remarkable similarities to various postmortem findings in the PFC of subjects with schizophrenia. For example, decreased cortical thickness, increased neuron density, and reductions in GAD_{67} mRNA expression have been reported in the heterozygous reeler mouse.

Glutamate Neurotransmission

Several lines of evidence from clinical studies suggest that glutamatergic neurotransmission may also be deficient in schizophrenia.[15] For example, phenylcyclidine (PCP) and ketamine, which are noncompetitive antagonists of the NMDA subtype of glutamate receptor, may transiently induce in control subjects positive and negative symptoms and some cognitive deficits that are similar to those present in schizophrenia. These drug-induced symptoms occur in adults, but rarely in children. This has been suggested to mimic the delayed age of onset of schizophrenia. Furthermore, ketamine has been reported to exacerbate positive and negative symptoms and cognitive dysfunction in subjects with schizophrenia, and this exacerbation can be reversed by treatment with clozapine. Conversely, treatment with glycine, which facilitates NMDA receptor function by binding to a modulatory site, and D-cycloserine, a selective partial agonist at the glycine modulatory site, have been reported to improve positive and negative symptoms and cognitive dysfunction in subjects with schizophrenia. Together, these clinical observations suggest that NMDA receptors may be hypofunctional in schizophrenia.

Animal models lend further support to the NMDA receptor hypofunction hypothesis in schizophrenia. For example, chronic PCP treatment in rats and monkeys results in impairments in cognitive performance and reduced social interactions. Furthermore, mutant mice that express only 5% of an essential subunit of the NMDA receptor, NMDAR1, also exhibit increased stereotypy and reduced social interactions, and these behaviors can be improved by treatment with haloperidol or clozapine.

Multiple mechanisms have been proposed by which NMDA receptor hypofunction may be involved in the pathophysiology of schizophrenia. For example, Jentsch and Roth describe how chronic administration of NMDA receptor antagonists to rats and monkeys results in a reduction in cortical dopamine neurotransmission, particularly in the prefrontal cortex, but an increase in subcortical dopaminergic activity.[16] These observations may be consistent with current views of the dopamine hypothesis of schizophrenia that deficient PFC activity of dopamine contributes to the cognitive features of the disorder, whereas hyperfunctional subcortical dopamine may be critical for psychosis. In addition, Olney and Farber hypothesize that hypofunction of NMDA receptors in schizophrenia primarily is manifested by reduced NMDA receptor-mediated activation of GABA neurons, and, consequently, reduced inhibition of excitatory neurons.[17] Disinhibited excitatory neurons then release excessive glutamate that overactivates other glutamate receptor subtypes, resulting in psychotic and cognitive dysfunction as well as neurodegenerative effects including cell death in subjects with schizophrenia. In addition, in rats treated with NMDA receptor antagonists, neurodegenerative consequences do not appear until after puberty, similar to the delayed onset of schizophrenia. However, both pyramidal neurons and inhibitory neurons express NMDA receptors, and no studies have yet demonstrated a selective alteration in NMDA receptors in cortical inhibitory neurons in schizophrenia.

In contrast to clinical evidence and experimental animal models that support the hypothesis of NMDA receptor hypofunction in schizophrenia, genetic studies fail to find evidence of linkage between schizophrenia and polymorphisms of the NMDAR1 subunit (an obligate subunit in NMDA receptors) or with any of the multiple metabotropic glutamate receptors subunits. Furthermore, multiple postmortem studies have not provided consistent evidence of altered NMDA receptor expression in schizophrenia.[15] For example, radiolabeled-ligand binding studies in the frontal cortex of subjects with schizophrenia have reported no changes in NMDA receptor binding. Also, studies of mRNA expression of the NMDAR1 subunit have yielded inconsistent results, finding a decrease, no change, or even an increase in frontal cortex. However, these studies lacked the sensitivity to determine whether NMDA receptors are selectively altered in inhibitory neurons but not pyramidal neurons, as implied by the Olney and Farber hypothesis.[17] Studies of the other major types of ionotropic glutamate receptors, AMPA and kainate, and of metabotropic glutamate receptors in schizophrenia have also generally been negative with one notable exception: in the hippocampus and medial temporal lobe, several studies have reported decreased mRNA and protein expression of the AMPA receptor GluR1 and GluR2 subunits. Interestingly, the NMDA receptor requires an initial depolarization event, such as that caused by activation of AMPA receptors located in the same synapse, in order to remove the voltage-dependent Mg^{++} blockade of the NMDA receptor Na^+ channel. Thus, the hypothesized NMDA receptor hypofunction in schizophrenia may, at least in theory, result from reduced AMPA-mediated depolarization in hippocampus and medial temporal lobe. To summarize, although current clinical observations and the use of animal models have built an intriguing case in support of NMDA receptor hypofunction in schizophrenia, direct evidence of disturbances in NMDA receptor expression in the brains of subjects with schizophrenia remains elusive.

GENETIC VARIATION

The genetic liability to schizophrenia appears to be transmitted in a polygenic, nonmendelian fashion. A number of chromosomal loci have been found to be associated with schizophrenia, including 22q11-13, 6p, 13q, and 1q21-22.[18] Interestingly, several of these loci contain genes that have well-delineated neurobiologic functions, including genes that regulate some of the molecular systems discussed in the preceding section. However, these observations have not yet been converted into reliable single gene findings through the use of positional cloning approaches. In addition, although linkage studies in general have proved to be difficult to replicate in subsequent cohorts of subjects, this phenomenon may highlight the genetic complexity of schizophrenia, with different subtypes or etiologies of schizophrenia produced by different fundamental molecular defects.

Consequently, it is not possible at present to point to single genes that have been unequivocally implicated as susceptibility factors for schizophrenia. However, the following four interesting examples, illustrating different strategies for identifying candidate genes, warrant attention.

COMT

In order to identify susceptibility genes for this disorder, one approach is to examine the *effect* of allelic variations in genes whose protein products may contribute to the regulation of normal brain processes that are deficient in schizophrenia, such as cognitive functioning.[5] For example, the dopamine neurotransmitter system plays a critical role in working memory function in the PFC, and several lines of evidence suggest that allelic variations in catechol-O-methyltransferase (COMT), a major enzyme involved in the metabolic degradation of dopamine, may contribute to the liability of schizophrenia.[5] For example, microdeletions of chromosome 22 q11, the locus of the COMT gene, have been reported in approximately 2% of subjects with schizophrenia. Furthermore, patients with velocardiofacial syndrome, which involves variable deletions of 22q11, have an increased prevalence of psychotic symptoms and schizophrenia. Finally, linkage studies of loci at 22q12-13, which is nearby, though not identical, to the locus for COMT, have also found associations with schizophrenia.

One of the multiple polymorphisms of the COMT gene has been demonstrated to profoundly affect the ability of COMT to metabolize dopamine. A single guanine to adenosine transition results in a change in amino acids from valine (val) to methionine (met) at codon 108 or 158 (for the soluble and membrane-bound forms of COMT, respectively). The met-containing COMT enzyme has 25% of the activity of val-containing COMT, resulting in drastic reduction in dopamine metabolism in the met-containing COMT enzyme, and, consequently, increased amounts of dopamine. Weinberger and colleagues have hypothesized that the presence of the high activity val-containing COMT allele, which results in lower dopamine levels, may contribute to impaired cognitive function in schizophrenia.[5] Indeed, COMT appears to be primarily responsible for the majority of dopamine metabolism in the PFC, but not in other brain regions, such as the striatum. For example, in COMT knockout mice, dopamine levels are elevated by over 200% in frontal cortex but not in striatum or hypothalamus. Furthermore, Weinberger and colleagues demonstrated that individuals with schizophrenia who are homozygous for the val genotype commit more perseverative errors on the Wisconsin Card Sort Task (which assesses working memory and other executive functions) than heterozygotes or individuals homozygous for the met genotype.[5] This is consistent with other studies demonstrating that a reduction in dopamine in the PFC impairs working memory function. In addition, the val/val genotype is associated with more perseverative errors on the Wisconsin Card Sort Task than either the val/met genotype or the met/met genotype in normal control subjects as well. Furthermore, several family-based association studies utilizing the transmission disequilibrium test have reported weak, yet significant, associations between the val-containing COMT allele and schizophrenia

However, several lines of evidence suggest, at most, a limited role of COMT in schizophrenia. For example, numerous case-control association studies have consistently failed to find an association between the val-containing COMT allele, or other COMT polymorphisms, and schizophrenia. Furthermore, studies suggesting an association between the high activity val-containing COMT allele and schizophrenia seem to contradict other studies suggesting that deletion of the COMT gene, such as in velocardiofacial syndrome, may be associated with schizophrenia. Finally, the high prevalence of the val-containing COMT allele in normal human populations suggests that the val-containing COMT allele may play a minor role, at most, in the pathology of schizophrenia. To our knowledge, analyses of the protein and mRNA expression of COMT in frontal cortex have not been conducted yet in postmortem brain tissue samples from subjects with schizophrenia, so it is unclear whether alterations in the gene expression of COMT may be associated with schizophrenia.

α_7 Nicotinic Receptor

A large body of literature has documented the presence of sensory gating abnormalities in individuals with schizophrenia. That is, affected individuals appear to have deficits in the ability to gate, or internally screen, sensory stimuli, such that an "undifferentiated and involuntary tide of sensory data sweep away the stable constructs of reality."[19] In humans, the gating of auditory stimuli is evidenced as a decrement in the evoked electroencephalographic response to the second of two consecutive auditory stimuli. Specifically, when two paired tones are delivered 500 msec apart, the amplitude of the P50 auditory evoked potential (a positive response that occurs 50 msec after a tone) to the second tone normally decreases to less than 40% of the P50 following the first tone. In contrast, in over 75% of individuals with schizophrenia, and in about 50% of their unaffected family members, the response to the second tone fails to show this normal decrease in amplitude and may actually increase.

This deficit in the P50 is transmitted as autosomal dominant in families with schizophrenia, suggesting that the power of genetic analyses for this phenotype would be increased relative to schizophrenia itself. Indeed, Freedman and colleagues found that this trait was linked to a dinucleotide repeat polymorphism (D15S1360) located at chromosome 15q14.[20] Evidence for linkage of the locus to schizophrenia was also positive, but not as strong, and as expected, attempts to replicate the linkage to schizophrenia have produced both positive and negative findings.

The relevance of this locus for the pathophysiologic mechanism of auditory gating deficits, and possibly for the pathogenesis of schizophrenia, is supported by the fact that the CHRNA7 gene for the α_7 subunit of the nicotinic acetylcholine receptor (nAChR) is located <120kb from the dinucleotide marker. The nAChR, a ligand-gated ion channel, is a pentameric structure in the plasma membrane composed of two types of subunits (α_{2-9} and β_{2-4}) that differ by the presence, in the α subunits, of specific amino acids in the N-terminal region that mediate ligand binding. The genomic structure for the human CHRNA7 includes partial duplication, with duplicated exons 5 to 10 located 1Mb proximal to the full-length gene on chromosome 15. The function of the partial duplication remains to be determined.

Several lines of evidence, in both humans and animal models, support a role for the nAChR α_7 subunit in the pathophysiology of sensory gating deficits in schizophrenia.[21] In humans, the binding of α-bungarotoxin, which probably corresponds to nAChRs containing the α_7 subunit, is reduced in the postmortem hippocampus and other brain regions of individuals with schizophrenia. In addition, the P50 deficit is improved by nicotine in both subjects with schizophrenia and their unaffected family members. However, in contrast to control subjects who show an upregulation of nicotinic receptors in association with smoking, individuals with schizophrenia exhibit lower binding at every level of smoking history. Furthermore, in sensory gating paradigms in rats, the N40 wave is thought to be the analogue of the human P50. Interestingly, both administration of specific antagonists of the α_7 nAChR and use of antisense oligonucleotides complementary to the α_7 translation start site blocked gating of the N40 wave in rats.

These observations are of particular clinical interest because smoking and other uses of nicotine-containing tobacco products are much more common in schizophrenia than in the general population, and individuals with schizophrenia appear to extract more nicotine from each cigarette than individuals without schizophrenia. These observations suggest that individuals with schizophrenia use tobacco excessively as a means of self-medication. That is, by stimulating deficient α_7-containing nAChRs, they are able to transiently reduce the subjective distress associated with sensory gating disturbances. However, how the apparent inherited liability at chromosome 15q14 is translated into the functional deficit remains unclear. Both the underexpression and early developmental overexpression of the CHRNA7 gene have been hypothesized.

RGS4

Genes that contribute to the inherited susceptibility for schizophrenia may be expected to share several properties: (1) a protein product that appears likely to play a role in the pathophysiology of the illness and in the pathways that are affected by therapeutic interventions, (2) an mRNA that shows altered expression levels across the brain in the disease state, and (3) a chromosomal locus strongly implicated in linkage and association studies. Recent studies suggest that the gene for RGS4, a member of the family of Regulators of G-protein Signaling proteins, represents such a candidate. First, like other RGS proteins, RGS4 plays a critical role in modulating

G-protein pathway signaling by attaching to the activated GTP-bound G-α proteins of G-protein-coupled neurotransmitter receptors (GPCRs) where they act as GTP-ase activating proteins and thus shorten the duration of G-protein mediated intracellular signaling. Different RGS family members have distinct anatomical distributions in the brain, although RGS expression patterns have not been linked to specific neurotransmitter systems. However, many neurotransmitter systems that have been implicated in the pathophysiology of schizophrenia, such as GABA, glutamate, and dopamine, utilize GPCRs that are regulated by RGS proteins, and at least some of these GPCRs are the targets of antipsychotic drugs.

Second, a recent microarray study revealed a robust and consistent decrease in cortical levels of the *RGS4* transcript in schizophrenia, whereas other RGS or G-protein signaling components did not exhibit significant transcript changes.[22] Furthermore, *RGS4* transcript levels were not altered in subjects with major depressive disorder or in monkeys treated chronically with the antipsychotic agent haloperidol in a manner that mimics clinical use, and subjects with alcoholism were reported to have increased mRNA levels of *RGS4*. Together, these findings suggest that decreased *RGS4* mRNA levels may not be a common feature of all psychiatric disorders, or the result of treatment or comorbid conditions that frequently accompany schizophrenia.

Third, *RGS4* is located at chromosome 1q21-22, a locus recently implicated in schizophrenia.[23] It has been found that of the 70 genes mapped to the 1q21-22 locus represented on the platform used in the microarray study, only *RGS4* exhibited altered expression across multiple schizophrenic subjects. This finding supports, to some degree, the idea that variants in *RGS4* may contribute to these inheritance patterns. However, sequence-based analysis of the coding region of *RGS4* in these schizophrenic subjects did not report informative polymorphisms or mutations.

To determine whether altered *RGS4* expression reflects a primary inherited abnormality in schizophrenia, Chowdari and colleagues conducted genetic association studies in over 1400 subjects using *RGS4* polymorphisms.[24] They surveyed a genomic region of approximately 300 kb and detected associations for four SNPs localized to a 10-kb span at *RGS4*. The global association tests for haplotypes bearing all four SNPs suggested that the transmission distortion was unlikely to be due to chance alone, especially when all family-based samples were considered, but its mechanism and specificity for schizophrenia require further study.

WKL1

A third strategy for identifying susceptibility genes is to study families with multiple affected individuals who share a clinical subtype of schizophrenia that appears to be more homogeneous than the broader disorder. This approach has been used to identify a novel gene in a German family with a subtype of schizophrenia termed periodic catatonia. Catatonia, a nonspecific clinical syndrome that may occur in several psychiatric disorders, refers to psychomotor disturbances that may involve either a pronounced decrease in spontaneous movements and activities (e.g., muteness, rigidity, waxy flexibility) or an abnormal increase in activity (e.g., talking and shouting continuously). Although not included in the Diagnostic and Statistical Manual of Mental Disorders IV, periodic catatonia was identified as a subtype of schizophrenia by the German psychiatrist Karl Leonhard. Leonhard described periodic catatonia as an independent disorder with considerable hereditary loading that was characterized clinically by alternating hyperkinetic and akinetic states, with hallucinations and delusions present early in the course of illness.

In 12 multiplex pedigrees, a genome scan revealed significant linkage to periodic catatonia on chromosome 15q15, and evidence of suggestive linkage on chromosome 22q13.[25] The latter observation was primarily supported by a single large family, and within this family a novel gene called *WKL1* was identified at the 22q13 locus. *WKL1*, which probably encodes a cation channel distantly related to the shaker potassium channel subfamily, was found to have a 1121 cytosine to adenine transversion that produced a missense mutation of leu to met in the region probably corresponding to the transmembrane portion of the ion channel. In the pedigree, 7 of 17 family members who were heterozygous for the mutation had periodic catatonia, whereas none of the 6 family members homozygous for the wild-type gene were affected. This finding suggests a role for the mutation in the development of periodic catatonia. It is an important finding since it is the only example of a putative schizophrenia susceptibility gene for which a mutation and a specific clinical phenotype cosegregate with such strength. However, since over half of the individuals carrying the mutated allele did not manifest the clinical syndrome, other genetic and/or environmental factors must also be required for the appearance of periodic catatonia.

WKL1 may also serve as an informative example of a gene defect that is rare but makes a major contribution to a distinctive phenotype of a subtype of a heterogeneous disorder such as schizophrenia. Interestingly, mutations in other potassium-channel encoding genes (e.g., *KCNA1*, *KCNQ2-3*) lead to episodic ataxia/myokymia and neonatal epilepsy, clinical syndromes that may bear some pathophysiologic relationships to the distinguishing motor features of periodic catatonia. These phenotypic similarities suggest that the *WKL1* mutation more likely contributes to the psychomotor component of periodic catatonia than to the psychotic symptoms and cognitive deficits that are common to schizophrenia in general.

IMPLICATIONS FOR UNDERSTANDING THE ETIOPATHOGENESIS OF SCHIZOPHRENIA

The epidemiologic data regarding risk factors for schizophrenia and the examples of disease-related alterations in molecular systems and individual genes summarized in this chapter provide a framework for considering how complex interactions among genetic and environmental factors (probably of multiple types) may contribute to alterations in cascades of molecular systems in the brain that can, in turn, give rise to the multiple phenotypic features of schizophrenia.[4]

First, it is clear that there is a genetic predisposition for the development of schizophrenia. Although rare mendelian forms of the illness may exist, most affected individuals probably carry some combination of allelic variations (the number of combinations may be large) in a variety of genes, such as those for COMT, α_7 nAChR, and RGS4, each of which contributes some liability for different phenotypic features of the illness. The presence of the predisposing alleles for a given gene alone is not sufficient to manifest the illness, but does contribute to its heritability. In addition, this combination of inherited factors would also likely contribute to secondary alterations in the expression of other genes whose protein products play an essential role in the types of brain functions that are disturbed in schizophrenia.

Second, these altered patterns of gene expression may be influenced, or perhaps even triggered, by adverse environmental events occurring during particular sensitive periods of development, such as the prenatal, perinatal, and adolescence time frames, when rapid changes take place in different aspects of brain structure-function. Thus, individual differences in the manifestation (or lack thereof) of disease characteristics in response to a particular environmental event would depend upon the susceptibility conferred by the allelic variations associated with schizophrenia.

Third, the combination of functional disturbances related to inherited factors and the altered patterns of gene expression due to the interaction of genetic and environmental factors may have a cumulative effect producing additional disturbances in later developmental processes. These downstream consequences in specific brain circuits may translate subtle disturbances in motor, cognitive, and social function evident early in life into the presence of the full clinical syndrome later in life in those who subsequently develop schizophrenia.

Although clearly incomplete, some of the findings discussed in this chapter illustrate this view of the etiopathogenesis of schizophrenia. As described previously, allelic variations in RGS4 may represent one example of inherited susceptibility factors for schizophrenia. The associated decrease in RGS4 mRNA expression, and the presumed resulting decrease in RGS4 protein levels, would have as a functional consequence alterations in the duration and timing of information transfer at the neural connections formed by the subpopulations of neurons that express RGS4. This type of alteration in synaptic function would be predicted to lead to changes in the expression of a number of other genes whose protein products contribute to synaptic function, especially if the RGS4-mediated alterations in synaptic function were present during developmental periods in which the maturation of synaptic connections is particularly sensitive to experience-driven activity. Consistent with this hypothesis, genes encoding proteins that contribute to the mechanics of presynaptic function exhibit decreased expression in the PFC of subjects with schizophrenia, and evidence of molecular and functional alterations in the major excitatory and inhibitory neurotransmitter systems of the cerebral cortex are present in schizophrenia. Furthermore, these alterations in synaptic function are associated with decreased expression of genes that regulate specific aspects of the metabolic activity essential for neurotransmission. Together, these alterations within the circuitry of the PFC, in concert with reduced PFC dopamine levels due to val-COMT and/or other inherited liabilities, may represent the neural basis for some of the cognitive deficits present in schizophrenia.

Clearly, however, conversion of this type of proposal into an integrated understanding of the etiopathogenesis of schizophrenia rests upon a number of factors including (1) identification of the full spectrum of genetic liabilities for the illness; (2) development of tractable model systems that permit testing of the pathophysiologic processes that may link specific genetic and environmental factors with altered molecular systems found in schizophrenia; and (3) establishment of relationships between a given constellation of genetic and molecular features and phenotypes of the illness.

REFERENCES

1. Lewis DA, Lieberman JA: Catching up on schizophrenia: Natural history and neurobiology. Neuron 2000;28:325–334.

2. Frangou S, Murray RM: Schizophrenia, 2nd ed. London, Martin Dunitz, 2000.

3. Gottesman II: Schizophrenia Genesis: The Origins of Madness. New York, Freeman, 1991.

4. Lewis DA, Levitt P: Schizophrenia as a disorder of neurodevelopment. Ann Rev Neurosci 2002;25: 409–432.

5. Weinberger DR, Egan MF, Bertolino A, et al: Prefrontal neurons and the genetics of schizophrenia. Biol Psychiatry 2001;50:825–844.

6. Lewis DA: Is there a neuropathology of schizophrenia? Neuroscientist 2000;6:208–218.

7. Selemon LD, Goldman-Rakic PS: The reduced neuropil hypothesis: A circuit based model of schizophrenia. Biol Psychiatry 1999;45:17–25.

8. Mirnics K, Middleton FA, Lewis DA, Levitt P: Analysis of complex brain disorders with gene expression microarrays: Schizophrenia as a disease of the synapse. Trends Neurosci 2001;24:479–486.

9. Middleton FA, Mirnics K, Pierri JN, et al: Gene expression profiling reveals alterations of specific metabolic pathways in schizophrenia. J Neurosci 2002;22: 2718–2729.

10. Lewis DA, Pierri JN, Volk DW, et al: Altered GABA neurotransmission and prefrontal cortical dysfunction in schizophrenia. Biol Psychiatry 1999;46: 616–626.

11. Benes FM, Berretta S: GABAergic interneurons: Implications for understanding schizophrenia and bipolar disorder. Neuropsychopharm 2001;25:1–27.

12. Volk DW, Pierri JN, Fritschy JM, et al: Reciprocal alterations in pre- and postsynaptic inhibitory markers at chandelier cell inputs to pyramidal neurons in schizophrenia. Cerebral Cortex 2002;12:1063–1070.

13. Reynolds GP, Zhang ZJ, Beasley CL: Neurochemical correlates of cortical GABAergic deficits in schizophrenia: Selective losses of calcium binding protein immunoreactivity. Brain Res Bull 2001;55:579–584.

14. Costa E, Davis J, Grayson DR, et al: Dendritic spine hypoplasticity and downregulation of reelin and GABAergic tone in schizophrenia vulnerability. Neurobiol Dis 2001;8:723–742.

15. Goff DC, Coyle JT: The emerging role of glutamate in the pathophysiology and treatment of schizophrenia. Am J Psychiatr 2001;158:1367–1377.

16. Jentsch JD, Roth RH. The neuropsychopharmacology of phencyclidine: From NMDA receptor hypofunction to the dopamine hypothesis of schizophrenia. Neuropsychopharm 1999;20:201–225.

17. Olney JW, Farber NB: Glutamate receptor dysfunction and schizophrenia. Arch Gen Psychiatry 1995;52:998–1007.

18. Riley BP, McGuffin P: Linkage and associated studies of schizophrenia. Am J Med Genet 2000;97: 23–44.

19. Braff DL, Geyer MA: Sensorimotor gating and the neurobiology of schizophrenia: Human and animal model studies. In Schulz SC, Tamminga CA (eds): Schizophrenia: Scientific Progress. New York, Oxford University Press, 1989.

20. Freedman R, Leonard S, Gault JM, et al: Linkage disequilibrium for schizophrenia at the chromosome 15q13-14 locus of the α7-nicotinic acetylcholine receptor subunit gene (CHRNA7). Am J Med Genet 2001;105:20–22.

21. Weiland S, Bertrand D, Leonard S: Neuronal nicotinic acetylcholine receptors: From the gene to the disease. Behav Brain Res 2000;113:43–56.

22. Mirnics K, Middleton FA, Stanwood GD, et al: Disease-specific changes in regulator of G-protein signaling 4 (RGS4) expression in schizophrenia. Mol Psychiatry 2001;6:293–301.

23. Brzustowicz LM, Hodgkinson KA, Chow EWC, et al: Location of a major susceptibility locus for familial schizophrenia on chromosome 1q21-q22. Science 2000;288:678–682.

24. Chowdari KV, Mirnics K, Semwal P, et al: Association and linkage analyses of RGS4 polymorphisms in schizophrenia. Hum Mol Gen 2002;11: 1373–1380.

25. Meyer J, Huberth A, Ortega G, et al: A missense mutation in a novel gene encoding a putative cation channel is associated with catatonic schizophrenia in a large pedigree. Mol Psychiatry 2001;6:302–306.

CHAPTER 74

Obsessive-Compulsive Disorder and Tourette Syndrome

Paul J. Lombroso

Marcos T. Mercadante

Larry Scahill

Obsessive-compulsive disorder (OCD) is a heterogeneous disorder. The best-studied subgroup of OCD consists of OCD patients with Tourette syndrome (TS). Although the co-occurrence of TS and OCD has been noted since their earliest description, multiple lines or research since the 1980s suggest that some forms of OCD are etiologically related to TS.[1,2] The etiologic relationship between TS and OCD has emerged through the combined efforts of epidemiologists, geneticists, clinical trial researchers, experts in the neural pathways that connect the cortex with the basal ganglia, and neuroimmunologists interested in brain-based autoimmune phenomena. Although considerable effort has been devoted to isolating the genes associated with TS and OCD, none have been found to date. Earlier work suggests that TS is caused by alterations at a single autosomal locus, but the underlying genetics now appear to be more complex. This chapter presents a summary of the current state of knowledge concerning the relationship between OCD and TS and their etiology.

CLINICAL FEATURES

OCD is characterized by recurrent and intrusive thoughts or images (obsessions) that are usually accompanied by intentional repetitive behaviors (compulsions). The compulsions are often performed to relieve the obsessional worry or the anxiety caused by the obsessions. In order to meet the current diagnostic criteria for OCD (DSM-IV), the obsessions or compulsions, or both, must be time consuming and cause marked distress.

This clinical presentation has been the basis for the classification of OCD as an anxiety disorder. Authors have proposed a dimensional approach to classifying OCD subtypes as defined by factor analysis.[3] These include (1) aggression and checking, (2) symmetry and ordering/arranging, (3) contamination and cleaning, and (4) hoarding. In addition, a subgroup of OCD patients perform compulsions in response to sudden urges or tactile sensations. Unlike the classic obsessive-compulsive sequence associated with many OCD patients in whom mounting anxiety is punctuated by the repetitive behavior, these patients report that their behaviors are driven by the need to achieve a sense of completeness or a "just right" feeling.[2]

It may be useful to conceptualize OCD as a spectrum of disorders from obsessions with no accompanying behaviors to compulsions with few accompanying thoughts. It is noteworthy that in children, the onset of compulsions often precedes the onset of obsessions.[4] In addition, a greater prevalence of tics and tic-like compulsions in early-onset OCD patients has been reported. The term *tic-like compulsions* refers to touching, tapping, rubbing, blinking, and staring rituals. These tic-like compulsions are more common in OCD patients with a history of tics. In some cases, these tic-like compulsions may be difficult to distinguish from complex tics. In other cases, however, it is clear that these repetitive habits are performed to relieve the distress caused by an obsession rather than prompted by a perceptional urge.[2]

Tic disorders are characterized by sudden, repetitive movements or vocalizations that are similar to some aspects of normal behavior. They are classified with respect to their type (motor or phonic), and their duration (transient or chronic). Approximately 10% to 12% of children have transient tics. By convention, the diagnosis of a transient tic disorder is used when tics are present for less than 12 months. Tics that persist beyond 12 months are classified as chronic tic disorder. If both motor and phonic tics are present for more than 12 months, the disorder is known as Tourette syndrome. Chronic tic disorders may be as common as 4% in children of school age, whereas TS occurs in an estimated 1 to 3 per 1000 children.[5]

Tic disorders typically begin in childhood with a mean age of onset at 7 years. Symptoms vary from one individual to the next and within the same individual over time. In many cases, tics begin with eye blinking or facial movements and progress to involve additional muscles of the face, neck, and shoulders. Phonic tics usually begin 1 to 2 years after the motor tics and consist of throat clearing, grunting, or repetitive sniffling. More complex vocalizations, including swearing (coprolalia), echolalia, and the utterance of nonsense syllables, do not occur in all cases. These more dramatic vocalizations occur in fewer than 25% of patients. There has been an appreciation for sensory phenomena that typically precede tics. These *auras* are described variously as an itch, pressure, or an urge, and some patients describe this experience as intermediate between voluntary and involuntary. Although they are not able to refrain from performing the tic, some patients describe a sense of giving in to the urge to relieve the sensation.

Most individuals with TS report that their tics vary over time and that they occur in bouts. The worst period for many patients is the first decade after the illness begins, with the majority reporting a significant reduction in symptoms as they pass through adolescence. Nonetheless, a substantial minority of patients are chronically disabled with paroxysms of tics that continue into adulthood.[6]

A hallmark of TS is that tic symptoms often increase in frequency and intensity during periods of fatigue or stress. Lifetime tic severity may also be influenced by perinatal exposures that presumably exert a negative influence on early brain development. Other environmental exposures that may influence the severity of tics include stimulant medications, steroids, and (proposed), recurrent infections. These observations have led researchers to consider a stress-diathesis model for TS in which the interaction of inherited genetic vulnerability factors with cumulative environmental stressors during critical periods of brain development lead to the severity of the illness.[7]

Clinically ascertained cases of TS are associated with a variety of other disorders. For example, more than 60% of patients referred to clinicians have problems with inattention, impulsiveness, and hyperactivity. These children may warrant a separate diagnosis of attention deficit with hyperactivity disorder (ADHD). As many as 30% of individuals with TS have sufficiently severe obsessive-compulsive symptoms to warrant an additional diagnosis of OCD. Well over 50% of patients, however, describe some obsessive-compulsive symptoms that do not meet diagnostic criteria for OCD. Several studies report high rates of aggressiveness, depression, learning disabilities,

and anxiety disorders in TS probands. Some researchers have wondered if these clinically referred cases reflect an ascertainment bias in that children with more that one illness are often referred to clinics for assessment and treatment. Surveys in community samples, however, have also observed a higher frequency of ADHD among children with TS than is normally seen in the community.[5]

NEURAL PATHWAYS

The basal ganglia are a group of forebrain structures that serve as a way station for neural pathways projecting from the cerebral cortex to the thalamus and back to the cortex. These parallel pathways appear to be somatotopically organized and minimally overlapping as they interconnect cortex, basal ganglia, globus pallidus, substantia nigra, and thalamus. They carry neural signals related to motor, somatosensory, cognitive, and emotional functions. Current understanding of the pathophysiology of TS and OCD suggests that a disruption of one or more of these pathways at any level disrupts the entire loop. Moreover, it has been proposed that the types of symptoms expressed depend on where and how the disruption occurs.

The striatum, composed of the caudate nucleus and putamen, is a functional subdivision of the basal ganglia (Fig. 74–1). It receives excitatory glutamatergic input from virtually all regions of the cortex. The input from

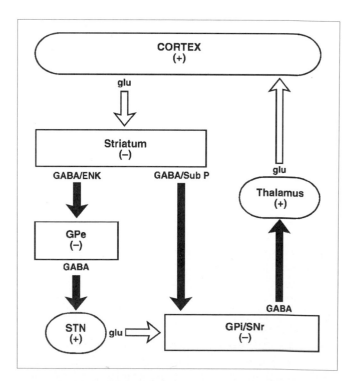

FIGURE 74–1. Simplified diagram of circuitry within the basal ganglia. Excitatory pathways are indicated by the *open arrows*, and inhibitory pathways are indicated by the *filled arrows* (see text for details).

the cortex is topographically organized, and the vast majority of striatal neurons (the medium spiny neurons) have large dendritic arborizations that probably permit some overlap in the cortical inputs. In addition to this excitatory projection from cortex, the striatum receives major dopaminergic input from the substantia nigra pars compacta.

The glutamatergic and dopaminergic inputs converge on the spines of the medium spiny neurons. Glutamatergic synapses from the cortex make synaptic contact on the tips of these spines, whereas the dopaminergic synapses from the substantia nigra make contact with spine shafts. The close proximity of the two synaptic inputs suggests a functional relationship, and there is considerable evidence that the dopamine input is able to modulate the excitatory glutamatergic input from the cortex.

The consensus is that the primary function of the striatum is to integrate the excitatory projections from a variety of cortical areas and modulate the excitatory outputs of the thalamus back to the cortex. Modulation of the thalamus is thought to occur through two pathways, one direct and one indirect (see Fig. 74–1). The direct pathway consists of the inhibitory GABAergic pathways from the striatum to the medial globus pallidus which, when activated, tend to promote thalamic excitatory output to the cortex. This occurs as the striatum reduces the GABAergic inhibitory projections from the globus pallidus internal segment and from the substantia nigra pars reticulata to the thalamus.

Through an indirect pathway, the striatum diminishes the excitatory output from thalamic projections to the cortex. The subthalamic nucleus provides excitatory glutamatergic projection to the globus pallidus internal segmental and substantia nigra pars reticulata. Increased activity of the subthalamic nucleus increases the excitatory input to the globus pallidus and substantia nigra pars reticulata. The latter two nuclei are thereby activated and reduce excitatory thalamic output to the cortex. In summary, the direct pathway promotes excitatory output to "drive" the cortex, whereas the indirect pathway has the opposite effect on the cortex.

Immunocytochemical analyses reveal additional levels of striatal organization. The striatum is composed of two compartments that are differentiated by specific neurochemical markers such as acetylcholinesterase. Acetylcholinesterase staining reveals patch-like areas of lighter staining, called *striosomes*, within more heavily stained regions called the *matrix*. These two compartments receive distinctive synaptic projections. In primates, the striosomes receive synaptic input primarily from the orbitofrontal and cingulate cortex, as well as from the basolateral nucleus of the amygdala. Many of the sensory, motor, and associative areas of the neocortex project primarily to neurons of the matrix. Thus, the matrix receives synaptic input from a larger area of the cortex than do the striosomes. The output pathways are

also distinct. The striosomes project to the substantia nigra pars compacta via an inhibitory, GABAergic pathway. The matrix projects to the globus pallidus and the substantia nigra pars reticulata via direct and indirect pathways. Over 95% of striatal projection neurons originate in medium-sized spiny neurons that can be subdivided according the neuropeptides they contain (e.g., enkephalin, substance P).[8]

Mink[9] suggested a model of normal basal ganglia function that is useful in understanding the pathophysiology of TS. The model proposes that tonically active inhibitory outputs emerging from the basal ganglia act as a brake on motor pattern generators in the cortex and brain stem. When an individual wants to make a particular movement, two events must occur. A specific movement or motor pattern emerges from the basal ganglia output neurons and projects to competing motor pattern generators to increase their firing rate and thereby apply a higher degree of inhibition on these competing movement patterns. At the same time, other basal ganglia output neurons that are part of the desired motor pattern generator decrease their firing rate, removing the tonic inhibition of those neurons and releasing the brake for the desired movement. Movement initiation is thereby enabled, whereas other unwanted movements are inhibited. The projections of the striatum to globus pallidus internal segment and substantia nigra pars reticulata form the electrophysiologic basis for activation of specific neurons in a central region while surrounding neurons are inhibited. This center-surround pattern is maintained in the thalamus and in the thalamocortical excitatory projections.

According to this model, the pathophysiology of TS is due to inappropriate activation of neurons in the striatum, which leads to failed inhibition of a specific neuron in the globus pallidus. This abnormal inhibition leads to activation of discrete thalamic neurons and activation of their cortical targets. The resulting unwanted motor patterns lead to tics and possibly compulsive behaviors. The model is consistent with the notion that repetitive symptoms in TS and OCD result from an impairment in the inhibitory control of cortico-striatal-thalamo-cortical loops.

NEUROIMAGING

In vivo neuroimaging studies such as functional MRI (fMRI), positron emission tomography (PET), and single positron emission computerized tomography (SPECT) have also been used to determine whether alterations can be found in cortico-striato-thalamo-cortical circuits in these disorders. Functional MRI studies evaluate metabolic differences in brain following the completion of a mental operation. Neuroimaging techniques have been applied to the study of OCD in both children and adults since the 1990s. Structural imaging studies, though not uniform in their findings, suggest greater volumes in the orbitofrontal cortex. One pediatric study showed enlarged anterior cingulate volumes in OCD patients when compared with controls. By contrast, this structural difference has not been observed in adult OCD patients.

Beginning with the work of Baxter and colleagues, significant functional differences in cortico-striato-thalamo-cortical and limbic circuits have been found in several studies. Decreased metabolic activity in caudate, orbitofrontal cortex, and anterior cingulate following successful treatment with an SSRI or cognitive-behavioral therapy has been replicated by several investigators further supporting the role of these pathways.[10] Investigators have also used PET or fMRI techniques during symptom provocation paradigms to evaluate areas of activation associated with OCD. These studies consistently show increased metabolic activity in orbitofrontal cortex, right caudate, and anterior cingulate, again implicating failed inhibition of cognitive and sensory stimuli in cortico-striato-thalamo-cortical and limbic systems in the pathophysiology of OCD.[11]

Some investigators are using functional imaging techniques with OCD subjects performing specific cognitive tasks that rely on cortico-striato-thalamo-cortical pathways. In a series of investigations, Rauch and colleagues have shown that OCD patients show deficient right striatal activation during the performance of a sequential learning task when compared with controls.[11] The task involves measurement of reaction time to visual cues presented in an undisclosed pattern while the subject is in the scanner. To the extent that the subject learns the pattern, reaction time will improve. This sort of implicit learning has been shown to rely on right-sided cortico-striato-thalamo-cortical pathways. The relative absence of right striatal activation in OCD patients when compared with controls confirms a role of these parallel circuits in OCD and provides a model for future investigation.

The pathophysiology of TS has long been presumed to involve anatomic and functional disturbances of the basal ganglia. This presumption is based on clinical observations in TS (e.g., the effectiveness of D2 blockers for the treatment of tics) and preclinical studies on basal ganglia function. Neuroimaging studies in TS samples support the presence of abnormal basal ganglia morphology in TS, but the findings have not been consistent. This failure to replicate specific findings is probably due to sample differences and small samples in these studies. Basal ganglia volumes were measured on high resolution magnetic resonance images acquired in 154 TS and 130 healthy children and adults. Repeated measures analyses tested hypotheses concerning regional specificity, age effects, and abnormal asymmetries in the TS basal ganglia. In contrast to earlier reports, the caudate nucleus volumes were significantly smaller in both TS children and adults. Lenticular nucleus volumes also were smaller in TS adults and in TS children, but this was true only of those individuals with a diagnosis of comorbid OCD. Moreover, regional volumes did not correlate significantly with the severity of tic, OCD, or ADHD symptoms.[12]

In a separate analysis of the same data set, Peterson found that TS subjects have larger volumes in prefrontal and parieto-occipital cortical regions, and smaller inferior occipital volumes.[13] The increased orbitofrontal and parieto-occipital cerebral volumes were significantly associated with tic severity in adults but not in children, suggesting potential age differences. Taken together, the findings from these studies support the presumed disturbance in cortico-striato-thalamo-cortical circuitry; however, age effects require additional study.

Functional neuroimaging studies of subjects with TS have also supported a model that suggests alterations in these circuits.[13] Most studies included only adults. Sample sizes are generally small, ranging from 3 to 20 TS patients with similar number of controls. Perhaps because of the small sample sizes, several of these studies found no difference in D2 receptor systems in TS patients when compared with controls. Others identified increases in the number of DA transporter, perhaps reflecting a compensatory response to heightened synaptic dopamine levels, or increased postsynaptic D2 receptor density, which would be consistent with the supersensitivity model of TS.

In a study of tic suppression in adults with TS, there were significant changes in metabolic activity in the basal ganglia and thalamus and in anatomically connected cortical regions. Of interest in this study was that the increase in metabolic activity in the right caudate and decreased activity in related subcortical regions during active tic suppression was negatively correlated with tic severity. As tic severity increased, these signal changes decreased, suggesting that tics are caused by failure of inhibitory systems.[12]

NEUROCHEMISTRY

A large body of evidence suggests the involvement of a complex neurotransmitter network in the pathophysiology of OCD. The major neurotransmitters studied include serotonin, dopamine, glutamate, and gamma-amino butyric acid (GABA). Substantial evidence supports the role of serotonin in the pathophysiology of OCD. Both the frontal cortex and the basal ganglia are rich in serotonin (5-HT) receptors, and compared with other antidepressant agents selective serotonin reuptake inhibitors (SSRI) are the best treatment for OCD. It is still unclear whether improvement with SSRIs is due to direct action on the serotonin pathways or the downstream effects of serotonin on other neurotransmitter systems. Given that as many as 30% to 40% of OCD patients show partial or no response to these drugs, serotonin reuptake blockade is probably not the only mechanism involved in OCD.

It has been suggested that the anti-obsessive effects of these drugs are distinct from their antidepressant effects. Some researchers contend that the antidepressive effects of SSRIs are associated with desensitization at the terminal serotonin autoreceptors in the frontal cortex, which occurs approximately 3 weeks after SSRIs are initiated. By contrast, the impact on the orbito-frontal cortex may take up to 8 weeks and is thought to be related to relief of the OCD symptoms.[14]

Support for disturbances in the dopamine pathways in TS is based on the evidence that D2 receptor antagonists can suppress tics. The dopamine hypothesis for TS proposes a relative increase in dopamine transmission in TS patients. This may be due to an increased number of postsynaptic dopamine receptors, an increase in the affinity of these receptors for dopamine, or an abnormality in presynaptic function that leads to excessive phasic release of dopamine.[15] TS-related abnormalities in other neurotransmitter systems have been suggested. Noradrenergic and GABAergic systems in TS have been implicated because of the therapeutic effects of α2-adrenergic agonists and the benzodiazepines, although the latter class of medications shows only modest effects on tics.[16] The role for the opioid system is suggested by postmortem immunohistochemical findings showing a decrease in dynorphin within the striatum of TS patients, but this finding has yet to be replicated.

The evidence for an abnormality in dopamine pathways is the most persuasive. The vast majority of TS patients respond dramatically to agents that block dopamine D2 receptors. Up to 80% of patients taking these drugs report a clinically meaningful improvement in tic symptoms. Moreover, tics may worsen on exposure to stimulants, which are known to increase central dopaminergic activity. Withdrawal from neuroleptic treatment is often difficult to accomplish because tic symptoms rebound. This rebound is presumably due to heightened receptor sensitivity and/or up-regulation of postsynaptic DA receptors. Additional support for the involvement of dopamine comes from studies showing elevated levels of homovanillic acid, a major breakdown product of dopamine, in the cerebrospinal fluid of TS subjects compared with normal controls.[17]

Taken together, these studies suggest that TS is associated with a relative dopaminergic imbalance arising from an excessive amount of dopamine release, oversensitive dopamine receptors, or a poorly functioning reuptake system, but these are unlikely to be complete explanations. For example, a similar argument has been proposed for the etiology of schizophrenia, where the therapeutic response of postsynaptic dopamine blockers and the aggravation of symptoms with psychostimulants are well documented. However, the positive response to clozapine, a drug with minimal D2 blockade, in schizophrenia indicates that the dopamine hypothesis is incomplete for schizophrenia and may be for TS as well.

The dopamine hypothesis can be examined with PET. An increase in affinity or numbers of postsynaptic dopamine receptors in TS patients would be associated with an increase in binding to radioactive ligands. Several studies have found no differences in dopamine receptor bindings among TS subjects, whereas a study among monozygotic twins discordant for tic symptoms found an increase in dopamine receptor binding in the more severely affected twin.[17]

GENETICS

Family studies are often the first step when investigating whether a particular disorder has a higher frequency among family members than the general population. These types of analyses look for genetic and environmental factors that may contribute to the expression of an illness. Twin studies are a form of family analysis that attempts to tease apart the contribution of genetic and environmental factors in vulnerable individuals. These studies take advantage of the fact that monozygotic twins are genetically identical and, when reared together, share nearly identical environments. Dizygotic twins, in contrast, share approximately 50% of their genes, while also sharing nearly identical environments. One can predict that if an illness is completely dependent on genetic factors, then monozygotic twins will have a concordance of 100%, whereas dizygotic twins will have a significantly lower concordance. Genetic studies among OCD and TS subjects suggest that both genetic and environmental factors play a critical role in the etiology and expression of symptoms.

Twin studies of OCD patients demonstrate a higher concordance among monozygotic (75%) compared with dizygotic (30%) pairs. A large study of OCD patients and their families indicates that some forms of OCD are familial and associated with tics, some forms are familial and not related to tics, and still other forms are not related to tics and do not appear to be familial.[18] Considering the heterogeneous character of OCD, researchers expected a polygenic model. However, segregation analyses of a large sample of OCD proband families suggest that a major gene is involved in the pathophysiology of OCD and that a mendelian-dominant model can explain its inheritance.[19] In another study, OCD phenotypes were defined by factor analysis and reported a single major gene of effect for the factor consisting of symmetry and ordering compulsions. Interestingly, the need for symmetry and ordering compulsions are more common in tic-related forms of OCD. This study, which compared OCD subjects with controls, rejected a polygenic model in the segregation analysis after probands were reclassified according to OCD symptom factor scores.[3]

Linkage analysis is the next step in isolating genes that contribute to symptoms in these disorders. Unfortunately, these techniques, which have been used successfully to isolate a large number of genes responsible for various neurologic disorders, have proved much less successful for psychiatric disorders such as OCD. In the case of TS, studies using traditional linkage strategies have excluded the involvement of over 80% of the genome. This failure suggests that several genes might be involved in the expression of OCD, because traditional linkage studies are known to become less informative when more than one gene is involved.

Candidate genes have been examined in association studies, where a number of affected individuals in a single family are typed for specific gene variants. Obvious choices for candidate genes include those involved in the neurotransmitter pathways associated with the basal ganglia. This would include genes that encode enzymes that produce or metabolize monoamines, genes that code for receptor proteins, and genes associated with specific neurotransmitter compartments, such as the monoamine transporters.

One candidate gene that is potentially associated with OCD is the gene for catechol-O-methyltransferase (COMT). A functional polymorphism in the coding region of the COMT gene may be associated with OCD probands, especially in males, although this finding has not been confirmed.[20] Another candidate gene is monoamine oxidase A. Polymorphisms for this gene are associated with different levels of enzymatic activity.[21] A candidate gene for early-onset OCD encodes a glutamate transporter. This gene, however, showed no functional mutations in families of seven OCD probands included in the genome scan by Veenstra-VanderWeele and colleagues.[22]

The original description of TS included a familial pattern of expression. More systematic family studies published in the late 1970s described an increase in the frequency of tic disorders in the first degree relatives of TS subjects. The rate of TS among relatives of TS probands is between 10% and 15%, approximately 10-fold higher than the rate found in the general population. Pauls suggests that OCD is part of the TS spectrum of disorders because in families harboring a vulnerability gene, males were more likely to express TS and females were more likely to develop OCD.[23]

Twin studies showed a significant difference in the concordance for monozygotic (90%) and dizygotic twins (20%). Environmental factors contribute to some degree, as the concordance is not 100% for monozygotic twins. Examination of medical records showed lower birth weights among affected co-twins in monozygotic twins discordant for tic symptoms, suggesting that prenatal factors might contribute to the expression of symptoms later in life. In another series of concordant monozygotic twins, the more severely affected co-twin had lower birth weight.[23]

Segregation analyses indicate that the tendency to inherit TS and chronic motor tics is transmitted vertically as a single gene of major effect. Indeed, the data in some studies are consistent with an autosomal dominant locus with sex-specific penetrance. Other researchers, however, were unable to reject a multifactorial or polygenic model, suggesting that TS is the result of multiple genes acting together. Additional studies have provided evidence for a mixed model, as well as an intermediate, model, of inheritance. It is likely that the differing models reflect differences in ascertainment, data collection methods (e.g., from direct interviews of all family members versus obtaining family history from a single informant), and the different assumptions were made during data analyses.[17]

A systematic linkage study of the entire human chromosome has begun in several laboratories using highly polymorphic markers. To date, over 80% of the human genome has been excluded. These studies assume that the same gene is involved in TS in all the families being studied. As with OCD, however, genetic heterogeneity within these pedigrees would make it very difficult, if not impossible, to localize a gene using traditional linkage analysis techniques.

Several additional strategies have been used to deal with the technical difficulties associated with genetic heterogeneity. One has been the analysis of families in which a specific chromosomal abnormality is found in an affected proband with TS. Several translocations have been described on chromosome 18, and additional karyotypes of other probands point to abnormalities on chromosomes 9 and 22. Investigators are now attempting to determine whether gene(s) at the translocation site have been disrupted as a result of the chromosomal rearrangements.

Given the difficulty of localizing TS genes with traditional linkage approaches, family-based association strategies have also been used, with a number of genes relating to neurotransmitters implicated in the etiology of TS. These include the various dopamine receptors, the dopamine transporter, dopamine β-hydroxylase, prodynorphin, pro-opiomelanocortin, tyrosine hydroxylase, gastrin-releasing peptide, and the serotonin receptor gene. Surprisingly, each of these loci has been excluded as the gene conferring susceptibility for TS.[23]

The Tourette Syndrome Association International Consortium on Genetics, a worldwide consortium of researchers, focused on the genetics of TS, and adopted the sib-pair method to investigate genetic linkage in TS. In this method, investigators attempt to identify shared genes in a large sample of affected siblings. Such studies in TS show that chromosomes 4 and 8 have high maximum likelihood scores in multipoint analyses. An earlier family study of TS probands in an isolated South African population found an association between TS and markers on chromosomes 11, 14, 20, and 21. Unfortunately, none of the regions identified overlapped with the regions of interest in the sib-pair genome scan.[23] A third genome scan using multigenerational TS families showed a significant tendency for linkage with regions on chromosome 19, and these regions were also found to be positive in the sib-pair study, although the magnitude of the association was lower than for the regions on chromosomes 4 and 8.

ANIMAL MODELS

An animal model of OCD or TS would be of considerable value. With this tool, researchers could examine environmental and genetic interactions, confirm neurologic substrates, and search for more effective medical treatments. This effort has largely been limited to animals exhibiting repetitive behaviors. A quinpirole rat preparation has been suggested as a model for checking behaviors, because rats exposed to this dopamine agonist perform considerably more checking than normal rats.[24] In addition, the acral lick dermatitis model, a self-injurious grooming behavior found in dogs, has been proposed as a good animal model for OCD. The strongest evidence for this comes from the amelioration of symptoms after SSRI treatment.[25] However, due to the difficulties in analyzing the meaning of these animal behaviors, these models continue to remain controversial. Furthermore, repetitive behavior models may be better suited for TS than OCD.

More promising animal models for TS have emerged. Administering drugs that activate the dopamine pathways can promote repetitive behaviors called *stereotypies*. Amphetamine, apomorphine, and cocaine are the drugs most commonly used in this model. Such drugs promote the release of dopamine into the synapse and block the dopamine reuptake at the presynaptic terminal. At low doses, rodents increase locomotor activity. As the dosage is increased, stereotypies emerge. Although all of these drugs enhance dopamine function in striatum, the mechanism of action differs slightly. Stereotypies induced through these dopaminergic mechanisms appear to require an intact nigrostriatal pathway because lesions in this pathway, or the administration of neuroleptic medications that functionally block dopamine in the striatum, attenuate the production of stimulant-induced stereotypies.

Psychostimulants and apomorphine lead to a robust induction of immediate early genes (IEGs) in striatal neurons that are believed to participate in the movement-enhancing direct pathway. IEGs are transcription factors that regulate the expression of other genes. The proteins encoded by these genes are necessary for responding appropriately to the incoming signal. Immunohistochemical studies indicate that stimulants produce a predictable pattern of gene induction within the two striatal compartments. IEG induction, however, is more prominent in neurons within striosomes compared with neurons in the matrix. Moreover, the relative amount of IEG induction in the two compartments is the best predictor of the degree of stereotypy caused by amphetamine, apomorphine, or cocaine. Despite the differences in mechanism of action, all three drugs induce stereotypies and all three drugs produce IEG induction in a greater striosome-to-matrix pattern. These gene induction patterns appear to reflect the activity of neurons in the cortico-striatal circuit and imply that an imbalance of activity in neurons within the striosome versus the matrix is responsible for the observed repetitive movements.[26] It would be of interest to determine the patterns of IEG induction in neurons that lie on a single pathway of the cortico-striatal-thalamo-cortical loops.

A new animal model is based on the proposed autoimmune hypothesis. The autoimmune hypothesis emerged following the observation of increased prevalence of OCD in Sydenham chorea patients, which is a late manifestation of rheumatic fever associated with an earlier streptococcal infection. When an epidemic of streptococcal pharyngitis occurred in Providence, Rhode Island, tic disorders increased among affected children. Swedo and colleagues then proposed the existence of a subgroup of children with tics or OCD, or both, now known by its acronym PANDAS.[27] Pediatric autoimmune neuropsychiatric disorder associated with streptococcal infections is defined by the following five criteria: (1) the presence of a tic disorder and/or OCD consistent with DSM-IV; (2) prepubertal onset of neuropsychiatric symptoms; (3) history of a sudden onset of symptoms and/or an episodic course with abrupt symptom exacerbation interspersed with periods of partial or complete remission; (4) evidence of a temporal association between onset or exacerbation of symptoms and a streptococcal infection; and (5) adventitious movements (e.g., motoric hyperactivity and choreiform movements) during symptom exacerbation.

The proposed pathophysiology in this subgroup of patients is based on the molecular mimicry hypothesis, which suggests that vulnerable individuals respond to streptococcal infections in the normal fashion by producing antibodies to fight the infection. However, the antibodies then cross-react with previously unaffected tissues in the host causing neurologic damage. This model suggests that neuronal function is compromised when epitopes within the CNS are recognized by autoantibodies in a manner analogous to the sequence of events proposed for Sydenham chorea. Evidence for this hypothesis comes from a single study demonstrating dramatic therapeutic benefit in TS and/or OCD patients treated with plasmapheresis. Several other laboratories have now shown evidence for autoantibodies in the blood serum of a subgroup of TS and OCD patients.[17]

Studies from two independent laboratories have demonstrated that stereotypies can be induced in rodents by infusing their striatum with serum from affected individuals with high levels of antineural autoantibodies. These studies show that stereotypies are not induced after infusing serum from normal controls or from TS patients with low levels of antineural autoantibodies (Fig. 74–2). Because a third laboratory was unable to reproduce these results, additional research is necessary to determine whether autoantibodies, in fact, play a role in some cases of TS and OCD.[17]

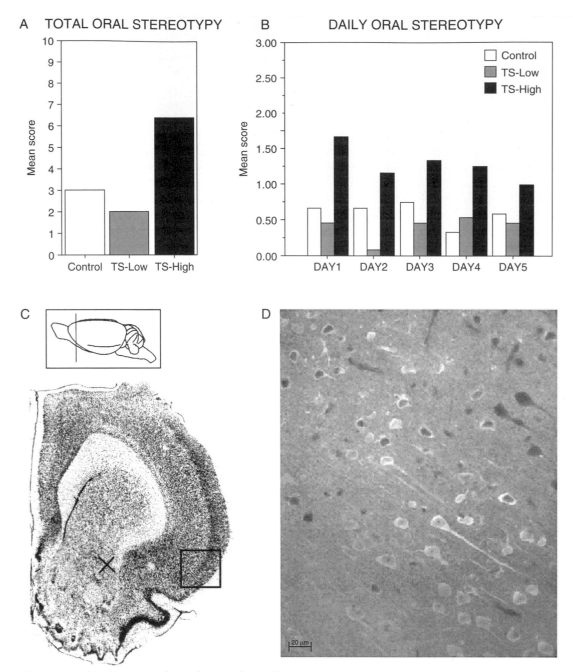

FIGURE 74–2. Induction of stereotypies after infusion of sera from TS patients into the ventrolateral striatum of rats. Sera were selected for the presence of either high or low levels of autoantibodies as determined by antineural immunofluorescence patterns on rat striatal cryostat sections. Three groups were tested: a control, a TS group with low autoantibody levels, and a TS group with high levels of autoantibodies. Total oral stereotypies *(A)* or daily oral stereotypy scores more than 5 days *(B)* are shown. The site for the infusion of sera is indicated by the *X* in *C*. A representative example of the neural immunofluorescence pattern from a nearby cortical region, (indicated by the box in *C*), is shown in *D*. (Adapted with permission from Taylor JR, Morshed S, Parveen S, et al: An animal model of Tourette's syndrome. Am J Psychiatry 2002;159:657–660.)

THERAPY

Pharmacologic and Other Treatments for OCD.
Current pharmacologic treatments, particularly the serotonin reuptake inhibitors, alleviate OCD symptoms in most, but not all, OCD patients. Cognitive-behavior therapy (CBT) based on exposure and response preven-tion is the psychological treatment of choice. In pediatric patients, family members are often involved in the patient's rituals, thus family education is an essential component of the treatment plan. Family and patient organizations can provide valuable education and support for OCD patients and their families.

The introduction of serotonin reuptake inhibitors, such as clomipramine and, later, the selective serotonin reuptake inhibitors (SSRIs) was an important advance in pharmacologic treatment for OCD. A series of clinical trials in both children and adults showed conclusively that clomipramine was not only superior to placebo, it was also superior to desipramine, a drug in the same chemical class that is devoid of serotonin reuptake properties. Since the introduction of clomipramine, even more specific serotonin reuptake inhibitors have been released. Although these drugs are a tremendous advance, only about 60% of the OCD patients treated with SSRIs show a positive response, suggesting that systems in addition to serotonin pathways are involved in the pathophysiology.

Several additional SSRIs are now available, including fluoxetine, fluvoxamine, sertraline, paroxetine, and citalopram. Of these, all but citalopram have been evaluated in placebo-controlled studies in children. The SSRIs have several features in common, permitting a few similar treatment guidelines. First, albeit with some variation, these drugs have relatively long half-lives. Thus, the dosing should move up gradually to avoid over shooting the optimal dose. Second, again to varying degrees, each of these drugs is subject to drug-drug interactions. For example, fluoxetine and paroxetine are potent inhibitors of the 2D6 pathway in the liver. Combined use of fluoxetine with a drug that relies on the 2D6 pathway, such as risperidone, will effectively increase the dose of the second drug. Third, these drugs appear to produce similar results. For example, placebo-controlled studies in children show only a 25% to 30% difference over placebo. Fourth, each of these drugs has a relatively long time to take effect, such that an adequate trial may take 8 to 10 weeks. In view of these considerations, clinicians should educate patients and families about appropriate expectations for pharmacotherapy.

To date, no studies have shown dramatic differences in the efficacy of various SSRIs, but one meta-analysis suggests that clomipramine is the most effective serotonin-reuptake inhibitor for OCD (Table 74–1).[28] Clomipramine requires close clinical supervision due to its wide spectrum of side effects, and the need for periodic electrocardiograph examinations and drug level moni-

toring. The usual dose begins at 25 mg or 50 mg a day, with gradual increases up to a maximum of 200 mg/d in children and 300 mg/d in adults. A single dose should not be higher than 150 mg. Clomipramine is also vulnerable to drug-drug interactions. For example, inhibition of the cytochrome P450 (CYP3A4) by erythromycin can result in toxic levels of clomipramine. By contrast, the SSRIs do not require routine ECGs or serum drug levels. Common side effects of the SSRIs include gastrointestinal complaints, sexual dysfunction, sedation, and behavioral activation. Behavioral activation induced by SSRIs appears to be especially common in children. The serotonergic syndrome, which includes hypertension, hyperthermia, myoclonus, and changes in mental status, is rare. This risk increases dramatically if the SSRIs are given in combination with monoamine oxidase inhibitors.

Given the percentage of patients who do not respond to serotonin-reuptake inhibitor agents, additional strategies for refractory cases are of great interest. Augmenting SSRIs has been attempted with a number of drugs, but few have been successful. To date, only haloperidol and risperidone have been shown to be effective in placebo-controlled studies when added to an SSRI in refractory OCD. In both of these studies, patients were randomly assigned to receive placebo or the antipsychotic medication in addition to ongoing SSRI treatment. In some of the severe and refractory cases, neurosurgical procedures such as cingulotomy has been proposed, following failure with all other treatment modalities including behavioral, family, and pharmacologic therapies.

Pharmacologic Treatments for TS. Several medications have been used for the treatment of tics, but only a few have been adequately tested in placebo-controlled studies.[16] The goal of treatment is to achieve a balance between adequate tic control and minimizing side effects, rather than tic eradication.

Two neuroleptics have been considered the most effective medications. Haloperidol and pimozide have been compared in several studies. In general, it has been found that the efficacy of both drugs is similar, although haloperidol has been associated with a higher frequency of side effects. Given its potency as a postsynaptic D2

TABLE 74–1. Dose Range, Half-Life, and Metabolic Pathways of Serotonin Reuptake Inhibitors

Drug	Starting Dose	Dose Range (mg)	Half-Life	Primary Enzymatic Pathway	Enzymatic Inhibition
Clomipramine	25	50–300	32 hours	CYP2D6, CYP2C19	None
Fluoxetine	5–10	20–80	1–4 days	CYP2D6, CYP3A3/4	CYP2D6
Sertraline	12.5–25	50–200	24 hours	CYP3A3/4	CYP2D6 (mild)
Fluvoxamine	12.5–25	50–300	16 hours	CYP1A2	CYP2D19, CYP1A2
Paroxetine	10–20	10–50	24 hours	CYP2D6	CYP2D6
Citalopram	5–10	10–40	33 hours	CYP2D6	CYP2D6 (mild)

receptor blocker, haloperidol is effective at low doses (e.g., 0.5 to 2.0 mg/d). The typical side effects include sedation, dysphoria, cognitive dulling, weight gain, and extrapyramidal symptoms, such as dystonia, dyskinesia, and akathisia. Pimozide has been used within a dose range from 0.5 to 4 mg/d. In this dose range, QT prolongation is unlikely; however, at higher doses or in combination with drugs that inhibit CYP3A4, this is an important consideration.

Atypical neuroleptics have also been tried for tic treatment. Tiapride and sulpiride, unavailable in the U.S. market, have shown positive results in controlling tics; however, both drugs require more study to confirm their effectiveness. Risperidone, a D2 and 5HT2 blocking agent, has been found effective in tic treatment in open-label and randomized double-blind trials. With a dose range between 1.0 to 3.0 mg/d, in two divided doses, this drug has been associated with low frequency of extrapyramidal effects, but drowsiness and weight gain are common. Ziprasidone, also a D2 and 5HT2 blocking agent, has a unique receptor profile with 5-HT1A-agonist properties and modest norepinephrine and serotonin reuptake blocking effects, suggesting that it may have additional anxiolytic and antidepressant effects. At least one placebo-controlled study showed the efficacy of this agent in controlling tics with low frequency of side effects and no weight gain. This agent was delayed in its entry to the marketplace owing to FDA concern about QTc prolongation. Although additional study persuaded the FDA to approve the drug, cardiac monitoring during the dose adjustment and periodically thereafter is probably warranted.[16]

Non-neuroleptic agents are also available for treatment of tics. Clonidine, an α-2-agonist antihypertensive agent, was first introduced as a tic treatment by Donald Cohen and colleagues in the 1970s. It is typically prescribed in a dose range of 0.10 mg to 0.3 mg/d, divided into three to four times per day. Despite the inconsistent results reported in the literature, clonidine is commonly used in children with TS, due to concerns about long-term exposure to neuroleptics, such as tardive dyskinesia. Guanfacine, another α2-agonist, has been introduced for TS treatment and was helpful for the treatment of ADHD in children with tics in a placebo-controlled study. The transdermal nicotine patch has been proposed as an alternative to neuroleptics such as haloperidol. Despite these claims, a placebo-controlled trial failed to show any added benefit of the nicotine patch when added to haloperidol.

Several other medications have been tried with varying success in their capacity to suppress tics. These drugs include the dopamine agonist, pergolide; the dopamine depleting agent, tetrabenazine; the muscle relaxant, baclofen; the antiandrogen drug, flutamide; and the antidystonia injection, botulinum. Of these, pergolide and botulinum toxin are emerging as possibly effective, but more study is needed. Although not well studied, clonazepam is unlikely to be effective as a monotherapy. Baclofen has been evaluated only in one small study and showed modest results. The anti-androgen drug, flutamide, is of interest on theoretical grounds but was not effective in a placebo-controlled study.

FUTURE DIRECTIONS

Research on TS and OCD is likely to build on some of the findings presented in this chapter. Immunologic, neuroimaging, neurochemical, and family genetic studies will continue to clarify the underlying pathophysiology of these disorders. Moreover, longitudinal clinical investigations into the phenomenology and natural history may provide additional clues on the biologic processes involved. The field would also benefit from the development of animal models that will allow investigators to explore specific hypotheses. New psychopharmacologic agents with better side effect profiles will require testing. Through these combined efforts, we will eventually come to a more complete understanding of the neurobiologic mechanisms involved in TS and OCD.

Acknowledgments

This work was supported in part by the Fundação de Amparo à Pesquisa do Estado de São Paulo, Brazil, to Dr. Mercadante (99/08560-6), the RUPP Program Project (LS), and the NIMH to Dr. Lombroso (MH 01527). The authors thank Virginia W. Eicher for helpful discussions.

REFERENCES

1. King RA, Leckman JF, Scahill L, Cohen DJ: Obsessive-compulsive disorder, anxiety, and depression. In Leckman JF, Cohen DJ (eds): Tourette's Syndrome—Tics, Obsessions, Compulsions. New York, John Wiley & Sons, 1999, pp 43–62.

2. Miguel EC, Rosário-Campos MC, Shavitt RG, et al: The tic-related obsessive-compulsive disorder phenotype. In Cohen DJ, Jankovic J, Goetz CG (eds): Tourette Syndrome. Philadelphia, Lippincott Williams & Wilkins, 2001, 43–55.

3. Leckman JF, Zhang H, Alsobrook JP, Pauls DL: Symptom dimensions in obsessive-compulsive disorder: Toward quantitative phenotypes. Am J Med Genetics 2001;105:28–30.

4. Eichstedt JA, Arnold SL: Childhood-onset obsessive-compulsive disorder: A tic-related subtype of OCD? Clin Psychol Rev 2001;21:137–158.

5. Scahill L, Tanner C, Dure L: The epidemiology of tics and Tourette syndrome in children and adolescents. Adv Neurol 2001;85:261–271.

6. Leckman JF, Peterson BS, King RA, et al: Phenomenology of tics and natural history of tic disorders. In Cohen DJ, Jankovic J, Goetz CG (eds): Tourette Syndrome. Philadelphia, Lippincott Williams & Wilkins, 2001, pp 1–14.

7. Leckman JF, Riddle MA: Tourette's syndrome: When do habit-forming systems form habits of their own? Neuron 2000;28:349–354.

8. Graybiel AN, Canales JJ: The neurobiology of repetitive behaviors: Clues to the neurobiology of Tourette syndrome. In Cohen DJ, Jankovic J, Goetz CG (eds): Tourette Syndrome. Advances in Neurology. Philadelphia, Lippincott Williams & Wilkins, 2001, pp 123–134.

9. Mink J: Neurobiology of basal ganglia circuits. In Cohen DJ, Jankovic J, Goetz CG (eds): Tourette Syndrome. Philadelphia: Lippincott Williams & Wilkins, 2001, pp 113–122.

10. Saxena S, Brody AL, Schwartz JM, Baxter LR: Neuroimaging and frontal-subcortical circuitry in obsessive-compulsive disorder. Br J Psychiatry 1998;35:26–37.

11. Rauch SL, Whalen PJ, Curran T, et al: Probing striato-thalamic function in obsessive-compulsive disorder and Tourette syndrome using neuroimaging methods. In Cohen DJ, Jankovic J, Goetz CG (eds): Tourette Syndrome. Philadelphia, Lippincott Williams & Wilkins, 2001, pp 207–224.

12. Peterson BS, Staib L, Scahill L, et al: Regional brain and ventricular volumes in Tourette syndrome. Arch Gen Psychiatry 2001;58:427–440.

13. Peterson BS: Neuroimaging studies of Tourette syndrome: A decade of progress. In Cohen DJ, Jankovic J, Goetz CG (eds): Tourette Syndrome. Philadelphia Lippincott, Williams & Wilkins, 2001, pp 179–196.

14. Mansari M, Bouchard C, Blier P: Alteration of serotonin release in the guinea pig orbito-frontal cortex by selective serotonin reuptake inhibitors. Relevance to treatment of obsessive-compulsive disorder. Neuropsychopharmacology 1995;13:117–127.

15. Singer HG, Wendlandt JT: Neurochemistry and synaptic neurotransmission in Tourette syndrome. In Cohen DJ, Jankovic J, Goetz CG (eds): Tourette Syndrome. Philadelphia, Lippincott Williams & Wilkins, 2001, pp 163–178.

16. Scahill L, Chappel PB, King RA, Leckman JF: Pharmacologic treatment of tics disorders. Child Adolesc Psych Clin North Am 2000;9:99–117.

17. Lombroso PJ, Leckman JF: Tourette's syndrome and tic-related disorders in children. In Charney D, Bunney B, Nestler E, (eds): Neurobiological Foundations of Mental Illness. New York, Oxford University Press, 1999, pp 779–787.

18. Pauls DL, Alsobrook JP 2d: The inheritance of obsessive-compulsive disorder. Child Adolesc Psychiatr Clin North Am 1999;8:481–496.

19. Nestadt G, Lan T, Samuels J, et al: Complex segregation analysis provides compelling evidence for a major gene underlying obsessive-compulsive disorder and for heterogeneity by sex. Am J Hum Genet 2000;67:1611–1616.

20. Schindler KM, Richter MA, Kennedy JL, et al: Association between homozygosity at the COMT gene locus and obsessive compulsive disorder. Am J Med Genet 2000;96:721–724.

21. Camarena B, Rinetti G, Cruz C, et al: Additional evidence that genetic variation of MAO-A gene supports a gender subtype in obsessive-compulsive disorder. Am J Med Genet 2001;105:279–282.

22. Veenstra-VanderWeele J, Kim SJ, Gonen D, et al: Genomic organization of the SLC1A1/EAAC1 gene and mutation screening in early-onset obsessive-compulsive disorder. Mol Psychiatry 2001;6:160–167.

23. Pauls D: Update on the genetics of Tourette syndrome. In Cohen DJ, Jankovic J, Goetz CG (eds): Tourette Syndrome. Philadelphia, Lippincott Williams & Wilkins, 2001, pp 281–293.

24. Szechtman H, Eckert MJ, Tse WS, et al: Compulsive checking behavior of quinpirole-sensitized rats as an animal model of obsessive-compulsive disorder (OCD): Form and control. BMC Neurosci 2001;2:4–19.

25. Wynchank D, Berk M: Fluoxetine treatment of acral lick dermatitis in dogs: A placebo-controlled randomized double blind trial. Depress Anxiety 1998; 8:21–23.

26. Canales JJ, Graybiel AM: A measure of striatal function predicts motor stereotypy. Nat Neurosci 2000;3:377–383.

27. Swedo SE, Leonard HL, Garvey M, et al: Pediatric autoimmune neuropsychiatric disorders associated with streptococcal infections: Clinical description of the first 50 cases. Am J Psychiatry 1998;155:264–271.

27a. Taylor JR, Morshed S, Parveen S, et al: An animal model of Tourette's syndrome. Am J Psychiatry 2002;159:657–660.

28. Greist JH, Jefferson JW, Kobak KA, et al: Efficacy and tolerability of serotonin transport inhibitors in obsessive-compulsive disorder. A meta-analysis. Arch Gen Psychiatry 1995;52:53–60.

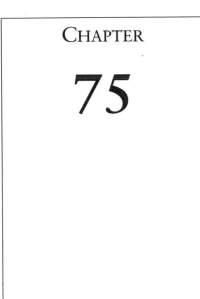

CHAPTER

75

Molecular and Genetic Bases of the Addictions

John C. Crabbe, Jr.
Kristine M. Wiren

CLINICAL FEATURES AND DIAGNOSTIC EVALUATION

Addiction is not a medical term, and the range of disorders that should be included varies according to the beliefs of the beholder. Nonetheless, its lay usage and dictionary definitions reflect the common belief that at its core is a behavioral surrender to habitual behavior that is self-destructive. As with most psychiatric disorders, attempts to define diagnostic boundaries must employ terms and constructs from entirely different languages, those seeking to describe biologic sources of influence and those (more familiar to the lay public) describing intrapsychic events whose basis is unknown. The term *addiction* does not appear in the *Diagnostic and Statistical Manual–IV* employed by psychiatrists and psychologists for differential diagnosis, but in that manual, "substance use disorders" (including alcohol-use disorders and other abused-drug disorders) would be on nearly everyone's list of addictions, and disorders such as bulimia nervosa, pathologic gambling, and several others would certainly make the list for many.[1]

Although other addictive behaviors are occasionally discussed, we have focused this review on drug addiction for several reasons. The majority of data on genetic contributions to addictive behaviors relates to drug dependence. In addition, this allows us to consider the neurobiologic evidence in greater depth. The substantial neurobiologic insights reviewed in the next section have been derived almost entirely from studies employing genetic animal models, in which many of the key features of addiction have been modeled successfully in mice and rats. This has been possible because drugs, given by the experimenter in a controlled setting at measured doses to genetically defined subjects, exert their effects in increas-

ingly well understood pharmacologic pathways, often via specific receptors localized in the brain. Many pharmacologic tools (e.g., antagonist drugs) and genetic manipulations are available to the experimenter.

Once the global boundaries of the addictions have been agreed on, to ascertain genetic contributions will require, as for any complex trait, that specific diagnostic heterogeneities and comorbidities can be differentiated and measured. The ultimate goal of genetic studies is to identify specific genes, and for these complex traits there are many contributing genes, each apparently conferring only a relatively small degree of risk for or protection against diagnosis. Finding any such gene presents a large signal-to-noise problem, largely because of the small effect it has, but also because genes interact with each other. For example a gene possessed by the specific individual whose risk is being assessed might itself be irrelevant to diagnosis, yet could potentiate the risk conferred by a specific other gene (i.e., having two risk-promoting genes might increase actual risk 10-fold).

Even within the substance abuse and dependence diagnoses, the path is not clear. The National Institute on Alcohol Abuse and Alcoholism defines alcoholism on their web site as synonymous with alcohol dependence, and as including four symptoms—craving, loss of control, physical dependence, and tolerance. These symptoms include both physical sequelae of chronic drug use, accessible to an observer, and internal feelings and thoughts about ability to control one's behavior. There is a high comorbidity between alcoholism and smoking, as well as between alcohol abuse and misuse of other drugs. These comorbidities appear to reflect the influence of some genes in common, a condition known as pleiotropism; yet, each abused substance also shows evidence for individualized genetic risk as well. Depression and substance abuse are highly comorbid, and some personality traits may predispose to addictive behaviors.

More problematic yet for genetic analyses, twin and family studies have consistently shown that about half of addiction risk is statistically attributable to genes. This means that the other half of an individual's risk is coming from putatively nongenetic, environmental factors such as personality, family, peers, social class, and cultural influences, all of which can be protective against or increase risk of substance abuse. Inevitably, an individual's genotype, with its specific risk promoting or protective genes, interacts with all the aforesaid environmental conditions to produce individual risk, which of course will change developmentally as gene actions and environmental milieu change. The picture is not entirely bleak, however. In some instances, genetic studies have helped to refine diagnostic issues. For example, a long-standing belief by the public that an "addictive personality" exists is often invoked to "explain" a wide variety of maladaptive habits (if not outright overindulgences). Systematic studies reveal little support for a genetic basis for this postulated disorder.[1]

In the following sections, we will point the reader to reviews of the human molecular genetic evidence regarding addiction risk and discuss some examples. We will review theories of the neurobiologic bases of drug dependence, most of which have studied dysregulation in the brain circuits underlying both normal and pathologic reward. We will focus on genetic animal models because such models have been directed toward multiple aspects relevant to understanding drug dependence. The targets of such models take pharmacology as their template, and include the initial response of a naive organism to a drug; the neuroadaptation that accompanies chronic drug administration, which can be either reduced (tolerance) or increased (sensitization) sensitivity; drug dependence, which is inferred from the characteristic withdrawal symptoms that occur when the drug is removed; the reinforcing effects of the drug (which include craving in humans, but which may be either positive or negative); and the area of pharmacokinetics, which describes metabolism and elimination of the drug. An interesting area of activity in genetic animal model research has been the identification of other factors that may be of relevance, such as anxiety-like behavior and stress responses. We will consider exciting findings in the role of individual differences in gene expression and their potential application to the emerging field of pharmacogenomics.

MOLECULAR THEORIES

Features Modeled in Animals

Animal models of addiction have greatly aided the understanding of mechanisms underlying drug addiction. Classes of drugs that are commonly abused include sedative-hypnotics (alcohol), psychomotor stimulants (cocaine and amphetamine) and opiates, as well as other drugs that do not fit easily into these classes (e.g., nicotine). Animals and humans will readily self-administer these drugs, demonstrating that they constitute positive reinforcers during acute administration. Much progress has been made identifying and characterizing the neuronal circuits and mechanisms that mediate the acute reinforcing effects of drugs of abuse, particularly as a result of analyses using rodent animal models.

One consequence of acute administration shared by all of these classes of drugs is enhancement of the release of dopamine in the extended amygdala, which may be an important mediator of the acute reinforcing effects of these drugs. A central feature of drug addition is a progression from acute voluntary intake of drug to compulsive, chronic drug use in vulnerable individuals.[2] To further complicate the situation, drug addiction is a stubborn and intractable problem in that even after extended periods of abstinence, the risk of relapse to renewed drug use is high.[3]

Two main types of brain responses to chronic drug administration have been described—neuronal adaptations that are believed to represent homeostatic responses to the continued presence of the drug; and changes in synaptic plasticity associated with specific learned behaviors associated with drug taking and drug-related stimuli.[2] Such brain responses occur at the cellular, biochemical, and molecular level and are evidenced as morphologic and functional changes in specific brain structures and even substructures. It has been hypothesized that the persistence of the risk of relapse may reflect the altered pattern of neuronal connectivity and thus responsiveness that results from these changes.

Homeostatic Changes and Neuronal Adaptations

As described earlier, drug addition in both humans and animal models can be characterized by compulsive drug taking, the continued inability to limit intake and the subsequent development of drug dependence. A defining aspect of drug dependence is the emergence and elaboration of a constellation of symptoms after the abrupt cessation of drug use collectively termed withdrawal. Some drugs, such as alcohol and barbiturates, but not all, give rise to clear physical symptoms as severe as life-threatening seizures. All addictive drugs can produce emotional or other intrapsychic withdrawal symptoms such as anxiety, dysphoria, and anhedonia. The behavioral withdrawal syndrome thus appears to result from compensatory neuronal cellular adaptations that occur during chronic drug administration. In response to the potent neuronal stimulation that results from the continued presence of abused drugs, such long-term stable neuronal adaptation acts to maintain organismal homeostasis and reduce drug effects (tolerance). With abrupt discontinuation of drug administration, these neuronal adaptations are both unmasked and now unrestricted to produce withdrawal symptoms that are in the opposite direction of those produced by the drug. One example is the neuronal hyperexcitability that is evidenced during alcohol withdrawal. Another is the dysphoria accompanying withdrawal, which has been termed "reward dysregulation."[2] These dysregulations of homeostasis are thought to involve the nucleus accumbens and the ventral tegmental area-accumbens (mesolimbic) system. The nucleus accumbens is an integral part of the extended amygdala.

Synaptic Plasticity and Associative Learning

Molecular mechanisms normally involved in associative learning include stimulation of dopamine D1 receptors, the activation of the cAMP/PKA/CREB signal transduction pathway, a transient burst of altered gene expression, and subsequent synaptic rearrangements and altered neuronal connectivity that result. There is substantial and growing evidence that activation of adenylyl cyclase with the downstream activation of protein kinase A (PKA) and cAMP binding protein (CREB) plays a significant role in the chronic effects of abused drugs.[3,4] Enhanced phosphorylation of downstream intracellular targets, such as potassium channels, results in increased neurotransmitter concentrations resident in the synapse. After drug administration, gene expression differences would follow the activation of CREB in the network of genes with 5' CRE regulatory elements. One example discussed later is the upregulation of prodynorphin expression in the nucleus accumbens. This cascade of changes is dependent on new RNA and protein synthesis and is associated with structural changes in the brain that may result from regulation of cell adhesion molecules such as nerve cell adhesion molecule (NCAM).

There is an abundance of opioid receptors and processed peptides in both the nucleus accumbens and ventral tegmental area. The presence of serotonin and its receptors and their convergence with dopamine- and serotonin-containing fibers also suggests interaction of these multiple neurotransmitter systems. In addition, GABA, glutamate and acetylcholine have all been suggested to be involved in behavioral responses to drugs of abuse. Reviews of the multiplicity of structural and functional changes accompanying chronic drug administration and withdrawal indicate that the specific changes seen depend to some degree on which drug is studied, but the broad pattern of dysregulation of these classic reward pathway components is similar.[2–4]

HUMAN MOLECULAR AND GENETIC DATA

Classic Genetic Methods: Twins, Families, Adoptees, and Genetic Epidemiology

Given the complex interplay of genetic and environmental factors that predispose individuals to addiction, most work has concentrated on unraveling these contributions to find evidence for genetic influences. Comorbidity for the various addictive behaviors has been demonstrated in twins and other biologic relatives, and environmental factors inferred by further comparisons with adoptees. Substantial genetic influence has been demonstrated for risk of alcoholism, substance abuse (especially smoking), eating disorders, and other potential representatives of the class of addictive behaviors.[1] An increasing recognition of the value of epidemiologic studies for identifying clusters of risk-related traits has been shown. Some twin studies have been particularly helpful in defining comorbidities more clearly, for example by demonstrating that alcoholism and drug dependence share common genetic influences as well as some individual factors predisposing to genetic risk.

Twin and family studies can identify traits with common genetic or environmental influence, or both, and can assess gene-environment interaction as well. Thus, they will facilitate our deeper understanding of the genetic etiology of addictive behavior. The generally small number of subjects in such studies makes it difficult for them by themselves to locate relevant genes (but see later).

Molecular Genetic Studies—Association and Linkage

As the Human Genome Project accumulated more and more information about the specific DNA sequences in the human genome, the power and precision of genetic mapping studies were enhanced manifold. Genetic mapping studies attempt to correlate genetic markers (i.e., sequences of DNA that have been localized to specific locations in the genome, such as the mid-region of chromosome 6) with the trait being mapped (e.g., diagnosis) across specific groups of individuals. Co-occurrence of specific markers with the trait suggests that a gene of which the marker sequence is a part, or a separate gene reasonably close by on the same chromosome (i.e., linked), is synthesizing a gene product that directly or indirectly enhances risk. Because many hundreds of comparisons are made in these kinds of analyses, there is a high false-positive rate for identifying such associations or linkages. Further, because addictions are polygenic traits, each gene thus mapped exerts a small risk enhancement or protection, so there is a correspondingly low statistical power to detect linkage.

Despite the intrinsic difficulties, many hundreds of linkage and association studies have been performed for alcoholism, drug dependence, and the sundry other addictive disorders. Positive findings are beginning to appear, particularly for those disorders under more intense scrutiny, such as alcoholism and smoking.[5,6] Most of these studies search the surrounding genomic area for a likely "candidate gene," one whose function is known, as the possible cause of the genetic effect.

Candidate genes are nominated based on previously existing biologic data, such as a study that identified a marker near the serotonin 5-HT$_{1B}$ receptor gene in two populations of impulsive-aggressive alcoholics.[7] It is not currently known whether the "candidate genes" nominated by linkage and association studies in fact contribute to the disorders being mapped. This inferential problem is shared by studies using animal models, and because the solutions are conceptually similar, we will discuss the next steps in a later section.

Enhancing the Power of Human Genetic Mapping Studies

There are several approaches currently underway for solving the problems of low signal-to-noise that bedevil gene mapping studies. Obviously, population sizes can be increased, but this is very expensive and may not increase power very much. The use of "endophenotypes" (or intermediate phenotypes) has become very popular. In recognition of the comorbidity of many traits (and, more simply, the pleiotropic effects of genes on multiple traits that are assumed to contribute to and complicate the disentanglement of such comorbidity), it has been suggested that biologic phenotypes be sought that are "closer to the gene." One such example is the abnormal P300 sensory evoked potential characterizing alcoholics and their offspring. On the assumption that the collection of genes contributing to abnormal P300 responses will be simpler than that contributing to the complex trait, alcoholism, mapping studies have identified quantitative trait loci (QTLs), or loci, where a gene or genes influencing P300 must reside.

Similarly, a long-term epidemiologic study demonstrated decades ago that college-aged men with a positive family history for alcoholism were less sensitive than those without to the effect of an acute dose of alcohol to induce body sway and subjective intoxication. In a follow-up study many years later, family history predicted alcoholism diagnosis, but the sensitivity to acute ethanol effects was a far better predictor of alcoholism, accounting for most of the individual differences in susceptibility to alcoholism. The low sensitivity to alcohol trait was subsequently mapped to specific genetic markers.[8]

The discovery of single nucleotide polymorphisms (SNPs) has fueled much discussion of their potential as a new generation of markers, and some successes in mapping complex traits have been reported. Use of this new marker system is not without disadvantages (e.g., the map of SNPs in the genome is less well articulated than that for standard multi-base DNA markers, the sheer number of SNPs is overwhelming, and so on). The potential for using SNPs to classify dependent subjects in the interests of targeting subsequent therapies individually has also been proposed.[6]

More powerful designs (e.g., the transmission disequilibrium test and its variants) can increase detection power and are increasingly used. Additionally, statistical genetic methods are being developed to deal with gene-gene interactions. By conditioning a gene's effects on the genotype at another locus, genetic signal can be enhanced. Although such methods are computationally difficult and lead to great increases in the numbers of comparisons made, they may reveal genetic effects when those effects are masked by the presence of other genes. An interesting and thoughtful paper proposed a synthetic approach in an attempt to combine the strengths of classic twin designs with those of family-based linkage and association studies, and proposed the value of such an approach for gene mapping studies as well.[9]

A Case of Protective Genes: ADH and ALDH Polymorphisms

Alcoholism is one of the longest-studied complex traits in human genetics, and the findings with alcohol metabolizing enzymes offer an interesting illustration of the hope awaiting genetic studies.[5] Ethyl alcohol is metabolized rapidly to acetaldehyde, which causes many symptoms including nausea, facial flushing, dizziness, and headaches. The enzymatic conversion is effected by the enzyme alcohol dehydrogenase (ADH) and many ADH alleles are distributed in human populations. Most humans then rapidly convert the acetaldehyde to acetate and carbon dioxide, innocuous products that are excreted, because they possess variant alleles for the aldehyde dehydrogenase (ALDH) gene that lead to synthesis of an efficient ALDH protein. There is a variant allele for the ALDH gene that leads to a slow-metabolizing form of the protein, ALDH2*2, and this allele is present at high frequencies in southeast Asian gene pools. When an individual heterozygous (or, more strikingly, homozygous) for ALDH2*2 drinks alcohol, he or she rapidly accumulates acetaldehyde and frequently experiences the unpleasant resulting symptomatology. It has been shown that individuals possessing one or two slow-ALDH alleles are protected against developing alcoholism. After years of population-based screening studies, a single Asian alcoholic was finally found to be an ALDH2*2 homozygote. The variant ALDH allele therefore offers a substantial degree of protection against alcoholism.[5] There is a similar polymorphism in ADH that reduces alcoholism risk, but to a lesser degree, perhaps 20%.

It is an interesting feature of these findings that disulfiram has long been used as a pharmacotherapy for alcoholism under the trade name Antabuse. Disulfiram is an ALDH inhibitor, so an individual taking this drug chronically experiences the flushing, nausea, and so on, after drinking alcohol, just as if he or she were genetically protected by a variant enzyme. The treatment has seen limited use because it has been difficult to get patients to comply with their medication schedule, but it is not entirely without efficacy.

Thus, genetic analyses can identify candidates for pharmacotherapy that may be helpful for their addictions. The use of the long-acting opioid agonists (methadone and certain of its derivatives) to blunt the reinforcing effects of heroin is another case where targeting a drug's obvious pharmacologically relevant sites has seen success. Many years have been spent in pursuit of a drug that would pharmacologically "antagonize" the effects of cocaine or methamphetamine, or both, with little to show for the efforts. It is not unreasonable to hope that including genetic analyses in the search for pharmacotherapies will lead to the next generation of effective drugs.

GENETIC ANIMAL MODELS

Why Study Nonhuman Animals?

Humans are a very messy species for genetic studies. They have few offspring, small families, the generation time is inconveniently long, they breed with whomever they please, and ascertaining the genetic specifics of their ancestry is difficult. To overcome these problems requires very large population sizes with consequent enormous expense. There is a long history of application of genetic animal models to the study of addiction genetics. The advantages are obvious—on every feature named earlier, rodents are far more desirable subjects than are humans. The price, of course, is that rodent behavior can never model the full spectrum of any complex behavioral trait expressed in humans. There are species-specific differences in physiology, behavior, social structure, and their interactions that ensure that an animal model can never be isomorphic with the human trait (or diagnosis) it targets. Human-mouse genetics are quite similar, and the two species appear to share more than 80% homology for groups of linked genes because of syntenic conservation due to shared ancestry. That is, knowing where a particular gene is in the genome of one species will predict about 80% of the time where the homologous gene is in the other. Genetic animal models have, therefore, taken the initial, reductionistic approach of attempting to model the various contributing features of complex traits separately, and have had increasing success.

Classic Genetic Animal Model Methods

Selective Breeding

Recognition of the power of behavior genetic analysis led to its very early application to the study of alcohol-related traits. In the late 1940s, rats were bred to drink alcohol solutions in preference to water at the University of Chile. This successful application of one of the oldest methods in agricultural genetics, selective breeding, led to many successive and more modern applications. There are now one-half dozen sets of rat lines, and mouse lines as well, that differ genetically in their willingness to ingest rather large amounts of alcohol.[1]

One of the features of selective breeding is that breeding for one trait leads to the development of differences in many other traits as well. This is because any given gene does not exert a single effect, but rather has many upstream effects on a variety of traits, a phenomenon termed *pleiotropy*. Genetically high-drinking rats will self-administer intoxicating doses of alcohol under some circumstances. They have been found to have an array of behavioral and neurochemical differences as compared with lines selected to avoid alcohol solutions.[10] For example, genetic preferrers appear to be less sensitive to the aversive effects of alcohol, to be more sensitive to the motor stimulant and electroencephalographic effects of ethanol, and to develop more persistent tolerance. High alcohol consumption appears to be associated with low brain serotonin, which is interesting in that specific serotonin reuptake inhibitors are currently showing some signs of clinical efficacy in the treatment of alcoholism.[10]

Many lines of rats and mice have been genetically selected for high and low sensitivity to many important effects of abused drugs (e.g., sensitivity, development of tolerance, dependence, and withdrawal symptoms). The targeted drugs include most of those widely abused. Selected lines have been used in many studies to further our understanding of the neurobiologic changes that accompany chronic drug administration.[11]

The powerful tool of genetic selection has been used principally in the substance abuse area of the addictions. Some attempts have been made to develop lines differentially genetically predisposed to traits thought to be highly comorbid with the addictions. For example, anxiety, impulsivity, antisocial behavior, and depression can be modeled in rat and mouse behavioral assays, although these behavioral assays have a bit more than the usual level of difficulty in convincing nonbelievers they possess face validity. For example, rats have been bred for high or low anxiety-related behaviors using such laboratory assays, and the high-scoring rats have been reported to drink more alcohol than the low-scoring line. Given the intrinsic power of this method to assess genetic polymorphisms, it might well be worthwhile to develop additional lines of mice or rats that differ in some of the other traits correlated with drug abuse susceptibility in humans.

Inbred Strains

One of the most straightforward genetic animal model systems is to examine existing genetic variation. Conveniently, there exist more than 100 inbred strains of mice and many of rats. All same-sex members of such a strain (say, C57BL/6 mice) are like monozygotic twins, and possess two copies of the same allele at all genes. If many strains are compared for a trait under controlled environmental conditions, any mean differences among the strains can be attributed straightforwardly to their genetic differences. Beginning in the late 1950s, C57BL/6 strain mice were shown to prefer to drink alcohol solutions, whereas other strains, such as DBA/2, were nearly complete teetotalers. C57BL/6 mice will apparently readily self-administer nearly all drugs of abuse with great avidity, as has been made clear in many subsequent studies comparing strains for alcohol and drug sensitivity, tolerance, dependence or withdrawal severity, or both, and propensity to self-administer drugs.[12]

Strain comparisons are returning to favor as it becomes more apparent to the neuroscience community that the information gleaned is cumulative. Because the genotypes of each strain remain nearly invariant over time, studies conducted 40 years ago are still informative today. We have thus learned a great deal about a few common inbred strains. The specific genes that lead to the strain differences, however, have remained anonymous, because the large numbers of alleles for any gene represented in a multi-strain survey make genotyping difficult and expensive.

One boost to strain surveys is a new initiative spearheaded by The Jackson Laboratory, the Mouse Phenome Project. By supplying up to 40 inbred strains to willing phenotypers, and assembling a relational database containing the resulting behavioral and physiologic data, centralized access to strain data will vastly improve in the next few years. One very powerful use of this database will be to enable correlational analyses of the strain's average phenotypes. Such analyses have already taught us much about codetermination of genetic influence. For example, mouse strains that are efficient at learning to inhibit a signaled nose poke response were those that had low ethanol consumption when offered a choice between ethanol and water. Similarly, high alcohol-preferring strains tend to show minimal withdrawal severity after chronic ethanol intake. Together, these studies might be interpreted to mean that being able to avoid alcohol self-administration is a consequence of a genetic predisposition to experience severe withdrawal coupled with the ability to inhibit responding. Given the difficulties of mapping mouse behavioral assays directly to human traits mentioned earlier, this would be quite an interpretational stretch from the data, but it could suggest informative experiments to test the hypothesis.

Quantitative Trait Locus Mapping

Inbred strains, selected lines, and various other genetically specified populations have been used in studies analogous to the association and linkage studies described earlier with human populations. The proximal goals of these studies are first to locate in the genome a region, a quantitative trait locus (QTL), harboring a gene that affects the trait to be mapped, and then to refine that genomic map until a single gene or cluster of genes can be proved to be responsible for the effect on the trait. Of course, each QTL generally accounts for only a small proportion of the variability in the complex behavioral traits

contributing to addiction, so this is a difficult task. The more long-term goals of QTL mapping projects are then to move to human populations for studies of the homologous, or orthologous gene, and use information about the biologic effects of the gene's product to help design therapeutic agents or other therapies. These efforts were undertaken in the early 1990s and have succeeded for several complex traits of importance to medicine.[13] For addiction-related traits, no QTL has yet been tracked to a responsible gene.

Many addiction-related traits have been targeted for QTL mapping studies. As with most genetic animal model studies in this domain, alcohol-related responses are overrepresented in the QTL work. Traits for which there are significant QTL associations include alcohol preference drinking, acute and chronic alcohol withdrawal, place preference and taste aversion conditioned by alcohol, and acute alcohol induced hypothcrmia, locomotor stimulation, and sedation. Other QTLs have been mapped for several responses to morphine, cocaine-induced seizures, and withdrawal from pentobarbital. These traits and their QTLs, as well as progress toward high-resolution mapping of some of the QTLs have been discussed elsewhere.[1]

Currently, QTL fine mapping involves the development of congenic strains. In a congenic strain, a very small sequence of DNA on a chromosome is moved from one genetic background to another, inbred background. This is accomplished by examining genetic markers surrounding the QTL and searching for rare cases where a recombination has occurred—that is, during cell division, when an exchange of chromosomal material has occurred, termed a *crossover*, between one of the markers and the QTL. Gradually, with continued breeding, this leads to a narrowing of the confidence interval of DNA sequence surrounding a mapped QTL until only a single gene remains. If a congenic strain containing a single introduced gene differs on the trait versus the background strain, the remaining gene must be responsible for the QTL and the QTL has become a QT gene.[14]

Random Mutagenesis

QTL mapping relies on studying the existing polymorphisms in the genome. It seeks to associate possession of a particular allele at a particular gene with a high or low score on the trait. An alternative is to create many mutations at random throughout the genome, and then to screen the mutagenized mice (actually, their offspring) to see whether behavioral outliers can be detected. This process of random mutagenesis is now usually induced by treatment of males with the chemical N-ethylnitrosourea, or ENU. There are several large projects currently underway whose goals are to identify many hundreds of such mutants, and several projects have included behavioral screens for alcohol or drug sensitivity. Many studies also screen for assays for traits thought to be comorbid, such as anxiety or impulsivity, but none has progressed to the stage of identifying the mutation affecting an addiction-related trait.[14]

Targeted Mutagenesis

The most important advance in genetic animal model studies during the 1990s was the maturation of the technology for manipulating the genome directly. By introducing altered genetic material directly into the germ line of mice, investigators have produced many hundreds of mouse strains in which a specific gene is overexpressed, underexpressed, or for which the gene product is nonfunctional (i.e., a null mutant or knockout). The genes targeted for such manipulations were selected based on the scientific evidence regarding the biologic underpinnings of the trait. In the addictions, most such targets were neurotransmitters, their enzymes of metabolism, receptors, or transporters, particularly those of importance to the mesostriatal dopaminergic "reward" pathways that have been shown to be important for addictive drugs in particular. As more understanding of the intracellular messages triggered by receptor interactions has been developed, these signaling proteins have also been targeted.

Production of null mutants is currently the standard technology for direct genetic manipulation. The list of null mutants in which addiction traits have been shown to be affected is long and growing weekly. Many lists of targeted genes are available (e.g., http://165.112.78.65/KOS/KOSearch.taf?function=form [see reference 15]), and links to such lists can be found at http://www.ibngs.org/links.html. Use of these model strains will continue to be invaluable, especially as the tissue-specific and conditionally expressed generation of genetically altered mice become more widely used. These strains can have expression of the targeted gene restricted to particular brain regions, and have gene expression turned on or off at particular developmental stages, thereby reducing many of the interpretational difficulties with the first generation of null mutants.

Transgenic Overexpression

As noted previously, there is a large body of evidence implicating involvement of cAMP-PKA signaling in the mesolimbic reward pathway. One strategy that has been employed to characterize the contribution of PKA activity in the reward pathway is to employ genetically altered mice. Transgenic overexpression of a wild-type allele driven by a brain-specific promoter can complement results obtained with mice with targeted disruption of the same gene. Transgenic mice can also be constructed using genes that have been mutated to be either constitutively active or to act as an interfering mutant (dominant negative) to reduce activity of the endogenous product. As an example of this kind of approach, heterozygous mice

with targeted disruption of one Gsa allele have been studied, and show increased sensitivity to the sedative or hypnotic effects, or both, of alcohol and decreased alcohol consumption.[16] Likewise, different mice with reduced neuronal downstream PKA activity, in which a dominant negative isoform of the regulatory subunit of PKA is expressed in forebrain under control of CaMKIIa promoter, also demonstrate reduced alcohol consumption and increased sensitivity to the sedative or hypnotic effects, or both, of ethanol. In contrast, a third line of mice with increased PKA as a result of transgenic overexpression of a constitutively active form of Gsa (with reduced GTPase activity) show reduced sensitivity to the sedative or hypnotic effects, or both, of alcohol. Taken together, results obtained with such genetically modified mice to produce opposite phenotypes provide strong and converging evidence of the involvement of a specific pathway in the measured behavioral response.

ROLE OF GENE EXPRESSION

Substantial data support the observation that both acute and chronic drug administration results in changes in the expression of many different genes in the central nervous system—what may be termed a drug-regulated network. With chronic drug abuse, some of these changes and the cellular consequences are quite long-lived, even after extended periods of abstinence and, perhaps, for a lifetime.

The mechanism(s) mediating drug-related changes in gene expression remain elusive, particularly for alcohol. Because no identified receptor exists to mediate alcohol effects on cellular machinery, both direct effects and indirect effects involving other signaling cascades have been invoked. Two areas of investigation into the role of gene expression in drug addiction are currently quite active: individual, pre-existing differences in gene expression that, in the presence of drug, may predispose to addiction vulnerability; and changes in gene expression after drug administration that may mediate aspects of drug dependence and the severity of withdrawal, and may also lead to increased risk of relapse after a period of abstinence. The importance of identifying these networks in specific brain regions lies in the potential involvement of such drug-induced changes in mediating many of the adverse events related to chronic drug use. The vulnerability to relapse subsequent to withdrawal and even the development of addiction itself may be the result of brain region-specific and long-lived "neuroadaptive" changes in gene expression.[3] Thus, results from these challenging studies may find application to the emerging field of pharmacogenomics.

In this section, we will focus on expression differences in the central nervous system that result from acute and chronic ethanol administration as a paradigm for drug-regulated gene expression. Because of space limitations, we will not discuss naive differences in gene expression that may be predisposing factor(s) important in alcoholism liability, which have been covered in an excellent review.[10] We will also not discuss translational and post-translational modifications of existing mRNA and proteins, the identification of which will require employing a proteomic strategy as outlined later. Such regulation may be a significant factor influencing protein abundance and activity that mediates behavioral and metabolic responses to chronic drug administration, particularly in large postmitotic cells such as neurons. The reader is instead encouraged to evaluate relevant data in a review by Lang and colleagues.[17]

The effect of drug administration on gene expression can be evaluated with a variety of methodological approaches. Such techniques can be subdivided on a theoretic basis into those that directly characterize and quantify expression of a manageable number of mRNA transcripts of known sequence based on potential involvement in drug-related responses, and those that globally screen the transcriptosome for expression differences—that is, they screen without bias tens of thousands of genes, even fragments of sequence.

Investigation of Candidate Genes

The first approach has been termed *candidate gene* analysis because these sequences are characterized only after previous results implicate their importance, thus identifying the specific mRNAs as candidates for mediating behavioral responses to drug administration. Many of these genes represent the target proteins for different drugs of abuse. Because changes in expression after chronic administration of drug are oftentimes opposite in direction to changes observed after acute administration, it has been proposed that long-lived neuroadaptive changes in expression are the result of and in opposition to the acute (rewarding) effects of the drug. Because gene regulation by drug administration may be temporally linked in this fashion, it is important to identify expression differences in both settings.

Changes in expression after acute or chronic drug exposure have been quantified for a defined set of known genes using Northern analysis, RNase protection analysis (RPA), or a variety of reverse-transcription polymerase chain reaction (RT-PCR) approaches. Broad classes of proteins whose transcripts have been characterized as drug-regulated represent traditional candidate genes. These include both ligand-gated and G-protein–coupled neurotransmitter receptor subunits and neurotransmitter transporters genes, transcription factors, including immediate early genes such as the c-*fos* family and cAMP-response element binding protein (CREB), components of signaling cascades, such as protein kinase C (PKC) and A (PKA), adenylyl cyclase and G-protein subunits, and certain neuropeptides such as prodynorphin, vasopressin, and brain-derived neurotrophic factor.[18]

Perhaps the best evidence for direct involvement of drug-regulated changes in gene expression in behavioral responses to drug administration may be that of changes in cAMP systems, including CREB-regulated prodynorphin expression.[3] After both alcohol and cocaine exposure, prodynorphin expression has been shown to be upregulated in specific brain areas associated with drug reward, including nucleus accumbens. This upregulation can be mediated by changes in CREB expression and phosphorylation. Thus, elevation of CREB leads to altered gene expression, including increased prodynorphin, and negative kappa-opioid receptor activation, for which prodynorphin is a ligand. Direct blockade of either CREB expression with viral-mediated gene transfer of a dominant-negative CREB or of negative kappa-opioid receptor activation with the antagonist norBNI alters signs of dysphoria/depression and aversion observed during cocaine withdrawal,[19] directly implicating CREB pathway involvement in drug-induced dysphoria.

Analysis of Global Changes in Gene Expression

Analysis of gene expression differences that allow for global characterization is particularly useful for neurobehavioral syndromes such as drug addiction, because simple single gene effects are unlikely to be the sole underlying mechanism. Many genes, and combinations of genes, will probably be involved to give rise to clinical syndromes of addiction. Techniques that have been employed to screen globally for expression differences without bias, and thus to identify novel genes, include subtraction hybridization, mRNA differential display, serial analysis of gene expression (SAGE), and gene chip or microarray analysis.

Early studies characterizing changes in expression after chronic ethanol administration employed material isolated from cultured cells, analyzed by subtractive hybridization studies that enriched the pool of regulated RNA. Heat shock proteins, molecular chaperones, and mitochondrial genes were identified as differentially regulated.[20] Differential display analysis, a technique that allows for direct visualization of all gene expression patterns, has been employed to analyze brain expression after chronic ethanol exposure in rodent models. In these studies, mitochondrial and chaperone genes were also identified as targets for ethanol. One series of investigations has focused on the changes in gene expression caused by cocaine and amphetamine, which has led to the discovery of a novel class of neuropeptides derived from the CART gene (cocaine and amphetamine-related transcript).[21]

Currently, the most powerful and challenging approach to global screening is to employ a gene chip that contains arrays of tens of thousands of DNA sequences on a solid substrate. Complex RNA probes are simultaneously hybridized to a complementary sequence on the chip; quantification of the hybridization pattern thus identifies gene expression differences between two samples. These kinds of analyses are still in their infancy, but some interesting trends are emerging. Gene chip studies comparing human alcoholic samples from frontal cortex to matched controls have confirmed some subtractive hybridization and differential display observations, particularly with respect to chaperone proteins.[22] Somewhat surprisingly, a major system influenced by a lifetime of drug abuse comprised many myelin-related genes. These data illustrate the power of bioinformatic analysis, that is, when several genes that have impact on a particular pathway or system are identified as regulated by drug administration, the more likely the finding is to be biologically meaningful. Animal models are being employed in expression array studies as well. One study reported changes in expression of several genes related to intracellular signaling cascades, including multiple protein kinases, in nuclear accumbens tissue taken from primates exposed to cocaine for over a year.[23] Another experiment used a rodent model derived from a genetic selection for alcohol sensitivity. Comparison of untreated, whole brain tissue revealed 41 genes differentially expressed out of more than 18,000 nonredundant mouse cDNA clones in lines selected for high versus low alcohol sensitivity.[24]

Interestingly, in studies to date, the most robustly regulated genes are not neurotransmitter system components or genes that had been previously examined as likely candidates. Many, if not most, of the genes now recognized as regulated were not anticipated to be important or even involved in drug-mediated responses. This is both the great benefit and the daunting challenge of an unbiased approach. Understanding the significance of these unanticipated changes in gene expression in a larger context, and the role played by the translated proteins as a network in a brain region-specific fashion, remains a significant challenge for future studies.[18,21]

It should be noted that the focus of work thus far has been at the level of the gene, that is, DNA. The gene products and gene proteins accomplish the neurobiologic business of the organism, and expression of a gene does not necessarily translate directly into production of a functional protein. The new field of proteomics, in which complex patterns of protein expression are analyzed, is widely touted as the next frontier for expression-based analyses. Because of the complexity of proteins and their frequent post-translational processing or alternative splicing into multiple active forms, or both, studies of protein expression, which are directly analogous to the gene-based approaches just discussed, are even more complex.

THERAPY

Existing Therapy

Addictions treatment strategies are varied and often applied in combination. For example, using a broad definition, there are many forms of psychotherapy frequently offered to those addicted to alcohol, drugs, or those seeking relief from other maladaptive behavioral patterns characterizing addiction. These include the familiar 12 step self-help programs, psychosocial therapies such as motivational enhancement therapy, brief interventions, behavior therapies that manipulate the reinforcements derived from drug use, psychodynamic therapies, cognitive-behavioral therapy, and multiple forms of couples, family, group, and community-targeted therapies. Clinicians can distinguish many forms and variants in addition to these. Nearly all medical disorders are currently treated with drugs, and the addictions are no exception. Although psychotherapy is sometimes offered alone, it is usually coupled with a drug. The drugs used include disulfiram inhibitors (Antabuse, discussed earlier, for alcoholism), specific serotonin reuptake inhibitors and other drugs affecting serotonin function (e.g., fluoxetine, sertraline, ondansetron), opioid agonists (methadone, *l*-acetyl-α-methadol [LAAM]) and antagonists (naltrexone), nicotine replacement, and acamprosate, a drug affecting NMDA receptors. In addition, there are many complementary, or alternative, medical treatments applied to the addictions, including acupuncture, yoga, and herbal therapies. These alternative therapies are often administered in conjunction with more routine medical treatment and are being used by more and more people. As they are generally not studied in a scientifically controlled design, their efficacy is difficult to evaluate.

To an increasing extent, different treatment modalities are being offered in combination, for example, multiple drugs with different actions combined with psychotherapy, or using vouchers in a community reinforcement approach for patients on methadone maintenance. Self-treatment with herbal preparations can be problematic because these preparations can influence the metabolism of medically prescribed drugs. Because we are neither clinicians nor involved in human subjects research, our opinion is derived from the literature rather than from experience. It appears to us that nearly all of the conventional therapies will help a percentage of the individuals who try them, on the order of 20% to 25% in most large, controlled studies. It has proved difficult to predict who will be helped by which therapy, and the majority of addicted patients seeking therapy of any sort will not succeed in remaining abstinent for at least a year. Thus, although there is clear value to the existing therapies, there is also ample room and need for improvement.

Prospects for Genomically Driven Therapies

Pharmacogenomics is the term given to the emerging field that seeks to use genetic information to discover new drugs as therapeutic targets and to individualize their application based on an individual's genetic fingerprint. It has assumed the knowledge from the field of study long known as *pharmacogenetics*, which has sought to identify the polymorphisms in drug enzymes and receptors that result in genetically based, individual differences in drug metabolism and begun to build on that knowledge. A useful review of the field[25] describes the central feature of pharmacogenomics as its orientation toward looking at groups of genetic polymorphisms which may be used to predict both the efficacy and the toxicity of a drug for an individual. There are no known cases, to date, where this method has been applied to addiction-related traits, but the enterprise is a logical extension of the wealth of Human Genome Project-driven genomic data that is accumulating. Major pharmaceutical companies have applied this logic as well as discoveries derived from QTL mapping and gene expression studies, described earlier, in attempts to identify novel targets for treatment of complex trait disorders. A slightly absurd example might illustrate the general idea. For example, a gene expression array experiment might show that a large group of genes involved in histamine metabolism, catabolism, and function (e.g., enzymes, receptors) showed greatly increased or decreased expression in animals chronically treated with alcohol. This would be a very surprising result, because our understanding of the likely neurobiologic targets that are dysregulated by chronic alcohol include GABA, NMDA, catecholamines, and serotonin systems, but not histaminergic systems. The hope is that this might lead to a clinical trial treating alcoholics with a specific histaminergic receptor antagonist drug, and a cure for alcoholism. The target pathway would never have been identified using the usual neurobiologic approaches, which mostly look where the past light was, that is, in the already-suspect systems.

Major pharmaceutical companies are avidly pursuing characterizing many complex disease traits using this strategy, including asthma and hypertension, to give examples. There has been a historical, and continuing, major lack of interest by these companies in pursuing the addictions, which we find very puzzling. Given the very high prevalence of addiction (about 1 in 10 U.S. males is a diagnosed alcoholic, never mind the many who are undiagnosed, and smoking prevalence remains at about 20% of U.S. adults), and the fact that most of the addicted are gainfully employed and could thus pay for their drug treatment, it is troubling that these disorders have not been the subject of greater interest.

CONCLUSIONS AND FUTURE DIRECTIONS

Molecular and genetic studies of complex diseases have experienced spectacular progress in the last few years, much of it enabled by the proliferation of the genomic sciences. Both knowledge of the genome, and the ability to manipulate it, have contributed to this progress. Nonetheless, progress has been greatest for those disorders with simpler genetic structure, that is, those in which a gene or a few genes have a striking effect on risk. The addictions are in many ways paradigmatic for complex psychiatric disorders. Their very high prevalence and diversity mirrors, and is probably due in part to, their complex genetics. As we have emphasized in this chapter, a great advantage to studies of the addictions is a historical wealth of genetic animal models, which have offered many insights into the neuroadaptive dysregulation that accompanies the descent into an addicted state. Experience has given us a clear idea of the strengths and weaknesses of the various genetic animal models.[13]

Important advances would include development of additional animal models not only for ethanol seeking and relapse, but also for the effects of ethanol on emotional states. Whereas many aspects of addictive behavior have been modeled in the laboratory, some of the key features of these disorders remain little studied. For example, the best predictors of eventual substance abuse are a family history, and the age at which use was initiated. We know a great deal about the interactions of genetic predisposition and their modulation by environmental factors in humans, but the limited power of human genetic studies has made it very difficult to trace these influences to specific genes. Given this knowledge, it is troubling that there is so little work in experimental neuroscience devoted to exploring the developmental onset of the addictions, in particular the risk factors—biologic, behavioral, and genetic—that distinguish animals that will go on to display addictive behavior. The potential interaction with other drugs of abuse, such as nicotine, is an important issue because of comorbidity. An underexplored area is the contribution of gender to multiple aspects of drug abuse, including severity and sites of organ damage, addiction liability, and risk of relapse.

Additionally, confirmation of brain regional differences in expression and functional significance of those changes needs to be established. Changes in receptor subunit assembly at the protein level at distinct, discrete sites has not been reliably established. Further characterization of post-translational changes in brain expression (phosphorylation and targets of kinases or CREB) or in receptor function through changes in subcellular routing and distribution (membrane, cytoskeletal, or internalization) will also be important.

Another area that is currently insufficiently studied is the complexity of the interactions across the levels of genes, their proteins, and environmental influences. It will not be enough merely to produce lists of expressed genes, or proteins, that accompany an addicted state. Rather, the combined, interactive influence of these factors should be explored systematically at the whole organism level, whose most integrated expression is behavior, a perspective that has been called *behavioral genomics*.[1] The new tools of bioinformatics, which are currently largely confined to data at the level of proteins and genes, will need to be married to the sophisticated multivariate statistical methods of epidemiology and to the behavioral sciences. Only after this advance will we achieve a behavioral genomics perspective allowing discernment of pathways that lead from genetic risk to addictive or addiction-free behavior. This is a large challenge, but the basic data are in place and the tools are being improved.

Acknowledgments

Preparation of this chapter was supported by grants from the Department of Veterans Affairs, the National Institute on Alcohol Abuse and Alcoholism, the National Institute on Drug Abuse, and the National Institute on Diabetes and Digestive and Kidney Diseases.

REFERENCES

1. Crabbe JC: Genetic contributions to addiction. Annu Rev Psychol 2002;53:435–452.

2. Koob GF, Le Moal M: Drug addiction, dysregulation of reward, and allostasis. Neuropsychopharmacology 2001;24:97–129.

3. Nestler EJ: Molecular basis of long-term plasticity underlying addiction. Nat Rev Neurosci 2001;2:119–128.

4. Hyman SE, Malenka RC: Addiction and the brain: The neurobiology of compulsion and its persistence. Nat Rev Neurosci 2001;2:695–703.

5. Enoch MA, Goldman D: The genetics of alcoholism and alcohol abuse. Curr Psychiatr Rep 2001;3:144–151.

6. Walton R, Johnstone E, Munafo M, et al: Genetic clues to the molecular basis of tobacco addiction and progress towards personalized therapy. Trends Mol Med 2001;7:70–76.

7. Lappalainen J, Long JC, Eggert M, et al: Linkage of antisocial alcoholism to the serotonin 5-HT$_{1B}$ receptor gene in 2 populations. Arch Gen Psychiatr 1998;55:989–994.

8. Schuckit MA, Edenberg HJ, Kalmijn J, et al: A genome-wide search for genes that relate to a low level of response to alcohol. Alcohol Clin Exp Res 2001;25:323–329.

9. Jacob T, Sher KJ, Bucholz KK, et al: An integrative approach for studying the etiology of alcoholism and other addictions. Twin Res 2001;4:103–118.

10. McBride WJ, Li TK: Animal models of alcoholism: Neurobiology of high alcohol-drinking behavior in rodents. Crit Rev Neurobiol 1998;12:339–369.

11. Browman KE, Crabbe JC, Li TK: Genetic strategies in preclinical substance abuse research. In Bloom FE, Kupfer DJ (eds): Psychopharmacology: A Fourth Generation of Progress (CD-ROM version 3). Philadelphia, Lippincott Williams & Wilkins, 2000. http://www.acnp.org/citations/GN401000077.

12. Crabbe JC, Harris RA (eds): The Genetic Basis of Alcohol and Drug Actions. New York, Plenum Press, 1991.

13. Phillips TJ, Belknap JK, Hitzemann RJ, et al: Harnessing the mouse to unravel the genetics of human disease. Genes Brain Behav 2002;1:14–26.

14. Belknap JK, Hitzemann R, Crabbe JC, et al: QTL analysis and genome-wide mutagenesis in mice: Complementary genetic approaches to the dissection of complex traits. Behav Genet 2001;31:5–15.

15. Buck KJ, Crabbe JC, Belknap JK: Alcohol and other abused drugs. In Pfaff DW, Berrettini WH, Joh TH, Maxson SC (eds): Genetic Influences on Neural and Behavioral Functions. Boca Raton, Fla., CRC Press, 2000, pp 159–183.

16. Wand G, Levine M, Zweifel L, et al: The cAMP-protein kinase A signal transduction pathway modulates ethanol consumption and sedative effects of ethanol. J Neurosci 2001;21:5297–5303.

17. Lang CH, Frost RA, Kumar V, Vary TC: Impaired myocardial protein synthesis induced by acute alcohol intoxication is associated with changes in eIF4F. Am J Physiol Endocrinol Metab 2000;279: E1029–E1038.

18. Reilly MT, Fehr C, Buck KJ: Alcohol and gene expression in the central nervous system. In Moussa-Moustaid N, Berdanier CD (eds): Nutrient-Gene Interactions in Health and Disease. Boca Raton, Fla., CRC Press, 2001, pp 131–162.

19. Pliakas AM, Carlson RR, Neve RL, et al: Altered responsiveness to cocaine and increased immobility in the forced swim test associated with elevated cAMP response element-binding protein expression in nucleus accumbens. J Neurosci 2001;21:7397–7403.

20. Thibault C, Lai C, Wilke N, et al: Expression profiling of neural cells reveals specific patterns of ethanol-responsive gene expression. Mol Pharmacol 2000;58:1593–1600.

21. Kuhar MJ, Joyce A, Dominguez G: Genes in drug abuse. Drug Alcohol Depend 2001;62:157–162.

22. Lewohl JM, Wang L, Miles MF, et al: Gene expression in human alcoholism: Microarray analysis of frontal cortex. Alcohol Clin Exp Res 2000;24: 1873–1882.

23. Freeman WM, Nader MA, Nader SH, et al: Chronic cocaine-mediated changes in non-human primate nucleus accumbens gene expression. J Neurochem 2001;77:542–549.

24. Xu Y, Ehringer M, Yang F, Sikela JM: Comparison of global brain gene expression profiles between inbred long-sleep and inbred short-sleep mice by high-density gene array hybridization. Alcohol Clin Exp Res 2001;25:810–818.

25. Evans WE, Johnson JA: Pharmacogenomics: The inherited basis for interindividual differences in drug response. Annu Rev Genomics Hum Genet 2001;2:9–39.

CHAPTER 76

Autism

M.L. Cuccaro

K.H. Lewis

Margaret A. Pericak-Vance

Autism is a neurodevelopmental disorder characterized by significant disturbances in social, communicative, and behavioral functioning. Onset of autism is in early childhood (usually younger than 3 years of age) with symptoms continuing throughout life. The cause or causes of autism are still unknown. The severe impairment and associated behavioral problems in autism confer a profound burden on the patients, their parents, and their families. Thus, ongoing research to dissect autism etiology, which could eventually result in successful therapeutic intervention, is critical.

CLINICAL FEATURES AND DIAGNOSTIC EVALUATION

Clinical Features

Basic Aspects. The Pervasive Developmental Disorders (PDDs), of which autism is the most common (see later for prevalence estimates) and best known, represent one of the most intensely studied groups of complex neurodevelopmental disorders. The diagnostic classification of Pervasive Developmental Disorders derives from the observation that the impairments in socialization, communication, and play "pervade" all aspects of a child's life and arise from a developmental disability. The PDDs are defined by impairments in each of three categories: (1) social reciprocity or relatedness; (2) communication; and (3) behavior.

The core deficit in autism, impairment in reciprocal social interaction, assumes various forms. In essence, individuals with a PDD fail to acquire the basic skills necessary to manage basic social demands and successfully develop social relationships. This difficulty results from a wide range of impairments that are reflected in four categories: (1) nonverbal behaviors (e.g., gaze, gestures, facial expression); (2) inability to develop peer relationships appropriate to the developmental level; (3) failure to share pleasure with others; and (4) lack of social-emotional reciprocity. The means available to quantify these social deficits are limited; therefore, clinical judgments regarding reciprocal social skills are usually qualitative and rely on examiner impressions of social competence based on a combination of history and observation.

The criteria for impaired communication also consist of four behaviorally defined categories: (1) delay or lack of language and gestures; (2) failure to initiate or sustain conversations; (3) the presence of stereotyped, repetitive, or idiosyncratic language; and (4) impaired imaginary and imitative play. Because communication and language features are more easily quantified using standard measures, these features are often used to distinguish between diagnostic groups within the PDDs (e.g., autism or autistic disorder and Asperger disorder [ASPD]). However, even within one PDD diagnostic group, communication and language features may vary widely because not all four categories are required for a diagnosis. For example, diagnosis may be based on the presence of delay or lack of development in spoken language as opposed to conversation impairments.

The third set of diagnostic criteria within the PDDs consists of repetitive behaviors and restricted interests. The criteria consist of four categories of behaviors: (1) circumscribed interests and preoccupations; (2) adherence to routines or rituals; (3) repetitive motor mannerisms; and (4) persistent interest in objects or parts of objects that deviates from standard use. Although essential to PDD diagnosis, these features may also be heavily influenced by level of developmental disability. Evidence to support this is seen in the high frequency of repetitive behaviors in individuals with developmental disabilities or mental retardation, or both, without a PDD. Developmental disability is found in a majority of children with a PDD (approximately 60% to 70%), but the level of disability varies widely, from very mild to severe. Repetitive behaviors occur more frequently in individuals with autism and low developmental functioning than they do in higher functioning individuals with autism.

Clinical Disorders. DSM-IV identifies five distinct PDDs: Autistic Disorder, Asperger Disorder, Rett Disorder, Childhood Disintegrative Disorder, and Pervasive Developmental Disorder, Not Otherwise Specified.[1]

Autistic Disorder, or autism, is defined by features from each of the three core areas described earlier (social, communicative, and behavioral) with clear evidence of onset before three years of age. The criteria for ASPD are identical to those of autism with two notable exceptions: normal acquisition of language and intact cognitive developmental abilities. Normal language acquisition is defined as development of single words by 2 years of age and phrase speech by 3 years of age. *Pervasive Developmental Disorder, Not Otherwise Specified (PDD-NOS)* is a subthreshold diagnosis applied in those cases where there is impairment of social interaction, communication, or stereotyped behavior patterns or interest, or both, but where full features for autism or another PDD are not met. This "subthreshold" category is thus defined implicitly, that is, no specific guidelines for diagnosis are provided. The heterogeneity of this group, as well as the absence of a formal set of diagnostic criteria, has impeded research around this diagnosis.

Rett Disorder (RTT) and *Childhood Disintegrative Disorder (CDD)* are more clinically distinct disorders. Both are marked by normal developmental periods followed by catastrophic decline in all developmental skills. RTT is an X-linked disorder caused by mutations in the methyl-CpG-binding protein 2 (MeCP2) gene. RTT usually affects females and was thought to be lethal in males. Several reports have identified male patients with RTT and mutations in the MeCP2 gene. The hallmark of classic RTT is a brief period of apparently normal development followed by deceleration in head growth (acquired microcephaly), loss of purposeful hand use, and characteristic hand stereotypies. Loss of language and impaired social reciprocity are common along with progression to moderate to severe mental retardation. *Childhood Disintegrative Disorder* (CDD) has a longer period of normal development that may last until 4 years of age or later, during which there are no apparent signs of the disorder. As in RTT, this period is followed by a significant loss of social, communicative, and adaptive skills. The resulting clinical picture is characterized by severe impairments in reciprocal social interaction, communication, and repetitive behaviors as well as mental retardation.

Phenotype and Diagnosis

Autism and the other PDDs are clinically defined disorders. Determination of diagnosis relies on careful delineation of developmental and behavioral patterns, as well as observation of social, communicative, and behavioral phenomena. There are no biologic markers or tests that result in a positive indicator for the disorder. This leads to potential difficulties in diagnosis and identification. For example, variations across, as well as within, individuals over time complicate diagnosis during different points in development. This is especially true in younger children because delays in language or development may be confused with a PDD. Impairments in social and communicative functioning, although clear in the definitional criteria, are sometimes difficult for the clinician to determine. Impairments in social functioning may stem from various difficulties ranging from anxiety to oppositionality or negativism. Further complications arise from the fact that social impairment occurs in multiple disorders and blurs diagnostic boundaries. A useful distinction between the non-PDDs and the PDDs is the extent to which the social difficulties are primary (e.g., autism) versus secondary (e.g., social problems in a disruptive behavior-disordered individual who lacks friends due to his or her aggressive behaviors).

Overlap between social, communicative, and behavioral functioning has also hampered phenotype clarification. Differentiation among the PDDs is confounded by the interrelationships among the core domains. For instance, greater communication problems or the presence of repetitive and stereotyped behaviors are associated with increased social deficits. Efforts to develop a quantitative basis for the PDDs will succeed only if we can disentangle these domains.

Diagnostic difficulties have also resulted from use of a categorical system in which autism and the other PDDs are considered discrete entities. There is now growing acceptance of the conceptualization of autism as a spectrum disorder rather than a categorical disorder. The term *autism spectrum disorders* (ASD) now appears as commonly as Pervasive Developmental Disorders (PDD), although it is not included in official diagnostic nomenclature. ASD is a broader conceptualization in which autism is viewed as one point on a continuum of disorders in which social-communicative functioning is disturbed. The different PDDs are believed to vary along a continuum of severity. In this model, given the different disorders within the PDDs (or along the spectrum), a hierarchical approach to diagnosis is used in which certain diagnoses take precedence. For instance, in the absence of regressive phenomena, autism is the diagnosis of choice. This hierarchy was implemented in order to avoid assignment of different diagnoses over the course of development.

The relationship between the upper and lower boundaries of the spectrum and autism remains unclear. This highlights the problems associated with behavioral heterogeneity. Individuals who receive a diagnosis of autism may be very different. The meaningfulness of these differences is poorly understood. There has been limited success in linking behavioral differences or phenotypic variation to etiology or treatment. These complications also seriously impede efforts to identify the genetic factors that contribute to autism, as the phenotypic variation strongly suggests significant genotypic variability as well.

Epidemiology. Population-based studies of autism prevalence over the past two decades have varied from a rate of 1 per 1000 to 6.0 per 1000 for children with ASDs. Bertrand et al[2] suggest that the growing numbers of children identified with autism and related disorders may be due to earlier underestimates of prevalence or, alternatively, an increased rate over the past 2 decades. Using sophisticated case detection methodology, Bertrand et al found prevalence rates of four cases per 1000 children for children who met full criteria for autism and 6.7 cases per 1000 for ASD children. The differences in rates from earlier studies may be the result of more comprehensive case-finding methods and changes in the diagnostic criteria for autism. There has also been the suggestion that environmental factors may be partially responsible for the increase in prevalence. Although environmental factors have been linked with autism in some instances (e.g., exposure to rubella) there has not been any evidence to suggest that environmental factors pose a public health concern.

In the prevalence estimates, Fombonne[3] reports that the prevalence of autism is one per 1000 whereas the larger group of ASDs is six per 1000. In addition, examination of time trends revealed that the prevalence of ASDs did not change according to year of birth. Similar studies have described prevalence rates in younger populations of 57.9 per 10,000 and 62.6 per 10,000, respectively, for ASDs. Croen and colleagues[4] found that increased administrative incidence of autism in eight progressive birth cohorts in California were paralleled by a nearly identical decrease in the prevalence rate of mental retardation. They concluded that changes in diagnostic practices account for the observed increases in number of children diagnosed with autism.

Autism, like other neurodevelopmental disorders, occurs more commonly in males. Current estimates suggest a male to female ratio of 3 or 4:1. However, gender differences vary as a function of intellectual function. Fombonne reports that in individuals with autism without mental retardation, the male to female ratio is 6:1; when moderate to severe mental retardation is present the male to female ratio is approximately 1.7:1. Clearly, although females are affected in lower numbers relative to males, they tend to demonstrate a more severe clinical picture.

CLINICAL DIAGNOSTIC PROCEDURES AND METHODS

Increased emphasis on diagnostic clarification has spurred the development of diagnostic procedures. Autism is a behaviorally defined diagnosis based on a thorough developmental history in conjunction with behavioral observations. Evolution of the formal diagnostic criteria has been accompanied by development of diagnostic and classification methods. Three general categories of instruments have been developed: informant interviews, observational procedures, and checklists and rating scales.

Interview Methods

Autism Diagnostic Interview-Revised (ADI-R). The ADI-R is a standardized, investigator-based interview designed with the goal of reliable diagnostic differentiation between autism and non-autism in individuals with mental ages older than 18 months.[5] The ADI-R is directly linked to DSM-IV and ICD-10 diagnostic criteria. The standard ADI-R consists of 111 items and usually takes 2 to 3 hours to administer, using the parent or other caregiver as primary informant. A shorter clinical version is available but has not been subjected to comparable reliability and validity studies to date. The ADI-R consists of a series of developmentally organized questions and parallels a standard diagnostic assessment interview. ADI-R administration requires careful inquiry and description of behavioral phenomena that allow the examiner or investigator to rate the behavior in question with respect to presence and severity. Individual ADI-R items are scored on a 0 to 3 scale (usually rating behaviors from absent to constantly present), and used to complete a 41-item algorithm. The algorithm is divided into subscales corresponding to the three central domains affected in the PDDs: (1) reciprocal social interaction; (2) communication; and (3) restricted and repetitive behaviors or interests and stereotyped patterns. Reliability and validity is excellent. Although the ADI-R is able to distinguish autism from nonautism, there are difficulties with further discriminations (i.e., within the PDDs).[5]

Diagnostic Interview for Social and Communicative Disorders. The Diagnostic Interview for Social and Communicative Disorders (DISCO) is a clinical interview similar in scope and purpose to the ADI-R (i.e., an investigator based instrument).[6] The DISCO is primarily intended to elicit information relevant to the broad autistic spectrum to provide a context for clinical assessment of development across different domains, as well as assessment of disabilities and specific needs. The DISCO differs from the ADI-R in several ways. The ADI-R is primarily a clinical research diagnostic tool, whereas the DISCO is primarily a clinical procedure. The DISCO is dimensional in nature and, as such, is concerned with the spectrum of disorders, whereas the ADI-R is categorical. The DISCO is based on a *bottom up* approach, in which any information related to autism is collected and patterns are identified. It is independent of diagnostic formulations. The ADI-R is based on a *top down* approach, in which individuals who meet only the criteria for the disorder are identified. The DISCO provides broader coverage, not only to the autistic spectrum but also to other conditions, such as attention deficit disorder, hyperactivity, obsessive-compulsive disorder, Tourette syndrome, and catatonia—all of which have potential overlap with autism. The DISCO takes a trained examiner approximately 3 hours to administer to a parent or caregiver. The DISCO is primarily a clinical instrument but can be used for research. Algorithms are available that allow an experienced clinician to differentially diagnose individuals within the autistic spectrum using the DISCO. Reliability and validity indices are acceptable.[6]

Observational Methods

Autism Diagnostic Observation Schedule-Generic (ADOS-G).[7] The Autism Diagnostic Observation Schedule-Generic (ADOS-G) is a semistructured, standardized assessment of social interaction, communication, play, and imaginative use of materials. One of four different ADOS-G modules is administered over a 30-to 45-minute period. Module selection is based on level of expressive language and age. The ADOS-G allows for the creation of different social contexts for individuals of different skill levels. This provides opportunities to diagnose and classify younger and lower-functioning individuals. The goal of the ADOS-G is to elicit spontaneous behaviors in standardized contexts. Clinician ratings of select social and communication skills observed during performance of the various items serve as the basis for the diagnostic algorithm. This algorithm is used to differentiate between autism, non-autism pervasive developmental disorder, and not-autism.

The ADOS-G consists of codings made from a single observation and does not include information about history or functioning in other contexts. This means that the ADOS-G *alone* cannot be used to arrive at a diagnostic determination. For example, to receive a DSM-IV or ICD-10 diagnosis of autism, an individual must show evidence of restricted or repetitive behaviors and evidence of abnormalities manifest before 36 months of age. If an individual showed restricted, repetitive behaviors on the ADOS-G, this would increase the likelihood of a diagnosis of autism, but other historical information, such as that provided by the ADI-R, would be required. Reliability and validity studies have demonstrated acceptable standards. The ADOS-G has proved useful for both clinical and research purposes. In particular, the ADOS-G provides important current information, which assists in diagnostic classification as well as phenotype delineation.

Screening Tool for Autism in Toddlers (STAT). The STAT is an empirically derived measure designed for early identification of autism.[8] The STAT is a relatively brief (20 to 30 minutes), interactive measure that can identify children in need of more extensive and specialized follow-up diagnostic testing. The STAT contains a wide variety of interactional items and consists entirely of items that do not require language comprehension. The STAT is suitable for a broader age range but has been validated for children between 24 and 35 months of age. Stone and colleagues examined the validity of the STAT as a Stage 2 (used to differentiate children with autism from those with other developmental disorders) screening instrument in a clinic-based sample of two-year-old children referred for suspected developmental disorders.[8] The diagnostic algorithm resulted in a sensitivity of .83 and a specificity of .86, which are well within acceptable limits. As with any study of younger children, they point out that criterion-related validity is not possible and the standard consists of clinical diagnosis.[8] The STAT represents an important research tool to allow for the study of critical features that predict autism at later ages as well as the investigation of developmental change in phenotype.

Checklist and Rating Scale Methods

Checklist for Autism in Toddlers (CHAT). The CHAT is a brief screening procedure designed to prospectively identify autism in children 18 months of age.[9] The CHAT assesses behaviors typically impaired in young children with autism including pretend play, protodeclarative pointing, and gaze monitoring. The CHAT is completed on the basis of parental report (nine items) and observation elicited under direct testing (five items). Observation items are intended to verify parent or caregiver report. The CHAT assesses nine different developmental areas with specific failures indicative of autism. The CHAT is best used as a two-stage screener but suffers from low sensitivity. The CHAT is an important clinical tool but offers research benefits similar to the STAT in identifying social and behavioral features that are predictors of autism.

Autism Screening Questionnaire (ASQ). The ASQ is a 40-item checklist that is completed by the primary caregiver.[10] The ASQ is intended as a screening tool for presence of a pervasive developmental disorder (PDD). Items are based on the revised version of the ADI algorithm for diagnosis of autism. Similar to the ADI-R, the questions focus on qualitative deviance rather than developmental delay or impairment and, where the latter is likely to affect codings, the questions focus on the four- to five-year age period. Otherwise the questions concern lifetime manifestations. Items are simply scored as present or absent and a total score calculated. No considerations are made for individuals with language versus no language, as scores for individuals with autism with and without language were found to be broadly comparable and the proportions of individuals with scores at or above the cutoff of 15 were similar for the two groups. The ASQ differentiates well between autism and mental retardation and between autism and non-PDD diagnoses other than mental retardation. The most satisfactory differentiation is provided by the total ASQ score with scores of 15 or more as the standard optimal cutoff. The ASQ may provide researchers with an index of severity to allow for differentiation of subgroups within larger samples of individuals with autism.

Childhood Autism Rating Scale (CARS). The CARS is a clinician- or teacher-completed scale that utilizes either direct observation or parent information.[11] The CARS consists of 15 items that are rated from 1 to 4, with use of midpoints. These ratings are summed to yield a total score that is compared to cutoff scores derived from an initial sample of individuals with autism. The CARS has been used with the entire age range. The CARS, although useful as a screening instrument, bears little relation to current diagnostic criteria, and samples a wide range of different behaviors often found in people with autism, including several sensory-based items. The CARS has high sensitivity (.93). The CARS has also been used to index severity of autism, which allows for more careful study of the autism spectrum.

COGNITIVE CHARACTERISTICS, FUNCTIONS, AND FEATURES

Autism is characterized by selective cognitive impairments. No specific pattern of cognitive performance has been consistently identified across the diagnostic group. This lack of consistency most likely reflects the wide variability in expression of autism. Nevertheless, identification of patterns of cognitive performance can add to clinical characterization and phenotype description. In addition, studies have demonstrated that individuals with autism and their family members may share certain cognitive patterns. The study of cognitive impairments in autism has focused on a number of different domains including cognitive intellectual abilities, executive functioning, theory of mind, and central coherence. The most frequently studied cognitive characteristics are cognitive intellectual skills and executive functioning.

Cognitive Intellectual Abilities. A majority of individuals with autism have measured intellectual abilities below established cutoffs for mental retardation. Estimates have suggested that 60% to 75% of individuals diagnosed with autism fall in the mentally retarded range.

Nonetheless, this feature appears to be a crucial attribute or dimension along which to stratify groups. There is tremendous heterogeneity in the cognitive developmental functioning of individuals with autism, from those persons with developmental indices in the severe class of mental retardation (i.e., developmental levels three standard deviations below the norm) to those who have measured scores in the very superior range (in excess of three standard deviations above the norm). In addition to this intragroup variability in cognitive developmental functioning, there is evidence that suggests that people with autism display performance inconsistencies. This feature is often used to aid in differential diagnosis (i.e., cognitive profiles of persons with autism are uneven, whereas individuals with mental retardation are frequently evenly depressed). A number of different measures are used to estimate cognitive abilities. This involves both measures that cover a broad range of abilities, including verbal and nonverbal abilities, as well as those that focus on nonverbal skills alone. Although individuals with autism demonstrate better performances on nonverbal measures, caution is warranted in inferences based on such tests alone.

Executive Functions. Executive functions (EF) consist of several different processes such as planning, abstraction, flexibility, sustained attention, and inhibition. Individuals with autism have demonstrated impairments across multiple studies of EF. However, Liss and coworkers suggest that individuals with autism have specific EF impairments—particularly in perseverance under conditions of increased difficulty and planning.[12] In a study of high-functioning individuals with autism they found increased perseverative errors in the autism sample.[12] However, this impairment disappeared when verbal abilities were statistically controlled. Similarly, a significant relationship between EF measures and adaptive functioning was mediated by verbal abilities. Klinger and Renner suggest that EF measures may be of clinical value.[13] However, the lack of consistency across age groups, the failure of this deficit to account for behavioral features, the presence of EF deficits in other clinical groups, and variability among individuals with autism suggests that EF is not a robust cognitive dimension in autism.

Adaptive Functioning

Adaptive deficits, particularly in the socialization domain, represent a consistent weakness in autism. Measures of adaptive function such as the Vineland Adaptive Behavior Scales (VABS) have been used as diagnostic procedures, as well as to clarify phenotype.[14] Individuals with autism display clear differences in social adaptive functioning relative to individuals with varied developmental disorders across measures of adaptive skills. Gillham and colleagues examined individuals with autism relative to individuals with PPD-NOS and a developmentally delayed group.[15] The autism group showed significantly worse performance than either comparison group across the major VABS domains (socialization, daily living skills, and communication) as well as more maladaptive behaviors. Further, Gillham and coworkers noted that social impairment is far more important than deviant or unusual behaviors in diagnostic determination or classification. Liss and associates examined adaptive behavior as a function of autistic symptomatology, IQ, and severity (high- vs. low-functioning) in autistic and developmentally disordered controls matched for age and IQ.[16] Their findings suggest that autistic symptoms and behaviors interfere with adaptive skill development only in higher-functioning individuals. Lower levels of cognitive functioning inhibit the development of adaptive behavior and basic skills in individuals with autism. Carter and colleagues developed special VABS population norms for use in autism.[17] The supplementary norms permit delineation of both unique profile and scatter in autism and address the lack of discriminatory effectiveness in lower functioning individuals (i.e., floor effect). The supplementary norms were divided into four norm groups based on age (<10 years of age and >10 years of age) and language status (mute or verbal). The use of the supplementary norms will enhance clinical efforts because it provides an additional point of comparison that is more suited to autism as opposed to the national norms or special population norms. From a research perspective, the supplementary norms introduce a new method for stratification of individuals into meaningful groups.

Subtypes

The use of subgroups in clinical and genetic studies is useful as a means to reduce heterogeneity and increase power. For instance, in autism increased LOD (logarithm of the odds) scores have been found in linkage studies when probands were stratified on the basis of language development. Beglinger and Smith suggest four different subtype categories which have evolved in autism: (1) social interaction or communication; (2) intellectual or adaptive functioning, (3) medical features; or (4) combinations of the above.[18] These subtypes have been developed using either an empirical/statistical approach or a conceptual/clinical one.

The best example of a conceptual/clinical approach is Wing social typology, in which three subtypes were described. The aloof subtype consists of children who reject most social contact and demonstrate severe impairment in verbal and nonverbal communication, as well as all-encompassing repetitive behaviors and activities. The passive subtype is composed of children who fail to demonstrate spontaneous social initiations but who will accept the overtures of others. This group has better imitative and communicative abilities. The active-but-odd group often initiate social overtures but in a one-sided

and peculiar fashion. This group has difficulties with basic social conventions. Several studies have documented the validity of Wing social subtypes with the aloof and active-but-odd reflecting the ends of the continuum. However, it is not clear to what extent the subtypes simply reflect developmental functioning (i.e., age and IQ). Alternate social subtypes were identified using factor analysis of features gathered from diagnostic measures. The three factors from both the ADOS-G and ADI-R consisted of affective reciprocity, joint attention, and theory of mind. According to Beglinger and Smith, the affective reciprocity factor may be basic to social behavior in autism.[18] Other useful subtype methods or approaches use developmental level, typically based on intellectual or adaptive level. The combination of multiple variables using cluster or factor analytic methods has yielded consistent findings of three or four different subtypes that are similar to Wing social subtypes. In addition, the influence of developmental level is also significant. Based on their review, Beglinger and Smith conclude that reliable subgroups are derived from both clinical and statistical methods with developmental level, social functioning, and repetitive behaviors accounting for the most variance.[18] The number of subtypes appears to be three or four depending on whether it is a social subtype or a scheme based on multiple features. Beglinger and Smith propose a continuum of autism in which four subgroups are present.[18] The defining features are developmental level, social features, and repetitive behaviors. Certainly, subtypes represent a strategy for increasing our understanding of differences among individuals with autism, although the groupings tend to be highly interdependent. Further, the various studies have employed a wide variety of methods as the basis for subgroups. There is limited study of the relationship of subgroups to different variables in autism such as response to treatment, course, and prognosis in a noncircular fashion.

PATHOLOGY

Structural and functional brain abnormalities have been identified across a number of studies. This is consistent with the conception of autism as a neurodevelopmental disorder. Studies of direct examination of neuropathology in autism have suggested increased brain weight, changes in Purkinje cells, and developmental abnormalities of the inferior olive as common findings.[19] Positive findings of increased head circumference and increased brain volume have been noted but with no clear etiological mechanism. Neuroimaging studies have raised a number of questions around structural brain changes in autism. Studies of neural structures in autism have described hypoplasia in the cerebellum and hippocampus, reduced parietal volume, thinning of the corpus callosum, and abnormal brain volume. Quantitative MRI studies of young children with autism over time suggests substantial brain growth following birth. MRI measures at 2 to 3 years of age revealed 90% of the children to have larger brain volumes than normal controls. Comparison of adolescents with autism to normal controls revealed no such differences. These results may reflect abnormal regulation of brain growth as a mechanism in the development of autism. Boddaert and Zilbovicius reviewed functional neuroimaging studies (PET, SPECT, and MRI) of individuals with autism.[20] Early studies were inconclusive, in part because of methodologic limitations, such as low-resolution imaging.

Investigators have found evidence of bitemporal hypoperfusions with involvement of the bilateral superior temporal gyrus, as well as frontal regions of the brain. Studies of functional brain imaging during auditory stimulation suggest abnormal activation patterns of the left frontal cortex. PET studies using cognitive paradigms indicate responses reflective of disorganized neural circuits. According to Boddaert and Zilbovicius, activation studies using fMRI showed similar disorganization as clear differences in brain activation were apparent relative to normal controls. This is well illustrated in a study examining fMRI during facial processing, which supported previous findings that the activation of fusiform gyrus, a consistent finding in normal individuals, is absent or weak in autistic individuals. Facial processing in autistic subjects occurred in aberrant or individualized regions such as the frontal cortex or primary visual cortex. This abnormal activation pattern was noted in the context of a reduced amygdala structure.

Associated Medical Conditions. Autism can occur in the presence of various neuropsychiatric, neurologic, and genetically determined conditions. A survey of such co-occurrences cited in the literature reveals numerous associations including tuberous sclerosis, fragile X syndrome, Joubert syndrome, Moebius syndrome, fetal valproate syndrome, neuroaxonal dystrophy, Down syndrome, Cohen syndrome, Chiari malformation, Myhre syndrome, Cowden syndrome, schizophrenia, hypomelanosis of Ito, and Smith-Lemli-Opitz syndrome. Chromosomal abnormalities occur in a number of individuals as well (see review by Wassink and Piven) including 22q11, interstitial deletion of chromosome 13, and isodicentric 15.[21] It is likely that the various syndromes and disorders do not result in autism per se. Rather, they may give rise to social and communication problems that are phenotypically similar to autism. These findings have implications for clinical and research efforts in that it is crucial to rule out a number of different disorders before diagnosis of autism or PDD. In addition, it is not clear to what extent autism is a comorbidity in some instances or a product of the neurodevelopmental disruption associated with the disorder in other instances. Not all individuals with the various disorders or syndromes demonstrate autism or PDD features. It has long been believed that various disorders cannot be diagnosed in the presence of autism (e.g., ADHD). However, a review

of the literature indicates that Tourette disorder, attention deficit hyperactivity disorder, mood disorders, and anxiety disorders have been successfully examined with respect to the co-occurrence of autism. The extent to which such disorders can be reliably diagnosed in individuals with autism remains unclear.

A link has been proposed between the measles, mumps, rubella vaccine (MMR) and ASDs. However multiple studies, both in the UK and North America, have failed to detect any relationship between MMR vaccination and ASDs.[22,23] There was no support for the hypothesis that MMR or measles-containing vaccines cause autism at any time after vaccination, including assessment of increased risk associated with second exposures to MMR vaccine. In addition, no relationship was found between MMR, bowel problems, and autism using a population study with case note review method where the latter was linked to independently recorded vaccine data. This remains a highly controversial issue.

BIOCHEMCIAL (ENZYMATIC) FINDINGS

Candidate Neurobiologic Pathways

Numerous neurologic systems have been suggested to play a role in the etiology of autism.

Serotonin (5-hydroxytryptamine, 5-HT) in Autism. Involvement of serotonin pathways in autism was first suspected after an early report in 1961 of serotonin in the blood of some patients with autism. Subsequent studies have provided further intriguing data and are described in detail in a thorough review.[24] The primary evidence implicating serotonin in autism is summarized subsequently.

Multiple studies indicate that elevation of serotonin occurs in the blood of about 25% of individuals with autism; these elevated serotonin levels are because of a corresponding elevation in platelets that contain 99% of blood serotonin. A positive correspondence has been found between serotonin levels in individuals with autism and unaffected parents and siblings. Treatment of affected individuals with potent inhibitors of the serotonin transporter mechanism has been shown in some cases to reduce restricted and repetitive behaviors. The primary source of serotonin synthesis in the body is enterochromaffin cells in the intestinal mucosa. Knockout mice with null mutations of the serotonin transporter have gastrointestinal disturbances not unlike those reported in autism. Disruption of normal serotonin levels in developing rodent models results in altered neuronal outgrowth with neuroanatomic and behavioral effects similar to that seen in human autism. Depletion of tryptophan, which leads to reduced serotonin synthesis and neurotransmission, causes worsening of anxiety and repetitive behaviors in greater than 50% of adults with autism. In addition, positron emission tomography (PET) imaging studies using α[¹⁴C]methyl-L-tryptophan reveal decreased serotonin synthesis in the brains of children with autism compared to controls during early childhood development.

Serotonin in Development. The role serotonin is thought to play in the development of organized structures in the cortex increases the likelihood that serotonin is implicated in the pathophysiology of autism. Levels of serotonin, serotonin reuptake sites, and receptors are all higher during brain development, compared to adult levels. Fluctuations, either up or down, in 5-HT levels during development can result in altered synaptic connectivity in sensory cortical regions. Studies in the mouse have revealed that the thalamocortical projections to cortex are transiently serotoninergic, expressing genes for *VMAT2* and SERT. 5-HT is acquired by these afferents from the 5-HT released by the ascending raphe projections. The thalamocortical afferents can then utilize the 5-HT as a "borrowed" neurotransmitter. This transient serotoninergic character of sensory inputs to cortex is of great interest because disrupted serotoninergic availability, as modeled in the MAOA and 5HTT (SERT) knockout mice, alters the structure of the barrel cortex.

Genetic Evidence for Serotonin Involvement. Of the serotonin-related genes, the most research to date has been done on *SLC6A4*, which encodes the serotonin transporter (SERT or HTT). Numerous studies describing analysis of the SERT gene in various neuropsychiatric disorders have focused on an insertion/deletion polymorphism (HTTLPR) in the promoter and a variable number tandem repeat (VNTR) within intron 2 (HTTINT2). Both variants have been proposed to affect transcription at the SERT locus. Several transmission disequilibrium test (TDT) studies using these two markers have failed to yield any consistent association of the SERT gene with autism. However, a detailed analysis of SERT haplotypes in a large data set has not been performed.

The International Molecular Genetic Study of Autism Consortium (IMGSAC) follow-up genomic screen reported maximum multipoint LOD scores of 2.34, with sex-specific analysis suggesting an excess sharing of paternal alleles at HTTINT2 in the SERT gene locus (*SLC6A4*) on chromosome 17q11.[25] Parental-specific multipoint LOD scores were 2.32 (paternal) and 0.16 (maternal). This finding suggests a parental sex-specific effect, possibly related to imprinting. Parental-specific effects at *SCL6A4* are supported by findings of similar non-mendelian inheritance of a C57BL/6J-specific alcohol dependence quantitative trait locus (QTL) in mouse. The QTL co-localizes to a small genomic interval including the mouse SERT ortholog. Imprinting at the SERT locus is an example of the type of complicating analytical factor not taken into account in most published studies.

Serotonin: Receptors, Signaling, and Metabolism. The physiologic effects of serotonin are mediated by interaction with 5-HT receptors, of which there are currently 15 known receptor subtypes. In-depth discussion of serotonin-related proteins, and their background related to possible role in autism, has been reviewed previously.[24] Among these subtypes are the 5-HT₂ family of serotonin receptors, consisting of the 5-HT₂A, 5-HT₂B and 5-HT₂C receptors, all of which are coupled to the heterotrimeric G-protein G_q (3). SERT and 5-HT₂A receptors are expressed in platelets. 5-HT₁A Receptors are important in neurotrophic actions of serotonin during development. In addition to 5-HT receptors, enzymes involved in serotonin biosynthesis (*TPH*; tryptophan hydroxylase), trafficking in the cell (*VMAT2*; vesicular monoamine transporter 2), and metabolism (*MAOA*; monoamine oxidase A) are keys to the regulation of serotonin levels. These all then represent important candidates for effects in serotoninergic pathways.

GABA. GABA is the primary inhibitory neurotransmitter in adult brain, but during development, GABA acts as an excitatory neurotransmitter, due to high intracellular chloride concentration in immature neurons. This different developmental role for GABA makes it a more likely candidate for involvement in autism. In brain, GABA acts on the GABA_A receptor complex, a heteropentameric structure forming a central chloride channel. Twenty different receptor subunit genes have been characterized in mammals. In addition to providing binding sites for GABA, the GABA_A receptor contains sites for several therapeutic agents and drugs, including benzodiazepines, barbiturates, anesthetics, and alcohols. Binding studies using labeled ligands in human children and nonhuman primates indicate that GABA_A receptor density is greatest early in life. Two studies indicate a significant decrease in GABA_A receptor density in autism. PET imaging in vivo using [¹¹C] flumazenil (FMZ) shows decreased binding in children with autism compared to controls. Data have also been presented showing a significant decrease in GABA_A receptors in hippocampus from autism brains compared to control brains. Mutations have been reported for the *GABRG2* gene in two families with epilepsy phenotypes. Epilepsy or seizure disorders are seen in a significant fraction of autistic subjects. Three GABA_A receptor subunit genes are located in the 15q11-q13 region, a region which is duplicated in a small percentage of autistic subjects, and findings of linkage disequilibrium have been reported for *GABRB3* in this cluster.

Other Candidate Systems

Glutamate. There is some evidence of a role for genes affecting the glutamate systems in autism. First, studies have found significant linkage and linkage disequilibrium at the GLUR6. Second, a mutation of the δ2GluR (*GRIK2*) gene has been observed in the *Lurcher* phenotype in mice. *Lurcher* is inherited as a semi-dominant phenotype characterized by ataxia resulting from selective, cell-autonomous apoptosis of cerebellar Purkinje cells during postnatal development. Analysis of these mice reveals behavioral and motor phenotypes similar to some findings in human autism.

Reelin. Postmortem neuroanatomic studies of human autism brain tissue have identified several abnormalities similar to those found in the *Reeler* mouse.[19] The *Reeler* allele is a recessive deletion mutation; affected animals have a reeling and ataxic gait. The reelin protein is a secreted glycoprotein that acts as a signaling molecule with important roles in neural development. One report has described significant association of autism with alleles and haplotypes including a polymorphic GGC triplet repeat in the 5' untranslated region.[26]

Elevated Neuropeptides. Nelson and colleagues studied the levels of a number of neuropeptides in archived neonatal blood of children who went on to develop autism.[27] Brain-derived neurotrophic factor (BDNF), neurotrophin 4/5 (NT4/5), vasoactive intestinal peptide (VIP), and calcitonin gene-related peptide (CGRP) all showed significantly higher levels compared to controls.

Oxytocin/Vasopressin. Oxytocin (OT) is implicated in maternal behavior, separation anxiety, sexual behavior, and other measures of affiliation. A connection to autism was first suggested by a report of altered plasma OT levels in patients with autism. Subsequent analysis confirmed a substantial decrease in OT and showed a highly significant increase in the ratio of OT-X to OT, where OT-X is the OT-C-terminal extended peptide. 20% to 30% of patients with autism show elevated levels of uric acid, the end product of purine metabolism. Significant increases in de novo purine synthesis in these patients have also been observed.[28] These findings together indicate the possibility that abnormalities in purine metabolism may play a role in some forms of autism.

IMMUNOCHEMICAL FINDINGS

No systematic study has been done, to date, to provide any complete analysis of immune abnormalities in autism. However, significant histochemical abnormalities have been widely reported in individuals with autism. All of the reported abnormalities occur more frequently in autistic subsets than in controls, yet none appear to cosegregate completely with autism or even to occur in a majority of children with autism. Possible reasons for these varied immunologic findings are discussed subsequently.

Evidence has been found for an immunologic role in the pathogenesis of autism based on abnormal histochemical findings in the blood of various subsets of patients with autism as compared to controls. Korvatska

and colleagues summarize findings, which include changes in lymphocyte subsets, i.e., abnormalities of T cells, B cells, natural killer (NK) cells, and macrophages; alterations in serum immunoglobulin classes and subclasses and cytokine production; the presence of autoantibodies to neural antigens; and possible genetic linkage to the major histocompatibility complex (MHC) regions. The incidence of autoimmune disorders in close family members of patients with autism is higher than for the families of controls.

Studies have presented further evidence of immunologic alterations in people with autism. Excessive innate immune responses have been found in the majority of children with developmental regression and autism spectrum disorders as compared to a control group. Immunohistochemistry was performed on children with autistic spectrum disorders and bowel symptoms. This study found a distinct lymphocytic colitis, with increased basement membrane thickness and mucosal gamma delta T cell density, increased CD8(+) density, and increased intraepithelial lymphocyte numbers as compared to control groups without GI symptoms, with ileal lymphoid nodular hyperplasia (LNH), with Crohn's disease, and with ulcerative colitis. A study was performed to determine whether autism is accompanied by an activation of the inflammatory response system (IRS), whose products, such as proinflammatory cytokines, may induce or contribute to some of the behavioral symptoms of autism. The results suggest that autism may be accompanied by an activation of the monocytic and Th-1-like arm of the IRS, leading to increased production of interleukin-1 receptor antagonist (IL-1RA) and interferon (IFN)-gamma.

Numerous observations of abnormalities in lymphocyte subsets, potentially associated with autoimmune or abnormal immunologic responses, in autism patients are another interesting finding. In a study of soluble interleukin-2 (sIL-2), interleukin-2 receptor (sIL-2R), T8 antigen and interleukin-1 (sIL-1) in autistic children, sIL-2 and T8, but not sIL-2R or sIL-1, were significantly increased in the sera compared to controls and other children with mental retardation. Children with autism have also been shown to have a lower percentage of helper-inducer cells and a lower helper:suppressor ratio, with both measures inversely related to the severity of symptoms. A deficiency of suppressor-inducer (CD4 + CD45RA) T cells has been reported in autism patients compared to controls. Additional studies have described immunoglobulin A deficiencies in a subset of autism patients, findings of alterations and incomplete or partial T cell activation, and abnormal opioid-immune reactions in autistic children. A monoclonal antibody to D8/17, which identifies a B lymphocyte antigen, is greatly elevated in patients with autism. Severity of repetitive behaviors significantly correlates with D8/17 expression, and D8/17-positive patients have significantly higher compulsion scores than D8/17-negative patients.

Although a large number of immunologic and biochemical abnormalities have been reported in autism patients, it must be kept in mind that most of these studies have involved very small numbers of affected patients and controls. In addition, the standards and procedures used to verify the diagnosis of autism are not consistent across studies and, in many cases, are not as stringent or as well described as one would wish.

Neurotransmitter abnormalities and immune abnormalities are the only consistent findings in autism other than neurobehavioral symptoms, leading to speculation about linkage between the two systems. Korvatska and colleagues suggest a number of broad hypotheses for consideration in the ongoing effort to elucidate the pathogenesis of autism.[29] For instance, abnormal neurotransmitter metabolism may be responsible, in part, for the wide-ranging immunologic abnormalities found in children with autism. Another possibility is that immune dysfunction affects the CNS (perhaps supported by the findings of anti-brain antibodies and the clustering of autoimmune disorders in families with autism), and is possibly an aberrant immune response to developmentally expressed antigens in susceptible individuals. The reverse must also be considered, as an inherent CNS defect could trigger a broad spectrum of immune responses that may vary significantly between individuals, a result that would be consistent with the findings in patients with autism. Immune alterations are frequent findings in other neuropsychiatric conditions as well. Another hypothesis would involve parallel changes occurring in both the immune system and the CNS in the course of the disease, either because of a deficiency present only in these two systems or because of a more complex systemic condition originating elsewhere.

MOLECULAR-GENETIC DATA

The genetic basis of autism is currently unknown. There is convincing evidence, however, that genetics plays a significant role in the etiology of autism. Refinements in diagnostic methods and criteria, as discussed earlier, are an encouraging development that promises to greatly aid the search for the genetic basis of autism. However, the extreme phenotypic heterogeneity, wide spectrum of symptoms, and presumed genetic heterogeneity, combined with our current lack of understanding of the pathogenesis or neurobiology of autism, complicate genetic research. Nevertheless, since the 1990s the pace of genetic research in autism has accelerated exponentially. Numerous genomic screens and candidate gene studies have been undertaken. Current research points to the probability of not only genetic heterogeneity but also epistatic effects of multiple genes in autism.

Epidemiologic data from several studies have consistently implicated genetic factors in the etiology of autism.[3] Pooled estimates of concordance rates for monozygotic (MZ) versus dizygotic (DZ) twins are 64% MZ and approximately 3% DZ. Heritability estimates for autism range from over 90% to 100%. Sibling recurrence risk ratio (λ_s) estimates range from 75 to 100. This estimate is at least 10-fold higher than that seen in other complex genetic disorders such as schizophrenia ($\lambda_s = 10$), multiple sclerosis ($\lambda_s = 20$), and Alzheimer disease ($\lambda_s = 4$ to 5); many of these disorders, especially Alzheimer disease, have benefited greatly from genetic studies. The consensus of studies suggests that there are anywhere from 3 to 10 loci underlying the genetic forms of autism.[30] Given the high λ_s, it may seem surprising that more progress has not been made on finding the genes involved in autism. Indeed, if we hypothesize four genes of equal additive effect in autism, the λ_s for each locus would be 37.5, and the genes should be identifiable even in relatively small data sets. However, the rapid decrease in λ_s with increasing degree of relationship in autism suggests an epistatic interaction of these multiple loci.[30] Four genes of equal *multiplicative* effect would have a λ_s of only 3.5 each. Although such genes are harder to detect, simulations suggest that geneticists have high power to detect genes under complex models with gene-specific effects of λ_s approximately 2.

Genomic Screens in Autism

There have been at least seven genome screens in autism to date (Table 76–1).[31–37] An updated analysis based on a genomic screen by the International Molecular Genetic Study of Autism Consortium (IMGSAC) from 1998 was published in 2001.[38] Evaluation of the significance of the various genomic screens is a complicated matter. Although some of the regions identified as interesting overlap, many do not. This may be, in part, because of different methodologies across the various screens, including but not limited to, differences in diagnostic criteria and differences in statistical methods. Interesting linkage findings (defined as a MLOD [LOD score maximized over the genetic models tested, allowing for heterogeneity] or two-point or multipoint MLS [maximum LOD score for sib pair data] greater than 1.00 or a p value greater than or equal to 0.05 on any linkage test) from all seven screens and the IMGSAC follow-up analysis are summarized in Table 76–1 and are briefly discussed subsequently.

IMGSAC reported the first genome screen with 316 microsatellite markers on 99 white families from Europe and the United States.[31] They identified regions on six chromosomes, 4, 7, 10, 16, 19, and 22, with a critical level of multipoint MLS (MMLS) greater than 1.00. Chromosome 7q gave the highest score with an MMLS of 2.53 near markers D7S530 and D7S684. An area on chromosome 16p near the telomere was the next most significant region with an MMLS of 1.99. Subsequent analyses from IMGSAC included evidence for an MMLS equal to 2.20 on chromosome 2 and an MMLS greater than 2.00 on chromosome 17.[38] Philippe and associates performed a genomic screen in 51 multiplex autism families using affected sib pair analysis.[32] Eleven interesting regions were identified in this screen using a critical level of *p*-value less than or equal to 0.05: 2q, 4q, 5p, 6q, 7q, 10q, 15q, 16p, 18q, 19p, and Xp. The most significant peak was close to marker D6S283 (MMLS = 2.23). In another genomic screen, Risch and coworkers identified locations with MMLS greater than 1.00 on 1p, 7q, 13q, 17p, and 18p using 90 multiplex families.[33] The Collaborative Linkage Study of Autism (CLSA) reported a genomic screen in 75 multiplex autism families. Their strongest linkages were to chromosomes 13 and 7.[37] CLSA peak markers were D13S800 with an MLOD of 3.00 and D7S1813 with an MLOD of 2.20. Buxbaum and colleagues reported their strongest evidence for linkage from their two-stage genomic screen of 95 autism families to be on chromosome 2q with an MLOD of 1.96.[34]

Several critical regions emerged from Shao and coworkers' genomic screen by the Collaborative Autism Team (CAT) that are consistent with the regions reported by other autism groups.[36] The most interesting results for the CAT data set are on chromosomes 2, 3, 7, 15, 19, and X. The region on chromosome 2 overlaps with those reported by the IMGSAC study.[31,32,34] The 7q region identified by Shao and associates appears to overlap with results from the IMGSAC study, the CLSA, and the Paris group.[31,32,37] The IMGSAC study gave their peak score as MLS values of 2.53 on chromosome 7q32-35.[31] The increased LOD scores from their subsequent investigation with a dense set of markers further supported 7q as an autism susceptibility region.[38] The peak on chromosome 7 from the Paris group was also on this region.[32] On chromosome 15, Philippe and colleagues identified a potential susceptibility region, with positive results for three adjacent markers, which may overlap with our identified region 15q11-q13.[32] Regions on 19 and X potentially overlap with those reported by IMGSAC, the Paris group, and Liu's group.[32,35] Additionally, Shao and associates revealed a unique region on chromosome 3 as potentially involved in autism susceptibility.[36] The X chromosome findings are of interest because of the increased male:female ratio of 3 to 4 to 1 seen in autism, which has been described in both simplex and multiplex autism families.[39] Despite this abnormal sex ratio, previous studies of X-linkage in autism have concluded that if X-linked transmission exists, it is likely to account for only a subset of autism families.[40,41] The genomic screen data suggest the possibility that a subset of families may be X-linked.

Refining Phenotype

One of the most exciting approaches applied to autism research is the use of phenotypic data to enhance the process of gene discovery. Although these studies are in their infancy, the potential for success using this approach is great.

The presence of genetic heterogeneity complicates the search for genes in any genetic disorder, especially a complex disorder. In autism, phenotypic heterogeneity further confounds the issue. With the wide acceptance of standard diagnostic tools, principally the ADI-R, researchers now have a consistent set of diagnostic criteria with which to determine phenotype.[42] However, the variation in clinical features that fall under the autism diagnosis remains extreme. Researchers have begun to explore ways of increasing power to detect genetic linkage in autism by incorporating the rich phenotypic information available into the genetic analysis. This exploitation of phenotypic information can be used to increase the power of available data sets as well as to define a more homogeneous subset.

Piven has argued strongly that the inclusion of the broader autism phenotype, or BAP, which includes relatives of probands who exhibit some autistic-like clinical features but fall well short of the diagnostic criteria, is crucial to expanding sample size.[43] According to Piven, preliminary results suggest that the different factors combining to produce the diagnosis of autism may index independent genetic effect in both the BAP and autism.[43] Therefore, samples may include BAP affecteds to increase sample size and then may segregate for particular traits in order to decrease phenotypic, and hopefully genetic, heterogeneity.

Lord and colleagues have emphasized the need to segregate samples by the three autism content areas (social reciprocity, communication, and restricted or repetitive interests and behaviors) in order to reflect the range of "behavioral phenotypes" that are present in the autism spectrum disorders.[44] They also note the need to control for developmental level, something that small samples sizes have, so far, made impossible. They suggest two specific methods to develop in order to use the available data more efficiently: (1) derive a factor score using items from the ADOS-G modules, and (2) develop latent class analysis using ADOS-G scores, standard ADI-R algorithm score, and ADI-R algorithm computed for correct status.[44]

Buxbaum and coworkers published a report of a genomic screen whose data were reanalyzed after segregating for delayed onset of phrase speech (phrase speech delay, PSD).[34] Their results support the hypothesis that phenotypic segregation may increase power to detect linkage in autism. They found significant increase in their results for regions on chromosome 2 when they selected for PSD families. This was the first practical demonstration that phenotypic heterogeneity in autism may indeed reflect genetic heterogeneity. Shao and associates confirmed these findings in an independent data set.[45]

To explore the power of including as affected those family members who display the BAP, parental structural language phenotype information was incorporated into

TABLE 76–1. Summary of Linkage Results in Genome Screens for Autism

Chr	CAT (Shao et al.) 2002[i]	AGRE (Liu et al.) 2001[ii]	Buxbaum et al. 2001[iii]	Philippe et al. 1999[ii]	Risch et al. 1999[iv]	CLSA (Barrett et al.) 1999[iii]	IMGSAC 1998[iv]	IMGSAC 2001[iv]
1p					D1S1675 149.20cM 2.15			
2q	D2S2215 134.5cM 1.16 (MLOD) D2S116 198.6cM 1.30 (MLS)		D2S319 7.6cM 1.20dom D2S335 175.9cM 1.20dom D2S364 186.2cM 2.25dom					D2S1351 111.43cM MLS=1.60 D2S2188 206.39cM 3.74
3	D3S3680 36.1cM 1.51 (MLS)							
4							D4S412-CFTR 3.0–125.5cM 1.55	
5q		D5S2494 45–69cM 2.55	D5S406 11.9cM 1.46rec					
6q				Near D6S283 132.8cM 2.23				
7p					D7S1876 10.72 cM 1.01			
7q	D7S495 144.7cM 1.38 (MLOD)	D7S523 123cM 1.02 D7S483 165cM 2.13				D7S1813 104cM 2.2	D7S530–D7S684 136.4–149.6cM 2.53	D7S477 119.60cM 3.20
8q		D8S1179 134cM 1.66						D8S261 38.84cM 1.12
9			D9S283 94.9cM 1.09dom					D9S164 140.25cM 1.09 D9S1826 141.87cM 1.46 D9S158

Chr					
10				D10S197–D10S201 50.5–105.9cM 1.36	142.07cM 1.36 D10S197 53.66cM 1.08 D10S208 64.29cM 1.43 D10S201 116.63cM 1.22
13q			D13S800 5.5cM 3.0 D13S217–D13S1229 19cM 2.3		
15q	GABRA3 14.6cM 1.47 (MLOD) D1S659 43.5cM 1.50 (MLOD)		D15S118 41.1cM MLS=1.10		
16p		D16S2619 28cM 1.91		D16S407–D16S3114 16.7–21.8cM MLS=1.51	D16S407 16.70cM 1.59 D16S3114 21.80cM 2.12 D16S3102 23.10cM 2.93 HTTINT2 45.37cM 2.34
17p			D17S1876 13.2cM 1.21		
18q			D18S878 ND 1.00		
19p	D19S425 59.6cM 1.21 (MLS)	D19S433 52cM 2.46	D19S226 24.1cM 1.37		
22				D22S264–D22S280 4.0–25.0cM 1.39	
Xq	DXS6789 62.5cM 2.54 (MLS) DxS1047–q tel 82cM 2.67				

For screens reporting results for multiple data sets, results given in this table are for the complete data set in the study.
iParametric LOD (MLOD) score determined by LINKAGE or two-point MLS determined by ASPEX.
iiMultipoint maximum LOD score determined by MAPMAKER/SIBS.
iiiMaximal multipoint heterogeneity LOD score determined by GENEHUNTER.
ivMultipoint maximum LOD score as determined by ASPEX.

linkage analysis for autism on chromosomes 7q and 13q. Results demonstrated that language phenotype might be genetically relevant to chromosome 7q linkage. Linkage signals were particularly amplified in families where both probands had severe language delay and parents reported structural language difficulties. These results support previous reports of linkage to chromosome 7q.

Further support for phenotypic segregation, as well as for a specific language region on chromosome 7q, were provided by further analysis of data from the Autism Genetic Resource Exchange (AGRE) genomic screen.[46] Alarcon and colleagues performed nonparametric linkage analysis in 152 families, focusing on three language-related traits from the ADI-R.[42] Results demonstrated evidence for a quantitative trait locus for age at first word on chromosome 7q between markers D7S1824 and D7S3058. IMGSAC also refined their linkage analysis data for the D7S524-D7S482 region on chromosome 7q by including additional families, fine mapping of the region with a high density of markers, and allelic association studies. The IMGSAC data showed peak linkage at D7S477.

CANDIDATE GENE STUDIES

Chromosome 7 Studies

As a result of the linkage findings on chromosome 7, candidate gene studies have also emerged. Reports suggest two genes, WNT2 (wingless-type MMTV integration site-2) at 7q31[21] and RELN (Reelin) at 7q22,[26] influence genetic risk in autism. Both genes are also good functional candidates. The WNT2 gene is one of more than a dozen WNT genes that are active during human development. WNT genes encode several signaling proteins with regulatory roles in embryonic patterning, cell proliferation, and cell determination. The WNT signaling pathway also includes several receptors that are expressed in both developing and mature nervous systems. Because autism is a developmental disorder that affects the nervous system, one could hypothesize that a change in a WNT protein might contribute to the development of autism. Wassink and coworkers reported finding that variations of the WNT2 gene were associated with autism (p = 0.013).[21] They found the association was stronger when they examined the genes of a subset of people with autism and severe language delays consistent with other studies on chromosome 7 that suggest that language delay could play a role in autism. They also found two non-conservative missense mutations that segregate with autism in two families.

Using two different but complementary methods of family-based association analysis, the pedigree disequilibrium test (PDT) and Transmit (TMT), McCoy and associates tested patients for genetic association with two WNT2 variants in the 5'UTR and 3'UTR regions of WNT2. No significant association was found between autism and the WNT2 genotypes. The coding region of WNT2 was also tested for the two reported autism mutations (T G in the signal domain of Exon 1 of WNT2 [Leu5Arg] and C T change in Exon 5 [Arg299Trp]) and failed to identify these WNT2 mutations in the data set. These data suggest that the WNT2 gene is not a major contributor to genetic risk in autism.[47]

RELN regulates neuronal migration during brain development. In mice, RELN also has been suggested to be involved in schizophrenia. Several research groups are currently studying the role of the human RELN in brain development and human disease. Persico and coworkers found certain variations in the size of the trinucleotide repeat (>10 repeats) occur more often in individuals *with* autism than in individuals *without* autism.[26] This finding suggests that RELN, containing a larger repeat length polymorphism, may be associated with some cases of autism.

In addition, McCoy and associates examined the association of a 5'UTR polymorphism in RELN ($[GCC]_n$) in a data set that included both the CAT multiplex and singleton families and 90 AGRE multiplex families.[47] PDT and TMT analysis of the combined data found no evidence for association (p = 0.35, p = 0.07, respectively). However, examining the AGRE families independently resulted in support of association to RELN (p = 0.005 [PDT]; p = 0.009 [TMT]). Follow-up analyses in RELN in an expanded data set and using single nucleotide polymorphisms (SNPs) resulted in further evidence of association between autism and RELN. The most significant association was detected on exon 44 (PDT p-value = 0.003) and the 5'UTR repeat (PDT p-value = 0.03) from this expanded data set. The two-locus haplotype with these two polymorphisms was overrepresented in affected individuals (TMT p < 0.001) (Shao and colleagues, unpublished data). These data suggest that additional analysis of the RELN gene is necessary in order to elucidate its potential involvement as an autism risk gene.

Chromosome 15 Studies

Evidence for the localization of an autism gene to chromosome 15q11-q13 is based on cytogenetics, linkage analysis, and association studies. Cytogenetic reports have found patients affected with autism associated with duplications of the 15q11-q13 region. Duplications of 15q11-q13 and autism or atypical autism have been found to segregate with maternal inheritance of the duplication, whereas paternal inheritance did not. This, in conjunction with several other reports of maternally derived duplications leading to autistic-like symptoms, has led to the suggestion that maternally derived duplications of the critical chromosome 15 region lead to autism or atypical autism, whereas paternally derived duplications yield a normal phenotype.[48]

The second line of evidence for an autism candidate gene on chromosome 15 is linkage to 15q11-q13 in some autism families. Linkage has been detected with parametric LOD scores of 2.5 for D15S156, 1.6 for D15S219, and 1.4 for GABRβ3, which are distal to the Prader-Willi syndrome (PWS) and Angelman syndrome (AS) regions. Affected relative pair analysis resulted in a p-value of 0.02 for D15S219 and a peak MLS of 1.1 at D15S156.[49] There is additional evidence for association with autism in this region, including reports of linkage disequilibrium between autism and a marker in β-subunit of the γ-aminobutyric acid A (GABA) receptor gene complex, GABRβ3 155CA-2 (p = .0014). Studies of the GABA gene complex have also shown significant evidence of linkage disequilibrium in the γ3 subunit of GABR. These results strengthen the hypothesis, already suggested by cytogenetic results, that the 15q11-13 region harbors a genetic susceptibility factor for autism.

Additional Candidate Gene Studies

Several functional candidate genes continue to arouse interest and evaluations have been published of adenosine deaminase (ADA) Asp8Asn polymorphism, 5-HTTLPR, and GXAlu tetranucleotide repeat in intron 27b of the NF1 gene.

ADA: Significantly elevated levels of the low-activity Asn allele of the ADA gene have been found in autism probands relative to controls in a case control study. ADA is an enzyme involved in purine metabolism. Defects in this metabolic pathway have been hypothesized to be involved in *purine autism*, a version of autism where patients show hyperuricosuria.

NF1: No association has been found between the (AAAT)$_6$ allele of the GXAlu tetranucleotide repeat in intron 27b of the NF1 gene and autism. This novel allele had previously been reported in 4 of 85 autistic patients, or 4.7%, but a later study did not find this allele in any of 204 autistic probands or 200 controls.

5-HT: Serotonin metabolism has also sparked considerable interest as having a role in autism. Elevated serotonin levels have been found consistently in 30% to 50% of autistic patients. Hollander and Pallanti have suggested that 5-HT$_{1DB}$ be explored as an autism candidate gene because this gene has been implicated in obsessive-compulsive disorder (OCD).[50] A higher rate of OCD in first-degree relatives of autistic probands has been reported and elevated levels of 5-HT1D sensitivity have been correlated with higher levels of severe repetitive behaviors in autistic patients. Hollander and Pallanti suggest that one component of 5-HT function, 5-HT1D sensitivity, may influence heterogeneity in autism.[50] Evidence has been found for association to autism of functional polymorphisms in the serotonin transporter promoter region (5-HTTLPR). A significant excess of the long/long 5-HTTLPR genotype has been observed, as was preferential transmission of the long allele of the 5-HTTLPR.

Cytogenetic Abnormalities

Several specific chromosomal abnormalities have also been associated with autism, including fragile sites (Xp28, Xp22, 19q23, and 6q26), sex chromosome abnormalities (Y, XYY, XXX, and XY mosaicism), and autosomal anomalies (9qh+, trisomy 21, chromosome 7 rearrangements, partial duplication of chromosome 15, and chromosome 18 anomalies). All involve single families or small numbers and many have associated dysmorphology not included in the diagnostic criteria for PDDs. The most frequent of these anomalies has been the chromosome 15 q11-q13 duplication or inversion, or both, which has been found in at least 20 independent autism patients. In many cases the new arrangements are thought to be maternal in origin. There is no evidence that chromosomal abnormalities account for more than a very small fraction of autism cases.

ANIMAL MODELS

No complete animal model of autism currently exists, and because of the heterogeneous nature of the disease it is unlikely that one will be developed in the near future. Research has focused on models of significant component symptoms or characteristics of autism, based on hypotheses about the pathophysiology of the disease. Investigators have looked at viral infections that may model neurologic impairments in autism and alterations in serotoninergic pathways that may mimic those observed in many children with autism. These findings are summarized in detail in a review by Andres.[51]

A rat model for various neurodevelopmental psychopathologic disorders, including schizophrenia and autism, has been constructed by lesioning of the basolateral and central amygdala or central hippocampus in rats. When lesioning occurred early in development, a variety of behavioral disturbances resulted; when lesioning occurred later in life only deficits in social behaviors developed. These results suggest that amygdala and hippocampus damage early in life results in enduring behavioral disturbances. This model has not been evaluated for its particular applicability to autism.

Another developmental brain injury model is rats infected neonatally with Borna disease virus (BDV), who display social behavior deficits. This model may be useful in studying the pathophysiologic mechanisms of the gene-environment interaction that may contribute to the wide variability in autism phenotype; however the infection is not a precise model for neurologic damage.

GS guinea pigs are a guinea pig strain with cerebellar and corticocerebral abnormalities that may be similar to those reported in some human patients with autism. Behavioral tests to determine if the GS guinea pigs represent a useful animal model for autism found that the animals do exhibit autistic-like behavior patterns, including motor stereotypy, lack of exploration and response to environment, and poor social interaction.

A rat hyperserotonemic model is being developed by treating developing rat pups with a serotoninergic antagonist. The treated pups display some of the behavioral and metabolic features associated with autism: overreactivity to auditory or sensory stimuli, altered motor skills, lack of separation anxiety from their dam, decreased alternation in spontaneous alternation tasks, and metabolic abnormalities. This provides further support for the hypothesis that the serotoninergic pathways play a role in autism or in some subset of cases of autism.

Models for abnormalities in the nonapeptides oxytocin and vasopressin are also under investigation, including mice lacking the oxytocin gene that fail to develop social memory and Brattleboro rats that have a spontaneous vasopressin deficiency and show reduced social memory and deficiencies in other cognitive functions.

THERAPY

Treatment of autism and the PDDs has shown great promise-particularly early intervention and neurobiologic interventions. Equally important advances have been made in the arenas of behavioral and educational interventions.

Early Intervention

Early intervention for children with autism encompasses a range of different approaches that endeavor to provide intensive programming aimed at ameliorating the language, adaptive, cognitive, social, play, and behavioral difficulties typical of this group. Several features consistently are found in effective preschool programs, including similar curriculum content, intensive supportive teaching environments with programmed generalization, emphasized predictability and routine, highly structured settings, transition planning, family involvement, behavioral shaping strategies, and intensive efforts (e.g., number of hours per week).

Embedded within the early intervention approach is home-based, intensive applied behavior analysis. This approach merits special mention given the intensity with which it is sought by parents and caregivers. This demand has led to development of a range of programs being offered as approximations of the original programs (e.g., home-based model developed by UCLA or Rutgers groups). The model programs are highly structured and led by individuals with expertise in applied behavior analysis and young children with autism. Weiss[52] found that intensive behavioral intervention was effective and Smith[53] found that children with autism showed greater benefit from intensive applied behavioral intervention as

compared to parent training only. Gains were evident in intelligence, visual-spatial skills, language, and academics, although not adaptive functioning or a measure of behavior problems. In a related study, Smith and colleagues found that a parent-directed, intensive early intervention program for young children with autism resulted in initial positive gains; however, these gains dissipated and they suggested that the change in status was a function of reduced consistency and frequency of consultation.[54] Bibby and coworkers[55] studied children in home-based programs in which consultants and parents had variable training. The investigators noted that in the absence of oversight from trained and experienced consultants, outcomes were well below those obtained in other studies. There is a strong suggestion that the competency of supervision and consultation, as well as its frequency, has a significant impact on outcome for young children with autism.

A review by Delprato examined outcomes of language-based interventions for young children with autism (traditional operant behavioral procedures vs. normalized interventions).[56] The main conclusion was that in all eight studies with language criterion responses, normalized language training was more effective than discrete-trial training. Furthermore, in both studies that assessed parental affect, normalized treatment yielded more positive affect than discrete-trial training.

Eikeseth and associates obtained positive results for intensive applied behavior analysis in older children (ages 4 to 7) conducted in a school setting.[57] This intervention resulted in significant gains across standardized measures of cognitive, language and adaptive functioning. Although treatment was not provided as early as in other studies, the authors point out that intervention at this later age range may represent the initial point of treatment contact for many children with autism.

Psychopharmacologic Interventions

Several reviews have explored the efficacy of pharmacologic interventions in autism. Volkmar reports on the issues that complicate understanding of treatment effects in autism research, including behavioral heterogeneity, difficulty interpreting results in lower functioning or younger individuals, and over-interpretation of case study findings.[58] Pharmacologic interventions have focused on three major neurochemical systems in autism: dopaminergic, serotoninergic, and those involving the neuropeptides. Outcome studies have relied on behavior observations, other informants, and clinical ratings of global improvements. According to Volkmar, it is often the case that the best responses to treatment involve associated symptoms rather than the core features of autism. Dopamine receptor agonists (neuroleptics) have been studied extensively with reductions in stereotypy and withdrawal noted. In an effort to reduce extrapyramidal side effects, dopamine antagonists (atypical neuroleptics) such as clozapine, olanzapine, and risperidone have been studied in autism. Improvements have been described including reduced aggression, improved global functioning, and reduced side effects. However, weight gain, particularly with risperidone, has been a complicating factor for use in children with autism. Stimulants, dopamine agonists, have been used to target hyperactivity in autism with mixed results. Any benefits are offset by a high potential for adverse effects such as exacerbation of stereotypies. Serotonin reuptake inhibitors (SRIs) have been widely used to target obsessive-compulsive and repetitive behaviors in autism. The most widely used agents, clomipramine, fluvoxamine, and fluoxetine have demonstrated effectiveness in reducing repetitive phenomena as well as self-injury and aggression and in improving social relatedness.

One encouraging development is the creation of the Research Units on Pediatric Psychopharmacology (RUPP) Autism Network. This multisite group has addressed the complex issues involved in developing assessment strategies for measuring change in psychopharmacology studies. This has been accomplished by using measures that are sensitive to individual change over a wide spectrum of treatment responses and side effects. These measures are used in conjunction with careful instrument selection and adaptation as well as flexible administration techniques. This group published a large-scale multisite, randomized, double-blind trial of risperidone.[59] In this study, the investigators examined efficacy over an 8-week period in a group of 101 children with autism ranging in age from 5 to 17 years. Clear gains were evident in reducing behavior problems common to autism, such as tantrums, self-injury, and aggression. No differences were found between the risperidone and placebo groups on core social communication symptoms. This effort is promising and points to the possibility that evidence-based interventions can be used to address problem behaviors that often mitigate behavioral- and language-based treatments.

Not surprisingly, a number of other medications have been studied in autism. These include antiviral agents (amantadine chloride), anticonvulsants (lamotrigine), and histamine blockers (famotidine). One agent that has been studied extensively is secretin, a gastrointestinal peptide hormone that stimulates pepsinogen secretion by the stomach and inhibits the secretion of acid by the stomach. It stimulates the secretion of bicarbonate by the pancreas and the liver and is used in the diagnosis of certain gastrointestinal and pancreatic disorders. There are no indications for use in children with neurodevelopmental disorders. Initial clinical reports indicated substantive changes in social and language behavior following single dose administration to children with autism. However, randomized, double-blind, placebo-controlled, crossover studies have not yielded significant findings apart from slight changes in activity and affect. This was true for studies in which secretin was administered in a single dose or on two occasions. Two studies confirmed the lack of an appreciable effect for use of secretin in children with autism. Carey and colleagues noted a lack of reliable meaningful improvement to single dose synthetic secretin in a double-blind, placebo-controlled crossover study.[60] However, Kern and associates in a double-blind, placebo-controlled crossover study evaluated the effect of a single dose of intravenous porcine secretin on measures of behavior and language in children with autism.[61] In contrast to previous studies, a subgroup of children, those with active chronic diarrhea, showed a positive response to secretin. This response was seen in reduced aberrant behaviors and improved language. Children without diarrhea showed no changes in behavior. These findings highlight the importance of looking to subgroups within autism.

Advances in neurobiologic studies suggest that immunologic and metabolic interventions may be of increasing importance. Evidence regarding the association between metabolic abnormalities and autism points to the role of various metabolic derangements. Although metabolic problems are not believed to explain a large percentage of autism cases, conventional metabolic interventions have potential value for subgroups of children. Further study is warranted, with special attention to the genetic basis of metabolic difficulties. Evidence for immunologic abnormalities has prompted development of numerous biologic therapies (e.g., intravenous immune globulin or IVIG), as well as dietary interventions. In a review of the published literature regarding the use of gluten- or casein-free diets, Knivsber and colleagues describe consistent positive results (i.e., reduction of autistic behavior and improved social and communication skills).[62]

CONCLUSION AND FUTURE RESEARCH DIRECTIONS

Autism is a complex lifelong neurodevelopmental disorder that we now know affects more children than previously suspected. There is evidence to suggest that autism is one point on a spectrum of disorders in which social, communicative, and behavioral anomalies result in significant impairment. Intensive efforts to identify the biologic, genetic, and environmental basis of autism has advanced rapidly. Improvements in clinical methods have clarified the phenotype and allowed for construction of meaningful subgroups within the PDDs. Intervention and treatment methods have also moved forward. Psychosocial interventions have demonstrated effectiveness. Pharmacologic and other biologic therapies have shown equal promise in reducing the range of problem behaviors seen in children with autism.

The etiology of autism is now ripe for dissection using statistical methods and molecular genetic tools. The long-range goal is to identify all major, moderate, and epistatic genetic effects in autism. The isolation of the genes for autism and related disorders, and the dissection of how these genes interact, will result in new therapeutic interventions and hold tremendous potential in the coming years.

Future research aimed at reducing behavioral heterogeneity through identification of clinical and biologic subtypes will be crucial for the dissection of genetic etiology. The use of performance-based measures and the development, or adaptation of, measures that have broader application for individuals with autism will be essential to characterizing clinical and behavioral patterns within the PDDs for use in phenotype construction. The identification of biologic subtypes is also an important avenue for study in that it will allow for elucidation of mechanisms that contribute to clinical state.

REFERENCES

1. American Psychiatric Association. Diagnostic and Statistical Manual of Mental Disorders (DSM-IV). Washington, D.C., American Psychiatric Press, 1994.

2. Bertrand J, Mars A, Boyle C, et al: Prevalence of autism in a United States population: The Brick Township, New Jersey, investigation. Pediatrics 2001; 108:1155–1161.

3. Fombonne E: Epidemiological trends in rates of autism. Mol Psychiatry 2002;7 Suppl 2:S4–S6.

4. Croen LA, Grether JK, Selvin S: Descriptive epidemiology of autism in a California population: Who is at risk? J Autism Dev Disord 2002;32:217–224.

5. Lord C, Pickles A, McLennan J, et al: Diagnosing autism: Analyses of data from the Autism Diagnostic Interview. J Autism Dev Disord 1997;27: 501–517.

6. Leekam SR, Libby SJ, Wing L, et al: The Diagnostic Interview for Social and Communication Disorders: Algorithms for ICD-10 childhood autism and Wing and Gould autistic spectrum disorder. J Child Psychol Psychiatry 2002;43:327–342.

7. Lord C, Risi S, Lambrecht L, Cook EH Jr, et al: The autism diagnostic observation schedule-generic: A standard measure of social and communication deficits associated with the spectrum of autism. J Autism Dev Disord 2000;30:205–223.

8. Stone WL, Coonrod EE, Ousley OY: Brief report: Screening tool for autism in two-year-olds (STAT): Development and preliminary data. J Autism Dev Disord 2000;30:607–612.

9. Baron-Cohen S, Wheelwright S, Cox A, et al: Early identification of autism by the CHecklist for Autism in Toddlers (CHAT). J R Soc Med 2000;93: 521–525.

10. Berument SK, Rutter M, Lord C, Pickles A: Autism screening questionnaire: Diagnostic validity. Br J Psychiatry 1999;175:444–451.

11. Schopler E, Reichler RJ, Renner BR: The childhood autism rating scale. Los Angeles, Western Psychological Services, 1988.

12. Liss M, Fein D, Allen D, et al: Executive functioning in high-functioning children with autism. J Child Psychol Psychiatry 2001;42:261–270.

13. Klinger LG, Renner P. Performance-based measures in autism: Implications for diagnosis, early detection, and identification of cognitive profiles. J Clin Child Psychol 2000;29:479–492.

14. Sparrow SS, Balla D, Cicchetti D: Vineland Adaptive Behavior Scales, Interview Edition, Survey Form. Circle Pines, Minn, American Guidance Service, 1984.

15. Gillham JE, Carter AS, Volkmar FR, Sparrow SS: Toward a developmental operational definition of autism. J Autism Dev Disord 2000;30:269–278.

16. Liss M, Harel B, Fein D, et al: Predictors and correlates of adaptive functioning in children with developmental disorders. J Autism Dev Disord 2001;31: 219–230.

17. Carter AS, Volkmar FR, Sparrow SS, et al: The Vineland adaptive behavior scales: Supplementary norms for individuals with autism. J Autism Dev Disord 1998;25:287–302.

18. Beglinger LJ, Smith TH: A review of subtyping in autism and proposed dimensional classification model. J Autism Dev Disord 2001;31:411–422.

19. Kemper TL, Bauman M: Neuropathology of infantile autism. J Neuropathol Exp Neurol 1998;57: 645–652.

20. Boddaert N, Zilbovicius M: Functional neuroimaging and childhood autism. Pediatr Radiol 2002; 32:1–7.

21. Wassink TH, Piven J, Vieland VJ, et al: Evidence supporting WNT2 as an autism susceptibility gene. Am J Med Genet 2001;105:406–413.

22. Taylor B, Miller E, Lingam R, et al: Measles, mumps, and rubella vaccination and bowel problems or developmental regression in children with autism: Population study. BMJ 2002;324:393–396.

23. Farrington CP, Miller E, Taylor B: MMR and autism: Further evidence against a causal association. Vaccine 2001;19:3632–3635.

24. Cook EH, Leventhal BL: The serotonin system in autism. Curr Opin Pediatr 1996;8:348–354.

25. International Molecular Genetic Study of Autism Consortium (IMGSAC). Further characterization of the autism susceptibility locus AUTS1 on chromosome 7q. Hum Mol Genet 2001;10:973–982.

26. Persico AM, D'Agruma L, Maiorano N, et al: Reelin gene alleles and haplotypes as a factor predisposing to autistic disorder. Mol Psychiatry 2001;6:150–159.

27. Nelson KB, Grether JK, Croen LA, et al: Neuropeptides and neurotrophins in neonatal blood of children with autism or mental retardation. Ann Neurol 2001;49:597–606.

28. Page T: Metabolic approaches to the treatment of autism spectrum disorders. J Autism Dev Disord 2000;30:463–469.

29. Korvatska E, Van de Water J, Anders TF, Gershwin ME: Genetic and immunologic considerations in autism. Neurobiol Dis 2002;9:107–125.

30. Jorde LB, Hasstedt SJ, Ritvo ER, et al: Complex segregation analysis of autism. Am J Hum Genet 1991;49:932–938.

31. International Molecular Genetic Study of Autism Consortium. A full genome screen for autism with evidence for linkage to a region on chromosome 7q. Hum Mol Genet 1998;7:571–578.

32. Philippe A, Martinez M, Guilloud-Bataille M, et al: Genome-wide scan for autism susceptibility genes. Paris Autism Research International Sibpair Study. Hum Mol Genet 1999;8:805–812.

33. Risch N, Spiker D, Lotspeich L, et al: A genomic screen of autism: Evidence for a multilocus etiology. Am J Hum Genet 1999;65:493–507.

34. Buxbaum JD, Silverman JM, Smith CJ, et al: Evidence for a susceptibility gene for autism on chromosome 2 and for genetic heterogeneity. Am J Hum Genet 2001;68:1514–1520.

35. Liu J, Nyholt DR, Magnussen P, et al: A genomewide screen for autism susceptibility loci. Am J Hum Genet 2001;69:327–340.

36. Shao Y, Wolpert CM, Raiford KL, et al: Genomic screen and follow-up analysis for autistic disorder. Am J Med Genet 2002;114:99–105.

37. Barrett S, Beck JC, Bernier R, et al: An autosomal genomic screen for autism. Collaborative linkage study of autism. Am J Med Genet 1999;88:609–615.

38. International Molecular Genetic Study of Autism Consortium. A genomewide screen for autism: Strong evidence for linkage to chromosomes 2q, 7q, and 16p. Am J Hum Genet 2001;69:570–581.

39. McLennan JD, Lord C, Schopler E: Sex differences in higher functioning people with autism. J Autism Dev Disord 1993;23:217–227.

40. Hallmayer J, Spiker D, Lotspeich L, et al: Male-to-male transmission in extended pedigrees with multiple cases of autism. Am J Med Genet 1996;67:13–18.

41. Hallmayer J, Hebert JM, Spiker D, et al: Autism and the X chromosome. Multipoint sib-pair analysis. Arch Gen Psychiatry 1996;53:985–989.

42. Lord C, Rutter M, Le Couteur A: Autism Diagnostic Interview-Revised: A revised version of a diagnostic interview for caregivers of individuals with possible pervasive developmental disorders. J Autism Dev Disord 1994;24:659–685.

43. Piven J: The broad autism phenotype: A complementary strategy for molecular genetic studies of autism. Am J Med Genet 2001;105:34–35.

44. Lord C, Leventhal BL, Cook EH, Jr: Quantifying the phenotype in autism spectrum disorders. Am J Med Genet 2001;105:36–38.

45. Shao Y, Raiford KL, Wolpert CM, et al: Phenotypic homogeneity provides increased support for linkage on chromosome 2 in autistic disorder. Am J Hum Genet 2002;70:1058–1061.

46. Alarcon M, Cantor RM, Liu J, et al: Evidence for a language quantitative trait locus on chromosome 7q in multiplex autism families. Am J Hum Genet 2002;70:60–71.

47. McCoy PA, Shao Y, Wolpert CM, et al: No association between the WNT2 gene and autistic disorder. Am J Med Genet 2002;114:106–109.

48. Wolpert CM, Menold MM, Bass MP, et al: Three probands with autistic disorder and isodicentric chromosome 15. Am J Med Genet 2000;96:365–372.

49. Bass MP, Menold MM, Wolpert CM, et al: Genetic studies in autistic disorder and chromosome 15. Neurogenetics 2000;2:219–226.

50. Hollander E, Pallanti S: 5-HT(1D) function and repetitive behaviors. Am J Psychiatry 2001;158:972–973.

51. Andres C: Molecular genetics and animal models in autistic disorder. Brain Res Bull 2002;57:109–119.

52. Weiss MJ: Differential rates of skill acquisition and outcomes of early intensive behavioral intervention for autism. Behav Int 1999;14:3–22.

53. Smith T, Groen AD, Wynn JW: Randomized trial of intensive early intervention for children with pervasive developmental disorder. Am J Ment Retard 2000;105:269–285.

54. Smith T, Buch GA, Gamby TE: Parent-directed, intensive early intervention for children with pervasive developmental disorder. Res Dev Disabil 2000;21:297–309.

55. Bibby P, Eikeseth S, Martin NT, et al: Progress and outcomes for children with autism receiving parent-managed intensive interventions. Res Dev Disabil 2002;23:81–104.

56. Delprato DJ: Comparisons of discrete-trial and normalized behavioral language intervention for young children with autism. J Autism Dev Disord 2001;31:315–325.

57. Eikeseth S, Smith T, Jahr E, Eldevik S. Intensive behavioral treatment at school for 4- to 7-year-old children with autism. A 1-year comparison controlled study. Behav Modif 2002;26:49–68.

58. Volkmar FR: Pharmacological interventions in autism: Theoretical and practical issues. J Clin Child Psychol 2001;30:80–87.

59. McCracken JT, McGough J, Shah B, et al: Risperidone in children with autism and serious behavioral problems. N Engl J Med 2002;347:314–321.

60. Carey T, Ratliff-Schaub K, Funk J, et al: Double-blind placebo-controlled trial of secretin: Effects on aberrant behavior in children with autism. J Autism Dev Disord 2002;32:161–167.

61. Kern JK, Van Miller S, Evans PA, Trivedi MH: Efficacy of porcine secretin in children with autism and pervasive developmental disorder. J Autism Dev Disord 2002;32:153–160.

62. Knivsber AM, Reichelt KL, Nodland M. Reports on dietary intervention in autistic disorders. Nutr Neurosci 2001;4:25–37.

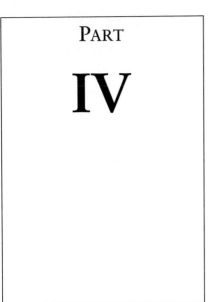

PART

IV

A NEUROLOGIC GENE MAP

CHAPTER

77

A Neurologic Gene Map

Roger N. Rosenberg

Anita Harding[†]

Antonio V. Delgado-Escueta

Susan T. Iannaccone

TABLE 77–1. A Neurologic Gene Map

Chromosome/Region	Gene/Disease Locus
1cen-q32	Muscle phosphofructokinase/glycogenosis VII
* 1p	Childhood absence evolving to juvenile myoclonic epilepsy
1p12	Neurofilament, heavy polypeptide-like
1p13	Adenosine monophosphate deaminase 1/myopathy
1p13	Beta-nerve growth factor
1p13	N-ras oncogene
* 1p13.3-p21	Paroxysmal dystonic choreoathetosis (DYT9)
* 1p15	Late infantile neuronal ceroid lipofuscinoses
1p21	Glycogen storage disease
* 1p21-q21	Spinocerebellar ataxia (SCA19); dominant
1p21-qter	Actin, alpha chains
1p22-p21	Zellweger syndrome, Type II
1p31	Dihydrolipoyl transacylase/maple syrup urine disease
* 1p31.3-p35	Glucose transporter deficiency (Glut-1), autosomal dominant
1p32	Infantile neuronal ceroid lipofuscinoses (Finnish type); Haltia-Santavuori disease; CLN1; palmitoyl-protein thioesterase; recessive
* 1p32	Park10; late onset susceptibility locus
* 1p33-p35	Dominant hearing loss (GJB3, connexin B3 protein)
1p34	Alpha-L-fucosidase-1/fucosidosis
1p34	Uroporphyrinogen decarboxylase/porphyria cutanea tarda
* 1p35-36	Rigid spine syndrome (RSMD1); selenoprotein N(SEPN1) defect
* 1p35-36	Hereditary motor and sensory neuropathy, axonal form; CMT 2A; kinesin superfamily motor protein KIF1B
* 1p35-36	Early onset Parkinson disease; recessive, (Park6)

*Added in the 3rd edition.
†Deceased

(*Continued*)

TABLE 77–1. (*Continued*)

Chromosome/Region		Gene/Disease Locus
*	1p35-p36	Rigid spine syndrome
*	1p36	Parkinson disease (Park7); recessive; sumoylation
*	1p36	Park9
*	1p36.1	Schwarz-Jampel syndrome; perlecan (HSPG2)
*	1p36.13-p36.32	Primary torsion dystonia; dominant; incomplete penetrance; DPYT13; cervical/cranial dystonia
	1p36.2-p36.1	Neuroblastoma III
*	1p36.3	5,10-methylenetetrahydrofolate reductase deficiency; hyperhomocysteinemia
	1q	Usher syndrome 2
	1q	Xeroderma pigmentosum A
*	1q11-q23	Limb girdle muscular dystrophy 1B; dominant; lamins A and C
*	1q21	Lipoid proteinosis; Urbach-Wiethe disease; ECMI
	1q21	Glucocerebrosidase/Gaucher disease
*	1q21	Charcot-Marie-Tooth disease, type 2C
	1q21.2-q23	Hereditary motor and sensory neuropathy I; myelin P0 protein type (CMT1B) (1 family with axonal neuropathy)
	1q21-q23	ATPase, Na+/K+, alpha$_2$ polypeptide
	1q21-q23	Nemaline myopathy, α tropomyosin slow
	1q22-q25	ATPase, Na+/K+, beta polypeptide
	1q31-q32	Hypokalemic, periodic paralysis (hypo PPI)-alpha subunit of the dihydropyridine receptor/calcium channel
*	1q31-q42	Early onset Alzheimer's disease; presenilin 2; Volga-Germans; dominant
*	1q32	Malignant hyperthermia susceptibility 5; CACNA1S
*	1q42	Congenital muscular dystrophy 1B
*	1q42.1	Nemaline myopathy; α-actin
*	1q42.1-q42.2	Chédiak-Higashi syndrome; recessive CHS-1
*	2	Familial temporal lobe epilepsy with hippocampal scleroses and Interleukin (IL)-1β, IL-1α, and IL-1 receptor antagonist gene
	2p	Carbamoylphosphate synthetase (CPS) I/CPS I deficiency
	2p12-q11	Neurofilament, light polypeptide-like 1
*	2p13	Limb girdle muscular dystrophy 2B; dysferlin; Miyoshi myopathy
*	2p13	Parkinson disease; Park3 (dominant with reduced penetrance)
	2p21	Holoprosencephaly-2
*	2p21-p24	Hereditary spastic paraplegia; autosomal dominant; dementia; (SPG4); spastin; cytosolic protein, binds to microtubules
	2p23	Pro-opiomelanocortin
	2p24	N-myc oncogene
*	2q	Autosomal dominant partial epilepsy with variable foci
*	2q	Autistic disorder
	2q	Desmin
	2q	Glutamate decarboxylase
	2q12-q11	Diazepam-binding inhibitor
*	2q13-q14	Protein C deficiency; associated with ischemic stroke
	2q12-q21	Sodium channel type II, alpha polypeptide
*	2q21	Xeroderma pigmentosum; type B; recessive; ERCC3

TABLE 77–1. (*Continued*)

Chromosome/Region	Gene/Disease Locus
* 2q21.2-q22	Nebulin; nemaline myopathy
2q21-q32	Muscle nicotinic ACHR, alpha subunit
* 2q22-q23	NURR1 gene; nuclear receptor super family gene; homozygous polymorphism in Intron 6 increases risk for Parkinson disease.
* 2q23-q31	Generalized epilepsies with febrile seizures plus (possibly generalized epilepsy with febrile seizures) SCN1A mutation; severe myoclonic epilepsy of Dravet; (FEB3)
* 2q24-q32	Congenital myasthenic syndrome; slow channel; alpha subunit acetylcholine receptor (AChR)
* 2q24-34	Hereditary spastic paraplegia; dominant; SPG13; heat shock protein 60; Hsp60 mitochondrial chaperonin (Cpn60)
* 2q31	Tibial muscular dystrophy (Udd)
2q32-qter	Muscle nicotinic ACHR, gamma subunit
* 2q33-35	Juvenile amyotrophic lateral sclerosis, recessive; type 2; putative GTPase regulator; Alsin
2q33-qter	Cerebrotendinous xanthomatosis
2q33-qter	Muscle nicotinic ACHR, delta subunit
* 2q35	Desmin myopathy; desmin
* 2q35-q35	Paroxysmal dystonic choreoathetosis (Mount-Reback syndrome) (DYT8)
* 2q37	Bethlem myopathy; collagen 6a3
* 3	Frontotemporal dementia (FTD 3)
* 3p11.1-p11.2	Protein S deficiency; associated with ischemic stroke
3p21.1-p21.1	Spinocerebellar ataxia type 7 with retinal dystrophy; (SCA 7) (CAG repeat) dominant
* 3p14.2-p12.1	Idiopathic generalized epilepsy with generalized spike waves
3p14.3	Wernicke-Korsakoff syndrome, susceptibility to
3p21	Pyruvate dehydrogenase, E_1 beta subunit/pyruvate dehydrogenase deficiency
3p24	Retinoic acid receptor, beta
* 3p24.2	Acetylcholinesterase deficiency; collagenic tail (Col Q) of AChR.
* 3p24.2-p26	Familial moyamoya disease
* 3p25	Limb girdle muscular dystrophy 1c; caveolin-3
* 3p25	Xeroderma pigmentosum; type C; recessive; x pcc
* 3q25.2-q27	Cerebral cavernous malformations (CCM3)
3p26-p25	von Hippel-Lindau disease (VHL 1 and 2); type 1-retinal angiomas, CNS
3pter-3p21	Beta-galactosidase l/GMs gangliosidosis
3q	Usher syndrome type 3
* 3q	Myotonic dystrophy (DM2)
* 3q13-q22	Hereditary motor and sensory neuropathy, axonal form (CMT 2B)
* 3q13.1	Malignant hyperthermia susceptibility 4
* 3q21	Myotonic dystrophy type 2; CCTG repeat; intronic; zinc finger protein 9 (ZNF9)
3q21-q24	Rhodopsin/retinitis pigmentosa 4, dominant
* 3q23-q25	Ceruloplasmin; aceruloplasminemia with parkinsonism and iron deposition in basal ganglia; ataxia syndrome, with hypoceruloplasminemia
3q24-q25	Dandy-Walker anomaly
* 3q26	Chloride channel gene 2; voltage-gated chloride channel; idiopathic generalized epilepsy; CLCN2
* 3q27-q28	Hereditary spastic paraplegia; recessive; SPG14
3q28	Somatostatin
4p13-p12	GABA A receptor, $alpha_2$ and $beta_1$ subunits

TABLE 77–1. *(Continued)*

	Chromosome/Region	Gene/Disease Locus
*	4p14-p16.3	Parkinson disease; UCH-L 1 gene; (also Park5) (dominant); ubiquitin hydrolase
*	4p15	Parkinson disease, recessive; Park4
	4p15.3	Quinoid dihydropteridine reductase/deficiency; phenylketonuria syndrome
	4p16.3	Huntington disease, CAG repeats
	4p16.3	Hurler and Hurler-Scheie syndrome
	4p16-q23	ATPase, Na+/K+, beta polypeptide-like 1
	4q11-q13	Alpha-fetoprotein
*	4q12	Limb girdle muscular dystrophy 2E; beta-sarcoglycan
*	4q21-q23	Dominant Parkinson disease (alpha-synuclein)
	4q21-q23	Mucolipidosis II, III
	4q22-q23	Pyruvate dehydrogenase, E_1 alpha peptide-like
*	4q24	Susceptibility locus for migraine with aura
	4q25	Epidermal growth factor
*	4q34-q35	Progressive external ophthalmoplegia; dominant; adenine nucleotide translocator 1; with multiple mtDNA deletions
	4q35-qter	Facioscapulohumeral dystrophy 1A; dominant; (1B?)
*	5	Cockayne syndrome A; recessive; CKN1 (ERCC8)
	5	GM2 activator protein/GM2 gangliosidosis, AB variant
*	5p	Malignant hyperthermia susceptibility 6
	5p11-q13	Arylsulfatase B/Maroteaux-Lamy syndrome
	5p13-p12	Growth hormone receptor
	5q11.2-q13.2	Dihydrofolate reductase/deficiency
*	5q12	Susceptibility locus for stroke
	5q12.2-q13.3	Acute and chronic childhood spinal muscular atrophy; survival motor neuron peptide; types 1, 2, 3
	5q11.2-q13.3	Schizophrenia
	5q11-q13	Maroteaux-Lamy syndrome
	5q13	Hexosaminidase B/Sandhoff disease
*	5q14-q15	Familial febrile seizures (FEB4)
	5q23	Diphtheria toxin sensitivity
*	5q23-q33	Charcot-Marie-Tooth disease type 4c
*	5q31	Limb girdle muscular dystrophy 1A; myotilin; dominant
	5q31-q32	Beta$_2$-adrenergic receptor, surface
	5q31-q32	Glucocorticoid receptor
*	5q31-q33	Spinocerebellar ataxia 12; dominant; brain specific regulatory subunit of protein phosphatase 2A; CAG expansion (>30 CAG repeats in affected)
*	5q33	Beta-synuclein
*	5q33	Limb girdle muscular dystrophy 2F; delta sarcoglycan
	5q33-q35	Hereditary hyperkplexia (familial startle syndrome)-dominant glycine receptor
	5q33-q35	Platelet-derived growth factor receptor, beta chain
*	5q33.1	Primary systemic carnitine deficiency; sodium ion dependent carnitine transporter
*	5q34	Generalized epilepsy with febrile seizures plus (GEFS+)
*	6p11	Juvenile myoclonic epilepsy (E_1M_1)
	6p21.1-cen	Retinitis pigmentosa, peripherin related

TABLE 77–1. (*Continued*)

	Chromosome/Region	Gene/Disease Locus
	6p21.3	Major histocompatibility complex
	6p21.3	Neuraminidase 1/possibly sialidosis
	6p-21.3	Juvenile myoclonic epilepsy
	6p22.3	Schizophrenia, dysbindin
	6p22-p21	Branch chain keto acid dehydrogenase E1/maple syrup urine disease
	6p23-p21.1	Prolactin
*	6p23-p24	Spinocerebellar ataxia type 1; SCA1, CAG repeat; ataxin-1; dominant
*	6p25.2	Parkinson disease; parkin
	6pter-p21	Tubulin, beta polypeptide
	6pter-p23	Mitochondrial malic enzyme 2
*	6q2	Congenital muscular dystrophy 1A; laminin a2/merosin
	6q23	Arginase /argininemia
	6q24ᵃ	Limb-girdle muscular dystrophy 1D
*	6q24	Progressive myoclonus epilepsy (EPM2A); Lafora disease; laforin (tyrosine phosphatase); recessive; EPM2B (Lafora disease type 2, linkage to D6S311 and D6S471)
*	6q24-q27	Vasoactive intestinal polypeptide
*	6q25.2-q27	Recessive juvenile Parkinson (mutant parkin) (Park2); ubiquitin protein ligase
*	6q25-qter	Fucosidosis; recessive; type 2; FUCA2
*	6q27	Spinocerebellar ataxia type 15; CAG repeat
	7cen-q11.2	Myosin, heavy polypeptide 5
	7p13	Greig cephalopolysyndactyly syndrome
	7p13-p12	Epidermal growth factor receptor
*	7p13-p15	Cerebral cavernous malformations (CCM2)
	7p13-p12.3	Myopathy due to phosphoglycerate mutase deficiency
*	7p14	Hereditary motor and sensory neuropathy, axonal form; CMT 2D
	7p15.1-p13	Retinitis pigmentosa-9
	7p21.3	Craniosynostosis (some families)
*	7p21.3 p15.1	Spinocerebellar ataxia (SCA21); dominant
	7pter-q22	Actin, cytoskeletal
	7pter-q22	Argininosuccinate lyase/argininosuccinicaciduria
	7pter-q22	Neuropeptide Y
	7q	Cavernous malformations of the brain
*	7q	Limb girdle muscular dystrophy 1E
	7q	Retinitis pigmentosa-10
	7q11.23	Zellweger syndrome-1
*	7q21-q22	Cerebral cavernous malformations (CCM1) (Krit 1 gene)
*	7q21-q22	Malignant hyperthermia susceptibility 3; CACNL2A
*	7q21-q31	Myoclonus-dystonia syndrome, dominant; E-sarcoglycan (SGCE) gene; DYT11
	7q21.2-q22	Beta-glucuronidase/mucopolysaccharidosis VII
*	7q22-q32	Spinocerebellar ataxia (SCA18); dominant
	7q31-q35	Myotonia congenita, dominant (Thomsen disease); (chloride channel gene 1) (muscle chloride channel)
	7q36	Holoprosencephaly-3

(*Continued*)

TABLE 77–1. (*Continued*)

Chromosome/Region	Gene/Disease Locus
* 8p	Neuroregulin-1; Risk factor for schizophrenia
8p	Progressive epilepsy with mental retardation; recessive; Finland
* 8p11-p12	Adolescent-onset idiopathic generalized epilepsies with generalized spike-waves (Non-juvenile myoclonic epilepsy; random grand mal and juvenile absence seizures)
8p11-q21	Retinitis pigmentosa I
* 8p-21	Distal, neuronal form of Charcot-Marie-Tooth disease, recessive or dominant; neurofilament light chain
* 8p21-p22	Adult onset idiopathic torsion dystonia; dominant; incomplete penetrance; cranial-cervical dystonia; DYT 6
* 8p22-pter	Recessive microcephaly (MCPH1) (DYT6)
* 8p23	Juvenile neuronal ceroid lipofuscinosis; CLN 7; recessive; Turkish variant
* 8q	Amyotrophic lateral sclerosis; recessive
* 8q12-q13	Hereditary spastic paraplegia; autosomal recessive (SPG-5)
8q13	Corticotropin-releasing hormone
8q13.1-q13.3	Friedreich ataxia; vitamin E-deficient type; alpha tocopherol transport protein defect
* 8q13-q21	Familial febrile seizures (FEB1)
* 8q13-q21.1	Charcot-Marie-Tooth disease type 4A; ganglioside-induced differentiation-associated protein 1
* 8q22.1-q24.1	Spinocerebellar ataxia; type 16
* 8q23-q24	Hereditary spastic paraplegia; SPG 8; dominant
8q23-q24	Proenkephalin
* 8q23.3-q24.1	Benign adult familial myoclonic epilepsy and mental retardation; CLN 8
* 8q24	Benign familial neonatal convulsions (EBN2) – KCNQ3 mutation
* 8q24	Childhood absence epilepsy with or without grand mal (ECA1)
* 8q24	Epidermolysis bullosa with muscular dystrophy; plectin
9	Coproporphyrin oxidase/coproporphyria
* 9p13	Ataxia with oculomotor apraxia (AOA) with hypoalbuminemia; histidine triad (HIT) superfamily; polynucleotide kinase 3′ phosphatase; aprataxin (APTX)
* 9p1-q1	Distal myopathy with rimmed vacuoles; hereditary inclusion body myopathy (Nonaka)
* 9p12-p13	Hereditary inclusion body myopathy; UDP-N-acetylglucosamine-2-epimerase/N-acetylmannosamine kinase (GNE) gene; recessive
9p13	Galactose-1-phosphate uridyltransferase/galactosemia
* 9q13.2	Nemaline myopathy; beta-tropomyosin
9q13-q21.1	Friedreich ataxia; frataxin; GAA intronic repeats; recessive; may be heterozygous with a point mutation; iron transport protein deficiency in mitochondria
* 9q21	Autosomal recessive chorea-acanthocytosis
* 9q21-q22	Autosomal dominant amyotrophic lateral sclerosis; frontotemporal dementia
* 9q31	Fukuyama muscular dystrophy; fukutin
* 9q31	Walker-Warburg muscular dystrophy
* 9q31-q33	Familial dysautonomia; inhibitor of kappa light polypeptide gene enhancer in B cells, kinase complex-associated protein
* 9q31-q33	Limb-girdle muscular dystrophy type 2H; putative E3-ubiquitin-ligase gene
* 9q31-q34.1	Limb-girdle muscular dystrophy 2H
9q32-q34	Torsion dystonia (some families), dominant; DYT 1; ATP-binding protein; Torsin A; 3bp deletion of GAG
* 9q32-q34.1	Xeroderma pigmentosum, complementation group; type A; recessive X PAC

TABLE 77–1. (*Continued*)

Chromosome/Region	Gene/Disease Locus
9q33	Sequin/amylin neuropathy, Finnish type
* 9q33-q34	Spastic paraplegia; dominant; SPG19
* 9q33-q34.1	Rendu-Osler-Weber syndrome I dominant; ENG
* 9q34	Nonprogressive recessive ataxia; mental retardation
9q34	Argininosuccinate synthetase/citrullinemia
* 9q34	Autosomal dominant juvenile amyotrophic lateral sclerosis; ALS 4
* 9q34	Cerebellar ataxia with oculomotor apraxia
9q34	Dopamine-beta-hydroxylase
9q34	Porphyria, acute hepatic
9q34.1-q34.2	Tuberous sclerosis (some families); hamartin
10	Glycoprotein neuraminidase/sialidosis
10	Mitochondrial ATPase
* 10q	Temporal lobe epilepsy with auditory symptoms
* 10q	Autosomal dominant Alzheimer disease
* 10q11	Cockayne syndrome B; recessive; ERCC6
* 10q21	Charcot-Marie-Tooth disease type 4E; early growth response 2; congenital hypomyelinating neuropathy; dominant
* 10q23.2	Hereditary motor-sensory neuropathy-Russe; dominant
* 10q23.3-q24.3	Progressive external ophthalmoplegia; dominant; twinkle; with multiple mtDNA deletions
10q23.3-q24.1	Infantile-onset spinocerebellar ataxia of Nikali, et al.
* 10q23.3-q24.1	Hereditary spastic paraplegia; dominant; SPG 9
10q23-q24	Glutamate dehydrogenase
10q24-q26	Adrenergic alpha$_2$ receptor
* 10q24.1-q25.1	Intermediate Charcot-Marie-Tooth disease; dominant
* 11	Best macular degeneration (bestrophin)
11p	Major affective disorder type 1
11p	Usher syndrome type 1C
* 11p11-q11	Spinocerebellar ataxia type 5: (SCA5); CAG repeat; dominant
* 11p12-p11	Xeroderma pigmentosum; type E; recessive; DBB2
* 11p15	Variant juvenile neuronal ceroid lipofuscinosis; Jansky-Bielschowsky disease; tripeptidyl peptidase (TPP1); (CLN2)
11p15.4-15.1	Niemann-Pick disease Types A and B
11p15.5	Tyrosine hydroxylase (recessive dopa responsive dystonia)
11q	Pyruvate carboxylase
11q	Usher syndrome 1C
* 11q12-q14	Spastic paraplegia; dominant; SPG17; amyotrophy of hand muscles; Silver syndrome
* 11q13.2-q13.4	Spinal muscular atrophy with respiratory distress type 1 (SMARD1); immunoglobulin μ-binding protein-2 (IGHMBP2); recessive
* 11q13	Autosomal recessive congenital deafness (Myosin 7A gene) (MY07A gene)
11q13.5	Usher syndrome type 1B
* 11q13	Distal spinal muscular atrophy
11q13-q13.2	Muscle glycogen phosphorylase/McArdle disease
* 11q13-q21	Spinal muscular atrophy with retinal dystrophy

(*Continued*)

Table 77–1. (*Continued*)

	Chromosome/Region	Gene/Disease Locus
	11q14-q21	Tyrosinase
	11q14-q23	Tuberous sclerosis (some families)
*	11q21-q23	Desmin myopathy; alpha-β-crystallin (CRYαβ)
*	11q22	Charcot-Marie-Tooth disease type 4B; myotubularin-related protein 2
	11q22-q23	Dopamine D2 receptor; myoclonus-dystonia syndrome; dominant
	11q23	Ataxia telangiectasia
	11q23	Tuberous sclerosis-2
	11q23.2qter	Porphobilinogen deaminase/acute intermittent porphyria
	11q23-q24	Apolipoprotein Al/amyloid neuropathy, Iowa type
	11q23-q24	Neural cell adhesion molecule
	12p	Dominant episodic ataxia (EA1)-K+ channelopathy; KCNA1
*	12p11.2-q13.1	Parkinson disease (Park8); dominant
	12p13	Gamma neuronal enolase 2
*	12p13	Autosomal dominant hereditary spastic ataxia (SAX 1)
*	12p13.31	Dentato-rubro-pallido-luysian atrophy; CAG repeat; "Haw River" syndrome; atrophin binds to a TATA-binding protein which is a cofactor for cAMP-responsive element binding (CREB) protein-dependent transcriptional activation (Tsuji); CREB is inhibited
*	12q11-q14	Rendu-Osler-Weber syndrome II; dominant; ACVRLK 1
*	12q13	Hereditary spastic paraplegia; dominant; SPG 10
*	12q13	Congenital muscular dystrophy; integrin-7 (ITG A7)
	12q22-q24.1	Tuberous sclerosis (some families)
	12q22-q24.2	Phenylalanine hydroxylase/phenylketonuria
	12q22-qter	Short and medium-chain acyl CoA dehydrogenase/lipid storage myopathy
*	12q23-q24.1	Spinocerebellar ataxia type 2 (SCA2); CAG repeat; ataxin-2; dominant
*	12q24	Amyotrophic lateral sclerosis; dominant; hereditary motor neuronopathy
	13q	Hereditary spastic paraplegia; SPG 20-Spartin
*	13p22	Finnish late infantile neuronal ceroid lipofuscinosis
*	13q11	Autosomal recessive congenital deafness (connexin-26, gap junction protein beta$_2$ gene)
*	13q11	Spastic ataxia 2 Charlevoix-Saguenay, recessive
*	13q12-q13	Limb girdle muscular dystrophy; 2C; gamma-sarcoglycan
	13q14.2	Retinoblastoma
	13q14.2-q21	Wilson disease; ATP7β gene
*	13q21	Spinocerebellar ataxia, type 8 (SCA 8); CTG repeat; dominant; ataxin 8
	13q21-q31 (or pter-q13)	ATPase, Na+/K+, alpha polypeptide-like 1
*	13q21-q32	Late infantile neuronal ceroid-lipofuscinosis (Finnish type); (CLN5); Novel transmembrane protein of unknown function; recessive
*	13q33	Xeroderma pigmentosum; type G; recessive; ERCC5
	13q34	Ataxia; dominant; fibroblast growth factor 14 gene
	14	Dominant distal myopathy
	14q	Dopa-responsive dystonia; T$_4$ biopterin type
	14q	Hereditary spastic paraplegia; autosomal dominant
*	14q	Idiopathic basal ganglia calcification
	14q	Protoporphyrin oxidase/variegate porphyria
	14q	Usher syndrome 1A

TABLE 77–1. (*Continued*)

Chromosome/Region	Gene/Disease Locus
* 14q	Spasticity, recessive; complicated with mental retardation, macular pigmentation and distal amyotrophy (Kjellin syndrome)
* 14q	Spastic paraparesis and epilepsy (SPG 15)
* 14q	Hereditary benign chorea
* 14q	Amyotrophic lateral sclerosis; dominant
14q11.1-q13	Holoprosencephaly-4
14q11.2-q13	Oculopharyngeal muscular dystrophy; poly (A) binding protein 2 (PABP 2; GCG repeat)
* 14q11.2-q24.3	Dominant spastic paraparesis (SPG3); SPG3A (GTPase)
14q12	Central core disease
* 14q22.1-q22.2	Dopa-responsive dystonia (GCH-1); (GTP cyclohydrolase 1 gene)(DYT5) (Segawa syndrome, recessive)
14q24.3	Early onset Alzheimer disease, familial Alzheimer disease; dominant; presenilin 1
* 14q24.3-q32.1	Machado-Joseph disease (SCA3) CAG repeat; MJD-ataxin (3); dominant
14q32	Usher syndrome-1A
14q32.3	Brain creatine kinase
14q32.33	Immunoglobulin heavy chain gene cluster
15	Marfan syndrome
15	Xeroderma pigmentosum, complementation group F
* 15q	Epilepsy, dysmorphic face, mental retardation, temporal lobe malformation; 15q trisomy (chromosome 12–15 translocation)
* 15q	Amyotrophic lateral sclerosis; dominant
* 15q	Spastic paraparesis; recessive; SPG11; mental retardation; arm weakness; dysarthria; nystagmus
15q11	Dyslexia (some families)
* 15q11.1	Hereditary spastic paraplegia, autosomal dominant, SPG 6
15q11-q12	Angelman and Prader-Willi syndromes
* 15q13-q15	Hereditary spastic paraplegia, recessive; SPG 11
* 15q14	Centrotemporal spikes in families with rolandic epilepsy
* 15q14	Juvenile myoclonic epilepsy
* 15q14-q21.3	Spinocerebellar ataxia; type II
* 15q15	Periodic catatonia susceptibility (partial schizophrenia)
* 15q15-q21.1	Limb girdle muscular dystrophy 2A; calpain-3
* 15q15-q22	Autosomal recessive juvenile amyotrophic lateral sclerosis; ALS 5
* 15q21-q23	Variant late infantile neuronal ceroid lipofuscinosis; membrane spanning proteins; CLN 6
15q22-qter	Muscle pyruvate kinase
* 15q22-q26	Progressive external ophthalmoplegia; dominant; polymerase gamma; with multiple mtDNA deletions
15q23-q24	Hexosaminidase A/Tay-Sachs disease; GM2 gangliosidosis
* 15q24	Autosomal dominant nocturnal frontal lobe epilepsy; acetylcholine receptor
* 15q24	Dominant nocturnal frontal lobe epilepsy
* 16p12	Batten disease; juvenile neuronal ceroid lipofuscinosis; recessive; CLN-3; novel transmembrane protein of unknown function
* 16p12-q12	Autosomal recessive rolandic epilepsy with paroxysmal exercise-induced dystonia and writer's cramp
* 16p12-q12	Familial infantile convulsions and paroxysmal choreoathetosis

(*Continued*)

TABLE 77–1. (*Continued*)

Chromosome/Region	Gene/Disease Locus
* 16p13	Autosomal recessive idiopathic myoclonic epilepsy of infancy
16p13	Tuberous sclerosis (some families); tuberin
* 16p13.3-p13.13	Xeroderma pigmentosum; type F; recessive; ERCC4
* 16q12.2-q21	Bilateral frontoparietal polymicrogyria (BFPP)
* 16q22.1	Spinocerebellar ataxia type 4; dominant; CAG repeat
* 16q24.3	Autosomal recessive spastic paraplegia; SPG-7; paraplegin; mitochondrial protein
* 16q24.1	Giant axonal neuropathy; recessive; gigaxonin; GAN
17	Gamma actin
* 17p11.2-p12	Hereditary motor and sensory neuropathy (HMSN) Type I (most families), trisomy; PMP22 protein type (CMT 1A)
* 17p12-p11	Congenital myasthenic syndrome; slow channel; muscle nicotinic receptor AChR, beta subunit
* 17p13	Congenital myasthenic syndrome; slow channel; epsilon subunit acetylcholine receptor (AChR); also fast channel
* 17p13.1	Dominant inclusion body myopathy (IBM3)
17p13.1	Tumor protein pS3
17p13.3	Miller-Dieker syndrome, lissencephaly; beta subunit of platelet activating factor; Acetylhydrolase, brain isoform Ib
17pter-p11	Myosin, heavy chain cluster
17q11.2	von Recklinghausen neurofibromatosis (NF1); neurofibromin type
* 17q11.2-q24	Malignant hyperthermia susceptibility 2; ?SCN 4A
* 17q12	Limb girdle muscular dystrophy 2G; telethonin
* 17q12-q21.33	Limb girdle muscular dystrophy 2D; alpha-sarcoglycan
* 17q21.3	Dominant spastic paraparesis (SPG4) (CAG repeats)
17q21-q22	Disinhibition-dementia-parkinsonism-amyotrophy complex (Lynch-Wilhelmsen type); dominant; mutation in the *tau* gene
17q21-q22	Nerve growth factor receptor
17q22-q24	Growth hormone
17q23	(Pompe disease) acid alpha-glucosidase/acid maltase deficiency
17q23.1-q25.3	Hyperkalemic periodic paralysis (SCN4 A gene) (muscle sodium channel alpha subunit); paramyotonia congenita
* 17q25	Familial moyamoya disease
* 18p	Focal dystonia (DYT7); adult onset; dominant; incomplete penetrance; torticollis
18pter-q11	Holoprosencephaly-1
* 18q11-q12	Niemann-Pick disease type C; intracellular cholesterol trafficking; NP–type *Dis* allelic
18q11.2-q12.1	Transthyretin/familial amyloid polyneuropathy, several types
* 18q21	Amyotrophic lateral sclerosis (dominant)
* 18q21.1	Dominant spastic paraparesis (CAG repeats) (SPG4)
18q22.1	Tourette syndrome
18q22-18qter	Myelin basic protein; multiple sclerosis susceptibility
19	Malignant hyperthermia (muscle ryanodine receptor)
19cen-q13.1	Lysosomal alpha-D-mannosidase B/mannosidosis
19cen-q13.2	Late onset familial Alzheimer disease–apolipoprotein E (2, 3, 4) locus
19p	Mannosidosis
* 19p	Familial febrile seizures (FEB2)

TABLE 77–1. (*Continued*)

	Chromosome/Region	Gene/Disease Locus
*	19p12-p13.2	Intermediate Charcot-Marie-Tooth disease; dominant
*	19p13	Dominant episodic ataxia-2, acetazolamide responsive; expanded CAG repeats; CA^{++} channel alpha$_1$-subunit gene; CACNL1A4; absence epilepsy
	19p13	Hereditary hemiplegic migraine; linked to dominant episodic ataxia; spinocerebellar ataxia type 6; dominant; CAG repeat
*	19q	Amyotrophic lateral sclerosis; dominant
	19q12	Cerebral arteriopathy with subcortical infarcts and leukoencephalopathy; CADASIL; notch 3
*	19q13	Dystonia; rapid onset; parkinsonism; dominant; incomplete penetrance; DYT 12
	19q12-13.2	Poliovirus sensitivity
	19q12-13.2	Ryanodine receptor/malignant hyperthermia
*	19q12-q13.1	Central core disease; ryanodine receptor
*	19q13	Generalized epilepsies with febrile seizures; SCN1β mutation
*	19q13	Benign familial infantile convulsions
*	19q13	Malignant hyperthermia susceptibility 1; ryanodine receptor
*	19q13	Hereditary spastic paraplegia; dominant; SPG12
	19q13.1	Myelin-associated glycoprotein
	19q13.1-q13.2	Maple syrup urine disease-1
*	19q13.1-q13.3	Charcot-Marie-Tooth disease type 4F; periaxin
	19q13.2-q13.3	Muscle creatine kinase
*	19q13.2-13.3	Xeroderma pigmentosum, type D; recessive; ERCC2
*	19q13.3	Limb girdle muscular dystrophy 2I
	19q13.3	Myotonic dystrophy; CTG repeat; myotonin protein kinase (DM1)
*	19q13.3-q14.4	Spinocerebellar ataxia type 13
*	19q13.4	Spinocerebellar ataxia type 14
*	19q13.4	Nemaline myopathy; troponin T
*	19q13.4-ter	Spinocerebellar ataxia 14
*	19q31	Central core disease with rods; ryanodine receptor
	20p11.22-p11.21	Cystatin C/Icelandic amyloid angiopathy
	20p11.23-qter	Growth hormone releasing factor
*	20p13	Neuroaxonal dystrophy; pantothenate kinase gene (PANK2)
	20pter-p12	Prion protein/inherited spongiform encephalopathies; Creutzfeldt-Jacob disease; Gerstmann-Sträussler-Scheinker disease types
*	20q	KCNQ2; benign familial neonatal convulsions (EBN1)
*	20q13.2	Autosomal dominant nocturnal frontal lobe epilepsy; NACHR-α4 subunit mutation
	20q13.2	Pituitary tumor, growth-hormone secreting hormone
	20q13.2-q13.3	Benign neonatal convulsions (EBN1) (Nicotinic acetylcholine receptor)
*	21q	Autosomal dominant amyotrophic lateral sclerosis (SOD1)
	21q21.2	Dutch hereditary cerebral hemorrhage; amyloid precursor protein gene (codon 693)
	21q21.2	Early-onset familial Alzheimer disease; amyloid precursor protein gene (codons 670–671, 692, 717)
*	21q22.1	Multiple carboxylase deficiency; HLCS
	21q21.3-q22.05	Schizophrenia, chronic
	21q22.1-q22.2	Amyotrophic lateral sclerosis (some families); Cu/Zn superoxide dismutase (SOD1) (ALS 1)

(Continued)

TABLE 77–1. *(Continued)*

	Chromosome/Region	Gene/Disease Locus
*	21q22.3	Unverricht-Lundborg disease; progressive myoclonus epilepsy (EPM1); cystatin B
*	21q22.3	Bethlem myopathy; collagen 6a1–6a2
*	21q22.3	Homocystinuria; cystathionine β synthase deficiency
	22	Catecholamine-O-methyltransferase
	22pter-q11	Alpha-L-iduronidase/Hurler and Scheie syndromes
	22q	Transcobalamin II deficiency
*	22q11.2	Microdeletion syndrome (aspects of DiGeorge syndrome, velocardiofacial syndrome, conotruncal anomaly of face syndrome (Takao syndrome) (catecholamine-O-methyltransferase gene–COMT); bipolar symptoms
*	22q11-q12	Familial partial epilepsy with variable foci
	22q11-q13	Thyrotropin-stimulating hormone receptor
	22q12.2	Bilateral acoustic neurofibromatosis (NF2)
	22q13.31-qter	Arylsulfatase A/metachromatic leukodystrophy
*	22q13.32-qter	Mitochondrial neurogastrointestinal encephalopathy (MNGIE)
*	22q13-qter	Spinocerebellar ataxia type 10 (SCA10); dominant; ATTCT repeat
	22q12.1-ql3.1	Neurofilament, heavy polypeptide
	22q12.3-qter	Meningioma
*	22q13	Bipolar disorder
	22q13.1-q13.2	Cytochrome P450 IID/debrisoquine sensitivity
*	22q13.33	Catatonic schizophrenia; cation channel mutation (putative)
	22q13-qter	Neuroaxonal dystrophy
*	Xp11-p12	X-linked amyotrophic lateral sclerosis
*	Xp11.2-p11.3	Arthrogryposis and spinal muscular atrophy
	Xp11.21-cen	Incontinentia pigmenti type 1
	Xp11.3-p11.23	Monoamine oxidase B
	Xp11.3-p11.23	Monoamine oxidase A
*	XP11.4-Xpter	Infantile spasms syndrome
	Xp11.4-p11.3	Norrie disease
	Xp11.4-p11.2	Retinitis pigmentosa type 2
*	Xp11-11.4-p21.1	X-linked mental retardation without dysmorphic features and epilepsy
	Xp21.1	Kell blood group precursor/McLeod syndrome
	Xp21.1	Ornithine transcarbamylase/deficiency
	Xp21.1-p11.4	Retinitis pigmentosa 3
	Xp21.2	Duchenne and Becker muscular dystrophies; dystrophin
	Xp21.3-p21.2	Retinitis pigmentosa 6
	Xp22	Aicardi syndrome
	Xp22	Ocular albinism; 2 types
	Xp22.1	Pyruvate dehydrogenase E_1 alpha polypeptide/pyruvate dehydrogenase
	Xp22.1-p21.2	Glycine receptor
	Xp22.2	X-linked HMSN2
	Xp22.2-p22.1	Retinoschisis
	Xp22.32	Kallmann syndrome
*	Xp24-q26	Charcot-Marie-Tooth disease type 2x; Ionescu syndrome

TABLE 77–1.　(*Continued*)

Chromosome/Region	Gene/Disease Locus
Xq	Ataxia and dementia syndromes
* Xq11.2	Spastic paraplegia; SPG 16
* Xq11-q12	Kennedy disease (X-linked spinobulbar muscular atrophy; androgen receptor; CAG repeat
Xq11-q13	X-linked HMSN1, dominant
* Xq12-q13	Menkes disease; copper transporting P-type membrane ATPase (MNK)
* Xq13	Charcot-Marie-Tooth disease type X; connexin32
* Xq13.1	X-linked dystonia parkinsonism syndrome (DYT3)
Xq21	Dystonia/parkinsonism (Filipino type)
Xq21	Mental retardation of the Snyder-Robinson type
Xq21.1-q21.2	Choroideremia
Xq21.3-q22	Alpha-galactosidase A/Fabry disease
* Xq21.3-q22	Mohr-Tranebjaerg syndrome, sensorineural deafness, dystonia, mental retardation, cortical blindness (DFN-1/MTS)
Xq21.3-q22	Myelin proteolipid protein/Pelizaeus-Merzbacher disease
* Xq22	Hereditary spastic paraplegia (SPG-2) (myelin proteolipid protein)
Xq22.2	X-linked HMSN 3; connexin 32 protein type; recessive
* Xq22.3-q23	X-linked lissencephaly and subcortical band heterotopia; double cortex syndrome; double cortin gene (DCX)
Xq25-q26.1	Lowe oculocerebral syndrome
Xq26	Hypoxanthine-guanine phosphoribosyltransferase/Lesch-Nyhan syndrome
Xq27	Paraneoplastic cerebellar degeneration-related protein
Xq27.3	Fragile X mental retardation syndrome; CCG repeats
Xq27.3-q28	Emery-Dreifuss muscular dystrophy (emerin type)
Xq27.3-q28	Iduronate 2-sulfatase/Hunter syndrome
Xq27-q28	Centronuclear myopathy
Xq27-q28	Incontinentia pigmenti 2
Xq27-q28	Major affective disorder 2
* Xq27-q28	Rett syndrome; methyl-CpG binding protein2 (MECP2); occurs almost exclusively in women
* Xq28	Incontinentia pigmenti; NEMO/IKBKG
Xq28	Adrenoleukodystrophy, adrenoleukomyeloneuropathy
Xq28	Deutan and protan color blindness
Xq28	Fragile X type E; GCC repeats
* Xq28	Spastic paraplegia; SPG1; L1 CAM
* Xq28	Spastic paraplegia; SPG2; proteolipid protein; PLP; intrinsic myelin protein
Xq28	Hydrocephalus, aqueductal stenosis type
Xq28	Myotubular myopathy; myotubularin
Xq28	γ amino butyric acid (GABA) A receptor alpha$_3$ subunit
Xql2cen-q22	Bulbospinal neuronopathy of Kennedy; androgen receptor; CAG repeats
Xql2-q22	X-linked spastic paraplegia

Index

Note: Page numbers followed by f refer to figures; page numbers followed by t refer to tables.